HAMRIC AND HANSON'S

ADVANCED PRACTICE NURSING

An Integrative Approach

EDITION

6

HAMRIC AND HANSON'S

ADVANCED PRACTICE NURSING

An Integrative Approach

MARY FRAN TRACY, PhD, RN, APRN, CNS, FAAN
Associate Professor
School of Nursing
University of Minnesota
Nurse Scientist
University of Minnesota Medical Center
Minneapolis, Minnesota

EILEEN T. O'GRADY, PhD, RN, ANP
Certified Nurse Practitioner and Wellness Coach
Owner, The School of Wellness
McLean, Virginia

ELSEVIER

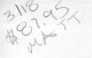

ELSEVIER

3251 Riverport Lane
St. Louis, Missouri 63043

HAMRIC and HANSON'S ADVANCED PRACTICE NURSING: ISBN: 978-0-323-44775-1
AN INTEGRATIVE APPROACH, SIXTH EDITION

Notices

Practitioners and researchers must always rely on their own experience and knowledge in evaluating and using any information, methods, compounds or experiments described herein. Because of rapid advances in the medical sciences, in particular, independent verification of diagnoses and drug dosages should be made. To the fullest extent of the law, no responsibility is assumed by Elsevier, authors, editors, or contributors for any injury and/or damage to persons or property as a matter of products liability, negligence or otherwise, or from any use or operation of any methods, products, instructions, or ideas contained in the material herein.

Previous editions copyrighted 2014, 2009, 2005, 2000, and 1996.

Library of Congress Cataloging-in-Publication Data

Names: Tracy, Mary Fran, editor. | O'Grady, Eileen T., 1963- editor.
Title: Hamric and Hanson's advanced practice nursing : an integrative
  approach / [edited by] Mary Fran Tracy, Eileen T. O'Grady.
Other titles: Advanced practice nursing (Hamric) | Advanced practice nursing
Description: Sixth edition. | St. Louis, Missouri : Elsevier, [2019] | Preceded by Advanced practice
  nursing : an integrative approach / [edited by] Ann B. Hamric, Charlene M. Hanson, Mary Fran Tracy,
  Eileen T. O'Grady.
  5th ed. 2014. | Includes bibliographical references and index.
Identifiers: LCCN 2017055231 | ISBN 9780323447751 (pbk. : alk. paper)
Subjects: | MESH: Advanced Practice Nursing
Classification: LCC RT82.8 | NLM WY 128 | DDC 610.73–dc23 LC record available at
  https://lccn.loc.gov/2017055231

Executive Content Strategist: Lee Henderson
Content Development Manager: Lisa Newton
Senior Content Development Specialist: Danielle M. Frazier
Publishing Services Manager: Julie Eddy
Book Production Specialist: Clay Broeker
Design Direction: Renee Duenow

Printed in the United States of America

Last digit is the print number: 9   8   7   6   5   4   3   2   1

Working together
to grow libraries in
developing countries

www.elsevier.com • www.bookaid.org

I would like to dedicate this book

to my advanced practice nurse colleagues

who are inspirational as they strive every day

to provide optimal care for patients.

I'm extremely grateful to my family and friends who were

a constant source of support throughout the project.

MFT

I dedicate this book to my beloved profession,

to nurses everywhere who care deeply about the human condition,

and of course, to my one and only Humayun,

who listened patiently to my editing and other woes.

Also, to my teenage sons Liam and Conor

who keep it real. And funny.

EO

The editors would also like to dedicate this edition to Ann Hamric and Charlene Hanson.

We are grateful for their foresight, their vision, and the passion they convey

for the advanced practice nurse role. We are thankful for their previous mentoring

and for the consultation they specifically provided for this current edition.

Contributors

Anne W. Alexandrov, PhD, RN, AGACNP-BC, CNS, ANVP-BC, NVRN-BC, CCRN, FAAN
Professor
College of Nursing
University of Tennessee Health Science Center
Memphis, Tennessee
Professor
College of Nursing
Australian Catholic University
Sydney, Australia
NET SMART
Health Outcomes Institute
Fountain Hills, Arizona

Cynthia Arslanian-Engoren, PhD, MSN, BSN, FAAN
Associate Professor
School of Nursing, Department of Health Behavior and
     Biological Sciences
University of Michigan
Ann Arbor, Michigan

Melissa D. Avery, PhD, CNM, FACNM
Professor
School of Nursing
University of Minnesota
Minneapolis, Minnesota

Denise Bryant-Lukosius, BScN, MScN, PhD
Associate Professor
School of Nursing and Department of Oncology
Co-Director
Canadian Centre for APN Research
McMaster University
Clinician Scientist and Director
Canadian Centre of Excellence in Oncology APN
Juravinksi Hospital and Cancer Centre
Hamilton, Canada

Karen A. Brykczynski, PhD, RN, FNP, FAAN
Home Health Nurse
Largo, Florida
Professor (retired)
School of Nursing
University of Texas Medical Branch
Galveston, Texas

Maureen Cahill, BSN, MSN, APN-CNS
Senior Policy Adviser
Regulation
National Council of State Boards of Nursing
Chicago, Illinois

Margaret Faut Callahan, CRNA, PhD, FNAP, FAAN
Provost
Health Sciences Division
Loyola University
Chicago, Illinois

Michael Carter, DNSc, DNP
University Distinguished Professor
College of Nursing
University of Tennessee Health Science Center
Memphis, Tennessee
Adjunct Clinical Professor of Geriatrics
College of Medicine
University of Arkansas for Medical Sciences
Little Rock, Arkansas
Adjunct Professor
School of Nursing, Midwifery, and Paramedicine
Curtin University
Perth, Australia

Anne Z. Cockerham, PhD, CNW, WHNP-BC, CNE
Associate Dean for Academic Affairs
Frontier Nursing University
Hyden, Kentucky

Cindi Dabney, BSN, MSNA, DNP
Assistant Director of Didactic Education
Anesthesia Option
University of Tennessee Health Science Center
Memphis, Tennessee

Lynne M. Dunphy, PhD, APRN, FNP-BC, FAAN, FAANP
Associate Dean for Practice and Community Engagement
Professor
Christine E. Lynn College of Nursing
Florida Atlantic University
Boca Raton, Florida

Margaret M. Flinter, MSN, PhD
Senior Vice President and Clinical Director
Community Health Center, Inc.
Middletown, Connecticut

Mikel Gray, PhD, FNP, PNP, CUNP, CCCN, FAANP, FAAN
Professor
Department of Urology and Department of Acute and
     Specialty Nursing Care
School of Nursing
University of Virginia
Charlottesville, Virginia

Jane Guttendorf, DNP, CRNP, ACNP-BC, CCRN
Assistant Professor
School of Nursing, Department of Acute/Tertiary Care
University of Pittsburgh
Acute Care Nurse Practitioner
Department of Critical Care Medicine
University of Pittsburgh Medical Center, UPMC Presbyterian
Pittsburgh, Pennsylvania

Ann B. Hamric, PhD, MS, BSN
Professor Emeritus
School of Nursing
Virginia Commonwealth University
Richmond, Virginia

Charlene M. Hanson, EdD, RN, FNP-BC, FAAN
Professor Emerita and Family Nurse Practitioner
Nursing
Georgia Southern University
Statesboro, Georgia

Gene E. Harkless, BSN, MSN, DNSc
Associate Professor
Nursing
University of New Hampshire
Durham, New Hampshire

Marilyn Hravnak, RN, PhD, CRNP, BC, FCCM, FAAC
Professor
School of Nursing
University of Pittsburgh
Pittsburgh, Pennsylvania

Jean E. Johnson, PhD, RN, FAAN
Dean Emerita
School of Nursing
George Washington University
Washington, District of Columbia

Arlene W. Keeling, PhD, RN, FAAN
Centennial Distinguished Professor and Associate Director
Eleanor Crowder Bjoring Center for Nursing
Historical Inquiry
School of Nursing
University of Virginia
Charlottesville, Virginia

Ruth M. Kleinpell, PhD, RN, APRN-BC, FAAN, FAANP, FCCM
Assistant Dean for Clinical Scholarship
Professor
Vanderbilt University School of Nursing
Nashville, Tennessee
Professor
Rush University College of Nursing
Chicago, Illinois

Michael J. Kremer, PhD, CRNA, CHSE, FNAP, FAAN
Professor and Director
Nurse Anesthesia Program
Rush University College of Nursing
Co-Director
Rush Center for Clinical Skills and Simulation
Rush University Medical Center
Chicago, Illinois

Brigid Lusk, PhD, RN, FAAN
Adjunct Clinical Professor
College of Nursing
University of Illinois at Chicago
Chicago, Illinois

Carole L. Mackavey, DNP, MSN, RN, FNP-C
Assistant Professor and Co-Director, FNP Track
Family Health/SON
University of Texas Health Science Center at Houston
Houston, Texas

Kathy S. Magdic, DNP, ACNP-BC
Assistant Professor
Acute-Tertiary Care
University of Pittsburgh
Pittsburgh, Pennsylvania

Nancy Munro, MN, CCRN, ACNP-BC, FAANP
Senior Acute Care Nurse Practitioner
Critical Care Medicine Department
National Institutes of Health
Bethesda, Maryland

Eileen T. O'Grady, PhD, RN, ANP
Certified Nurse Practitioner and Wellness Coach
Owner, The School of Wellness
McLean, Virginia

Geraldine S. Pearson, PhD, PMH-CNS, FAAN
Associate Professor
Psychiatry, Child/Adolescent Division
University of Connecticut School of Medicine
Farmington, Connecticut

Susanne J. Phillips, DNP, APRN, FNP-BC
Clinical Professor
Nursing Science
University of California, Irvine
Irvine, California

Laura Reed, MSN, DNP
Assistant Professor
Advanced Practice and Doctoral Studies
University of Tennessee Health Science Center
Memphis, Tennessee

Melissa A. Saftner, PhD, CNM, RN
Clinical Associate Professor
School of Nursing
University of Minnesota
Minneapolis, Minnesota

Jeanne Salyer, PhD, RN
Associate Professor
Adult Health and Nursing Systems
Virginia Commonwealth University School of Nursing
Richmond, Virginia

Sue Sendelbach, PhD, RN, FAAN, FAHA
Director of Nursing Research (retired)
Abbott Northwestern Hospital
Minneapolis, Minnesota

Katherine E. Simmonds, MS, MPH, WHNP-BC
Assistant Professor
School of Nursing
Track Coordinator of Women's Health and Adult
Gerontology/Women's Health NP Specialties
MGH Institute of Health Professions
Charlestown, Massachusetts

Mary Fran Tracy, PhD, RN, APRN, CNS, FAAN
Associate Professor
School of Nursing
University of Minnesota
Nurse Scientist
University of Minnesota Medical Center
Minneapolis, Minnesota

S. Brian Widmar, PhD, RN, ACNP-BC, CCRN, FAANP
Director, Adult-Gero Acute Care NP Specialty
School of Nursing
Vanderbilt University
Nashville, Tennessee

Marisa L. Wilson, DNSc, MHSc, RN-BC, CPHIMS, FAAN
Associate Professor and Specialty Track Coordinator Nursing
    Informatics
Family, Community, and Health Systems
University of Alabama at Birmingham School of Nursing
Birmingham, Alabama

Lucia Wocial, BA, BS, MS, PhD
Nurse Ethicist
Fairbanks Center for Medical Ethics
Indiana University Health
Adjunct Assistant Professor
School of Nursing
Indiana University
Indianapolis, Indiana

Frances Kam Yuet Wong, BSN, MEd, PhD
Professor
School of Nursing
Hong Kong Polytechnic University
Hong Kong, China

Reviewers

Deborah Becker, PhD, ACNP, BC, CHSE, FAAN
Practice Associate Professor of Nursing
Director, Adult Gerontology Acute Care Nurse Practitioner
    Program
Biobehavioral and Health Science Department
University of Pennsylvania, School of Nursing
Philadelphia, Pennsylvania

Angela P. Clark, PhD, RN, ACNS-BC, FAAN, FAHA
Associate Professor Emerita
School of Nursing
University of Texas at Austin
Austin, Texas

Michelle L. Edwards, DNP, APRN, FNP, ACNP, FAANP
System Vice President, Advanced Practice
National Clinical Enterprise
Catholic Health Initiatives
Englewood, Colorado

Loretta C. Ford, EdD, PNP, FAAN, FAANP
Professor and Dean Emerita
School of Nursing
University of Rochester
Rochester, New York

Lynn Gallagher-Ford, PhD, RN, DPFNAP, NE-BC
Director
Center for Transdisciplinary Evidence-Based Practice
College of Nursing
Ohio State University
Columbus, Ohio

Deborah B Gardner, PhD, RN, FAAN, FNAP
Health Policy and Leadership Consultant
Gardner and Associates, LLC
Honolulu, Hawaii

Laurie K. Glass, RN, PhD, FAAN
Professor Emerita and Director
Center for Nursing History
College of Nursing
University of Wisconsin—Milwaukee
Milwaukee, Wisconsin

Ann B. Hamric, PhD, RN, FAAN
Professor Emeritus
School of Nursing
Virginia Commonwealth University
Richmond, Virginia

Charlene M. Hanson, EdD, RN, FNP-BC, FAAN
Professor Emerita
Georgia Southern University
Family Nurse Practitioner
School of Nursing
Georgia Southern University
Statesboro, Georgia

Catherine Horvath, DNP, CRNA
Assistant Professor
School of Nursing and Health Studies
Georgetown University
Washington, District of Columbia

Lynda A. Mackin, PhD, AGPCNP-BC, CCNS
Health Science Clinical Professor
Physiological Nursing
University of California San Francisco School of Nursing
San Francisco, California

Tim Porter-O'Grady, DM, EdD, APRN, FAAN, FACCWS
Senior Partner, Health Systems
TPOG Associates, Inc.
Adjunct Professor, SON
Emory University
Registered Mediator and Arbitrator
Clinical Wound Specialist, Mercy Care
Atlanta, Georgia
Professor of Practice, CONHI
Arizona State University
Phoenix, Arizona
Professor of Practice and Leadership Scholar, CON
Ohio State University
Columbus, Ohio

Joanne K. Singleton, PhD, RN, FNP-BC, CNL, FNAP,
FNYAM
Professor
Graduate Studies
College of Health Professions, Lienhard School of Nursing
Pace University
New York, New York

Margaret C. Slota DNP, RN, FAAN
Associate Professor; Director, DNP Program
School of Nursing and Health Studies
Georgetown University
Washington, District of Columbia

Sheila Cox Sullivan, PhD, RN, VHA-CM
Director/Research, EBP and Analytics
Office of Nursing Services
Department of Veterans Affairs
Washington, District of Columbia

Lisa Summers, MSN, DrPH, FACNM
Deputy Director
DNP Program
School of Nursing
Yale University
New Haven, Connecticut

Carol Taylor, PhD, RN
Professor of Medicine and Nursing
Senior Clinical Scholar, Kennedy Institute of Ethics
Department of Advanced Nursing Practice
Georgetown University School of Nursing and Health
     Studies
Washington, District of Columbia

Preface

Revision of this sixth edition of *Advanced Practice Nursing: An Integrative Approach* has provided an opportunity for reflection during this unique time of health care evolution in the United States to see how far advanced practice nursing has come since the first edition of this book by Hamric, Spross, and Hanson in 1996. Editing this book also makes it clear that advanced practice nursing has unbounded opportunities for growth into the future—many of these yet to even be imagined. Advanced practice registered nurses (APRNs) are being seen as increasingly valuable, both inside and outside of nursing. Many events have aligned to contribute to this recognized value of APRNs: the Institute of Medicine's *The Future of Nursing* report (2010) and its update, *Assessing Progress on the IOM Future of Nursing Report* (2015); increasing shortages of providers, particularly in underserved areas; increased access to health care created by the Patient Protection and Affordable Care Act (ACA, 2010); a focus on improving and ensuring patient safety and quality care; an aging population with multiple chronic health conditions requiring providers skilled in the coordination of care for these complex patients; a recognition that social circumstances such as education, income level, and access to quality food and water determine health; and an increasing emphasis on preventative health care that goes beyond the provision of medical care alone. The collaboration of APRN professional organizations along with the American Association of Colleges of Nursing and the National Council of State Boards of Nursing to develop the Consensus Model for APRN Regulation (2008) has resulted in APRNs being more cohesive in presenting consistent messaging and speaking with a unified voice.

At the time of publication of the previous edition (2014), the Consensus Model was still relatively new. In the time since, APRNs and professional organizations have gained increasing clarity on how to optimize use of the model to promote changes in APRN regulation and standardize APRN educational curricula. As of this writing, APRNs in more than half of the United States have gained full practice authority (National Council of State Boards of Nursing, 2017); yet even in those states, there are still barriers to full practice (e.g., inability to pronounce death, limiting of scope of practice by hospitals and health systems). Further, while the Veterans Administration granted full practice authority to APRNs (United States Department of Veterans Affairs, 2016), they only granted it to three of the four APRN roles, withholding the authority from CRNAs. It is situations like these that highlight the ongoing need for all APRNs to continue to speak with one voice, expressing the value of APRNs as a whole while still recognizing the uniqueness added by each of the APRN roles.

The number of Doctor of Nursing Practice (DNP) programs continues to explode, rapidly increasing the number of DNP graduates in the nation's workforce. The DNP-prepared APRN brings a strong set of leadership skills and the expertise to embed evidence into all kinds of practices, which is very beneficial to society. On the other hand, we know the DNP-prepared APRN has created continuing APRN role confusion. Many people inside and outside of nursing confuse the DNP as a new role within nursing versus a degree. This book continues to provide clarity on the four specific APRN roles within the APRN umbrella term, regardless of degree type. As advanced practice education continues to evolve, we would hope the confusion of terms will dissipate.

Purpose

The purpose of this book is to continue to promote the clarion call for nursing leaders, educators, and practicing clinicians to seek integrated understanding of APRNs. It explores how they are prepared and the evolving opportunities for the roles that they will create and assume given the developing health care landscape. This sixth edition continues to collate the latest trends and evidence regarding APRN competencies, roles, and challenges in today's environment. However, there is still significant work ahead to solidify within and outside the profession the value-added benefit of APRNs as direct care providers and leaders—an imperative for patient safety and quality care around the globe.

Underlying Premises

Readers may notice a change in terms, with the use of "advanced practice registered nurse" (APRN) in this edition versus "advanced practice nurse" (APN) in previous editions. There were several reasons for this change in terms: (1) APRN is increasingly becoming more common as the standard lexicon within and outside of nursing; (2) to differentiate between the increasingly standardized roles of APRNs in the United States versus the use of the term APN for international roles, which, of necessity, are more varied due to significant differences between countries; and (3) to attempt to provide more clarity between the traditional use of *advanced practice nursing* for APRN roles versus *advanced nursing practice,* which is used for all nurses who are obtaining DNP degrees, not just APRNs. Transition to the APRN term should not imply that the editors are viewing these APRN roles only through a regulatory lens. On the contrary, we continue to advocate, as did the previous editors, that advanced practice nursing is viewed in the broadest sense in this book—encompassing the entire professional understanding and enactment of APRN roles, with patients and families at the center of their purpose of existence.

It is assumed that health care policy is an ongoing process, made up of small and large revisions over decades. Many health care polices in the United States are being debated and altered, and unintentional consequences are being discovered; therefore, the policy issues surrounding APRNs are, of necessity, living, moving, and ever-changing. The purpose of this book is also to make clear the ongoing APRN policy issues in the United States, knowing that incrementalism can make it difficult to write with certitude around any health care policy. Moreover, the international community, who may have a more centralized system, could benefit from knowing about our health policy issues so that they can make strategic decisions on pitfalls to avoid, such as having collaboration legislated.

Finally, each APRN student comes to a graduate program with a background in nursing. Human caring and compassion for others lies at the heart of nursing. While caring is not laid out as a core APRN competency, it is assumed that each student who comes to the APRN role already embodies the Nursing Code of Ethics, Provision 1: "The nurse practices with compassion and respect for the inherent dignity, worth, and unique attributes of every person" (American Nurses Association, 2015). Human caring and showing of compassion are covered in the Direct Clinical Practice and Guidance and Coaching chapters, both more fully and at an advanced practice level.

Organization

This edition continues the tradition of extensive updating and revision based on the most current evidence available. The editors and authors have incorporated content up until the final feasible moment in order to provide readers with the latest changes in regulatory, credentialing, and professional issues impacting APRNs. Exemplars have been updated throughout the book, and Key Summary Points have been added to the end of each chapter to emphasize the key takeaways for readers. In Part I, "Historical and Developmental Aspects of Advanced Practice Nursing," Chapter 2 has incorporated new conceptual models, including international models, to continue to provide examples for connecting conceptual models to actual APRN practice. In addition, Chapter 6 has been significantly revised to provide an update on the status of international APN roles and the challenges for the roles in all regions of the world. While advanced practice nursing is significantly different between the United States and other countries, there is much we can do to collaborate and learn from each other. In Part II, "Competencies of Advanced Practice Nursing," the seven competencies are outlined—Direct Clinical Practice, Guidance and Coaching, Consultation, Evidence-Based Practice, Leadership, Collaboration, and Ethical Decision Making; they continue to stand the test of time as the foundational core for all APRN roles. Chapter 8 has been extensively revised to reflect the increasing importance of APRN guidance and coaching in context of the focus on helping patients and families achieve health. In Part III, "Advanced Practice Roles: The Operational Definitions of Advanced Practice Nursing," each of the APRN role chapters has been updated to highlight the unique niche APRNs fill in exhibition of the core competencies through each of the specific roles. This is particularly reflected in context of the implications of the Consensus Model, the changing health care policy environment, and increasing numbers of DNP-prepared APRNs. Of note in Part IV, "Critical Elements in Managing Advanced Practice Nursing Environments," Chapter 19 has been revised to provide an overall context of policy implications for APRNs and the need for APRNs to be engaged in advocacy at all levels. Chapter 20 includes more information on entrepreneurship and intrapreneurship. Chapter 23 continues to be a rich resource for evidence demonstrating the outcomes of APRNs.

Audience

This book is intended for graduate nursing students, practicing APRNs, educators, administrators, and nursing leaders. The book will be a resource for graduate students as they learn to incorporate theory, research, policy, and practice skills into their developing roles. It provides an understanding of the common threads among APRN roles, the unique contributions of each role, and the holistic advanced skills distinct to APRNs as compared with other non-nurse providers.

This book will be useful to practicing APRNs as an update for a health care environment that is constantly changing. It provides a foundation for practice and an opportunity to self-assess for areas of strength and areas for growth throughout one's APRN career. APRNs can use pertinent sections of the book with administrators to highlight role functions and documented outcomes of APRNs and how optimization of each role can be envisioned and implemented.

For educators, the book continues to serve as a comprehensive resource for use in educational APRN program curricula. Instructor resources available with this book include slides with content that corresponds to each chapter as well as each of the images in the book. In addition, a new instructor resource with this edition will be a test bank of questions. These Evolve resources can be accessed at http://evolve.elsevier.com/Hamric/

Approach

The Editors extend a sincere and grateful thank you to the book's contributors. It has been an even more challenging endeavor to complete this sixth edition revision during these chaotic and uncertain times in the US health care environment. It, at times, seems as if the focus of health care legislation and policy is changing on a daily basis. It has taken thoughtful consideration on the part of each author to determine how to update the chapters with meaningful detail, while still conveying the key points for the current and future practice of APRNs, notwithstanding the exact contextual changes that are yet unknown.

Regardless of the eventual result of US health care policy and enactment, quality and holistic patient care will always be the focus of APRN practice. APRNs are here to stay, and bringing all APRNs under the same umbrella is a powerful way to strengthen our ability to write our own script. *The strength of the wolf is in the pack.*

Transitions

In closing, it is with deep gratitude that we want to acknowledge the transition in editors with this edition.

The fifth edition was Ann Hamric's last as the senior editor of this text. Ann writes: "In both its rewards and challenges, envisioning and 'birthing' the first five editions of this book has been a highlight of my professional career. When we began this enterprise, the profession had not agreed on educational or certification requirements to be considered an APN, or whether APNs needed to maintain a direct clinical practice. There was no integrative understanding that advanced practice nursing included midwifery or nurse anesthesia. Now, all these features of advanced practice nursing are well established. Watching the international growth of advanced practice nursing and interacting with international colleagues who are using this work to advance practice in their own countries has been very gratifying. I am deeply indebted to the other editors and all our contributors over the editions for the joy of creating a work that has stood the test of time and provided leadership for understanding this critically important level of nursing practice. Many of those who wrote with us in the various editions have become personal friends as well as valued colleagues. This work has immeasurably enriched my life on many levels, and I am very grateful to have had a part in shaping advanced nursing through this book."

Charlene Hanson has also retired as editor for the book while continuing in a mentoring and support role. Chuckie writes, "When I came to the new conceptualization for this textbook in 1993, it was with the idea that as an editor I would help to integrate the APN roles of nurse practitioner, nurse midwife, and nurse anesthetist into the seminal CNS work of Hamric and Spross. It has been a fine journey, with rich rewards, working through exciting and challenging times with wonderful colleagues. I have watched health care and advanced practice nursing significantly advance with each new edition, fondly known by students as 'The Hamric Book.' Helping graduate students here and abroad to find their niche as competent, resourceful APNs has been a high point of my career. My heartfelt thanks to all who have made this journey possible for me. I look forward to seeing where we are headed in the future."

Mary Fran Tracy
Eileen T. O'Grady

References

American Nurses Association. (2015). *Code of ethics for nurses with interpretive statements.* Silver Spring, MD: Author.

APRN Joint Dialogue Group. (2008). Consensus model for APRN regulation: Licensure, accreditation, certification & education. Retrieved from http://www.aacn.nche.edu/education-resources/APRNReport.pdf.

Institute of Medicine. (2011). *The future of nursing: Leading change, advancing health*. Washington, DC: National Academies Press.

Institute of Medicine. (2015). Report in brief: Assessing progress on the Institute of Medicine report *The Future of Nursing*. Retrieved from http://www.nationalacademies.org/hmd/~/media/Files/Report%20Files/2015/AssessingFON_releaseslides/Nursing-Report-in-brief.pdf.

National Council of State Boards of Nursing. (2017). Implementation status map. Retrieved from https://www.ncsbn.org/5397.htm.

Patient Protection and Affordable Care Act, 42 U.S.C. § 18001 (2010).

United States Department of Veterans Affairs. (2016). VA grants full practice authority to advance practice registered nurses. Retrieved from https://www.va.gov/opa/pressrel/pressrelease.cfm?id=2847.

Contents

PART II
Competencies of Advanced Practice Nursing

PART IV
Critical Elements in Managing Advanced Practice Nursing Environments

Highlights From the History of Advanced Practice Nursing in the United States

Brigid Lusk • Anne Z. Cockerham • Arlene W. Keeling

> *"You measure the size of the accomplishment by the obstacles you had to overcome to reach your goals."*
>
> —*Booker T. Washington*

CHAPTER CONTENTS

This chapter sets the stage for the rest of the book. Nurses who ventured into advanced practice roles in the years before certification and accreditation and legislation need to have their stories told. More than that, these stories provide continuity to guide us through to our current practice and provide a basis for our current thinking. Awareness of the history of advanced practice nursing is a necessary foundation for effecting changes in practice and policy. Fortunately, these stories also make for fascinating reading.

This chapter covers selected highlights of the history of advanced practice nursing in the United States from the late 19th century to the present (Box 1.1). It examines four established advanced practice roles—certified registered nurse anesthetists (CRNAs), certified nurse-midwives (CNMs), clinical nurse specialists (CNSs), and nurse practitioners (NPs)—in the context of the social, political, and economic environment of the time and within the context of the history of medicine, technology, and science. Legal issues and issues related to

1915   Lakeside Hospital School of Anesthesia opens in Cleveland, Ohio

1925   Kentucky Committee for Mothers and Babies, precursor to Frontier Nursing Service, founded

1931   American Association of Nurse Anesthetists (AANA) founded

1941   American Association of Nurse-Midwives (AANM) founded

1945   AANA develops and implements Certified Registered Nurse Anesthetists certification examination

1954   Master's Program in Psychiatric Nursing started at Rutgers University—first Clinical Nurse Specialist education program

1955   American College of Nurse-Midwives (ACNM) founded

1965   Pediatric Nurse Practitioner certification program opens in Colorado

1969   Merger of ACNM and AANM

1973   National Association of Pediatric Nurse Practitioners founded

1984   All states recognize nurse-midwifery

1985   American Academy of Nurse Practitioners (AANP) founded

1995   National Association of Clinical Nurse Specialists founded

1995   American College of Nurse Practitioners (ACNP) founded

2002   Acute Care Nurse Practitioners join the AANP

2004   American Association of Colleges of Nursing recommends that all advanced practice nurses earn Doctor of Nursing Practice degree

2013   American Association of Nurse Practitioners founded through merger of AANP and ACNP

gender and health care workforce are considered. Although sociopolitical and economic context is critical to understanding nursing history, only historical events specifically relevant to the history of advanced practice nursing are included. Readers may consult the references of this chapter for further information.

The Doctor of Nursing Practice (DNP) degree, introduced by the American Association of Colleges of Nursing (AACN) in 2004, was aimed at ensuring a strong educational preparation for advanced practice registered nurses (APRNs). Initially, this initiative was developed in response to the reality of ever-increasing curricular requirements in master's degree programs throughout the country (Keeling, Kirchgessner, & Brodie, 2010). As originally proposed by the AACN (2014), the DNP would standardize practice entry requirements for all APRNs by the year 2015, assuring the public that each APRN would have had 1000 supervised clinical hours prior to entering the practice setting. Moreover, the proposed curriculum for DNPs would include competencies deemed essential for nursing practice in the 21st century (AACN, 2006). The year 2015 has now come and gone but the issue of requiring the practice doctorate remains unsettled. Discussion surrounding the DNP as assessed by each of the four major APRN professional bodies is covered at the end of each section of this chapter.

A brief comment on terminology: The use of the term *specialist* in nursing can be traced to the turn of the 20th century, when it was used to designate a nurse who had completed a postgraduate course in a clinical specialty area or who had extensive experience and expertise in a particular clinical practice area. With the introduction of the NP role during the 1960s and 1970s, the terms *expanded role* and *extended role* were used, implying a horizontal movement to encompass expertise from medicine and other disciplines. The more contemporary term *advanced practice,* which began to be used in the United States in the 1980s, reflects a more vertical or hierarchical movement encompassing graduate education within nursing, rather than a simple expansion of expertise by the development of knowledge and skills used by other disciplines. Since the 1980s, the term *advanced practice nurse* (APN) has increasingly been used to delineate CRNAs, CNMs, CNSs, and NPs. In the last decade, state nurse practice acts have gradually adopted the term *advanced practice registered nurse*. These professional and regulatory influences served to unite the advanced practice specialty roles conceptually and legislatively, thereby promoting collaboration and cohesion among APRNs.

Nurse Anesthetists

The roots of nurse anesthesia in the United States can be traced to the late 19th century, shortly after the use of certain gasses to induce unconsciousness was discovered. Thatcher (1953) cited contemporary accounts of two instances of nurses giving anesthesia as early as the American Civil War (1861–1865). In 1863, following the Battle of Gettysburg, a Mrs. John Harris set out from Baltimore with "chloroform and stimulants" and ministered "as much as in her power to the stream of wounded" (Moore, 1866; cited in Thatcher, 1953, p. 33). In the second instance, taken from *The Medical and Surgical History of the War of the Rebellion* (1883): "More chloroform was added and reapplied by a nurse in attendance (the surgeon having stepped aside for a moment)" (Thatcher, 1953, p. 34). Jolly, in her history of Roman Catholic nuns during the same war, cited further instances of nuns administering anesthesia (Jolly, 1927).

The administration of chloroform was a relatively simple procedure in which the anesthetizer poured the drug over a cloth held over the patient's nose and mouth; several early nursing texts included instructions for anesthetic administration (Box 1.2). However, one of these, Nicholas Senn's *A Nurse's Guide to the Operating Room,* gave a real sense of the hazards involved. He wrote:

> Usually complete anesthesia is preceded by a stage of excitement of variable duration. … The patient shouts, prays, swears, sings, cries, laughs, or fights, according to his temperament, habits, religious belief, occupation or social position in life. Tonic and clonic spasms, irregular respiration and cyanosis are some of the alarming symptoms. (Senn, 1905, p. 90)

Yet nurses typically gave anesthesia only when a physician was unavailable. This was very likely when surgery was performed in private houses, when a nurse could well be the only other trained person present (Adams Hampton, 1893; Senn, 1905; Weeks-Shaw, 1902). Following the increasingly scientific and specialized nature of giving anesthesia, the practice became the prerogative of physicians, although there arose notable exceptions.

Anesthesia at Mayo Clinic

At St. Mary's Hospital in Rochester, Minnesota, Dr. William Worrall Mayo was among the first physicians in the country to recognize and formally train nurse anesthetists. In 1889, Mayo hired Edith Granham to be his anesthetist and office nurse. Subsequently, he hired Alice Magaw (later referred to as the "mother of anesthesia"; Keeling, 2007). Magaw kept excellent records of her results and, in 1900, published them in the *St. Paul's Medical Journal.* Reporting her "Observations on 1,092 Cases of

 BOX 1.2 Instructions for Administration of Chloroform (1893)

A nurse is often called upon in private practice to administer an anæsthetic, as it is not possible at every operation to have sufficient medical assistance. (p. 331) … The forenoon is the best time to select for giving an anæsthetic, as the vital powers are in better condition, if the patient has had a good night and is not exhausted by nervous strain, pain, or work. The clothing should be light and warm, but loose about the neck and chest, and no corset or tight waist should be permitted, because the respiratory organs must have freedom of movement. … If the patient be a child, care should be taken to see that the mouth is quite empty, as there may be coins, buttons, or other articles stowed away in the mouth. (pp. 332–333)

… The nurse must also have at hand a hypodermic syringe (sterilized and in good order), whiskey or brandy, tincture of digitalis, a solution of strychnine, morphine, atropine, and aqua ammonia, as any of them may be called for. (p. 333) … Besides the anæsthetizer, if the patient is a woman, the nurse should always be present to give any necessary assistance, but a second or even a third person may be needed if there be much struggling. (p. 334)

Ether is probably given in this country oftener than any other anæsthetic, as there seems to be little danger to life under ordinary circumstances when it is carefully administered. … Speaking generally, chloroform is preferable for very young or very old patients. (p. 334) … In the early stages of the administration of ether the patient may suddenly stop breathing and the face become cyanosed; the cone should be at once removed, and pressure made upon the chest and sides once or twice, when the breathing will recommence. (p. 336)

From Adams Hampton, I. (1893). The administration of anæsthetics. In *Nursing: Its principles and practice* (Ch. 22, pp. 331–336). Philadelphia: Saunders.

Anesthesia from January 1, 1899 to January 1, 1900," she wrote:

> In that time, we administered an anesthetic 1,092 times; ether alone 674 times; chloroform 245 times; ether and chloroform combined, 173 times. I can report that out of this number, 1,092 cases, we have not had an accident; we have not had occasion to use artificial respiration once; nor one case of ether pneumonia; neither have we had any serious

renal results. Tongue forceps were used but once, the operation was on the jaw and it was quite necessary. (Magaw, 1900, p. 306)

Between 1899 and 1901, the family of Doctors Mayo added several other nurse anesthetists to their surgical teams. Soon, the Mayo Clinic would become world renowned for its nurse anesthesia training program.

Early Challenges

During the 1910s, nurse anesthetists faced obstacles as well as new opportunities. Early in the decade, as the specialty of anesthesia was on the rise, the medical profession began to question a nurse's right to administer anesthesia, claiming that these nurses were practicing medicine without a license. In 1911, the New York State Medical Society argued (unsuccessfully) that the administration of an anesthetic by a nurse violated state law (Thatcher, 1953). A year later, the Ohio State Medical Board passed a resolution specifying that only physicians could administer anesthesia. Despite this resolution, nurse anesthetist Agatha Hodgins established the Lakeside Hospital School of Anesthesia in Cleveland, Ohio, in 1915. The challenge culminated in a lawsuit brought against the Lakeside Hospital program by the state medical society. This lawsuit was unsuccessful and resulted in an amendment to the Ohio Medical Practice Act protecting the practice of nurse anesthesia. However, medical opposition to the practice of nurse anesthesia continued in Kentucky, and another lawsuit against nurse anesthetists was filed (*Frank et al. v. South et al.,* 1917). In that case, the Kentucky appellate court ruled that anesthesia provided by nurse anesthetist Margaret Hatfield did not constitute the practice of medicine if it was given under the orders and supervision of a licensed physician (in this case, Dr. Louis Frank). The significance of this decision was that the courts declared nurse anesthesia legal but "subordinate" to the medical profession. It was a landmark decision, one that would have lasting implications for nurse anesthetists' practice. Later in the century it would also have an impact on the practice of APRNs in all four roles (Keeling, 2007).

Growth of Nurse Anesthesia Practice

Opportunities for nurse anesthetists increased, albeit poignantly, when the United States entered World War I in 1917. That year more than 1000 nurses were deployed to Britain and France, including nurse anesthetists, some of whom had trained at the Mayo and Cleveland Clinics. The realities of the front were gruesome; shrapnel created devastating wounds and mustard gas destroyed lungs and caused profound burns (Beeber, 1990). The resulting need for pain relief and anesthesia care for the wounded soldiers created an immediate demand for nurse anesthetists' knowledge and skills (Keeling, 2007). The war also created opportunities for research, and physicians and nurses began investigating new methods of administering anesthesia. At the well-established Lakeside Hospital anesthesia program, Dr. George Crile and nurse anesthetist Agatha Hodgins experimented with combined nitrous oxide–oxygen administration. They also investigated the use of morphine and scopolamine as adjuncts to anesthesia.

After the war, opportunities for the employment of nurse anesthetists were mixed. For example, in 1922 Samuel Harvey, a Yale professor of surgery, hired Alice M. Hunt as an instructor of anesthesia with university rank at the Yale Medical School, a significant and prestigious appointment for a nurse (Thatcher, 1953). In contrast to Hunt's experience, however, many other nurse anesthetists struggled to find practice opportunities. Medicine was becoming increasingly complex, scientific, and controlled by organized medical specialties intent on preserving their spheres of practice, including anesthesia. Interprofessional conflict over disciplinary boundaries seemed inescapable.

It was soon clear that nurse anesthetists, too, needed to organize as a specialty. In 1931, at Lakeside Hospital, Hodgins established the National Association of Nurse Anesthetists (later renamed the American Association of Nurse Anesthetists [AANA]) and served as the organization's first president. At the first meeting of the association, the group voted to affiliate with the American Nurses Association (ANA). However, the ANA denied the request, probably because the ANA was afraid to assume legal responsibility for a group that could be charged with practicing medicine without a license (Thatcher, 1953).

The ANA's fears were not unfounded. During the 1930s, the devastation of the national economy made jobs scarce and the tension between nurse anesthetists and their physician counterparts continued, with more legal challenges to the practice of nurse anesthesia. In California, the Los Angeles County Medical Association sued nurse anesthetist Dagmar Nelson in 1934 for practicing medicine without a license; Nelson won. According to the judge, "The administration of general anesthetics by the defendant Dagmar A. Nelson, pursuant to the directions and supervision of duly licensed physicians and surgeons, as shown by the evidence in this case, does not constitute the practice of medicine or surgery" (McGarrel, 1934).

In response, Dr. William Chalmers-Frances filed another suit against Nelson that again resulted in a judgment for Nelson (*Chalmers-Frances v. Nelson,* 1936). In 1938, the physician appealed the case to the California Supreme Court, which again ruled in favor of Nelson. The case became famous. The courts established legal precedent—the practice of nurse anesthesia was legal and within the scope of nursing practice, as long as it was done under the guidance of a supervising physician. At that time there were 39 training programs for nurse anesthetists in the nation (Horton, 2007a).

While World War II provided opportunities for young nurses in Europe to learn the skills necessary to administer anesthesia, it also was the period in which anesthesia grew into a medical specialty (Waisel, 2001). In 1939, just before the United States entered the war, the first written examination for board certification in medical anesthesiology was given, but the specialty still sought legitimacy. Meanwhile, demands for anesthetists, advances in

the types of anesthesia available, and continuing education in the field increasingly stimulated physicians' interest in the specialty. In particular, the use of the new drug sodium pentothal required specialized knowledge of physiology and pharmacology, underscoring the emerging view that only physicians could provide anesthesia. In fact, the administration of anesthesia was becoming more complex, and anesthesiologists demonstrated their expertise not only in administering sodium pentothal but also in performing endotracheal intubation and regional blocks (Waisel, 2001). Clearly, medicine was strengthening its hold on the specialty.

At the same time, World War II increased the demand for anesthetists on the battlefield. Despite profound shortages of anesthetists early in the war, the US military would not grant nurse anesthetists a specific designation within the military, and experienced nurse anesthetists were required to accept general nurse status. Later, when shortages became even more severe, staff nurses were trained to administer anesthesia (Exemplar 1.1).

Shortly afterward the United States was again at war, this time with Korea, and once again war provided a setting in which opportunities abounded for nurse anesthetists. By the end of the decade, the army had established nurse anesthesia education

---

EXEMPLAR 1.1   Nurse Anesthetists in the 8th Evacuation Hospital, Italy, 1942–1945

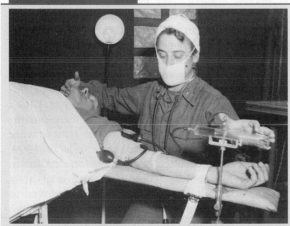

(Courtesy University of Virginia, Center for Nursing Historical Inquiry.)

During World War II, the University of Virginia sponsored the 8th Evacuation Hospital, a 750-bed mobile hospital a few miles from the front lines in North Africa

and Italy. Conditions were demanding and the work overwhelming; surgical teams sometimes operated around the clock despite air raids, heavy rains, and blackouts. There, Dorothy Sandridge Gloor, a young surgical nurse, was trained on the job to give anesthesia. The unit had only one trained anesthesiologist and two nurse anesthetists on staff, and it soon became apparent that more help was needed if the team was to keep up with the "endless stream of battle casualties requiring surgery" (Kinser, 2011, p. 11). Gloor and other nurse anesthetists worked side by side with the surgeons for 16-hour shifts, collaborating with their colleagues to save the injured soldiers. She learned new skills and the specialty knowledge necessary to deliver anesthesia, noting how she learned to start intravenous infusions and make critical observations of the patient on which to base the administration of anesthesia (Kinser, 2011). Working with patients to calm their fears prior to surgery, and explaining what would happen in the operating suite, Gloor and her colleagues demonstrated expertise in coaching the critically injured men. ◎

programs, including one at Walter Reed General Hospital, which graduated its first class in 1961—but this class consisted only of men. Later, the Letterman General Hospital School of Anesthesia in San Francisco also graduated an all-male class. This significant movement of men into a nursing specialty was unprecedented and would continue in the next decade when the United States entered the war in Vietnam.

As was the case in wars of other eras, the war in Vietnam (1955–1975) provided nurses with opportunities to stretch the boundaries of the discipline as they treated thousands of casualties in evacuation hospitals and aboard hospital ships. Not surprisingly, nurse anesthetists played an active role at the front, providing vital services in the prompt surgical treatment of the wounded. According to one account:

> The nurse anesthetist suddenly became a part of a new concept in the treatment of the severely wounded. The Dust-Off helicopter brings medical aid to severely wounded casualties who formerly would have died before or perhaps during evacuation. … Very often it is a nurse anesthetist who first is available to intubate a casualty, and by so doing may avoid the need for tracheostomy. (Jenicek, 1967, p. 348)

Opportunity was not without cost. Of the 10 nurses killed in Vietnam, two were nurse anesthetists (Bankert, 1989).

Reimbursement and Education

Reimbursement for CRNA practice is not clear cut. In fact, third-party payment had its own set of issues. Beginning in 1977, the AANA led a long and complex effort to secure third-party reimbursement under Medicare so that CRNAs could bill for their services. The organization would finally succeed in 1989. Meanwhile, the financial threat posed by CRNAs to physicians was the source of continued interprofessional conflicts with medicine. During the second half of the 20th century, tensions escalated, particularly in relation to malpractice policies, antitrust, and restraint of trade issues. In 1986, *Oltz v. St. Peter's Community Hospital* established the right of CRNAs to sue for anticompetitive damages when anesthesiologists conspired to restrict practice privileges. A second case, *Bhan v. NME Hospitals, Inc., et al.* (1985), established the right of CRNAs to be awarded damages when exclusive contracts were made between hospitals and physician anesthesiologists. Undeniably, CRNAs were winning the legal battles and overcoming practice barriers erected by hospital administrators and physicians.

Since the founding of the AANA in the early 1930s, the primary focus had been to improve educational standards. The leaders had stressed university affiliation and a standardized curriculum. The AANA's *Essentials of an Acceptable School of Anesthesiology for Graduate Registered Nurses* first came out in 1945. At the same time the AANA instituted mandatory certification for CRNAs. This formal credentialing of CRNAs specified the requirements that a nurse had to meet to practice as a nurse anesthetist, preceded credentialing of nurses in the other specialties, and marked a significant milestone. Five years later the AANA's plan for accreditation of anesthesia programs was approved, and the first accreditation of programs started in 1952 (Horton, 2007a).

The 1970s proved to be a difficult decade for nurse anesthetists. In 1972, years after the inception of nurse anesthesia as a specialty role, only four state practice acts specifically mentioned them. Nevertheless, some progress was made in interprofessional relations that year. The AANA and the American Society of Anesthesiologists issued a "Joint Statement on Anesthesia Practice," promoting the concept of the anesthesia team. However, in 1976 the Board of Directors of the American Society of Anesthesiologists voted to withdraw support from the 1972 statement, endorsing one that explicitly supported physician control over CRNA practice (Bankert, 1989). Meanwhile, the AANA continued to promote university affiliation, and by 1982 the AANA President and Board of Directors promoted the baccalaureate degree as an entry requirement for nurses entering anesthesia programs and master's degrees for graduates (Horton, 2007b).

The 1990s saw a significant growth in CRNA education programs, although many of the programs were very small. As the decade opened, there were 17 master's programs in nurse anesthesia; by 1999, there were 82 (Bigbee & Amidi-Nouri, 2000). In 2017, there are 120 accredited nurse anesthesia programs in the United States; 62 are approved to award a doctoral degree (AANA, 2017). Since 1998, all accredited programs in nurse anesthesia are required to be at the master's level (Horton, 2007b); however, they are not uniformly located in schools of nursing. Instead, they are housed in a variety of disciplines, including schools of nursing, medicine, allied health, and basic science. The University of Minnesota started the first post-baccalaureate DNP program for CRNAs in 2009 (Glass, 2009).

Following up on the AANA's long pursuit of education reflective of the complexities of modern anesthesia delivery, plans are in place for a clinical doctorate as entry to nurse anesthesia practice. In 2007, the AANA affirmed its support that the Doctor of Nurse Anesthesia Practice (DNAP) be the entry for nurse anesthesia practice by 2025 (AANA, 2007). Seven years later the Council on Accreditation for Nurse Anesthesia Programs approved trial standards for a practice doctorate for implementation in 2015. All students entering nurse anesthesia programs in and after 2022 must graduate with a doctoral degree (Council, 2015). Chapter 18 presents a discussion of the current CRNA role.

Nurse-Midwives

Unlike nurse anesthetists, who have only been practicing for 150 years or so, midwives have practiced since the beginning of time. Midwives entered the US through the slave trade or during waves of European immigration. These untrained or foreign-trained women lost much of the public's esteem as childbirth became medicalized in the late 19th and early 20th centuries. As Clara Noyes, an early nurse leader, wrote "the word 'midwife,' in America, at least, is one to which considerable odium is attached, and immediately creates a mental picture of illiteracy, carelessness and general filth" (Noyes, 1912, p. 466). With the rise of scientific medicine, coupled with the possibility of "twilight sleep" (through scopolamine and morphine), many upper and middle class urban white women began to use obstetricians to deliver their babies in hospital delivery rooms (Dawley, 2000; Rinker, 2000). Meanwhile, women in isolated communities throughout the country, particularly in rural settings, continued to rely on lay midwives well into the 20th century.

"Granny Midwives"

Granny midwives, as they were condescendingly called, were untrained African-American women who provided the vast majority of obstetric care in the racially segregated southern US states prior to the 1950s. Typically they were the only providers of care for most black Southern women at a time when few hospitals admitted black patients and there was no public funding to support physician attendance in the home. In rural southern states such as Mississippi, in which 50% of the population was black, most women (80% of African-American and 8% of white women) relied on these midwives to deliver their babies (Smith, 1994). In 1940s Arkansas, granny midwives attended approximately three fourths of all African-American births (Bell, 1993). Yet data from 1921 actually showed that the physicians' outcomes were no better than those of the lay midwives (Dawley, 2000).

Frontier Nursing Service Midwives

In 1925, nurse-midwife Mary Breckinridge founded the Frontier Nursing Service (FNS) in an economically depressed, rural mountainous area of southeastern Kentucky. British nurse-midwives and American public health nurses provided midwifery and nursing care through a decentralized network of nurse-run clinics (Breckinridge, 1981; Rooks, 1997). Because there were few roads in the mountainous region, the nurses traveled by horseback to attend births, carrying their supplies in saddlebags. One FNS nurse described the bags and their standing orders, or *Medical Routines,* whereby a physician committee supervised their practice:

> The whole of the district work of the FNS in the Kentucky mountains is done with the aid of two pairs of saddle-bags. ... In these bags we have everything needed for a home delivery. ... In one of the pockets we carry our *Medical Routines* which tells us what we may—and may not—do. A very treasured possession! (Summers, 1938, pp. 1183–1184)

Nurse-Midwifery: Early Education and Organization

In the early 20th century, national concern about high maternal-infant mortality rates led to heated debates surrounding issues of midwife licensure and control, and lay midwives were blamed. In 1914, Dr. Frederick Taussig, speaking at the annual meeting of the National Organization for Public Health Nursing (NOPHN) in St. Louis, proposed that the creation of "nurse-midwives" might solve the "midwife question" and suggested that nurse-midwifery schools be established to train graduate nurses (Taussig, 1914). Later in the decade, the Children's Bureau called for efforts to instruct pregnant women in nutrition and recommended that public health nurses teach principles of hygiene and prenatal care to so-called granny midwives (Rooks, 1997).

Aside from two tiny, short-lived nurse-midwifery schools (Manhattan Midwifery School in New York City and Preston Retreat Hospital in Philadelphia), about which little is documented, the earliest school

| EXEMPLAR 1.2 | Nurse-Midwife Maude Callen |

Maude Callen (1898–1990) was unknown outside her small South Carolina community until photojournalist W. Eugene Smith produced a 10-page photo essay on her for *Life Magazine* in December 1951. Callen's remarkable work as a nurse-midwife made a national impression. Two years later, in a follow-up article, the magazine wrote that readers had donated $18,500—enough to build a much-needed clinic.

Callen trained as a nurse at the Georgia Infirmary, the first hospital for African-Americans in the United States and one of the earliest to train African-American women as nurses. Callen and her husband then moved to Pineville, South Carolina, where Callen had accepted an appointment as a missionary nurse. Historian Darlene Clark Hine quoted a newspaper report: "Pineville was [twenty-two] miles from the nearest hospital or [ten miles to the local] doctor and people sent for Miss Maude when they became ill. She was available day and night" (2011, p. 133). During her first years in Pineville, after she was hired as a public health nurse,

Callen organized public health clinics, conducted prenatal classes, opened the county's first venereal disease clinic, and vaccinated children in schools. One former student gives a vivid picture of Callen as he remembered those days: "She came in to give us shots and we were afraid; there was a lot of running and hollering in the classroom. But she held us and did her job. She would dress so neat. She wore a gray uniform with a white collar and white shoes. She was a beautiful lady" (quoted in Clark Hine, 2011, p. 135). With support from the state division of maternal and child health, Callen attended the 6-month midwifery course offered by the Tuskegee School of Nurse-Midwifery in Alabama (Clark Hine, 2011). As the first African-American nurse-midwife in South Carolina, Callen taught annual midwifery institutes, was called out to assist with difficult births, and delivered more than 800 babies. A midwifery student remembered "I don't know what would have happened [to the people] if Miss Maude had not been there" (quoted in Clark Hine, 2011, p. 135). ◎

to educate nurse-midwives was the School of the Association for the Promotion and Standardization of Midwifery (APSM) in New York City (Burst & Thompson, 2003). Affiliated with the Maternity Center Association, the APSM opened in 1932. More commonly known as the Lobenstine Midwifery School, the APSM graduated its first class in 1933. In 1939, the entry of Britain into World War II proved to be the catalyst for the establishment of the second major school for nurse-midwifery in the United States. That year, the Kentucky FNS lost many of its British nurse-midwives when they returned to England to work; in response, FNS leader Mary Breckinridge established the Frontier Graduate School of Midwifery (Buck, 1940; Cockerham & Keeling, 2012).[a] A short-lived midwifery school, the Tuskegee School of Nurse-Midwifery, was opened in Alabama for African-American nurses and lasted from 1941 to 1946 (Exemplar 1.2). The aim was to reduce the high infant and maternal mortality in the southern US, but the school closed due to untenable working conditions leading to an inability to retain instructors (Varney & Thompson, 2016).

The establishment of a formal organization of practicing nurse-midwives, the American Association

of Nurse-Midwives (AANM), was key to midwifery development in the 1940s. The AANM was incorporated in 1941 under the leadership of Mary Breckinridge (News Here and There, 1942, p. 832). Three years later, in 1944, the NOPHN established a section for nurse-midwives within their organization. However, there were organizational issues for the midwives when the NOPHN was absorbed by the two other major nursing organizations in the early 1950s. The American College of Nurse-Midwives (ACNM) was founded in 1955. In 1969, upon the death of the AANM's long-time president, Mary Breckenridge, the AANM and the ACNM merged (Varney & Thompson, 2016).

Growth of Midwifery Practice

Public interest in natural childbirth that stemmed from the women's movement was particularly beneficial to the practice of nurse-midwifery in the 1970s; the demand for nurse-midwifery services increased dramatically during that decade. In addition, sociopolitical developments, including the increased employment of CNMs in federally funded health care projects and the increased birth rate resulting from baby boomers reaching adulthood, converged with inadequate numbers of obstetricians to foster the rapid growth of CNM practice (Varney, Kriebs, & Gegor, 2004).

[a]This program was for nurses who already had a degree in nursing (i.e., registered nurses) but was not a graduate program in the modern sense of the term.

In 1971 the ACNM, the American College of Obstetricians and Gynecologists, and the Nurses' Association of the American College of Obstetricians and Gynecologists issued a joint statement supporting the development and employment of nurse-midwives in obstetric teams directed by a physician. The joint statement, which was critical to the practice of nurse-midwifery, reflected some resolution of the interprofessional tension that had existed through much of the 20th century. However, it did not provide for autonomy for CNMs. Later in the decade, the ACNM revised its definitions of CNM practice and its philosophy, emphasizing the distinct midwifery and nursing origins of the role (ACNM, 1978a, 1978b). This conceptualization of nurse-midwifery as the combination of two disciplines, nursing and midwifery, was unique among the advanced practice nursing specialties. It served to align nurse-midwives with non-nurse midwives, thereby broadening their organizational and political base. Philosophically controversial, even within nurse-midwifery, the conceptualization created some distance from other APRN specialties that saw advanced practice roles as based solely in the discipline of nursing. This distinction would continue to isolate CNMs from some APRNs for the next several decades.

By the 1980s, the public's acceptance of nurse-midwives had further grown, and demand for their services had increased among all socioeconomic groups. In 1982, there were almost 2600 CNMs, most located on the East Coast. "Nurse-midwifery had become not only acceptable but also desirable and demanded. Now the problem was that, after years during which nurse-midwives struggled for existence, there was nowhere near the supply to meet the demand" (Varney, 1987, p. 31).

Another problem that intensified in the 1980s was the escalating cost of malpractice insurance. The critical issue for insurance companies at this time was the tension between covering a nurse-midwife's planned normal healthy practice, with minimal risk, against the possibility of a complex delivery outcome. The annual cost of nurse-midwives' malpractice insurance rose from $38 annually in 1982 to about $3500 annually in 1986. This huge increase occurred when midwives earned, on average, $23,000 a year (Langton & Kammerer, 1985). The price of insurance was impacted by where nurse-midwives practiced—in a hospital, birthing center, or private home. Attending a delivery in a private home was the most risky because midwives lacked any immediate medical support. Due to the cost of insurance, many CNMs gave up delivering babies altogether; others sought employment in physicians' offices, public health departments, and hospitals in which they could be covered by their employers' policies. Some forfeited coverage completely. In 1987, an Arizona study found that about 10% of CNMs were practicing without insurance (Xu, Lori, Siefert, Jacobson, & Ransom, 2008).

During the 1990s, increasing demand for CNM services resulted in a gradual expansion in the scope of nurse-midwifery practice. CNMs began to provide care to women with relatively high-risk pregnancies in collaboration with obstetricians in some of the nation's academic tertiary care centers (Rooks, 1997). During this decade, two practice models emerged: the CNM service model, in which CNMs were responsible for the care of a caseload of women determined to be eligible for midwifery care, and the CNM-physician team model. Nurse-midwives continued making progress in establishing laws and regulations needed to support their practice. However, the struggle for prescriptive authority continued until 2007, when Pennsylvania's nurse-midwives, the last in the country, finally received the right to prescribe (ACNM, 2007).

Reimbursement

Conflict with the medical profession arose as obstetricians perceived a growing threat to their practices. The denial of hospital privileges, attempts to deny third-party reimbursement, and state legislative battles over statutory recognition of CNMs ensued. In particular, problems concerning restraint of trade emerged. In 1980, the US Congress and the Federal Trade Commission conducted a hearing to determine the extent of the restraint of trade issues experienced by CNMs. In two cases, one in Tennessee and one in Georgia, the Federal Trade Commission obtained restraint orders against hospitals and insurance companies attempting to limit the practice of CNMs, in essence ensuring that CNMs could practice (Diers, 1991). Third-party reimbursement for CNMs was a second issue. In 1980, CNMs working under the Civilian Health and Medical Program of the Uniformed Services (CHAMPUS; now Tricare) for military dependents were the first to receive approval for reimbursement. Third-party payment for CNMs was also included under Medicaid. Statutory recognition by state legislatures was a third problem that would be addressed in the 1980s. By 1984, all 50 states had recognized nurse-midwifery in their state laws or regulations (Varney, 1987).

Nurse-Midwifery: Later Education

Much like nurse anesthetist programs had done before them, and indeed with help from the AANA, the midwifery organization acted to form an accrediting body; the first draft of their accreditation criteria appeared in 1962. Accreditation supported the midwives' aim to control their entry criteria and their professional education. Midwifery programs in the United States provided two different credentials: certificates and, later, master's degrees as midwifery programs emerged in university settings in the late 1950s. In 1966 accreditation criteria mandated that all nurse-midwifery programs had to be affiliated with a university (Varney & Thompson, 2016). In 2017, there were 40 master's programs in nurse-midwifery and just 7 post-baccalaureate DNP nurse-midwifery programs (AACN, 2017). In an interesting move, unlike other APRN professional organizations, the ACNM has stated that there is no evidence to support requiring a doctoral degree for entry into midwifery practice. They argue that current educational standards result in safe and positive outcomes for women and newborns. Therefore in 2012 the ACNM reaffirmed its 2007 position statement that the DNP is not required for entry into midwifery practice (ACNM, 2012). Current discussion of the nurse-midwifery APRN role is presented in Chapter 17.

Clinical Nurse Specialists

The clinical nurse specialist evolved out of the increasing complexity of nursing care. The use of the term *specialist* in nursing can be traced to the turn of the 20th century, when hospitals offered postgraduate courses in various specialty areas, including anesthesia, tuberculosis, operating room, laboratory, and dietetics. In the first issue of the *American Journal of Nursing,* in an article titled "Specialties in Nursing," Katherine Dewitt (1900) described specialty practice and the specialist's need for continuing education:

> Those who devote themselves to one branch of nursing often do so because of the keen interest they feel in it. The specialist can and should reach greater perfection in her sphere when she gives her entire time to it. Her studies should be continued in that direction, she should try constantly to keep up with the rapid advances in medical science. … The nurse who is a specialist can often supplement the doctor's work to a great extent. (p. 16)

The roots of the CNS role lie in the area of psychiatric nursing, which had its origins in the Quaker reform movement initiated earlier in mid-19th century England. In the United States, these Quaker reformers challenged the brutal treatment of the insane and advocated "moral treatment," emphasizing gentler methods of social control in a domestic setting (D'Antonio, 1991, p. 411).

Psychiatric Nursing Specialists

The first American training program for psychiatric nurses was founded in 1880 at McLean Hospital in Massachusetts (Critchley, 1985). According to Linda Richards, an 1873 graduate of the New England Hospital School of Nursing, the McLean Hospital maintained high standards and demonstrated "the value of trained nursing for the many persons afflicted with mental disease" (Richards, 1911, p. 109). Richards served as superintendent of nurses at the Taunton Insane Hospital for 4 years, beginning in 1899. She subsequently organized a nursing school for the preparation of psychiatric nurses at the Worcester Hospital for the Insane and finally went to the Michigan Insane Hospital in Kalamazoo, where she remained until 1909 (Richards, 1911). Because of this work, Richards is credited with founding the specialty of psychiatric nursing.

During the first decades of the 20th century, Harry Stack Sullivan's classic writings and the work of Sigmund Freud changed psychiatric nursing dramatically. The emphasis on interpersonal interaction with patients and milieu treatment supported the movement of nurses into a more direct role in the psychiatric care of hospitalized patients.

World War II influenced the specialty of psychiatric nursing because of an increased public awareness of psychiatric problems in returning soldiers (Critchley, 1985). During the 1940s, new treatments were introduced for the care of the mentally ill, including the widespread use of electroshock therapy, which required the assistance of nurses who had specialized knowledge and training. According to a 1942 *American Journal of Nursing* article, "Only the nurse skilled in her profession and with additional psychiatric background has a place in mental hospitals today" (Schindler, 1942, p. 861). By 1943, three postgraduate programs in psychiatric nursing had been established. As nurse educator Frances Reiter later reflected on her career, she recalled having first used the term *nurse clinician* in a speech in 1943 to describe a nurse with advanced "curative" knowledge and clinical competence committed to providing the highest quality of direct patient care (Reiter, 1966).

In 1946, after Congress passed the National Mental Health Act designating psychiatric nursing as a core discipline in mental health, federal funding for graduate and undergraduate educational programs and research became available. Psychiatric nursing became established as a graduate-level specialty, one that would lead the way for clinical nurse specialization in the next decade.

In 1954, Hildegarde E. Peplau, a professor of psychiatric nursing, established a master's program in psychiatric nursing at Rutgers University in New Jersey. Considered the first CNS education program, this program, and the growth of specialty knowledge in psychiatric nursing that ensued, provided support for psychiatric nurses to begin exploring new leadership roles in the care of patients with mental illness in inpatient and outpatient settings. Scholarship in psychiatric nursing also flourished, including Peplau's conceptual framework for psychiatric nursing. Her book, *Interpersonal Relations in Nursing: A Conceptual Frame of Reference for Psychodynamic Nursing* (1952), provided theory-based practice for the specialty. Clearly, the link between academia and specialization was becoming stronger and the psychiatric specialty was leading the way.

Coronary Care Nursing Specialists

Cardiac rhythms, constantly visualized on the newly developed bedside monitors, required educated nurses and thus called for another early nursing clinical specialty. With the establishment of the Bethany Hospital Coronary Care Unit (CCU) in Kansas City, Kansas, in 1962 and a second unit at the Presbyterian Hospital in Philadelphia, coronary care nursing emerged as a new clinical specialty. As CCUs proliferated across the country with the support of federally funded regional medical programs, nurses and physicians acquired specialized clinical knowledge in the area of cardiology. Together, these nurses and physicians discussed clinical questions and negotiated responsibilities (Lynaugh & Fairman, 1992). In so doing, CCU nurses also expanded their scope of practice. Identifying cardiac arrhythmias, administering intravenous medications, and defibrillating patients who had lethal ventricular fibrillation, CCU nurses blurred the invisible boundary separating the disciplines of nursing and medicine. These nurses were diagnosing and treating patients in dramatic lifesaving situations, thereby challenging the very definition of nursing that had been published by the ANA only a few years earlier (Keeling, 2004, 2007) (Box 1.3 and Exemplar 1.3).

Growth of Clinical Nurse Specialist Practice

The 1960s are most often noted as the decade in which clinical nurse specialization took its modern form. After the enactment of the Nurse Training Act of 1964, numerous CNS master's programs were created. Peplau (1965) contended that three social forces precede the development of areas of specialization: (1) an increase in specialty-related information, (2) new technologic advances, and (3) a response to public need and interest. In addition to shaping most nursing specialties, these forces had a particularly strong effect on the development of the psychiatric CNS role in the 1960s. The Community Mental Health Centers Act of 1963, as well as the growing interest in child and adolescent mental health care, directly enhanced the expansion of that role in outpatient mental health care.

A rapid proliferation of CNS programs and jobs, as well as an emerging role ambiguity and confusion that accompanied them, defined the 1970s for CNSs. During this decade, psychiatric CNSs continued to provide leadership in the educational and clinical arenas while federal funding from the Professional Nurse Traineeship Program provided fiscal support for new programs. In addition to psychiatric and coronary care specializations, the specialties of critical care and oncology nursing also grew during the 1970s. The American Association of Critical-Care Nurses, founded in 1969 as the American Association of Cardiovascular Nurses, addressed the continuing educational needs of new specialists in the areas of coronary care and intensive care nursing. Only 4 years later, after the ANA and American Cancer Society sponsored the first National Cancer Nursing Research Conference, a group of oncology nurses met to discuss the need for a national organization to support their specialty. Officially incorporated in 1975, the Oncology Nursing Society provided a forum for issues related to cancer nursing and supported the growth of advanced practice nursing in this specialty (Lusk, 2005; Oncology Nursing Society, 2011). The ANA officially recognized the CNS role in the mid-1970s, defining the CNS as an expert practitioner and change agent. The ANA's definition specified a master's degree as a requirement for the CNS (ANA Congress of Nursing Practice, 1974).

As with the other advanced nursing specialties of nurse anesthesia and midwifery, the development

BOX 1.3 American Nurses Association Defines Nursing Practice (c. 1950s)

The classic work of nurse scholar Virginia Henderson on scientifically based, patient-centered care laid the foundation for changes in nursing that would occur in the second half of the 20th century, including the development of APRNs. Influenced by Henderson and by Hildegarde Peplau, innovative nurses such as Frances Reiter at New York Medical College initiated a clinical nurse graduate curriculum designed to provide nurses with an intellectual clinical component based on a liberal arts education, in effect supporting a broader role for nurses (Fairman, 2001). However, although academic nursing was making strides toward establishing specialty education and expanding the nurse specialist's scope of practice, the ANA developed a model definition of nursing that would unduly restrict nursing practice for the next several decades. The definition, prepared in 1955 and adopted by many states, read as follows (ANA, 1955):

The practice of professional nursing means the performance for compensation of any act in the observation, care and counsel of the ill … or in the maintenance of health or prevention of illness … or the administration of medications and treatments as prescribed by a licensed physician. … The foregoing shall not be deemed

to include acts of diagnosis or prescription of therapeutic or corrective measures.

Although the ANA may simply have been seeking clarity in defining the discipline's boundaries, its exclusion of the acts of diagnosis and prescription stifled the development of advanced practice nursing. Discussing the impact of the ANA's restrictions on diagnosis and prescription, law professor Barbara Safriet (1992) argued: "Even at the time the ANA's model definition was issued … it was unduly restrictive when measured by then current nursing practice." Nurses had been assessing patients for more than 50 years. According to historian Bonnie Bullough (1984), "The fascinating thing about the disclaimer [regarding diagnosis and prescription] is that it was made *not* by the American Medical Association, but the American Nurses Association. … In effect, organized nursing surrendered without any battle over boundaries." The ANA's 1955 definition of nursing would restrict the expansion of nurses' scope of practice for the rest of the 20th century as the profession struggled with the dichotomy of care versus cure and of medical versus nursing diagnoses. In essence, the definition reversed years of hard-won gains in expanding the scope of nursing practice.

of the CNS role included early evaluation research that served to validate and promote this new role. Georgopoulos and colleagues (Georgopoulos & Christman, 1970; Georgopoulos & Jackson, 1970; Georgopoulos & Sana, 1971) conducted studies evaluating the effect of CNS practice on the nursing process and outcomes in inpatient adult health care settings. These and other evaluative studies (Ayers, 1971; Girouard, 1978; Little & Carnevali, 1967) demonstrated the positive effect of the CNS on improving nursing care and patient outcomes. Moreover, with the increasing demand from society to cure illness using the latest scientific and technologic advances, hospital administrators willingly supported specialization in nursing and hired CNSs, particularly in the revenue-producing intensive care units.

The CNS role remained the dominant APRN role in the 1980s, with CNSs representing 42% of all APRNs (US Department of Health and Human Services, 1996). The ANA's Social Policy Statement (ANA, 1980) clearly delineated the criteria required to assume the title of CNS and was of particular

significance to the maturation of the CNS role during this decade. According to that statement,

The specialist in nursing practice is a nurse who, through study and supervised clinical practice at the graduate level (master's or doctorate), has become expert in a defined area of knowledge and practice in a selected clinical area of nursing. … Upon completion of a graduate program degree in a university graduate program with an emphasis on clinical specialization, the specialist in nursing practice should meet the criteria for specialty certification through nursing's professional society. (ANA, 1980, p. 23)

By 1984, the National League for Nursing had accredited 129 programs for the preparation of CNSs. These new, clinically focused graduate programs were instrumental in developing and defining the CNS role. Concurrently, some nurse researchers once again studied the outcomes related to CNS practice. In 1987, for example, McBride and colleagues demonstrated that nursing practice, particularly in relation to documentation, improved as a result of

EXEMPLAR 1.3	Interprofessional Practice in the 1960s: Rose Pinneo and Lawrence Meltzer

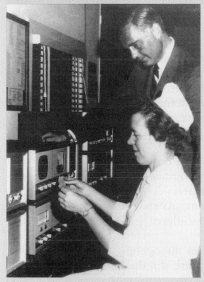

(Courtesy University of Virginia, Center for Nursing Historical Inquiry.)

In 1962, Dr. Lawrence Meltzer, of the Presbyterian Hospital in Philadelphia, proposed that the role of the nurse would be central to the new system of coronary care. The nurse would be present in the coronary care unit (CCU) 24 hours a day. When the research project began on January 15, 1963, about 8 months after the Hartford CCU opened in Kansas City, Meltzer immediately faced the challenge of staffing it. Rose Pinneo, RN, MSN, a graduate of both Johns Hopkins School of Nursing and the University of Pennsylvania, agreed to be the nursing director. In July 1963, 6 months after agreeing to accept the job, Pinneo, a small-framed, unassuming professional, took on the nursing leadership role in the new unit, implementing the new role for nurses (Pinneo, 1967).

In the CCUs in the 1960s, clinical expertise on the part of the nurse would be invaluable. As Pinneo described it, "The nurses' role is more complex than that of the usual hospital nurse", and she went on to explain it further:

> *Utilizing the unique combination of clinical assessment and cardiac monitoring, the nurse makes independent decisions. She determines those situations requiring her immediate intervention to save life prior to the physician's arrival or those situations that warrant calling the physician and waiting for his evaluation. It is in these precious moments that the patient's life may literally be in the hands of the nurse. (Pinneo, 1972, p. 4)*

Collaboration with physicians at the grassroots level would be key to the CCU nurses' success. Pinneo and other nurses who worked in the first CCUs worked closely with cardiologists (Keeling, 2004), and interprofessional on-the-job training was the norm. These changes in setting, technology, and expectations of the nurse exemplify stage I in the transition of specialties into advanced practice nursing (see Chapter 5).

The creation of the CCU initiated a new era for nurses. The changes that occurred in the clinical setting of the CCU helped establish collegial relationships between nurses and physicians that would be important for advanced practice registered nurses in the decades to follow. In intensive care units and CCUs, collaborative practice was essential. "Most importantly, nurses and physicians learned to trust each other" (Lynaugh & Fairman, 1992, p. 24). ◎

---

the introduction of a CNS in an inpatient psychiatric setting. However, at about that time, health care cost containment raised concerns about the future of the CNS role (Hamric, 1989).

Declining Demand for Clinical Nurse Specialists

By the late 1980s, many CNSs had shifted the focus of their practice away from the clinical area and instead focused on the educational and organizational aspects of the CNS role, such as orientation programs, in-service education, and administrative functions.

This shift was supported by the view that CNSs were too valuable to spend their time on direct patient care (Wolff, 1984). Meanwhile, others who continued to assert that the essence of the CNS role was clinical expertise were publishing articles and books on the topic (Hamric & Spross, 1983, 1989; Sparacino, 1990).

The increasing emphasis on cost containment in the 1980s produced legislative and economic changes that affected advanced practice nursing and the health care delivery system as a whole (Box 1.4). In particular, the establishment of a prospective payment system in 1983 was a landmark event. This payment

BOX 1.4   Access to Cost-Effective, Quality Health Care for All Americans

The need to provide cost-effective, quality health care to US citizens prompted the Senate Committee on Appropriations to request a report from the Office of Technology Assessment on the contributions of nurse practitioners (NPs), certified nurse-midwives (CNMs), and physician assistants in meeting the nation's health care needs. The 1986 report, entitled *Nurse Practitioners, Physician Assistants and Certified Nurse-Midwives: A Policy Analysis,* was based on an analysis of numerous studies that assessed quality of care, patient satisfaction, and physician acceptance. It concluded, "within their areas of competence NPs … and CNMs provide care whose quality is equivalent to that of care provided by physicians" (Office of Technology Assessment, 1986). However, while the Office of Technology Assessment was conducting this study, the American Medical Association House of Delegates, threatened by the possibility of competition from advanced practice registered nurses, passed a resolution to "oppose any attempt at empowering non-physicians to become unsupervised primary care providers and be directly reimbursed" (Safriet, 1992).

system, which used diagnosis-related groups to classify billing for hospitalized Medicare recipients, represented an effort to control rising costs by shifting reimbursement from payment for services provided to payment by case (capitation). As a result, hospital administrators put increasing pressure on nurses and physicians to save money by decreasing the length of time patients remained hospitalized. The emphasis on cost containment also heralded budget cuts for hospitals. The CNS role came under intense review at this time. CNSs were not obviously cost-effective or overtly essential to patient care. The outcomes of the CNS role had not been empirically tracked and the role was poorly defined. The result was the elimination of some CNS positions by the end of the decade.

The decade of the 1990s opened with cutbacks in employment opportunities for CNSs because of the financial problems in hospitals and closed with the federal government's recognition of Medicare reimbursement for CNS services. The cost of health care was a constant concern and, when President Clinton was elected in 1992, the country was in

serious need of health care reform. Determined to take a proactive stance in the movement, the ANA wrote its Agenda for Health Care Reform (ANA, 1992). The plan focused on restructuring the US health care system to reduce costs and improve access to care. Although the Clinton administration's efforts for reform failed, radical changes were made by the private sector, in which the once-dominant fee-for-service insurance plans were overtaken by managed care organizations (Safriet, 1998). The changing marketplace created new challenges for APRNs as they struggled not only with restrictive, outdated state laws on prescriptive authority, but also with "non-governmental, market-based impediments" to their practices (Safriet, 1998, p. 25). In this environment, APRNs continued to expand their roles, educational programs, and practice settings.

Nationwide, in the opening years of the 1990s, CNS programs were still the most numerous of all master's nursing programs, with more than 11,000 students enrolled (National League for Nursing, 1994). The largest area of specialization was adult health–medical-surgical nursing. However, with the increasing emphasis on primary care in the mid-1990s, the rapid growth of NP programs, the financial challenges faced by hospital administrators, and the introduction of the ACNP role in tertiary care centers, the number of CNS positions in hospitals declined sharply.

The 1996 National Sample Survey of Registered Nurses revealed that a significant number (7802) of CNSs were also prepared as NPs, educated to diagnose and treat health conditions (US Department of Health and Human Services, 1996). According to the National Sample Survey, these dual-role–prepared APRNs were more likely to be employed as NPs than as CNSs. By that time, of the 61,601 CNSs in the United States, only 23% were practicing in CNS-specific positions (US Department of Health and Human Services, 1996). This low percentage may have reflected the fact that CNSs accepted different positions—for example, as administrators or staff educators. It may also have reflected the decline in the number of CNS positions available because of budget cutbacks.

Clinical Nurse Specialist Education and Reimbursement

Education for CNS practice was complicated due to the number of specialties involved. In many specialties, existing certification examinations were targeted to nurses who were experts by experience, not graduates of master's programs that specifically trained them for specialty practice. Thus advanced-level certification for the CNS was slow to emerge. For example, it was not until 1995 that the Oncology Nursing Society administered the first certification examination for advanced practice in oncology nursing. A further complication was that not all states recognized these examinations for APRN regulatory purposes.

In 2013, there were 148 schools offering a master's degree as a CNS and 18 offering a post-baccalaureate DNP CNS. Enrollment, however, was low, totaling just over 2200 students (AACN, 2015). As of Spring 2016, CNSs could practice to the full extent of their education and training in 28 states and could practice in collaboration with a physician in an additional 13 states. The ability of CNSs to prescribe medications and durable medical equipment depended on state regulations, which gradually allowed prescriptive authority to more CNSs (NACNS, 2015a). CNSs are now authorized to prescribe without physician supervision in 20 states (NACNS, 2015b).The National Association of Clinical Nurse Specialists (NACNS) was formed in 1995, promoting organization of the role at the national level. Soon thereafter, the Balanced Budget Act of 1997 specifically identified CNSs as eligible for Medicare reimbursement (Safriet, 1998). The law, providing Medicare Part B direct payment to NPs and CNSs regardless of their geographic area of practice, allowed both types of APRNs to be paid 85% of the fee paid to physicians for the same services. Moreover, the law's inclusion and definition of CNSs corrected the previous omission of this group from reimbursement (Safriet, 1998). The possibility of reimbursement for services was an important step in the continuing development of the CNS role because hospital administrators would continue to focus on the cost of having APRNs provide patient care.

The creation of the NACNS, followed by third-party reimbursement for their services, represented two major steps for the CNS. The NACNS developed core competencies and criteria for the evaluation of CNS graduate programs and certificates. Practice competency varies by specialty and is the responsibility of over 20 professional organizations, although all must include the NACNS core competencies (NACNS, 2015c). In 2015, the NACNS endorsed the DNP as entry to practice for CNSs by 2030; previously they had been neutral on this question (NACNS, 2015c). Recent aspects of the CNS role are discussed in Chapter 14.

Nurse Practitioners

NPs provide care through diagnosis and treatment as well as addressing disease prevention and health management. The idea of using nurses to provide what we now refer to as primary care services dates to the late 19th century. During this period of rapid industrialization and social reform, public health nurses played a major role in providing care for poverty-stricken immigrants in cities throughout the country.

The Henry Street Settlement and Primary Care

In 1893, Lillian Wald, a young graduate nurse from the New York Training School for Nurses, established the Henry Street Settlement (HSS) House on the Lower East Side of Manhattan. Its purpose was to address the needs of the poor, many of whom lived in overcrowded, rat-infested tenements. For several decades, the HSS visiting nurses, like other district nurses, visited thousands of patients, with little interference in their work (Wald, 1922). The needs of this disadvantaged community were limitless. According to one account (Duffus, 1938):

> There were nursing infants, many of them with the summer bowel complaint that sent infant mortality soaring during the hot months; there were children with measles, not quarantined; there were children with ophthalmia, a contagious eye disease; there were children scarred with vermin bites; there were adults with typhoid; there was a case of puerperal septicemia, lying on a vermin-infested bed without sheets or pillow cases; a family consisting of a pregnant mother, a crippled child and two others living on dry bread … a young girl dying of tuberculosis amid the very conditions that had produced the disease. (p. 43)

In addition to making home visits, the HSS nurses saw patients in the nurses' dispensary in the settlement house. There they treated "simple complaints and emergencies not requiring referral elsewhere" (Buhler-Wilkerson, 2001). For a time, their work usually went unnoticed, but interprofessional conflict was inevitable. According to nurse historian Karen Buhler-Wilkerson (2001):

> As the number of ambulatory visits grew, the settlement risked attracting the unwelcome attention of the increasingly disagreeable "uptown docs." The New York Medical Society's recent success in

attaching a clause to the Nursing Registration Bill prohibiting nurses from practicing medicine gave the society a new opportunity to disrupt the settlement's neighborly activities. ... By 1904 ... Lavinia Dock [a colleague of Lillian Wald] wrote to Wald about doctors' concerns that nurses were "carrying ointments and even giving pills" outside the strict control of physicians. (p. 110)

To resolve this problem, the HSS nurses obtained standing orders for emergency medications and treatments from a group of Lower East Side physicians (Buhler-Wilkerson, 2001; Keeling, 2007). Nonetheless, conflicts with medicine surfaced again when the HHS nurses expanded their visits to areas of the city outside the Lower East Side. The situation came to a head with the collapse of the stock market in 1929, when uptown physicians apparently saw the nurses as an economic threat. That year, the Westchester Village Medical Group accused the nurses of practicing medicine. Angered by the accusation, Elizabeth MacKenzie, Associate Director of Nurses at the HSS, defended the HSS nurses in her reply (MacKenzie, 1929):

> My dear Dr. Black:
> Your letter ... addressed to Miss Elizabeth Neary, Supervisor of our Westchester Office, has been referred to me for reply. May I call the attention of your group to the fact that in administering the work in that office, Miss Neary does so as a representative of the HSS Visiting Nurse Service and in accord with definite policies in effect throughout the entire city-wide service. It has been the unvarying policy of the organization over the 35 years of its service to work in close cooperation with the medical profession doing nursing and preventive health work entirely and avoiding any semblance of the "practice of medicine" in competition with the doctors. ... We will call a meeting ... to which the members of your group will be invited for a frank discussion of our common problems.

Although the records about this meeting are no longer available, one can assume that the meeting happened and the nurses continued to practice because HSS remained active until the 1950s. Nonetheless, as is apparent in these two scenarios, from early in the 20th century there was evidence of interprofessional conflicts as nurses began to expand their scope of practice. There is also evidence of emerging collaboration between the professions as physicians and nurses negotiated solutions to the boundary problems. What is clear, even in those early years, is that nurses were considered "good enough" to care for the poor, whereas physicians would care for those who could pay.

The Frontier Nursing Service and Other Examples of Early Primary Care

In addition to providing midwifery services, FNS nurses in Leslie County, Kentucky, informally modeled what would later become the primary care NP role. During the 1930s, the FNS continued the work that Breckinridge had started in 1925, providing most of the primary health care needed by people living in rural Appalachia. Working out of eight centers that covered 78 square miles in remote mountainous regions, the FNS nurses had considerable autonomy. They made diagnoses and treated patients, dispensing herbs and medicines (including morphine) with the permission of their medical advisory committee. Working from standing orders written by that committee, the nurses also dispensed medicines such as aspirin, ipecac, cascara, and castor oil at their own discretion (FNS, 1948). That unprecedented autonomy in practice was not always recognized, however, even by the FNS nurses themselves. During an interview in 1978, FNS nurse Betty Lester reflected on her work as assistant field supervisor in Leslie County in the 1930s (Keeling, 2007):

> See, we nurses don't prescribe and we don't diagnose. We can make a tentative diagnosis and we can give that to the doctor, and if there's anything wrong then he'll tell us how to treat it. So they [the doctors] gave us this routine of things that we could use and the things we could do—and the things we couldn't do. (p. 49)

Lester denied the extent of the practice autonomy she had had. Like other registered nurses of the era, she had been socialized to defer to physicians' judgment and orders. So, recalling her practice later in her life, Lester acknowledged only that she and her colleagues had made "tentative" diagnoses. In reality, she had practiced on her own because there were few telephones in the isolated community and even fewer physicians available for personal consultation. For all practical purposes, the diagnoses she had made were the only diagnoses and the treatment she had given was the only treatment (Keeling, 2007).

During the 1930s, in addition to the FNS nurses, other nurses working among the poor in rural areas also practiced with exceptional autonomy. In particular, the Farm Security Administration (FSA) nurses "were given unusual latitude in their clinical roles"

(Grey, 1999, p. 94) in migrant health clinics across the United States. According to historian Michael Grey (1999), who chronicled the history of rural health programs established by President Franklin D. Roosevelt during the Great Depression, which began in 1929 and lasted through approximately 1940:

> With the verbal approval of the camp doctor, they [FSA nurses] could write prescriptions and dispense drugs from the clinic formulary. ... They staffed well baby clinics, coordinated immunization programs ... decided whether a sick migrant required referral to a physician ... and provided emergency care. (p. 94)

Like the FNS nurses, FSA nurses practiced according to standing orders issued by the FSA medical offices and approved by local physicians. As Dr. H. Daniels recalled in a 1984 interview, "Nurses functioned pretty autonomously. They were able to do a lot of what NPs do after a lot of training, but these nurses did it through experience" (Grey, 1999, p. 96). Essential to this practice autonomy for the FNS and FSA nurses was the tacit requirement that the patients be poor and marginalized and have little access to physician-provided medical care.

The same requirements held true for the field nurses working with the Bureau of Indian Affairs (BIA) in the first half of the 20th century, who often found themselves traveling the reservations alone, making diagnoses and treating patients. In addition to making home visits, BIA nurses conducted well-baby "nursing conferences," the initial intent of which was health education and disease prevention. In actuality, these conferences became what are referred to today as nurse-run clinics; Navajo mothers would bring in sick infants and children to be seen by the nurse (Keeling, 2007). Reporting on her work at Teec Nos Pas in the Northern Navajo region in May 1931, nurse Dorothy Williams described the reality of providing much-needed care of ear infections, sore throats, skin infections, and other commonly occurring problems. Williams referred to the conferences as "clinics":

> Five clinics held this week, three general and two baby clinics. Mothers bathed their babies and were given material to cut out and make gowns for baby. Preschool children were weighed, inspected and mothers advised about diets for underweights [sic]. ... Fifty treatments given (Williams, 2007).

Although the NP role had been modeled informally in the FNS in the 1930s, it was during the 1960s that the role was first described formally and implemented in outpatient pediatric clinics, originating in part as a response to a shortage of primary care physicians. As the trend toward medical specialization drew increasing numbers of physicians away from primary care, many areas of the country were designated underserved with respect to the numbers of primary care physicians. "Report after report issued by the AMA [American Medical Association] and the Association of American Medical Colleges decried the shortage of physicians in poor rural and urban areas" (Fairman, 2002, p. 163). At the same time, consumers across the nation were demanding accessible, affordable, and sensitive health care while health care delivery costs were increasing at an annual rate of 10% to 14% (Jonas, 1981).

Growth of Nurse Practitioner Practice

The event marking the inception of the modern NP role was the establishment of the first pediatric NP (PNP) program by Loretta Ford, RN, and Henry Silver, MD, at the University of Colorado in 1965. This demonstration project, funded by the Commonwealth Foundation, was designed to prepare professional nurses to provide comprehensive well-child care and manage common childhood health problems. The 4-month program, during which certified registered nurses were educated as PNPs without requiring master's preparation, emphasized health promotion and inclusion of the family. A study evaluating the project demonstrated that PNPs were highly competent in assessing and managing 75% of well and ill children in community health settings. In addition, PNPs increased the number of patients served in private pediatric practice by 33% (Ford & Silver, 1967). Like early nurse-midwife and nurse anesthetist studies, these positive findings demonstrated support for this new nursing role.

The PNP role was not without significant intra-professional controversy, particularly with regard to educational preparation. Early on, certificate programs based on the Colorado project rapidly sprang into existence. According to Ford (1991), some of these programs shifted the emphasis of PNP preparation from a nursing to a medical model. This was in contrast to the original University of Colorado demonstration project that stressed collaboration between nursing and medicine (Exemplar 1.4). As a result, one of the major areas of controversy in academia was over the fact that NPs made medical diagnoses and wrote prescriptions for medications, essentially stepping over the invisible medical

EXEMPLAR 1.4   **Loretta Ford: Cofounder, with Henry Silver, of the Nurse Practitioner Role**

There was a spirit of excitement, of anger, and of tremendous possibility in the United States of the 1960s. Americans marched for civil rights, President's Johnson's "War on Poverty" had begun, and people demanded access to health care. Within nursing, the American Nurses Association called for requiring the baccalaureate degree for entry into practice, while Dr. Loretta Ford, a nurse, and Dr. Henry Silver, a pediatrician, introduced the concept of the nurse practitioner.

Silver saw an unmet need for pediatric health care providers and he thought that appropriately educated nurses could offer it, but nurse educators were resistant. Then he met Loretta Ford. She was excited; she understood the potential of expanding care through allowing nurses to practice to the fullest extent of advanced nursing education (Pearson, 1985). The term *nurse practitioner* was coined, Ford later explained, because "So many nurses in a specialty were either teachers or administrators, not practitioners of nursing. We wanted to emphasize the clinical practice role" (Jacox, 2002, p. 162). "Abuse and misuse of nurses became obvious," she noted at another time. "Nurses were doing so many things. Mostly they were nursing the system, nursing the doctors, nursing the desk, nursing everything else but the patients" ("An interview with Dr. Loretta Ford," 1975, p. 10).

Ford consistently stated that nurse practitioners must align their professional stance with nursing and not focus on a medical orientation (Pearson, 1985). She argued that nurse practitioners should diagnose "within the context of the patient's health status, social qualities, physical characteristics, and economic realities: within the patient's personality and strength. … They must understand the importance of caring and compassion" (Pearson, 1999, pp. 25-6). To underscore this, Ford further argued that today's practitioners must know their history. "Maybe they know about Florence Nightingale, but they don't know all of the things that Florence Nightingale had as basic tenets of the nursing that she started" (O'Grady & Lusk, 2016).

Loretta Ford's career as a nursing exemplar mirrors advice she has given to today's nurses: "The future belongs to those who are committed, courageous, competent, compassionate—and to those with enough chutzpah to create their own destiny" (Jacox, 2002, p. 164). ◎

boundary into the realm of curing. Because of this, some nurse educators and other nurse leaders questioned whether the NP role could be conceptualized as being within the discipline of nursing, a profession that had historically been ordered to care (Reverby, 1987; Rogers, 1972).

While nursing professors debated the educational preparation of NPs (Keeling, 2007; Rogers, 1972), the NP role attracted considerable attention from professional groups and policymakers. Health policy groups such as the National Advisory Commission on Health Manpower issued statements in support of the NP concept (Moxley, 1968). At the grassroots level, physicians accepted the new role and hired NPs. The NP role had already appeared in the practice setting.

In the 1970s, NPs continued to enhance their visibility in the health care system, negotiating with physicians to expand their scope of practice and demonstrating their cost-effectiveness in providing quality care. Nevertheless, it was also a period characterized by intraprofessional conflict because some leaders in the nursing community continued to reject the role. In contrast, state legislatures increasingly recognized these expanded roles of registered nurses and a group of pro-NP nursing faculty, already teaching in NP programs, held their first national meeting in Chapel Hill, North Carolina, in 1974. This meeting would lay the foundation for the formation of the National Organization of Nurse Practitioner Faculties (NONPF).

In the early 1970s, US Department of Health, Education, and Welfare Secretary Elliott Richardson established the Committee to Study Extended Roles for Nurses. This group of health care leaders was charged with evaluating the feasibility of expanding nursing practice (Kalisch & Kalisch, 1986). They concluded that extending the scope of the nurse's role was essential to providing equal access to health care for all Americans. According to an editorial in the *American Journal of Nursing*, "The kind of health care Lillian Wald began preaching and practicing in 1893 is the kind the people of this country are still crying for" (Schutt, 1971, p. 53). The committee urged the establishment of innovative curricular designs in health science centers and increased financial support for nursing education. It also advocated standardizing nursing licensure and national certification and developing a model nurse practice law suitable for national application. In addition, the committee called for further research related to cost-benefit analyses and attitudinal surveys to assess the impact of the NP role. This report resulted in increased federal support for training programs for the preparation of several types of NPs, including family NPs, adult NPs, and emergency department NPs (Kalisch & Kalisch, 1986).

Controversy and Support for the Nurse Practitioner's Role

Conflict and discord about the NP role continued to characterize relationships between NPs and other nurses. Some academics who believed that NPs were not practicing nursing continued to pose resistance to the role (Ford, 1982). Nurse theorist Martha Rogers, one of the most outspoken opponents of the NP concept, argued that the development of the NP role was a ploy to lure nurses away from nursing to medicine, thereby undermining nursing's unique role in health care (Rogers, 1972). Subsequently, nurse leaders and educators took sides for and against the establishment of educational programs for NPs in mainstream master's programs. Over time, the standardization of NP educational programs at the master's level, initiated by the group of faculty who formed the NONPF, would serve to reduce intraprofessional tension.

Despite the resistance to NPs in nursing, physicians increasingly accepted NPs in individual health care practices. Working together in local practices, NPs and MDs established collegial relationships, negotiating with each other to construct work boundaries and reach agreement about their collaborative practice. "In the NP-MD dyad, negotiations centered on the NP's right to practice an essential part of traditional medicine: the process or skill set of clinical thinking ... to perform a physical examination, elicit patient symptoms, ... create a diagnosis, formulate treatment options, prescribe treatment and make decisions about prognosis" (Fairman, 2002, pp. 163–164). The proximity of a supervising physician was thought to be key to effective practice, and on-site supervision was the norm. Grassroots acceptance of the role was dependent on tight physician supervision and control of the protocols under which NPs practiced. That supervision was not without benefit to the newly certified, inexperienced NPs. According to Corene Johnson, "Initially, we had to always have a physician on site. ... I didn't resent that. Actually, I needed the backup" (Fairman, 2002, p. 164).

During the 1980s, the concept of advanced nursing practice began to be defined and used in the literature. In 1983, Harriet Kitzman, an associate professor at the University of Rochester, explored the interrelationships between CNSs and NPs (Kitzman, 1983). She used the term *advanced practice* throughout her discussion, applying the term not only to advanced education, but also to CNS and NP practice. She noted, "Recognition for advanced practice competence is already established for both NPs and CNSs through the profession's certification programs. ... advanced nursing practice cannot be setting-bound, because nursing needs are not exclusively setting-restricted" (Kitzman, 1983, pp. 284, 288). At about this time, the Council of Primary Health Care Nurse Practitioners and the Council of Clinical Nurse Specialists began to explore the commonalities of the two roles. In 1988, the councils conducted a survey of all NP and CNS graduate programs and identified considerable overlap in curricula. Subsequently, between 1988 and 1990, the two councils discussed a proposal to merge, and, in 1991, the Council of Nurses in Advanced Practice was formed. Unfortunately, the merger was short-lived because of the restructuring of the ANA during the early 1990s. Nevertheless, it was an important step in the organizational coalescence of advanced practice nursing (ANA, 1991). In 1984, an associate professor at the University of Wisconsin–Madison, Joy Calkin, proposed a model for advanced nursing practice, specifically identifying CNSs and NPs with master's degrees as APRNs (Calkin, 1984). By the end of the decade, the nursing literature was increasingly using the term. Published in 1996, the first edition of this text included CRNA and CNM roles as advanced practice nursing, reflecting an integrative vision of advanced practice that was increasingly being seen in the literature.

Although physicians and NPs collaborated at the local level, organized medicine began to increase its resistance to the NP role. One of the most contentious areas of interprofessional conflict involved prescriptive authority for nursing (Box 1.5). As one author so aptly noted, "Nursing's efforts to obtain the legal authority to prescribe may be seen as the second chapter in the struggle over the use of the word 'diagnosing' in Nurse Practice Acts" (Hadley, 1989, p. 291). Basically, prescriptive authority, regarded as a delegated medical act, was dependent on NPs' legal right to provide treatment. In 1971, Idaho became the first state to recognize diagnosis and treatment as part of the scope of practice of specialty nurses (Idaho Code § 54-1413, 1971).

BOX 1.5   The Fight for Nurse Practitioner Prescriptive Privileges

The fight for prescriptive authority for nurse practitioners (NPs) spanned the latter decades of the 20th century. By 1983, only Oregon and Washington granted NPs statutory, independent prescriptive authority. Other states granting prescriptive authority to NPs did so with the provision that a licensed physician directly supervises the NP. How prescriptions were handled depended on the availability of the physician, negotiated boundaries of the individual physician-NP team, and the state in which practice occurred. In some cases, that meant that physicians pre-signed a pad of prescriptions for the NP to use at her or his discretion; in remote area clinics, such as those in the Frontier Nursing Service, a physician would countersign NP prescriptions once a week and, in other cases, the physician would write and sign a prescription at the request of the NP. With the exception of the latter, these practices were of questionable legality (Keeling, 2007).

However, "As path-breaking as the statute was, it was still rather restrictive in that any acts of diagnosis and treatment had to be authorized by rules and regulations promulgated by the Idaho State Boards of Medicine and Nursing" (Safriet, 1992, p. 445). Moreover, the Drug Enforcement Act required that practitioners wishing to prescribe controlled substances obtain US Drug Enforcement Administration (DEA) registration numbers, and only those practitioners with broad prescriptive authority (e.g., physicians and dentists) could obtain these numbers.

Growth in Nurse Practitioner Numbers and Expanded Scope of Practice

Significant growth in the numbers of NPs in practice and the fight for prescriptive authority for NPs characterized the 1980s. NP practice increased immeasurably during this time as new types of NPs developed, the most significant of which were the emergency NP, neonatal NP, and family NP. By 1984, approximately 20,000 graduates of NP programs were employed, for the most part, in settings "that the founders envisioned" (Kalisch & Kalisch, 1986, p. 715): outpatient clinics, health maintenance organizations, health departments, community health centers, rural clinics, schools, occupational health

clinics, and private offices. By the late 1980s, however, based on their success in neonatal intensive care units, NPs with specialty preparation were increasingly being used in tertiary care centers (Silver & McAtee, 1988).

During this period, the multiple roles for NPs created competing interests that would affect their ability to speak with one voice on legislative issues. In an attempt to rectify this situation, the ANA established the Primary Health Care Nurse Practitioner Council. At about the same time, the American Academy of Nurse Practitioners was established in 1985 as the first organization for NPs from all specializations. In 1995 a competing NP organization was formed to serve as a "SWAT team" on policy during President Clinton's health care reform initiative. Named the American College of Nurse Practitioners, the new organization was seen as an umbrella organization to bring all the NP organizations together.

Throughout the 1980s, NPs worked tirelessly to convince state legislatures to pass laws and establish reimbursement policies that would support their practice. Interprofessional conflicts with organized medicine, and to a lesser extent with pharmacists, centered on control issues and the degree of independence the NP was allowed. These conflicts intensified as NPs moved beyond the physician extender model to a more autonomous one. In a seminal case, *Sermchief v. Gonzales* (1983), the Missouri medical board charged two women's health care NPs with practicing medicine without a license (Doyle & Meurer, 1983). The initial ruling was against the NPs but, on appeal, the Missouri Supreme Court overturned the decision, concluding that the scope of practice of APRNs could evolve without statutory constraints (Wolff, 1984). In essence, this case provided a model for new state nurse practice acts to address issues related to APRN practice with very generalized wording, a change that allowed for expansion in the roles and functions of APRNs.

In the early 1990s, federal legislation regulating narcotics in the Controlled Substances Act would be of major significance to NP progress in implementing prescriptive authority. As NPs began to gain prescriptive authority for controlled substances in different states, they required a parallel authority granted by the DEA. In 1991, the DEA first responded to this situation by proposing registration for "affiliated practitioners" (Definition and Exemption of Affiliated Practitioners for the Drug Enforcement Administration, 1991). This proposal called for those NPs who had prescriptive authority pursuant to a practice protocol or collaborative practice agreement to be assigned a registration number for controlled substances tied to the number of the physician with whom they worked. This proposal received much criticism specifically related to the restriction of access to health care and the legal liability of the prescribers, and the proposal was revoked in 1992. Later that year, the DEA amended its regulations by adding a category of "mid-level providers" (MLPs), who would be issued individual provider DEA numbers as long as they were granted prescriptive authority by the state in which they practiced. The MLP's number would begin with an M for mid-level provider, rather than an A or B. The MLP provision took effect in 1993, significantly expanding NPs' ability to prescribe.

Neonatal and Acute Care Nurse Practitioners

One of the newer types of NPs to emerge was the neonatal NP. Originating in the late 1970s in response to a shortage of neonatologists coinciding with restrictions in the total time pediatric residents could devote to neonatal intensive care, the neonatal NP was the forerunner of the acute care NP of the 1990s. These highly skilled, experienced neonatal nurses assumed a wide range of new responsibilities formerly undertaken by pediatric residents, including interhospital transport of critically ill infants and newborn resuscitation (Clancy & Maguire, 1995).

Like the earlier neonatal NP role, the adult acute care NP (ACNP) role grew in response to residency shortages in intensive care units, although this time the shortage was because of decreases in the number of residents available to work in the medical subspecialties. In addition, increasingly complicated tertiary care systems lacked coordination of care. Advanced practice nursing responded quickly to this need, building on the earlier work of Silver and McAtee (1988) to create a role that promoted quality patient care and nursing's leadership in health care delivery (Daly, 1997). University of Pennsylvania professors Anne Keane and Therese Richmond were among those who documented the emergence of the tertiary NP (TNP):

> The TNP is an advanced practice nurse educated at the master's level with both a theoretical and experiential focus on complex patients with specialized health needs. ... There is precedent for the NP in tertiary care. For example, neonatal nurse practitioners are central to the provision of care in many intensive care nurseries. ... It is our belief that the TNP can provide clinically expert specialized care in a holistic manner in a system that is often typified by fragmentation, lack of communication among medical specialists, and a loss of recognition of the patient and patient's needs as central to the care delivered. (Keane & Richmond, 1993, p. 282)

From 1992 to 1995, acute care nurse practitioner (ACNP) tracks in master's programs proliferated across the country. Soon, questions abounded concerning the content of the curriculum. To resolve these, educators met annually at ACNP consensus conferences, beginning in 1993. The ANA's Credentialing Center administered the first ACNP certification examination in December 1995. By 1997, there were 43 programs nationwide that prepared ACNPs at the master's or post-master's level (Kleinpell, 1997). In 2002, the ACNPs formally merged with the American Academy of Nurse Practitioners, with the goal of uniting primary care NPs and ACNPs under an umbrella organization. By this time, ACNPs were employed in multiple specialties, including cardiology, cardiovascular surgery, neurosurgery, emergency and trauma, internal medicine, and radiology services (Daly, 2002).

During this decade, the growth in the number of NP programs, increase in prescriptive authority for NPs, and autonomy that NPs found in their practice settings converged to make the NP role enticing, and increasing numbers of nurses who wanted to be APRNs chose the NP role. The problem was that there were a number of organizations speaking for the various types of NPs. The American Academy of Nurse Practitioners continued to be active after the American College of Nurse Practitioners was founded in 1995. In addition, PNPs formed the National Association of Pediatric Nurse Associates and Practitioners (NAPNAP), and nurses interested in women's health issues formed the Association of Women's Health, Obstetric and Neonatal Nurses (AWHONN). These groups soon offered their own certification examinations, in competition with those offered by the ANA's Credentialing Center. One thing that they did agree on, however, was education for practice. In August 1993, representatives of 63 of 66 tricouncil organizations attending a national nursing summit agreed to require master's education for the NP role (Cronenwett, 1995). In 2013 the American Academy of Nurse Practitioners and the American College of Nurse Practitioners merged to form the American Association of Nurse Practitioners (AANP, 2013a).

Nurse Practitioner Education

During the 1990s, the number of NPs increased dramatically in response to increasing demand, the national emphasis on primary care, and the concomitant decrease in the number of medical residencies in the subspecialties. In 1990, there were 135 master's degree and 40 certificate NP programs. Between 1992 and 1994, the number of institutions offering NP education more than doubled, from 78 to 158. In 1994, most institutions offered several tracks, which led to a total of 384 NP tracks in master's programs throughout the United States. By 1998, the number of institutions offering NP education again doubled, representing a total of 769 distinct NP specialty tracks (AACN, 1999; NONPF, 1997). Most of these programs were at the master's or post-master's level. In 2013, the number of institutions offering a master's NP degree was 368, while 92 colleges offered a post-baccalaureate DNP NP (AACN, 2015).

The NONPF has supported the concept of the DNP since its outset in 2002, and in 2015 it reaffirmed that support. The NONPF cautions, however, that it does not require NP educational programs to be at the doctoral level and indeed, in 2015, less than half of US NP programs were at that level (NONPF, 2015). Chapters 15 and 16 present discussions of NP roles.

Meanwhile there has been rapid growth in the number of DNP programs nationwide. According to the DNP Directory, in 2017, there were 303 DNP programs, with more than 124 new programs in the planning stage (AACN, 2017). A survey commissioned by the AACN (2014) showed that about 70% of schools offering APRN education continue to only offer at the Master's of Science in Nursing (MSN) level and others continue to offer the MSN while also offering the DNP. Thus the master's degree remains the dominant form of APRN education.

Conclusion

Providing care to people in underserved areas has, by default, been assigned to nursing throughout the 20th and early 21st centuries. Moreover, history is clear that the concept of expanding the scope of practice for nurses was inextricably entwined with that assignment. HSS visiting nurses cared for poor immigrants of the Lower East Side unopposed by physicians until physicians perceived them as a threat. FNS nurses made diagnoses and treated patients in remote areas of Appalachia with the full approval of the physician committee who supervised them, and BIA nurses cured, as best they could, Native Americans in their communities. In other cases, if one considers time as place, so-called after midnight nurses expanded their scope of practice by defibrillating patients in CCUs across the nation, and army nurses did whatever needed to be done on the battlefield (Keeling, 2004). Only when APRNs threatened physicians' practice and income did organized medicine accuse them of practicing medicine without a license. Moreover, organized nursing itself was responsible for resisting the expansion of the scope of practice of nursing. However, it is also clear that when nurses and physicians focused on providing quality care for their patients, they were capable of working collaboratively and interdependently throughout the 20th century.

Further analysis of the history of advanced practice nursing demonstrates the importance of evaluative research in documenting the contributions of APRNs to the health care system and patients' well-being. As evidenced by nurse anesthetist Alice Magaw's 1900 publication on outcomes, the early "APRNs" were particularly visionary in their use of data to document their effectiveness. Throughout the century, evaluative research based on measurable outcomes served as a tool for the profession to argue its position to health care policymakers and the medical profession (Brooten et al., 1986; Hamric, Lindbak, Jaubert, & Worley, 1998; Mitchell-DiCenso et al., 1996; Shah, Brutlomesso, Sullivan, & Lattanzio, 1997). As Beck (1995) stated, "It is inconsistent for a state medical association to maintain a position that quality health care is their objective … [while] … disregarding data demonstrating the positive impact of APNs on health care" (p. 15).

The powerful influence of organizational efforts also emerges as a theme. National organization has been key to progress for advanced practice nursing, particularly in the realms of policy and regulation. Within the development of each of the advanced practice specialties, several common features have emerged. Strong national organizational leadership has been clearly demonstrated to be of critical importance in enhancing the growth and protection of the specialty. Based on the experience of the two oldest specialties, nurse anesthesia and nurse-midwifery, the process of establishing an effective national organization has taken a minimum of 3 decades. The history of these specialties reveals that specialty organizations have also played a critical role in the credentialing process for individuals in the specialty. The strength, unity, and depth of the organizational development of the two oldest advanced nursing specialties continue to serve as models for the younger developing specialties.

An additional theme to emerge is the importance of professional unity regarding the requisite education of APRNs. Early in the 20th century, specialty education was considered to be postgraduate with a heavy component of on-the-job training; however, that education was commonly postdiploma, not postbaccalaureate, and did not result in a master's degree. These early programs were of variable length and quality. The establishment of credible and stable educational programs has been a crucial step in the evolution of advanced practice nursing. As educational programs moved from informal, institutionally based models with a strong apprenticeship approach to more formalized graduate education programs, the credibility of APRN roles has increased. State regulations also influenced the evolution of advanced practice as an increasing number of states mandated a master's degree as a prerequisite for APRN licensure.

The influence of interprofessional struggles is apparent in all the advanced specialties, with the possible exception of the CNS. The legal battles between nursing and organized medicine are long-standing, particularly in relation to the nurse anesthesia, nurse-midwifery, and nurse practitioner specialties. Most of these tensions have revolved around issues of control, autonomy, and economic competition. However, the issues are complex, with isolated examples of physician support of expanding nursing practice, such as physicians' support of early nurse anesthesia practice and Melzer's collaboration with Pinneo in expanding CCU nurse practice. In all, outcomes of the legal battles have mostly proven to be positive for nursing and have helped legitimize APRN roles.

Nurse anesthetists, nurse-midwives, and NPs have specifically challenged the boundaries between nursing and medical practice. When they did, organized medicine responded and, today, these predictable responses should not be unexpected or underestimated. According to Inglis and Kjervik (1993), "It should be noted that organized medicine, largely through lobbying, has played a central role in creating and perpetuating the states' contradictory and constraining provisions of APRN practice" (p. 196). However, multiple national organizations and government entities have now called for the APRN to be effectively utilized, particularly since the passage of the Affordable Care Act (ANA, 2016).

Controversy within the nursing community was also a strong theme as the specialties developed. CRNAs, and to some extent NPs, developed outside of mainstream nursing, whereas CNSs developed within the mainstream from the start. Nevertheless, each specialty has had to deal with resistance from other nurses. These intraprofessional struggles can be understood within the context of change—each of the APRN specialties represented innovations that challenged the status quo of the nursing establishment and the health care system.

Throughout the 20th and early 21st centuries, prescriptive authority for advanced practice nursing, inextricably linked to economic and boundary issues between medicine and nursing, has been a particularly volatile legislative issue. Today, in most states, NPs, CNMs, and CRNAs can prescribe drugs with varying degrees of physician involvement and supervision. Although CNSs can prescribe in many states, they have not received the full recognition that has been granted to the other APRN groups. In 1997, Medicare expanded reimbursement for APRNs to all geographical and clinical settings, allowing direct Medicare reimbursement to 85% of the physician rate (AANP, 2013b). Thus, despite a great deal of progress in the roles of APRNs, specifically through the Consensus Model (Stanley, 2009), over the last century and gradual changes in state legislation and third-party reimbursement, APRNs have not reached their full potential to fulfill US health care needs. Barriers to enhancement of prescriptive authority for APRNs include the following: (1) exclusive reimbursement patterns, (2) anticompetitive practices and resistance of organized medicine, (3) and variable state regulation and practice acts (Beck, 1995; Keeling, 2007).

Societal forces have clearly influenced the development of advanced practice nursing. Gender issues have affected all the specialties to some degree because of the unique position of nursing as a female-dominated profession. The specialties of nurse anesthesia and NP have been the exceptions, with more men entering these fields. Within nurse-midwifery, the status of women and women's health were powerful forces in the establishment and development of the specialty. The societal impact of war has served as a catalyst to the development of advanced practice nursing, education, and professional organizations. Finally, economic changes, particularly in relation to health care financing, have had a powerful effect on the development of advanced practice nursing. The dramatic growth of managed care systems in the 1990s, in particular, has presented new challenges and opportunities for APRNs related to reimbursement, scope of practice, and autonomy (Safriet, 1998). The Patient Protection and Affordable Care Act (2010) has led to more fundamental changes in health care financing and delivery and increased the need for APRN services (Lathrop & Hodnicki, 2014).

With unremitting changes in nursing and health care, it is apparent that APRN specialties will continue to evolve and diversify. As new roles emerge, the history of advanced practice nursing continues to be written. Today, particularly in light of the DNP initiative, the profession is at a critical juncture at which it must decide whether it will mandate doctoral-level preparation for all APRN roles. While there is agreement on master's-level preparation for all APRNs, disagreements about the requirement of the doctorate (Cronenwett et al., 2011) may continue to impede progress on the adoption of standardized educational criteria in the future. Undoubtedly, as law professor Safriet (1998) has argued, consistency in the definition of advanced practice nursing and in the criteria for licensure as an APRN is critical to autonomy in practice.

Thus what remains to be seen is whether the profession can unite on issues related to the definition of advanced practice nursing and standardized criteria for educational preparation to ensure that APRNs are permitted to practice with the autonomy experienced by other professionals. If that can be done, as the 2011 Institute of Medicine's *The Future of Nursing* report suggested, APRNs will make a significant contribution to the transformation of health care in the 21st century.

Key Summary Points

- Throughout the 20th and 21st centuries, APRNs have provided care to the underserved poor, particularly in rural areas of the nation. However, when that care competes with physicians' reimbursement for their services, there has been significant resistance from organized medicine and their supporters in state legislative bodies, which results in interprofessional conflict.
- Documentation of the outcomes of practice helped establish the earliest nursing specialties and continues to be of critical importance to the survival of APRN practice.
- The efforts of national professional organizations, national certification, and the move toward graduate education as a requirement for advanced practice have been critical to enhancing the credibility of advanced practice nursing. For example, the move toward a DNP for APRNs has been highly successful. From an initial 2004 American Association of Colleges of Nursing position statement advancing the concept of a clinical doctorate for APRNs, there were, in 2016, almost 300 sites offering the DNP.
- Intraprofessional and interprofessional resistance to expanding the boundaries of the nursing discipline continues to occur.
- Societal forces, including wars, the economic climate, and health care policy, have influenced APRN history.

References

To access the references for this chapter, use your smartphone's QR code reader to scan the code below, or go to http://booksite.elsevier.com/9780323447751.

Conceptualizations of Advanced Practice Nursing

Cynthia Arslanian-Engoren

> *"The truth is rarely pure, and never simple."*
>
> —*Oscar Wilde*

CHAPTER CONTENTS

Concepts, models, and theories are used by advanced practice registered nurses (APRNs) to elicit histories, perform physicals, plan treatment, evaluate outcomes, and develop interpersonal relationships, as well as to help patients and families improve their health, cope with illnesses, and die with dignity. All APRNs, regardless of their years of experience and practice, rely on common processes and language to communicate with colleagues about patient care and to explain clinical situations. As such, it is important that the nursing profession and APRNs understand the language of advanced practice

nursing to communicate it to each other, clients, and stakeholders.

Understanding the conceptualization of advanced practice nursing, APRN practice, similarities and differences among APRNs, and how APRNs contribute to affordable, accessible, and effective care is central to actualizing a patient-centered, interprofessional health care system that maximizes patient outcomes and minimizes negative consequences. Conceptualizations of advanced practice nursing include models and theories that guide the practice of APRNs. The use of theory is fundamental to the sound progress in any practice discipline. Common language and mutually understood conceptual and theoretical frameworks support communication, guide practice,

We wish to acknowledge the previous chapter author, Judith A. Spross, PhD, RN, FAAN, for her excellent work in previous editions.

and are used to evaluate practice, education, policy, and research.

Such a foundation is essential for APRNs given the proposed changes in the US health care system, as seen in the Patient Protection and Affordable Care Act (ACA) (2010), the *Consensus Model for APRN Regulation* (APRN Joint Dialogue Group, 2008), and *The Future of Nursing* (Institute of Medicine [IOM], 2011). Other forces driving a common understanding of APRNs are the increasing numbers of programs offering the Doctor of Nursing Practice (DNP) degree, accountable care organizations, and the promulgation of interprofessional competencies (Canadian Inter-professional Health Collaborative [CIHC], 2010; Health Professions Network Nursing and Midwifery Office, 2010; Interprofessional Education Collaborative [IPEC] Expert Panel, 2011), as well as recommendations to the US Congress to increase funding for interprofessional education and practice (National Advisory Council on Nurse Education and Practice, 2015).

In addition to efforts in the United States, nursing associations, councils, and regulatory agencies in other countries have clarified, established, and/or regulated APRN roles and practice (Canadian Nurses Association [CNA], 2007, 2008, 2009a, 2009b; ICN Nurse Practitioner/Advanced Practice Nursing Network, 2016; International Council of Nurses [ICN], 2009; Nursing and Midwifery Board of Australia, 2014). In countries in which APRN roles exist, in addition to studies of the distinctions among roles (Gardner, Chang, Duffield, & Doubrovsky, 2013; Gardner, Duffield, Doubrovsky, & Adams, 2016; Lowe, Plummer, O'Brien, & Boyd, 2012), APRN educational programs are being established, for example, in Israel (Kleinpell et al., 2014), mainland China (Wong et al., 2010), and Singapore (National University of Singapore Yong Loo Lin School of Medicine, 2016). Country-specific frameworks are being developed to clarify education, scope of practice, registration and licensing, and/or credentialing (Fagerström, 2009). Although contextual factors may differ from those in the United States, global opportunities exist for clarifying and advancing APRN practice specific to a country's culture, health system, professional standards, and regulatory requirements. A sample of conceptual and theoretical models of APRN practice from various countries is presented in this chapter along with US and international conceptualizations of APRN roles.

Professional organizations with interests in licensing, accreditation, certification, and educational (LACE) issues regarding APRNs also operate from a conceptualization of advanced practice nursing, whether implicit or explicit. In this chapter, models promulgated by APRN stakeholder organizations that describe the nature of advanced practice nursing and/or differentiate between advanced and basic practice, and selected models, including international, that have guided APRN practice are discussed. Problems associated with lack of a unified definition of advanced practice and imperatives for undertaking this important work exist. When practical, consensus on advanced practice nursing models should be beneficial for patients, society, and the profession. The APRN Consensus Model (APRN Joint Dialogue Group, 2008) and core competencies of APRN practice brought needed conceptual clarity to the regulation of advanced practice nursing in the United States. However, variations in scope of practice still remain between states in the United States (Pearson, 2014) and around the world (Kleinpell et al., 2014). Additionally, work is still needed to differentiate basic and advanced nursing practice and the practice of APRNs from that of other disciplines. Therefore the purposes of this chapter are as follows:

1. Lay the foundation for thinking about the concepts underlying advanced practice nursing by describing the nature, purposes, and components of conceptual models.
2. Identify conceptual challenges in defining and operationalizing advanced practice nursing.
3. Describe selected conceptualizations of advanced practice nursing.
4. Make recommendations for assessing existing models and developing, implementing, and evaluating conceptual frameworks for advanced practice.
5. Outline future directions for conceptual work on advanced practice nursing.

It is important to note that, because of the dynamic and evolving nature of health care and nursing organizations activities in this arena, nationally and globally, readers are encouraged to consult the websites cited in this chapter for up-to-date information.

Nature, Purposes, and Components of Conceptual Models

A conceptual model is one part of the structure of nursing knowledge. Ranging from most abstract to most concrete, this structure consists of metaparadigms, philosophies, conceptual models, theories, and empirical indicators (Fawcett & Desanto-Madeya, 2013). Traditionally, key concepts in the metaparadigm of nursing are humans, the environment, health, and nursing (Fawcett & Desanto-Madeya, 2013).

Fawcett and Desanto-Madeya (2013) described a conceptual model as "a set of relatively abstract and general concepts that address the phenomena of central interest to a discipline, the propositions that broadly describe these concepts, and the propositions that state relatively abstract and general relations between two or more of the concepts" (p. 13). In addition, they noted that a conceptual model is "a distinctive frame of reference ... that tells [adherents] how to observe and interpret the phenomenon of interest to the discipline" and "provide[s] alternative ways to view the subject matter of the discipline; there is no 'best' way" (p. 13). Although there is no best way to view a phenomenon, evolving a more uniform and explicit conceptual model of advanced practice nursing benefits patients, nurses, and other stakeholders (IOM, 2011) by facilitating communication, reducing conflict, and ensuring consistency of advanced practice nursing, when relevant and appropriate, across APRN roles, and by offering a "systematic approach to nursing research, education, administration, and practice" (Fawcett & Desanto-Madeya, 2013, p. 15).

Models may help APRNs articulate professional role identity and function, serving as a framework for organizing beliefs and knowledge about their professional roles and competencies, providing a basis for further development of knowledge. In clinical practice, APRNs use conceptual models in the delivery of their holistic, comprehensive, and collaborative care (Carron & Cumbie, 2011; Dunphy, Winland-Brown, Porter, Thomas, & Gallagher, 2011; Elliott & Walden, 2015; Musker, 2011). Models may also be used to differentiate among and between levels of nursing practice—for example, between staff nursing and advanced practice nursing (Gardner et al., 2013) and between clinical nurse specialists (CNSs), nurse-midwives, and nurse practitioners (NPs) (Begley et al., 2013).

Conceptual models are also used to guide research and theory development by focusing on a given concept or examining the relationships among select concepts to elucidate testable theories. For example, Gullick and West (2016) evaluated Wenger's Community of Practice framework to build research capacity and productivity for CNSs and NPs in Australia. Faculty, in the preparation of students for APRN roles, use conceptual models to plan curricula, to identify important concepts and their relationships, and to make choices about course content and clinical experiences (Perraud et al., 2006; Wong et al., 2010).

Fawcett and Graham (2005) and Fawcett, Newman, and McAllister (2004) have challenged us to think about conceptual questions of advanced practice:

- What do APRNs do that makes their practice "advanced"?
- To what extent does incorporating activities traditionally done by physicians qualify nursing practice as "advanced"?
- Are there nursing activities that are also advanced?

Because direct clinical practice is viewed as the central APRN competency, this begs the question: What does the term *clinical* mean? Does it refer only to hospitals or clinics? These questions are becoming more important given the APRN Consensus Model and given the role that APRNs are expected to play across the continua of health care as a result of ongoing changes to health care legislation. From a regulatory standpoint, the emphasis on a specific population as a focus of practice will lead, when appropriate, to reconceptualizing curricula to ensure that graduates are prepared to succeed in new or revised certification examinations. Hamric and Tracy (see Chapter 3) have noted that although some APRN competencies (e.g., collaboration) may be performed by nurses in other roles, the expression of these competencies by APRNs is different. For example, although all nurses collaborate, a unique aspect of APRN practice is that APRNs are authorized to initiate referrals and prescribe treatments that are implemented by others (e.g., physical therapy). Innovations and reforms arising from changes in health care legislation will ensure that APRNs are explicitly engaged in the delivery of care across care settings, including in nursing clinics and palliative care settings, and as full participants in interprofessional teams. Changes in regulations and in the delivery of health care may be the impetus that leads to new or revised conceptualizations of advanced practice nursing (e.g., defining theoretical and evidence-based differences between the care provided by APRNs and other providers and clinical staff, the role of APRNs in interprofessional teams, and specialization and subspecialization in advanced practice nursing). Working together, nursing leaders and health policymakers will be able to design a health care system that delivers high-quality care at reasonable cost, based on disciplinary and interdisciplinary competencies, outcomes, effectiveness, efficacy, and efficacy.

In addition to a pragmatic reevaluation of advanced practice nursing concepts based on the evolution of APRN regulation and health care reform, important theoretical questions are being raised about the conceptualization of advanced practice nursing. Issues range from the epistemologic, philosophical, and ontologic underpinnings of advanced practice (Arslanian-Engoren, Hicks, Whall, & Algase, 2005) and the extent to which APRNs are prepared to apply nursing theory to their practices (Algase, 2010; Arslanian-Engoren et al., 2005; Karnick, 2011) to the questions about the nature of advanced practice knowledge, discerning the differences between and among the notions of specialty, advanced practice, and advancing practice (Allan, 2011; Christensen, 2009, 2011; MacDonald, Herbert, & Thibeault, 2006; Thoun, 2011).

In summary, questions arising from a changing health policy landscape and from theorizing about advanced practice nursing underscore the need for well thought-out, robust conceptual models to guide APRN practice. Conceptual clarity of advanced practice nursing, what it is and is not, is important not only for patients and those in the nursing profession but also for interprofessional education (CIHC, 2010; Health Professions Network Nursing and Midwifery Office, 2010; IPEC Expert Panel, 2011) and practice (American Association of Nurse Anesthetists [AANA], 2012). Conceptual clarity of advanced practice nursing will also inform the creation of accountable care organizations and support efforts to build teams and systems in which effective communication, collaboration, and coordination will lead to high-quality care and improved patient, institutional, and fiscal outcomes.

Conceptualizations of Advanced Practice Nursing: Problems and Imperatives

Despite the usefulness and benefits of conceptual models, conceptual confusion and uncertainty remain regarding advanced practice nursing. One noted issue is the lack of a well-defined and consistently applied core stable vocabulary used for model building. Despite progress, this challenge remains. For example, in the United States *advanced practice nursing* is the term that is used, but the ICN and CNA use the term *advanced nursing practice.* Considerable variation is noted between the conceptual definition of advanced practice nursing and that of advanced nursing practice as used in Australia, Canada, New Zealand, the United States, Canada, and the United Kingdom (Stasa, Cashin, Buckley, & Donoghue, 2014). Adding to this opacity is the use of the term *advanced practitioner* to describe the role of non-APRN experts in the United Kingdom and internationally (McGee, 2009). The role and

functions of APRNs need to be clearly and consistently conceptualized.

The APRN Consensus Model (APRN Joint Dialogue Group, 2008) represents a major step forward in promulgating a uniform definition of advanced practice in the United States, for the purpose of regulation. However, the lack of a core vocabulary continues to make comparisons difficult because the conceptual meanings vary. Competencies are more commonly used to describe concepts of APRN practice, but reflection on and discussion of other terms such as *roles, hallmarks, functions, activities, skills,* and *abilities* continue and may contribute to the urgent need for clarification of conceptual models and a common language.

Few models of APRN practice address nursing's metaparadigm (person, health, environment, nursing) comprehensively. The problem in comparing, refining, or developing models is that concepts are often used without universal meaning or consensus and, occasionally, with no or inconsistent definitions. It is rightly anticipated that conceptual models of the field and its practice change over time. However, the evolution of advanced practice nursing and its comprehension by nurses, policymakers, and the public will be enhanced if scholars and practitioners agree on the use and definition of fundamental concepts of APRN practice.

Another challenge is the paucity of conceptual models describing the practice and outcomes of APRNs. Although the numbers of models are increasing, they remain small. Further compounding this issue is the scarcity of international and global models of APRN practice. Models are needed that address the diverse health and cultural needs of individuals, families, and communities worldwide.

Another issue is a lack of clarity in the conceptualizations that differentiate the clinical practice of APRNs from that of registered nurses (RNs) without graduate degrees in advanced practice. Conceptual models can help to identify key concepts and variables that distinguish the focus, levels of practice, and outcomes between and among nurses with different levels and types of academic preparation and specialty certification.

Of additional importance is clarifying and distinguishing the differences in practice of APRNs and physician colleagues. Some graduate APRN students may struggle with this issue as part of role development. The lack of conceptual clarity is apparent in advertisements that invite both NPs and physician assistants to apply for the same position. Organized medicine continues to expend resources trying to limit

or discredit advanced practice nursing, even as some physician leaders work on behalf of advocating for APRNs. Barriers to APRNs' ability to practice to the full extent of their education and training as recommended by the IOM (2011) may be the result of lack of conceptual clarity between nursing at the advanced practice level and the practice of medicine. To this end, the philosophical underpinnings of conceptual models of APRN practice need explication.

The emphasis on interprofessional education and practice is another issue in need of clarification. Interprofessional education and practice is central to accountable, collaborative, coordinated, and high-quality care. Graduate education of APRNs alongside other health professionals is beginning to take place. For example, at the University of Michigan, an interprofessional clinical decision-making course with graduate students from nursing (APRN students), pharmacy, dentistry, medicine, and social work is one of the first of its kind in the nation. Students learn together and from each other about their roles, preparation, and disciplinary foci (Sweet, Madeo, Fitzgerald, et al., 2017). The development of interprofessional competencies for health professionals (CIHC, 2010; Health Professions Network Nursing and Midwifery Office, 2010; IPEC Expert Panel, 2011) indicates the need for high-functioning, interprofessional teams of health care experts to maximize patient outcomes. The existence of interprofessional competencies and emergence of promising conceptualizations of interprofessional work are critical contextual factors for elucidating and advancing conceptualizations of advanced practice nursing (Barr, Freeth, Hammick, Koppel, & Reeves, 2005; Reeves et al., 2011). Conceptual models for APRN practice on interprofessional teams are needed to explicate the unique and critical contributions of APRNs to patient outcomes and system resources.

Among many imperatives for reaching a conceptual consensus on advanced practice nursing, most important are the interrelated areas of policymaking, licensing and credentialing, and practice, including competencies. In the policymaking arena, for example, not all APRNs are eligible to be reimbursed by insurers, and even those activities that are reimbursable are often billed incident to a physician's care, rendering the work of APRNs invisible. The APRN Consensus Model (APRN Joint Dialogue Group, 2008), the ACA (2010), and the IOM's call for changes to enable APRNs to work within their full scope of practice (IOM, 2011) will make it easier for US policymakers to recommend and adopt changes to policies and regulations that now constrain APRN practice, eventually making the contributions of APRNs to quality care visible and reimbursable. Agreement on vocabulary and concepts such as competencies that are common to all APRN roles will maximize the ability of APRNs to work within their full scope of practice.

Although some progress has been made, there are compelling reasons for continuing dialogue and activity aimed at clarifying advanced practice nursing and the concepts and models that help stakeholders understand the nature of APRN work and the contributions of APRNs. Reaching consensus on concepts and vocabulary will serve theoretical, practical, and policymaking purposes. As the work of health care reform and implementing interprofessional competencies, education, and practice moves forward, there will be opportunities for the profession to conceptualize advanced practice nursing more clearly. Box 2.1 presents outcomes that come from clarification and consensus on conceptualization of the nature of advanced practice nursing.

Conceptualizations of Advanced Practice Nursing Roles: Organizational Perspectives

Practice with individual clients or patients is the central work of the field; it is the reason for which nursing was created. The following questions are the kinds of questions a conceptual model of advanced practice nursing should answer:

- What is the scope and purpose of advanced practice nursing?
- What are the characteristics of advanced practice nursing?
- Within what settings does this practice occur?
- How do APRNs' scopes of practice differ from those of other providers offering similar or related services?
- What knowledge and skills are required?
- How are these different from those of other providers?
- What patient and institutional outcomes are realized when APRNs deliver care? How are these outcomes different from those of other providers?
- When should health care systems employ APRNs, and what types of patients particularly benefit from APRN care?
- For what types of pressing health care problems are APRNs a solution in terms of improving outcomes, quality of care, and cost-effectiveness?

BOX 2.1 **Clarification and Consensus on Conceptualization of the Nature of Advanced Practice Nursing**

1. Clear differentiation of advanced practice nursing from other levels of clinical nursing practice.
2. Clear differentiation between advanced practice nursing and the clinical practice of physicians and other non-nurse providers within a specialty.
3. Clear understanding of the roles and contributions of advanced practice registered nurses (APRNs) on interprofessional teams, enabling employers to create teams and accountable care organizations that can meet institutions' clinical and fiduciary outcomes.
4. Clear delineation of the similarities and differences among APRN roles and the ability to match APRN skills and knowledge to the needs of patients.
5. Regulation and credentialing of APRNs that protect the public and ensure equitable treatment of all APRNs.
6. Clear articulation of international, national, state, and local health policies that do the following:
   a. Recognize and make visible the substantive contributions of APRNs to quality, cost-effective health care and patient outcomes.
   b. Ensure the public's access to APRN care.
   c. Ensure explicit and appropriate mechanisms to bill and pay for APRN care.
7. A maximum social contribution by APRNs in health care, including improvement in health outcomes and health-related quality of life for the people to whom they provide care.
8. The actualization of practitioners of advanced practice nursing, enabling APRNs to reach their full potential, personally and professionally.

Of the conceptual models presented in this chapter, some are more narrowly focused than others, and some are more homogeneous or mixed with respect to the phenomenon studied. Models may be seen as micromodels in terms of the unit of analysis or as metamodels incorporating a number of conceptual frameworks. Still other models explain systems and the relationships between and among systems. All these foci are important, depending on the purposes to be served. However, in the development of conceptual models, the phenomenon to be modeled must be carefully defined. For example, a model may encompass the entire field of advanced practice nursing or be confined to distinctive concepts (e.g., collaborative practice between APRNs and physicians or the difference between APRN practice and the practice of non-APRN nurses). If a phenomenon and its related concepts are not clearly defined, the model could be so inconsistent as to be confusing or so broad that its impact will be diluted.

In addition to describing concepts and how they are related, assumptions about the philosophy, values, and practices of the profession should be reflected in conceptual models. The discussion of conceptualizations of advanced practice nursing is guided by these assumptions:

1. Each model, at least implicitly, addresses the four elements of nursing's metaparadigm: persons, health and illness, nursing, and the environment.
2. The development and strengthening of the field of advanced practice nursing depends on professional agreement regarding the nature of advanced practice nursing (a conceptual model) that can inform APRN program accreditation, credentialing, and practice.
3. APRNs meet the needs of society for advanced nursing care.
4. Advanced practice nursing will reach its full potential to the extent that foundational conceptual components of any model of advanced practice nursing framework are delineated and agreed on.

Consensus Model for Advanced Practice Registered Nurse Regulation

In 2004, an APRN Consensus Conference was convened to achieve consensus regarding the credentialing of APRNs (APRN Joint Dialogue Group, 2008; Stanley, Werner, & Apple, 2009) and the development of a regulatory model for advanced practice nursing. Independently, the APRN Advisory Committee for the National Council of State Boards of Nursing (NCSBN) was charged by the NCSBN Board of Directors with a similar task of creating a future model for APRN regulation and, in 2006, disseminated a draft of the APRN Vision Paper (NCSBN, 2006), a document that generated debate and controversy. Within a year, these groups came

together to form the APRN Joint Dialogue Group, with representation from numerous stakeholder groups, and the outcome was the APRN Consensus Model (APRN Joint Dialogue Group, 2008).

The APRN Consensus Model includes important definitions of roles, titles, and population foci. Furthermore, it defines specialties and describes how to make room for the emergence of new APRN roles and population foci within the regulatory framework. A timeline for adoption and strategies for implementation were put forth, and progress has been made in these areas (see Chapter 22 for further information; only the model is discussed here). Fig. 2.1 depicts the components of the APRN Consensus Model, the four recognized APRN roles and six population foci. The term *advanced practice registered nurse* refers to all four APRN roles. An APRN is defined as a nurse who meets the following criteria (APRN Joint Dialogue Group, 2008):

- Completes an accredited graduate-level education program preparing him or her for one of the four recognized APRN roles and a population focus (see discussion in Chapter 3)
- Passes a national certification examination that measures APRN role and population-focused competencies and maintains continued competence by national recertification in the role and population focus

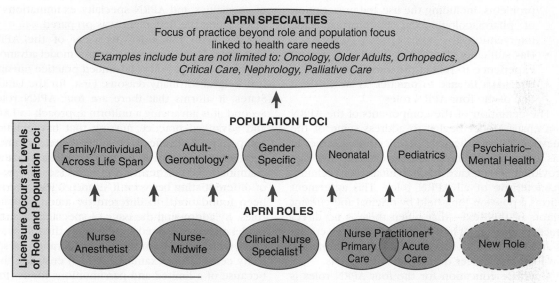

FIG 2.1 Consensus model for APRN regulation. This model was based on the work of the APRN Consensus Work Group and the NCSBN APRN Advisory Committee. *(From APRN Joint Dialogue Group. [2008]. Consensus model for APRN regulation. Retrieved from http://www.aacn.nche.edu/education-resources/APRNReport.pdf.)* *The population focus *Adult-Gerontology* encompasses the young adult to the older adult, including the frail elderly. APRNs educated and certified in the Adult-Gerontology population are educated and certified across both areas of practice and will be titled Adult-Gerontology CNP or CNS. In addition, all APRNs in any of the four roles providing care to the adult population (e.g., Family or Gender Specific) must be prepared to meet the growing needs of the older adult population. Therefore the education program should include didactic and clinical education experiences necessary to prepare APRNs with these enhanced skills and knowledge.
†The clinical nurse specialist (CNS) is educated and assessed through national certification processes across the continuum from wellness through acute care.
‡The certified nurse practitioner (CNP) is prepared with the acute care CNP competencies and/or the primary care CNP competencies. At this point in time the acute care and primary care CNP delineation applies only to the Pediatrics and Adult-Gerontology CNP population foci. Scope of practice of the primary care or acute care CNP is not setting-specific but is based on patient care needs. Programs may prepare individuals across both the primary care and acute care CNP roles. If programs prepare graduates across both roles, the graduate must be prepared with the consensus-based competencies for both roles and must successfully obtain certification in both the acute and the primary care CNP roles.

- Possesses advanced clinical knowledge and skills preparing him or her to provide direct care to patients; the defining factor for *all* APRNs is that a significant component of the education and practice focuses on direct care of individuals
- Builds on the competencies of RNs by demonstrating greater depth and breadth of knowledge and greater synthesis of data by performing more complex skills and interventions and by possessing greater role autonomy
- Is educationally prepared to assume responsibility and accountability for health promotion and/or maintenance, as well as the assessment, diagnosis, and management of patient problems, including the use and prescription of pharmacologic and nonpharmacologic interventions
- Has sufficient depth and breadth of clinical experience to reflect the intended license
- Obtains a license to practice as an APRN in one of the four APRN roles

The definition of the components of the APRN Consensus Model begins to address some of the questions about advanced practice posed earlier in this chapter. An important agreement was that providing direct care to individuals is a defining characteristic of all APRN roles. This agreement affirms a position long held by original and current editors of this text—that when there is no direct practice component in the role, one is not practicing as an APRN. It also has important implications for LACE and for career development of APRNs.

Graduate education for the four APRN roles is described in the Consensus Model document. It must include completion of at least three separate, comprehensive graduate courses in advanced physiology and pathophysiology, physical health assessment, and advanced pharmacology (the "three Ps"), consistent with requirements for the accreditation of APRN education programs. In addition, curricula must address three other areas—the principles of decision making for the particular APRN role, preparation in the core competencies identified for the role, and role preparation in one of the six population foci.

The Consensus Model asserts that licensure must be based on educational preparation for one of the four existing APRN roles and a population focus, that certification must be within the same area of study, and that the four separate processes of LACE are necessary for the adequate regulation of APRNs (APRN Joint Dialogue Group, 2008; see Chapter 22).

The six population foci displayed in Fig. 2.1 include the individual and family across the life span as well as adult/gerontologic, neonatal, pediatric, women's health/gender-specific, and psychiatric/mental health populations. Preparation in a specialty, such as oncology or critical care, cannot be the basis for licensure. Specialization "indicates that an APRN has additional knowledge and expertise in a more discrete area of specialty practice. Competency in the specialty area could be acquired either by educational preparation or experience and assessed in a variety of ways through professional credentialing mechanisms (e.g., portfolios, examinations)" (APRN Joint Dialogue Group, 2008, p. 12). This was a critical decision for the group to reach, given the numbers of specialties and APRN specialty examinations in place when the document was prepared.

Even with this brief overview of the APRN Consensus Model, one sees how this model advanced the conceptualization of advanced practice nursing. It is helpful for many reasons. First, for the United States, it affirms that there are four APRN roles. Second, it is advancing a uniform approach to LACE and advanced practice nursing that has practical and policymaking effects, including better alignment between and among APRN curricula and certification examinations. Furthermore, it addresses the issue of differentiating between RNs and APRNs and has been foundational to differentiate among nursing roles. By addressing the issue of specialization, the model offers a reasoned approach for the following: (1) avoiding confusion from a proliferation of specialty certification examinations; (2) ensuring that, because of a limited and parsimonious focus (four roles and six populations), there will be sufficient numbers of APRNs for the relevant examinations to ensure psychometrically valid data on test results; and (3) allowing for the development of new APRN roles or foci to meet society's needs.

Although there are a number of noted strengths of the Consensus Model, there are also limitations. First, competencies that are common across APRN roles are not addressed beyond defining an APRN and indicating that students must be prepared "with the core competencies for one of the four APRN roles across at least one of the six population foci" (APRN Joint Dialogue Group, 2008, p. 10). The model leaves it to the different APRN roles to develop their own core competencies.

In addressing specialization, the model also leaves open the issue of the importance of educational preparation, in addition to experience, for advanced practice in a specialty. Two years after the 2004

APRN consensus conference, the American Association of Colleges of Nursing (AACN, 2006) put forth the Essentials of Doctoral Education for Advanced Nursing Practice. The Essentials established the DNP, the highest practice degree and the preferred preparation for specialty nursing practice. The AACN called for doctorate-level preparation of APRNs by the year 2015. DNP preparation for entry to practice has been endorsed by the AANA (2007), the National Association of Clinical Nurse Specialists (2015), and the National Organization of Nurse Practitioner Faculties (NONPF, 2015). However, the American College of Nurse-Midwives (ACNM, 2015) has not endorsed the DNP as a requirement for entry into practice for CNMs, instead supporting the completion of a graduate degree program requirement for certification and entry into clinical practice.

Although experience in an area is certainly a factor that leads to the emergence of new specialties, experience alone may be insufficient for the APRN who specializes in oncology or critical care (or another specialty) to achieve desired outcomes in timely and cost-effective ways. These are specialties in which the population's needs are many and complex and the scope of research knowledge is similarly broad and deep. These are important areas of conceptualization that need to be addressed by the American Nurses Association (ANA) and specialty professional nursing organizations, rather than by a group with a regulatory focus.

Numerous efforts are underway to implement this model in the United States. The NCSBN has an extensive toolkit to help educators, APRNs, and policymakers implement the new APRN regulatory model (NCSBN, 2015). The work undertaken to produce the APRN Consensus Model (APRN Joint Dialogue Group, 2008) illustrates the power of interorganizational collaboration and is a promising example of how a model can, as Fawcett and Desanto-Madeya (2013) have suggested, reduce conflict and facilitate communication within the profession, across professions, and with the public.

American Nurses Association

As the only full-service professional organization representing the interests of the 3.6 million RNs in the United States through its constituent and state nurses associations and its organizational affiliates, the ANA and its constituent organizations have also been active in developing documents that address advanced practice nursing. Two of these are particularly important for the contemporary conceptualizations of advanced practice nursing. Since 1980, the ANA has periodically updated its Social Policy Statement (ANA, 2010b). Specialization has consistently been identified as a concept that differentiates advanced practice nursing from basic nursing practice. The most recent edition of the policy notes that specialization ("focusing on nursing practice in a specific area, identified from within the whole field of professional nursing"; ANA, 2010b, p. 17) can occur at basic or advanced levels and that APRNs use additional specialized knowledge and skills obtained through graduate education in their practices. According to this statement, advanced nursing practice "builds on the competencies of the registered nurse and is characterized by the integration and application of a broad range of theoretical and evidence-based knowledge that occurs as part of graduate nursing education" (ANA, 2010b, p. 18). In this document, APRNs are defined as RNs who hold master's or doctoral degrees and are licensed, certified, and/or approved to practice in their roles by state boards of nursing or regulatory oversight bodies. APRNs are prepared through graduate education in nursing for one of four APRN roles (NPs, certified registered nurse anesthetists [CRNAs], NMs, CNSs) and at least one of six population foci (family/individual across the life span, adult/gerontology, neonatal, pediatrics, women's health/gender-related health, psychiatric/mental health) (ANA, 2010b). These definitions of specialization and advanced practice are consistent with the APRN Consensus Model.

The ANA also establishes and promulgates standards of practice and competencies for RNs and APRNs. Six standards of practice and 10 standards of professional performance are described in the second edition of *Nursing: Scope and Standards of Practice* (ANA, 2010a). Each standard is associated with competencies. Of the 16 total standards, all but one (Standard 11, "Communication") outlines additional competencies for APRNs compared with RNs. For example, Standard 5, "Implementation," addresses the consultation and prescribing responsibilities of APRNs and Standard 12, "Leadership," addresses the mentoring and role development responsibilities of APRNs. It is in the description of the competencies that APRN practice and the practice of nurses prepared in a specialty at the graduate level are differentiated from RN practice.

In addition to these documents, the ANA, together with the American Board of Nursing Specialties (ABNS), convened a task force on Clinical Nurse Specialist competencies. For many reasons, including the recognition that developing psychometrically sound certifications for numerous specialties, especially for CNSs, would be difficult as the profession moved toward implementing the APRN Consensus Model, the ANA and ABNS convened a group of stakeholders in 2006 to develop and validate a set of core competencies that would be expected of CNSs entering practice, regardless of specialty (National Association of Clinical Nurse Specialists [NACNS]/National CNS Core Competency Task Force, 2010). This work is discussed later in this chapter in the section on the NACNS.

American Association of Colleges of Nursing

Over the last decade, the AACN has undertaken two nursing education initiatives aimed at transforming nursing education. In 2006, the AACN called for APRN preparation to be at the doctoral level in practice-based programs (DNP), with master's level education being refocused on generalist preparation (e.g., clinical nurse leaders, staff, and clinical educators). Clinical nurse leaders are not APRNs (AACN, 2005, 2012; Spross et al., 2004) and therefore are not included in this discussion of conceptualizations. Through these initiatives, and to the extent that the AACN and Commission on Collegiate Nursing Education influence accreditation, the DNP is becoming

the preferred degree for most APRNs. The growth of DNP education has advanced considerably. In 2006, there were 20 DNP programs; in 2016, there were 289, with an additional 128 DNP programs in the planning stage (AACN, 2015). Enrollments in and graduation from DNP programs have also risen substantially (AACN, 2016).

The DNP Essentials (AACN, 2006) are composed of eight competencies for DNP graduates (Box 2.2). For APRNs, "Essential VIII specifies the foundational practice competencies that cut across specialties and are seen as requisite for DNP practice" (AACN, 2006, p. 16; see Box 2.3). Recognizing that DNP programs also prepare nurses for non-APRN roles, the AACN acknowledged that organizations representing APRNs are expected to develop Essential VIII as it relates to specific advanced practice roles and to "develop competency expectations that build upon and complement DNP Essentials 1 through 8" (AACN, 2006, p. 17). These Essentials affirm

 BOX 2.2   Essentials of Doctoral Education for Advanced Nursing Practice

   I. Scientific underpinnings for practice
  II. Organizational and systems leadership for quality improvement and systems thinking
 III. Clinical scholarship and analytical methods for evidence-based practice
  IV. Information systems and technology and patient care technology for the improvement and transformation of health care
   V. Health care policy for advocacy in health care
  VI. Interprofessional collaboration for improving patient and population health outcomes
 VII. Clinical prevention and population health for improving the nation's health
VIII. Advanced nursing practice

From American Association of Colleges of Nursing. (2006). The essentials of doctoral education for advanced nursing practice. Retrieved from http://www.aacn.nche.edu/publications/position/DNPEssentials.pdf.

 BOX 2.3   Essential VIII: Advanced Nursing Practice Competencies

1. Conduct a comprehensive and systematic assessment of health and illness parameters in complex situations, incorporating diverse and culturally sensitive approaches.
2. Design, implement, and evaluate therapeutic interventions based on nursing science and other sciences.
3. Develop and sustain therapeutic relationships and partnerships with patients (individual, family, or group) and other professionals to facilitate optimal care and patient outcomes.
4. Demonstrate advanced levels of clinical judgment, systems thinking, and accountability in designing, delivering, and evaluating evidence-based care to improve patient outcomes.
5. Guide, mentor, and support other nurses to achieve excellence in nursing practice.
6. Educate and guide individuals and groups through complex health and situational transitions.
7. Use conceptual and analytical skills in evaluating the links among practice, organizational, population, fiscal, and policy issues.

From American Association of Colleges of Nursing. (2006). The essentials of doctoral education for advanced nursing practice (pp. 16–17). Retrieved from http://www.aacn.nche.edu/publications/position/DNPEssentials.pdf.

that the advanced practice nursing core includes the "three Ps" (three separate courses)—advanced health/physical assessment, advanced physiology/pathophysiology, and advanced pharmacology—and is specific to APRNs. The specialty core must include content and clinical practice experiences that help students acquire the knowledge and skills essential to a specific advanced practice role. These requirements were reconfirmed in the Consensus Model (APRN Joint Dialogue Group, 2008).

The DNP has been described as both a "disruptive innovation" (Hathaway, Jacob, Stegbauer, Thompson, & Graff, 2006) and a natural evolution for NP practice. The DNP has been endorsed as entry for APRN practice by three of the four professional association/organizations representing APRNs, with the exception of the ACNM (2015). As a result of national DNP discussions, APRN organizations have promulgated practice competencies for doctorally prepared APRNs (e.g., ACNM, 2011c; CNS Practice Doctorate Competencies Taskforce of the NACNS, 2009). The NONPF (2012) now has one set of core competencies for NPs. Organizational positions on doctoral education are briefly explored in the discussion of APRN organizations later in this chapter.

Although not a conceptual model per se, the AACN's publication *The Essentials of Doctoral Education for Advanced Nursing Practice* (2006) addresses concepts and content now evident in other documents that address standards of APRN practice and education. The fact that Essential VIII affirms a set of common competencies across APRN roles is an important contribution to conceptual clarity about advanced practice in the United States. Because these Essentials, with the exception of Essential VIII, are intended to address DNP preparation for any nursing role, the contribution of this document to conceptual clarity regarding advanced practice nursing specifically is limited, and its broad definition can lead to further confusion. With the evolution of the DNP, more conceptual clarity may be gained regarding advanced practice nursing and the role of APRNs. However, it is possible that the rapid expansion of this degree will contribute to less clarity in the short term about the nature of advanced nursing practice and the centrality of direct care of patients to APRN work, particularly because the DNP will also prepare nurses for other, nonclinical nursing roles. A discussion of APRN organizations' conceptualization of APRN practice follows, along with a discussion of the extent to which their responses to the DNP influence conceptual clarity on advanced practice nursing.

National Organization of Nurse Practitioner Faculties

The mission of the NONPF is to provide leadership in promoting quality NP education. Since 1990, the NONPF has fulfilled this mission in many ways, including the development, validation, and promulgation of NP competencies. As of 2012, there is only one set of NP core competencies (NONPF, 2012). A brief history of the development of competencies for NPs is presented here, in part because their development has influenced other APRN models.

In 1990, the NONPF published a set of domains and core competencies for primary care NPs based on Benner's (1984) domains of expert nursing practice and the results of Brykczynski's (1989) study of the use of these domains by primary care NPs (Price et al., 1992; Zimmer et al., 1990). Within each domain were a number of specific competencies that served as a framework for primary care NP education and practice.

After endorsing the DNP as entry-level preparation for the NP role, and consistent with the recommendations in the APRN Consensus Model (APRN Joint Dialogue Group, 2008), new NP core competencies were developed in 2011 and amended in 2012, with core competency content developed in 2014 (NONPF, 2011, 2012, 2014). Each of the nine core competencies is accompanied by specific behaviors that all graduates of NP programs, whether master's or DNP prepared, are expected to demonstrate. Population-specific competencies for specific NP roles, together with the nine core competencies, are intended to inform curricula and ensure that graduates will meet certification and regulatory requirements.

From a conceptual perspective, these NP core and population-specific competency documents are notable for several reasons: (1) the competencies for NPs were developed collaboratively by stakeholder organizations; (2) empirical validation is used to affirm the competencies; (3) overall, the competencies are conceptually consistent with statements in the APRN Consensus Model, the DNP Essentials (AACN, 2006), and the ANA's *Nursing: Scope and Standards of Practice* (ANA, 2010a); and (4) the revised competencies are responsive to society's needs for advanced nursing care and the contextual factors that will shape NP practice for at least the next decade. In the amended 2011 NONPF competencies (NONPF, 2011, 2012), there is an emphasis on practice that is not in the APRN

Consensus Model (APRN Joint Dialogue Group, 2008)—patient-centered care, interprofessional care, and independent or autonomous NP practice, clearly responsive to health care reform initiatives, are addressed.

National Association of Clinical Nurse Specialists

The NACNS published the *Statement on Clinical Nurse Specialist Practice and Education* in 1998, revised it in 2004, and is currently working on the next iteration, which is not yet published at the time of this chapter. Although acknowledging the early conceptualization of CNS practice as subroles proposed by Hamric and Spross (1983, 1989), this conceptualization failed to adequately differentiate CNS practice from that of other APRNs. The NACNS statement was put forth to resolve the ambiguity about this foundational APRN role. Three spheres of influence are posited: patient, nurses and nursing practice, and organization or system, each of which requires a unique set of competencies (NACNS, 2004; see Fig. 2.2). The statement also outlined expected outcomes of CNS practice for each sphere and competencies that parallel those of the nursing process.

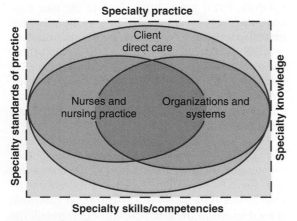

FIG 2.2 National Association of Clinical Nurse Specialists model. CNS practice conceptualized as core competencies in three interacting spheres is shown, as actualized in specialty practice and guided by specialty knowledge and standards. The reader should note that this model predates the Consensus Model of APRN Regulation and the definitions of specialization and population foci in the Consensus Model. *(From National Association of Clinical Nurse Specialists. [2004]. Statement on clinical nurse specialist practice and education [2nd ed.]. Harrisburg, PA: Author.)*

Thus CNSs have sphere-specific competencies of assessment, diagnosis, intervention, and evaluation.

As work on the APRN Consensus Model neared completion, the NACNS and the APRN Consensus Work Group asked the ANA and the ABNS to "convene and facilitate the work of a National CNS Competency Task Force," using a standard process to develop nationally recognized education standards and competencies (NACNS/National CNS Competency Task Force, 2010, p. 3). The process of developing and validating the competencies is described in the document. Fig. 2.3 illustrates the model of CNS competencies that emerged from this work, a synthesis of the NACNS' spheres of influence, Hamric's seven advanced practice nursing competencies, and the Synergy model. Subsequently, new criteria for evaluating CNS education programs were developed, based on the competencies (Validation Panel of the NACNS, 2011). The APRN Consensus Model has impacted certification for CNS roles more than any other APRN role.

The 2004 statement and the new CNS competencies are not entirely parallel. Some aspects of the 2004 statement were more comprehensive with regard to theoretical elements (e.g., inclusion of assumptions and theoretical roots in nursing). The 2010 document has an appendix that includes definitions of key concepts (e.g., nurses and nursing practice, spheres of influence, and competencies). An underlying assumption of these core competencies, which has empirical validation (e.g., Lewandowski & Adamle, 2009), is that CNSs have an impact on patients, nursing practice, and organizational outcomes. From a conceptual standpoint, the CNS competencies document brought needed clarity on several fronts: (1) ensuring that all CNSs would be eligible for credentialing under the APRN Consensus Model so that CNSs could take a psychometrically valid examination on their core competencies, because examinations could not be developed for every existing area of specialization; (2) advancing the work of the NACNS in ensuring consistency among programs preparing CNSs; and (3) because CNSs' work often looks very different from that of other APRNs (e.g., fewer responsibilities for prescribing but more responsibilities for clinical and systems leadership), facilitating the profession's ability to speak about what is common across APRN roles. At least two areas will need further clarification. One is the relationship between the 2004 statement and the 2010 competencies, because both documents are available and CNS authors still refer to the 2004 statement. Both are being used, which is understandable; there is content in the statement that is not in

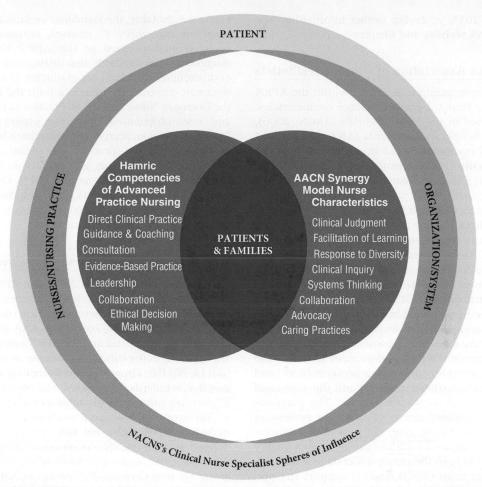

PATIENT

Hamric
Competencies
of Advanced
Practice Nursing

Direct Clinical Practice
Guidance & Coaching
Consultation
Evidence-Based Practice
Leadership
Collaboration
Ethical Decision
Making

PATIENTS
& FAMILIES

AACN Synergy
Model Nurse
Characteristics

Clinical Judgment
Facilitation of Learning
Response to Diversity
Clinical Inquiry
Systems Thinking
Collaboration
Advocacy
Caring Practices

NURSES/NURSING PRACTICE

ORGANIZATION/SYSTEM

NACNS's Clinical Nurse Specialist Spheres of Influence

FIG 2.3 NACNS model of CNS competencies. *(From National Association of Clinical Nurse Specialists/National CNS Competency Task Force. [2010]. Clinical nurse specialist core competencies: Executive summary 2006–2008. Retrieved from http://www.nacns.org/docs/CNSCoreCompetenciesBroch.pdf.)*

the new competencies document, including, in addition to the 2004 competencies, relevant history, a description of CNS practice, and recommendations for graduate programs. The second area will be the ongoing need for clarity regarding specialty as defined in the Consensus Model (the population focus, not specialization, is the basis for regulation). From a regulatory standpoint, it would seem that a CNS's specialty is his or her population focus as defined in the Consensus Model.

Initially the NACNS published a white paper describing a position of neutrality regarding the DNP as an option for CNS education (NACNS, 2005). However, the NACNS did develop core competencies for doctoral-level practice, recognizing that some CNSs would pursue advanced clinical

doctorates (CNS Practice Doctorate Competencies Taskforce of the NACNS, 2009). Three years later, the NACNS (2012) published a *Statement on the APRN Consensus Model Implementation,* outlining the importance of grandfathering currently practicing CNSs and monitoring the implementation of the Consensus Model to ensure that its adoption would not negatively affect the ability of CNSs to practice.

In June of 2015, the NACNS issued a position statement endorsing the DNP as entry into practice for CNSs by 2030. Within this position statement, the NACNS stated support for "CNSs who pursued other graduate education to retain their ability to practice within the CNS role without having to obtain the DNP for future practice as an APRN after 2030"

(NACNS, 2015, p. 2). For further information, see the NACNS website and Chapter 14.

American Association of Nurse Anesthetists

CRNAs are recognized as APRNs within the APRN Consensus Model. Advanced practice competencies, as described in the DNP Essentials (AACN, 2006), the ANA Scope and Standards (ANA, 2010a), and the APRN competencies identified in this text, are evident in the official statements of the AANA (2010, 2013a, 2013b). These statements include scopes of practice, standards for practice, and ethics. Chapter 18 provides a thorough discussion of CRNA practice.

The CRNA's scope and standards of practice are defined in two separate documents from the AANA: *Scope of Nurse Anesthesia Practice* (2013a) and *Standards for Nurse Anesthesia Practice* (2013b). The *Scope of Nurse Anesthesia Practice* addresses the responsibilities of CRNAs performed in collaboration with other qualified health care providers, while the *Standards for Nurse Anesthesia Practice* describe the minimum rules and responsibilities of professional CRNA practice. The Scope document addresses the professional role; education, accountability and leadership; anesthesia practice; and the value and future of nurse anesthesia practice. The purposes of the 11 Standards are to: (1) assist the profession in evaluating CRNA care, (2) provide a common foundation on which CRNAs can develop a quality practice, (3) help the public understand what they can expect from CRNAs, and (4) support and preserve the basic rights of patients. The *Scope of Nurse Anesthesia Practice* and *Standards for Nurse Anesthesia Practice* provide descriptions that can be characterized as clinical competencies or responsibilities (e.g., managing a patient's airway)—the direct clinical practice of CRNAs.

Initially, the AANA did not support the DNP for entry into CRNA practice and established a task force to evaluate doctoral preparation further. Subsequently, the AANA issued a position statement (2007) requiring doctoral preparation for nurse anesthesia practice by the year 2025. However, the position statement does not specify the type of doctoral degree. This likely reflects the diversity of existing practice doctorates for nurse anesthesia practice in addition to the DNP, such as Doctor of Nurse Anesthesia Practice and Doctor of Management of Practice in Nurse Anesthesia (Dreher, 2011; Hawkins & Nezat, 2009). In 2015, the Council on Accreditation of Nurse Anesthesia Educational Programs revised its 2004 accreditation standards for nurse anesthesia

education. Notably, the standards include a requirement for the "three P" courses, consistent with requirements specified in the APRN Consensus document. The standards also distinguish between competencies expected for graduates of a practice doctorate program (referencing both the DNP and the Doctor of Nurse Anesthesia Practice as examples) and research-oriented doctorate programs (e.g., Ph.D.). In addition, accreditation standards have been developed for the practice doctorate in nurse anesthesia (Council on Accreditation of Nurse Anesthesia Educational Programs, 2015). Competencies within these documents align with those in the DNP Essentials (AACN, 2006), referred to as "commonly accepted national standards."

American College of Nurse-Midwives

Certified nurse-midwives (CNMs) are APRNs who are recognized in the APRN Consensus Model. Advanced practice competencies, described in the DNP Essentials (AACN, 2006), the ANA Scope and Standards (ANA, 2010a), and the APRN competencies are apparent in the official statements of the ACNM (2011a, 2011b). These statements include scopes of practice, standards for practice, and ethics. Chapter 17 presents a thorough discussion of CNM practice.

The scope of practice for CNMs (and certified midwives [CMs] who are not nurses) has been defined in four ACNM documents: *Definition of Midwifery and Scope of Practice of Certified Nurse-Midwives and Certified Midwives* (ACNM, 2011a), the *Core Competencies for Basic Midwifery Practice* (ACNM, 2012a), *Standards for the Practice of Midwifery* (ACNM, 2011b), and the *Code of Ethics* (ACNM, 2013). The core competencies are organized into 16 hallmarks describing the art and science of midwifery and the components of midwifery care. The components of midwifery care include professional responsibilities, midwifery management processes, fundamentals, and care of women and of the newborn, within which are prescribed competencies. According to the definition, "CNMs are educated in two disciplines: nursing and midwifery" (ACNM, 2011a, p. 1). Competencies "describe the fundamental knowledge, skills and behaviors of a new practitioner" (ACNM, 2012a, p. 1). The hallmarks, components, and associated core competencies are the foundation on which midwifery curricula and practice guidelines are based.

In addition to the competencies, there are eight ACNM standards that midwives are expected to meet (ACNM, 2011b) and a code of ethics (ACNM, 2013).

The standards address issues such as qualifications, safety, patient rights, culturally competent care, assessment, documentation, and expansion of midwifery practice. Three ethical mandates related to the ACNM mission of midwifery to promote the health and well-being of women and newborns within their families and communities are identified in the ethics code.

As of 2010, CNMs entering practice must earn a graduate degree, complete an accredited midwifery program, and pass a national certification examination (see Chapter 17 for detailed requirements; ACNM, 2011a); the type of graduate degree is not specified. The ACNM does recognize the value of doctoral education as a valid and valuable path for CNMs, as evidenced by a statement on the practice doctorate in midwifery, including competencies (ACNM, 2011c). Although not cited, these competencies align with those in the DNP Essentials (AACN, 2006); the ACNM recognizes that there are other paths for a practice doctorate in midwifery. At the present time, the ACNM (2015) does not support the DNP as a requirement for entry into nurse-midwifery practice. Reasons cited are: (1) midwifery practice is safe, based on the rigor of their curriculum standards and outcome data; (2) there is inadequate evidence to justify the DNP as a mandatory educational requirement for CNMs; and (3) the costs of attaining such a degree could limit the applicant pool and access to midwifery care (ACNM, 2012b). Midwifery organizations have recently addressed the aspects of the 2008 Consensus Model that they support and identified those aspects that are of concern (ACNM, Accreditation Commission for Midwifery Education, & American Midwifery Certification Board, 2011).

International Organizations and Conceptualizations of Advanced Practice Nursing

In this section, issues of a common language and conceptual framework for advanced practice nursing are addressed. International perspectives on advanced practice nursing are covered more extensively in Chapter 6.

The ICN Nurse Practitioner/Advanced Practice Nursing Network (2016) defines a nurse practitioner/advanced practice nurse as "a registered nurse who has acquired the expert knowledge base, complex decision-making skills and clinical competencies for expanded practice, the characteristics of which are shaped by the context and/or country in which s/he is credentialed to practice." A master's degree is recommended for entry level (ICN Nurse Practitioner/Advanced Practice Nursing Network, 2016). Key concepts include educational preparation, the nature of practice, and regulatory mechanisms. The statement is necessarily broad, given the variations in health systems, regulatory mechanisms, and nursing education programs in individual countries.

In 2008 the CNA published *Advanced Nursing Practice: A National Framework,* which defined advanced nursing practice, described educational preparation and regulation, identified the two APRN roles (CNS and NP), and specified competencies in clinical practice, research, and leadership. In addition, they have issued position statements on advanced nursing practice (CNA, 2007) that affirm the key points in the national framework document and define and describe the roles and contributions to health care of NPs (CNA, 2009b) and CNSs (CNA, 2009a). In 2010 the CNA published a Core Competency Framework for NPs, which included the incorporation of theories of advanced practice nursing. The CNA (2013) is also leading efforts not only to distinguish the role of the CNS from that of the NP, but to strengthen the role of the CNS, which includes ICN competencies.

Furthermore, leaders have undertaken an evidence-based, patient-centered, coordinated effort (called a decision support synthesis) to develop, implement, and evaluate the advanced practice nursing roles of the CNS and NP in Canada (DiCenso et al., 2010), a process different from the one used to advance these roles in the United States. This process included a review of 468 published and unpublished articles and interviews conducted with 62 key informants and four focus groups that included a variety of stakeholders. The purpose of this work was to "describe the distinguishing characteristics of CNSs and NPs relevant to Canadian contexts"; identify barriers and facilitators to effective development and use of advanced practice nursing roles; and inform the development of evidence-based recommendations that individuals, organizations, and systems can use to improve the integration of advanced practice nurses into Canadian health care (DiCenso et al., 2010, p. 21). The European Specialist Nurses Organisations (2015) defined 10 core (generic) competencies of CNS practice in Europe. The competencies address clinical role, patient relationship, patient teaching/coaching, mentoring, research, organization and management, communication and teamwork, ethics and decision making, leadership/policymaking, and public health. The competencies were developed to clarify the role of the CNS and include advanced knowledge in anatomy, physiology, pathophysiology and pharmacology, similar to the APRN Consensus Model. It is expected that CNSs will collaborate with other health professionals to deliver high-quality patient care to ensure safety, quality of care, and equity of access to promote health and prevent disease.

Section Summary: Implications for Advanced Practice Nursing Conceptualizations

From this overview of organizational statements that clarify and advance APRN practice, it is clear that, nationally and internationally, stakeholders are actively defining advanced practice nursing. Progress in this area includes global agreement that this level of clinical nursing practice is advanced and builds on basic nursing education. As such, it requires additional education and is characterized by additional competencies and responsibilities. In the United States, the consensus on an approach to APRN regulation was critical for the following reasons: (1) clarifying what is an APRN and the role of graduate education and certification in licensing APRNs, (2) ensuring that APRNs are fully recognized and integrated in the delivery of health care, (3) reducing barriers to mobility of APRNs across state lines, (4) fostering and facilitating ongoing dialogue among APRN stakeholders, and (5) offering common language regarding regulation.

Although there may not be unanimous agreement on the DNP as the requirement for entry into advanced practice nursing, the promulgation of the document fostered dialogue nationally and within APRN organizations on the clinical doctorate (whether or not it is the DNP) as a valid and likely path for APRNs to pursue. As a result, each APRN organization has taken a stand on the role of the clinical doctorate for those in the role and has developed or is developing doctoral-level clinical competencies. In doing so, it appears that the needs of their patients, members, other constituencies, and contexts have been considered. Until the time when a clinical doctorate becomes a requirement for entry into practice for all APRN roles, the development of doctoral-level competencies for APRN roles will help stakeholders distinguish between master's- and clinical doctorate-prepared APRNs with regard to competencies.

Although important differences exist between roles and across countries, a common identity for APRNs resulting from policy and regulatory initiatives would facilitate communication within and outside the profession, consistent with assertions by Styles (1998) and Fawcett and Desanto-Madeya (2013) on the purposes of models. There are important

differences among APRN organizations regarding such issues as doctoral preparation, which is also consistent with Fawcett and Desanto-Madeya's (2013) assertion that there is not one best model.

The level of consensus regarding regulation in the United States reflects considerable and laudable progress, paving the way for policies and health care system transformations that will enable APRNs to be able to more fully ensure access to health care and improve its quality. The processes that have led to this juncture in the United States have required openness, civility, a willingness to disagree, and wisdom. Finally, there are at least two different approaches (collaborative policymaking in the United States and an evidence-based approach in Canada) to determine how best to assess contributions of APRNs and develop ways to integrate APRNs more fully into health care infrastructures in order to maximize their benefits to patients and populations. The global APRN community can examine these processes for insights on how to adapt them to suit their particular context.

The organizational models described address professional roles, licensing, accreditation, certification, education, competencies, and clinical practice. The descriptive statements about APRN roles and competencies demonstrate the common elements that exist across all APRN roles. These include a central focus on and accountability for patient care, knowledge and skills specific to each APRN role, and a concern for patient rights. The published definitions, standards, and competencies offer models against which similarities and differences among APRN roles and practices can be distinguished, educational programs can be developed and evaluated, and knowledge and behaviors can be measured for certification purposes. These will also assist practitioners to understand, examine, and improve their own practice, and develop job descriptions. As advanced practice nursing moves forward in the United States and globally, the profession will continue to define situations in which a conceptual consensus, as well as alternative conceptualizations, will serve the public and the nursing profession.

Conceptualizations of the Nature of Advanced Practice Nursing

The APRN role-specific models promulgated by professional organizations raise several questions, such as:

- What is common across APRN roles?
- Can an overarching conceptualization of advanced practice nursing be articulated?

- How can one distinguish among basic, expert, and advanced levels of nursing practice?

Several authors have attempted to discern the nature of advanced practice nursing and address these questions. The extent to which all APRN roles are considered is not always clear; some only focus on CNS and NP roles.

Select frameworks are presented here that address the nature of advanced practice nursing. From the present review of a number of frameworks, the concepts of roles, domain, and competency are among those most commonly used to explain advanced practice nursing. However, meanings are not consistent. Hamric's model, which uses the terms *roles* and *competencies*, is the only one that is integrative—that is, it explicitly considers all four APRN roles. Because it is integrative, has remained relatively stable since 1996, has informed the development of the DNP Essentials (AACN, 2006) and CNS competencies, and is widely cited, it is discussed first, enabling the reader to consider the extent to which important concepts are addressed by other models. Otherwise, the models are discussed in chronologic order and include examples from both US and international conceptual models of APRN practice.

Hamric's Integrative Model of Advanced Practice Nursing

One of the earliest efforts to synthesize a model of advanced practice that would apply to all APRN roles was developed by Hamric (1996). Hamric, whose early conceptual work was done on the CNS role (Hamric & Spross, 1983, 1989), proposed an integrative understanding of the core of advanced practice nursing, based on literature from all APRN specialties (Hamric, 1996, 2000, 2005, 2009, 2014; see Chapter 3). Hamric proposed a conceptual definition of advanced practice nursing and defining characteristics that included primary criteria (graduate education, certification in the specialty, and a focus on clinical practice with patients) and a set of core competencies (direct clinical practice, collaboration, guidance and coaching, evidence-based practice, ethical decision making, consultation, and leadership). This early model was further refined, together with Hanson and Spross in 2000 and 2005, based on dialogue among the editors. Key components of the model (Fig. 2.4) include the primary criteria for advanced nursing practice, seven advanced practice competencies with direct care as the core competency on which the other competencies depend, and environmental and contextual factors

that must be managed for advanced practice nursing to flourish.

The revisions to Hamric's original model highlight the dynamic nature of a conceptual model, and that essential features remain the same. Models are refined over time according to changes in practice, research, and theoretical understanding. The inherent stability and robustness of Hamric's model are noteworthy, particularly in light of the many potentially transformative advanced practice nursing initiatives being developed. This model forms the understanding of advanced practice nursing used throughout this text and has provided the structure for each edition of the book. Hamric's model has been used by contributors to this text to further elaborate specific competencies such as guidance and coaching (Spross, 2009; see Chapter 8), consultation (see Chapter 9), and ethical decision making (see Chapter 13). It has also informed the development of the DNP Essentials (AACN, 2006) and the revised CNS competencies and is widely cited in the advanced practice literature, which provides further evidence of its contribution to conceptualizing advanced practice nursing.

In addition, integrative literature reviews provide further support for Hamric's integrative conceptualization of advanced practice nursing. Mantzoukas and Watkinson's (2007) literature review sought to identify "generic features" of advanced nursing practice; seven generic features were identified: (1) use of knowledge in practice, (2) critical thinking and analytic skills, (3) clinical judgment and decision making, (4) professional leadership and clinical inquiry, (5) coaching and mentoring, (6) research skills, and (7) changing practice. The first three generic features are consistent with the direct care competency in Hamric's model; these three characteristics seem directly related to clinical practice, which supports direct care as a central competency. The remaining four features are consistent with the three competencies of leadership, guidance and coaching, and evidence-based practice competency in Hamric's model.

Similarly, an integrative literature review of CNS practice by Lewandowski and Adamle (2009) affirmed the direct care, collaboration, consultation, systems leadership, and coaching (patient and staff education) competencies in Hamric's model. Ten countries were represented in their review, and their findings were organized using NACNS's three spheres of influence. Within the first sphere, management of complex or vulnerable populations, they found three essential characteristics—expert direct care, coordination of care, and collaboration. In the sphere of educating

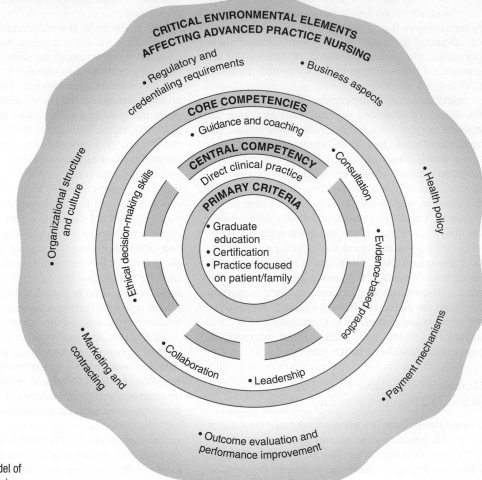

FIG 2.4 Hamric's model of advanced practice nursing.

and supporting interdisciplinary staff, substantive areas of CNS practice were education, consultation, and collaboration. Within the system sphere of influence, CNSs facilitate innovation and change. These findings lend support for the integration of Hamric's model with the NACNS model of CNS core competencies (NACNS/National CNS Competency Task Force, 2010).

Conceptual Models of APRN Practice: United States Examples

Fenton's and Brykczynski's Expert Practice Domains of the CNS and NP

Some of the early work describing the practice domains of APRNs (CNSs and NPs) was conducted by Fenton (1985) and Brykczynski (1989), using

Benner's model of expert nursing practice (Benner, 1984). To fully appreciate their contributions to the understanding of advanced practice, it is important to highlight some of Benner's key findings about nurses who are experts by experience. Although Benner's seminal work, *From Novice to Expert* (1984), has been used in the conceptualization of advanced practice nursing, it is important to note that Benner has not studied advanced practice nurses; her model was based on the expert practice of clinical nurses. Fenton's and Brykczynski's studies represent an extension of Benner's findings and theories to advanced practice nursing.

The early work of Benner and associates informed the development of the first NONPF competencies, graduate curricula in schools of nursing, models of practice, and the standards for clinical promotion.

A noted contribution of this early work was that it "put into words what they had always known about their clinical nursing expertise but had difficulty articulating" (Benner, Tanner, & Tesla, 2009). It is perhaps this impact that led to the sustained integration of Benner's studies of experts by experience into the APRN literature, including descriptions and development of competencies.

Through the analysis of clinical exemplars discussed in interviews, Benner (1984) derived a range of competencies that resulted in the identification of seven domains of expert nursing practice. Within this lexicon, these domains are a combination of roles, functions, and competencies, although the three were not precisely differentiated. The seven domains are the helping role, administering and monitoring therapeutic interventions and regimens, effective management of rapidly changing situations, diagnostic and monitoring function, teaching and coaching function, monitoring and ensuring the quality of health care practices, and organizational and work role competencies.

Fenton (1985) and Brykczynski (1989) each independently applied Benner's model of expert practice to APRNs, examining the practice of CNSs and NPs, respectively. Fenton and Brykczynski (1993) jointly compared their earlier research findings to identify similarities and differences between CNSs and NPs. They verified that nurses in advanced practice were indeed experts, as defined by Benner, showing they were experts by more than experience alone. They identified additional domains and competencies of APRNs (Fig. 2.5). Across the top of Fig. 2.5 are the seven domains identified by Benner and the additional domain found in CNS practice (Fenton, 1985), that of consultation provided by CNSs to other nurses (rectangular dotted box, top right). Under this box are two new CNS competencies (hexagonal boxes). The third (rounded) box is a new NP competency identified by Brykczynski in 1989. In this study of NPs, Brykczynski identified an eighth domain (the management of health and illness in ambulatory care settings) and recognized it as a qualitatively different expression from the first two domains identified by Benner. For NPs, the new competencies were a result of the integration of the diagnostic-monitoring and administering-monitoring domains.

The figure also reveals new CNS and NP competencies identified by Fenton and Brykczynski's work. New CNS competencies were identified under the organization and work role domain (e.g., providing support for nursing staff) and the helping role, in addition to the consulting domain and competencies. New NP competencies were noted in seven of the eight domains (e.g., detecting acute or chronic disease while attending to illness under the diagnostic-administering domains). By examining the extent to which APRNs demonstrate the seven domains found in experts by experience and uncovering differences, the findings offer insight into the differences between expert and advanced practice. In addition, Fenton and Brykczynski's work also described ways in which the CNS and NP roles may differ with regard to practice domains and competencies.

These early findings suggest that a deeper understanding of advanced practice could be beneficial to understanding and conceptualizing advanced nursing practice. Benner's methods could be applied to studies of advanced practice nursing, with the following aims: (1) to confirm Fenton and Brykczynski's findings in CNS and NP roles and identify new domains and competencies across all four APRN roles, (2) to understand how APRN competencies develop in direct-entry graduate and RN graduate students, and (3) to compare the non–master's-prepared clinician's competencies with the APRN's competencies to distinguish components of expert versus advanced practice nursing. Studies focused on how APRNs acquire expertise in APRN and interprofessional competencies could inform future conceptualizations of advanced practice nursing.

Calkin's Model of Advanced Nursing Practice

Calkin's model (1984) was the first to explicitly distinguish the practice of experts by experience from advanced practice nursing of CNSs and NPs. Calkin developed the model to help nurse administrators differentiate advanced practice nursing from other levels of clinical practice in personnel policies. The model proposed that this could be accomplished by matching patient responses to health problems with the skill and knowledge levels of nursing personnel. In Calkin's model, three curves were overlaid on a normal distribution chart. Calkin depicted the skills and knowledge of novices, experts by experience, and APRNs in relation to knowledge required to care for patients whose responses to health care problems (i.e., health care needs) ranged from simple and common to complex and complicated (Fig. 2.6). A closer look at Fig. 2.6A, shows that patients have many more human responses (the highest and widest curve) than a beginning nurse would have the knowledge and skill to effectively manage. The impact of experience is illustrated in Fig. 2.6B. The highest and widest curve is effectively the same, but

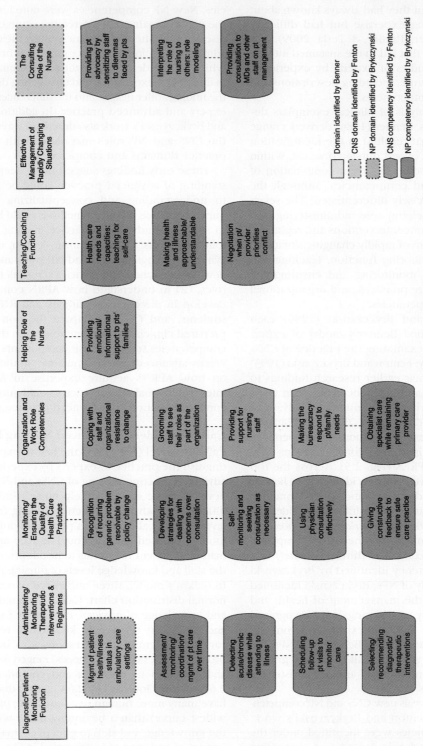

FIG 2.5 Fenton's (1985) and Brykczynski's (1989) expert practice domains of the CNS and NP. *Mgmt*, Management; *pt*, patient. *(From Fenton, M. V., & Brykczynski, K. A. [1993]. Qualitative distinctions and similarities in the practice of clinical nurse specialists and nurse practitioners. Journal of Professional Nursing, 9[6], 313–326.)*

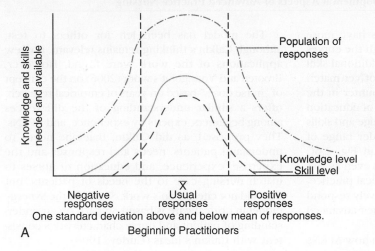

A Beginning Practitioners

Y-axis: Knowledge and skills needed and available

Labels:
- Population of responses
- Knowledge level
- Skill level

X̄

Negative responses — Usual responses — Positive responses

One standard deviation above and below mean of responses.

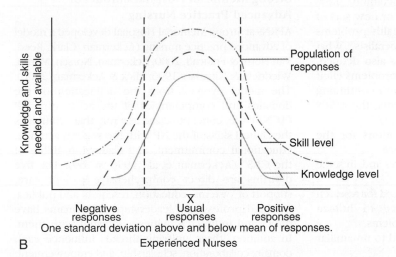

B Experienced Nurses

Y-axis: Knowledge and skills needed and available

Labels:
- Population of responses
- Skill level
- Knowledge level

X̄

Negative responses — Usual responses — Positive responses

One standard deviation above and below mean of responses.

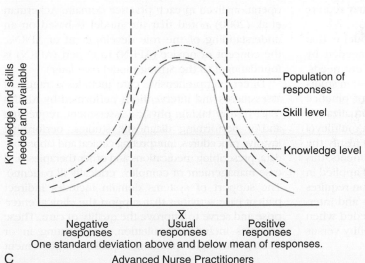

C Advanced Nurse Practitioners

Y-axis: Knowledge and skills needed and available

Labels:
- Population of responses
- Skill level
- Knowledge level

X̄

Negative responses — Usual responses — Positive responses

One standard deviation above and below mean of responses.

FIG 2.6 Calkin's model of advanced nursing practice. Patient responses correlated with the knowledge and skill of (A) beginning practitioners, (B) experienced nurses, and (C) advanced practice nurses (APNs). *(From Calkin, J. D. [1984]. A model for advanced nursing practice.* Journal of Professional Nursing, 14, *24–30.)*

because of experience, expert nurses have more knowledge and skill. However, although the curves are higher and somewhat wider, the additional skill and knowledge of expert nurses do not yet match the range of responses they may encounter in the patients. In Fig. 2.6C, APRNs, by virtue of education and experience, do possess the knowledge and skills that enable them to respond to a wider range of human responses. The three curves in Fig. 2.6C are parallel each other, suggesting that even as less common human responses arise in clinical practice, APRNs are able to creatively and effectively respond to these unusual problems because of their advanced knowledge and skills.

Calkin used the framework to explain how APRNs perform under different sets of circumstances—when there is a high degree of unpredictability, new conditions, new patient population, or new sets of problems, and a wide variety of health problems requiring the services of "specialist generalists." What APRNs do in terms of functions was also defined. For example, when patients' health problems elicit a wide range of human responses with continuing and substantial unpredictable elements, the APRN should do the following (Calkin, 1984):

- Identify and develop interventions for the unusual by providing direct care.
- Transmit this knowledge to nurses and, in some settings, to students.
- Identify and communicate the need for research or carry out research related to human responses to these health problems.
- Anticipate factors that may lead to unfamiliar human responses.
- Provide anticipatory guidance to nurse administrators when the changes in the diagnosis and treatment of these responses may require altered levels or types of resources.

A principal advantage of Calkin's model is that the skills, education, and knowledge needed by nurses are considered in relation to patient needs. It provides a framework for scholars to use in studying the function of APRNs in a variety of practice situations and should be a useful conceptualization for administrators who must maximize a multilevel interprofessional workforce and need to justify the use of APRNs. In today's practice environments, this conceptualization could be modified and applied in other settings based on whether a situation requires an APRN or RN and which mix of intra- and interprofessional staff and support staff is needed when settings have a high degree of predictability versus those that have high clinical uncertainty.

The model has been left for others to test; although Calkin's thinking remains relevant, no new applications of the work were found. However, Brooten and Youngblut's work (2006) on the concept of "nurse dose," based on years of empirical research, offers a similar understanding of the differences among beginners, experts by experience, and APRNs. They proposed, as did Calkin, that one needs to understand patients' needs and responses and the expertise, experience, and education of nurses to match nursing care to the needs of patients, but they did not cite Calkin's work. Similarly, the Synergy model in critical care is based, in part, on an understanding of patient and nurse characteristics consistent with Calkin's ideas (Curley, 1998).

Strong Memorial Hospital's Model of Advanced Practice Nursing

APRNs at Strong Memorial Hospital developed a model of advanced practice nursing (Ackerman, Clark, Reed, Van Horn, & Francati, 2000; Ackerman, Norsen, Martin, Wiedrich, & Kitzman, 1996; Mick & Ackerman, 2000). The model evolved from the delineation of the domains and competencies of the acute care NP (ACNP) role, conceptualized as a role that "combines the clinical skills of the NP with the systems acumen, educational commitment, and leadership ability of the CNS" (Ackerman et al., 1996, p. 69). The five domains are direct comprehensive patient care, support of systems, education, research, and publication and professional leadership. All domains have direct and indirect activities associated with them. In addition, three unifying threads influence each domain: collaboration, scholarship, and empowerment, which are illustrated as circular and continuous threads (Ackerman et al., 1996), (Fig. 2.7). These threads are operationalized in each practice domain. Ackerman et al. (2000) noted that the model is based on an understanding of the role development of APRNs; the concept of novice (APRN) to expert (APRN) is foundational to the Strong model (see later).

Direct comprehensive care includes a range of assessments and interventions performed by APRNs (e.g., history taking, physical assessment, requesting and/or performing diagnostic studies, performing invasive procedures, interpreting clinical and laboratory data, prescribing medications and other therapies, and case management of complex, critically ill patients). The support of systems domain includes indirect patient care activities that support the clinical enterprise and serve to improve the quality of care. These activities include consultation, participating in or leading strategic planning, quality improvement

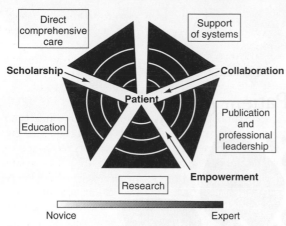

FIG 2.7 The Strong Memorial Hospital's model of advanced practice nursing. *(From Ackerman, M. H., Norsen, L., Martin, B., Wiedrich, J., & Kitzman H. J. [1996]. Development of a model of advanced practice. American Journal of Critical Care, 5, 68–73.)*

initiatives, establishing and evaluating standards of practice, precepting students, and promoting APRN practice. The education domain includes a variety of activities (e.g., evaluating educational programs, providing formal and informal education to staff, educating patients and families, and identifying and disseminating educational resources). The research domain addresses the use and conduct of research, while the publication and professional leadership domain includes APRN functions involved with disseminating knowledge about the ACNP role, participating in professional organizations, influencing health and public policy, and publishing. APRNs are expected to exert influence within and outside their institution.

The unifying threads of collaboration, scholarship, and empowerment are attributes of advanced practice that exert influence across all five domains and characterize the professional model of nursing practice. Collaboration ensures that the contributions of all caregivers are valued. APRNs are expected to create and sustain a culture that supports scholarly inquiry, whether it is questioning a common nursing practice or developing and disseminating an innovation. APRNs support the empowerment of staff, ensuring that nurses have authority over nursing practice and opportunities to improve practice.

The Strong model is a parsimonious model that has many similarities with other advanced practice conceptualizations. For example, its domains are consistent with the competencies delineated in Hamric's model. However, unlike Hamric's model, which posits direct care as the central competency

that informs all other advanced nursing practice competencies, all domains of practice in the Strong model, including direct care, are considered "mutually exclusive of each other and exhaustive of practice behaviors" (Ackerman et al., 1996, p. 69).

It is notable that this model was the result of a collaborative effort between practicing APRNs and APRN faculty members. One could infer that such a model would be useful for guiding clinical practice and planning curricula, two of the purposes of conceptual models outlined earlier in this chapter. The Strong model has informed studies of advanced practice nursing in critical care since its publication (e.g., Becker, Kaplow, Muenzen, & Hartigan, 2006; Chang, Gardner, Duffield, & Ramis, 2010; Mick & Ackerman, 2000). Further work by Gardner et al. (2013) in Australia used the Strong model to delineate the practice of APRNs (Grade 7) from the practice of registered nurse/midwife roles (Grade 5) and to delineate and define advanced practice nursing (Gardner et al., 2016). Ackerman, Mick, and Witzel (2010) have proposed an administrative model for managing APRNs and a central leadership model for hospital-based NPs (Bahouth et al., 2013).

Texas Children's Hospital Transformational Advanced Professional Practice (TAPP) APRN Model

The Strong Memorial Hospital model has also influenced the development of the Texas Children's Hospital transformational advanced professional practice (TAPP) APRN model (Elliott & Walden, 2015) (Fig. 2.8). To better reflect the current conceptualization of the APRN role, two additional domains of professional practice were added to the Strong model: quality and safety, and credentialing and regulatory practice. Professional ethics was also added as a unifying conceptual strand.

The essence of the APRN role within this model is direct, comprehensive, family-centered care. The TAPP model includes this single patient care domain along with six professional development domains: organizational priorities; quality and safety; evidence-based practice and research; education; transformational professional practice; and credentialing and regulatory practice. The model recognizes that the amount of time and effort APRNs devote to the execution of the six professional development domains may vary dependent on needs of the system, patient population, and strengths and interest of individual APRNs.

An added strength of the TAPP model is the description of APRN practice along three continuums: clinical expertise, health, and role. The clinical

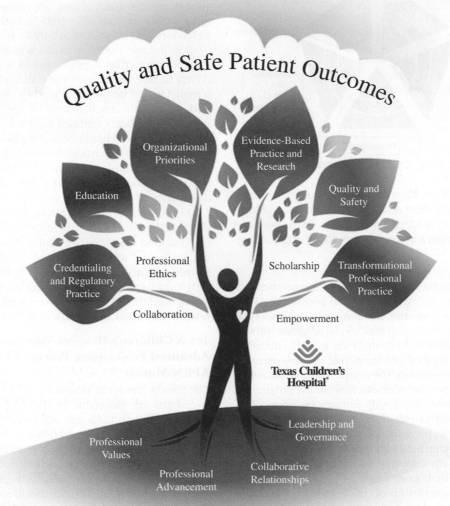

FIG 2.8 Elliott and Walden's transformational advanced professional practice model. *(From Elliott, E. D., & Walden, M. [2015]. Development of the transformational advanced professional practice model.* Journal of the American Association of Nurse Practitioners, 27*[9], 479–487.)*

expertise continuum is reflective of the Benner (1984) model of expert practice (novice to expert), with expertise varying dependent on years of APRN and specialty experience and differing roles. The health continuum includes APRN care for patients who are healthy; for those who have common, stable or chronic health conditions; and for those who have complex, acute, critical, or rare health conditions. The role continuum of professional practice ranges

from dependent on colleagues and mentors to assume a more independent role in each of the patient care and professional domains of practice.

Although the authors indicate the model can be easily adapted to all four APRN roles, they also include physician assistants, thereby diluting the emphasis on models that conceptualize the unique practice of APRNs. In addition, because the NONPF core competencies (Thomas, Crabtree, Delaney, et al.,

2011) were used along with the APRN Consensus Model (APRN Joint Dialogue Group, 2008) to develop the TAPP model, future work should test the appropriateness of this model for APRN roles in other than NP roles.

Shuler's Model of NP Practice

The historical importance of Shuler's model as an early NP model is briefly discussed here (Shuler & Davis, 1993a). Readers should refer to the original article to see the full model.

Shuler's experience integrating nursing and medical knowledge skills into the NP role led to the development of a conceptual model that would illuminate the unique contributions and expanded role of NPs. Shuler's Nurse Practitioner Practice Model is a complex systems model that is holistic and wellness oriented. It is definitive and detailed in terms of how the NP-patient interaction, patient assessment, intervention, and evaluation should occur (Shuler & Davis, 1993a). Table 2.1 outlines key model constructs and related theories. Knowing that these familiar concepts are embedded in this comprehensive model may help readers appreciate its potential usefulness.

Shuler's model is intended "to impact the NP domain at four levels: theoretical, clinical, educational, and research" (Shuler & Davis, 1993a). The model addresses important components of advanced practice nursing: (1) nursing's metaparadigm (person, health, nursing, and environment); (2) the nursing process; (3) assumptions about patients and NPs;

and (4) theoretical concepts relevant to practice. The model could be characterized as a network or system of frameworks.

Clinical application of Shuler's model is intended to describe the NP's expanded nursing knowledge and skills "into medicine," the benefits for NP and patient, and a framework whereby NP services can be evaluated (Shuler & Davis, 1993b). Shuler and Davis (1993b) published a lengthy template for conducting a visit. Although it is difficult to imagine ready implementation into today's busy NP practices, Shuler and colleagues' clinical applications of the model have been published by Shuler (2000), Shuler and Davis (1993b), and Shuler, Huebscher, and Hallock (2001). In the current health care environment, the Circle of Caring model (Dunphy, Winland-Brown, Porter, Thomas, & Gallagher, 2011) may be more useful for addressing some of the issues that led Shuler to create her model—integrating nursing and skills traditionally associated with medicine while learning the NP role, and retaining a nursing focus while providing complex diagnostic and therapeutic interventions.

Conceptual Models of APRN Practice: International Examples

SickKids APRN Framework

A conceptual model of APRN (CNS and NP) practice was developed in Canada for the care of children and adolescents (LeGrow, Hubley, & McAllister, 2010). The model was informed by four other models: the Strong

---

TABLE 2.1   Model Constructs and Underlying Theoretical Concepts Included in Shuler's Model of Nurse Practitioner Practice

Model Constructs	Holistic Patient Needs	Nurse Practitioner–Patient Interaction	Self-Care	Health Prevention	Health Promotion	Wellness
Underlying theoretical concepts	Basic needs Wellness activities Health and illness Psychological health Family Culture Social support Environmental health Spirituality	Contracting Role modeling Self-care activities Teaching/learning Culture Family Social support Environmental health	Wellness activities Preventive health activities Health promotion activities Compliance Problem solving Teaching/learning Contracting Culture Family Social support Environmental health	Primary prevention Secondary prevention Tertiary prevention Preventive health behavior Family Culture Environmental health	Health promotion behavior Wellness Family Culture Environmental health Social support	Self-care activities Wellness activities Disease prevention activities Health promotion activities Family Culture Social support Environmental health Spirituality Contracting Teaching/learning

From Shuler, P. A., & Davis, J. E. (1993a). The Shuler nurse practitioner practice model: A theoretical framework for nurse practitioner clinicians, educators, and researchers, Part 1. *Journal of the American Academy of Nurse Practitioners, 5,* 11–18.

Memorial Hospital model (King & Ackerman, 1995; Mick & Ackerman, 2000); the Illness Beliefs Model (Wright, Watson, & Bell, 1996); the Five Practices of Exemplary Leadership (Kouzes & Posner, 2002); and the CNA (2000) Advanced Nursing Practice National Framework, which includes APRN competencies. SickKids is a family-centered model that was designed to capture the essence of the pediatric APRN role in five domains: pediatric clinical practice, research and scholarly activities, interprofessional collaboration, education and mentorship, and organization and system management. It is applicable to various pediatric practice settings across the continuum of care from the community to the hospital.

The model has been implemented throughout the organization. It has provided a common language for the conceptualization of the APRN role, to establish common expectations and competencies, establish professional development opportunities, and develop a competency-based performance evaluation. This is a promising model to conceptualize the APRN role. However, research is needed to assess the ability of the model to evaluate the impact and outcomes of pediatric APRN practice.

Model of Exemplary Midwifery Practice

In 2000, Kennedy introduced a model of exemplary midwifery practice to identify essential characteristics, specific outcomes, processes of care provided, and their relationship to specific health outcomes of women and/or infants (Fig. 2.9). The development of the model was informed by critical and feminist theories and a Delphi study using input from recipients of midwifery care and exemplary midwives, not all of whom were master's or doctorally prepared APRNs.

The model is schematically presented as three concentric spheres. The inner sphere describes three dimensions of exemplary midwifery practice: therapeutics, caring, and the profession. Therapeutics illustrates how and why midwives choose and use specific therapies. Caring depicts how the midwife demonstrates care for and about the client, and the dimension of the profession examines how exemplary practice might be enhanced and accepted. The middle sphere of the model depicts five processes of exemplary midwifery practice: support for the normalcy of birth, vigilance and attention to detail, creation of a setting that is respectful and reflects the woman's needs, respect for the uniqueness of the woman and family, and updates on knowledge, personal and peer review and balance of professional personal life. Lastly, the outer sphere depicts five qualities of exemplary midwifery practice: (1)

exceptional clinical skills and judgment, knowledge of self and limits, clinical objectivity, confidence, intelligence and intellectual curiosity; (2) commitment to empowering women, integrity and honesty, humility, realistic, gentle, warmth, nurturing and understanding and supportive; (3) commitment to the profession, accountability, motivation, love of the work of midwifery; (4) commitment to family-centered care, tolerance, nonjudgmental, compassion, interest in others, flexibility; and (5) belief in the normalcy of birth, commitment to the health of women and families, patience, maturity, wisdom, persistence, positive outlook, and calm.

Although laudable efforts have been made to develop a conceptual model of exemplary midwifery practice, additional work is needed. For example, conceptual and operational definitions of the multiple concepts and the relationships among and between them need further clarification. In addition, because not all CNM participants in this study were educated and trained as APRNs, the model needs to be examined and tested in APRN-prepared CNMs to evaluate its utility and it ability to guide APRN CNM practice and improve outcomes for women and their families.

Conceptual Framework of ACNP Role and Perceptions of Team Effectiveness

A conceptual framework from Canada by Kilpatrick, Lavoie-Tremblay, Lamothe, Ritchie, and Doran (2013) was developed using cross-case analysis to describe key concepts that affect ACNP role enactment, boundary work, and perceptions of team effectiveness (Fig. 2.10). The development of the conceptual framework was influenced by the conceptual framework of Sidani and Irvine (1999) for evaluating the NP role in the acute care setting and the Donabedian (1966, 2005) model of quality care that incorporates structures, processes, and outcomes.

Presented as multiple concentric circles, this conceptual framework has three central process dimensions at its core: ACNP role enactment, boundary work, and perceptions of team effectiveness. There is a bidirectional relationship proposed between the central process dimensions. Key concepts are identified within each central process dimension and include medical and advanced practice nursing and role (ACNP role enactment process dimension); creating space, loss, trust, interpersonal dynamics, and time (Boundary Work process dimension); and decision making, communication, cohesion, care coordination, problem solving, and a focus on patient/family (Perceptions of Team Effectiveness process dimension). Although key concepts are

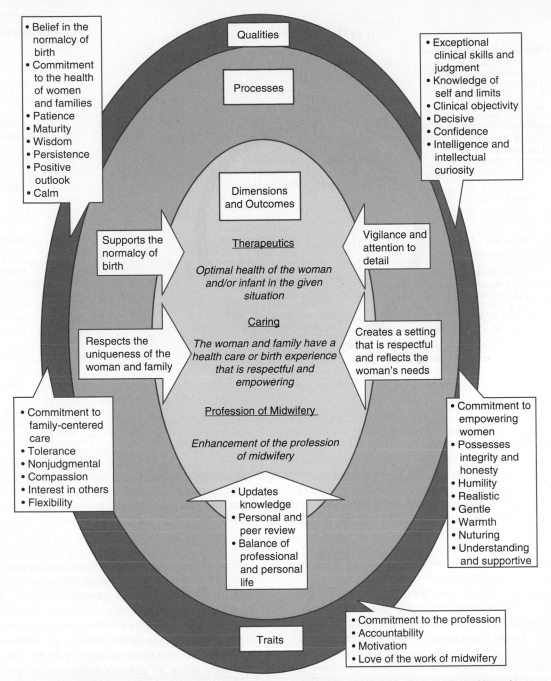

FIG 2.9 Kennedy's abstract model of the dimensions of exemplary midwifery practice. *(From Kennedy, H. P. [2000]. A model of exemplary midwifery practice: Results of a Delphi study.* Journal of Midwifery & Women's Health, *45[1], 4–19.)*

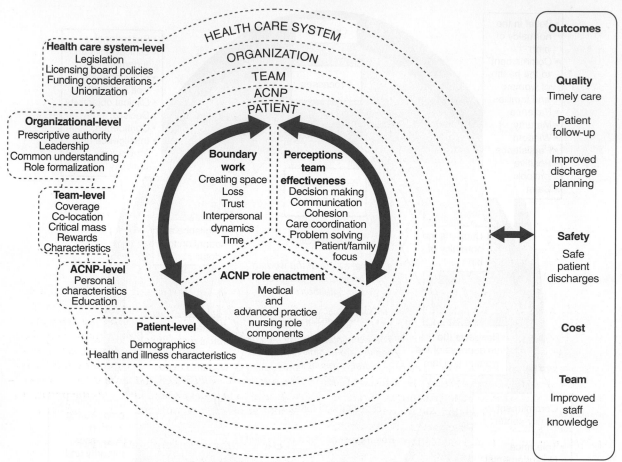

FIG 2.10 Kilpatrick et al.'s conceptual framework of ACNP role enactment, boundary work, and perceptions of team effectiveness. *(From Kilpatrick, K., Lavoie-Tremblay, M., Lamothe, L., Ritchie, J. A., & Doran, D. [2013]. Conceptual framework of acute care nurse practitioner role enactment, boundary work, and perceptions of team effectiveness.* Journal of Advanced Nursing, 69*[1], 205–217.)*

identified, the conceptual and operational definitions of these concepts are not presented.

Moving outward from the core of the conceptual framework are five concentric rings representing different layers of the structural dimensions (Patient, ACNP, Team, Organization, and Health care System) that affect the central process dimensions. The proximity of the layers is important: the closer the structural layer is to the core, the more the direct effect is on the central process dimensions. Dotted lines between the process and structural dimension represent the bidirectional relationship between the dimensions. Outcomes indicators include quality (timely care, patient follow-up, improved discharge planning); safety (safe patient discharges); cost; and team improved staff knowledge.

Given the recent emphasis on teamwork and the enactment of highly functioning interprofessional teams to achieve improved patient outcomes, this framework is timely and novel because it focuses on the impact of ACNPs on teamwork. Future work should focus on the measurement of outcomes specific to and reflective of APRN care in light of the current scope of practice legislation, organizational support for the role, and patient and family perceptions of team effectiveness.

Model for Maximizing NP Contributions to Primary Care

Poghosyan, Boyd, and Clarke (2016) have proposed a conceptual model to optimize full scope of practice for NPs in primary care (Fig. 2.11). After completing

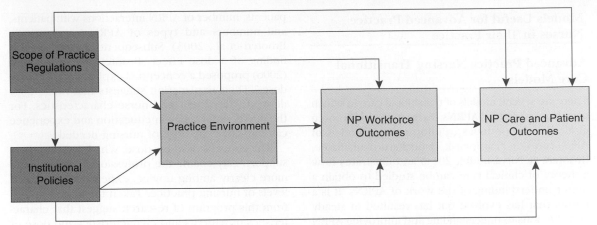

FIG 2.11 Poghasyan, Boyd, and Clark's proposed model for maximizing contributions to primary care. *(From Poghosyan, L., Boyd, D. R., & Clarke, S. P. [2016]. Optimizing full scope of practice for nurse practitioners in primary care: A proposed conceptual model. Nursing Outlook, 64[2], 146–155.)*

a thorough review of the literature, the authors developed a comprehensive model describing potential factors that affect NP care and patient outcomes. Three factors were identified: scope of practice regulations, institutional policies, and practice environments. Scope of practice regulations is defined as regulations across the United States that vary from state to state (despite competency-based educational preparation and national certification examinations) that create barriers to NPs' abilities to practice to their full education and training, thereby creating barriers to optimal NP practice (e.g., hospital admitting privileges, recognition of primary care provider status, prescribing autonomy). Institutional policies are described as idiosyncratic differences between organizations even within the same state or jurisdiction that negatively impact an NP's ability to deliver patient care. These include restriction in NP practice beyond state legislation or regulation. Practice environments that support NP practice are defined as those that promote high-quality patient care and maximize the effectiveness and utility of primary care NPs. Positive practice environments promote favorable relationships between NPs and physicians and NPs and administration that support independent NP practice. Additionally, effective communication, similar vision and prioritization of care and teamwork support a favorable practice environment for primary care NPs. Lastly, negative issues that affect NP workforce outcomes include high workloads, complex patients, rapidly changing administrations, and organization structures. These negative issues can lead to job stress, job dissatisfaction, burnout, and turnover.

The authors are commended on their work to develop a conceptual model to optimize full scope of practice for primary care NPs. As the authors noted, additional research is needed to fully understand the impact of restricted scope of practice and institutional policies on NP care and patient outcomes. Although the relationships between and among the variables will need to be tested, the model holds the potential to inform policy, practice, and patient outcomes.

Section Summary: Implications for Advanced Practice Nursing Conceptualizations

When one considers conceptualizations of advanced practice nursing described by professional organizations and individual authors, similarities and differences emerge. Many conceptual models address competencies that APRNs must possess. All are in agreement that the direct care of patients is central to APRN practice. Most models affirm two or more competencies identified by Hamric, and some models emphasize some competencies more than others. Some models (e.g., the Calkin and Strong models) address the issue of skill mix as it relates to APRNs, an issue of concern to administrators who hire APRNs. A notable difference across models is the extent to which the concept of environment as it relates to APRN practice is addressed. Another noted difference in the models is that only the Hamric model addresses all four APRN roles (CNS, CRNA, CNM and NP). In the next section, selected models that APRNs may find useful as they develop and evaluate their own practices are described.

Models Useful for Advanced Practice Nurses in Their Practice

Advanced Practice Nursing Transitional Care Models

There are several models of transitional care in which care is provided by APRNs. Early work by Brooten et al. (1988) continues to inform these models of APRN care (e.g., Partiprajak, Hanucharurnkul, Piaseu, Brooten, & Nityasuddhi, 2011) and illustrates how a theory of clinical care can be studied to obtain a better understanding of the work of APRNs. It is a model that has evolved but has resulted in steady contributions to understanding and improving APRN practice. This theoretical and empirical steadfastness has had a significant influence on the new policies evolving as the United States undergoes health care reform.

Using a conceptual model proposed by Doessel and Marshall (1985), Brooten et al. integrated this framework into their evaluation of outcomes of APRN transitional care with different clinical populations. APRN transitional care was defined as "comprehensive discharge planning designed for each patient group plus APN home follow-up through a period of normally expected recovery or stabilization" (Brooten et al., 2002, p. 370). Brooten's model was intended to address outlier patient populations (e.g., those whose care, for clinical reasons, was likely to cost more). Across all studies, care was provided by NPs and/or CNSs whose clinical expertise was matched to the needs of the patient population. In these studies, APRN care was associated with improved patient outcomes and reduced costs.

Research by Brooten, Naylor, and others (Bradway et al., 2012) who have studied transitional care by APRNs has provided empirical support for several elements important to a conceptualization of advanced practice nursing. In a summary of the studies conducted, the investigators identified several factors that contribute to the effectiveness of APRNs: content expertise, interpersonal skills, knowledge of systems, ability to implement change, and ability to access resources (Brooten, Youngblut, Deatrick, Naylor, & York, 2003). This finding provides empirical support for the importance of the APRN competencies of direct care, collaboration, coaching, and systems leadership.

Two other important findings were the existence of patterns of morbidity within patient populations and an apparent dose effect (i.e., outcomes seemed to be related to how much time was spent with patients, number of APRN interactions with patients, and numbers and types of APRN interventions; Brooten et al., 2003). Subsequently, based on this finding of a dose effect, Brooten and Youngblut (2006) proposed a conceptual explanation of "nurse dose." Their explanation suggests that nurse dose depends on patient and nurse characteristics. For the nurse, differences in education and experience can influence the dose of nursing needed.

The concept of nurse dose, which has empirical support, may enable the profession to differentiate more clearly among novice, expert, and advanced levels of nursing practice. Taken together, findings from this program of research suggest that characteristics of patients and characteristics and dose of APRN interventions are important to the conceptualization of advanced practice nursing. Finally, the fact that this program of research has used NPs and CNSs to intervene with patients provides support for a broad conceptual model of APRN practice that encompasses APRN characteristics, competencies, patient factors, environment, and other concepts that can inform role-specific models.

Although there have been other studies of APRNs providing transitional care, Brooten's work is highlighted because of the additional analyses that were done and the ultimate influence on health policy of this program of research (e.g., Naylor, Aiken, Kurtzman, Olds, & Hirschman, 2011). The findings help to understand the APRN characteristics and interventions that contributed to the success of the interventions and a model of care that evolved from the skilled care provided by APRNs.

The impact of the research conducted by Naylor, Bowles, et al. (2011) using the Translational Care Model, in which APRNs are the primary coordinators of care, provide home visits, and collaborate with the patient, family caregivers, and health care colleagues (physicians, nurses, social workers, and other health team members), is evident in many of the provisions of the ACA and its implementation (Naylor, 2012). The Community-Based Care Transitions Program was created by Section 3026 of the ACA and is being implemented by the Centers for Medicare & Medicaid Services Partnership for Patients (2017).

Dunphy and Winland-Brown's Circle of Caring: A Transformative, Collaborative Model

A central premise of Dunphy and Winland-Brown's model (1998) is that the health care needs of individuals, families, and communities are not being met in a health care system dominated by medicine in which medical language (i.e., the International Classification of Diseases, 10th Revision, Clinical Modification [ICD-10-CM] codes) is the basis for reimbursement. They proposed the Circle of Caring to foster a more active and visible nursing presence in the health care system and to explain and promote medical-nursing collaboration. Dunphy and Winland-Brown's transformative model (Dunphy, Winland-Brown, Porter, Thomas, & Gallagher, 2011; Fig. 2.12) is a synthesized problem-solving approach to advanced practice nursing that builds on nursing and medical models (Dunphy & Winland-Brown, 1998).

The authors argued that a model such as theirs is needed because nursing and medicine have two different traditions, with the medical model being viewed as reductionistic and the nursing model being regarded as humanistic. Neither model, by itself, provided a structure that allowed APRNs to be recognized for their daily practice and the positive patient health outcomes that can be attributed to APRN care. The model's authors viewed the development of nursing diagnoses as an attempt to differentiate nursing care from medical care, but because few nursing diagnoses are recognized by current reimbursement systems, the nursing in APRN care was rendered invisible.

The Circle of Caring model was proposed to incorporate the strengths of medicine and nursing in a transforming way. The conceptual elements are the processes of assessment, planning, intervention, and evaluation, with a feedback loop. Integrating a

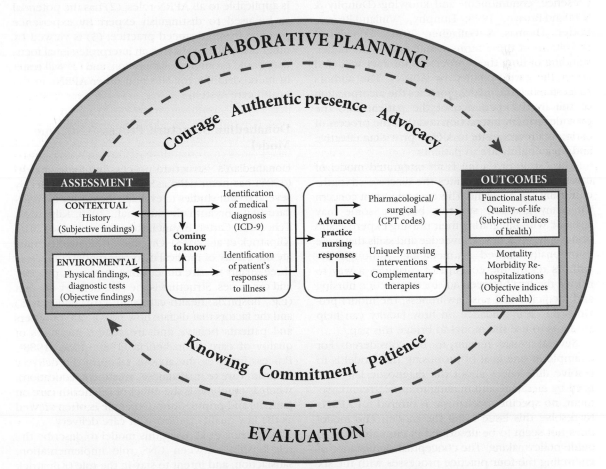

FIG 2.12 Dunphy and Winland-Brown's Circle of Caring model. *NP*, nurse practitioner. *(From Dunphy, L. M., Winland-Brown, J. E., Porter, B. O., Thomas, D. J., & Gallagher, L. M. [2011]. Primary care in the twenty-first century: A circle of caring. In L. M. Dunphy, J. E. Winland-Brown, B. O. Porter, & D. J. Thomas [Eds.]. Primary care: The art and science of advanced practice nursing [3rd ed., pp. 3–18]. Philadelphia: FA Davis.)*

nursing model with a traditional medical model permits the following to occur:

- The assessment and evaluation are contextualized, incorporating subjective and environmental elements into traditional history taking and physical examination.
- The approach to therapeutics is broadened to include holistic approaches to healing and makes nursing care more visible.
- Measured outcomes include patients' perceptions of health and care, not just physiologic outcomes and resource use.

The assessment-planning-intervention-evaluation processes in linear configuration are encircled by caring. Caring is actualized through interpersonal interactions with patients and caregivers to which NPs bring patience, courage, advocacy, authentic presence, commitment, and knowing (Dunphy & Winland-Brown, 1998; Dunphy, Winland-Brown, Porter, Thomas, & Gallagher, 2011). Conceptual definitions of these terms would add to the understanding of how these processes interact with and affect the care provided by APRNs. The authors suggested that the model promotes the incorporation of the lived experience of the patient into the provider-patient interaction and that the process of caring is a prerequisite to APRNs providing effective and meaningful care to patients.

The Circle of Caring is an integrated model of caregiving that incorporates the discrete strengths of nursing and medicine. This is an important concern for many graduate students because some may struggle with integrating their nursing expertise and philosophy with new knowledge and skills that were traditionally viewed as medicine. Although the authors regard the concept of caring as a way to bridge the gap between advanced practice nursing and medicine and raise awareness, the model provides no clear guidance on how faculty can help students to use the model to bridge this gap.

Several issues remain to be considered. For example, if one goal of proposing the model is to resolve differences about the diagnostic language used by medicine and nursing to obtain reimbursement, no specific mechanism is offered for APRNs to resolve this issue using the model. The model does not seem to be described in enough detail to guide policymaking. The conceptual significance of encircling the four practice processes with the six caring processes is unclear, although the primary care textbook by Dunphy, Winland-Brown, Porter, and Thomas (2011) devotes a chapter to caring in the NP role (Boykin & Schoenhofer, 2011). Given

today's health policy context, the value of this model, with its emphasis on the APRN-patient relationship and caring processes, could inform practice evaluation and research on APRN practices. For example, the Circle of Caring model has been used for the development of an online risk assessment of mental health (McKnight, 2011), evaluation of medication adherence (Palardy & March, 2011), and neonatal transport (Thomas, 2011). In addition, the primary care textbook (Dunphy, Winland-Brown, Porter, & Thomas, 2011) is informed by their Circle of Caring model.

Given the emphasis on interprofessional education and efforts to distinguish advanced practice nursing from medical practice, empirical testing of this model is warranted. This testing would help determine whether the model has the following features: (1) is applicable to all APRN roles; (2) has the potential to be used to distinguish expert by experience practice from advanced practice; (3) is viewed by other disciplines as having an interprofessional focus that would promote collaboration; and (4) will result in more visibility for NPs and other APRNs in the health care system.

Donabedian Structure/Process/Outcome Model

Donabedian's structure/process/outcome model (2005) has been used as the conceptual model by several recent studies to evaluate the quality of APRN care (e.g., Bryant-Lukosius et al., 2016; Kilpatrick, Tchouaket, Carter, Bryant-Lukosius, & DiCenso, 2016; Kilpatrick et al., 2013). Originally designed to evaluate the quality of medical care, this model compasses three quality-of-care dimensions: structure, process, and outcomes. Structure is the care delivery context (e.g., hospitals, health care staff, cost, equipment) and the factors that dictate how health care providers and patients behave and are system measures of quality of care (Donabedian, 1980, 1986, 1988). Process involves the actions taken in the delivery of health care (e.g., diagnosis, treatment, education), whereas outcome is the effect of the health care on patients and populations. Outcome is often viewed as the key quality indicator of care delivery.

Kilpatrick et al. used this model to describe the relationship between CNS role implementation, satisfaction, and intent to stay in the role (Kilpatrick et al., 2016) and to evaluate team effectiveness when an ACNP is added to the health care team (Kilpatrick et al., 2013). The model provided the framework to examine outcomes and barriers to CNS practice in Canada and the frequency with which components of the CNS role (clinical, education, research, leadership, scholarly and professional development, and consultation) were enacted. Findings indicate that CNS role components of clinical and research, along with balanced scholarly and professional development and consultation activities, were associated with role satisfaction. Additional research is needed to determine if implementation of the CNS role influences intention to remain in or actual departure from the role.

Guided by the Donabedian model, Bryant-Lukosius et al. (2016) developed an evaluation framework to inform decisions about the effective utilization of APRNs in Switzerland (Fig. 2.13). An international group of stakeholders (e.g., APRNs, APRN educators, administrators, researchers) from Canada, Germany, Switzerland, and the United States convened to develop and refine the framework. The developed framework is deliberately broad and flexible to respond to the evolving APRN roles in Switzerland. Key concepts of the model are introduction stage, implementation, and long-term sustainability. The introduction stage includes the type of APRN and corresponding competencies. The implementation stage focuses on the resources (policies, education, funding) to support the different APRN roles and promote the optimal utilization and implementation of the role. Long-term sustainability focuses on long-term benefits and impact of APRN roles (consumers, system, providers) in Switzerland. Because the role of the APRN is in its early stage, the authors have indicated their plan to engage in concerted efforts with policymakers and other stakeholders to actively involve them in its use and application. Several resources have been developed to actualize this (e.g., toolkit, evaluation plan template).

Recommendations and Future Directions

Given the variety of conceptualizations and inconsistency in terminology, it is not surprising that APRN students and practicing APRNs would find the conceptualization of advanced practice nursing confusing. The challenge for APRNs (students and practicing nurses) is to find a model that works for them, that enables them to understand and evaluate their practices and attend to the profession's efforts to create a coherent, stable, and robust conceptualization of advanced practice nursing.

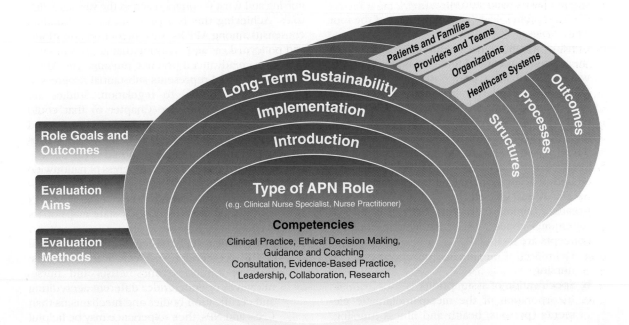

FIG 2.13 Bryant-Lukosius education framework matrix—key concepts for evaluating advanced practice nursing roles. *(From Bryant-Lukosius, D., Spichiger, E., Martin, J., Stoll, H., Kellerhals, S. D., Fliedner, M., et al. [2016]. Framework for evaluating the impact of advanced practice nursing roles.* Journal of Nursing Scholarship, 48*[2], 201–209.)*

Conceptualizations of Advanced Practice Nursing

This overview of extant models of advanced practice nursing is necessarily cursory, primarily focused on western literature (Canada, Europe, United States). Although there is some agreement on selected elements of advanced practice, differences remain regarding the conceptualization of the ARPN. To promote a unified conceptualization of advanced practice nursing, the following recommendations are put forth:

1. Conduct a rigorous content analysis of the statements published by national and international professional organizations that describe the advanced practice nursing of recognized APRNs (CNMs, CNSs, CRNAs, certified NPs). This would be a natural evolution of the work done by the APRN Consensus Work Group, the NCSBN APRN Advisory Committee, the CNA, and others to inform future work. As part of this analysis, an assessment of the extent to which nursing's metaparadigmatic concepts are integrated into statements about the nature of advanced practice nursing should be undertaken.

2. Conduct a content analysis of statements that address advanced practice nursing promulgated by specialty organizations.

3. Review recent role delineation studies of the four APRN roles.

4. Conduct a comprehensive integrative review of the advanced practice literature, building on the work of Mantzoukas and Watkinson (2007) and Lewandowski and Adamle (2009). This could be modeled on the work of Reeves et al. (2011) and their conceptualization of interprofessional education, identifying concepts and relationships that need further development.

5. Synthesize results to collaboratively propose a definition of advanced practice nursing to be used nationally and globally.

6. Create a common structure for organizational statements about APRNs that ensures nursing concepts are included:
   a. Definition of nursing and advanced practice nursing
   b. Specification of assumptions
   c. Incorporation of the metaparadigmatic elements (persons, health and illness, nursing, environment) into scopes and introductions to key documents
   d. Referencing documents such as the ANA's social policy statement and the ICN's statements on nursing

7. Implement a structure for developing statements that define advanced practice nursing to explicate the foundational and philosophical underpinnings of each organization's approach to defining advanced practice nursing.

8. Use the results from recommendations 1 through 5 above to inform revisions of the DNP Essentials (AACN, 2006), standards, and other documents that address APRN LACE issues for APRN roles. Future revision of documents regarding APRNs should be informed by a clear conceptualization of advanced practice nursing and empirical evidence.

9. Because the terms *advanced practice nursing* and *advanced nursing practice* are being used to refer to APRN work in different ways in the United States versus internationally, revisit the work on definitions of these terms done by Styles (1998) and Styles and Lewis (2000) and clarify these definitions as they relate to APRNs.

Consensus Building Around Advanced Practice Nursing

A priority for the profession is a collaboratively developed conceptualization of advanced practice nursing and what is common across the various APRN roles. Achieving this is a prerequisite for building consensus among APRNs, stakeholder organizations, and policymakers and ensuring that all patients will benefit from advanced practice nursing. The APRN Consensus Model represents substantial progress in this area with regard to regulation. Studies are underway worldwide (see Chapter 6) that could inform efforts to refine conceptualizations of advanced nursing practice. Ongoing development of consensus on advanced practice nursing should involve:

- Periodic updates on the progress of nationwide implementation of the regulatory model—successes and challenges (note that the NCSBN periodically updates state-by-state maps on its website).

- Communication between national and global APRN accrediting and certification bodies. Because US nurse anesthetists and nurse-midwives operate under different accrediting and certification bodies and mechanisms than CNSs and NPs, their experience may be helpful in countries in which nurses and midwives are regulated separately, or where nurse anesthesia is not a practice role.

- Consensus of common terms used in documents describing APRN practice.

It is evident from this review that there is still a need for common language to describe advanced practice nursing. Clear articulation and consensus of the conceptual differences among terms such as *essentials, competencies, hallmarks,* and *standard of care* is needed among the various users within the profession and among other stakeholders. The responses of the AANA, ACNM, NACNS, and NONPF to the DNP initiative and concerns about selective implementation of the APRN Consensus Model are likely to influence the evolution of advanced practice nursing in the next decade. The extent to which we reach agreement within the profession will affect policy related to advanced practice and whether the public recognizes and requests the services of APRNs. Disagreement on the nature and credentialing of advanced practice nursing should be resolved by continued efforts to foster true consensus by:

- Addressing the legitimate concerns of these organizations (e.g., impact on access to care, concerns about certification or grandfathering existing APRNs)
- Establishing priorities for negotiation and resolution by stakeholder groups and initiating a process to find common ground and address disagreements
- In the face of disagreements, working toward agreement on a common identity to facilitate public understanding of APRN roles

These consensus-building efforts are needed if our profession is to remain attractive to new nurses and new APRNs and to make room for evolving APRN roles.

Consensus on Key Elements of Practice Doctorate Curricula

Several authors have expressed concern that, because the DNP is a practice degree and not a research degree, it may not be demanding enough with regard to theory and research methods, which may be just as important for evaluating practice and testing practice models as they are in nursing Ph.D. programs. Although the ACNM does not currently support the practice doctorate for entry into practice and the AANA has delayed endorsing doctoral preparation for entry into practice until 2025 and the NACNS until 2030, APRN organizations have prepared doctoral-level competencies that are consistent with those proposed in the DNP. One question that will need to be addressed is whether regulations will specify which type of nursing practice doctorate will be needed when, and if, a

doctorate becomes the entry-level credential for all APRNs because, as Dreher (2011) has noted, there are other practice doctorates in nursing.

Research on Advanced Practice Nurses and Their Contribution to Patients, Teams, and System Outcomes

Theory-based research on APRNs' contributions to improved patient outcomes and cost-effectiveness is needed to inform and validate the conceptualizations of advanced practice nursing. Increased knowledge about advanced practice nursing is critical (see Chapter 23). The worth of any service depends on the extent to which practice meets the needs and priorities of health care systems, the public policy arena, and society in general. In addition to research that links advanced practice nursing with outcomes, the following recommendations are put forth:

1. Promising conceptual models of advanced practice nursing should be refined based on research that validates key concepts and tests theoretical propositions associated with these models.
2. Studies are needed to examine advanced practice nursing across APRN roles and between physician and APRN practices with regard to processes and outcomes. Studies conducted across APRN roles can determine whether the assumption that a core set of competencies is used by all APRNs is valid, and the activities that differentiate one APRN role from another. The studies of APRN and physician practice can identify the factors that distinguish APRN practice from physician practice as a basis for understanding differences in outcomes and developing proposals to optimally use each provider to achieve high-quality, patient-centered, cost-effective care.
3. As conceptualizations of interprofessional teams evolve, the roles and contributions of APRNs and their interdisciplinary colleagues to outcomes need examination.

When there is a better empirical understanding of the similarities and differences across APRN roles and between physicians and APRNs, this knowledge must be packaged and presented to colleagues in other disciplines, policymakers, and the public. These data will be key to educating physician colleagues, health care consumers, and policymakers about the meaning and relevance of advanced practice nursing to the health of our society.

Conclusion

Consensus regarding a conceptual model of advanced practice nursing is needed to guide practice, research, and public policy. The future of advanced practice nursing depends on the extent to which practice meets the needs and priorities of society, health care systems, and the public policy arena. A stable, robust model of advanced practice nursing will serve to guide the development of advanced practice nursing and ensure that patients will have access to APRN care.

Issues, limitations, and imperatives related to conceptualizing advanced practice nursing have been identified in this review of conceptual models of APRN practice. The nursing profession, nationally and internationally, remains at a critical juncture with regard to advanced practice nursing. In each country in which APRNs practice, the need to move forward with a unified voice on this issue is urgent if APRNs and the nursing profession as a whole are to fulfill their social contract with the individuals, institutions, and communities. A unified conceptualization of advanced practice nursing focuses the efforts of the profession on preparing APRNs, promulgating policies, and fostering research to enable the realization of the outcomes, including maximizing the social contribution of APRNs to the health needs of society and promoting the actualization of APRNs.

Key Summary Points

- Conceptualizations of advanced practice nursing include models and theories that guide the practice of APRNs.
- Conceptual models can and do differentiate practice among and between levels of nursing practice and between APRNs and other health care providers.
- National and international efforts are underway to develop a unified consensus on the conceptualization of advanced practice nursing.
- Conceptual consensus is needed to clarify concepts and models that help stakeholders understand the nature of APRNs' work and their contributions to patient and system outcomes.

References

To access the references for this chapter, use your smartphone's QR code reader to scan the code below, or go to http://booksite.elsevier.com/ 9780323447751.

A Definition of Advanced Practice Nursing

Ann B. Hamric • Mary Fran Tracy

"Nothing is more powerful than an idea whose time has come"
—*Victor Hugo*

CHAPTER CONTENTS

This chapter considers two central questions that provide the foundation for this text:

- Why is it important to define carefully and clearly what is meant by the term *advanced practice nursing?*
- What distinguishes the practices of advanced practice registered nurses (APRNs) from those of other nurses and other health care providers?

Advanced practice nursing is considered here as a concept, not a role, a set of skills, or a substitution for physicians. Rather, it is a powerful idea, the origins of which date back more than a century. Such a conceptual definition provides a stable core understanding for all APRN roles (see Chapter 2), it promotes consistency in practice that can aid others in understanding what this level of nursing entails, and it promotes the achievement of value-added patient outcomes and improvement in health care delivery processes. Advanced practice nursing is a relatively new concept in nursing's evolution (see Chapter 1). Although debates and dissension are

necessary and even healthy in forging consensus, ultimately the profession must agree on the key issues of definition, education, credentialing, and practice. Such agreement is critically important to the survival, much less the growth, of advanced practice nursing. In the international context, although these issues may be defined differently by different countries, in-country standardization is likewise essential. In this chapter, advanced practice nursing is defined and the scope of practice of APRNs is discussed. Various APRN roles are differentiated and key factors influencing advanced practice in health care environments are identified. The importance of a common and unified understanding of the distinguishing characteristics of advanced practice nursing is emphasized.

The advanced practice of nursing builds on the foundation and core values of the nursing discipline. APRN roles do not stand apart from nursing; they do not represent a separate profession, although references to "the nurse practitioner (NP) profession," for example, are seen in the literature. It is the nursing core that contributes to the distinctiveness seen in APRN practices as compared to non-nursing providers such as physician assistants. According to the American Nurses Association (ANA, 2010), nursing practice has seven essential features:

> ... provision of a caring relationship that facilitates health and healing; attention to the range of human experiences and responses to health and illness within the physical and social environments; integration of assessment data with knowledge gained from an appreciation of the patient or the group; application of scientific knowledge to the processes of diagnosis and treatment through the use of judgment and critical thinking; advancement of professional nursing knowledge through scholarly inquiry; influence on social and public policy to promote social justice; and, assurance of safe, quality, and evidence-based practice. (p. 9)

These characteristics are equally essential for advanced practice nursing. Core values that guide nurses in practice include advocating for patients; respecting patient and family values and informed choices; viewing individuals holistically within their environments, communities, and cultural traditions; and maintaining a focus on disease prevention, health restoration, and health promotion (ANA, 2015a; Friberg & Creasia, 2011; Hood, 2014). These core professional values also inform the central perspective of advanced practice nursing.

Efforts to standardize the definition of advanced practice nursing have been ongoing since the 1990s (American Association of Colleges of Nursing [AACN], 1995, 2006; ANA, 1995, 2003, 2010; Hamric, 1996, 2000, 2005, 2009, 2014; National Council of State Boards of Nursing [NCSBN], 1993, 2002, 2008). However, full clarity regarding advanced practice nursing has not yet been achieved, even as this level of nursing practice spreads around the globe. The growing international use of APRNs with differing understandings in various countries has only complicated the picture (see Chapter 6). Different interpretations of advanced practice (AACN, 2006; ANA, 2013), debates about who is and is not an APRN, and discrepancies in educational preparation for APRNs remain issues for the international community, even as efforts are underway by the International Council of Nurses to develop a standardized definition of advanced practice nursing (A. Scanlon, personal communication, December 2016).

In spite of this lack of clarity (Dowling, Beauchesne, Farrelly, & Murphy, 2013; Pearson, 2011; Ruel & Motyka, 2009), emerging consensus on key features of the concept is increasingly evident. The definition developed by Hamric has been relatively stable throughout the six editions of this book. The primary criteria used in this definition are now standard elements used in the United States and, increasingly, elsewhere to regulate APRNs. Similarly, consensus is growing in understanding advanced practice nursing in terms of core competencies. Even authors who deny a clear understanding of the concept propose competencies—variously called attributes, components, or domains—that are generally consistent with, although not always as complete as, the competencies proposed here.

It is important to distinguish the conceptual definition of advanced practice nursing from regulatory requirements for any APRN role (NCSBN, 2008). Of necessity, regulatory understandings focus on the more basic and measurable primary criteria of graduate educational preparation, advanced certification in a particular population focus, and practice in one of the four common APRN roles: nurse practitioner (NP), clinical nurse specialist (CNS), certified registered nurse anesthetist (CRNA), and certified nurse-midwife (CNM). This approach is clearly seen in the APRN definition outlined in the *Consensus Model for APRN Regulation* (APRN Joint Dialogue Group, 2008) and has been very helpful and influential in standardizing state requirements for APRN licensure across the United States. Although necessary for regulation, however, this approach does not constitute an adequate understanding of advanced practice nursing. Limiting the profession's understanding of advanced practice nursing to regulatory definitions can lead to a reductionist approach that results in a focus on a set of concrete skills and activities, such as diagnostic acumen or prescriptive authority. Understanding the advanced practice of the nursing discipline requires a definition that encompasses broad areas of skilled performance (the competency approach). As Chapter 2 notes, conceptual models and definitions are also useful for providing a robust framework for graduate APRN curricula and for building an APRN professional role identity.

Distinguishing Between Specialization and Advanced Practice Nursing

Before the definition of advanced practice nursing can be explored, it is important to distinguish between specialization in nursing and advanced practice nursing. Specialization involves the development of expanded knowledge and skills in a selected area within the discipline of nursing. All nurses with extensive experience in a particular area of practice (e.g., pediatric nursing, trauma nursing) are specialized in this sense. As the profession has advanced and responded to changes in health care, specialization and the need for specialty knowledge have increased. Thus few nurses are generalists in the true sense of the word (Kitzman, 1989). Although family NPs traditionally represented themselves as generalists, they are specialists in the sense discussed here because they have specialized in one of the many facets of health care—namely, primary care. As noted in Chapter 1, early specialization involved primarily on-the-job training or hospital-based training courses, and many nurses continue to develop specialty skills through practice experience and continuing education. Examples of currently evolving specialties include genetics nursing, forensic nursing, and clinical transplant coordination. As specialties mature, they may develop graduate-level clinical preparation and incorporate the competencies of advanced practice nursing for their most advanced practitioners (Hanson & Hamric, 2003; also see Chapter 5); examples include critical care, oncology nursing, and palliative care nursing.

The nursing profession has responded in various ways to the increasing need for specialization in nursing practice. The creation of specialty organizations, such as the American Association of Critical-Care Nurses and the Oncology Nursing Society, has been one response. The creation of APRN roles—the CRNA and CNM roles early in nursing's evolution and the CNS and NP roles more recently—has been another response. A third response has been the development of specialized faculty, nursing researchers, and nursing administrators. Nurses in all these roles can be considered specialists in an area of nursing (e.g., education, research, administration); some of these roles may involve advanced education in a clinical specialty as well. However, they are not necessarily advanced practice nursing roles.

Advanced practice nursing includes specialization but also involves expansion and educational advancement (ANA, 1995, 2003, 2015b; Cronenwett, 1995). As compared with basic nursing practice, APRN practice is further characterized by the following: (1) acquisition of new practice knowledge and skills, particularly theoretical and evidence-based knowledge, some of which overlaps the traditional boundaries of medicine; (2) significant role autonomy; (3) responsibility for health promotion in addition to the diagnosis and management of patient problems, including prescribing pharmacologic and nonpharmacologic interventions; (4) the greater complexity of clinical decision making and leadership in organizations and environments; and (5) specialization at the level of a particular APRN role and population focus (ANA, 1996, 2015b; NCSBN, 2008).

It is necessary to distinguish between specialization as understood in this chapter and the term *population focus*. The framers of the Consensus Model for APRN regulation were interested in licensing and regulating advanced practice nursing in two broad categories. The first was regulation at the level of role—CNS, NP, CRNA, or CNM. The second category was termed *population focus* and, although not explicitly defined, six population foci were identified: family and individual across the life span, adult-gerontology, pediatrics, neonatal, women's health and gender-related, and psychologic and mental health. These foci are at different levels of specialization; for example, family and individual across the life span is broad, whereas neonatal is a subspecialty designation under the specialty of pediatrics. Therefore population focus is not synonymous with specialization and should not be understood in the same light. As the Consensus Model states:

> Education, certification, and licensure of an individual must be congruent in terms of role and population foci. APRNs may specialize but they cannot be licensed solely within a specialty area. *In addition, specialties can provide depth in one's practice within the established population foci.* … Competence at the specialty level will not be assessed or regulated by boards of nursing but rather by the professional organizations. (APRN Joint Dialogue Group, 2008, p. 6)

Distinguishing Between Advanced Nursing Practice and Advanced Practice Nursing

The terms *advanced practice nursing* and *advanced nursing practice* have distinct definitions and cannot be seen as interchangeable. In particular, recent definitions of advanced nursing practice do not clarify the clinically focused nature of advanced practice nursing. For example, the third edition of *Nursing's Social Policy Statement* defines the term *advanced nursing practice* as "characterized by the integration and application of a broad range of theoretical and evidence-based knowledge that occurs as part of graduate nursing education" (ANA, 2010, p. 9). This broad definition has evolved from the AACN's *Position Statement on the Practice Doctorate in Nursing*

(AACN, 2004), which recommended doctoral-level educational preparation for individuals at the most advanced level of nursing practice. The Doctor of Nursing Practice (DNP) position statement (AACN, 2004) advanced a broad definition of advanced nursing practice as the following:

> … any form of nursing intervention that influences health care outcomes for individuals or populations, including the direct care of individual patients, management of care for individuals and populations, administration of nursing and health care organizations, and the development and implementation of health policy (p. 3).

A definition this broad goes beyond advanced practice nursing to include other advanced specialties not involved in providing direct clinical care to patients, such as administration, policy, informatics, and public health. One reason for such a broad definition was the desire to have the DNP degree be available to nurses practicing at the highest level in many varied specialties, not only those in APRN roles. A decision was reached by the original task force (AACN, 2004) that the DNP degree was not to be a clinical doctorate, as was advocated in early discussions (Mundinger et al., 2000) but, rather, a practice doctorate in an expansive understanding of the term *practice*. The AACN's *The Essentials of Doctoral Education for Advanced Nursing Practice* (2006) distinguishes between roles with an aggregate, systems, and organizational focus (characterized as "advanced specialties") and roles with a direct clinical practice focus (APRN roles of CNS, NP, CRNA, and CNM), while recognizing that these two groups share some essential competencies. It is important to understand that the DNP is a *degree,* much as is the Master's of Science in Nursing (MSN), and not a *role;* DNP graduates can assume varied roles, depending on the specialty focus of their program. Some of these roles are not APRN roles as advanced practice nursing is defined here.

Although the AACN has made attempts to be clear about the terms *advanced nursing practice* and *advanced practice nursing* in their statements on DNP education, this is a difficult distinction to understand. The nuances in the differences between these terms have not been clear to nurses in education and practice, professionals outside of nursing, and, at times, even DNP graduates themselves. As a result, the specific distinctions between the advanced specialties (such as administration) and APRN roles continue to require clarification. The current confusion in the United States also has global implications because the international community prefers *advanced nursing practice* when referring to direct care roles that are comparable to US APRN roles (Staser, Cashin, Buckley, & Donoghue, 2014).

Advanced practice nursing is a concept that applies to nurses who provide direct patient care to individual patients and families. As a consequence, APRN roles involve expanded clinical skills and abilities and require a different level of regulation than non-APRN roles. These skills afford APRNs unique perspectives in making broader practice decisions for individuals and populations specifically in their specialty areas. This text focuses on advanced practice nursing and the varied roles of APRNs. Graduate programs that prepare students for APRN roles will have different curricula from those preparing students for administration, informatics, or other specialties that do not have a direct practice component (AACN, 2006).

Defining Advanced Practice Nursing

As noted, the concept of advanced practice nursing continues to be defined in various ways in the nursing literature. The CINAHL Database (2016) defines advanced practice broadly as anything beyond the staff nurse role: "The performance of additional acts by registered nurses who have gained added knowledge and skills through post-basic education and clinical experience." As noted with the DNP definition, a definition this broad incorporates many specialized nursing roles, not all of which should be considered as advanced practice nursing.

Advanced practice nursing is often defined as a constellation of four roles: the NP, CNS, CNM, and CRNA (NCSBN, 2002, 2008; Stanley, 2011). For example, the third edition of *Nursing: Scope and Standards of Practice* does not provide a definition of advanced practice nursing but uses a regulatory and role-based definition of APRNs:

> A nurse who has completed an accredited graduate-level education program preparing her or him for the role of certified nurse practitioner, certified registered nurse anesthetist, certified nurse-midwife, or clinical nurse specialist; has passed a national certification examination that measures the APRN-, role-, and population-focused competencies; maintains continued competence as evidenced by recertification; and is licensed to practice as an APRN. (ANA, 2015b, p. 2–3)

In the past, some authors discussed advanced practice nursing only in terms of selected roles such as the NP and CNS roles (Lindeke, Canedy, & Kay, 1997; Rasch & Frauman, 1996) or the NP role exclusively (Hickey, Ouimette, & Venegoni, 2000; Mundinger, 1994). Defining advanced practice nursing in terms of particular roles limits the concept and denies the unfortunate reality that some nurses in the four APRN roles are not using the core competencies of advanced practice nursing in their practice. These definitions are also limiting because they do not incorporate evolving APRN roles. Thus although such role-based definitions are useful for regulatory purposes, it is preferable to define and clarify advanced practice nursing as a concept without reference to particular roles.

Core Definition of Advanced Practice Nursing

The definition proposed in this chapter builds on and extends the understanding of advanced practice nursing proposed in the first five editions of this text. Important assertions of this discussion are as follows:

- Advanced practice nursing is a function of educational and practice preparation and a constellation of primary criteria and core competencies.
- Direct clinical practice is the central competency of any APRN role and informs all the other competencies.
- All APRNs share the same core criteria and competencies, although the actual clinical skill set varies depending on the needs of the APRN's specialty patient population.

A definition should also clarify the critical point that advanced practice nursing involves advanced nursing knowledge and skills; it is not a medical practice, although APRNs perform expanded medical therapeutics in many roles. Throughout nursing's history, nurses have assumed medical roles. For example, common nursing tasks such as blood pressure measurement and administration of chemotherapeutic agents were once performed exclusively by physicians. When APRNs begin to transfer new skills or interventions into their repertoire, these become nursing skills, informed by the clinical practice values of the profession.

Actual practices differ significantly based on the particular role adopted, the specialty practiced, and the organizational framework within which the role is performed. In spite of the need to keep job descriptions and job titles distinct in practice settings, it is critical that the public's acceptance of advanced practice nursing be enhanced and confusion decreased. As Safriet (1993, 1998) noted, nursing's future depends on reaching consensus on titles and consistent preparation for title holders. The nursing profession must be clear, concrete, and consistent about APRN titles and their functions in discussions with nursing's larger constituencies: consumers, other health care professionals, health care administrators, and health care policymakers.

Conceptual Definition

Advanced practice nursing is the patient-focused application of an expanded range of competencies to improve health outcomes for patients and populations in a specialized clinical area of the larger discipline of nursing. [a]

In this definition, the term *competencies* refers to a broad area of skillful performance; seven core competencies combine to distinguish nursing practice at this level. Competencies include activities undertaken as part of delivering advanced nursing care directly to patients. Some competencies are processes that APRNs use in all dimensions of their practice, such as collaboration and leadership. At this stage of the development of the nursing discipline, competencies may be based in theory, practice, or research. Although the discipline is expanding its research-based evidence to guide practice, an expanded ability to use theory also is a key distinguishing feature of advanced practice nursing. In addition, a strong experiential component is necessary to develop the competencies and clinical practice expertise that characterize APRN practice. Graduate education and in-depth clinical practice experiences work together to develop the APRN.

The definition also emphasizes the patient-focused and specialized nature of advanced practice nursing. APRNs expand their capability to provide and direct care, with the ultimate goal of improving patient and specialty population outcomes; this focus on outcome attainment is a central feature of advanced practice nursing and the main justification for differentiating this level of practice. Finally, the critical importance of ensuring that any type of advanced practice is grounded within the larger discipline of nursing is made explicit.

Certain activities of APRN practice overlap with those performed by physicians and other health care

---

[a]The term *patient* is intended to be used interchangeably with *individual* and *client*.

professionals. However, the experiential, theoretical, and philosophical perspectives of nursing make these activities advanced nursing when they are carried out by an APRN. Advanced practice nursing further involves highly developed nursing skill in areas such as guidance and coaching, as well as the performance of select medical interventions. Particularly with regard to physician practice, the nursing profession needs to be clear that advanced practice nursing is embedded in the nursing discipline—*the advanced practice of nursing is not the junior practice of medicine.*

Advanced practice nursing is further defined by a conceptual model integrating three primary criteria and seven core competencies, one of them central to the others. This discussion and the chapters in Part II of this text isolate each of these core competencies to clarify them. The reader should recognize that this is only a heuristic device for clarifying this conceptualization of advanced practice nursing. In reality, these elements are integrated into an APRN's practice; they are not separate and distinct features. The concentric circles in Figs. 3.1 through 3.3 represent the seamless nature of this interweaving of elements. In addition, an APRN's skills function synergistically to produce a whole that is greater than the sum of its parts. The essence of advanced practice nursing is found not only in the primary criteria and competencies demonstrated, but also in the synthesis of these elements into a unified composite practice that conforms to the conceptual definition just presented.

Primary Criteria

Certain criteria (or qualifications) must be met before a nurse can be considered an APRN. Although these baseline criteria are not sufficient in and of themselves, they are necessary core elements of advanced practice nursing. The three primary criteria for advanced practice nursing are shown in Fig. 3.1 and include an earned graduate degree with a concentration in an advanced practice nursing role and population focus, national certification at an advanced level, and a practice focused on patients and their families. As noted, these criteria are most often the ones used by states to regulate APRN practice because they are objective and easily measured (see Chapter 22).

Graduate Education

First, the APRN must possess an *earned graduate degree with a concentration in an APRN role.* This graduate degree may be a master's or a DNP. Advanced

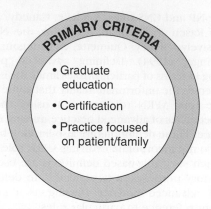

FIG 3.1 Primary criteria of advanced practice nursing.

practice students acquire specialized knowledge and skills through study and supervised practice at the graduate level. Curricular content includes theories and research findings relevant to the core of a particular advanced nursing role, population focus, and relevant specialty. For example, a CNS interested in palliative care will need coursework in CNS role competencies, the adult population focus, and the palliative care specialty. Because APRNs assess, manage, and evaluate patients at the most independent level of clinical nursing practice, all APRN curricula contain specific courses in advanced health and physical assessment, advanced pathophysiology, and advanced pharmacology (the so-called "three Ps"; AACN, 1995, 2006, 2011). Expansion of practice skills is acquired through faculty-supervised clinical experience, with master's programs requiring a minimum of 500 clinical hours and DNP programs requiring 1000 hours. As noted earlier in the ANA definition, there is consensus that a master's education in nursing is a baseline requirement for advanced practice nursing; nurse-midwifery was the latest APRN specialty to agree to this requirement (American College of Nurse-Midwives [ACNM], 2009).

Why is graduate educational preparation necessary for advanced practice nursing? Graduate education is a more efficient and standardized way to inculcate the complex competencies of APRN-level practice than nursing's traditional on-the-job or apprentice training programs (see Chapter 5). As the knowledge base within specialties has grown, so too has the need for formal education at the graduate level. In particular, the skills necessary for evidence-based practice and the theory base required for advanced practice nursing mandate education at the graduate level.

Some of the differences between basic and advanced practice in nursing are apparent in the following: the range and depth of APRNs' clinical knowledge; APRNs' ability to anticipate patient responses to health, illness, and nursing interventions; their ability to analyze clinical situations and explain why a phenomenon has occurred or why a particular intervention has been chosen; the reflective nature of their practice; their skill in assessing and addressing nonclinical variables that influence patient care; and their attention to the consequences of care and improving patient outcomes. Because of the interaction and integration of graduate education in nursing and extensive clinical experience, APRNs are able to exercise a level of discrimination in clinical judgment that is unavailable to other experienced nurses (Spross & Baggerly, 1989).

Professionally, requiring at least master's-level preparation is important to create parity among APRN roles so that all can move forward together in addressing policymaking and regulatory issues. This parity advances the profession's standards and ensures more uniform credentialing mechanisms. Moving toward a doctoral-level educational expectation may also enhance nursing's image and credibility with other disciplines. Decisions by other health care providers, such as pharmacists, physical therapists, and occupational therapists, to require doctoral preparation for entry into their professions provided compelling support for nursing to establish the practice doctorate for APRNs to achieve parity with these disciplines (AACN, 2006). Nursing has a particular need to achieve greater credibility with medicine. Organized medicine has historically been eager to point to nursing's internal differences in APRN education as evidence that APRNs are inferior providers.

The clinical nurse leader (CNL) role represents a new and different understanding of the master's credential. Historically, master's education in nursing was, by definition, specialized education (see Chapter 1). However, the master's-prepared CNL is described as an "advanced generalist", a staff nurse with expanded leadership skills at the point of care (AACN, 2007). The AACN's revision of *The Essentials of Master's Education in Nursing* (2011) was developed for this generalist practice, whereas the DNP Essentials (AACN, 2006) are aligned more with the understanding of advanced practice nursing described here. Even though CNLs have expanded leadership skills and graduate-level education, they are clearly not APRNs. APRN graduate education is highly specialized and involves preparation for an expanded scope of practice, neither of which characterizes CNL education. The existence of generalist and APRN specialty master's programs has the potential to confuse consumers, institutions, and nurses alike; it is incumbent on educational programs to clearly differentiate the curricula for generalist CNL versus specialist APRN roles to avoid role confusion for these graduates. It is likewise important that CNL graduates understand that they are not APRNs.

The AACN's proposed 2015 deadline for APRNs to be prepared at the DNP level was heavily debated (Cronenwett et al., 2011) and was not realized, even though the number of DNP programs increased dramatically (from 20 programs in 2006 to 289 in 2015 with an additional 128 new DNP programs in the planning stages (AACN, 2016). Master's-level programs that prepare APRNs are continuing at this point in time.

Certification

The second primary criterion that must be met to be considered an APRN is professional certification for practice at an advanced level within a clinical population focus. The continuing growth of specialization has dramatically increased the amount of knowledge and experience required to practice safely in modern health care settings. National certification examinations have been developed by specialty organizations at two levels. The first level that was developed tested the specialty knowledge of experienced nurses and not knowledge at the advanced level of practice. More recently, organizations have developed APRN-specific certification examinations in a specialty. CNM and CRNA organizations were farsighted in developing certifying examinations for these roles early in their history (see Chapter 1). As regulatory groups, particularly state boards of nursing, increasingly use the certification credential as a component of APRN licensure, the certification landscape continues to change. As noted, the Consensus Model has mandated regulation of APRNs at a role and population focus level (APRN Joint Dialogue Group, 2008), accelerating the development of more broad-based APRN certification examinations.

National certification at an advanced practice level is an important primary criterion for advanced practice nursing. Continuing variability in graduate curricula makes sole reliance on the criterion of graduate education insufficient to protect the public. Although standardization in educational requirements for each APRN role has improved over the last decade, it is difficult to argue that graduate education alone can provide sufficient evidence of competence for regulatory purposes. National certification examinations provide a consistent standard that must be met by each APRN to demonstrate beginning competency for an advanced level of practice in his or her role. Certification also enhances title recognition in the regulatory arena, which promotes the visibility of advanced practice nursing and enhances the public's access to APRN services.

It is critically important that certifying organizations work to clarify the certification credential as appropriate only for currently practicing APRNs. Given the centrality of the direct clinical practice component to the definition of advanced practice nursing, certification examinations must establish a significant number of hours of clinical practice as a requirement for maintaining APRN certification. Some faculty and nursing leaders who do not maintain a direct clinical practice component in their positions have been allowed to sit for certification examinations and represent themselves as APRNs. Statements such as "Once a CNS, always a CNS," which are heard with NPs and CNMs as well, perpetuate the mistaken notion that an APRN title is a professional attribute rather than a practice role. Such a misunderstanding is confusing inside and outside of nursing; by definition, these individuals are no longer APRNs.

As noted, the Consensus Model focuses regulatory efforts on these broad role and population foci rather than on particular specialties, although some specialties are represented (e.g., neonatal NPs). This decision not to recognize established APRN certification examinations in specialties such as oncology or critical care for state licensure purposes has challenged the CNS role more than other APRN specialties. The American Nurses Credentialing Center (ANCC) has become the dominant certifying organization for State Board of Nursing–supported CNS examinations. The number of examination options for CNSs has significantly decreased as the Consensus Model is being implemented; the ANCC website (www.nursecredentialing.org) maintains a listing of currently available CNS examinations. It is likely that the types of APRN certification examinations offered will evolve in the Consensus Model transition period (ANCC, 2016). Even though APRN regulation is becoming more standardized, a need exists for the continued development of specialty examinations at the advanced practice nursing level, particularly for CNS specialties; as it stands now, many CNSs have to take the broad-based certification examination recognized by their state in addition to an APRN-level specialty certification examination necessary for their practice. Another unintended consequence of the limitations set by recognizing only six population foci is that educational programs have closed CNS concentrations given the lack of a sanctioned

certification examination in the specialty. Although other factors also influenced these decisions, not recognizing specialty examinations for regulatory purposes is a key factor in these closures.

The limited population foci sanctioned at present can be seen as a first step in standardizing regulation; the Consensus Model report noted the expectation that additional population foci would evolve. Even with these transitional issues, the Consensus Model represents an important standardization of APRN regulation and has helped cement the primary criterion of certification as a core regulatory requirement for APRN licensure.

Practice Focused on Patient and Family

The third primary criterion necessary for one to be considered an APRN is a practice focused on patients and their families. As noted in describing DNP graduates, the AACN DNP Essentials Task Force differentiated APRNs from other roles using this primary criterion. They noted two general role categories (AACN, 2006): "roles which specialize as an advanced practice nurse (APN) with a focus on care of individuals; and roles that specialize in practice at an aggregate, systems, or organizational level. This distinction is important as APRNs face different licensure, regulatory, credentialing, liability, and reimbursement issues than those who practice at an aggregate, systems, or organizational level" (p. 17). This criterion does not imply that direct practice is the only activity that APRNs undertake, however. APRNs also educate others, participate in leadership activities, and serve as consultants (Bryant-Lukosius et al., 2016; Ruel & Motyka, 2009); they understand and are involved in practice contexts to identify and effect needed system changes; they also work to improve the health of their specialty populations (AACN, 2006). However, to be considered an APRN role, the patient/family direct practice focus must be primary.

Historically, APRN roles have been associated with direct clinical care. Recent work is solidifying this understanding. The Consensus Model (APRN Joint Dialogue Group, 2008) has made clear that the provision of direct care to individuals as a significant component of their practice is *the* defining factor for all APRNs. The centrality of direct clinical practice is further reflected in the core competencies presented in the next section.

Why limit the definition of advanced practice nursing to roles that focus on clinical practice to patients and families? There are many reasons. Nursing is a practice profession. The nurse-patient interface is at the core of nursing practice; in the final analysis, the reason that the profession exists is to render nursing services to individuals in need of them. Clinical practice expertise in a given specialty develops from these nurse-patient encounters and lies at the heart of advanced practice nursing. Ongoing direct clinical practice is necessary to maintain and develop an APRN's expertise. Without regular immersion in practice, the cutting edge clinical acumen and expertise found in APRN practices cannot be sustained.

If every specialized role in nursing were considered advanced practice nursing, the term would become so broad as to lack meaning and explanatory value. Distinguishing between APRN roles and other specialized roles in nursing can help clarify the concept of advanced practice nursing to consumers, other health care providers, and even other nurses. In addition, the monitoring and regulation of advanced practice nursing are increasingly important issues as APRNs work toward more authority for their practices (see Chapter 22). If the definition of advanced practice nursing included nonclinical roles, development of sound regulatory mechanisms would be impossible.

It is critical to understand that this definition of advanced practice nursing is not a value statement but, rather, a differentiation of one group of nurses from other groups for the sake of clarity within and outside the profession. Some nurses with specialized skills in administration, research, and community health have viewed the direct practice requirement as a devaluing of their contributions. Some faculty who teach clinical nursing but do not themselves maintain an advanced clinical practice have also thought themselves to be disenfranchised because they are not considered APRNs by virtue of this primary criterion. Perhaps this problem has been exacerbated with use of the term *advanced* because this term can inadvertently imply that nurses who do not fit into the APRN definition are not advanced (i.e., are not as well prepared or highly skilled as APRNs).

No value difference exists between nurses in non-APRN specialties and APRNs; both groups are equally important to the overall growth and strengthening of the profession. The profession must be able to differentiate its various roles without such differentiation being viewed as a disparagement of any one group. Thus it is critical to understand that this definition of advanced practice nursing is not a value statement but a differentiation of one group of nurses from other groups for the sake of clarity

within and outside the profession. We must be able to say what advanced practice nursing is not, as well as what it is, if we are to clarify the concept. As the ANA (1995) has noted, all nurses—whether their focus is clinical practice, educating students, conducting research, planning community programs, or leading nursing service organizations—are valuable and necessary to the integrity and growth of the larger profession. However, all nurses, particularly those with advanced degrees, are not the same, nor are they necessarily APRNs. Historically, the profession has had difficulty differentiating itself and has struggled with the prevailing lay notion that "a nurse is a nurse is a nurse." This antiquated view does not match the reality of the health care arena, nor does it celebrate the diverse contributions of all the various nursing roles and specialties.

Seven Core Competencies of Advanced Practice Nursing

Direct Clinical Practice: The Central Competency

As noted earlier, the primary criteria are necessary but insufficient elements of the definition of advanced practice nursing. Advanced practice nursing is further defined by a set of seven core competencies that are enacted in each APRN role. The first core competency of direct clinical practice is central to and informs all of the others (see Fig. 3.2). In one sense,

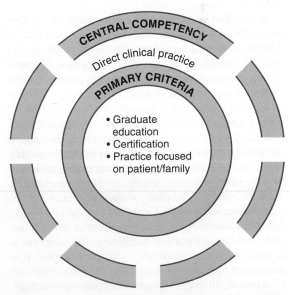

FIG 3.2 Central competency of advanced practice nursing.

it is "first among equals" of the seven core competencies that define advanced practice nursing. Although APRNs do many things, excellence in direct clinical practice provides the foundation necessary for APRNs to execute the other competencies, such as consultation, guidance and coaching, and leadership within organizations.

However, clinical expertise alone should not be equated with advanced practice nursing. The work of Patricia Benner and colleagues (Benner, 1984; Benner, Hooper-Kyriakidis, & Stannard, 1999; Benner, Tanner, & Chesla, 1996) is a major contribution to an understanding of clinically expert nursing practice. These researchers extensively studied expert nurses in acute care clinical settings and described the engaged clinical reasoning and domains of practice seen in clinically expert nurses. Although some of the participants in this research were APRNs (in the most recent report [Benner et al., 1999], 16% of the nurse participants were APRNs), most were nurses with extensive clinical experience who did not have APRN preparation. Calkin (1984) has characterized these latter nurses as "experts by experience." (See Chapter 2 for a discussion of Calkin's conceptual differentiation between levels of nursing practice.) Benner and colleagues did not discuss differences in the practices of APRNs as compared with other nurses that they have studied. They stated that " 'Expert' is not used to refer to a specific role such as an advanced practice nurse. Expertise is found in the practice of experienced clinicians and advanced practice nurses" (Benner et al., 1999, p. 9).

Although clinical expertise is a central ingredient of an APRN's practice, the direct care practice of APRNs is distinguished by six characteristics: (1) use of a holistic perspective, (2) formation of therapeutic partnerships with patients, (3) expert clinical performance, (4) use of reflective practice, (5) use of evidence as a guide to practice, and (6) use of diverse approaches to health and illness management (see Chapter 7). These characteristics help distinguish the practice of the expert by experience from that of the APRN. APRN clinical practice is also informed by a population focus (AACN, 2006) because APRNs work to improve the care for their specialty patient population, even as they care for individuals within the population. As noted, experiential knowledge and graduate education combine to develop these characteristics in an APRN's clinical practice. It is important to note that the "three Ps" that form core courses in all APRN programs (pathophysiology, pharmacology, and physical assessment) are not separate competencies in this understanding, but provide baseline knowledge and skills to support the direct clinical practice competency.

The specific content of the direct practice competency differs significantly by specialty. For example, the clinical practice of a CNS dealing with critically ill children differs from the expertise of an NP managing the health maintenance needs of older adults or a CRNA administering anesthesia in an outpatient surgical clinic. In addition, the amount of time spent in direct practice differs by APRN specialty. CNSs in particular may spend most of their time in activities other than direct clinical practice (see Chapter 14). Thus it is important to understand this competency as a central defining characteristic of advanced practice nursing rather than as a particular skill set or expectation that APRNs only engage in direct clinical practice.

Additional Advanced Practice Nurse Core Competencies

In addition to the central competency of direct clinical practice, six additional competencies further define advanced practice nursing regardless of role function or setting. As shown in Fig. 3.3, these additional core competencies are as follows:

- Guidance and coaching
- Consultation
- Evidence-based practice
- Leadership
- Collaboration
- Ethical decision making

These competencies have repeatedly been identified as essential features of advanced practice nursing. In addition, each role is differentiated by some unique competencies (see the specific role chapters in Part III of this text). The nature of the patient population receiving APRN care, organizational expectations, emphasis given to specific competencies, and practice characteristics unique to each role distinguish the practice of one APRN group from others. Each APRN role organization publishes role-specific competencies on their websites: the National Association of Clinical Nurse Specialists (NACNS) for CNSs (www.nacns.org); the National Organization of Nurse Practitioner Faculties (NONPF) for NPs (www.nonpf.org); the ACNM for CNMs (www.acnm.org); and the American Association of Nurse Anesthetists for CRNAs (www.aana.com). There is a dynamic interplay between the core APRN competencies and each role; role-specific expectations grow out of the core competencies and

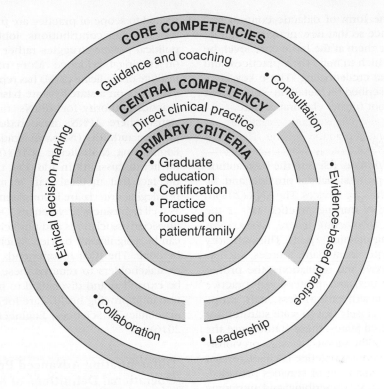

FIG 3.3 Core competencies of advanced practice nursing.

similarly serve to inform them as APRNs practice in a changing health care system. In addition, competencies promoted by other professional groups become important to the understanding of advanced practice nursing; for example, the Interprofessional Education Collaborative competencies on interprofessional practice are helping to shape the understanding of collaboration (Interprofessional Education Collaborative Expert Panel, 2011; see Chapter 12).

It is also important to understand that each of the competencies described in Part II of this text have specific definitions in the context of advanced practice nursing. For example, leadership has clinical, professional, and systems expectations for the APRN that differ from those for a nurse executive or staff nurse. These unique definitions of each competency help distinguish practice at the advanced level. Similarly, certain competencies are important components of other specialized nursing roles. For example, collaboration and consultation are important competencies for nursing administrators. The uniqueness of advanced practice nursing is seen in the synergistic interaction between direct clinical practice and this constellation of competencies. In Fig. 3.3, the openings between the central practice

competency and these additional competencies represent the fact that the APRN's direct practice skill interacts with and informs all the other competencies. For example, APRNs consult with other providers who seek their practice expertise to plan care for specialty patients. They are able to provide expert guidance and coaching for patients going through health and illness transitions because of their direct practice experience and insight.

The core competencies are not unique to APRN practices. Physicians and other health care providers may have developed some of them. Experienced staff nurses may master several of these competencies with years of practice experience. These nurses are seen as exemplary performers and are often encouraged to enter graduate school to become APRNs. What distinguishes APRN practice is the *expectation* that every APRN's practice encompasses all these competencies and seamlessly blends them into daily practice encounters. This expectation makes APRN practice unique among that of other providers.

These complex competencies develop over time. No APRN emerges from a graduate program fully prepared to enact all of them. However, it is critical that graduate programs provide exposure to each competency in the form of didactic content and practical experience so that new graduates can be prepared to utilize them at the basic core level, be given a base on which to build their practices, and be tested for initial credentialing. These key competencies are described in detail in subsequent chapters and are not further elaborated here.

Scope of Practice

The term *scope of practice* refers to the legal authority granted to a professional to provide and be reimbursed for health care services. The ANA (2015b) defined the scope of nursing practice as "... the description of the *who, what, where, when, why,* and *how* of nursing practice" (p. 2). This authority for practice emanates from many sources, such as state and federal laws and regulations, the profession's code of ethics, and professional practice standards. For all health care professionals, scope of practice is most closely tied to state statutes; for nursing in the United States, these statutes are the nurse practice acts of the various states. As previously discussed, APRN scope of practice is characterized by specialization; expansion of services provided, including diagnosing and prescribing; and autonomy to practice (NCSBN, 2008). The scopes of practice also differ among the various APRN roles; various APRN organizations have provided detailed and specific descriptions for their particular role. Carving out an adequate scope of APRN practice authority has been a historic struggle for most of the advanced practice groups (see Chapter 1), and this continues to be a hotly debated issue among and within the health professions. Significant variability in state practice acts continues, such that APRNs can perform certain activities in some states, notably prescribing certain medications and practicing without physician supervision, but may be constrained from performing these same activities in other states (NCSBN, 2016). The Consensus Model's proposed regulatory language can be used by states to achieve consistent scope of practice language and standardized APRN regulation (APRN Joint Dialogue Group, 2008).

Although almost 2 decades old, a report by the Pew Health Professions Commission (Finocchio, Dower, Blick, Gragnola, & Taskforce on Health Care Workforce Regulation, 1998) remains relevant today. The Taskforce noted that the tension and turf battles between professions and the increased legislative activities in this area "clog legislative agendas across the country." These battles are costly and time-consuming and lawmakers' decisions related to scope of practice are frequently distorted by campaign contributions, lobbying efforts, and political power struggles rather than being based on empirical evidence. More recently, while the Institute of Medicine (IOM) has reported that progress continues on a state-by-state basis in achieving full practice authority for APRNs, there are still many states where APRNs have reduced or restricted practice authority (National Academies of Sciences, Engineering, & Medicine, 2016) (see Chapter 22 for further discussion). In addition, the IOM highlights the fact that medical staff member and hospital privileging criteria are inconsistent due to state laws as well as business preferences. Opposition by some physician associations and physicians is ongoing and can be a significant barrier. Much work remains to be done. The IOM recommends that the coalition of stakeholders to remove these barriers needs to be expanded and diversified to increase collaboration in improving health care for patients (National Academies of Sciences, Engineering, & Medicine, 2016).

Differentiating Advanced Practice Roles: Operational Definitions of Advanced Practice Nursing

As noted earlier, it is critical to the public's understanding of advanced practice nursing that APRN roles and resulting job titles reflect actual practices. Because actual practices differ, job titles should differ. The following corollary is also true—if the actual practices do not differ, the job titles should not differ. For example, some institutions have retitled their CNSs *clinical coordinators* or *clinical educators,* even though these APRNs are practicing consistently with the practices of a CNS. This change in job title renders the CNS practice less clearly visible in the clinical setting and thereby obscures CNS role clarity. As noted, differences among roles must be clarified in ways that promote understanding of advanced practice nursing, and the Consensus Model (APRN Joint Dialogue Group, 2008) clarifies appropriate titling for APRNs.

Workforce Data

It is difficult to obtain accurate numbers for APRNs by role, particularly for those prepared as CNSs. The US Bureau of Labor Statistics has separate classifications for NPs, CRNAs, and CNMs in their Standard Occupational Classification listing, so some data are collected when the Bureau does routine surveys.

⊚ TABLE 3.1	Number of APRNs by Category		
APRN Role	Numbers	Source	Website
Nurse Practitioner	>234,000	American Academy of Nurse Practitioners National NP Database	www.aanp.org/all-about-nps/np-fact-sheet
Clinical Nurse Specialist	>72,000	National Association of Clinical Nurse Specialists	www.nacns.org/docs/APRN-Factsheet.pdf
Certified Registered Nurse Anesthetist	>50,000	American Association of Nurse Anesthetists	www.aana.com/ceandeducation/becomeacrna/ Pages/Nurse-Anesthetists-at-a-Glance.aspx
Certified Nurse-Midwife	11,500	American College of Nurse-Midwives	www.midwife.org/Essential-Facts-about-Midwives

However, CNSs are not listed as a separate role in the classification system; rather the role is subsumed under the general registered nurse (RN) classification. The Bureau of Labor Statistics has refused to add a CNS classification despite repeated attempts to convince them otherwise. Therefore the latest APRN role numbers are based on the respective organizational data for consistency (Table 3.1).

It is essential to have accurate tracking of APRN numbers by distinct role as well as by geographic distribution and basic demographic statistics. Gathering data only on select APRN roles or as subcategories of the RN role diminishes the profession's ability to actively and appropriately advocate for patients on a national level for needed care that can best be provided by APRNs.

Four Established Advanced Practice Nurse Roles

Advanced practice nursing is applied in the four established roles and in emerging roles. These APRN roles can be considered to be the operational definitions of the concept of advanced practice nursing. Although each APRN role has the common definition, primary criteria, and competencies of advanced practice nursing at its center, each has its own distinct form. Some of the distinctive features of the various roles are listed here. Differences and similarities among roles are further explored in Part III of this text.

The NACNS (2004) has distinguished CNS practice by characterizing "spheres of influence" in which the CNS operates. These include the patient/client sphere, the nurses and nursing practice sphere, and the organization/system sphere (see Chapter 14). A CNS is first and foremost a clinical expert who provides direct care to patients with complex health problems. CNSs not only learn consultation processes, as do other APRNs, but also function as formal

consultants to nursing staff and other care providers within their organizations. Developing, supporting, and educating nursing staff and other interprofessional staff to improve the quality of patient care is a core part of the nurses and nursing practice sphere. Managing system change in complex organizations to build teams and improve nursing practices, and effecting system change to enable better advocacy for patients, are additional role expectations of the CNS. Expectations regarding sophisticated evidence-based practice activities have been central to this role since its inception.

NPs, whether in primary care or acute care, possess advanced health assessment, diagnostic, and clinical management skills that include pharmacology management. Their focus is expert direct care, managing the health needs of individuals and their families. Incumbents in the classic NP role provide primary health care focused on wellness and prevention; NP practice also includes caring for patients with minor, common acute conditions and stable chronic conditions (see Chapter 15). The acute care NP (ACNP) brings practitioner skills to a specialized patient population within the acute care setting. The ACNP's focus is the diagnosis and clinical management of acutely or critically ill patient populations in a particular specialized setting. Acquisition of additional medical diagnostic and management skills, such as interpreting computed tomography and magnetic resonance imaging scans, inserting chest tubes, and performing lumbar punctures, also characterize this role (see Chapter 16).

The CNM (see Chapter 17) has advanced health assessment and intervention skills focused on women's health and childbearing. CNM practice involves independent management of women's health care. CNMs focus particularly on pregnancy, childbirth, the postpartum period, and neonatal care, but their practices also include family planning, gynecologic care, primary health care for women through menopause, and treatment of male partners for sexually transmitted infections (ACNM, 2012). The CNM's focus is on providing direct care to a select patient population.

CRNA practice (see Chapter 18) is distinguished by advanced procedural and pharmacologic management of patients undergoing anesthesia. CRNAs practice independently, in collaboration with physicians, or as employees of a health care institution. Like CNMs, their primary focus is providing direct care to a select patient population. Both CNM and CRNA practices are also distinguished by well-established national standards and certification examinations in their specialties.

These differing roles and their similarities and distinctions are explored in detail in subsequent chapters. It is expected that other roles may emerge as health care continues to change and new opportunities become apparent. This brief discussion underscores the rich and varied nature of advanced practice nursing and the necessity for retaining and supporting different APRN roles and titles in the health care marketplace. At the same time, the consistent definition of advanced practice nursing described here undergirds each of these roles, as will be seen in Part III of this text.

Critical Elements in Managing Advanced Practice Nursing Environments

The health care arena is increasingly fluid and changeable; some would even say it is chaotic. Advanced practice nursing does not exist in a vacuum or a singular environment. Rather, this level of practice occurs in an increasing variety of health care delivery environments. These diverse environments are complex admixtures of interdependent elements, as noted in Fig. 3.4. The term *environment* refers to any milieu in which an APRN practices, ranging from a community-based rural health care practice for a primary care NP to a complex tertiary health care organization for an ACNP. Certain core features of these environments dramatically shape advanced practice and must be managed by APRNs in order for their practices to survive and thrive (Fig. 3.4). Although not technically part of the core definition of advanced practice nursing, these environmental features are included here to frame the understanding that APRNs must be aware of these key elements in any practice setting. Furthermore, APRNs must be prepared to contend with and shape these aspects of their practice environment to be able to enact advanced practice nursing fully.

The environmental elements that affect APRN practice include the following:
- Managing reimbursement and payment mechanisms
- Dealing with marketing and contracting considerations
- Understanding legal, regulatory, and credentialing requirements
- Understanding and shaping health policy considerations
- Strengthening organizational structures and cultures to support advanced practice nursing
- Enabling outcome evaluation and performance improvement

With the exception of organizational structures and cultures, Part IV of this text explores these elements in depth. Discussion of organizational considerations is presented in Chapter 4 and woven throughout the chapters in Part III.

Common to all these environmental elements is the increasing use of technology and the need for APRNs to master various new technologies to improve patient care and health care systems. The ability to use information systems and technology and patient care technology is an essential element of master's and DNP curricula (AACN, 2006, 2011). Electronic technology in the form of electronic health records, coding schemas, communications, Internet use, and provision of care across state lines through telehealth practices is changing health care practice. These changes, in turn, are reshaping all seven APRN core competencies. Proficiency in the use of new technologies is increasingly necessary to support clinical practice, implement quality improvement initiatives, and provide leadership to evaluate outcomes of care and care systems (see Chapter 24).

Managing the business and legal aspects of practice is increasingly critical to APRN survival in the competitive health care marketplace. All APRNs must understand current reimbursement issues, even as changes related to the Patient Protection and Affordable Care Act (2010) are being debated. Payment mechanisms and legal constraints must be managed, regardless of setting. Given the increasing competition among physicians, APRNs, and nonphysician providers, APRNs must be prepared to market their services assertively and knowledgeably. Marketing oneself as a new NP in a small community may look different from marketing oneself as a CNS in a large health system, but the principles are the same. Marketing considerations often include the need to advocate for and actively

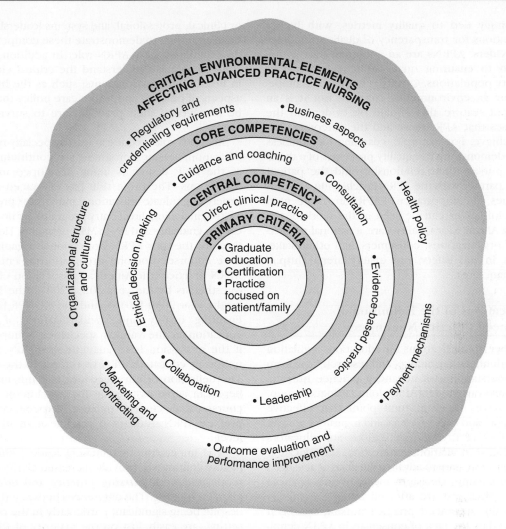

FIG 3.4 Critical elements in advanced nursing practice environments.

create positions that do not currently exist. Contract considerations are much more complex at the APRN level and all APRNs, whether newly graduated or experienced, must be prepared to enter into contract negotiations.

Health policy at the state and federal levels is an increasingly potent force shaping advanced practice nursing; regulations and policies that flow from legislative actions can enable or constrain APRN practices. Variations in the strength and number of APRNs in various states attest to the power of this environmental factor. Organizational structures and cultures, whether those of a community-based practice or a hospital unit, are also important facilitators of or barriers to advanced practice nursing;

APRN students must learn to assess and intervene to build organizations and cultures that strengthen APRN practice. Finally, APRNs are accountable for the use of evidence-based practice to ensure positive patient and system outcomes. Measuring the favorable impact of advanced practice nursing on these outcomes and effecting performance improvements are essential activities that all APRNs must be prepared to undertake because continuing to demonstrate the value of APRN practice is a necessity in chaotic practice environments.

Special mention must be made of health care quality. As quality concerns have escalated, more attention is being focused on quality metrics for all settings (see Chapter 24). Reimbursement is being increasingly tied to quality metrics, with higher expectations for transparency of quality outcomes by providers. APRNs are an important part of the solution to ensuring quality outcomes for their specialty populations. Quality is not itself a competency or an environmental element, but it is an important feature that should be evident in the processes that APRNs use and the outcomes that they achieve. For example, coaching for wellness should demonstrate the quality processes of a therapeutic nurse-patient relationship and the patient being a partner with the APRN in achieving wellness outcomes. The importance of APRN involvement in quality initiatives can be seen in the work of the Nursing Alliance for Quality Care, a national partnership of organizations, consumers, and other stakeholders in the safety and quality arena (http://www.naqc.org).

Implications of the Definition of Advanced Practice Nursing

A number of implications for education, regulation and credentialing, practice, and research flow from this understanding of advanced practice nursing. The Consensus Model (APRN Joint Dialogue Group, 2008) makes the important point that effective communication between legal and regulatory groups, accreditors, certifying organizations, and educators (licensing, accreditation, certification, and education [LACE]) is necessary to advance the goals of advanced practice nursing. Decisions made by each of these groups affect and are affected by all the others. Historically, advanced practice nursing has been hampered by the lack of consensus in APRN definition, terminology, educational and certification requirements, and regulatory approaches. The Consensus Model process, by combining stakeholders from each of the LACE areas, took a giant step forward toward the profession's achieving needed consensus on APRN practice, education, certification, and regulation.

Implications for Advanced Practice Nursing Education

Graduate programs should provide anticipatory socialization experiences to prepare students for their chosen APRN role. Graduate experiences should include practice in all the competencies of advanced practice nursing, not just direct clinical practice. For example, students who have no theoretical base or guided practice experiences in consultative skills

or clinical, professional, and systems leadership will be ill-equipped to demonstrate these competencies on assuming a new APRN role. In addition, APRN students need to understand the critical elements in health care environments, such as the business aspects of practice and health care policy that must be managed if their practices are to survive and grow.

All APRN roles require at least a specialty master's education; master's programs are continuing even as the DNP degree is being developed in many institutions. The profession has embraced a wide variety of graduate educational models for preparing APRNs, including direct-entry programs for non-nurse college graduates and RN-to-MSN programs. However, three of the four APRN professional organizations have endorsed doctoral preparation as entry into APRN practice (the American Association of Nurse Anesthetists by the year 2025 [2007], the NACNS by the year 2030 [2015], and the NONPF [2015]). Ensuring quality and standardization of APRN education in the various specialties is imperative if the profession is to guarantee a highly skilled, uniformly educated APRN workforce to the public. The definition of advanced practice nursing used here can serve as a guide for developing quality courses and clinical practice experiences that prepare APRN students to practice at an advanced level.

It is imperative that nursing leaders and DNP faculty continue to provide increased clarity for the terms *advanced nursing practice* and *advanced practice nursing*. The differences between the two, despite being significant particularly in the practice setting, are easily lost on the majority of RNs and even non-APRN DNP graduates. Lack of clarity about this distinction has created ongoing problems as DNP graduates prepared in non-APRN roles confuse their combined graduate preparation and their RN clinical experience with being an APRN. This type of confusion about roles within nursing only perpetuates the ongoing lack of clarity when communicating with physicians and policymakers (Carter et al., 2013; Carter, Lavis, & MacDonald-Rencz, 2014) and compromises the progress that APRNs have made in the practice arena.

Implications for Regulation and Credentialing

Significant progress has been made toward an integrative view of APRN regulation over the past decade, culminating in the LACE regulatory framework detailed in the Consensus Model. In particular, the primary criteria of graduate education, advanced certification, and focus on direct clinical practice for all APRN roles proposed in Hamric's definition have been affirmed as the key elements in regulating and credentialing APRNs (APRN Joint Dialogue Group, 2008). Such internal cohesion can go a long way toward removing barriers to the public's access to APRN care.

The Consensus Model has been an important unifying force within the APRN community. The regulatory clarity in this document has increasingly been seen in other national statements, and the work was highlighted in the IOM report on *The Future of Nursing* (IOM, 2011). The NCSBN has embarked on the "APRN Campaign for Consensus," a nationwide effort to have this model enacted in all the states. However, as of 2017, only 16 states have fully implemented the Consensus Model into legislation (NCSBN, 2017).

The IOM report also has given rise to action coalitions, funded by the AARP Foundation and the Robert Wood Johnson Foundation, in numerous states (Campaign for Action, 2017). The Campaign for Action has a dual focus, implementing solutions to the challenges facing the nursing profession and strengthening nurse-based approaches to transform how Americans receive quality health care. Although the Campaign for Action is broader in scope than just advanced practice nursing, many of the solutions for transforming health care involve APRNs being able to practice to the full extent of their education. It is critically important for all APRNs to be aware of and involved in these efforts.

One implication for credentialing flows from the diverse specialty and role base of advanced practice nursing. APRNs must practice and be certified in the specific population focus and role for which they have been educated. APRNs who wish to change their specialty, population focus, or APRN role need to return to school for education targeted to that area. The days are past when a primary care NP could take a job in a specialized acute care practice without further education to prepare for that specialty. This issue of aligning APRN job expectations with education and certification is not always well understood by practice environments, educators, or even APRNs themselves. However, the need to ensure congruence among particular APRN specialties and roles and education, certification, and subsequent practice has been identified by regulators, and more stringent regulations regarding this issue have been promulgated (NCSBN, 2008).

Implications for Research

As noted in Chapter 10, one of the core competencies of advanced practice nursing is the use of evidence-based practice in an APRN's practice and in changing the practice environment to incorporate the use of evidence. The practice doctorate initiative identified the increased need for leadership in evidence-based practice and for application of knowledge to solve practice problems and improve health outcomes as reasons for moving to the DNP degree for APRN practice (AACN, 2006). If research is to be relevant to health care delivery and to nursing practice at all levels, APRNs must be involved. APRNs need to recognize the importance of advancing the profession's and health care system's knowledge about effective patient care practices and to realize that they are a vital link in building and translating this knowledge into clinical practice.

Related to this research involvement is the necessity for more research differentiating basic and advanced practice nursing and identifying the patient populations that benefit most from APRN intervention. For example, there is compelling empirical evidence that APRNs can effectively manage chronic disease—preventing or mitigating complications, reducing rehospitalizations, and increasing patients' quality of life. This evidence is presented in the chapters in Part III of this text and in Chapter 23. Linking advanced practice nursing to specific patient outcomes remains a major research imperative for this century. It is interesting to note the increasing research being conducted in international settings as more countries implement advanced practice nursing and study the effectiveness of these new practitioners; discussions of this research are woven throughout the chapters of this book.

Similarly, research is needed on the outcomes of the different APRN educational pathways in terms of APRN graduate experiences and patient outcomes. Such data would be invaluable in continuing to refine advanced practice education. Outcomes achieved by graduates from DNP programs need similar study in comparison to master's-level APRN graduates; in critiquing the need for the DNP degree, Fulton and Lyon (2005) noted the absence of research data on whether there are weaknesses in current master's-level graduates.

Finally, it is incumbent upon DNP faculty to ensure that APRNs understand their role in evidence-based practice vis-à-vis research. In fact, faculty themselves continue to struggle with knowledge and understanding of evidence-based practice and its use in the completion of the scholarly DNP project (AACN, 2015; Dols, Hernandez, & Miles, 2017). Translational, evidence-based practice change, and quality improvement projects are the proper foci for DNP projects; such projects require a complex skill set that is the focus of DNP evidence-based practice courses. DNP students are not sufficiently educated in the particulars of the formal research process to be prepared to conduct independent research successfully, and faculty have an important responsibility to assist the student to identify an appropriate topic. Unfortunately, it is not uncommon to encounter APRN DNP projects that are not an implementation of evidence-based practice or a clinical change project to bring research evidence to influence practice, but rather involve the conduct of a research study. The DNP-prepared APRN is an evidence-based practice expert who evaluates and generates internal evidence, translates research into sustainable practice changes, and uses research to make practice decisions that improve the quality of patient care (AACN, 2006; Melnyk, 2016). Without this important understanding, nursing runs the risk of implying that advancing the science of nursing through research no longer requires PhD preparation. Such a misunderstanding could lead practice institutions to hire DNP graduates with the intention that they conduct rigorous independent research. It could also substantially delay the translation of research findings into clinical practice.

Implications for Practice Environments

Because of the centrality of direct clinical practice, APRNs must hold onto and make explicit their direct patient care activities. They must also articulate the importance of this level of care for patients. In addition, it is important to identify those patients who most need APRN services and ensure that they receive this care.

APRN roles require considerable autonomy and authority to be fully enacted. Practice settings have not always structured APRN roles to allow sufficient autonomy or accountability for achievement of the patient and system outcomes that are expected of advanced practitioners. It is equally important to emphasize that APRNs have expanded responsibilities—expanded authority for practice requires expanded responsibility for practice. APRNs must demonstrate a higher level of responsibility and accountability if they are to be seen as legitimate providers of care and full partners on provider teams responsible for patient populations. This willingness

to be accountable for practice will also promote consumers' and policymakers' perceptions of APRNs as credible providers in line with physicians.

The APRN leadership competency mandates that APRNs serve as visible role models and mentors for other nurses (see Chapter 11). Leadership is not optional in APRN practice; it is a requirement. APRNs must be a visible part of the solution to the health care system's problems. For this goal to be realized, each APRN must practice leadership in his or her daily activities. In practice environments, APRNs need structured time and opportunities for this leadership, including mentoring activities with new nurses.

New APRNs require a considerable period of role development before they can master all the components and competencies of their chosen role, which has important implications for employers of new APRNs. Employers should provide experienced preceptors, some structure for the new APRN, and ongoing support for role development (see Chapter 4 for further recommendations).

As a result of government titling, it is becoming common in the practice setting to label APRNs (as well as physician assistants) as "mid-level providers." The very use of this term for an APRN implies a hierarchical (and therefore a "less than") structure for all of nursing. If the APRN is "mid-level," then the implication is that the physician is at the top and the RN is thus positioned at the bottom of the care provider structure (Boyle, 2011). This is contrary to the reality that all health care providers bring unique and valued expertise to the care of patients; the professional leading the care at any given point in a patient's health encounter is dependent on the needs of the patient and the provider with the corresponding expertise. It is important that APRNs distinguish their roles from this unfortunately named category.

Finally, APRN roles must be structured in practice environments to allow APRNs to enact advanced nursing skills rather than simply substitute for physicians. It is certainly necessary for APRNs to gain additional skills in medical diagnosis and therapeutic interventions, including the knowledge needed for prescriptive authority. However, *advanced practice nursing is a value-added complement to medical practice, not a substitute for it.* This is particularly an imperative in the primary care arena; it may well be that substituting APRNs for physicians in classic, medically driven primary care configurations is not the best use of APRN skills. Because APRN competencies include those of partnering with patients, use of evidence, and coaching skills, APRNs may be more effectively used in wellness programs, working with chronically ill patients to strengthen their self-management and adherence, and designing and implementing educational programs for patients with complex management needs. New sustainable business models are needed that are more collaborative and configure teams in innovative ways to minimize fragmentation of care and make the best use of the APRN as a value-added complement to the traditional medical team.

As physician shortages increase, particularly the number of physicians prepared in family practice and the new hospitalist practices, this distinction between advanced practice nursing and medical practice must be clear in the minds of employers, insurers, and APRNs themselves. As advanced practice nursing evolves, it is becoming clear that APRNs represent a choice and an alternative for patients seeking care. Consequently, understanding what APRNs bring to health care must be articulated to multiple stakeholders to enable informed patient choice. A competency-based definition of advanced practice nursing aids in this articulation, so that APRNs are not just seen as physician substitutes.

Conclusion

Since the first edition of this text in 1996, substantial progress has been made toward clarifying the definition of advanced practice nursing. This progress is enabling APRNs, educators, administrators, and other nursing leaders to be clear and consistent about the definition of advanced practice nursing so that the profession speaks with one voice.

This is a critical juncture in the evolution of advanced practice nursing as national attention on nursing and recommendations for nursing's central role in redesigning the health care system are increasing. APRNs must continue to clarify that the advanced practice of nursing is not the junior practice of medicine but represents an important alternative practice that complements rather than competes with medical practice. In some cases, patients need advanced nursing and not medicine; identifying these situations and matching APRN resources to patients' needs are important priorities for transforming the current health care system. APRNs must be able to articulate their defining characteristics clearly and forcefully so that their practices will survive and thrive amidst continued cost cutting in the health care sector.

For a profession to succeed, it must have internal cohesion and external legitimacy, and it must have them at the same time (Safriet, 1993). Clarity about the core definition of advanced practice nursing and recognition of the primary criteria and competencies necessary for all APRNs enhance nursing's internal cohesion. At the same time, clarifying the differences among APRNs and showcasing their important roles in the health care system enhance nursing's external legitimacy.

Key Summary Points

- The advanced practice of nursing is not the junior practice of medicine; advanced practice nursing is a complement to, not a substitution for, medical practice.
- There is a clear and distinct difference between the terms *advanced practice nursing* and *advanced nursing practice,* and this difference needs to continue to be clearly elucidated, especially as the terms are used on a global basis.
- The three primary criteria of an earned graduate degree with a concentration in an advanced practice nursing role and population focus, national certification at an advanced level, and a practice focused on patients and their families are necessary but not sufficient to define advanced practice nursing.
- The DNP is an academic *degree,* not a *role.*
- All APRNs share the same core criteria and competencies, although the actual clinical skill set varies, depending on the needs of the APRN's specialty patient population.

References

To access the references for this chapter, use your smartphone's QR code reader to scan the code below, or go to http://booksite.elsevier.com/ 9780323447751.

Karen A. Brykczynski • *Carole L. Mackavey*

---

*"Where the needs of the world and your talents cross, there lies your
vocation."*

—*Aristotle*

CHAPTER CONTENTS

This chapter explores the complex processes of advanced practice registered nurse (APRN) role development, with the objectives of providing the following: (1) an understanding of related concepts and research; (2) anticipatory guidance for APRN students; (3) role facilitation strategies for new APRNs, APRN preceptors, faculty, administrators, and interested colleagues; and (4) guidelines for continued role evolution. This chapter consolidates literature from all the APRN specialties—including clinical nurse specialists (CNSs), nurse practitioners (NPs), certified nurse-midwives (CNMs), and certified registered nurse anesthetists (CRNAs)—to present a generic process relevant to all APRN roles. Some of this literature is foundational to understanding issues of role development for all APRN roles and, although dated, remains relevant. This chapter has been expanded to include international APRN role development experiences. To reflect the literature indicating that APRN role transition occurs as two distinct processes, the discussion is separated into (1) the educational component of APRN role acquisition and (2) the occupational or work component

of role implementation. This division in the process of role development is intended to clarify and distinguish the changes occurring during the role transitions experienced during the educational period (role acquisition) and the changes occurring during the actual performance of the role after program completion (role implementation). Strategies for enhancing APRN role development are described. The chapter concludes with summary comments and suggestions to facilitate future APRN role development and evolution.

Role development in advanced practice nursing is described here as a process that evolves over time. The process is more than socializing and taking on a new role. It involves transforming one's professional identity (Benner, 2011; Jarvis-Selinger, Pratt, & Regehr, 2012) and the progressive development of the seven core advanced practice competencies (see Chapter 3). The scope of nursing practice has expanded and contracted in response to societal needs, political forces, and economic realities (Levy, 1968; Safriet, 1992; see Chapter 1). Historical evidence suggests that the expanded role of the 1970s was common nursing practice during the early 1900s among public health nurses (DeMaio, 1979; see Chapter 1). However, the core of nursing is not defined by the tasks nurses perform. This task-oriented perspective is inadequate and disregards the complex nature of nursing.

Perspectives on Advanced Practice Nurse Role Development

Professional role development is a dynamic ongoing process that, once begun, spans a lifetime. The concept of graduation as commencement, whereby one's career begins on completion of a degree, is central to understanding the evolving nature of professional roles in response to personal, professional, and societal demands (Gunn, 1998). Professional role development literature in nursing is abundant and complex, involving multiple component processes, including the following: (1) aspects of adult development; (2) development of clinical expertise; (3) modification of self-identity through initial socialization in school; (4) embodiment of ethical comportment (Benner, Sutphen, Leonard, & Day, 2010); (5) development and integration of professional role components; and (6) subsequent resocialization in the work setting. Similar to socialization for other professional roles, such as those of attorney, physician, teacher, and social worker, the process of becoming an APRN involves aspects of adult development and professional socialization. The professional socialization process in advanced practice nursing involves identification with and acquisition of the behaviors and attitudes of the advanced practice group to which one aspires (Waugaman & Lu, 1999, p. 239). This includes learning the specialized language, skills, and knowledge of the particular APRN group, internalizing its values and norms, and incorporating these into one's professional nursing identity and other life roles (Cohen, 1981).

Novice-to-Expert Skill Acquisition Model

Acquisition of knowledge and skill occurs in a progressive movement through the stages of performance from novice to expert, as described by Dreyfus and Dreyfus (1986, 2009), who studied diverse groups, including pilots, chess players, and adult learners of second languages. The skill acquisition model has broad applicability and can be used to understand many different skills, ranging from playing a musical instrument to writing a research grant. The most widely known application of this model is Benner's (1984) observational and interview study of clinical nursing practice situations from the perspective of new nurses and their preceptors in hospital nursing services. Although this study included several APRNs, it did not specify a particular education level as a criterion for expertise. As noted in Chapter 3, there has been some confusion about this criterion. The skill acquisition model is a situation-based model, not a trait model. Therefore, the level of expertise is not an individual characteristic of a particular nurse but is a function of the nurse's familiarity with a particular situation in combination with his or her educational background. This model could be used to study the level of expertise required for other aspects of advanced practice, including guidance and coaching, consultation, collaboration, evidence-based practice, ethical decision making, and leadership.

Fig. 4.1 shows a typical APRN role development pattern in terms of this skill acquisition model. A major implication of the novice-to-expert model for advanced practice nursing is the claim that even experts can be expected to perform at lower skill levels when they enter new situations or positions. Hamric and Taylor's report (1989) that an experienced CNS starting a new position experiences the same role development phases as a new CNS graduate, only over a shorter period, supports this claim. The same pattern can be expected with new Doctor of Nursing Practice (DNP) graduates; they experience similar role development phases upon assuming a new DNP position, but they go through phases more quickly because they are informed by broader education and experience (Glasgow & Zoucha, 2011).

The overall trajectory expected during APRN role development is shown in Fig. 4.1; however, each APRN experiences a unique pattern of role transitions and life transitions concurrently. For example, a professional nurse who functions as a mentor for new graduates may decide to pursue an advanced degree as an APRN. As an APRN graduate student, she or he will experience the challenges of acquiring a new role, the anxiety associated with learning new skills and practices, and the dependency of being a novice. At the same time, if this nurse continues to work as a registered nurse, his or her functioning in this work role will be at the competent, proficient, or expert level, depending on experience and the situation. On graduation, the new APRN may experience a limbo period during which she or he is no longer a student and not yet an APRN, while searching for a position and meeting

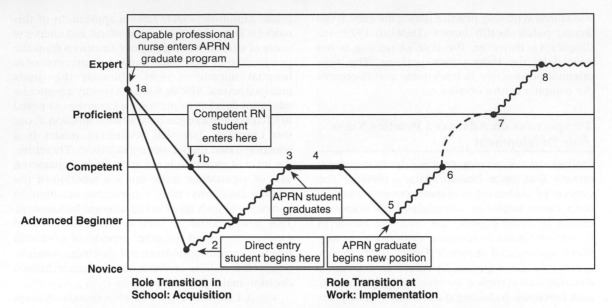

FIG 4.1 Typical APRN role development pattern. *1a,* APRN students may begin graduate school as proficient or expert nurses. *1b,* Some enter as competent RNs, with limited practice experience. Depending on previous background, the new APRN student will revert to novice level or advanced beginner level on assuming the student role. *2,* A direct-entry APRN student or non-nurse college graduate student with no experience would begin the role transition process at the novice level. *3,* The graduate from an APRN program is competent as an APRN student but has no experience as a practicing APRN. *4,* A limbo period is experienced while the APRN graduate searches for a position and becomes certified. *5,* The newly employed APRN reverts to the advanced beginner level in the new APRN position as the role trajectory begins again. *6,* Some individuals remain at the competent level. There is a discontinuous leap from the competent to the proficient level. *7,* Proficiency develops only if there is sufficient commitment and involvement in practice along with embodiment of skills and knowledge. *8,* Expertise is intuitive and situation specific, meaning that not all situations will be managed expertly. (See text for details.) Note: Readers may refer to the Dreyfus skill acquisition model for further details (Benner, 1984; Benner, Tanner, & Chesla, 2009; Dreyfus & Dreyfus, 1986, 2009). For the purpose of illustration, this figure is more linear than the individualized role development trajectories that actually occur.

certification requirements (see Chapter 22). Once in a new APRN position, this nurse may experience a return to the advanced beginner stage as he or she proceeds through the phases of role implementation. Even after making the transition to an APRN role, progression in role implementation is not a linear process. As Fig. 4.1 indicates, there are discontinuities, with movement back and forth as the trajectory begins again. Years later, the APRN may decide to pursue yet another APRN role or obtain a DNP. The processes of role acquisition, role implementation, and novice-to-expert skill development will again be experienced—although altered and informed by previous experiences—as the postgraduate student acquires additional skills and knowledge. Role development involves multiple,

dynamic, and situational processes, with each new undertaking being characterized by passage through earlier transitional phases and with some movement back and forth, horizontally or vertically, as different career options are pursued.

Direct-entry students who are non-nurse college graduates and APRN students with little or no experience as nurses before entry into an APRN graduate program would be expected to begin their APRN role development at the novice level (see Fig. 4.1). Some evidence indicates that although these inexperienced nurse students may lack the intuitive sense that comes with clinical experience, they avoid the role confusion associated with letting go of the traditional registered nurse (RN) role that is commonly reported with experienced nurse students

(Heitz, Steiner, & Burman, 2004). This finding has implications for APRN education as the profession moves toward the DNP as the preferred educational pathway for APRN preparation (American Association of Colleges of Nursing [AACN], 2006).

Another significant implication of the Dreyfus model (Dreyfus & Dreyfus, 1986, 2009) for APRNs is the observation that the quality of performance may deteriorate when performers are subjected to intense scrutiny, whether their own or that of someone else (Roberts, Tabloski, & Bova, 1997). The increased anxiety experienced by APRN students during faculty on-site clinical evaluation visits or during videotaped testing of clinical performance in simulated situations is an example of responding to such intense scrutiny. A third implication of this skill acquisition model for APRNs is the need to accrue experience in actual situations over time, so that practical and theoretical knowledge are refined, clarified, personalized, and embodied, forming an individualized repertoire of experience that guides advanced practice performance. As the profession encourages new nurses to move more rapidly into APRN education, students, faculty, and educational programs must search for creative ways to incorporate the practical and theoretical knowledge necessary for advanced practice nursing. Discussing unfolding cases is a useful approach for teaching the clinical reasoning in transition that is so essential for clinical practice (Benner et al., 2010; Day, Cooper, & Scott, 2012).

Role Concepts and Role Development Issues

This discussion of professional role issues incorporates role concepts described by Hardy and Hardy (1988) and Schumacher and Meleis (1994), along with the concept that different APRN roles represent different subcultural groups within the broader nursing culture (Leininger, 1994). Building on Johnson's (1993) conclusion that NPs have three voices, Brykczynski (1999a) described APRNs as tricultural and trilingual. They share background knowledge, practices, and skills of three cultures—biomedicine, mainstream nursing, and everyday life. They are fluent in the languages of biomedical science, nursing knowledge and skill, and everyday parlance. Some APRNs (e.g., CNMs) are socialized into a fourth culture as well, that of midwifery. Others are also fluent in more than one everyday language.

The concepts of role stress and strain discussed by Hardy and Hardy (1988) are useful for understanding

the dynamics of role transitions (Table 4.1). Hardy and Hardy described *role stress* as a social structural condition in which role obligations are ambiguous, conflicting, incongruous, excessive, or unpredictable. *Role strain* is defined as the subjective feeling of frustration, tension, or anxiety experienced in response to role stress. The highly stressful nature of the nursing profession needs to be recognized as the background within which individuals seek advanced education to become APRNs (Aiken, Clarke, Sloan, Sochalski, & Silber, 2002; Dionne-Proulz & Pepin, 1993). Role strain can be minimized by the identification of potential role stressors, development of coping strategies, and rehearsal of situations designed for application of those strategies. However, the difficulties experienced by neophytes in new positions cannot be eliminated. As noted, expertise is holistic, involving embodied perceptual skills (e.g., detecting qualitative distinctions in pulses or types of anxiety); formation of character, identity, and ethical judgment; shared background knowledge; and cognitive ability. A school-work, theory-practice, ideal-real gap will remain because of the nature of human skill acquisition, which occurs over time, and the undetermined nature of situations in actual practice, which requires engaged situated reasoning and consideration of patient preferences, practice standards, costs, clinical outcomes, and numerous other aspects that vary with each situation.

Bandura's (1977) social cognitive theory of self-efficacy may be of interest to APRNs in terms of understanding what motivates individuals to acquire skills and what builds confidence as skills are developed. Self-efficacy theory—a person's belief in his or her ability to succeed—has been used widely to further understanding of skill acquisition with patients (Burglehaus, 1997; Clark & Dodge, 1999; Dalton & Blau, 1996). Self-efficacy theory has also been applied to mentoring APRN students (Hayes, 2001) and training health care professionals in skill acquisition (Parle, Maguire, & Heaven, 1997). Attention to varied learning styles, different neurocognitive processes involved in learning, and APRN students as adult learners is important for teaching (Burns, Beauchesne, Ryan-Krause, & Sawin, 2006; Kumar, Fathima, & Mohan, 2013).

Role Ambiguity

Role ambiguity (see Table 4.1) develops when there is a lack of clarity about expectations, a blurring of responsibilities, uncertainty regarding role implementation, and the inherent uncertainty of existent

TABLE 4.1   **Selected Role Concepts**

Concept	Definition	Examples
Role stress	A situation of increased role performance demand	Returning to school while maintaining work and family responsibilities. The expectation of increased workload (number of patients seen). Keeping up with rapidly changing technology. Coping with restrictions related to payment system limitations.
Role strain	Subjective feeling of frustration, tension, or anxiety in response to role stress	Feeling of decreased self-esteem when performance is below expectations of self or significant others.
Role stressors	Factors that produce role stress	Financial, personal, or academic demands and role expectations that are ambiguous, conflicting, excessive, or unpredictable.
Role ambiguity	Unclear expectations, diffuse responsibilities, uncertainty about subroles	Recent graduates' uncertainty about role expectations. Some degree of ambiguity exists in all professional positions because of the evolving nature of roles and expansion of skills and knowledge.
Role incongruity	A role with incompatibility between skills and abilities and role obligations or between personal values and self-concept and role obligations	An adult nurse practitioner in a role requiring pediatric skills and knowledge. Difficulty of incorporating holistic nursing aspects of care into medical model.
Role conflict	Occurs when role expectations are perceived to be mutually exclusive or contradictory	Role conflict between advanced practice registered nurses (APRNs) and other nurses and between APRNs and physicians.
Role transition	A dynamic process of change over time as new roles are acquired	Changing from a staff nurse to an APRN role. Advancing from a master's-prepared APRN to a Doctor of Nursing Practice–prepared APRN.
Role insufficiency	Feeling inadequate to meet role demands	New APRN graduates experiencing feelings of inadequacy as a result of increased workload expectations and electronic health records documentation requirements. Change from solo practice or clinic to hospital requirements through mergers and acquisitions.
Role supplementation	Anticipatory socialization	Role-specific educational components in a graduate program (e.g., interviewing a practicing APRN or a clinical preceptorship experience with an APRN).

Adapted from Hardy, M. E., & Hardy, W. L. (1988). Role stress and role strain. In M. E. Hardy & M. E. Conway (Eds.), *Role theory: Perspectives for health professionals* (2nd ed., pp. 159–239). Norwalk, CT: Appleton & Lange; and Schumacher, K. L., & Meleis, A. I. (1994). Transitions: A central concept in nursing. *Image: The Journal of Nursing Scholarship, 26,* 119–127.

knowledge. According to Hardy and Hardy (1988), role ambiguity characterizes all professional positions. They have noted that role ambiguity might be positive in that it offers opportunities for creative possibilities. It can be expected to be more prominent in professions undergoing change, such as those in the health care field. To avoid uncertainty about roles in interprofessional educational experiences and promote successful interprofessional practice, a focus on the following key components is important: awareness of one's own professional role, understanding the professional roles of others, leadership skills, principles of teamwork, and conflict negotiations skills and knowledge (MacDonald et al., 2010). Role ambiguity has been widely discussed in relation to the CNS role (Bryant-Lukosius et al., 2010; Hamric,

2003; see also Chapter 14), but it is also a relevant issue for other APRN roles (Kelly & Mathews, 2001), particularly as APRN roles evolve (Stahl & Myers, 2002).

Role Incongruity

Role incongruity is intrarole conflict, which Hardy and Hardy (1988) described as developing from two sources. Incompatibility between skills and abilities and role obligations is one source of role incongruity. An example of this is an adult APRN hired to work in an emergency department with a large percentage of pediatric patients. Such an APRN will find it necessary to enroll in a family NP or pediatric NP program to gain the knowledge necessary to eliminate this role incongruity. This is a growing issue as NP roles become more specialized. Another source of role incongruity is incompatibility among personal values, self-concept, and expected role behaviors. An APRN interested primarily in clinical practice may experience this incongruity if the position that she or he obtains requires performing administrative functions. An example comes from Banda's (1985) study of psychiatric liaison CNSs in acute care hospitals and community health agencies. She reported that they viewed consultation and teaching as their major functions, whereas research and administrative activities produced role incongruity.

Role Conflict

Role conflict develops when role expectations are perceived to be contradictory or mutually exclusive. APRNs may experience conflict with varying demands of their role as well as intraprofessional and interprofessional role conflict.

Intraprofessional Role Conflict

APRNs experience intraprofessional role conflict for a variety of reasons. The historical development of APRN roles has been fraught with conflict and controversy in nursing education and nursing organizations, particularly for CNMs (Varney, 1987), NPs (Ford, 1982), and CRNAs (Gunn, 1991; see also Chapter 1). Relationships among these APRN groups and nursing as a discipline have improved markedly in recent years, but difficulties remain (Fawcett, Newman, & McAllister, 2004). The degree to which APRN roles demonstrate a holistic nursing orientation as opposed to a more disease-specific medical orientation remains problematic (see additional discussion under Interprofessional Role Conflict, later).

Communication difficulties that underlie intraprofessional role conflict occur in four major areas: (1) at an organizational level, (2) in educational programs, (3) in the literature, and (4) in direct clinical practice. Kimbro (1978) initially described these communication difficulties in reference to CNMs, but they are relevant for all APRN roles. The fact that CNSs, NPs, CNMs, and CRNAs each have specific organizations with different certification requirements, competencies, and curricula creates boundaries and sets up the need for formal lines of communication. Communication gaps occur in education when courses and textbooks are not shared among APRN programs, even when more than one specialty is offered in the same school. Specialty-specific journals are another formal communication

barrier because APRNs may read primarily within their own specialty and not keep abreast of larger APRN issues. In clinical settings, some APRNs may be more concerned with providing direct clinical care to individual patients, whereas staff nurses and other APRNs may be more concerned with 24-hour coverage and smooth functioning of the unit or institution. These differences may set the stage for intraprofessional role conflict.

During the 1980s and 1990s, when there was more confusion about the delineation of roles and responsibilities between RNs and NPs, RNs would sometimes demonstrate resistance to NPs by refusing to take vital signs, obtain blood samples, or perform other support functions for patients of NPs (Brykczynski, 1999b; Hupcey, 1993; Lurie, 1981), and they were not admonished by their supervisors for these negative behaviors. These behaviors are suggestive of horizontal violence (a form of hostility), which may be more common during nursing shortages (Thomas, 2003). Roberts (1983) first described horizontal violence among nurses as oppressed group behavior wherein nurses who were doubly oppressed as women and as nurses demonstrated hostility toward their own less powerful group, instead of toward the more powerful oppressors. Recognizing that intraprofessional conflict among nurses is similar to oppressed group behavior can be useful in the development of strategies to overcome these difficulties (Bartholomew, 2006; Brykczynski, 1997; Farrell, 2001; Freshwater, 2000; Roberts, 1996; Rounds, 1997). According to Rounds (1997), horizontal violence is less common among NPs as a group than among RNs generally. Over the years, as the NP role has become more accepted by nurses, there appear to be fewer cases of these hostile passive-aggressive behaviors, often currently referred to as bullying, toward NPs. However, they have been reported in APRN transition literature (Heitz et al., 2004; Kelly & Mathews, 2001). Heath (2014) identified courage as a key factor to address bullying, including "courage to stand up to a bully in a nonthreatening manner and courage to speak up if bullying is witnessed or experienced" (p. 441).

One way to address these issues would be to include APRN position descriptions in staff nurse orientation programs. Curry claimed (1994) that thorough orientation of staff nurses to the APRN role, including clear guidelines and policies regarding responsibility issues, is an important component of successful integration of NP practice in an emergency department setting; this is also applicable to other roles and settings. Another significant strategy for minimizing intraprofessional role conflict is for the new APRN, and APRN students, to spend time getting to know the nursing staff to establish rapport and learn as much as possible about the new setting from those who really know what is going on—the nurses. This action affirms the value and significance of nurses and nursing and sets up a positive atmosphere for collegiality and intraprofessional role cooperation and collaboration. In Kelly and Mathews' study (2001) of new NP graduates, such a strategy was exactly what new NPs regretted not having incorporated into their first positions.

Interprofessional Role Conflict

Conflicts between physicians and APRNs constitute the most common situations of interprofessional conflict. Major sources of conflict for physicians and APRNs are the perceived economic threat of competition, limited resources in clinical training sites, lack of experience working together, and the historical hierarchy. The relationship between anesthesiologists and CRNAs is an exemplar of ongoing conflict and clearly depicts interprofessional role conflict between physicians and APRNs (Exemplar 4.1).

One way to promote positive interprofessional relationships is to provide education and practice experiences that include APRN students, medical students, and both physician and APRN faculty to enhance mutual understanding of both professional roles (Kelly & Mathews, 2001). Developing such interprofessional educational experiences is difficult because of different academic calendars and clinical schedules. However, these obstacles can be overcome if these interdisciplinary activities are considered essential for improved health care delivery and if they have sufficient administrative support (Wynia, Von Kohorn, & Mitchell, 2012).

The issues of professional territoriality and physician concern about being replaced by advanced practice nurses were reported by Lindblad, Hallman, Gillsjö, Lindblad, and Fagerström (2010) from an ethnographic study of the first four graduates in 2005 from the first CNS program in Sweden. The CNSs and general practitioners agreed that the usefulness of the CNSs would have been greater if they had been able to prescribe medications and order treatments. After working with the CNSs, the general practitioners saw them more as an additional resource and complement rather than a threat. By 2009, there were 16 CNSs working in the new role in primary health care. The numbers of advanced practice nurses have increased gradually in Sweden. A study by Altersved, Zetterlund, Lindblad, and Fagerström (2011) indicates that the CNS is recognized as a resource to increase accessibility to more holistic primary care; however, the barriers of limited autonomy and lack of prescriptive authority need to be addressed to further role development.

The complementary nature of advanced practice nursing to medical care is a foreign concept for some physicians, who view all health care as an extension of medical care and see APRNs simply as physician extenders. This misunderstanding of advanced practice nursing underlies physicians' opposition to independent roles for nurses because they believe that APRNs want to practice medicine without a license (see Chapters 1 and 3). In fact, numerous earlier studies of APRN practice have demonstrated that advanced practice roles incorporate a holistic approach that blends elements of nursing and medicine (Brown, 1992; Brykczynski, 1999a, 1999b; Fiandt, 2002; Grando, 1998; Johnson, 1993). However, when APRNs are viewed by physicians as direct competitors, it is understandable that some physicians would be reluctant to be involved in assisting with APRN education (National Commission on Nurse Anesthesia Education, 1990). In addition, some nurse educators have believed that physicians should not be involved in teaching or acting as preceptors for APRNs. Improved relationships between APRNs and physicians will require redefinition of the situation by both groups.

The advocacy of the Interprofessional Education Collaborative Expert Panel (2011) for an interprofessional vision for all health professionals and the recommendation by the Institute of Medicine (2003) that the health professional workforce be prepared to work in interdisciplinary teams underscore the imperative of interprofessional collaboration (see Chapter 12). Competency in interprofessional collaboration is critical for APRNs because it is central to APRN practice (Farrell, Payne, & Heye, 2015). This content is incorporated into the leadership and interprofessional partnership components of *The Essentials of Doctoral Education for Advanced Nursing Practice* (AACN, 2006). Some interesting research has emerged on this issue in Canada and Europe. A participatory action research study conducted in British Columbia, Canada, indicated that NPs viewed collaboration as both a philosophy and a practice: "They cultivated collaborative relations with clients, colleagues, and health care leaders to address concerns of role autonomy and role clarity, extend holistic client-centered care and team capacity, and create strategic alliances to promote

EXEMPLAR 4.1 | **Interprofessional Role Conflict: The Case of Certified Registered Nurse Anesthetists and Anesthesiologists**

For many years, nurse anesthetists have provided high-quality anesthesia care in a variety of settings. They are the primary anesthesia providers in rural US hospitals, as noted on the American Association of Nurse Anesthetists (AANA) website (www.aana.com). According to the AANA (2016), more than 49,000 certified registered nurse anesthetists (CRNAs) provide quality anesthesia care to more than 65% of all patients undergoing surgical or other medical interventions that necessitate the services of an anesthetist (see Chapter 18). The fact that nurse anesthetists predated the first physician anesthesiologists by many years (see Chapter 1) may partly explain why the relationship between anesthesiologists and CRNAs has historically been interpreted by anesthesiologists as one of direct competition, thus creating an adversarial stance. Over the years, this relationship might be characterized as a cold war with overt offensives mounted periodically by anesthesiologists.

In 1970, CRNAs outnumbered anesthesiologists by a ratio of 1.5:1. By 2000, anesthesiologists outnumbered CRNAs (Blumenreich, 2000). Currently there are equal numbers of CRNAs and anesthesiologists; however, an anesthesiologist shortage and a surplus of CRNAs is predicted by 2020 (Conover, 2015; Jordan, 2011). This is one of the factors underlying conflicts over CRNA autonomy (see the AANA website, www.aana.com, for updates on this issue). Another factor is the decision made by the Centers for Medicare and Medicaid Services, after study of the available evidence in 1997, to reimburse nurse anesthetists directly under Medicare (Kleinpell, 2001). In response, anesthesiologists and the American Medical Association launched a major campaign against CRNA autonomy in the operating room, claiming that supervision of CRNAs by physicians is essential for public safety (Federwisch, 1999; Kleinpell, 2001; Stein, 2000; see also Chapter 18). Despite the very active political action committee of the American Nurses Association, the struggle with physicians over limiting the scope of practice of CRNAs is ongoing and reflects the experiences of other advanced practice nurse groups as well. An example of this continuing struggle is the Scope of Practice Partnership (SOPP), a coalition formed by the American Medical Association with other physician organizations to mount initiatives to limit the scope of practice of nonphysician clinicians (Waters, 2007). SOPP funds investigations into the educational preparation and licensure requirements of health care providers with the goal of opposing autonomous practice. SOPP targets all nonphysician providers (Lindeke & Thomas, 2010).

A current issue of role delineation and conflict is the anesthesiologists' efforts to categorize CRNAs and anesthesiologist assistants (AAs) on the same level as mid-level clinicians. Both are nonphysician anesthetists; however, the fundamental difference is that an AA works under the direct supervision of the physician and is trained using the medical model of education. The relationship between nonphysician anesthesia providers mimics the adversarial relationship that previously existed between physician assistants and nurse practitioners. Collegial relationships among the nonphysician providers may be more beneficial for both groups. The American Academy of Anesthesiologist Assistants (2016) website identifies 10 accredited programs for AAs in the United States, and 1800 practicing AAs. There are 114 accredited CRNA programs and approximately 40,000 practicing CRNAs (AANA, 2016). CRNAs are currently educated at the Master's of Science in Nursing level; however, this is changing. By 2025, all CRNAs will be required to have a doctorate for entry into practice (AANA, 2007). Thus the CRNA is achieving what nursing has been struggling with for the past few decades. The quality of care and patient safety provided by the CRNA has been well documented in peer-reviewed journals (AANA, 2016). Physicians still continue to verbalize the need for supervision, quoting patient safety and ignoring the evidence. Role acceptance is an ongoing issue for all advanced practice registered nurses. Progress is being made, but active participation and a strong voice are still needed to bring about the much-needed change. ◎

---

innovation and system change" (Burgess & Purkis, 2010, p. 300). Of particular importance is the fact that the NP participants described themselves as being nurses first and practitioners second. This is significant because when role emphasis is on physician replacement and support rather than on the patient-centered, health-focused, holistic nursing orientation to practice, the nursing components of the role become less valued and invisible (Bryant-Lukosius, DiCenso, Browne, & Pinelli, 2004). Medically driven and illness-oriented health systems tend to devalue these value-added components of APRN roles, and reimbursement mechanisms for including these aspects of care are lacking.

Fleming and Carberry (2011) reported on a grounded theory study of expert critical care nurses transitioning to advanced practice in an intensive care unit setting in Scotland. Initial perceptions were that the advanced practice nursing role was closely aligned with medical practice, but later perceptions supported earlier studies that the advanced practice nursing role was characterized by an integrated, holistic, patient-centered approach to care, which was close to the medical model but different because it was carried out within an expert nursing knowledge base. The authors determined that further research is needed to explore the outcomes of this integrated practice. This is the research imperative for advanced practice nursing—to demonstrate the impact of the holistic nursing approach to care on patient outcomes.

Nurse-midwives have been in the forefront of developing collaborative relationships with physicians for many years. All APRN groups would benefit from attention to the progress that CNMs have made in collaboration with physicians. The joint practice statement of the American College of Obstetricians and Gynecologists (ACOG) and the American College of Nurse-Midwives (2011) can be used as a model for other APRN groups. It highlights key principles for improving communication, working relationships, and seamlessness in the provision of women's health services (see also the American College of Nurse-Midwives website, www.acnm.org). Problems with previous joint practice statements were that they included varying interpretations of physician supervision. The Executive Summary of the Task Force for Collaboration in Practice and Implementing Team-based Care released by the ACOG in 2016 defines team-based care as involving at least two health care providers working collaboratively with patients as full participants, with health care providers functioning to the full extent of their education, certification, and experience (ACOG, 2016).

Role Transitions

Role transitions are defined here as dynamic processes of change that occur over time as new roles are acquired (see Table 4.1). The middle-range transitions theory of Meleis, Sawyer, Im, Hilfinger-Messias, and Schumacher (2000) has been widely used in both undergraduate and graduate education. It can be helpful for understanding and addressing the situational transitions associated with APRN role development. Five essential factors influence role transitions (Schumacher & Meleis, 1994): (1) personal meaning

of the transition, which relates to the degree of identity crisis experienced; (2) degree of planning, which involves the time and energy devoted to anticipating the change; (3) environmental barriers and supports, which refer to family, peer, school, and other components; (4) level of knowledge and skill, which relates to prior experience and school experiences; and (5) expectations, which are related to such factors as role models, literature, and media. The role strain experienced by individuals in response to role insufficiency (see Table 4.1 for definitions) that accompanies the transition to APRN roles can be minimized, although certainly not completely prevented, by individualized assessment of these five essential factors, development of strategies to cope with them, and rehearsal of situations designed for application of these strategies. Entering graduate school may be associated with a ripple effect of concurrent role transitions in family, work, and other social arenas (Klaich, 1990).

Advanced Practice Nurse Role Acquisition in Graduate School

The personal meaning of role transitions has been a major focus of APRN role development literature over the years, with alterations in self-identity and self-concept emerging as a consistent theme and role acquisition experiences sometimes described as identity crises (Roberts, Tabloski, & Bova, 1997). Studies of APRN role acquisition in school are outlined in Table 4.2.

In their study of NP students, Roberts et al. (1997) reported findings similar to those observed decades earlier by Anderson, Leonard, and Yates (1974). The description by Anderson et al. (1974) of NP students' progression from dependence to interdependence being accompanied by regression, anxiety, and conflict was found to be similar to observations made by Roberts et al. (1997) in graduate NP students over a period of 6 years (see Table 4.2). For many years, we (the authors) and our NP faculty colleagues have observed similar role transition processes in teaching role and clinical courses for graduate NP students. In a discussion of role transition experiences for neonatal NPs (NNPs), Cusson and Viggiano (2002) made the important point that even positive transitions are stressful.

Roberts et al. (1997) identified three major areas of transition as students progressed from dependence to interdependence: (1) development of professional competence, (2) change in role identity, and (3) evolving relationships with preceptors and faculty.

TABLE 4.2	APRN Student Role Transition Studies in School: Role Acquisition[a]		
Researchers	Method	Participants	Noteworthy Findings
Anderson, Leonard, & Yates (1974)	Descriptive observational study	NP students in a graduate program, a postbaccalaureate certificate program, and a continuing education program University of Minnesota	Four-stage process of NP role development: 1. Complete dependence 2. Developing competence 3. Independence 4. Interdependence
Roberts, Tabloski, & Bova (1997)	Descriptive study of observations of students and written clinical journals	100 NP students over 6 years University of Massachusetts	Four-stage transition process identified by Anderson et al. (1974) was validated in this study.
Steiner, McLaughlin, Hyde, Brown, & Burman (2008)	Descriptive correlational questionnaire	208 FNP graduates Wyoming and Idaho	Follow-up to Heitz et al. (2004) study to validate educational phase findings. Preceptor guidance was found to be a greater positive force than faculty guidance.
Spoelstra & Robbins (2010)	Descriptive qualitative thematic analysis	24 MSN students in first semester Role course Michigan	Overarching theme: the essence of nursing Three subthemes: 1. Importance of building a framework for advanced nursing practice 2. Importance of direct care 3. Importance of professional leadership supported by ethical values
Fleming & Carberry (2011)	Grounded theory	Two cohorts: 5 critical care nurse advanced practice trainees in first cohort; 4 in second cohort Intensive care units Scotland	Transition occurred in four areas: 1. Finding a niche 2. Coping with pressures 3. Feeling competent 4. Internalizing the role

[a]Studies are listed in chronological order.
FNP, Family nurse practitioner; *MSN*, Master's of Science in Nursing; *NP*, nurse practitioner.

The lowest level of competence coincided with the highest level of role confusion. This occurred at the end of the first semester and the beginning of the second semester in the three-semester program examined. Roberts et al. observed that the most intense transition period typically occurred at the end of the students' first clinical immersion experience.

Roberts et al. (1997) described the first transition as involving an initial feeling of loss of confidence and competence accompanied by anxiety. Initial clinical experiences were associated with the desire to observe rather than provide care, the inability to recall simple facts, the omission of essential data from history taking, feelings of awkwardness with patients, and difficulty prioritizing data. The students' focus at this time was almost exclusively on acquiring and refining assessment skills and continued development of physical examination techniques. By the end of the first semester, students reported returning feelings of confidence and the regaining of their former competence in interpersonal skills. Although

they were still tentative about diagnostic and treatment decisions, students reported feeling more comfortable with patients as some of their basic nursing abilities began to return.

Transitions in nursing role identity occurring during the first two stages were associated with feelings of role confusion. Students were dismayed at how slowly and inefficiently they were performing in clinical situations and reported feelings of self-doubt and lack of confidence in their abilities to function in the real world of health care. They sought shortcuts in attempts to increase their efficiency. They reported profound feelings of responsibility regarding diagnostic and treatment decisions and, at the same time, increasingly realized the limitations of clinical practice when they were confronted with the real-life situations of their patients. They recalled finding it easy to second-guess physicians' decisions in their previous nursing roles, but now they found those decisions more problematic when they were responsible for making them. They joked about feeling like adolescents. This is the point that Cusson and Viggiano (2002) were making when they commented, in reference to NNPs, that the infant really does look different when viewed from the head of the bed rather than the side of the bed. They explained that "rather than taking orders, as they did as staff nurses, neonatal NPs must synthesize incredibly complex information and decide on a plan of action. Experienced neonatal nurses often guide house staff regarding care decisions and writing orders to match the care that is being given. However, the shift in responsibility to actually writing the orders can be very intimidating" (p. 24).

Roberts et al. (1997) observed that a blending of the APRN student and the former nurse developed during stage II of the transition process as students renewed their appreciation for their previous interpersonal skills as teachers, supporters, and collaborators and again perceived their patients as unique individuals in the context of their life situations. Students developed increased awareness of the uncertainty involved in the process of making definitive diagnostic and treatment decisions. In spite of current attempts to reduce diagnostic and treatment uncertainty through evidence-based practice, a basic degree of uncertainty is still inherent in clinical practice. Although these insights served to demystify the clinical diagnostic process, the students' anxiety about providing care increased. Learning about strategies to cope with clinical decision making in situations of uncertainty, such as ruling out the worst case scenario, seeking consultation, and monitoring patients closely with phone calls and follow-up visits, can decrease anxiety and promote increased confidence (Brykczynski, 1991).

The transition in the relationships between students and preceptors and students and faculty in the study by Roberts et al. (1997) involved students feeling anxious that they were not learning enough and would never know enough to practice competently. Students felt frustrated and perceived that faculty and preceptors were not providing them with all the information they needed. During the third stage, as they felt more confident and competent, students began to question the clinical judgments of their preceptors and faculty. This process is thought to help students advance from independence to interdependence—the last stage of the transition process. Much of the conflict at this juncture appeared to derive from students' feelings of "ambivalence about giving up dependence on external authorities" (Roberts et al., 1997, p. 71) such as preceptors and faculty and assuming responsibility for making independent judgments based on their own assessments from their clinical and educational experiences and the literature. The relevance of these role acquisition processes for other APRN roles has not been reported. This is an area in which research would be helpful.

Fleming and Carberry's (2011) qualitative study of critical care nurse advanced practice trainees in Scotland provides confirmation of the experiences described here. They noted the trainees' feelings of inadequacy associated with moving from expert to novice and their anxiety and frustration over dealing with the role ambiguity of moving into a hybrid nursing and medical role. After a 12-month period, the trainees found their role "characterized by an integrated holistic patient-centered approach to care" (p. 74).

Until recently, the literature on APRN role acquisition in school has focused exclusively on individuals who were already nurses. A commonly held assumption among nurses is "the more clinical experience, the better" for acquiring the necessary knowledge and skill to take on complex APRN roles. At least 1 year of nursing practice is typically preferred for admission to APRN programs. The process of role acquisition for students in direct-entry APRN master's programs that admit non-nurse college graduates may differ because these individuals were not functioning as nurses before they entered the program. For additional information regarding this topic, the reader is referred to the qualitative study reported by Rich and Rodriguez (2002). In their qualitative study of family nurse practitioner (FNP) role transition, Heitz et al. (2004) found differences in role acquisition experiences between FNP students who were inexperienced nurses and FNP students who were experienced nurses. Feelings of insecurity, inadequacy, vulnerability, and being overwhelmed were typical, but role confusion was reported primarily by the more experienced RN students as they went through the process of letting go of the RN role and taking on the FNP role. It will be interesting to observe whether this finding holds true for students transitioning from the Bachelor of Science in Nursing to the DNP.

Strategies to Facilitate Role Acquisition

The anticipatory socialization to APRN roles that occurs in graduate education is analogous to a process that Kramer (1974) described for undergraduate RNs called "immunization." This same process is referred to as role supplementation in transitions theory

(Schumacher & Meleis, 1994). The overall objective is to expose students to as many real-life experiences as possible during the educational program to minimize reality shock and role insufficiency on graduation and initial role implementation. Role content can be incorporated into APRN curricula in a variety of ways, including: (1) in the overall framework for designing an APRN curriculum; (2) in a specific role course (see, e.g., Spoelstra & Robbins, 2010); (3) as part of specific assignments; and (4) in role seminars that span an entire curriculum. Hamric and Hanson (2003) asserted that it is an ethical mandate for all APRN educators, regardless of specialty, to provide graduates with up-to-date knowledge of professional role and regulatory issues in addition to concentration on clinical competence. The importance of explicit role preparation for the complex and challenging roles of graduates of DNP programs is recognized in the curriculum proposed by the AACN (2006). If there is not a separate role course, careful attention must be paid to this curriculum component so that it does not become integrated out of existence.

Specific strategies for facilitating role acquisition can be categorized according to three major purposes: (1) role rehearsal; (2) development of clinical knowledge and skills, including strategies for dealing with uncertainty; and (3) creation of a supportive network (Table 4.3). Rites of passage can be useful for signifying advancement to a new level of practice and set the stage for role rehearsal. The Willow Ceremony is a rite of passage developed at the University of Wyoming to commemorate beginning an APRN program (Burman, Hart, Conley, Caldwell, & Johnson, 2007). For adequate role rehearsal, APRN students should experience all aspects of the core competencies (see Chapter 3) directly while faculty and fellow students are available to help them process or debrief these experiences. Faculty can help students by identifying role acquisition periods of high stress in their particular program so that support can be built in during those periods. APRN students should be cautioned that other nurses, physicians, other providers, and administrators in the work setting may value only clinical expertise and not the other core competencies. Strategies for enhancing understanding of how the core competencies are embedded in each APRN role include preparation of short-term and long-term goals to use as guides in the development of professional portfolios, analysis of existing position descriptions, and development of the ideal position description. These are also helpful for guiding students in their search for an initial APRN position.

Clinical Knowledge Development

The development of clinical knowledge and skills for APRN role acquisition can be promoted by planning for realistic clinical experiences with the support of faculty and preceptors nearby. Steiner, McLaughlin, Hyde, Brown, and Burman (2008) pointed out the importance of teaching students how to learn and how to use resources to find out what they need to know. Emphasis on realism and a holistic situational perspective are important in clinical experiences for helping students understand that the complex clinical judgments involved in APRN assessment and management of patient situations over time are not simply technical medical knowledge but a hybrid of nursing and medical knowledge and experience. Teaching and learning experiences for all the APRN role components should integrate elements of research and theory and be incorporated into specialty APRN courses to build on the knowledge gained in the traditional graduate core and clinical support courses in the curriculum. New APRN graduates can benefit from familiarity with role transition processes by not expecting to be able to demonstrate all APRN role components fully and expertly immediately on graduation.

Clinical mentoring by preceptors is an important component of ensuring realistic clinical learning experiences and socialization into advanced practice nursing roles (AACN, 2015b; Burns et al., 2006; Donley et al., 2014). APRN student enrollment has increased markedly in the face of APRN faculty shortages, and APRN students enter clinical training experiences across the curriculum with varied skill levels (AACN, 2015). Identifying qualified and available preceptors is challenging and time consuming for faculty and support staff (Multi-discipline Clerkship/Clinical Training Site Survey, 2014). Students are matched with qualified APRN and non-nurse preceptors to provide learning opportunities, ensure development of required clinical skills, and foster the team concept. Course objectives, the advanced practice essentials (whether master's or doctoral), core competencies for the specific APRN role, and a preceptor learning agreement provide the basic structure and overall direction for faculty, preceptors, and students. Clinical faculty are responsible for conducting site visits and convening clinical conferences to evaluate learning. APRN course faculty are responsible for student, clinical faculty, preceptor, and clinical site evaluation and overall maintenance of high-quality educational standards. APRN students are linked with preceptors for one-on-one guidance in developing clinical skills and judgment. This

TABLE 4.3	Strategies to Promote APRN Role Acquisition in School	
Purpose	**Strategies**	**Implementation**
Role rehearsal	Rite of passage	Ceremony to signify moving into development of a new role.
	Role course	Provide overall framework for APRN role development and begin anticipatory guidance role development thread for entire program.
	Directly experience all core skills	Faculty and students monitor experience in all core competencies.
	Create professional marketing portfolio	Prepare an electronic portfolio containing, for example, philosophy of care, résumé, clinical experiences, ideal position description, salary data, certification details, and APRN brochures.
	Lifelike role negotiation seminar	Invite interprofessional guests.
	Identify with a role model or mentor	Develop mentee relationship with an APRN and maintain contact throughout the APRN program.
	Burning question interviews	Develop a list of important questions to ask APRNs relevant to future role satisfaction.
	Panel discussions	Faculty and students can plan discussion with various panels to increase understanding of issues such as potential positions available, practice settings, and other health team members.
	Critical incident presentations	Prepare an in-depth self-evaluation of a role conflict situation experienced in learning the APRN role and share this with peers and faculty.
	Interprofessional educational experiences	Shared courses in, for example, assessment, pharmacology, ethical and legal issues, and service learning experiences.
Develop clinical knowledge and skills	Realistic clinical immersion experiences	Clinical experiences need to reflect the real world of practice as much as possible.
	Clinical conferences	Discussion of clinical experiences with faculty and peers promotes clinical understanding.
	Clinical situation narrative seminars	Share full contextual details of situations to promote understanding of aspects of embedded clinical practice knowledge.
	Case study analysis	Clinical examples make classroom learning more concrete and memorable.
	Clinical logs	Maintain an electronic log of all patients seen, with pertinent details such as age, diagnosis, interventions, and outcomes.
	Final clinical preceptorships	A final semester of clinical practice helps put it all together.
	Faculty practice	Maintenance of faculty clinical competence enhances the credibility of APRN faculty.
Create a support network	Establish a peer support system	Join local, state, and national APRN groups.
	Share self- and peer evaluations	Learn to be comfortable with giving and receiving feedback for improvement.
	Faculty-student-preceptor social functions	Foster an APRN-supportive environment among faculty, clinicians, students, staff, and administrators.
	Establish a pattern for continuing education	Subscribe to selected APRN journals, participate in APRN conferences, and keep a record of continuing education hours.
	Create a virtual community	Establish electronic mail, social media, and Internet connections.
	Establish a self-monitoring system	Select a framework for self-evaluating role performance to keep track of progress in role transition over time.
	Form a self-care program	Develop health care practices to maintain and improve health, such as stress management, getting adequate sleep, rest, exercise, and a nutritious diet.

Adapted from Brykczynski, K. A. (2000). Chart 1-6: Strategies to promote NP role acquisition in school. In P. Meredith & N. M. Horan (Eds.), *Adult primary care* (p. 16). Philadelphia: WB Saunders.

apprenticeship model of education is time intensive and costly (AACN, 2015b).

All of these challenges require APRN educational programs to explore new and alternative models for providing clinical training, including increased use of low- and high-fidelity simulation to support clinical experiences and to evaluate students, and increased attention to interprofessional practice (AACN, 2015b). In 2012, the Centers for Medicare and Medicaid Services (CMS) launched the Graduate Nurse Education Demonstration project to increase the numbers of primary care NPs in an effort to address the increasing need for access to primary care providers (CMS, 2012). The CMS provided reimbursement for eligible hospitals to participate in the demonstration project in five major cities (Hospital of the University of Pennsylvania, Philadelphia, PA; Duke University Hospital, Durham, NC;

Scottsdale Healthcare Medical Center, Scottsdale, AZ; Rush University Medical Center, Chicago, IL; and Memorial Hermann-Texas Medical Center Hospital, Houston, TX). The hospitals partnered with accredited advanced practice nursing programs and reimbursed preceptors for training NP students (American Association of Nurse Practitioners [AANP], 2012). Project funding had already started decreasing by 2016, and a current concern is that preceptors may now expect reimbursement (CMS, 2015). Incentivizing community preceptors with educational opportunities, documentation of preceptor hours for recertification, and library access may motivate participation in the student-preceptor collaborative relationship (AACN, 2015b; Donley et al., 2014). Collaboration between schools of nursing and health care agencies in developing more formal systems of rewards and benefits that facilitate professional development and career mobility for preceptors is imperative for enhancing their recruitment and retention (AACN, 2015a; Donley et al., 2014).

Anticipatory planning for the first APRN position after program completion is important. In the current cost-constrained environment, the pressure to be cost-effective and to make an impact on health outcomes is greater than ever, but studies have shown that the initial year of practice is one of transition (Brown & Olshansky, 1998; Kelly & Mathews, 2001) and that an APRN's maximum potential may not be realized until after approximately 5 or more years in practice (Cooper & Sparacino, 1990). Reports of the transition experiences of new NP graduates during their first year after graduation suggest that the first position can be critical in terms of solidifying the NP's career (Brown & Olshansky, 1997; Heitz et al., 2004; Kelly & Mathews, 2001; Steiner et al., 2008). Preparation of students for assuming APRN roles on graduation should be a collaborative effort of students, faculty, and preceptors. The need for position descriptions that clearly outline roles and responsibilities has been emphasized as essential for smooth role transition (Cooper & Sparacino, 1990; Hamric & Taylor, 1989; McMyler & Miller, 1997). The transition to the first position is a process, not an event, that may take 6 months to 2 years (Steiner et al., 2008). It needs to be a focus of role content in APRN programs (Hamric & Hanson, 2003; Hunter, Bormann, & Lops, 1996).

Finally, and perhaps most importantly, an overall strategy for enhancing APRN clinical knowledge and skill is for faculty to maintain competency in clinical practice. Clinical competency enhances the faculty's ability to evaluate students clinically, discuss clinically relevant examples in classes, serve as preceptors for students, and evaluate the care provided in clinical preceptorship sites. The clinical competence of faculty is important to prevent a wide gap between education and practice, enhance faculty credibility, and foster realistic expectations for new APRN graduates.

Developing a Supportive Network

Establishing a peer support system, planning social functions with faculty and preceptors, and creating a virtual community can facilitate the development of a support network. The importance of forming a support network was emphasized by study findings (Kelly & Mathews, 2001; Kleinpell-Nowell, 2001). Computer literacy is critical for networking and access to the high-quality materials available on websites, in literature searches, and on smartphones. Students need expanded informatics skills and understanding of emerging technologies, including genetics and genomics, less invasive diagnostic tools and treatments, three-dimensional printing, robotics, biometrics, electronic health records, computerized provider order entry, and clinical decision support, to enhance their ability to practice (Huston, 2013). Neurocognitive theory provides evidence-based approaches to improving learning incorporating a wide variety of multimedia tools. Instructional design has added visual comprehension through videos, simulation, and interactive programs (Anderson, Love, & Tsai, 2014).

The establishment of a system for self-directed learning activities during the first few years after program completion forms the basis for maintaining competence throughout one's career (Gunn, 1998). The formation of a process for lifelong learning should be initiated during the APRN educational program as students create a computer-based, self-monitoring system that includes clinical and role transition experiences over time to serve as a reality check or timetable. On graduation, continuing education program attendance could be incorporated into this monitoring system to facilitate compilation of necessary documentation for certification, along with ongoing self-evaluation and role development. This information can be incorporated into students' online portfolios to centralize all career materials in one place.

Students need to be encouraged to develop and maintain self-care practices during their stressful educational experiences that they can continue when they move into the challenges of the practice arena.

Faculty can serve as role models for healthy lifestyles and incorporate analysis of self-care practices into assignments to aid students in developing improved well-being. Students invariably develop renewed appreciation from these self-care assignments for how difficult it is to change health habits, and they can share knowledge they gain from these learning experiences with peers and patients.

Advanced Practice Nursing Role Implementation at Work

After successfully emerging from the APRN educational process, new APRN graduates face yet another transition, from the student role to the professional APRN role, referred to as role implementation in this text (see Fig. 4.1). APRN graduates can be expected to experience attitudinal, behavioral, and value conflicts as they move from the academic world, in which holistic care is highly valued, to the work world, in which organizational efficiency is paramount. Anticipatory guidance is needed for role transition yet again. The process of APRN role implementation is another situational transition (Schumacher & Meleis, 1994) that is described here as a progressive movement through three or four phases or stages. In the APRN role development literature the term *phase* is used by some and the term *stage* is used by others (Poronsky, 2013). After checking several dictionaries, it is clear that the terms are synonymous and can be used interchangeably. One term is often favored over another in different fields; for example, in pharmacology drug trials are referred to in different phases whereas in human development the term *stage* is preferred. For the discussion here, the terms *phase* and *stage* are used as cited in the different studies (Table 4.4).

Hamric and Taylor (1989) described seven phases of CNS role development (see Table 4.4). There is general agreement that significant overlap and fluidity exist among the phases; however, for purposes of discussion they are considered sequentially. Of 42 CNSs in their first positions for 3 years or less, 40 experienced progression through the first three phases (identical to the first three phases identified by Baker [1979]). Most of the CNS respondents went through these three phases within 2 years. Phase 1, the orientation phase, is characterized by enthusiasm, optimism, and attention to mastery of clinical skills. Phase 2, the frustration phase, is associated with feelings of conflict, inadequacy, frustration, and anxiety. Arena and Page (1992) identified the imposter phenomenon as a feature of CNS practice

that could interfere with effective role implementation. In retrospect, it appears that the imposter phenomenon is one of the distressing features of the frustration phase. Phase 3, implementation, involves role modification in response to interactions with others and development of more realistic perspective as role expectations are adjusted.

CNSs with more than 3 years of experience described their role development experiences in terms very different from Baker's (1979) phases. Content analysis of these data led to a description of four additional phases (see Table 4.4). Experienced CNSs identified the integration phase, which was characterized by "self-confidence and assurance in the role, high job satisfaction, an advanced level of practice, and signs of recognition and respect for expertise within and outside the work setting" (Hamric & Taylor, 1989, p. 56). Only 10% of the CNSs with less than 5 years of experience in the role met the criteria for this phase, whereas 50% of those with more than 6 years of experience could be categorized as being in this phase. The integration phase was typically reached after 3 to 5 years in the CNS role. This fourth phase of integration—thought to be reached only after successful transition through the earlier phases—is characterized by refinement of clinical expertise and integration of role components appropriate for the particular situation.

Llahana and Hamric (2011) studied the role development experiences of diabetes specialist nurses (DSNs) in Great Britain who were not all master's prepared, although most held postgraduate qualification in diabetes care. Their findings indicated that role development phases were similar to those in Hamric and Taylor's earlier study (see Table 4.4). The anxiety experienced during the additional transition phase identified when an experienced DSN moved to a different practice site was related to orienting to a new work setting rather than to knowledge or competence in the role.

Hamric and Taylor (1989) also described three negative phases not evident in previous literature. The frozen phase is described as being associated with frustration, anger, and lack of career satisfaction. Restructuring of role responsibilities and changing organizational expectations characterize the reorganization phase. The complacent phase is characterized by comfort, stability, and maintenance of the status quo. Unlike the integration phase, these additional phases share a negative, nonproductive character. It is of interest that there was a higher proportion of nurses in negative phases (58%) in the British study (Llahana & Hamric, 2011) than

TABLE 4.4 APRN Role Transition Studies in Practice: Role Implementation[a]

Researchers	Method	Participants	Noteworthy Findings
Baker (1979)	Retrospective interviews	4 CNSs California	Four-phase role development: 1. Orientation 2. Frustration 3. Implementation 4. Reassessment
Hamric & Taylor (1989)	Questionnaire	100 CNSs US national	Seven-phase role development: 1. Orientation 2. Frustration 3. Implementation 4. Integration 5. Frozen 6. Reorganization 7. Complacent
Brown & Olshansky (1997)	One-year longitudinal grounded theory	35 FNPs first year in practice Washington	Four-stage transition: 1. Laying the Foundation 2. Launching 3. Meeting the Challenge 4. Broadening the Perspective
Kelly & Mathews (2001)	Focus group	21 recent NP graduates Illinois	Lack of control over workload Lack of support from nurses and physicians Loss of previous relationships Role ambiguity Difficulty incorporating holistic care and health promotion Personal satisfaction, increased confidence and autonomy Network of supportive peers helpful for coping with demands
Heitz, Steiner, & Burman (2004)	Grounded theory Telephone interviews	9 recent FNP graduates Western US	Role transition occurs in two phases. Phase 1 occurs in graduate school. • Faculty guidance was found to be a dominant force. • Greater role confusion was experienced by students with more RN experience prior to entering the program. Phase 2 occurs in practice over a 6-month to 2-year period following graduation.
Chang, Mu, & Tsay (2006)	Qualitative Inquiry	10 acute care NPs during first year of practice Taiwan	Findings similar to Brown & Olshansky (1997) study However, only three phases were described as follows: 1. Role ambiguity—similar to "Laying the Foundation" 2. Role acquisition—similar to "Launching" 3. Role implementation—covers both "Meeting the challenge" and "Broadening the perspective"
Cusson & Strange (2008)	Descriptive qualitative survey questionnaire	70 NNPs from 1 to 28 years in NNP practice; mean 13.9 years 21 US states	Four themes described as follows: 1. Ambivalence re: adequacy of preparation for role 2. Transition to NNP role described as difficult, uncomfortable, and stressful 3. Making it as a real NNP—1 year was a consistent benchmark 4. Helpers and hinderers—support of neonatologists, staff nurses, and unit managers was helpful Poor professional behavior of some staff nurses and other NNPs hindered role implementation.

Continued

TABLE 4.4   **APRN Role Transition Studies in Practice: Role Implementation[a]—cont'd**

Researchers	Method	Participants	Noteworthy Findings
Sullivan-Bentz et al. (2010)	Descriptive qualitative focused ethnography Narrative analysis	23 recent NP graduates during first year of practice 21 co-participants (physicians and NPs) Ontario, Canada	Brown & Olshansky's (1997) four-stage transition model formed the conceptual framework for the study. Findings from this study reflected many of the findings from the earlier study. By the end of the first year, NPs transitioned from feeling overwhelmed to feeling confident in their new role.
Glasgow & Zoucha (2011)	Descriptive and interpretive phenomenology	9 DNP graduates: 3 faculty, 4 practice, 1 dual faculty and practice, 1 executive roles Pennsylvania and New Jersey	Shared themes: 1. Changing context of DNP role: uncertainty, misunderstanding, tension 2. Feelings of confidence and empowerment in making decisions more autonomously 3. Finding one's way and responding to opportunity
Llahana & Hamric (2011)	Questionnaire based on Hamric & Taylor (1989) questionnaire	334 DSNs nationwide in UK	Validated experience of all 7 role development phases from Hamric & Taylor (1989) study by at least one DSN. An eighth phase, "transition," was identified for experienced DSNs who moved from one practice setting to another after having moved through the implementation and integration phases.
Desborough (2012)	Grounded theory	7 NPs in interviews; 5 of these in focus group Australia	Five major themes: 1. Developing clinical practice guidelines 2. Collaborating with the multidisciplinary team 3. Developing legitimacy and clinical credibility 4. Communicating 5. Transitioning to practice

[a]Studies are listed in chronological order.

CNSs, Clinical nurse specialists; *DSNs,* diabetes specialist nurses; *FNP,* family nurse practitioner; *MSN,* Master's of Science in Nursing; *NNP,* neonatal nurse practitioner; *NP,* nurse practitioner.

reported in the original Hamric and Taylor (1989) study (27%). One might speculate that APRNs experiencing these negative phases would be more vulnerable to position changes in today's cost-constrained health care system.

APRN role development processes are further delineated by findings from Brown and Olshansky's (1997) study of the role transition experiences of novice NPs during their first year of practice. Their characterization of this role transition process as moving from "limbo to legitimacy" is supported by Cusson and Strange's (2008) finding that 1 year in practice constituted a consistent benchmark for NNPs moving from ambivalence to "making it as a real NNP" and by Sullivan-Bentz et al.'s (2010) observation that NPs transition from feeling overwhelmed to feeling confident by the end of the first year of practice. The four-stage process identified by Brown and Olshansky (1997) is outlined in Table 4.4. The first stage, laying the foundation, was not described in previous literature. During this stage, new graduates take certification examinations, obtain necessary recognition or licensure from state boards of nursing,

and look for positions. This stage has been shortened because of the availability of online certification examinations.

The second stage, launching, was defined as beginning with the first NP position and lasting at least 3 months. During this stage, the new graduate NP experiences the anxiety associated with the crisis of confidence and competence that accompanies taking on a new position and the return to the advanced beginner skill level (Benner, Tanner, & Chesla, 2009; Dreyfus & Dreyfus, 1986, 2009). As the advanced beginner becomes increasingly aware of the number of elements relevant to actual performance in the role, he or she may become overwhelmed with the complexity of the skills required for the role and exhausted by the effort required for mastery. New NPs in Kelly and Mathews' (2001) study described similar experiences of exhaustion and frustration with lack of control over time. This is the at-work version of the crisis of confidence and competence experienced during stage 1 of the in-school role acquisition process (Roberts et al., 1997).

The feeling of being "an imposter" or "a fake," described by Brown and Olshansky (1997), Arena and Page (1992), and Huffstutler and Varnell (2006), was first reported in the psychologic literature in reference to high-achieving women (Clance & Imes, 1978). Clinical symptoms associated with this phenomenon—generalized anxiety, lack of self-confidence, depression, and frustration—are commonly reported by APRNs experiencing the frustration phase or launching stage. It is related to feeling unable to meet one's own expectations and those of others (Clance & Imes, 1978) and feelings of inadequacy and constantly being tested (Arena & Page, 1992). This phenomenon is typically a temporary experience associated with taking on a new role or beginning a new job. The Heitz et al. (2004) study related similar role transition experiences of self-doubt, disillusionment, and turbulence and also reported that engaging in positive self-talk was helpful. They suggested that issues of gender and age may underlie differing perceptions of personal commitments and sacrifices as obstacles to surmount in role transition.

Although Brown and Olshansky (1997, 1998) did not relate their findings about NP role transition to Hamric and Taylor's (1989) findings about CNS role development, there appear to be many similarities in the results of the two studies. The characteristics of Brown and Olshansky's launching stage are similar to those described by Hamric and Taylor for the frustration phase. Brown and Olshansky's third stage, meeting the challenge, is associated with feelings of regaining confidence and increasing competence. This stage has much in common with Hamric and Taylor's implementation phase, which is noted for returning optimism and enthusiasm as expectations are realigned. Brown and Olshansky's last stage, broadening the perspective, is characterized by feelings of legitimacy and competency as NPs. This last stage is similar to Hamric and Taylor's fourth phase of integration, during which the role is expanded and refined. The majority of NP role transition studies have been conducted with recent graduates; therefore, there are scant data to indicate whether or not NPs move on to the fourth phase of integration or develop any of the negative phases identified by Hamric and Taylor (1989) with CNSs or Llahana and Hamric (2011) with DSNs.

Rich (2005) investigated the relationship between duration of experience as an RN and NP clinical skills in practice among NPs who graduated within 4 years from three universities in the Northeast.

These graduates, 150 NPs, completed the self-report instrument assessments of their clinical skills (a response rate of 21%), and 60% of the collaborating physicians completed assessments of their NP clinical skills. Findings from the NP self-report data indicated that duration of practice experience as an RN was not correlated with level of competency in NP practice skills. "An unexpected finding was that there was a significant negative correlation between years of experience as an RN and NP clinical practice skills as assessed by the collaborating physicians" (Rich, 2005, p. 55). Data describing which role development phases the NP participants were experiencing or had experienced would have been helpful for enhancing understanding of the findings. The finding that collaborating physicians rated the NPs as more clinically competent than the NPs rated themselves (Rich, 2005) would be expected for NPs in the frustration phase or launching stage (see Table 4.4). Inclusion of assessments of role development and clinical competency in APRN follow-up studies would be helpful for building on the existing knowledge base.

Whether the frozen, reorganization, and complacent phases are distinct developmental phases or variations of the implementation and integration phases, they are clearly negative resolutions for APRNs and their organizations. APRNs should engage in periodic self-assessment so that they recognize beginning signs associated with these phases, such as feelings of anger or dissatisfaction, conflict between self-goals and those of the organization or supervisor, feeling pressure to change one's APRN role in ways that are incongruent with one's concept of the role, and feelings of complacency. Early recognition of problems and taking proactive steps to adapt to organizational changes can help prevent or ameliorate the negative feelings associated with these phases.

APRNs can keep track of their role transition process by setting specific time-limited goals, forming peer networks, and seeking out mentors. Further analysis of the relationships between the stages and phases of transitions during role implementation described here and outlined in Table 4.4 is needed. The relevance of these frameworks for transition processes experienced by other APRNs also needs study. It is promising to see some studies building on previous research. Further refinement of these findings could lead to their incorporation into APRN teaching, research, and practice and provide support for health care policy changes.

Summary Observations on Transition Studies Following Graduation

Examination of the findings from the diverse studies of APRN role transition following graduation in Table 4.4 leads to some important observations. Most studies are of recent APRN graduates and findings fairly consistently indicate a three-phase or three-stage process moving from advanced beginner competency to competency or proficiency during the first year of practice in terms of the novice-to-expert framework; from limbo to legitimacy in the Brown and Olshansky (1997) work; from frustration to implementation in the Baker (1979) and Hamric and Taylor (1989) work; or from ambiguity to role implementation in Chang, Mu, and Tsay's (2006) work. These studies indicate that the first year of APRN practice is commonly associated with a significantly difficult process of transition.

APRN programs are designed to prepare graduates for beginning, entry-level clinical competency. The questionnaire study conducted by Hart and Macnee (2007) at two national NP conferences found that 51% of NPs perceived that they were only somewhat or minimally prepared for actual practice. The demands of the current health care system can be overwhelming for new APRNs coping with the transition to practice. Clinical residency programs have been developed recently to address role transition issues of new APRN graduates (Bush & Lowry, 2016; Flinter, 2012; Sargent & Olmedo, 2013; Thabault, Mylott, & Patterson, 2015). They are typically a year in length and are designed to enhance new graduate transition into practice, promote quality patient care, and increase NP retention and satisfaction. Flinter (2012) pointed out the need to advocate for federal funding to support graduate APRN residency training. The fact that graduate NP residents are licensed and certified and their services are billable can help to offset some of the costs of such programs.

Strategies to Facilitate Role Implementation

The phases described by Hamric and Taylor (1989) are used here to structure discussion of strategies to facilitate transitions during APRN role implementation (Table 4.5). The clinical residency programs for new graduates noted earlier constitute an overall approach for enhancing transition through the first three phases of postgraduate role implementation and ending with the fourth phase, integration. A national collaboration of NP organizations has recommended that these postgraduate programs be referred to as "fellowships" rather than "residencies" to minimize confusion because they are not required for entry into practice, as are clinical residencies for physicians (AANP NP Roundtable, 2014).

Orientation Phase

The importance of being patient and recognizing that it takes time to develop fully in a new APRN role was stressed by NPs in Kleinpell-Nowell's surveys (1999, 2001). A strategy to facilitate role implementation for all APRNs during the orientation phase is development of a structured orientation plan (Goldschmidt, Rust, Torowicz, & Kolb, 2011). Sharrock, Javen, and McDonald (2013) described the contribution of clinical supervision to support nurses transitioning into new advanced practice roles. Brown and Olshansky (1997, 1998) noted the importance of clarification of values, needs, and expectations and of recognition that transitional experiences are time-limited. They also noted the importance of anticipatory guidance and realizing that these transition experiences follow a common pattern in new graduates. An APRN in a new position, whether experienced in the role or not, needs to be aware of the importance of being informed about the organizational structure, philosophy, goals, policies, and procedures of the agency.

Networking was emphasized by NPs in Kleinpell-Nowell's surveys (1999, 2001; see also Kleinpell, 2005). Peer support within and outside of the work setting is important, as noted by Hamric and Taylor (1989). New NPs stressed the importance of getting to know other nurses in the work setting, gaining their respect, and forming key alliances with them to enhance optimal functioning in their new position (Kelly & Mathews, 2001). Designating a more experienced APRN in the work setting as a mentor can be helpful and provide support for any APRNs new to a position (Sullivan-Bentz et al., 2010). APRNs who serve as preceptors for students can be particularly effective mentors for new graduates (Hayes, 2005). The importance of careful selection of a mentor was reported by NPs in the study by Kelly and Mathews (2001). Additional strategies suggested for networking within the system include developing peer support groups, being accessible to colleagues by phone or email, and getting involved in interdisciplinary groups (Sullivan-Bentz et al., 2010). APRNs should be encouraged to join local APRN groups for peer support, legislative and political updates, and networking opportunities. Numerous Internet sites are also available for networking, as noted earlier.

TABLE 4.5	Strategies to Promote APRN Role Implementation in Practice
Transition Phase	**Strategy**
Orientation	Follow a structured orientation plan
	Circulate literature on APRN roles
	Network with peers
	Identify role model or mentor
	Join local, state, and national APRN groups
	Identify your expectations
Frustration	Schedule debriefing sessions with experienced APRN
	Discuss your expectations and how they fit in real-world application
	Plan for longer patient appointments initially
	Schedule administrative time
	Collaborate with other providers
	Learn time-saving tips
	Engage in positive self-talk
	Practice well-being habits of self-care
Implementation	Reassess demands, priorities, goals—modify expectations
	Schedule a 6-month evaluation
	Collaborate with other specialties—seek opportunities to co-treat with other specialties
	Learn from repetitive practice
	Learn ways to manage uncertainty
	Assemble mobile clinical resource applications
Integration	Schedule a 12-month evaluation
	Plan for role refinement and expansion
	Continue intraprofessional and interprofessional collaboration
	Continue debriefing sessions
	Continue seeking verification and feedback from colleagues

Adapted from Table 4.4: Phases of Advanced Practice Nurse Role Development and Table 4.5: Transition Stages in First Year of Primary Care Practice. In: Brykczynski, K. A. (2014). Role development of the advanced practice nurse. In A. B. Hamric, C. M. Hanson, M. F. Tracy, & E. T. O'Grady (Eds.). *Advanced practice nursing: An integrative approach* (5th ed., pp. 98–100). St. Louis: Elsevier Saunders.

Page and Arena (1991) recommended that CNSs schedule and devote the major portion of their time during the orientation phase to direct patient care to solidify the clinical expert role. They also suggested making appointments with nursing leaders, physicians, and other health care professionals during this phase to garner administrative support. They recommended distributing business cards and making the job description available for discussion. They also counseled new CNSs to withhold suggestions for change until they have had the opportunity to assess the system more fully. When a new APRN joins the staff of an organization, the administrator should send a letter describing the APRN's background experiences and new position to key people in the organization.

Frustration Phase

Hamric and Taylor (1989) observed that the frustration phase might come and go and may overlap other phases. They noted that painful affective responses are typical of this difficult phase. They

suggested that monthly sessions for sharing concerns with a group of peers and an administrator might facilitate movement through this phase. Strategies identified as helpful for energizing movement from the frustration phase to the implementation phase include the following: obtaining assistance with time management (Allen, 2001); participating in support groups to ameliorate feelings of inadequacy; engaging in discussions for conflict resolution and role clarification (Desborough, 2012); reassessing priorities and setting realistic expectations; and focusing on short-term, visible goals.

Page and Arena (1991) suggested keeping a work portfolio to document activities so that APRN progress is more readily visible and accessible. This can be an expansion of the online portfolio and self-monitoring system initiated during the APRN program. Brown and Olshansky (1997) noted that organized sources of support such as phone calls, seminars, planned meetings with mentors, and scheduled time for consultation can significantly decrease feelings of anxiety. They noted that recognition of the discomfort arising from moving from expert back to novice and the realization that previous expertise can be valuable in the new role may help reduce feelings of inadequacy. They suggested that new APRNs request reasonable time frames for initial patient visits because novices take longer than experienced practitioners, and this may be key to successful adjustment to a new position.

Implementation Phase

During this phase, it is important for the APRN to reassess demands and expectations to prevent feeling overwhelmed. Priorities may need to be readjusted and short-term goals may need to be reformulated. Brown and Olshansky (1997, 1998) observed that competence and confidence are fostered through repetition. They also recommend scheduling a formal evaluation after approximately 6 months in which feedback about areas of strength and those needing improvement can be ascertained. Strategies mentioned as important during this time include seeking administrative support through involvement in meetings, maintaining visibility in clinical areas, and developing in-service programs with input from staff (Page & Arena, 1991). After some time in the implementation phase, APRNs may plan and execute small-scale projects to demonstrate their effectiveness in their new role.

Integration Phase

Hamric and Taylor's (1989) survey data indicated that CNSs maximize their role potential during the integration phase, which typically occurs after 3 years in practice. Satisfactory completion of the earlier phases appears to be essential for passage into this phase. One strategy for enhancing and maintaining optimal role implementation during this phase is having a trusted colleague who can act as a safe sounding board for "feedback, constructive criticism, and advice" (Hamric & Taylor, 1989, p. 79). During this phase, it is important to have a plan to guide continued role expansion and refinement, such as the portfolio mentioned earlier. Seeking appointment to key committees is important to increase recognition of APRNs in the organization. Administrative support and constructive feedback from a trusted mentor continue to be important. Development of a promotional system that offers professional advancement in the APRN practice role through additional benefits or financial incentives remains a challenge for practitioners and administrators.

International Experiences With Advanced Practice Nurse Role Development and Implementation: Lessons Learned and a Proposed Model for Success

Over the last 20 years, as advanced practice nursing (APN[a]) roles have been introduced in other countries, there has been increasing interest in their role development and implementation internationally. There is more variability in advanced practice nursing internationally in terms of educational standards, scope of practice, credentialing, and the like. The Canadian experience provides significant lessons learned and suggestions for successful APN role implementation worldwide (Canadian Nurses Association, 2006). CNS and NP roles have existed in Canada for 40 years, but their implementation has been sporadic because of numerous system-level factors (DiCenso et al., 2010b; Sangster-Gormley, Martin-Misener, Downe-Wamboldt, & DiCenso, 2011). A decreased demand for APN roles in Canada resulted from many factors, including lack of legislative and regulatory authority of APN roles, multiple titles and conflicting definitions, absence of reimbursement mechanisms, opposition from the medical profession, and inconsistent curriculum requirements, which subsequently led to the gradual closure of most NP and CNS programs by the late 1980s (Sangster-Gormley et al., 2011). Recently there has been renewed interest in APN roles as a way to promote changes in the Canadian health care system (DiCenso et al., 2010b). Hurlock-Chorostecki, Forchuk, Orchard, Van Soeren, and Reeves (2014) investigated the role of NPs in Ontario hospitals and found that they contribute to building cohesive interprofessional teamwork. Doetzel, Rankin, and Then (2016) explored barriers and facilitators to NP practice in Canadian emergency departments with the goal of promoting their utilization in emergency department fast track units.

Although external factors such as supports and barriers were addressed, the major focus of APN role development and implementation research has been on the micro level, with a focus on personal experiences of the individual clinician taking on a new role. A more comprehensive framework for role implementation developed in Canada is noteworthy in that it takes a macro perspective and involves stakeholders (e.g., administrators, patients, advocacy groups, support staff, professional organizations) in

[a]The acronym APRN is only used in the United States; therefore the acronym APN will be used for this international section of the chapter.

the APN role implementation process. It specifically addresses barriers to role implementation at the system, organizational, and practice setting levels (Bryant-Lukosius & DiCenso, 2004). The participatory, evidence-based, patient-focused process for APN role development, implementation, and evaluation (PEPPA) framework (Bryant-Lukosius & DiCenso, 2004) recognizes the complexity of the system factors involved in implementing a new role in an existing system. The PEPPA framework (Fig. 4.2) incorporates the principles of participatory action research "to promote more equitable distribution of power and enhance the contributions of nurses, patients, and other stakeholders in APRN role development" (Bryant-Lukosius & DiCenso, 2004, p. 531). It was developed to guide APN role implementation and has been used effectively in a variety of practice settings in Canada (Martin-Misener et al., 2010; McAiney et al., 2008; McNamara, Giguère, St.-Louis, & Boileau, 2009).

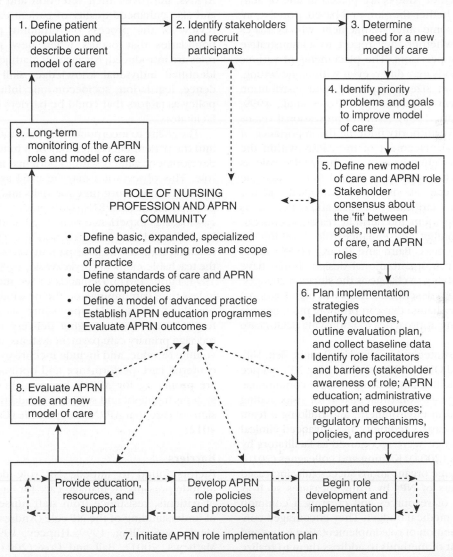

FIG 4.2 The participatory, evidence-based, patient-focused process for APRN role development, implementation, and evaluation (PEPPA) framework. *(From Bryant-Lukosius, D., & DiCenso, A. [2004]. A framework for the introduction and evaluation of advanced practice nursing roles. Journal of Advanced Nursing, 48, 532.)*

Facilitators and Barriers in the Work Setting

Facilitators

Aspects of the work setting exert a major influence on APRN role definitions and expectations, thereby affecting role ambiguity, role incongruity, and role conflict. The need for ongoing peer and administrative support is a theme throughout the literature on role development, beginning with the student experience and extending into practice. Administrative factors that should be considered include whether APRNs are placed in line or staff positions; whether they are unit-based, population-based, or in some other arrangement; who evaluates them; and whether they report to administrative or clinical supervisors. The placements of various APRN positions may differ, even within one setting, depending on size, complexity, and distribution of the patient population (Andrews et al., 1999; Baird & Prouty, 1989). Issues of professional versus administrative authority underlie the importance of the structural placement of the APRN within the organization. Effectiveness of the APRN role is enhanced when there is a mutual fit between the goals and expectations of the individual and the organization. Clarification of goals and expectations before employment and periodic reassessments can minimize conflict and enhance role development and effectiveness. Baird and Prouty (1989) maintained that the organizational design should have enough flexibility to change as the situation changes. Weiner (2009) described a theory of organizational readiness for change that can promote more flexible and promising approaches to improving health care delivery.

Practical strategies identified by Bonnel, Belt, Hill, Wiggins, and Ohm (2000) for initiating NP practice in nursing facilities included proactive communication, developing a consistent system for visits, setting up the physical environment, and building a team approach to care. Credibility and advanced clinical nursing practice were recognized as facilitators by Ball and Cox (2004). Keating and colleagues (2010) noted that some organizations successfully increased their numbers of NPs by using measures such as reallocation of resources and creating a common nursing and medical budget. They encouraged continued exploration of role implementation issues and development of methods to address them to realize the potential benefits of NP practice to the health care delivery system. DiCenso and colleagues (2010a) delineated standardization of requirements, adequate resources, interprofessional education, legislation and regulation, needs assessment and understanding of role, stakeholder involvement, and a Pan-Canadian approach as factors enabling role integration of advanced practice nurses in Canada. Doerksen (2010) reported on a study of professional development and mentorship needs of advanced practice nurses in Canada that identified needs for both formal and informal mentorship and administrative support as important for full role implementation. Sargent and Olmedo (2013) described a funded postgraduate residency program that facilitated role transition for APRNs, improved their retention and satisfaction, and also enhanced quality of patient care. In their review of the process of reframing professional boundaries that occurs when new professional roles are introduced, Niezen and Mathijessen (2014) identified individual knowledge, skill and confidence, legislation, socioeconomic influences, and policy as factors that could be barriers or potential facilitators.

The ability to incorporate teaching and counseling into the patient encounter may be a function of skill development gained with experience in the APRN role. This observation may be used as a rationale for structuring more time for visits and fewer total patients for new APRNs, with gradual increases in caseloads as experience is accrued. Older research has indicated that NPs incorporate counseling and teaching into the flow of patient visits—capturing the teachable moment (Brykczynski, 1999b; Johnson, 1993; Lurie, 1981). Demands to see more patients in less time can impinge on the possibility of incorporating more holistic aspects into patient encounters. Current and emerging delivery models that redesign primary care payment systems, moving from volume to value, and include incentives for patient-centered care performance and optimal outcomes are promising for APRNs because these payment systems highlight and support the additional dimensions of care that APRNs can provide (Calsyn & Lee, 2012).

Barriers

Factors found to impede NP role development include pressure to manage care for large numbers of patients, resistance from staff nurses, and lack of understanding of the NP role (Andrews, Hanson, Maule, & Snelling, 1999; Hupcey, 1993; Kelly & Mathews, 2001). Ball and Cox (2004) identified conflict, resistance, gender bias, political awareness, and established values as barriers to APRN role implementation. Keating, Thompson, and Lee

(2010) reported on a study of perceived barriers to progression and sustainability of NP roles in emergency departments 10 years after they were introduced in Victoria, Australia. The main barriers identified were lack of organizational support, legislative constraints, and lack of ongoing funding for advanced practice nursing education. Lack of structured orientation programs was considered a barrier to APRN role transition by Goldschmidt and colleagues (2011). Sargent and Olmedo (2013) recognized limited time for physicians and experienced APRNs to mentor new APRNs as an impediment to APRN role development. Role confusion, lack of specific practice guidelines, and remuneration issues were barriers noted by Doetzel, Rankin, and Then (2016) with APRNs in the emergency department. Other constraints operating in today's health care settings that affect not only APRNs but also other providers and office staff include new billing and coding guidelines, Health Insurance Portability and Accountability Act regulations, major health care reform with a focus on outcomes, monitoring for fraud and abuse, sexual harassment, and demands to integrate technology into practice.

Continued Advanced Practice Nurse Role Evolution

CNMs, CRNAs, NPs, and CNSs have attained positive recognition and support in clinical positions in many settings in the United States. However, in spite of the increasing familiarity and popularity of these APRN roles, some health care settings have used few, if any, APRNs and some staff members have had minimal experience working with APRNs. In some areas of the United States, physicians or physician assistants are preferred over APRNs. Even experienced APRNs can expect to encounter resistance to full implementation of their roles if they seek positions in institutions with no history of employing APRNs. Andrews and colleagues (1999) described their experiences introducing the NP role into a large academic teaching hospital. They delineated helpful strategies for marketing a new NP role to staff, patients, and the surrounding community, as well as ways to set up the necessary infrastructure to support the new role in the institution. They referred to this process as evolutionary.

The meaning of the evolution of established APRN roles varies according to the type of APRN role. The emphasis on cost containment in the health care delivery system led to the trend of having acute care NPs staff intensive care units to compensate for the

shortage of house staff physicians (Rosenfeld, 2001; Sechrist & Berlin, 1998). Then ACNP practice broadened from an intensive care unit focus to diverse settings including specialty clinics and private practice groups (Kleinpell, 2005; Kleinpell-Nowell, 2001). Evolution of APRN roles is also reflected in the expansion of practice to multiple areas or sites. Although responsibility for multiple areas in the same facility has been typical of many CNS roles for years, it is an evolutionary process for most other APRN roles. Multisite roles might signify practice responsibilities at different sites or multiple areas of responsibility in the same site, and they may combine inpatient and outpatient responsibilities (Stahl & Myers, 2002). Stahl and Myers' clinical practices (Exemplar 4.2) are models for APRN practice evolving to multiple sites, which constitutes a strategy for extending APRN resources and trying to use them more efficiently.

As individual APRNs mature into their respective roles and become more competent and confident in all role components, greater concentration on the unique nature of APRN practice can be expected. In their study of CNSs, Hamric and Taylor (1989) found that freedom to develop their unique APRN role, availability of feedback from a mentor, support to broaden their influence and take on new projects, and recognition of their contributions enabled experienced CNSs to stay energized in their clinical practice roles. As Peplau (1997) advocated, nurse leaders must emphasize what nurses do for patients. The claim that APRN practice incorporates active patient participation, patient education, family assessment, involvement and support, and community awareness and connections (Neale, 1999) needs to be documented. For example, Kelly and Mathews (2001) found that graduates with 1 to 7 years of experience as NPs found it difficult to adhere to ideals of holistic care and health promotion, given the pressures of the clinical situation.

Continued research that demonstrates positive outcomes of APRN care is essential for APRN practice to make an impact on health care policy (Brooten et al., 2002; Murphy-Ende, 2002; Russell, Vorder-Bruegge, & Burns, 2002; Ryden et al., 2000; see also Chapter 23). Rashotte (2005) advocated for dialogic forms of research to evoke the more holistic and humanistic aspects of what it means to be an APRN to complement the predominant instrumental and economic perspectives underlying most APRN research. Brykczynski's (2012) interpretive phenomenologic study of how NP faculty incorporate holistic aspects of care into teaching NP students is an

EXEMPLAR 4.2   **Evolving APRN Roles in Multisite Practices**

Expansion of practice to multiple sites is one way in which advanced practice registered nurse (APRN) practice is evolving, along with the integration of many health care delivery systems. Stahl is a clinical nurse specialist whose practice has evolved from the full range of clinical nurse specialist practice for four medical cardiac units at a tertiary care center to also include support primarily in education, consultation, and program development at two additional hospitals. Myers is an adult nurse practitioner who directs a hepatitis C program for a specialty physician group with 11 physicians at nine practice locations, and she also provides direct care for patients at four of the sites. Stahl and Myers (2002) relied on Quinn's (1996) wisdom for developing the leader within by expecting to "build the bridge as you walk on it" (p. 83) and learning "how to get lost with confidence" (p. 86). Their commitment to being continuous learners is a useful model for APRNs to follow as they experience the situational transitions that are inevitable as clinical practices evolve.

Self-mastery and commitment are the keys to meeting the needs of a multisite practice. Setting realistic expectations, maintaining healthy personal and professional boundaries, and establishing attainable goals can contribute to success in multisite practice. Practice challenges such as supervision and role requirements may differ from institution to institution. Inconsistency in electronic health records creates challenges for documentation. Several systems require users to attend training sessions, while others are not fully integrated or are simply cumbersome to navigate. Hospital mergers and or acquisitions of solo practice and community clinics impose regulatory requirements on the APRN that may not have previously existed. APRNs are required to apply for privileges to practice in hospitals. This mandated credentialing process can take up to 12 weeks and limit practice until completed. Additionally, the onboarding processes in different institutions present APRNs with multiple challenges in policy and procedures not usually present in solo practice.

Full practice authority has been granted to APRNs in federal programs, including the US Armed Forces, Indian Health Service, and Public Health Service systems, and in 24 states (National Council of State Boards of Nursing, 2016). Yet barriers preventing APRNs from practicing to the full extent of their education and training continue to exist (Hain & Fleck, 2014). The US Department of Veterans Affairs (VA) recently submitted a proposal granting APRNs full practice authority. There are over 5769 APRNs working within the VA system. On May 25, 2016, the VA proposed to amend its medical regulations to permit full practice authority of all VA-employed APRNs when they are acting within the scope of their VA employment (American Association of Colleges of Nursing, 2016; Brown, 2016; Federal Register, 2016; Japsen, 2016). The American Nurses Association, American Association of Nurse Anesthetists, American Association of Nurse Practitioners, and American Association Colleges of Nursing, along with state and local advanced practice organizations, rallied their members in positive response to this proposal. This national APRN campaign reached out to the public, asking for support and gaining recognition. This proposal was opposed by the American Medical Association and the American Society of Anesthesiologists (Brown, 2016).

In a press release on December 14, 2016, the VA announced that it was amending provider regulations to permit full practice authority to three roles of VA APRNs to practice to the full extent of their education, training, and certification, regardless of state restrictions that limit such full practice authority, except for applicable state restrictions on the authority to prescribe and administer controlled substances, when such APRNs are acting within the scope of their VA employment. Unfortunately, CRNAs were not included in the VA's full practice authority under the final rule (US Department of Veteran's Affairs, 2016). ◎

example of such dialogic research. More research activity and increasing involvement in the larger arena of health policy may also represent continuing role evolution for APRNs.

The DNP is another example of APRN role evolution. The DNP-prepared APRN brings an advanced skill set to health care with clear understanding of research and technology. DNP-prepared APRNs are educated to translate evidence into practice, promote collaboration and interprofessional teamwork, and advocate for change in health care policy to improve patient outcomes (Exemplar 4.3).

Evaluation of Role Development

Evaluation is fundamental to enhancing role implementation (see Chapter 24). Development of a professional portfolio to document APRN accomplishments can be useful for performance and impact (process and outcome) evaluation. Performance evaluation for

DNP: The Changing Face of Health Care

The Patient Protection and Affordable Care Act (2010) has had a significant impact on our health care system and has changed the face of primary care. Previously uninsured individuals with little or no health care in the last 10 to 20 years now have access to the health care system. This addition, along with an explosion of chronic illness coupled with the aging population, has resulted in an influx of patients presenting with complex clinical problems in primary care settings. The new face of health care supports the need for advanced clinical skills and leaders. Strong interprofessional collaboration is critical to successfully managing the current patient population. The doctor of nursing practice (DNP) responds to the need for advanced clinical skills and knowledge and increased collaboration with other disciplines at the systems level.

DNP programs continue to grow in numbers (currently 246 in the United States) as employers recognize the contributions made by doctorally prepared APRNs (American Association of Colleges of Nursing [AACN], 2015a). DNP practice continues to evolve as new DNP graduates enter the health care system. Nurse entrepreneur, nurse executive, clinical educator, and nurse informatist are some of the positions being filled by DNP graduates. The evolution of the DNP role has contributed to the expansion of DNP programs and the adaptation of existing DNP programs to meet the changing needs of the health care system. Many DNP programs have implemented specialization paths (executive, informatics, and education) to prepare students for the diverse opportunities available. The specialization pathway is in its infancy and is not consistent across the country. All accredited programs are guided by the eight DNP essentials established by the AACN (2006).

DNP preparation is empowering. Educated for professional leadership, the DNP-prepared APRN exemplifies the Institute for Healthcare Improvement's Triple Aim principles of improving the patient experience of care (including quality and satisfaction), improving the health of populations, and reducing the per capita cost of health care (O'Dell, 2016; Stiefel & Nolan, 2012). Bodenhiemer and Sinsky (2015) identified a concern with widespread health care provider burnout and dissatisfaction and have recommended revision of the Triple Aim to a Quadruple Aim. The Quadruple Aim adds improving the work life of health care providers as another essential principle for enhancing patient care. The DNP is prepared with increased clinical and advocacy skills on which he or she can capitalize to effect policy change and quality improvement in health care.

The new DNP-prepared APRN encounters a degree of uncertainty and anxiety while looking for the best career opportunity to demonstrate her or his advanced skills and knowledge (Glasgow & Zoucha, 2011). Many health professionals are unaware of the DNP-prepared APRN, and this degree has not achieved the level of equality expected with other practice doctorates as a result of role ambiguity, role conflict, and physician resistance. The lack of clarity adds to the role strain experienced by new DNP graduates. According to Glasgow and Zoucha (2011), the DNP is empowered with a broader perspective and an increased level of confidence, resulting in a decreased period of role transition. One might speculate that DNP-prepared APRNs move through the transitions in school and after graduation more quickly because of their advanced repertoire of both clinical and general life experience; however, further investigation is needed. DNP programs are growing, but individual DNPs will continue to face many challenges in the health care setting. The need for role clarity is paramount. As the number of DNP-prepared APRNs grows, their practice will continue to evolve and become more defined and accepted. DNP education is critical to advancing knowledge and clinical skills for advanced practice nurses (Hendricks-Ferguson, Akard, Madden, Peters-Herron, & Levy, 2015). The complexities of health care and advances in technology and research increase the need for the doctorally prepared APRN. ◎

APRNs should include self-evaluation, peer review, and administrative evaluation (Cooper & Sparacino, 1990; Hamric & Taylor, 1989). Use of a competency profile can be helpful for organizing evaluation in a dynamic way that allows for changes in role implementation over time as expertise, situations, and priorities change (Callahan & Bruton-Maree, 1994). APRNs can review the competency models available and select one to use for their ongoing competency profile (Sastre-Fullana, De Pedro-Gomez, Bennasar-Veny, Serrano-Gallardo, & Morales-Asencio, 2014). The competency profile can be used to assess performance in each of the core APRN competencies. APRN programs need to include content and skill development regarding self-evaluation and peer evaluation of role implementation so that individuals can learn to monitor their practice and identify difficulties early to avoid moving into negative developmental phases (Hamric & Hanson, 2003).

Outcome evaluation is important to demonstrate the effectiveness of each APRN role, to document the impact of APRN practice on quality of care, and to overcome APRN invisibility (O'Grady, 2008). Ongoing development of appropriate outcome evaluation measures, particularly for patient outcomes, is important (Bryant-Lukosius et al., 2016; Ingersoll, McIntosh, & Williams, 2000; see Chapter 23). The existence of a reward system to provide for career advancement through a clinical ladder program and accrual of additional benefits is particularly important for retaining APRNs in clinical roles. In less structured situations, APRNs can negotiate for periodic reassessments and salary increases through options such as profit sharing.

The evaluation process broadens to incorporate interprofessional review when APRN practice includes hospital privileges, prescriptive privileges, and third-party reimbursement. This expansion of the evaluation process has positive and negative aspects. Advantages to the review process associated with securing and maintaining hospital privileges include the many factors considered in the evaluation, the variety of perspectives, and the visibility afforded APRNs. APRNs should seek key positions on hospital review committees to promote APRN roles within the organization. A major difficulty in implementing interdisciplinary peer review is lack of interaction between and among the students of the various health professional groups during their formative educational programs. The resurgence of interest in developing and implementing interprofessional educational experiences between nursing students and medical students is encouraging (AACN, 2006; Hamric & Hanson, 2003; Institute of Medicine, 2003; Interprofessional Education Collaborative Expert Panel, 2011).

Conclusion

Role development experiences for APRNs are described as consisting of two distinct transition processes: the first is referred to here as role acquisition, which occurs in school, and the second as role implementation, which occurs in practice after graduation. The limits of the educational process in preparing graduates for the realities of the work world are acknowledged. Students, faculty, preceptors, and administrators need to be informed about the human skill acquisition process and its stages, processes of adult and professional socialization,

identity transformation, role acquisition, role implementation, and overall career development. Knowing (theoretical knowledge) and actually experiencing (practical knowledge) are different phenomena, but at least students and new graduates can be forewarned about the transition experiences in school and the turbulence that can be expected during the first year of practice. Anticipatory guidance for students can be provided through role rehearsal experiences, such as clinical preceptorships and role seminars. Students need to be encouraged to begin networking with practicing APRNs through local, state, and national APRN groups. This networking is especially important for APRNs who will not be practicing in proximity to other APRNs. Experienced APRNs and new APRN graduates can form mutually beneficial relationships.

Although anticipatory socialization experiences in school can facilitate role acquisition, they cannot prevent the transition that occurs with movement into a new position and actual role implementation. APRN programs should have a firm foundation in the real world. However, a certain degree of incongruence or conflict between academic ideals and work world reality will continue to exist (Ormond & Kish, 2001). APRNs must take a leadership role in guiding and directing planned change and guard against the mere maintenance of the status quo. Establishing mentor programs, structured orientation programs, and postgraduate fellowship programs for new APRNs in the work setting are ways to develop and maintain support for the positive developmental phases of role implementation and minimize role strain.

APRN role development has been described as dynamic, complex, and situational. It is influenced by many factors, such as experience, level of expertise, personal and professional values, setting, specialty, relationships with coworkers, aspects of role transition, life transitions, and organizational, system, and political realities. Frameworks for understanding APRN role development processes have been discussed, along with strategies for facilitating the dual transitions of role acquisition in school and role implementation upon graduation. Ongoing evolution of APRN roles in response to organizational and health care system changes and demands will continue. Future research studies to assess the applicability of this information to all APRN specialty groups are needed to further the understanding of APRN role development, guide educational and work setting innovations, and support health policy recommendations.

Key Summary Points

- Application of the Dreyfus Situational Model of Skill Acquisition to APRN role development depicts the acquisition of skills and knowledge as developing over time in stages from novice to expert, with the whole process evolving over time in cycles of progression and regression occurring as new skills and knowledge are acquired and new situations are encountered and mastered.
- APRN role development consists of two distinct processes: (1) Role acquisition is the process of APRN role transition that takes place during the APRN educational program. (2) Role implementation is the process of APRN role transition that occurs in the work setting following program completion.
- Conceptual understanding of role concepts and role development issues and familiarity with APRN research describing APRN role transition and implementation processes can enhance role acquisition and implementation experiences for individual APRNs, minimize the strain of role transitions, promote continued role evolution, and lead to educational innovations, improved health policy and regulations, and increased quality of health care.

References

To access the references for this chapter, use your smartphone's QR code reader to scan the code below, or go to http://booksite.elsevier.com/ 9780323447751.

Evolving and Innovative Opportunities for Advanced Practice Nursing

Jeanne Salyer

"The best way out is always through."

—Robert Frost

CHAPTER CONTENTS

Technologic advances and economic and socio-cultural conditions have sustained a climate of change in the health care environment, and opportunities for advanced practice nursing continue to emerge in the wake of these changes. As specialties have emerged, many new roles have evolved from specialty nursing practice and have expanded to incorporate some or all of the core attributes of advanced practice nursing (see Chapters 2 and 3). Some of these roles have clearly evolved as advanced practice roles, whereas others are in various stages of evolution. Not all specialties, however, will evolve into advanced practice roles, for a variety of reasons. For example, some specialties evolve away from the core definition of advanced practice nursing, which encompasses direct clinical practice and clinical expertise as essential ingredients. Other specialties, such as informatics and nursing administration, arise as specialties and remain as specialties because direct clinical practice is not a requisite role component.

The purpose of this chapter is to examine some currently evolving specialties and characterize stages in their continuing evolution from specialty nursing practice to advanced practice nursing. Some of these specialties have not yet fully evolved to an advanced level; however, movement within the specialty toward advanced practice may be accelerated as Doctor of Nursing Practice (DNP) programs target these specialties for development. The focus of the discussion is on the various specialties—not on particular advanced practice nursing roles, such as clinical nurse specialist (CNS), nurse practitioner (NP), certified nurse-midwife, or certified registered nurse anesthetist (CRNA). Specialties selected for inclusion in this discussion were chosen for one or more of the following reasons:

- The specialty has the potential to transition (or is transitioning) to the DNP.
- The specialty has the potential to evolve to advanced practice nursing, given the complexity of care required by the patient population, and direct care is likely to be a defining factor.

- The specialty has arisen as a result of scientific and/or technologic advances and the influence of these advances on the delivery of health care.
- The specialty is growing because of the rising incidence of health problems in the population.
- The specialty's patient population needs sophisticated care across settings in the complex health care environment.

Opportunities in these evolving specialties for advanced practice registered nurses (APRNs) are discussed and a framework for evaluating progress toward advanced practice status is presented. Exemplars provided by APRNs in the specialties were deliberately chosen to illuminate the added value of advanced practice competencies to these evolving specialties.

Patterns in the Evolution of Specialty Nursing Practice to Advanced Practice Nursing

Before discussing the evolution of specialty nursing practice into advanced practice nursing, it is important to make a distinction between the two as well as to clarify the use of the term *subspecialty* in this chapter. Specialization involves focusing on practice in a specific area derived from the field of professional nursing. Specialties can be further characterized as nursing practice that intersects with another body of knowledge, has a direct impact on nursing practice, and is supportive of the direct care provided to patients by other registered nurses (American Nurses Association [ANA], 2010a). As the profession of nursing has responded to changes in health care, the need for specialty knowledge has increased. For example, in the wake of the National Cancer Act of 1971, which was enacted as a consequence of the increasing incidence of cancer in the population and the need to advance national efforts in prevention and treatment, the oncology specialty became more widely recognized (Oncology Nursing Society [ONS], 2016). The ONS traces its origin to the first National Cancer Nursing Research Conference, supported by the ANA and American Cancer Society, in 1973, after which a small group met to discuss the need for a national organization to support their professional development. From these early efforts, this organization, which was incorporated in 1975, has become a leader in cancer care in the United States and around the world (ONS, 2016).

The classic specialties in nursing, now termed *populations* in the *Consensus Model for APRN Regulation* (APRN Joint Dialogue Group, 2008), have been pediatric (now termed *child health*), psychiatric and mental health, obstetrics (now termed *women's health*), community and public health, and medical-surgical nursing (now termed *adult health*). Specialties that have emerged within these populations include, for example, concentrations in adult and pediatric critical care, emergency, and oncology nursing. As a given specialty coalesces, nurses often form specialty nursing organizations out of clinicians' needs to share practice experiences and specialty knowledge. Some examples include the American Association of Critical-Care Nurses, the ONS, and the Association of Women's Health, Obstetric and Neonatal Nurses. Scope and standards of practice statements legitimize specialty designation and prompt efforts to provide opportunities for specialty education and certification. The efforts of the International Transplant Nurses Society (ITNS) to develop and approve a scope of practice statement, a core curriculum, and specialty certification in transplant nursing for registered nurses is just one example (ITNS/ANA, 2009; ANA/ITNS, 2016).

Advanced practice nursing includes but goes beyond population-focused specialization; it involves expansion, which legitimizes role autonomy, and advancement, characterized by the integration of a broad range of theoretical, research-based, and practical knowledge (ANA, 2010a; see Chapter 2). Thus advanced practice nursing reflects concentrated knowledge that offers the opportunity for expanded and autonomous practice based on a broader practical and theoretical knowledge base.

The term *specialty* suggests that the focus of practice is limited to parts of the whole (ANA, 2010b). For example, family NPs, who typically see themselves as generalists, have in fact specialized in one of the many facets of health care—namely, primary care. Subspecialization further delineates the focus of practice. In subspecialty practice, knowledge and skill in a delimited clinical area is expanded further. With this expanded knowledge and skill, there is potentially further advancement of theoretical, evidence-based, and practical knowledge in caring for a specific patient population base. Examples of subspecialty practices within the specialty of adult health nursing include diabetes, transplant, and palliative care nursing. Notably, most of the practice opportunities chosen for discussion in this chapter are subspecialty practices. This distinction between specialty and subspecialty is important, particularly for certification and regulatory reasons, and was codified when the National Council of State

Boards of Nursing (NCSBN) proposed the regulation of advanced practice nursing in terms of certification requirements at the broad population foci level (e.g., psychiatric and mental health, pediatrics, adult and gerontology), with specialty or subspecialty certification being voluntary (NCSBN, 2008). Regulatory considerations aside, the expansion of advanced practice nursing is increasingly occurring in specialty and subspecialty practice. Expanding these boundaries places APRNs on the cutting edge of clinical care delivery in a complex, ever-changing, health care environment. However, for the sake of consistency with the *Consensus Model for APRN Regulation* (APRN Joint Dialogue Group, 2008), in the remainder of this chapter, specialty and subspecialty practice are referred to as specialties.

From a historical perspective, the evolution of specialty nursing practice to advanced practice nursing follows a trajectory that has been described by several authors (Beitz, 2000; Bigbee & Amidii-Nouri, 2000; Hamric, 2000; Lewis, 2000; see Chapter 1). Hanson and Hamric (2003) synthesized these observations and characterized this evolution as having distinct stages (Table 5.1). Initially, in stage I, the specialty develops in response to changing patient needs, needs that are usually a result of new technology, new medical specialties, and/or changes in the health care workforce. For example, a lack of pediatric residents and the increasing number of neonatal intensive care units created an opportunity for the development of the neonatal NP role (DeNicola, Klied, & Brink, 1994; Honeyfield, 2009).

Stage II of development is characterized by progress to the point that organized training begins. This training is often institution-specific, on-the-job training that develops experts in the specialty. Some of these institution-specific programs develop into certificate programs; however, the content may not be standardized, and the quality of these specialty programs may vary. One example is the early transplant coordination role in major transplant centers (see "Clinical Transplant Coordination" later).

In stage III, the knowledge base required for specialty practice becomes more extensive and the scope of practice of the nurse with specialty training expands. There is growing recognition of the additional knowledge and skill needed for increasingly complex practice. It is not unusual at this stage to see APRNs migrate into an evolving specialty and further expand practice by infusing it with advanced practice core competencies, making the specialty resemble advanced practice and creating new calls for evolution to this higher level. This transition is clearly evident in wound, ostomy, and continence nursing (see "Wound, Ostomy, and Continence Nursing" later) as well as in palliative care nursing. Over time, pressure for the standardization of education and skills involved in the specialty arise from clinicians, the profession, and regulators. Certificate-level training programs move into graduate schools that assume responsibility for preparing nurses for these evolving specialties, improving standardization, elevating the status of the specialty, and fostering its emergence as an advanced practice role. In this third stage of the trajectory, graduate education

Stage	Description	Characteristics
I	Specialty begins	Specialty develops in practice settings; development driven by increasing complexity in care demands, new technology, changing workforce opportunities; on the job training, expansion of practice; not exclusively nursing
II	Specialty organizes	Organized training for specialty practice begins; institution-specific training develops; initially uses apprenticeship model; progresses to certificate training; specialty organization forms; certification examination develops but may not be nursing specific; reports appear on role of nurse in specialty
III	Pressures mount for standardization	Knowledge base grows; pressures mount for standardization, graduate education; knowledge base keeps growing, scope of practice expands for practitioners in the specialty; expanded practice leads to expanded regulatory oversight; leaders call for transition to graduate education and differentiated practice to standardize practice in the specialty; advanced practice registered nurses (APRNs) migrate to specialty or specialty nurses return to school; reports appear differentiating APRN role in the specialty
IV	Maturity and growing interprofessionalism	APRN practice in the specialty is well articulated, recognized by other providers; APRNs practice collaboratively with other practitioners in the specialty; APRNs are experts in the specialty or subspecialty; shared knowledge base with other health care professionals recognized; multidisciplinary certification examinations developed

TABLE 5.1 Four Stages in the Evolution of Advanced Practice Nursing

Adapted from Hanson, C. M., & Hamric, A. B. (2003). Reflections on the continuing evolution of advanced practice nursing. *Nursing Outlook, 51,* 203–211.

becomes an expected level of preparation (Hanson & Hamric, 2003).

Stage IV, initially described by Salyer and Hamric (2009), is characterized by mature and recognized APRN practice in the specialty, along with an emerging understanding of a shared interprofessional component. NPs in human immunodeficiency virus (HIV) practice who have attained certification as an HIV specialist, awarded by the American Academy of HIV Medicine, are an example of mature expert practitioners who share an interprofessional clinical knowledge base with physicians in this specialty.

It is important to note that these stages are dynamic and not mutually exclusive. It is not unusual for specialties to show characteristics of more than one stage simultaneously (e.g., graduate programs began to develop at the same time that most practitioners in the specialty were prepared in certificate programs). In addition, the duration of each stage may vary significantly by specialty. Thus, the evolution from specialty to advanced practice nursing can represent a natural maturation that should result from deliberate logical planning to strengthen the education and broaden the scope of practice of specialty nurses. Some of these roles evolve to fulfill the needs of specific patient populations or the needs of organizations. In some cases, changes in the legal recognition and regulation of practice also influence the movement toward advanced practice nursing. For example, the nurse-midwifery specialty moved toward requiring graduate-level educational preparation for their practitioners in response to the national movement among state boards of nursing to require this level of education for all APRNs. Complex and often controversial issues must be addressed before and during this evolutionary process (Box 5.1). In the following sections, the evolution of particular specialties to advanced practice nursing is described and these issues are discussed. Some of these specialties are struggling to evolve, and change is haphazard. Others are following a planned course of action and have emerged (or will soon do so) at the advanced practice level. All evolving specialties share two challenges—the need to gain support within and external to nursing for these roles and the need to clearly delineate their potential contributions in the health care environment.

Innovative Practice Opportunities (Stage I)

The initial stage of the evolution from specialty practice to advanced practice is characterized by

 BOX 5.1 **Issues in the Evolution of Specialty Nursing Practice to Advanced Practice Nursing**

- Defining the attributes of advanced practice in the specialty
- Delineating the core competencies of the specialty as encompassing the core competencies of advanced practice
- Delineating a vision of advanced practice that may step outside of nursing's traditional vision of what constitutes an advanced practice role and gaining support within the nursing and health care community for the role
- Standardizing curricula for achieving competency at the advanced practice level
- Clarifying certification and credentialing requirements
- Overcoming legal and regulatory issues that are barriers to patient and/or consumer access to advanced practice registered nurses (APRNs)
- Promoting recognition of APRNs and nursing as a profession
- Clarifying APRN role titles to be consistent and decrease confusion

Adapted from Hanson, C.M., & Hamric, A.B. (2003). Reflections on the continuing evolution of advanced practice nursing, *Nursing Outlook, 51,* 203–211.

the development of a specialty focus. Numerous examples are apparent in the history of nursing, which is replete with accounts of nursing's response to unmet patient needs. As a consequence, definable specialties emerge as nurses expand their practice to include the knowledge and skills necessary to meet the needs of patients requiring specialty care. Examples from our history include the specialty of enterostomal therapy nursing, now known as wound, ostomy, and continence (WOC) nursing, and forensic nursing, which has historically encompassed care provision in correctional facilities, psychiatric settings, and emergency departments as nurse examiners care for sexual assault and child abuse victims (Burgess, Berger, & Boersma, 2004; Doyle, 2001; Hutson, 2002; Maeve & Vaughn, 2001; McCrone & Shelton, 2001). As specialties begin to coalesce, the practice may not be viewed as a nursing role. For example, early enterostomal therapists were laypersons with ostomies. However, as the specialty evolved, the valuable contributions of nurses began to distinguish them from other care providers.

Several evolving roles in nursing are characterized as being innovative. Some of these roles do not reflect the core competencies of advanced practice nursing, and the role components differ significantly, in some cases, from those of an APRN. For example, if the focus of practice in forensic nursing had remained on the gathering of legal evidence, not on sustained clinical practice using advanced practice core competency elements, the role would not be evolving to an advanced practice level. Regardless, nurses functioning in these subspecialties, some of whom are APRNs, make unique contributions to the health of specific populations of patients. One such role to be explored as a stage I specialty is that of the hospitalist.

Hospitalist Practice

The development of the hospitalist movement over the past 20 years represents a break in the tradition of primary care physicians managing patients in inpatient and outpatient settings. In this model, inpatients are cared for by what is termed a *hospitalist physician*—a term coined by Wachter and Goldman (1996)—whose primary professional focus is the general medical care of hospitalized patients (Park & Jones, 2015). The hospitalist model, which is now expanding to include pediatric hospitalists, surgical hospitalists, neurologic hospitalists, obstetric-gynecologic hospitalists, orthopedic hospitalists and other specialty hospitalists (American Hospital Association [AHA]/AHA Physician Leadership Forum/Society of Hospital Medicine [SHM], 2012), has grown rapidly as a result of the role of managed care in organizations, increasing complexity of inpatient care, fragmentation of care, and pressures experienced by physicians in busy outpatient practices (AHA/AHA Physician Leadership Forum/SHM, 2012; Freed, 2004; SHM, 2016a; Wachter, 2004; Wachter & Goldman, 2016). In this model, inpatient management is voluntarily transferred by the outpatient physician to the hospitalist during the hospital admission and, on discharge, care is resumed by the outpatient physician.

The literature on hospitalist medicine discusses characteristics of hospitalists that are very similar to those of adult-gerontology acute care nurse practitioners (AG-ACNPs). This evolving paradigm of providers caring exclusively for acutely ill hospitalized patients provides opportunities for APRNs to work on the hospitalist team (Kleinpell, Hanson, Buchner, Winters, Wilson, & Keck, 2008; see Chapter 16). As part of a hospitalist team, which some suggest requires advanced training (Furfari, Rosenthal, Tad-y, Wolfe, & Glasheen, 2014), this APRN diagnoses acute and chronic conditions that may result in rapid physiologic deterioration or life-threatening instability, works collaboratively with a variety of health care professionals, promotes efficient use of resources, and provides quality care to achieve optimal cost-effective outcomes (American Association of Critical-Care Nurses, 2012; National Panel for Acute Care Nurse Practitioner Competencies, 2004). These specific functions illuminate the centrality of direct care practice of APRNs in this specialty. As the APRN hospitalist specialty continues to evolve, the added value of practice guided by acute care competencies has the potential to improve the quality of care received by hospitalized patients.

The SHM, with over 15,000 members, is a multidisciplinary organization (physicians, physician assistants [PAs], NPs). This organization is dedicated to supporting the growth and development of NPs and PAs in hospital medicine and recognizes the contributions of these providers and, through the Nurse Practitioner/Physician Assistant Committee, is developing initiatives and programs to promote and define the role of these providers in hospital medicine (SHM, 2016b). As the role of NPs and PAs continues to evolve, hospitalist practice will become more interprofessional, and APRNs and PAs will continue to be members of collaborative hospitalist teams to provide differentiated levels of care in the inpatient setting.

Commentary: Stage I

Hospitalist practice has clearly emerged as a specialty in medicine. Although NPs, particularly and most appropriately AG-ACNPs, are beginning to practice in this specialty, it is a stage I specialty for two reasons. First, the specialty is not yet recognized as a nursing specialty, and, although hospitalist practice for NPs has been defined by at least one state (Sullivan, 2009), describing unique distinctions between an APRN hospitalist and physician hospitalist has not yet been attempted. Second, APRN preparation for hospitalist practice is continuing to evolve as graduate nursing programs develop competency-based curricula more fully, with practica aimed at the development and refinement of knowledge and skills required for acute care, inpatient practice. One challenge for this stage I specialty is to clearly articulate the unique contributions that APRNs can bring to the care of hospitalized patients, which may decrease fragmentation of care and improve interprofessional collaboration and overall patient outcomes. In addition, graduate nursing programs offering acute care education can ensure that hospital practice, based on the identified competencies in hospital medicine (Dressler, Pistoria, Budnitz, McKean, & Amin, 2006) and AG-ACNP competencies (American Association of Colleges of Nursing, 2012), are incorporated into required clinical practica. The challenge to any APRN moving into this specialty is to maintain APRN competencies and avoid a practice that is strictly an extension of medical practice. This transition may be facilitated if acute care nursing organizations promote and support establishment of special interest groups to facilitate these transitions and collaborate with the SHM on the development of certification processes for those APRNs with appropriate national credentials (Exemplar 5.1).

Specialties in Transition (Stage II)

Stage II roles are characterized by progress in the evolution of the specialty to the point that organized training in the specialty begins. This training is often institution-specific, on-the-job training that develops experts in the specialty. The two roles discussed as demonstrating predominantly stage II characteristics but that may exhibit some characteristics of stage III are those of the clinical transplant coordinator (CTC) and forensic nurse (see Table 5.1).

Clinical Transplant Coordination

There is mounting evidence that the role of the CTC is evolving to the level of advanced practice nursing in response to patient care requirements in the referral and evaluation phase for patients, their families, and living donors, and in the pretransplant and posttransplant management phases of candidates and recipients. Specialty nurses with expertise in transplant nursing recognize the complex needs of these patients and many obtain graduate education to prepare themselves better to deal with the realities of transplant nursing. To the benefit of their patients, these coordinators have expanded the specialty by incorporating advanced practice core competencies.

Two organizations provide opportunities for ongoing education and preparation for certification for nurses who provide care for transplant patients, the North Atlantic Transplant Coordinators Organization (NATCO) and the ITNS. NATCO provides organized education in the specialty for clinical and procurement transplant coordinators (NATCO,

2016a) in preparation for certification by the American Board for Transplant Certification (2015). The ITNS, an organization focusing on the professional growth and development of the transplant clinician (ITNS, 2016), provides education on advances in transplantation and transplant patient care. The ITNS has published a core curriculum (Ohler & Cupples, 2007) and a scope and standards of practice statement (ANA/ITNS, 2016) for the specialty that incorporates core competencies. Unlike the NATCO core competencies for the advanced practice transplant professional (APTP), which define the APTP as a provider who is not a physician but is licensed to diagnose and treat patients in collaboration with a physician (NATCO, 2016b), the scope and standards of practice statement developed by the ITNS (ANA/ITNS, 2016) clearly addresses the scope of practice for transplant nurses, clinical and procurement transplant coordinators, and advanced practice transplant nurses, both NPs and CNSs. Building on the practice of the registered nurse generalist in transplant care and transplant nurse coordinator by demonstrating a greater depth and breadth of knowledge, greater synthesis of data and interventions, and significant role autonomy, which may include medical diagnosis and prescriptive authority, APRNs working in transplant centers integrate and apply a broad range of theoretical and evidence-based knowledge using specialized and expanded knowledge and skills (ITNS, 2016).

It can be argued that the complex needs of patients with end-stage organ disease require higher levels of clinical reasoning and analytic skills, such as those possessed by APRNs; however, to advance the CTC role (not just individuals in the role) to this higher level, attention to several issues is necessary. First and foremost, leaders in this specialty must systematically determine whether advanced practice core competencies (see Chapter 3) are required to enact the role fully or whether two levels of differentiated practice—generalist professional and APRN—should be defined. Second, the specialty's leadership must agree that the role is a nursing role. Because some CTCs are not nurses, making these decisions may disenfranchise many committed and experienced transplant professionals who are essential care providers. Similar to the different certifications in place for diabetes educators and advanced diabetes managers, a similar method of differentiation, recognizing the added value that advanced practice knowledge and skill brings to the CTC role, might serve to acknowledge the contributions of APRNs and other transplant professionals. Both the ITNS

EXEMPLAR 5.1   APRN Hospitalist[a]

The Hospital Medicine Nurse Practitioner Service at Strong Memorial Hospital, University of Rochester Medical Center, was started in 1995 as an initiative to reduce length of stay. Four nurse practitioners (NPs) were hired, along with a hospitalist, to start a short-stay unit. Patients included those with myocardial infarction rule-outs, new-onset atrial fibrillation, and simple cellulitis, as well as those needing observation after procedures. The NPs covered the unit 10 hours/day, 5 days/week, with fellows and other house staff covering the remaining hours (M. A. Terboss, personal communication, 2007).

Since its inception, the service has grown exponentially, primarily in response to the reduced number of medical resident positions and tighter restrictions on resident work hours by the Accreditation Council on Graduate Medical Education. In addition, the team's census grew along with the hospital census when two hospitals in the city closed. Other changes included an increase in patients, the addition of physician assistants to the team, and orthopedic surgery patients attended to by the Hospital Medicine Service. The service has expanded to cover patients on 15 patient care units, 24 hours/day, 7 days/week, including holidays.

The specialty of hospital medicine is relatively new, and therefore the role of the acute care nurse practitioner (ACNP) in a hospitalist role varies from hospital to hospital. At Strong Memorial, ACNPs have a variety of roles and responsibilities. They collaborate with the Hospital Medicine Division physicians and community-based primary care providers and share responsibility for examinations, documentation, order writing, and discharge planning. The ACNPs also follow patients admitted to subspecialty services, such as gastroenterology, nephrology, cardiology, and infectious diseases. Whereas the subspecialist attending physician or fellow may focus on the organ of interest, the ACNP independently manages comorbidities, updates families, and coordinates care, all of which provide a more holistic perspective to the patient's hospital stay.

Concrete defined tasks include admitting histories, physical examinations, orders, discharge instructions and summaries, and a daily visit with a progress note. ACNPs order and interpret diagnostic and laboratory tests, participate in multidisciplinary unit rounds, and update an electronic sign-out system for safer handoffs. Procedures such as line placement are usually provided by residents as part of their educational experience.

Many of the ACNP's responsibilities are less easily defined or measured. However, in these functions, the ACNP adds value to the care provided by the Hospital Medicine Service. They include coordination of care among the variety of consultants, other health professionals (e.g., physical therapists, nutritionists, social workers), and unit management. In addition, ACNPs update patients and families to maintain open communication and keep them informed of the care plan. They also orient new ACNPs to their role and mentor ACNP students. Most importantly, ACNPs collaborate with the bedside nurses and unit staff. Communication of updates, orders, and plans is essential to ensuring safe, timely, and quality care. The accessibility of the ACNP promotes collaboration and many opportunities for informal teaching. As APRNs, ACNPs are often the most knowledgeable about medication information, technology management, or even basic nursing care and can serve as resources for newer, less experienced nurses. Teaching and mentoring are important to ensure staff development and retention as well as safe patient care. The importance of these activities has been difficult to quantify. It has been and continues to be a challenge to the Hospital Medicine Service to measure these contributions and illustrate their value.

The future for ACNPs on hospital medicine teams is promising. The specialty is growing, along with the acuity of inpatients and the complexities of discharge planning, both of which ACNPs are well-suited to manage. ACNP programs are incorporating hospital medicine into their curricula and into clinical rotations. The ACNPs on the Hospital Medicine Service have precepted many of these students, some of whom have gone on to join our team. Many challenges are ahead, including finding ways to quantify our contribution in terms of quality of care, length of stay, and patient and staff satisfaction. Orienting new ACNPs to handle the complexity of these inpatients and recruiting for 24 hours/day, 7 days/week positions is also a challenge.

I find my role as an ACNP on the Hospital Medicine Service to be highly satisfying because I care for patients with a wide variety of health problems. I also have the opportunity every day to teach, learn, and make a difference for a patient or another nurse. Finally, it is very rewarding to work on a team of APRNs who are so dedicated to hospital medicine, providing excellent patient care and supporting and helping each other. I am proud to be an ACNP in hospitalist practice. ◎

[a]The author gratefully acknowledges Elizabeth Palermo, MS, RN, APRN-BC, Rochester, New York, for assistance with this exemplar.

and NATCO are moving in this direction by doing the following: (1) delineating the core competencies required for clinical and procurement transplant coordinators (ANA/ITNS, 2016; NATCO, 2016a); (2) developing a core curriculum for transplant nursing at the generalist level (Ohler & Cupples, 2007); and (3) as of 2004, initiating a certification examination for the clinical transplant nurse (certified clinical transplant nurse [CCTN]) (American Board for Transplant Certification, 2015). Institution-specific, on-the-job education and experience, attributes that characterize a stage II specialty, continue to be widely embraced in the specialty; however, efforts to provide more formalized education are now the standard.

Specialty certification is an issue for all evolving advanced practice nursing specialties. Educational institutions that prepare APRNs must consider the certification requirements and ensure that their graduates are eligible to sit for APRN certification examinations approved for legal recognition of an APRN role. Specialty certification offered by specialty organizations, although optional, demonstrates a knowledge base shared among clinicians in the specialty and improves clinical credibility.

The evolution toward advanced practice nursing for the CTC has been haphazard as a result of inattention to several issues. Most notably, the lack of recognition that the role requires advanced practice competencies and the lack of opportunities for advanced practice specialty certification may impede expansion into advanced practice nursing as an expectation of coordinator roles. The issue of specialty certification (at the generalist level) has been addressed, but no plans for advanced practice certification have been proposed, except for the APTP.

Clearly, however, there is a commitment to advanced practice nursing in transplantation and, given that commitment, more attention to these issues will be necessary for the CTC role to evolve to stage III.

Exemplar 5.2 demonstrates the complexity of care required for transplant candidates, recipients, and their families. In addition to expertise in advanced practice core competencies, the exemplar also highlights the skill of the APRN in dealing with systems issues—in the hospital and community—and staff education and coaching, both of which are important components of providing care to this challenging patient population. Collaboration as a member of a team of care providers affords the opportunity to advocate for patients and their family members and influence quality of care. Thus, the knowledge and expertise of advanced practice nurses could fully enable the potential of the CTC position.

Forensic Nursing

Forensic nursing has emerged as a specialty as a result of the severity of the national public health problems associated with violence. Recognition of the severity of these problems was first addressed in 1985 at the Surgeon General's Workshop on Violence and Public Health. In opening remarks, Dr. C. Everett Koop championed a multidisciplinary approach that addressed the prevention of violence and provision of better care for victims of violence. The severity of the problem was again addressed by the World Health Organization (WHO) in the *World Report on Violence and Health* (WHO, 2002). As the first comprehensive summary on the global impact of violence, it stated that more than

---

EXEMPLAR 5.2   **Clinical Transplant Coordinator**[a]

Organ transplantation remains the treatment of choice for end-stage disease involving the heart, kidney, liver, and lung. Additionally, transplantation of the bowel and pancreas are performed in select patients to treat intestine failure (whether function or surgical) and type 1 diabetes mellitus, respectively. In 2015, over 30,000 solid organ transplants were performed in the United States (Organ Procurement and Transplantation Network, 2016). The complexity of care, both before and after organ transplantation, requires that an interprofessional team provide care to the patient. Surgeons, physicians, social workers, pharmacists, nurses, advanced practice registered nurses (APRNs), and

psychologists evaluate and treat both the candidate and the organ recipient. The role of the transplant coordinator is to facilitate the care of the patient by collaborating with the interprofessional team and ensuring appropriate delivery of care. This process begins with initial referral to the transplant program, proceeds through the evaluation process and transplant surgery, and continues as long as the patient maintains care at the transplanting institution.

Currently, many transplant coordinators throughout the country are advanced practice nurses. Whether clinical nurse specialist or nurse practitioner, the APRN is prepared by advanced education to facilitate the

Continued

transplant evaluation process, determine patient acuity as well as the specific needs of the candidate, collaborate with colleagues on the interprofessional team, monitor changes in the candidate's health during the organ waiting period, facilitate the transplant procedure, assess the patient's health status during recovery from surgery, participate in care planning, and provide discharge teaching to the patient and family. Following discharge, the APRN coordinates care as required by the type of organ transplant (arrangement of biopsies, clinic visits, specialized testing) and serves as the patient's primary contact for health care access, whether by answering routine questions or determining the need for urgent treatment. Additionally, the role may involve many nonclinical responsibilities, such as education of health care team members, interaction with insurance providers, development of clinical protocols, regulatory reporting, participating in performance improvement activities, and research and publication.

As a heart transplant coordinator and APRN, I am able to integrate the core competencies of the role in order to provide optimum care to transplant candidates and recipients. One of my primary responsibilities is to provide expert coaching and advice to patients and family members, nursing staff, physicians, other members of the health care team, and members of the community. Education may be formal (in-service or conference presentations, mentoring students or new staff) or informal ("curbside" questions, telephone consultations). In my role I frequently consult with other providers such as surgeons, medical specialists, and mental health providers to be able to ensure optimal care for my patients. Providers who are unfamiliar with transplantation often seek out the assistance of the transplant coordinator to ensure that the plan of care is appropriate, that prescribed medications do not interfere with the immunosuppressive regimen, and that comorbidities and medication side effects are appropriately addressed. Additionally, I have had the opportunity to collaborate with colleagues from other institutions in the publication of specialty core curricula for the International Transplant Nurses Society as well as the American Association of Heart Failure Nurses.

Prior to discharge following heart transplantation, I teach patients and their caregivers about the immunosuppressive regimen—including dosing and side effects of medications, signs and symptoms of infection and/or rejection, and health promotion strategies (appropriate immunizations, age-appropriate cancer screening, and heart transplant surveillance). This information is reinforced during clinic visits and during other informal conversations as needed.

Successful transplantation requires collaboration among many disciplines. In fact, the Centers for Medicare and Medicaid Services and the United Network for Organ Sharing mandate an interprofessional care model. This interprofessional team consists of surgeons, physicians, nurses, social workers, psychologists, financial counselors, nutritionists, and pharmacists. At different times along the transplant continuum, each patient is reviewed by this team and the plan of care is developed or modified as necessary. The transplant coordinator often leads these team discussions as well as ensures that the appropriate team members have an opportunity to contribute information and expertise. At times these meetings can be contentious because opinions may differ, and the coordinator must guide the team to develop goals for a successful patient outcome. This may also include difficult decisions—ethical dilemmas regarding whether or not to offer heart transplantation. The discussions are difficult because there may not be another treatment option that would provide the patient with improved quality of life.

Optimal care of the heart transplant candidate and recipient is both evidence based and guideline directed; thus an understanding of the research process and the ability to translate research findings into clinical practice is essential. As a transplant coordinator I participate in research, both investigator-directed and multi-institutional protocols, as well as review and critique research manuscripts for publication.

In summary, the specialty of organ transplantation continues to grow because of the rising incidence of end-stage organ failure in the population. As an APRN heart transplant coordinator, my clinical role includes both direct and indirect care for and on behalf of a complex patient population. I am afforded the opportunity to enact the core competencies of advanced practice nursing because of the technologic advances in management of heart failure and the influence of these advances on care delivery. The added value of the knowledge of these core competencies enhances care for patients across the transplant continuum. ◎

[a]The author gratefully acknowledges Maureen Flattery, MS, RN, ANP-BC, Richmond, Virginia, for assistance with this exemplar.

1.6 million people were dying from violence every year and more were being injured and suffering mental health consequences. More recent information confirms the prominence of this public health problem as a leading cause of mortality, psychologic health effects, and lifelong disability (WHO, 2010).

In 1991, the ANA published a position statement on violence as a nursing practice issue and, in 1995, at the request of the International Association of Forensic Nurses (IAFN), they officially recognized forensic nursing as a specialty. In the wake of the ANA position statement, the American College of Nurse-Midwives (in 1995) and the Emergency Nurses Association (in 1996) issued similar statements (Burgess et al., 2004). The scope and standards of forensic nursing practice were initially published in collaboration with the IAFN in 1997 (IAFN/ANA, 1997). These standards were updated in 2009 (IAFN/ANA, 2009) and are in the process of being revised in 2017.

Since the 1970s, nurses have been formally recognized providers of health care services to victims of violence. Nurses have volunteered at rape crisis centers and, by the mid-1980s, were widely acknowledged for the expertise they had developed. In addition, nurses also were being recognized for their research competence. This combination of factors opened doors for nurses to collaborate with other health care providers, initiate courses and programs of research on victimology and traumatology, influence legislation and health care policy, and ultimately create a new specialty (Burgess et al., 2004). One organization, the Academy on Violence and Abuse, established in 2005 in response to the challenge issued by the Institute of Medicine (IOM, 2011b; see also Cohn, Salmon, & Stobo, 2002) to educate and train health professionals better about the often unrecognized health effects of violence and abuse, has worked extensively with multidisciplinary experts in violence and abuse prevention (e.g., nurses, dentists, social workers, psychologists, counselors, physicians). Their goal was to develop competencies at the level of the health care system, educational institution, and individuals to be a common starting point for profession-specific criteria regarding the skills, knowledge, and attitudes required for prevention (Ambuel et al., 2011). These efforts broaden the scope of influence of forensic nurses and offer opportunities to advance the specialty.

According to the ANA and IAFN, forensic nursing practice is the integration of nursing science, criminal justice, public health, forensic science, and phenomena related to violence and trauma across the life span in providing forensic health care to patients, families, communities, and populations (ANA/IAFN, 2015). Specialization in forensic nursing involves work with perpetrators and victims of interpersonal violence (sexual assault, elder abuse, domestic abuse/violence), death investigations, and legal and ethical issues. Forensic nurses work in concert with a collaborative, multidisciplinary group of professionals such as forensic psychiatric nurses, correctional nurses, emergency nurses, and trauma nurses, as well as a variety of other medical and law enforcement personnel. They may work for specialized hospital units (e.g., forensic psychiatric units), in emergency rooms, in medical examiners' offices, for law enforcement, as legal consultants, and for social services agencies. In addition, in collaboration with school nurses as a consequence of the increasing incidence of school violence, forensic nurses are becoming a significant line of defense for at-risk individuals, groups, agencies, and communities in efforts to reduce school violence (Jones, Waite, & Clements, 2012).

Like most stage II specialties, forensic nursing has traditionally been taught outside of formal education programs. Some of the earliest programs were institution-based programs preparing nurses as sexual assault nurse examiners (SANEs). The Commission for Forensic Nursing Certification, the successor to the Forensic Nursing Certification Board, was established in 2012 as an autonomous body to continue the Board's important work in advancing the certification programs of the IAFN. The Commission (IAFN, 2016a) offers three professional credentials: the adult/adolescent (SANE-A®) certification, the pediatric (SANE-P®) certification, and in collaboration with the American Nurses Credentialing Center (ANCC), the portfolio in advanced forensic nursing (AFN-BC). Newer education programs, such as those that prepare sexual assault forensic examiners (SAFEs) or forensic nurse examiners (FNEs), have expanded the scope of forensic nursing practice to include not only sexual assault incidents but also the gathering of forensic evidence in cases of domestic abuse or vehicular accident (IAFN, 2016b).

The trend of educating forensic nurses in certificate programs is changing as graduate nursing programs are established; thus forensic nursing is a specialty in transition. Similar to previous efforts to move WOC nursing into graduate nursing education programs (Gray, Ratliff, & Mawyer, 2000), forensic nursing has been taught at the graduate level in a few institutions for several years. Although certificate programs are sometimes the route to preparation, there are now several master's and DNP programs offering this specialty preparation.

Commentary: Stage II

Forensic nursing provides a different perspective on evolving specialties and is used here to illustrate a stage II practice that may become advanced practice, integrating multiple other specialties such as the family NP, psychiatric and mental health NP and CNS, and women's health NP. In stage II, the specialty becomes more organized and visible. Formal training programs develop, specialty organizations form, and certification moves beyond individual institution-based certificates for completion of training to national certification examinations. All these developments lend strength and credibility to the specialty and its practitioners. Although many forensic nurses are prepared in certificate programs, being a specialty in transition to advanced practice nursing presents some opportunities for this particular specialty to advance to a stage III practice.

One of the major challenges in stage II is demonstrating that the specialty is a nursing specialty. There are a number of evolving specialties, such as the previously mentioned advanced diabetes managers and clinical transplant coordinators, whose practitioners include non-nurses and nurses. Clearly, these roles cannot emerge as advanced practice nursing roles without clear distinctions being drawn between non-nursing practice and nursing practice in the specialty. Specialty organizations with members who are non–health care providers, such as NATCO, must face this challenge. In the case of transplantation, for example, recognition of an APRN level of practice or a sanctioning of practice at the APRN level for all specialty providers is evolving. For CTCs or other advanced practice nurses working with transplant candidates or recipients, a mechanism for certifying advanced practice transplant nurses (e.g., through the ITNS) is necessary to recognize nursing's essential role in transplantation, without diminishing the contributions of others who also provide essential care and services.

Emerging Advanced Practice Nursing Specialties (Stage III)

In the third stage of evolution to advanced practice, a specialty's knowledge base is growing and the scope of practice of nurses with specialty education is expanding. There is growing recognition of the additional knowledge and skills needed for increasingly complex practice in the specialty (Hamric, 2000). Pressures for standardization of education and skills required for specialty practice create incentives to move certificate-level training programs into graduate-level educational settings to increase standardization and raise the status of the specialty to an advanced practice level (Hanson & Hamric, 2003). According to Hanson and Hamric (2003), antecedents to legitimizing advanced practice must be addressed for a given specialty to evolve to advanced levels of practice (see Box 5.1). Two organizations are addressing the issues necessary to legitimize advanced practice in their specialties: the American Association of Nurse Anesthetists (AANA) for interventional pain practice and the Wound, Ostomy and Continence Nurses Society (WOCNS) for WOC nursing. Although these organizations have adopted differing approaches to advancing practice in their respective specialties, in each case the process was unified and proactive and depicts a framework that can guide other specialty organizations as they chart a course to advanced levels of practice.

Interventional Pain Practice

Millions of individuals suffer from acute or chronic pain every year, and the effects of pain exact a tremendous cost on our country in health care costs, rehabilitation, and lost worker productivity, as well as the emotional and financial burden it places on patients and their families (American Academy of Pain Medicine [AAPM], 2016a). According to the AAPM (2016a), pain affects more Americans than diabetes, heart disease, and cancer combined. Patients' unrelieved chronic pain problems often result in an inability to work and maintain health insurance. According to a recent IOM report, *Relieving Pain in America: A Blueprint for Transforming Prevention, Care, Education, and Research* (2011a), pain is a significant public health problem that costs society at least $560 to $635 billion annually, an amount equal to about $2000 for every person living in the United States. Much more needs to be done to meet the challenges of chronic pain management.

Because it is underrecognized and undertreated, the overall quality of pain management is and has been unacceptable to millions of patients with chronic pain. Pain management, particularly acute pain management, has been widely embraced in the inpatient and outpatient settings and is provided by a variety of health care professionals, including physicians, PAs, CRNAs, CNSs, and NPs. Interventional pain management, however, has emerged as the need to treat chronic pain has grown. APRNs as interventional pain practitioners face complex and often controversial issues that challenge the legitimacy of this practice.

One example is that of CRNAs who, in 1994, expanded their scope of practice to incorporate pain management specifically (AANA Board of Directors, 1994). In the wake of the 2001 Centers for Medicare and Medicaid Services policy, which allowed states to opt out of the reimbursement requirement that a surgeon or anesthesiologist oversee the provision of anesthesia by CRNAs, challenges to this option have been levied in several states to restrict more autonomous practice by these APRNs. It is the position of the American Society of Interventional Pain Physicians (Douglas, 2008; Huddleston, 2016) and the American Society of Anesthesiologists (2009) that interventional pain management is the practice of medicine. Thus actions have been taken in several states to restrict CRNA scope of practice in chronic pain management. Although the outcomes of these actions have been equivocal, in one response by the Federal Trade Commission (FTC) Office of Policy Planning, Bureaus of Economics and Competition, AANA directors replied to an invitation to comment on legislation that would regulate (restrict) providers of interventional pain management services. Insightful comments in this reply addressed the recent IOM report (2011a) that identified a key role for APRNs in improving access to health care and cautioned that restrictions on scope of practice have undermined nurses' ability to provide and improve general and advanced care (IOM, 2011a). Furthermore, the AANA expressed concerns that problems with access to these services may be especially acute for older patients with chronic pain as well as for rural and low-income individuals (AANA, 2011). Because a major component of the legislation addressed consumer protection, legislators were advised to investigate the need for the bill and its potential negative effects on cost, access, and consumer choice and, in the absence of safety concerns, reject the legislation (FTC, 2011). Similar issues have been addressed more recently (FTC, 2012), and concerns related to access and cost were raised—with suggestions to further review the impact of the proposed legislation. Notably, research has demonstrated no increase in adverse outcomes in opt-out or non–opt-out states as a consequence of CRNAs practicing without supervision (Dulisse & Cromwell, 2010).

Although these scope of practice issues are unresolved, attention to opportunities for interprofessional collaboration is essential for the pain interventionist role to grow and for APRNs to be recognized as competent providers. To be recognized for their role in chronic pain management, APRNs must be more visible in organizations such as the AAPM and the American Pain Society (APS). Both these organizations welcome providers from multiple disciplines, but nursing is underrepresented. The APS (2016) has reported that approximately 50% of its members are physicians and only 7.4% are nurses. Membership and participation in this organization would improve visibility, recognition, and colleagueship with others providing chronic pain management services. The AAPM (2016a) endorsed the collective benefits that professionals from a variety of disciplines can make to the specialty of pain management. Unlike the APS, the AAPM does offer a credentialing examination (AAPM, 2016b). There are two levels of credentialing—diplomate and fellow—both of which require 2 years of pain management practice prior to examination application. The diplomate credential requires a doctoral degree in a related health care field and the fellow credential requires a master's degree, also in a related health care field. A credentialing review committee determines eligibility to sit for the examination; administration, scoring, psychometric consultation, and analysis of the examination are conducted by an external agency. Although this credential would not be required for specialty practice in chronic pain management, obtaining this certification would ensure a common knowledge base and competencies among all disciplines. Because knowledge and competency have been addressed in challenges to scope of practice, which incorporates chronic pain management, this credential would ensure continuing education and upholding the standards of care in pain management practice. In addition to interdisciplinary certification encompassing core competencies of the specialty, voluntary subspecialty certification for nurse anesthetists in nonsurgical pain management (NSPM-C) through the National Board of Certification and Recertification of Nurse Anesthetists (2016)—initiated in January, 2015—would also establish credibility and promote recognition of practice in the specialty.

Wound, Ostomy, and Continence Nursing

WOC nursing, a specialty that developed in response to unmet patient needs after fecal or urinary diversion surgery, has evolved significantly since its inception in the 1960s. Historically, laypersons developed the subspecialty, dedicated exclusively to the care of ostomy patients (WOCNS, 1998). As health care changed and new patient needs arose, the original enterostomal therapy role evolved into a nursing specialty whose scope of practice expanded to include wound, skin, and continence care in addition to ostomy care. The WOCNS now recognizes four levels of care providers: WOC advanced practice registered nurse, WOC specialty nurse, foot care nurse, and wound treatment associate (Wound, Ostomy and Continence Nursing Certification Board [WOCNCB], 2016; Wound Treatment Associate Task Force, 2012). Thus the WOCNS and the WOCNCB differentiate among levels of care providers based on certification. The appropriate use of each level of wound care provider is endorsed (WOCNS, 2016).

The educational preparation for WOC nurses, which began as clinical training programs based heavily on experiential knowledge about ostomy management, has been provided in postbaccalaureate education programs. Some of these programs have begun to offer graduate-level course work in the specialty. Thus the content has been integrated to a limited extent into graduate curricula of some universities in the United States (Gray et al., 2000; WOCNS, 2016), and over time this trend has continued.

Eligibility for advanced practice certification in WOC nursing requires a registered nurse (RN) license and/or a license to practice as an APRN and a master's or higher degree in nursing in an advanced practice role (WOCNCB, 2016). These recent decisions by the WOCNCB to differentiate certification based on education clearly represent progress in addressing the added value of APRNs in this specialty. This is a critical decision point for this stage III specialty. Similar to the work done by the International Society of Nurses in Genetics (ISONG; see "Genetics Advanced Practice Nursing" later), who established levels of genetics knowledge, practice, and certification, WOC nursing has advocated for APRNs as having unique characteristics and contributions to make. These contributions reflect advanced practice core competencies obtained in graduate nursing education in addition to competencies attained in a specialty program aimed at preparing WOC nurses. The advanced practice certification builds on the entry-level certification and offers an incentive to entry-level WOC nurses to complete graduate nursing education as an APRN; it also further legitimizes the advanced practice of WOC nursing.

APRNs in the specialty may also wish to pursue additional recognition for advanced practice competency. Some nurses with graduate education in WOC nursing may seek certification as a wound management specialist (certified wound specialist [CWS]), a certification awarded to qualified clinicians through the American Board of Wound Management (2016) by the American Academy of Wound Management, a multidisciplinary organization; CNSs or NPs may seek certification as a urologic specialist by the certification board of the Society of Urologic Nurses and Associates (Certification Board for Urologic Nurses and Associates, 2016). In particular, the CWS certification recognizes a shared clinical knowledge base among professionals providing care to patients with complex wounds and may foster collaborative relationships that would further advance this specialty.

Commentary: Stage III

The stage III specialties discussed here are characterized by a growing knowledge base and an expanded scope of practice. For example, APRNs practicing as pain interventionists, most notably CRNAs, have expanded their scope of practice to incorporate advanced diagnostic and treatment knowledge and skills to make pain intervention more accessible. As a consequence, questions regarding their qualifications to provide these services have led to legal challenges. Some APRNs in this specialty, in addition to advanced practice certification, have responded to these challenges by seeking credentialing by multidisciplinary specialty organizations, a strategy that lends credibility to their practice. This barrier to evolution to a stage IV specialty is likely to be overcome as more APRNs transition to this specialty and demonstrate practice competencies. Exemplar 5.3 depicts an interprofessional collaborative practice and the CRNA's knowledge and expertise to deliver patient-centered, evidence-based care. To increase awareness of what can safely and competently be provided by CRNAs in pain management practice, these APRNs need to increase their visibility through membership in pain management specialty organizations and credentialing as pain practitioners, better positioning the specialty to emerge as a stage IV role.

WOC nurses have clearly differentiated basic professional practice from advanced practice in the specialty. However, attention to several issues is still necessary for the specialty to emerge fully at the advanced (stage IV) level (Box 5.2). For example, most WOC nurses are educated in certification

EXEMPLAR 5.3	Interventional Pain Practice[a]

The inception of PainCare in 1992 marked the beginning of interprofessional interventional pain management in the northern New England region of Maine, New Hampshire, and Vermont. This organization began to address a growing need for management of untreated chronic pain in underserved and remote regions of the northeast. Five certified registered nurse anesthetists (CRNAs) work as fully autonomous clinicians within this highly specialized practice setting; they provide comprehensive pain management services to those suffering from a wide variety of chronic pain conditions, many of whom have suffered for years without relief as the result of lack of access to specialized pain care.

In our pain management facility, the process of treating chronic painful conditions begins with meeting the patient during an initial office visit. The referral base for our patients includes specialty physicians (neurosurgical and orthopedic surgeons), primary care physicians, and nurse practitioners. This initial consultation entails taking a comprehensive and detailed medical and surgical history and performing a focused physical examination. At the conclusion of the initial office visit, we order the appropriate laboratory and imaging studies based on best evidence. Diagnostic studies may include electromyelography, ultrasound scanning, angiography, and/or bone scans. Because pain management is often interdisciplinary, we may make referrals to specialists such as neurologists, physiatrists, endocrinologists, oncologists, or orthopedic surgeons.

One of our roles as CRNA pain practitioners is to assimilate the findings from the patient's detailed medical history, extensively focused physical examination, and diagnostic testing. This is essential in identifying the causative pain generator and engaging an accurate treatment plan. Chronic pain can be difficult to treat and standard, conservative, and surgical treatments may prove unsuccessful. Prior surgical interventions often contribute to a patient's suffering. Furthermore, most patients who seek care at the pain center are currently taking prescription narcotics. Large doses of narcotics contribute significantly to tolerance issues. Side effects and systemic complications related to these potent medications are evident during the initial consultation with the patient. In these cases, pain relief is no longer forthcoming. The patient in chronic pain may experience many years of treatment and mistreatment prior to seeking care at our pain center.

Management of chronic pain requires a multimodal treatment plan. Once the process of patient counseling is initiated, it is our responsibility to initiate the discussion about realistic pain management expectations through patient education. Educating patients with regard to their pathology and treatment plan helps them gain a sense of control and understanding and places them as the central change agent. These chronic pain management patients are expected to attend all scheduled appointments and be active participants in the treatment plan. The patient must know that management of his or her pain will take time and that improving quality of life is a major goal of treatment.

As pain managers, we regularly make referrals as an integral component of clinical practice. Referrals may be made for one or a combination of the following: physical therapy, occupational therapy, chiropractic sessions, acupuncture, craniosacral therapy, and/or message therapy. We may refer obese or diabetic patients to nutritionists for counseling if it is thought that these conditions may be contributing to their pain. Additionally, therapeutic devices such as lumbar, thoracic, and cervical support braces, transcutaneous electrical nerve stimulation (TENS) units, or orthotics may be incorporated into the treatment plan for spine and extremity pain. Smoking cessation, biofeedback, and hypnosis may also play a role in effective pain management treatment plans.

Frequently, we see patients with coexisting psychiatric issues such as anxiety, depression, bipolar disorder, substance abuse, and posttraumatic stress disorder. Psychiatric professionals provide treatment and counseling as an essential part of an effective treatment plan. If a question of substance abuse arises, referrals for substance abuse evaluation and treatment are initiated. Our practice environment includes a comprehensive substance abuse program that plays an integral role in our interprofessional treatment facility.

An essential part of the practice includes medication management. Prescribing and selecting from a wide array of medications with various mechanisms of action contribute to the goal of relieving the patient's suffering. For example, opioids are prescribed for severe persistent pain and offer significant relief when other pharmacologic agents are not effective. On the other hand, more invasive procedures such as interventional injections may be used, which directly address causative pain generators. For example, during any given week, a pain manager may administer 40 to 50 cervical, thoracic, and lumbar epidural steroid injections; transforaminal injections; facet joint and medial branch nerve blocks

Continued

to the cervical, thoracic, and lumbar regions; stellate ganglion blocks; lumbar sympathetic blocks; hypogastric plexus blocks; occipital nerve blocks; intra-articular joint injections; and peripheral nerve blocks.

To improve accuracy and maximize safety, all invasive procedures are performed under direct fluoroscopic guidance to ensure accurate needle placement. Every interventional injectionist must be an expert with regard to imaging analysis and interpretation. CRNAs involved in pain management recognize the potential for serious and sometimes fatal complications related to these procedures. Profound and lasting pain relief, and quality and safety in practice, mandate that the pain practitioner be well trained in invasive and non-invasive pain management techniques as well as radiation safety.

Prior to independent practice, I was trained under the direct supervision of an anesthesiologist–interventional pain physician. Successful completion of interventional injection procedures under direct supervision and documentation of hundreds of procedures was required to be involved in this type of advanced practice. My clinical privileges were granted on written request and approved by the medical director and clinical board members. In 2009, I earned a Doctor of Nurse Anesthesia Practice (DNAP) degree that has further prepared me to incorporate best evidence into my clinical practice, contribute to nurse anesthesia scholarship, and assume various leadership roles. Additionally, I am certified with the American Academy of Pain Management as a Diplomate. This certification requires a doctoral degree, a 2-year practice in a pain management setting, recommendations from colleagues, and successful completion of a written certification examination. Additional study and training include participation in interventional pain cadaver conferences and completion of continuing education via the American Academy of Pain Management and the International Association for the Study of Pain.

The nurse anesthesia subspecialty of pain management is evolving in many exciting and innovative ways. For example, Excel Anesthesia and Pain Management Associates (EAPMA) is a group of CRNAs who provide training for university-based student registered nurse anesthetists (SRNAs) and other CRNA populations. Under Medicare guidelines, EAPMA CRNAs are able to bill for direct supervision and training of resident SRNAs. This unique billing arrangement is expected to enhance and expand CRNA pain practice. One US university has developed a specialized pain track for nurse anesthetists earning a clinical doctoral degree. Graduates of this program will qualify to sit for the AAPM certification examination. Members of EAPMA are also developing a separate certification examination for subspecialty pain management practice.

I believe the training and certification of CRNA pain managers is at an exciting turning point and will continue to establish itself. These well-trained and qualified pain practitioners will be a new generation of clinicians able to provide access to pain management services to underserved, critical access, and remote regions of the United States in which these services are currently unavailable. With over 400 patients under my care, I function autonomously in the role of pain manager. It is a true joy to practice in a setting where I am respected as an equal among interventional pain physicians, physiatrists, anesthesiologists, nurse practitioners, physician assistants, and primary care physicians. Almost all patients make significant progress in managing their chronic pain using an interprofessional treatment plan. Patients too often arrive at a pain center misunderstood and misdiagnosed, with their complaints deemed questionable. My role as pain manager at our facility is vital and serves an important public health function. The most gratifying part of my work is to witness patients who obtain pain relief for the first time in their lives. ◎

[a]The author gratefully acknowledges Russell Plewinski, DNAP, CRNA, DAAPM, Somersworth, New Hampshire, and Suzanne M. Wright, PhD, CRNA, Richmond, Virginia, for assistance with this exemplar.

programs. Only two accredited programs offer graduate credit for coursework toward clinical master's or doctoral degrees (DNP) (WOCNCB, 2016). Preparation in graduate or post-master's programs would standardize education and advance practice in the specialty. There are levels of practice in place that differentiate advanced practice nursing through their certification process. Thus this specialty is poised to emerge as a stage IV specialty as a result

of efforts clarifying certification and credentialing requirements and the initiation of advanced practice certification.

Established Advanced Practice Nursing Roles (Stage IV)

The fourth stage in the evolution of specialty practice to advanced practice is characterized by mature

BOX 5.2 **Questions to Address in Charting Specialty Evolution**

- Are advanced practice nursing competencies required to enact specialty practice fully, or are they an added value?
- What are the distinct advanced practice nursing roles within the specialty?
- How can the organization best recognize and value existing providers while moving to new expectations?
- How should certification and educational expectations be structured, especially if differentiating practice between non-APRNs and APRNs continues within the specialty?
- How should subspecialty certification within the context of advanced practice nursing regulation be addressed?
- How can the centrality of direct clinical practice be maintained?

specialties. APRNs practicing in these specialties are experts in the specialty, secure in understanding the unique contributions that they make in the direct care of patients. However, they embrace the notion that aspects of their practice are shared by experts from other disciplines essential to the care of their patients. Because of its origins in interprofessional practice, the advanced diabetes manager characterizes an established APRN role. APRNs in genetics have overcome obstacles to interdisciplinary practice through the development of interprofessional collaborative relationships and have also emerged as a stage IV APRN role.

Advanced Diabetes Manager

The rising incidence of diabetes mellitus has created new opportunities for APRNs. Advances in the science and technology of diabetes care and findings from two clinical research trials have redefined the roles of health care providers in diabetes care. Two classic studies, the Diabetes Control and Complications Trial (Diabetes Control and Complications Trial Research Group et al., 1993) and the United Kingdom Prospective Diabetes Study (United Kingdom Prospective Diabetes Study Group, 1998), have demonstrated the value of interprofessional teams consisting of dietitians, nurses, and pharmacists in the clinical management of those with diabetes mellitus. Before the results of these clinical trials were released, however, the American Association of Diabetes

Educators (AADE, 2004) published multidisciplinary scope and standards of practice guidelines, which were revised in 2005 (Martin et al., 2005). An advanced practice task force was established in 1993, and the dialogue among the three major disciplines constituting the membership of the association— nurses, dietitians, and pharmacists—and their credentialing bodies was initiated (Hentzen, 1994; Tobin, 2000). These collaborative efforts resulted in a definition of advanced practice in diabetes as the highest of various levels of practice used along the full continuum of diabetes care (Hentzen, 1994; Tobin, 2000). These levels are identified as the certified diabetes educator (CDE) and the board-certified advanced diabetes manager (BC-ADM) (Martin et al., 2005).

The CDE is a health care provider who meets educational and practice requirements, successfully completes the certification examination for diabetes educators, and is credentialed by the National Certification Board for Diabetes Educators. The CDE can provide the following: case management; diabetes education program development, coordination, and implementation; and referral to advanced practitioners, other health care team members, or community resources.

The BC-ADM, launched in 2000 as a result of unprecedented multiorganizational collaboration and initially credentialed by the ANCC, has been credentialed by the AADE since 2011. This advanced practice credential focuses on the management of diabetes, including prescribing medications, rather than on diabetes education; thus this credential distinguishes between two sets of skills (Daly, Kulkarni, & Boucher, 2001; Valentine, Kulkarni, & Hinnen, 2003). This level of credentialing is designed for licensed health care professionals, including registered dietitians, RNs, and registered pharmacists, as well as—more recently—PAs and physicians who hold graduate/advanced degrees and have recent clinical diabetes management experiences after they have been licensed. Currently, RNs make up the largest proportion of BC-ADMs (56.7%), followed by pharmacists (18.7%) and dietitians (9.5%) (J. Ricketts-Byrne, personal communication, 2016). Credentialing as a CDE is not required to take the advanced management examination.

Notably, the BC-ADM designation is unique. Although each discipline eligible for certification takes a different examination (Valentine et al., 2003), it was the first multidisciplinary approach to the certification of nurses, dietitians, and pharmacists ever developed by the ANCC (Daly et al., 2001;

Valentine et al., 2003). The fact that the ANCC agreed with the AADE's request to support the advanced-level examination for disciplines other than nursing to promote team collaboration and improve quality of care for individuals with diabetes represented the emergence of a new model of collaboration among practitioners who formerly may have competed for recognition by patient and consumer groups. The potential benefits of multidisciplinary certification include increased credibility with colleagues, patients and consumers, employers, and other health care professionals as a result of a shared knowledge base; differentiation of these providers as having advanced-level expertise in diabetes management; greater autonomy in the delivery of care and services; and improved reimbursement (Daly et al., 2001). In this multidisciplinary model, APRNs fill a niche in the care of these patients that facilitates self-care and achievement of treatment goals. Nurses constitute the largest group of health care professionals who deliver care to individuals with diabetes mellitus across the life span and in a variety of settings; therefore, graduate-level preparation for APRNs in diabetes management, consistent with American Diabetes Association standards, helps to fulfill the growing need for care providers in acute and primary care settings.

Genetics Advanced Practice Nursing

Mapping the human genome and the relevance of the Human Genome Project to health and disease have been revolutionizing the provision of genetic services specifically and health care generally. New genetic discoveries have made available an increasing number of genetic technologies for carrier, prenatal, diagnostic, and presymptomatic testing for genetic conditions. These discoveries are creating changes in the delivery of genetic services, the most immediate being the integration of genetics into the prevention and treatment, for example, of cardiovascular disease (Arnett et al., 2007; Santos et al., 2016), obesity (Walley, Blakemore, & Froguel, 2006; Yang, Kelly, & He, 2007), and cancer (Balmain, Gray, & Ponder, 2003; Karakasis, Burnier, Bowering, Oza, & Lheureux, 2016). Although brought to the forefront of public awareness by the mapping of the human genome, genetic services initially emerged out of a need for professionals who could provide genetic information, education, and support to patients and families with current and future genetic health concerns. Genetics experts in academic, medical, public health, and community-based settings have

traditionally provided these services. In each setting, genetics professionals, including medical geneticists, genetics counselors, and genetics APRNs, provide genetic services to patients and families. Working with other team members, genetics specialists obtain and interpret complex family history information, evaluate and diagnose genetic conditions, interpret and discuss complicated genetic test results, support patients throughout the genetic counseling process, and offer resources for additional individual and family support. Personalized medicine, an approach to care in which an individual's genomic information is used to tailor interventions to maximize health outcomes, is rapidly becoming a reality for several health conditions as a result of increased understanding of some of the most common health conditions (Feero & Guttmacher, 2014).

According to ISONG, the scope of genetics nursing practice is basic and advanced. At the basic level, genetics nurses are prepared to perform assessments to identify risk factors, plan care, provide interventions such as information, and evaluate for referral to genetic services. At the advanced level, master's-prepared nurses provide genetic counseling, case management, consultation, and evaluation of patients, families, resources, and/or programs (ANA/ISONG, 2016). Two levels of practice and recognition, which correspond to the scope of genetics nursing practice, currently exist: the genetics clinical nurse (GCN) and the advanced genetics nurse credential (AGN-BC). The credentials conferred by the ANCC mandate that specific educational, practice, and professional service requirements are met. The process is accomplished using a portfolio review. Eligibility for the AGN-BC certification requires the following: (1) hold a current, active RN license in a state or territory of the United States or hold the professional, legally recognized equivalent in another country; (2) practice the equivalent of at least 2 years full time as an RN; (3) have a graduate degree (master's, postgraduate certificate, or doctoral degree) in nursing; (4) have a minimum of 1500 practice hours in the specialty area of advanced genetics nursing in the past 3 years; and (5) have completed a minimum of 30 continuing education hours in genetics/genomics applicable to nursing within the last 3 years (ANCC, 2016). Currently, there are 82 nurses who hold AGN-BC certification (A. S. Kerber, personal communication, 2016).

Only four programs offer graduate-level genetic programs for nurses. Currently, educational preparation for APRNs occurs in master's programs in nursing. Although an increased focus on genetics has been occurring in graduate nursing programs as a result of recent revisions in the *Essentials of Master's Education in Nursing* (American Association of Colleges of Nursing, 2011), genetic content is usually obtained later in postbaccalaureate education programs or through continuing education courses. Regardless of the type of program or course, the course content must reflect the following: information in human genetics; molecular and biochemical genetics; ethical, legal, and social issues in genetics; genetic variations in populations; and clinical application of genetics, including genetic counseling to meet requirements for certification. Expectations for evidence-based practice, an advanced practice competency, which has the potential to transform health care because of integration of genetic knowledge, requires the knowledge acquired in graduate nursing education. In addition, the ethical decision-making skills of APRNs are important to this specialty. Because graduate nursing education preparation required for the AGN-BC credential places these nurses at the same level as other genetic services providers, such as genetics counselors, professional diversity and interprofessional collaboration are fostered.

The American Board of Genetic Counseling certifies some nurses; however, this avenue is not open to nurses unless they complete graduate education and clinical practice requirements in genetics medicine, human genetics, and/or genetic counseling. Nurses who wish to pursue graduate education solely in nursing are not eligible for this certification. Because the scope of practice for the advanced practice nurse in genetics is much broader than that of a genetics counselor, differentiation based on credentials is appropriate. In addition to counseling, the advanced practice nurse in genetics diagnoses and treats patients with a variety of clinical disorders (e.g., birth defects, chromosomal abnormalities, genetic disorders presenting in newborn, child, and adult muscular disorders, and intrauterine teratogen exposure) and inherited conditions. Because of the complexity of care required, collaboration among these professionals is necessary for appropriate genetics services delivery. Toward this end, the National Society of Genetic Counselors and ISONG jointly developed a position statement advocating a multidisciplinary collaborative approach to enhance the quality of genetic services and care (ISONG, 2006). These efforts by the ISONG have positioned the specialty to transition to a stage IV specialty as a result of collaborative efforts with genetics counselors who are master's prepared for their role (Exemplar 5.4).

Commentary: Stage IV

Caring for persons with diabetes has become complex, requiring the expertise and efforts of interprofessional teams. Because the nature of caring for patients with diabetes has historically required interdisciplinary collaboration, health care providers from these disciplines are secure in understanding the unique contributions that they make in patient management. They are experts—secure in their individual and shared clinical knowledge base—and embrace the challenges and opportunities inherent in interprofessional collaboration. This model of collaboration is somewhat unique and has been expertly developed by leaders in the AADE. The trajectory of change that was initiated in the early 1990s exemplifies the natural maturation of the specialty resulting from deliberate logical planning to strengthen the education and broaden the scope of practice of practitioners in this specialty. Similarly, and strategically, ISONG has made tremendous progress in defining roles for health care providers, including APRNs who are experts in genetics, fostering a collaborative relationship with genetic counselors and differentiating levels of practice within interprofessional teams.

Conclusion

As can be seen from Chapter 1, the evolution of specialties in nursing has a long and rich history that continues in the present. The progress made by members of specialty organizations that have evolved their specialties to advanced levels of practice (stages III and IV) can serve as examples for others that are struggling to evolve (stage II) or are newly emerging (stage I).

This chapter has examined each of these stages in the context of selected specialty groups and the evolving and innovative roles that characterize progression toward advanced practice nursing. Clearly, the ability to be deliberate in efforts to evolve the specialty speeds progress, as demonstrated by organizations such as the WOCN, AADE, and ISONG. Some specialties have evolved haphazardly. Others may not evolve into advanced practice nursing; without commitment from the nursing community and attention to the issues noted in Boxes 5.1 and 5.2, the move toward advanced practice nursing may be an unrealistic goal. It is important to recognize that progression to advanced levels of practice is neither inevitable nor necessary. For example, staff development educators are a respected specialty

EXEMPLAR 5.4   **Insights From Leaders in the Genetics Specialty**[a]

In 1976, the Genetic Diseases Act was passed by Congress and the Genetic Diseases Services Branch of the Office of Maternal Child Health, Health Services Administration, Department of Health and Human Services, was established. At that time, a small and academically diverse group of nurses was working with genetic programs in tertiary health care settings. They tended to come from practice backgrounds in pediatrics or obstetrics, which made sense because genetic services at that time were centered primarily on the delivery of prenatal diagnostic procedures and the evaluation of the dysmorphic child or the child with developmental delays. A relatively small number of master's-prepared genetics counselors also were working in similar settings. In the 1980s, however, medical geneticists started to employ or collaborate with nurses rather than counselors for a variety of reasons, including the limited number of counselors available and the broader scope of practice of nurses.

Differing perspectives emerged regarding basic requirements for certification and the appropriate credentialing body for awarding certification. Genetics counselors are required to have a degree from an approved master of science in genetic counseling program and are credentialed through the American Board of Medical Genetics (ABMG). In contrast, nurses advocated for a professional nursing organization as an appropriate credentialing body and graduate education in nursing as an acceptable educational route.

The number of genetics counselors increased faster than the number of genetics nurses in the 1980s. This led to the education meetings of the National Society of Genetic Counselors (NSGC) becoming focused on the learning needs of genetics counselors, not consistently and sufficiently addressing the issues that confronted genetics nurses. After the initial NSGC educational meetings, a bond was formed among those nurses working in genetics and monies were found to form the Genetics Nursing Network. In 1987, there was significant discussion among the members of the network regarding the benefits of establishing a formal professional organization for genetics nurses. The lack

of a professional group and the inability to obtain certification that would be recognized by the nursing profession led to the development of the International Society of Nurses in Genetics (ISONG). Membership in the organization continued to grow but the issue of certification remained unresolved. Nurses working in genetics had academic preparation ranging from diplomas to doctoral degrees. Some were already certified as genetics counselors and others were certified as nurse practitioners in their specialty area. After significant discussion by the membership of the ISONG, it was thought that the core knowledge required by genetics nurses was broader, but there was also the issue of recognition of a credential provided by a non-nursing organization being accepted by the nursing community. Also, it was understood that at that time there were not enough nurses to sit for a written examination to provide for test item validation. Therefore the Genetic Nursing Credentialing Commission was established to investigate alternatives that would address these issues. After extensive work, the Commission announced the establishment of the advanced practice nurse in genetics (APNG) credential and awarded the first credentials (by portfolio) in 2001. Currently the advanced genetics nurse credential (AGN-BC) is provided by the American Nurses Credentialing Center (2016).

As genetic knowledge has continued to develop, genetics has become an integral part of the education and clinical practice of all nurses. The ISONG has worked with the National Coalition for Health Professional Education in Genetics to develop competencies for health care professionals at the generalist and specialty levels and has collaborated with the American Nurses Association (2008) to publish these competencies, curricula guidelines, and outcome indicators specific to nurses. ISONG continues to grow and develop to meet the needs of nurses who are at any point on the novice to expert continuum and who focus on clinical practice, professional or consumer education, or research. ◎

[a]The author gratefully acknowledges Shirley Jones, PhD, RN, Louisville, Kentucky, and Judith Lewis, PhD, RN, Richmond, Virginia, for their assistance with this exemplar.

group within the nursing profession, yet their competencies are not consistent with those of advanced practice nursing (Hanson & Hamric, 2003). As specialties move through the stages described here, one important question for the specialty's

leadership is whether the specialty is best advanced by deliberate evolution to the advanced level of practice, development of differentiated levels of practice with distinct expectations and certifications, or continued development as a specialty (see Box

5.2). In these decisions, it is critically important to affirm the roles and value of all providers in the specialty, even as differentiation occurs for advancement and strengthening of specialty roles.

Concern over whether a specialty role is a shared nursing role (versus exclusively a nursing role) is an issue that will need to be examined in particular specialties. In the history of nursing, some roles have been characterized as sharing attributes with other types of health care providers. For example, some psychiatric CNSs attained their credentials to practice as licensed professional counselors. Other health care providers (e.g., counselors, psychologists) also receive this same credential, despite educational differences. Failure to acknowledge the value of multidisciplinary teams, shared knowledge, and overlapping expertise may limit opportunities for APRNs in the current health care environment and impede the advancement of specialties in the discipline. As a profession, nursing must embrace the notion that some roles are not exclusively nursing and must endorse differentiated practice models.

At the same time, the profession must define the advanced level of practice within the interprofessional model. This is critical for regulatory purposes, standardization of APRN competencies in the practice, and recognition by the public and insurers. In addition to the AADE, other specialty organizations (Table 5.2) certify health care providers who share a common knowledge base. These organizations are models of collaboration that communicate to consumers, other providers, third-party payers, and other stakeholders that there are national standards in the specialty that are upheld by these specialty care

TABLE 5.2 Specialty Organizations Offering Advanced-Level Certification

Specialty Organization	Credentialing Organization; Credential Awarded	Graduate Nursing Education Required?
American Academy of HIV Medicine[a]	American Academy of HIV Medicine; HIV Specialist	Implied (must be licensed as an NP)
Academy of Integrative Pain Management (formerly American Academy of Pain Management)[a]	Academy of Integrative Pain Management; APMP	Yes
American Board of Wound Management[a]	American Board of Wound Management; CWS	Yes (for diplomate or fellow status)
American Association of Critical-Care Nurses	AACN Certification Corporation; CCNS,[b] ACNPC,[b] ACNPC-AG, ACCNS-AG, ACCNS-P, ACCNS-N	Yes
American Association of Diabetes Educators[a]	American Association of Diabetes Educators; BC-ADM	No (master's in nursing or related field)
Association of Nurses in AIDS Care	HIV/AIDS Nursing Certification Board; AACRN	Yes
Hospice and Palliative Nurses Association	Hospice and Palliative Credentialing Center; ACHPN	Yes
International Society of Nurses in Genetics	American Nurses Credentialing Center; AGN-BC	Yes
International Nurses Society on Addictions	Addictions Nursing Certification Board; CARN-AP	No (master's in nursing or related field)
Oncology Nursing Society	Oncology Nursing Certification Corporation; AOCNS, AOCNP	Yes
Wound, Ostomy and Continence Nursing Society	Wound, Ostomy and Continence Nursing Certification Board; CWOCN-AP, CWCN-AP, COCN-AP, CCCN-AP	Yes
Society of Urologic Nurses and Associates	Certification Board for Urologic Nurses and Associates; CUNP	Yes (must already be NP)

AACRN, Advanced AIDS Certification Registered Nurse; *ACCNS-AG,* Acute Care Clinical Nurse Specialist–Adult-Gerontology; *ACCNS-N,* Acute Care Clinical Nurse Specialist–Neonatal; *ACCNS-P,* Acute Care Clinical Nurse Specialist–Pediatrics; *ACHPN,* Advanced Certified Hospice and Palliative Nurse; *ACNPC,* Acute Care Nurse Practitioner Certification; *ACNPC-AG,* Acute Care Nurse Practitioner–Adult-Gerontology; *AOCNP,* Advanced Oncology Certified Nurse Practitioner; *AOCNS,* Advanced Oncology Certified Clinical Nurse Specialist; *AGN-BC,* Advanced Genetics Nursing-Board Certified; *APMP,* Advanced Pain Management Practitioner; *BC-ADM,* Board Certified-Advanced Diabetes Management; *CARN-AP,* Certified Addictions Registered Nurse–Advanced Practice; *CCCN-AP,* Certified Continence Care Nurse–Advanced Practice; *CCNS,* Critical Care Clinical Nurse Specialist; *COCN-AP,* Certified Ostomy Care Nurse–Advanced Practice; *CUNP,* Certified Urologic Nurse Practitioner; *CWCN-AP,* Certified Wound Care Nurse–Advanced Practice; *CWOCN-AP,* Certified Wound Ostomy Continence Nurse–Advanced Practice; *CWS,* Certified Wound Specialist.
[a]Multidisciplinary membership.
[b]To conform with requirements of the Consensus Model for APRN Regulation (APRN Joint Dialogue Group, 2008), the CCNS and ACNPC exams are no longer offered, and these credentials are available now only as renewals.

providers. These multidisciplinary collaborative models represent a trend in health care that has given rise to a fourth stage in the evolution of advanced practice nursing. This stage is characterized by APRNs who are mature, expert practitioners in a specialty, secure in understanding the unique contributions that they make in the direct care of patients, yet embracing the notion that some aspects of their practice are shared by experts from other disciplines essential to the care of their patients.

The proliferation of role titles seen in evolving specialties requires special attention as APRNs begin practicing in the specialty. For example, within the transplant specialty, role titles such as clinical transplant coordinator, transplant coordinator, transplant nurse, transplant NP, and transplant CNS have been used in practice settings. The advanced practice role titles of CNS, NP, CRNA, and certified nurse-midwife need to be consistently applied to APRNs who are practicing in particular specialties to decrease role confusion. In addition, this consistency is important for promoting the recognition of advanced practice nursing within evolving specialties and the profession as a whole. For specialties that develop nonadvanced and advanced levels of practice, consistent titles are necessary to avoid confusion among providers and patients.

This is an extraordinarily interesting time in the history of the nursing profession. Opportunities and challenges for advanced practice nursing abound. What will the history books say about this period in the evolution and expansion of the nursing profession? As Hamric (2000) wrote in addressing the WOC specialty group, "[Our] hope is that they will say [we] clearly saw patients' needs and developed [our] skills to meet those needs; that [we] grasped the role opportunities that were possible and created new ones; and, most importantly, that [we] moved forward together" (p. 47).

Key Summary Points

- Professional and specialty organizations have been the driving force behind efforts to recognize and differentiate advanced practice nursing in a specialty or subspecialty.
- Although interprofessional practice characterizes advanced practice in all stages of evolution, mature specialties are characterized by *experts* in the specialty or subspecialty and a shared knowledge base with other health care professionals. Multidisciplinary certification examinations establish the credibility of these APRNs on interprofessional teams.
- Innovative opportunities for APRNs have extended into subspecialties within populations and more of these opportunities will exist as health care continues to evolve to higher levels of complexity.

References

To access the references for this chapter, use your smartphone's QR code reader to scan the code below, or go to http://booksite.elsevier.com/ 9780323447751.

International Development of Advanced Practice Nursing

Denise Bryant-Lukosius • Frances Kam Yuet Wong

> *"What you do makes a difference, and you have to decide what kind of difference you want to make."*
>
> —*Jane Goodall*

CHAPTER CONTENTS

Internationally, advanced practice nursing (APN) roles are on the threshold of new development and expansion that will include the first-time introduction of the roles in some countries and improved health systems integration in countries where roles are established. This chapter examines the current state, areas of progress, and new frontiers for APN role development within the global health care context. Evidence-based factors for facilitating the introduction of APN roles are explored and the next steps for supporting the global development of the roles are identified.

Advanced Practice Nursing Roles Within a Global Health Care Context

Defining Advanced Practice Nursing

There is international agreement that clinical practice involving the direct care of patients and families, groups, communities, or populations is a defining feature of APN roles and that these roles require an expanded range of competencies that include, but are in addition to, those for the basic practice of a registered nurse (Dowling, Beauchesne, Farrelly, & Murphy, 2013; Hamric, 2014; International Council of Nurses [ICN], 2008). The integration of clinical practice with competencies related to education, professional and organizational leadership, evidence-based practice, and research is what makes the roles advanced. However, just as the nursing profession is at different stages of development in countries around the world, so too is the development of APN roles. Reflecting the evolving nature of APN roles globally, the ICN (2008) broadly defines the nurse practitioner/advanced practice nurse[a] as a

> registered nurse who has acquired the expert knowledge base, complex decision-making skills and clinical competencies for expanded practice,

The authors gratefully acknowledge Joyce Pulcini for the previous edition of this chapter.

[a]In the United States there is a clear regulatory framework and role title of advanced practice registered nurse (APRN) for nurses working in nurse practitioner, clinical nurse specialist, nurse-midwife, or nurse anesthetist roles. In this chapter the term *advanced practice nurse (APN)* is used to reflect the international variability in APN role titling and regulation.

the characteristics of which are shaped by the context and/or country in which s/he is credentialed to practice. A master's degree is recommended for entry level. (p. 7)

Common features of APN roles include advanced education from an accredited program; formal licensure, registration, certification, and credentialing; integration of research, education, and management (leadership) with advanced clinical competencies; and regulatory mechanisms for autonomous and expanded scope of practice (ICN, 2016b). These features are consistent with the regulatory framework for the advanced practice registered nurse (APRN) in the United States related to licensure, accreditation, certification and education (LACE) (APRN Joint Dialogue Group, 2008). However, LACE features have more detailed role requirements rather than recommendations, as suggested by the ICN (2008, 2016b).

Global Deployment

Strong global demand for APN roles has been evident since 2001 and the launch of the ICN's International Nurse Practitioner/APN Network (INP/APNN) (Bryant-Lukosius & Martin-Misener, 2016). Internationally, few human resource systems are in place to monitor APN role deployment, and at country levels there are absent or inconsistent methods for identifying nurses in these roles. As such, the number of countries with APN roles is unknown but may range from 26 (Heale & Rieck-Buckley, 2015) to 68 (Roodbol, 2004). APN roles are found mainly in high-income countries, of which Canada, the United Kingdom, and the United States have the most established roles with decades of experience (see Chapter 1). In the last decade, APN roles have spread to other high-income countries such as South Africa and Singapore (Ayre & Bee, 2014; South African Nursing Council, 2012) and upper middle income countries like Jordan (Zahran, Curtis, Lloyd-Jones, & Blackett, 2012). There are few reports of APN roles in low- or middle-income countries.

In the last 6 years, interest in APN roles has intensified within the context of World Health Organization (WHO, 2010) strategic directions to meet 2015 Millennium Development Goals for improving global health. It was recognized that national health care systems could be improved by enhancing nursing roles to address provider shortages, overcome inequities through universal health coverage, and improve care quality.

Recommendations included establishing postbasic continuing nursing education programs to support advanced clinical practice (WHO, 2010); introducing specialized and APN roles to meet population health and health service needs, especially for primary health care (WHO, 2012); and developing career pathways for APN roles (WHO, 2015c).

Types of Advanced Practice Nursing Roles

In the United States, the regulatory framework for the APRN is specific to four certified roles: the nurse anesthetist (NA), nurse-midwife (NM), clinical nurse specialist (CNS), and nurse practitioner (NP) (APRN Joint Dialogue Group, 2008). The introduction of these longstanding roles varies in other countries, but internationally the CNS and NP roles are the most common types of APN roles (Delamaire & Lafortune, 2010; Heale & Rieck-Buckley, 2015). In the last 20 years, the nurse consultant (NC) has emerged as a new type of APN role (Baldwin et al., 2013).

Nurse-Midwife

Midwifery is one of the oldest health professions, dating back to the Stone Age (Barnawi, Richter, & Habib, 2013). As the profession evolved, a variety of sociocultural factors influenced the development of nursing and non-nursing midwifery roles, including NMs (have nursing and midwifery education), midwives (have midwifery but no nursing education), nurses, traditional birthing attendants, and generalist and specialist physicians. The International Confederation of Midwives (ICM, 2010) has developed competencies for basic midwifery practice that apply, but are not specific to, advanced roles. The education of NMs is variable, ranging from 2 to 6 years, with about half completing at least 4 years of training (United Nations Population Fund [UNFPA], 2014). This suggests that not all NMs have a master's degree as recommended by the ICN (2008) for APN roles. NMs who meet the ICM (2010) competencies have a scope of practice that includes prevention, health promotion, detecting complications, accessing medical care, and providing emergency measures within a primary health care framework. They work in varied settings, including the home, community, hospital, clinics, birthing centers, or health units.

Improving maternal-child health by expanding midwifery services, and in particular increasing the number of NMs and midwives, is a global priority (UNFPA, 2011). Major drivers are high maternal and infant morbidity and mortality rates, especially in low- and middle-income countries, as well as the increasing costs of medicalized care and growing use of unnecessary and expensive interventions such as cesarean sections (Renfrew et al., 2014). The importance of NMs and midwives for improving maternal-child care cannot be overstated. A report has shown that NMs and midwives with the appropriate education and who are regulated to meet ICM competencies for practice can deliver 87% of midwifery care (UNFPA, 2014). Since 2010, collaboration between the United Nations, the ICM, and the WHO led to a series of consensus meetings with agreement on strategic priorities and reporting on key indicators (Day-Stirk et al., 2014). As a result, there are more global workforce data on NMs compared to other types of APN roles. NMs make up about 5% of the midwifery workforce (UNFPA, 2014). Despite smaller numbers, NMs spend more time delivering sexual and reproductive health and maternal-newborn care compared to nurses and generalist physicians, accounting for 14% of full-time equivalents (UNFPA, 2014).

Nurse Anesthetist

Globally, the current status of NAs is not well described. In the last international surveys published 20 years ago, 107 countries were found to have nurses providing anesthesia care (McAuliffe & Henry, 1996, 1998). Survey results demonstrated the significant magnitude of anesthesia nursing across developed and developing countries. Nurses were involved in 83% of all procedures and were the sole provider for over 51% of procedures, especially in rural communities (McAuliffe & Henry, 1998). The education and scope of practice of NAs varies across countries and does not consistently meet requirements for APN roles in all situations. Country profiles provided by the International Federation of Nurse Anesthetists (2017) show that in the United States, Jamaica, France, and Sweden, the NA is an advanced role requiring graduate education. In other countries such as Cambodia, Congo, Ghana, Indonesia, Switzerland, and Tunisia, NAs require a postbasic nursing diploma or certificate taking 2 to 3 years to complete. In the United Kingdom, NAs complete a 9-month postbasic education program and function as anesthesia assistants, while in Taiwan they complete hospital-based training programs specific to each institution. In Brazil, China, Israel, and Spain, a regulatory framework for NAs does not exist and access to education is limited (Aaron & Andrews, 2016; Hu, Fallacaro, Jiang, Wang, & Ruan, 2013; Lemos & Peniche, 2016). Education programs in Nordic countries range from hospital-based training to master's degrees, but they have similar entry requirements (i.e., registered nurse with 1 or 2 years of work experience), and four out of the five countries have a protected title of NA (Jeon, Lahtinen, Meretoja, & Leino-Kilpi, 2015).

Nurse Practitioner

The NP role was first launched in the United States in 1965, followed by Canada and Jamaica in the mid-1970s, with the aim to improve people's health by increasing access to primary health care for vulnerable populations with high needs and those living in rural, remote, and underserved communities (Jamaica Association of Nurse Practitioners, 2016; Kaasalainen et al., 2010; Saver, 2015). In the 1980s, Canada and the United States introduced acute care NPs, beginning with a focus on neonatal care, to address shortages of physicians and to meet the complex care needs of acute and critically ill patients (Haut & Madden, 2015; Kilpatrick et al., 2010). Countries such as Australia (Carter, Owen-Williams, & Della, 2015), Ireland (Begley et al., 2010), the Netherlands (De Bruijn-Geraets, Van Eijk-Hustings, & Vrijhoef, 2014), New Zealand (Gagan, Boyd, Wysocki, & Williams, 2014), Sweden (Altersved, Zetterlund, Lindblad, & Fagerstrom, 2011), Taiwan (Chiu, Tsay, & Tung, 2015), Thailand (Hanucharurnkul, 2007), and the United Kingdom (East, Knowles, Pettman, & Fisher, 2015) introduced NPs in the 1990s and early 2000s. Exemplar 6.1 provides a profile of the NP role in Australia. The United States has 220,000 NPs, of which 83% are certified in primary care (American Association of Nurse Practitioners, 2016). Countries such as Australia (*n* = 1214), Canada (*n* = 4090), Ireland (*n* = 141), the Netherlands (*n* = 2749), and New Zealand (*n* = 142) have smaller numbers of NPs and fewer working in primary care compared to the United States, but trends indicate a growing number of NPs in this sector (Freund et al., 2015; Maier, Barnes, Aiken, & Busse, 2016). The settings where NPs work are also expanding to meet the health needs of aging populations and those with chronic conditions. NPs work in hospitals, outpatient clinics, group practices, public health, emergency departments, community health centers, hospices, and long-term care (American Association of Nurse Practitioners, 2016; Donald, Martin-Misener, et al., 2010; Donald et al., 2013; Kilpatrick et al., 2010; Maten-Speksnijder, Pool, Grypdonck, Meurs, & van Staa, 2015).

In countries with established roles (e.g., Australia, Canada, Ireland, Jamaica, the Netherlands, New

Margaret Adams, NP, PhD Candidate, and Glenn Gardner Professor, Queensland University of Technology

Nurse practitioner (NP) service in Australia is relatively new, with the first NP authorized in 2000. The NP title is protected by legislation and to gain NP endorsement, a registered nurse must demonstrate successful completion of an accredited Master of Nursing (Nurse Practitioner) degree and 3 years of experience working as an advanced practice nurse. In Australia, NP authorization is generic and there is no centralized register of specialty fields. In 2016, there were just under 1400 NPs across the country working in emergency departments, community and primary health, geriatric care, rehabilitation, and a range of acute care specialties. In 2010 the Australian government invested

nearly $60 million to expand the role of NPs in the health system, with legislative changes that enabled eligible NPs to access government-subsidized health care for their patients though the Medicare Benefits Schedule and the Pharmaceutical Benefits Scheme. Although access is currently limited to a small range of specified items, this move has had an important influence on the shift of NP service from almost exclusive employment in government-funded acute care facilities to the primary care context in a range of innovative service models. This belated but important expansion of NP service into the primary care sector in Australia is supported by education standards mandating a foundation of primary health care in an accredited master's degree. ◎

Zealand, and the United States) NPs are required to have a master's degree, but in other countries the education and regulatory requirements for NPs are evolving and varied (Heale & Rieck-Buckley, 2015). A distinguishing feature of NP roles is an expanded scope of practice with competencies in advanced health assessment, ordering diagnostic tests, communicating a diagnosis, prescribing treatments and medication, and performing procedures (Canadian Council of Registered Nurse Regulators, 2015; De Bruijn-Geraets et al., 2014; Gagan et al., 2014). There is some overlap in role responsibilities between NPs and CNSs, but due to their clinical expertise and expanded scope of practice, NPs tend to spend more time than CNSs providing direct clinical care (Donald, Bryant-Lukosius, et al., 2010; Gardner, Duffield, Doubrovsky, & Adams, 2016; National Council of State Boards of Nursing [NCSBN], 2007). The effectiveness of NPs is well established. Several systematic reviews show that when compared to standard care, NPs have similar or improved outcomes related to patient health, satisfaction with care, quality of care, and health care use (Donald et al., 2015; Martin-Misener et al., 2015; Stanik-Hutt et al., 2013).

Clinical Nurse Specialist

The CNS role was introduced in the United States, Canada, and the United Kingdom in the 1960s and 1970s in response to the rising complexity and specialization of health care and the need for clinical expertise, education, and leadership to improve care delivery and patient outcomes, develop nursing

practice, and support nurses at the point of care (Fulton, 2014; Kaasalainen et al., 2010; Leary et al., 2008). In the 1990s and 2000s, CNSs were further introduced in China, Hong Kong, Japan, New Zealand, the Republic of Korea, Taiwan, and Thailand (Kaur, 2014; Roberts, Floyd, & Thompson, 2011; Tian et al., 2014; Wongkpratoom, Srisuphan, Senaratana, Nantachiapan, & Sritanyarat, 2010). The United States has 70,000 CNSs, compared to 55,000 in the United Kingdom and 2000 in Canada (Kilpatrick et al., 2013; National Association of Clinical Nurse Specialists, 2016; Royal College of Nursing, 2012b). CNS education varies across countries, and this, coupled with inconsistent role titling, including the generic term *advanced practice nurse,* makes it difficult to discern specialized versus advanced CNS roles (Dury et al., 2014; Kilpatrick et al., 2013).

CNSs work in a variety of specialty areas that may be defined by a type of illness (e.g., cancer, cardiovascular disease), health needs (e.g., pain control, mental health), type of care (e.g., wound or critical care), setting (e.g., community), or age (e.g., neonatal, gerontology) (Bryant-Lukosius et al., 2010; Roberts et al., 2011; Vidall, Barlow, Crow, Harrison, & Young, 2011). Although CNSs were initially introduced in hospitals, the role has spread to provide specialized care for patients with complex and chronic conditions in outpatient, emergency department, home, community, and long-term care settings (Kilpatrick et al., 2013; Roberts et al., 2011; Tian et al., 2014; Vidall et al., 2011). Depending on the country, and unlike other types of APN roles,

CNSs may not have an expanded scope of practice that includes activities such as diagnosis or prescribing. Practice pattern studies illustrate the complexity of CNS work (Kilpatrick et al., 2013; Leary et al., 2008; Roberts et al., 2011). When compared to NPs, CNS are more likely to engage in multiple role activities (clinical, consultation, leadership, quality improvement, evidence-based practice, and research) and have greater involvement in nonclinical activities (Donald, Bryant-Lukosius, et al., 2010; Gardner et al., 2016; NCSBN, 2007). Positive patient health (e.g., survival rates) and health system (e.g., quality of care, service use, costs) outcomes resulting from CNS roles that complement or substitute for other health care providers are consistently reported in systematic reviews (Bryant-Lukosius, Carter, et al., 2015; Kilpatrick et al., 2014; Kilpatrick, Reid, et al., 2015; Newhouse et al., 2011).

Nurse Consultant

The NC role exists in Australia, the United Kingdom, and Hong Kong. The role was first introduced in Australia in 1986 and was modeled after the CNS role in the United States and the United Kingdom (O'Baugh, Wilkes, Vaughan, & O'Donohue, et al., 2007). Three grade levels differentiate increasing NC responsibilities across five role domains (clinical service and consultancy, clinical leadership, research, education, and clinical service planning); incremental work experience as a registered nurse (5–7 years) and specialty experience (0–5 years); and postbasic registration qualifications (New South Wales Department of Health, 2011). NC education in Australia is variable, ranging from a hospital certificate to a master's degree (Baldwin et al., 2013). In the United Kingdom, the NC role was introduced in the early 2000s and requires master's education and specialty experience. Role domains (direct care, professional leadership and consultancy, education and training, and service development) are similar to Australian NC roles (Gerrish, McDonnell & Kennedy, 2013). The NC sits at level 8 near the top of the nine-level nursing career framework in the United Kingdom (Royal College of Nursing, 2012a). In Hong Kong, the NC role was introduced in 2009 with similar requirements, including master's education and 8 years of experience in one of five clinical specialties (diabetes, renal, wound/stoma, psychiatry, and continence) (Lee et al., 2013). Role domains include clinical practice, academics, research, and leadership. NCs were introduced to retain experienced nurses in clinical practice by broadening the career path (Cashin, Stasa, Gullick, Conway, & Buckley, 2015;

Gerrish et al., 2013; Lee et al., 2013) and to improve the quality of care and outcomes for patients (Kennedy et al., 2011). Studies show that NCs manage complex patient and health care situations (Franks, 2014; Jannings, Underwood, Almer, & Luxford, 2010; Lee et al., 2013) and positively impact patient, health professional, organization, and systems outcomes (Cashin et al., 2015; Gerrish et al., 2013; Kennedy et al., 2011; Wong et al., 2017). These areas of impact are similar to those reported for CNSs in the United States (Lewandowski & Adamle, 2009). Similarities between the NC and CNS roles in the United States and Canada have been noted in literature reviews (Duffield, Gardner, Chang, & Catlin-Paull, 2009; Jokiniemi, Pietila, Kylma, & Haatainen, 2012).

New Frontiers and Future Role Expansion

There has been trendsetting growth in APN role development in Europe over the last decade. Sweden established an acute care NP education program in addition to an earlier focus on primary care (Jangland et al., 2014), and APN roles and education programs are emerging or established in Denmark, Finland, Iceland, and Norway (Hølge-Hazelton, Kjerholt, Berthelsen, & Thomsen, 2016; Oddsdottir & Sveinsdottir, 2011; Pill, Kolbaek, Ottmann, & Rasmussen, 2012; Wisur-Hokkanen, Glasberg, Makela, & Fagerstrom, 2015). The profile by Krista Jokiniemi describes the CNS role in Finland (Exemplar 6.2). In Spain, the advanced nurse specialist has been defined for midwifery, mental health, occupational health, geriatrics, pediatrics, and family/community nursing (Gonzalez Jurado, 2015), along with APN competencies for research and evidence-based practice, clinical and professional leadership, and care management (Sastre-Fullana, De Pedro-Gømez, Bennasar-Veny, Serrano-Gallardo, & Morales-Asencio, 2014). Innovative roles are also emerging to meet the needs of patients with complex comorbid conditions (del Rio Camara et al., 2015). In Switzerland, work has taken place to define (Morin, Ramelet, & Shaha, 2013), regulate (Swiss Association for Nursing Science, 2012), and evaluate APN roles (Bryant-Lukosius et al., 2016). The number of Swiss APN education programs has increased along with graduates working with varied patient populations (Imhof, Naef, Wallhagen, Schwarz, & Mahrer-Imhof, 2012; Kocher & Spichiger, 2014; Müller-Staub et al., 2015; Romain-Glassey et al., 2014; Serena et al., 2015).

APN roles are not formally recognized in Africa. However, in sub-Saharan countries such as Kenya (East, Arudo, Loefler, & Evans, 2014) and in South

| EXEMPLAR 6.2 | Profile on Emerging Advanced Practice Nursing Roles in Finland |

Krista Jokiniemi, Postdoctoral Fellow, University of Eastern Finland and McMaster University

Advanced roles for nurses emerged in Finland at the beginning of the 21st century with the introduction of the clinical nurse specialist (CNS) role. Other established advanced practice nursing (APN) roles include the nurse-midwife, nurse anesthetist, and more recently the nurse practitioner. Although there is a long history of specialist nursing practice and education in Finland, the concept of the advanced practice nurse at the national level is just beginning. There are no uniform national education programs, legislative or regulatory mechanisms, or protected titles in place for APN roles. Currently, there are close to 60 CNSs across the country working in inpatient units, clinics, and primary care. They develop specialized expertise through practice experience and master's degree education. CNSs operate in four distinct yet interrelated role spheres related to the patient, nursing, organization, and scholarship.

Within each sphere, six domains of advanced clinical practice, practice development, education, research, consultation, and leadership may be enacted depending on organizational needs, set goals, and skills of the individual practitioner. The main practice goal is to improve the quality of care, support staff and interprofessional teams in care provision, and foster the advancement of clinical nursing through scholarship. Strengthening APN roles is high on the health care agenda in Finland. Health care administrators have recognized the value of these roles for improving nursing practice, promoting evidence-based practices, strengthening the image of nursing, and increasing nursing recruitment and retention. To support the effective implementation of APN roles, it will be imperative to develop and validate competency descriptions, elaborate on role domain concepts, develop education curricula, and demonstrate the effectiveness of these innovative nursing roles. ◎

Africa (Duma et al., 2012) the roles are needed to improve population health, increase access to care, improve care quality, and develop the nursing workforce. Due to provider shortages, especially in primary care, nurses and NMs may acquire an expanded scope of practice similar to APN roles in other countries but without the benefit of graduate education (East et al., 2015; Ugochukwu, Uys, Karani, Okoronkwo, & Diop, 2013). In South Africa, master's-prepared advanced practice nurses are emerging in primary health care, midwifery, psychiatry, and pediatrics (Duma et al., 2012; South African Nursing Council, 2012; Temane, Poggenpoel, & Myburgh, 2014).

In Middle Eastern countries, APN roles have been introduced to expand, heighten the profile of, and modernize nursing and midwifery workforces. To overcome a reliance on foreign-trained nurses, countries such as Jordan (Zahran et al., 2012), Qatar (Hamad Medical Corporation, 2015), and Saudia Arabia (Brownie, Hunter, Aqtash, & Day, 2015) have launched graduate programs in critical care, maternal/newborn care, renal care, oncology, diabetes, and community health. Education programs for NMs, palliative care CNSs, and geriatric NPs have also been established in Israel (Aaron & Andrews, 2016; Livneh, 2011; Yafa, Dorit, & Shoshana, 2016). CNSs and family NPs are being introduced in Oman (Al-Maqbali, 2014; Almukhaini, Donesky, & Scruth, 2016).

English language publications do not fully describe APN role development in Asia, but several new education initiatives exist. They include APN graduate programs in Singapore and China (Ayre & Bee, 2014; Wong et al., 2010), an NP graduate program in Japan (Fukuda et al., 2014), and NP programs offering a Master's of Science degree in critical care and a postgraduate diploma in primary health care in India (Olabode, 2016). Needs related to improving care for aging populations, provider shortages, and chronic disease management were the main drivers for these programs. The profile by Frances Kam Yuet Wong describes APN role development in China (Exemplar 6.3).

The next frontier for introducing APN roles is Latin America, where few such roles exist (Bryant-Lukosius et al., 2017). Countries primed for APN roles are Brazil, Chile, Mexico, and Columbia. With support from the regional nurse advisor and from WHO Collaborating Centres in Primary Health Care in the United States and Canada, meetings have occurred to plan the introduction of APN roles (Pan American Health Organization [PAHO] & School of Nursing, McMaster University, 2015; PAHO & University of Michigan, 2016). Primary health care reform, access to health care, and universal health care coverage are the policy drivers for APN roles in the region. The profile by Consuelo Cerón Mackay describes APN role development in Chile (Exemplar 6.4).

| EXEMPLAR 6.3 | Profile on Advanced Practice Nursing Role Development in China |

Frances Kam Yuet Wong, Professor, Hong Kong Polytechnic University

China is a vast country consisting of 23 provinces, 5 autonomous regions, 4 municipalities, and 2 Special Administrative Regions (Hong Kong and Macau). Factors facilitating the introduction of advanced practice nursing (APN) roles include the national strategy to develop "Healthy China"; the national strategy to develop nursing, which highlights the importance of specialization in nursing practice; and elevation of the status of nursing from a second-class to first-class subject in 2011. With this change, nursing is more autonomous and university departments of nursing can admit postgraduate students. Many schools have introduced clinical master's degree programs that strengthen the preparation of advanced practice nurses. A challenge to introducing APN roles is the shortage of nurses. As of 2015, there were 3.2 million nurses in Mainland China, with a nurse-patient ratio of 2.36. This ratio is very low compared to other developed countries. Although there is a plan to increase the number of nurses, the sheer inadequacy in number will hamper the development of nursing at an advanced level. Another challenge is that structures to support APN roles (e.g., education, competencies) are not well established in the remote areas and less developed cities. Opportunities to develop APN roles are expanding with growing numbers of university-prepared nurses and increased access to graduate education. There are 58 master's and 10 doctoral nursing programs. There are also specific programs sending nurses overseas for specialty training.

The Guangdong Province illustrates progress in APN role development in China. From 2004 to 2005, the Hong Kong Polytechnic University provided a consultant course in collaboration with Nanfong Medical University to prepare advanced practice nurses in diabetes care, geriatrics care, intensive care, and infection control. From 2006 to 2011, 614 nurses were sent to Hong Kong for APN education in one of 13 different specialties (intensive care, orthopedics, operating room, geriatrics, midwifery, neonatal/pediatrics, renal, emergency room, cardiac, surgical, oncology, community, and psychiatric nursing). Guangdong now has a critical mass of advanced practice nurses to provide services and impact patient care. The Ministry of Health has also put policies and resources in place to support APN development, including accredited education programs, examination requirements, and employment conditions. ◎

In summary, APN role development has occurred mainly in high-income countries. Role expansion is now taking place in upper-middle (e.g., Brazil, China) and lower-middle (e.g., India, Kenya) income countries and may spread to lower-income countries such as Nepal and in Africa. APN roles are needed for strengthening the nursing and midwifery workforce, chronic disease prevention and management, and aging populations. Continued demand for APN roles in primary care is expected due to shortages of physicians (WHO, 2015b).

Facilitating the Introduction and Integration of Advanced Practice Nursing Roles

Contextual factors (e.g., sociopolitical, economic, geographic) influence the use of APN roles within health care systems, and barriers are often the absent mirror versions of facilitators (DiCenso et al., 2010). Table 6.1 highlights key facilitating factors, including pan-approaches and collaboration, funding and payment arrangements, systematic approaches to role planning, and the use and generation of evidence. Levels of engagement (international, national, and organizational) for successful APN role introduction and integration are examined for each factor.

Pan-Approaches and Collaboration

Pan-approaches are activities that span across jurisdictions. At the international level this may include activities involving more than one country, and at the national level activities that cut across regions within a country. National and international collaboration related to human resource policies and priorities, legislation and regulation, and competency development and education are strategic for jump starting the introduction and development of APN roles.

Human Resource Policies and Priorities

At the international level, policy priorities of the United Nations and the WHO have played a critical role in raising the profile and triggering actions for APN role development. For example, United Nations (2012) and WHO (2010) priorities to improve global health influenced the PAHO 52nd Directing Council's

EXEMPLAR 6.4   **Profile on Advanced Practice Nursing Roles in Chile**

Maria Consuelo Cerón Mackay, Director of the School of Nursing, Los Andes University, Chile

Interest in advanced practice nursing (APN) roles in Chile began in the late 1990s, when the School of Nursing of Universidad de los Andes recognized the need to develop clinical master's programs. At that time most graduate programs focused on developing nurses for an academic career. In 2001, a faculty member was sent to study in an APN program at New York University. On her return she was challenged to educate other faculty members about APN roles. The curriculum from New York University was used as a reference point, particularly for the clinical nurse specialist (CNS) role, because it was most suitable for Chilean health care needs focused on hospital care. In 2009, two faculty members visited the University of Pennsylvania, the University of California at San Francisco, and the Johns Hopkins School of Nursing to learn about APN education programs and to establish a support network. A memorandum of understanding was signed with the Institute for Johns Hopkins Nursing that allowed our students to spend 3 weeks at the Johns Hopkins Hospital to observe CNSs in action and develop their understanding of the role. Currently, the APN stream is a 2-year program, with the first year focused on theoretical

courses and the second on clinical practice. Physicians are acting as tutors for the students until enough CNSs have graduated to become mentors. In addition, a CNS from Johns Hopkins came to Chile for a week to provide intensive education for the students at a local hospital. The program is now 3 years old and has nine graduates. Although recruitment to the program is low, the CNS role is being successfully implemented in practice settings. Moreover, faculty members are sharing their APN education experiences as conference speakers nationally and in other Latin American countries. The invitation to participate at the 2015 Universal Access to Health and Universal Health Coverage APN Summit, organized by the Pan American Health Organization (PAHO) and the School of Nursing at McMaster University, encouraged me to begin the process to implement the nurse practitioner role. This meeting was crucial for guiding and speeding up the planning process. Main accomplishments include establishing a network among 11 nursing schools throughout Chile and developing partnerships with the Chilean Association of Schools of Nursing, the PAHO-Chile, the Ministry of Health, and the Chilean Association of Nurses, to work together to implement the nurse practitioner role in primary health care. ◎

TABLE 6.1   **Facilitating Factors for the Introduction and Integration of Advanced Practice Nursing Roles**

Facilitating Factors	International	National or Regional	Organization
Pan-Approaches and Collaboration			
• Human resource policies and priorities	X	X	
• Regulation	X	X	
• Education	X	X	
Funding and Payment Arrangements			
• To support the introduction of innovative advanced practice nursing roles and new models of care		X	X
Systematic Approaches to Role Planning		X	X
Use and Generation of Evidence	X	X	X

(2013) resolution on Human Resources for Health calling for the introduction of APN roles for primary health care in Latin American and the Caribbean (Cassiani & Zug, 2014). This resolution laid the foundation for APN role development and partnerships

between the PAHO, regional and international schools of nursing, and WHO Collaborating Centres.

A powerful example offering a template for international nursing and APN association leadership and health policy involvement in human resource planning is the collaboration between the ICM, the United Nations, and the WHO to improve the global midwifery workforce (Day-Stirk et al., 2014; UNFPA, 2011, 2014; WHO, 2015a). Through collaboration, agreement on midwifery workforce indicators and targets was established and implemented at national levels, resulting in a detailed data set used to evaluate and compare the impact of workforce policies and initiatives across countries. Early results showed improvement in educating and expanding the number of midwifery providers and in maternal-child health outcomes (UNFPA, 2014). The midwifery example is notable because of its success in workforce development in low- and middle-income countries where health needs are the greatest and where few APN roles exist. The ICM (2015) emphasized the essential role of national midwifery associations in workforce policy and decision making. Similarly, an ICN brief provided guidance on APN role development for national nursing associations (Bryant-Lukosius & Martin-Misener, 2016). A stronger role for nurses, including APN representatives, in international organizations such as the WHO is critical to inform human resource policy priorities and implementation strategies (Wong et al., 2015).

At the national level, health care contexts related to needs, policies, organization of services, the workforce, economics, and the societal role of women influence APN roles (Heale & Rieck-Buckley, 2015; Liu, Rodcumdee, Jiang, & Sha, 2015). National practice pattern studies can facilitate role integration by providing information to define APN roles, identify implementation barriers, and assess deployment in relation to policies for improving health (DiCenso et al., 2010; Gardner et al., 2016). The introduction of APN roles may be advantaged in countries with centralized health care governance and national health policies aligned with the roles. One example is Ghana, where national health human resource policies since 1995 have led to a steady increase in midwives (Matthews & Campbell, 2015). Qatar's National Cancer Strategy (2011–2016), with the goal for all cancer patients to be cared for by an oncology CNS (Qatar Supreme Council of Health, 2011), quickly led to the introduction of the role (Oxford Business Group, 2014). A systematic approach to introducing NM and NP roles occurred in Ireland, where the national health ministry worked closely with the national nursing council to deploy roles focused on priorities for health care reform (Begley et al., 2010). By 2009 and within 8 years, Ireland introduced over 120 APN roles, accounting for 0.2% of the nursing workforce (Delamaire & Lafortune,

2010). This is quite an accomplishment when compared to Canada, with just over 1600 NPs in 2008 making up 0.6% of the nursing workforce after 40 years of development. In Canada, responsibility for health care lies with 13 provinces and territories, resulting in disparate NP role deployment (DiCenso et al., 2010).

Regulation

The regulation of nursing is usually tied to health laws protecting public safety and promotes high-quality care by defining the scope and standards of practice, licensure, credentials, and educational requirements of the profession (ICN, 2013). Internationally, the regulatory requirements for APN roles are variable or absent in many countries (Aaron & Andrews, 2016; Carney, 2015; Heale & Rieck-Buckley, 2015; Maier, 2015). Legislative and regulatory policies embracing optimal scope of practice and full role autonomy without restrictions (e.g., physician supervision for practice or prescriptions) facilitate NP recruitment and retention and increase access to care, especially for rural and vulnerable populations (Barnes et al., 2016; Kuo, Loresto, Rounds, & Goodwin, 2013; Xue, Ye, Brewer, & Spetz, 2016). Regulatory mechanisms offering title protection and standardized education and competencies have been found to improve NP role clarity and implementation (Duffield et al., 2009; Lowe, Plummer, O'Brien, & Boyd, 2011). Conversely, the lack of regulation for CNS and other types of APN roles contributes to poor role clarity, variability in how roles are operationalized, and inability to monitor their workforce contributions, and may negatively impact role integration and sustainability (Duffield et al., 2009; East et al., 2015; Kilpatrick et al., 2013).

Reports of pan-approaches at the international level to improve APN regulation are few and would be an asset for guiding role introduction in low-income countries and those with new or emerging roles. The importance of international collaboration is illustrated by the Global Midwifery Twinning project involving the Royal College of Midwives in the United Kingdom and midwifery associations in Nepal, Cambodia, and Uganda (Ireland, van Teijlingen, & Kemp, 2015). The project was successful in building the capacity of midwives to lead and advocate for stronger midwifery associations, education, and regulation in these countries.

At national levels, pan-approaches to legislation and regulation in support of APN roles have been successful in Canada, the United States, New Zealand, and Wales for obtaining greater consistency in these policies, improving role understanding and implementation, and creating ways to monitor deployment across jurisdictions (Bryant-Lukosius et al., 2014; Goudreau, 2014; Kooienga & Carryer, 2015; NCSBN, 2008; Ryley & Middelton, 2015). In many countries, establishing a nursing regulatory framework will be an essential first step in establishing requirements for advanced practice. Ben Natan, Dmitriev, Shubovich, and Sharon (2013) found that the Israeli public was in favor of expanding nurses' scope of practice and authority. Engaging the public in the discourse may be an effective strategy to strengthen legislative and regulatory policies supportive of APN roles.

Competency Development and Education

Competencies are the knowledge, skills, judgment, and attributes required by advanced practice nurses to provide safe, ethical practice (Canadian Nurses Association, 2010). They are informed by a collective understanding of the APN role and provide the basis for entry-to-practice requirements and APN education curricula. Varied national interpretations of what an advanced practice nurse is have led to a perceived lack of role clarity internationally (Dowling et al., 2013). The ICN's (2008) competencies for the advanced practice nurse, along with recommendations for graduate education, provide nursing associations with a framework to develop competencies for their country and to lobby for these requirements (DiCenso et al., 2010). Studies conducted to examine APN roles across countries suggest that international convergence on defining and understanding APN roles may be occurring. Sastre-Fullana et al. (2014) conducted a review of APN competency frameworks and found agreement on 17 competencies across six types of APN roles in 26 countries. Research, clinical and professional leadership, mentoring and coaching, and expert clinical judgment were common role domains in 16 of 29 countries. Jokiniemi et al. (2012) found similar domains for CNS and NC roles in the United States, Australia, and Finland. In addition, the Advanced Practice Role Delineation tool discerns nurses practicing at an advanced level and differences in activities among varied APN roles (Gardner et al., 2016). There has also been a burst of activity in several countries to establish or refine competencies in order to clarify APN roles and strengthen role implementation (Canadian Nurses Association, 2015; Chang, Shyu, Tsay, & Tang, 2012; Lin, Lee, Ueng, & Tang, 2015; Maijala, Tossavainen, & Turunen, 2015; Nieminen, Mannevaara, & Fagerstrom, 2011).

At the international level, pan-initiatives may facilitate the consistency and quality of APN education across countries. For example, in addition to standards for practice and education, the International Federation of Nurse Anesthetists developed an approval process for schools, now completed by 14 education programs in nine countries (Horton, Anang, Riesen, Yang, & Bjorkelund, 2014). The Bologna process aims to standardize all professional education requirements across Europe. This process has accelerated the professionalization of nursing and creation of baccalaureate and master's education programs necessary to develop APN roles (Collins & Hewer, 2014).

At national levels, health policies, population health needs, and social factors influence the level and types of APN education (Liu et al., 2015). In many countries, APN role development is limited by a lack of education programs and master's-prepared faculty with APN experience (Heale & Rieck-Buckley, 2015). Partnerships between countries with emerging APN roles and schools of nursing in countries with established roles have occurred to address these education gaps. One such case is in Qatar, where the government partnered with the University of Calgary in Canada to develop undergraduate and graduate nursing education programs (Oxford Business Group, 2014). The leveling of APN education has become somewhat contentious with the requirement of the doctorate of nursing practice for APRNs in the United States (Ketefian & Redman, 2015). This is not an attainable goal in many countries where basic nursing education is being developed or where resources for graduate education are limited. At national levels it is important to keep in mind that a good fit between APN curricula and practice needs is key for optimal role implementation (Martin-Misener et al., 2010). There is limited research on APN education, but a few studies suggest that master's-prepared nurses implement their roles in a manner more consistent with APN standards of practice, compared to non–master's-prepared nurses (Kilpatrick et al., 2013; Pauley et al., 2004). At organizational levels, academic-clinical practice partnerships to provide mentorship and continuing education for advanced practice nurses can help to build their confidence, strengthen skills in underdeveloped areas such as research, and maintain competency (Bryant-Lukosius, 2015; Harbman et al., 2016).

Funding and Reimbursement Arrangements

Funding at national/regional and organizational levels is essential to introduce and expand the supply of advanced practice nurses to meet demands for health care. In the United States, new funding from the 2010 Patient Protection and Affordable Care Act has increased the number of APRNs providing primary care (Lathrop & Hodnicki, 2014). In Canada, provincial funding for Ontario NPs in primary, palliative, and long-term care enabled role expansion in these high-need areas (Bryant-Lukosius et al., 2014; Heale & Pilon, 2012; Ontario Ministry of Health and Long-Term Care, 2015). Similar expansion has not occurred for CNSs, acute care NPs, or NPs in anesthesia care in the absence of provincial funding. At an organizational level, advanced practice nurses are most often an operational cost as salaried employees. External funds or reallocated existing funds are required by organizations to introduce, maintain, or expand APN roles and may be difficult to obtain in challenging economic conditions (Gagan et al., 2014). Results of systematic reviews examining APN outcomes demonstrate that advanced practice nurses may reduce health care inefficiencies in 5 out of 10 areas identified by the WHO (Bryant-Lukosius et al., 2017). Using similar data to create a sound business case may help health care organizations identify efficiencies and cost savings that can be gained by the innovative use of APN roles and applied to offset salary costs.

Fee-for-service reimbursement models for advanced practice nurses exist in the United States and in Australia for primary care NPs (Carter et al. 2015). In the United States, pediatric and family NPs, NMs, and to a lesser extent NAs and CNSs can bill Medicaid and third-party payers such as insurance companies (American Nurses Association, 2016). Such models provide economic flexibility to increase access to care and introduce new services involving APN roles, especially for high-risk, low-income, and underserved populations (Barnes et al., 2016). The recruitment of advanced practice nurses is enhanced when policies ensure that they are reimbursed at the same funding level as physicians (Barnes et al., 2016). Reimbursement policies may partially explain differences among countries in the number of NPs making up the nursing workforce, as a crude indicator of health systems integration. Compared to other countries with established roles, the United States has a larger proportion of NPs in the nursing workforce (5.6% vs 1.5% or less) (Maier et al., 2016). Physician support is key for optimal NP role implementation and can be fostered by mitigating NP impact on physician income. Reimbursement models not reliant on physician fee-for-service reimbursement and that support collaboration with NPs are advantageous in that regard (DiCenso et al., 2010).

Systematic Approaches to Role Planning

APNs have been described as providing complex care interventions characterized by using multiple interacting competencies and having responsibilities for addressing difficult health care problems and improving outcomes for a variety of groups (e.g., patients, families, providers, teams, organizations, health systems) (Bryant-Lukosius, Israr, Charbonneau-Smith, & DiCenso, 2013). Several factors (e.g., competencies, education, regulation, legislation, funding) are required for successful role implementation. Numerous studies indicate that these factors are often not in place, resulting in serious challenges to APN role implementation and pointing to the need for more systematic approaches to role planning (Andregard & Jangland, 2014; Higgins et al., 2014; Jarosova et al., 2016; Lecocq, Mengal, & Pirson, 2015; Sangster-Gormley, Martin-Misener, Downe-Wamboldt, & DiCenso, 2011). One such approach is the PEPPA (Participatory, Evidence-Based, Patient-Focused Process for Advanced Practice Nursing) framework, offering a nine-step participatory, evidence-based, patient-focused, process for APN role development, implementation, and evaluation. The framework can be used by decision makers, researchers, educators, and nurses at national, regional, organizational, practice setting, or team levels to address barriers to effective APN roles related to role clarity, use of APN expertise, scope of practice, supportive practice environments, and ongoing development and evaluation (Bryant-Lukosius & DiCenso, 2004) (see Chapter 4). PEPPA incorporates principles for effective health human resource planning and has been used successfully to introduce APN and other provider roles in at least 16 countries (Boyko, Carter, & Bryant-Lukosius, 2016). Involving stakeholders (e.g., patient advocates, policymakers, managers, providers) early on in the process is essential for successful APN role implementation (Schober, Gerrish, & McDonnell, 2016). A major strength of PEPPA is the use of stakeholder engagement strategies to determine the need for and define the role, obtain role acceptance and support, and anticipate and resolve implementation barriers (Bryant-Lukosius et al., 2013). At organizational levels, health care administrators are pivotal for guiding the role planning and introduction process, and providing leadership and resources to support role implementation and evaluation (Carter et al., 2010; Elliott, Begley, Sheaf, & Higgins, 2016; Heale, Dickieson, Carter, & Wenghofer, 2014).

Use and Generation of Evidence

Linked with poor planning and the lack of systematic approaches to introducing APN roles is the fact that existing evidence is often not used to inform this process and that influential stakeholders (e.g., government policymakers, health care administrators, health care team members, and the public) at all health system levels (international, national, organizational) do not have a good understanding of the roles (Andregard & Jangland, 2014; DiCenso et al., 2010; Schober et al., 2016; Wisur-Hokkanen et al., 2015). To address these issues, PEPPA promotes the use of existing data for making decisions at each step of APN role development, and it is through this process that stakeholders become more knowledgeable and accepting of the roles. Other strategies are also required to engage and inform stakeholders. Conducting a stakeholder analysis is beneficial for identifying the levels of support, influence, and priorities of key decision makers (Bryant-Lukosius, 2009; Schober et al., 2016). APN champions can then be identified and leveraged to deliver evidence-based messages that are tailored to address the varied information needs of different stakeholders. Using multiple strategies to deliver tailored information in person and electronically, and in concise formats such as briefing notes, facilitates receipt of key messages by busy decision makers (Carter et al., 2014; Kilpatrick, Carter, et al., 2015). The INP/APNN is a special interest group of the ICN that supports APN role development by providing information and creating forums, such as a biannual conference, for information sharing and networking (ICN, 2016a). INP/APNN committees focus on issues related to practice, education, policy, and research and facilitate international surveys to examine APN role practice patterns (Heale & Rieck-Buckley, 2015; Pulcini, Jelic, Gul, & Loke, 2010).

Numerous systematic reviews of randomized controlled trials conducted over the past 35 years demonstrate the effectiveness of APN roles, especially in high-income countries (Bryant-Lukosius, Carter, et al., 2015; Bryant-Lukosius, Cosby, et al., 2015; Donald et al., 2013, 2015; Johantgen et al., 2012; Kilpatrick et al., 2014; Kilpatrick, Reid, et al., 2015; Martin-Misener et al., 2015; Morilla-Herrera et al., 2016; Newhouse et al., 2011; Stanik-Hutt et al., 2013; Swan, Ferguson, Chang, Larson, & Smaldone, 2015; Tsiachristas et al., 2015). Further research is needed on the cost-effectiveness of APN roles (Marshall et al., 2015), and guidelines to facilitate economic evaluations of these roles are being developed (Lopatina

et al., 2017). Given the consistency of evidence about their effectiveness, future research should focus on understanding the conditions, patient populations, and settings where APN roles are most effective for improving patient and health system outcomes (Bryant-Lukosius et al., 2013). The successful introduction of APN roles can also be informed by research to evaluate the effectiveness of implementation processes. Recently, the PEPPA framework was enhanced to support evaluations and the generation of meaningful data for effective decision making about APN roles at national, organizational, setting, and team levels (Bryant-Lukosius et al., 2016). Called PEPPA-Plus, the framework provides guidance and tools to address the information needs of different decision makers across three stages of APN role development (introduction, implementation, and long-term sustainability). At international and national levels, better health human resource data and agreement on indicators and targets for health systems integration for all types of APN roles will be essential to ensure their adequate supply and optimal deployment to areas of greatest need.

Next Steps in the Global Evolution of Advanced Practice Nursing Roles

Improving human resources for health will continue to be a global priority as outlined by the WHO's (2016) strategic plan, *Health Workforce 2030*. Strategic plan objectives and milestones related to investments in the health workforce, needs-based workforce planning, improved access and quality of education, and optimizing provider scopes of practice will benefit the global development of APN roles. Thus the next 15 years will provide exciting opportunities to expand the contribution of APN roles for improving global health. At the international level, nursing organizations and leaders can employ a variety of strategies to support the global development of APN roles, especially in countries where the roles do not exist or are just emerging. These strategies are summarized in Box 6.1. Strategies nursing organizations and leaders can use to support APN role development at country levels are summarized in Box 6.2.

Conclusion

To date, high-income countries have benefited the most from the introduction and expansion of APN roles. Despite substantial evidence of APN role effectiveness for improving health outcomes, increasing access and quality of care, and reducing the

BOX 6.1 **International-Level Strategies to Support the Global Development of Advanced Practice Nursing Roles**

- Leverage and share expertise and resources for APN education, practice, and policy across countries
- Improve role clarity by working toward greater consensus on role definitions and terminology, including delineation of specialized roles at an advanced level
- Support policies that build capacity and prevent the out-migration of nursing leaders, educators, researchers, and advanced practice nurses from countries where APN roles are just getting started

Adapted from Bryant-Lukosius and Martin-Misener (2016), Dury et al. (2014), Kooienga and Carryer (2015), Nardi and Diallo (2014), and the National Nursing Centres Consortium (2014).

 BOX 6.2 **Country-Level Strategies to Support Advanced Practice Nursing Role Development**

- Focus efforts on placing nurses at high-level policy decision-making tables to advocate for the APN role
- Advocate for systematic and evidence-based approaches to role development, implementation and evaluation
- Connect with key stakeholders around shared policy concerns to create conditions for healthcare organization and system transformational change
- Build consensus among stakeholders on health systems solutions that utilize APN roles
- Establish a knowledge translation plan to promote stakeholder awareness and understanding of APN roles and their benefits and to reduce barriers to role implementation
- Create communities of practice to develop advanced practice nurses

Adapted from Bryant-Lukosius and Martin-Misener (2016) and the National Nursing Centres Consortium (2014).

unnecessary use of costly acute care services, the overall integration of APN roles within health care systems is limited in most countries. Over the next decade, policy priorities to improve global health by strengthening the development and use of nursing expertise will create new prospects to expand the introduction of APN roles. Successful health systems integration of the next generation of APN roles will require pan-approaches, including international collaboration, greater attention to the use of systematic approaches, and collection and use of good data to identify implementation barriers and monitor role deployment and impact.

Key Summary Points

- There has been tremendous growth in the introduction of APN roles over the last decade. Population health needs for increased access to primary health care, care for the elderly, and chronic disease prevention and management will further drive role expansion.
- APN roles are an important strategy for developing and strengthening the nursing workforce to meet population health and health service needs.
- Systematic approaches to APN role development are essential for optimal role implementation and impact on outcomes.
- At international and national levels, ways to collect better APN role workforce data are needed to ensure an adequate supply of advanced practice nurses and their optimal deployment to areas of greatest need.

References

To access the references for this chapter, use your smartphone's QR code reader to scan the code below, or go to http://booksite.elsevier.com/ 9780323447751.

Direct Clinical Practice

Mary Fran Tracy

---

*"You can only lose something that you have, you cannot lose
something that you are."*

—*Eckhart Tolle*

Direct care is the central competency of advanced practice nursing. This competency informs and shapes the execution of the other six competencies. Direct care is essential for a number of reasons. To consult, collaborate, and lead clinical staff and programs effectively, an advanced practice registered nurse (APRN) must have clinical credibility. With the deep clinical and systems understanding that APRNs possess, they facilitate the care processes that ensure achievement of outcomes for individuals and groups of patients. Advanced practice occurs

within a health care system that is constantly changing—changing delivery models, reimbursement structures, regulatory requirements, population-based management, and even proposed changes in the basic educational requirements for advanced practice nurses through the Doctor of Nursing Practice (DNP) degree. The challenge that many APRNs face is how to maintain the characteristics of care that have helped patients achieve positive health outcomes and afforded APRN care a unique niche in the health care marketplace. Characteristics such as the use of a holistic perspective and formation of therapeutic partnerships with patients to co-implement individualized health care are challenged by cost containment strategies that emphasize standardization of care to achieve population-based outcome targets. Conversely, characteristics of APRN care such as health promotion, fostering self-care, and patient education are valued by practices offering care to patients because they result in an appropriate use of health care resources and sustain quality.

This chapter describes the direct clinical practice of APRNs and helps readers understand how it differs from the practice of experts by experience, describes strategies for balancing direct care with other competencies, and describes strategies for retaining a direct care focus. The six characteristics of APRN direct care practice are identified.

Direct Care Versus Indirect Care Activities

Direct care is the central APRN competency (see Chapter 3). The APRN is using advanced clinical judgment, systems thinking, and accountability in providing evidence-based care at a more advanced level than the care provided by the expert registered nurse (RN). The APRN is prepared to assist individuals through complex health care situations by the use of education, counseling, and coordination of care (American Association of Colleges of Nursing [AACN], 2006). Although an expert RN may, at times, demonstrate components of care that are at an advanced level, it is care that is gained through experience and is exemplary (not expected) at that level. Essentials I and II of DNP education for APRNs delineate that APRN-level care is demonstrated through advanced, refined assessment skills and implementation and evaluation of practice interventions based on integrated knowledge from a number of sciences, such as biophysical, psychosocial, behavioral, cultural, economic, and nursing science (AACN, 2006). Graduate-level APRN education provides a foundation for the evolution of practice over time as necessitated by health care and patients. This advanced level of practice is an expected competency of all APRNs, not an exemplary skill that is intermittently or inconsistently displayed by staff or expert nurses.

For the purposes of this chapter, the terms *direct care* and *direct clinical practice* refer to the activities and functions that APRNs perform within the patient-nurse interface. Depending on the focus of an APRN's practice, the patient may, and often does, include family members and significant others. The activities

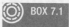 **BOX 7.1   Examples of Processes That Occur at the Point of Care**

- The patient-provider therapeutic partnership is established.
- Health problems become mutually understood through information gathering and effective communication.
- Health, recovery, or palliative goals are expressed by the patient.
- Management and treatment options are explored.
- Physical acts of diagnosis, monitoring, treatment, and pharmacologic and nonpharmacologic therapy are performed.
- Education, support, guidance and coaching, and comfort are provided.
- Decisions regarding future actions to be taken by each party are made.
- Future contact is planned.

that occur in this interface or as direct follow-up are unique because they are interpersonally and physically co-enacted with a particular patient for the purpose of promoting that patient's health or well-being. Many important processes transpire at this point of care (Box 7.1).

Advanced practice nursing activities occurring before and adjacent to the patient-nurse interface have a great influence on the direct care that occurs; however, they are not performed with an individual patient or their main purpose is tangential to the direct care of the patient. Activities such as collaboration, consultation, and mentoring of staff may all be occurring in relation to the direct care interface. It is often difficult to separate out these indirect care interventions, which are equally necessary for adequate fulfillment of the APRN role and care of the patient (Box 7.2). For example, when an APRN consults with another provider regarding the nature of a patient's condition or the care that should be recommended to a patient, the APRN is engaging in advanced clinical practice, but it is not direct care. Even though the APRN is accountable for the consultation, the primary purpose of that contact is to acquire information and understanding to use in formulating recommendations for the patient's direct care provider (see Chapter 9). Thus, according to the definition of direct care used in this chapter, the APRN is engaged in clinical practice but he or she is not providing direct care to the

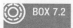 **BOX 7.2** **Examples of Advanced Practice Nurse Indirect Care Activities**

- Consultation with other health care providers (e.g., physicians, nurses, pharmacists)
- Discharge planning
- Care coordination
- Communication with insurance organizations
- Education of bedside nurses
- Unit rounds
- Researching evidence-based care guidelines
- Leading quality-of-care initiatives
- Support staff supervision
- Billing and coding
- Compliance monitoring
- Budget development and implementation

patient. The direct care role of the clinical nurse specialist (CNS) may not be as apparent to observers as it is for a nurse practitioner (NP), certified registered nurse anesthetist (CRNA), and certified nurse-midwife (CNM) because the CNS frequently shifts from direct to indirect activities depending on the situation and the providers involved. For the CNS, these shifts may occur during one patient encounter, and certainly across a day. Most APRNs will have a role in ensuring that others are providing quality and safe care through indirect practice (Exemplar 7.1).

APRN roles tend to diverge when comparing the amount of time spent in each of the direct care activities (Becker, Kaplow, Muenzen, & Hartigan, 2006; Verger, Marcoux, Madden, Bojko, & Barnsteiner, 2005). A research study by Oddsdottir and Sveinsdottir (2011) has demonstrated that CNSs spend most of their time in education and expert practice in the institutional domain; the authors recommended that the focus for CNSs needs to be on direct practice in the client/family domain. Critical care CNSs reported spending 36% of their time with nursing personnel, 21% with patient population work, and 17% on organizational and system work. Only 26% of their time was spent with individual patients, whereas acute care NPs spent 74% of their time with individual patients (Becker et al., 2006). This finding is consistent with other studies reporting that NPs spend more time on individual patient care and less time on indirect and service-related care (American Nurses Credentialing Center, 2004; Gardner, et al., 2010). Other studies have supported the finding that NPs and CNMs are spending most

of their time in direct care with patients (Holland & Holland, 2007; McCloskey, Grey, Deshefy-Longhi, & Grey, 2003; Rosenfeld, McEvoy, & Glassman, 2003; Swartz et al., 2003). There is no set formula as to how much time in direct care is "enough" or appropriate; however, direct care is a core competency and APRNs functioning in a clinical practice should spend at least some time over the balance of their role in direct care activities.

This delineation of direct and indirect practice is not intended to denigrate clinical activities that occur outside the patient-nurse interface—quite the contrary. These clinical activities and functions should be recognized as influencing what happens in the interface and as having a significant impact on patient outcomes. Because these other clinical activities significantly affect patient outcomes, they must be valued by the nursing community and health care systems. In the current environment of cost containment and technological development, all activities that enhance patients' health, recovery, and adjustment are critical components of care delivered by APRNs. Ball and Cox (2003), based on a study of CNSs and NPs, found that APRNs engage in a range of strategic activities, an excellent characterization of the direct and indirect but adjacent actions that make up the clinical practice of APRNs as depicted in exemplars throughout the chapter.

Researchers are beginning to understand the specific activities that constitute the direct care component of various advanced practice nursing roles. However, it is difficult to make generalizations about these activities because the APRNs in the studies noted previously had different roles and worked in different settings, with different populations. Different classification schemas were used to categorize APRN actions. For example, in some studies, investigators used the term *activities* to classify APRN actions; in others, the term *interventions* was used. The variability in terminology and definitions makes it difficult to compare results across APRN roles, settings, and populations. Nevertheless, a review of these studies yields some insights into the extent and nature of direct care activities in APRN roles.

Many direct care activities performed are similar across APRN roles, and preparation of all APRNs must include the "three Ps"—advanced *p*athophysiology, advanced health and *p*hysical assessment, and advanced *p*harmacology (AACN, 2011). Additional direct care activities that are similar across roles include patient and family education and counseling, ordering laboratory tests and medications, and

Direct Care

The care of patients with pulmonary hypertension is commonly managed in the outpatient environment. When those receiving continuous prostacyclin infusion therapy via tunneled central line come back to the hospital for treatment or testing, M.P., the cardiovascular clinical nurse specialist, completes a physical assessment of the patient's current condition and response to therapy.

Standard medical assessment of patient response to changes in prostacyclin therapy includes magnetic resonance imaging (MRI). Because the home infusion pump that delivers the medication cannot be taken into the MRI environment, and because disruption of the infusion can lead to significant complications (including rebound pulmonary hypertension), M.P. works directly with the patient to identify the safest method to continue therapy during the scan. After collecting information about the patient's medication, dose, and pump type, M.P. interviews the patient to assess: how the patient is feeling in response to current therapy; the longest period of time the patient has gone without the infusion medication; and how he or she tolerated the pause in therapy. The plan for continuing therapy during the MRI is established based on this data collection.

If the patient's infusion pump can function when adequate lengths of tubing are added to the basic infusion set to reach into the MRI area, leaving the pump outside the magnetic field, then M.P. works with the patient to either pre-prime the additional tubing at home or in the preparation area of MRI. Review of the plan for the study and answering the patient's questions and concerns with expertise eases the patient's concerns about undergoing the test.

If the patient's pump will not function appropriately with additional lengths of tubing, M.P. collaborates with a pharmacist experienced in the use of intravenous prostacyclins. M.P. and the pharmacist establish an appropriate concentration of medication to be used during the test, calculate the rate needed to achieve the same dose as the patient has been receiving at home, and order both the medications to use during the test and a syringe of medication in the same concentration as the home concentration to use in repriming the patient's central line. After reviewing with the patient the steps to be taken, M.P. helps the patient to convert to the hospital-based infusion prior to the MRI, then assists with conversion back to the home pump at the end of the study. Using advanced assessment skills, M.P. assesses the patient's tolerance of these transitions as well as any side effects he or she may experience during the transitions.

Advanced clinical assessment and planning skills are critical in managing patients in this population. Complex care planning, early identification of complications if they occur, and the ability to safely resolve those issues exemplify the importance of the advanced practice registered nurse's role in care of this very challenging patient population.

Indirect Care

The medical intensive care unit acute care nurse practitioner (ACNP) was approached by an experienced staff nurse who was struggling to develop an interpersonal relationship with the family of a complex, critically ill patient. The family was very anxious and was having difficulty synthesizing the information that the staff nurse was trying to provide to them.

Rather than intervene directly with the family, the ACNP recognized that this would be a good opportunity for the staff nurse to develop and expand her skills at interpersonal relationship building. The ACNP explored with the nurse the interventions that she had already attempted and reviewed with her the literature regarding family stressors in critical care, family needs, and the goal of assessing and addressing what the family perceives as their educational and care needs. Armed with this information, the nurse felt comfortable in working with the family to assess their priority educational and psychosocial needs to obtain the resources and information they needed.

The ACNP could have intervened by establishing a direct relationship with the family, which would have been providing direct care. In this case, however, she determined that it was more important to assist the staff nurse in the development of the relationship as a growth opportunity and to help the nurse form an ongoing partnership with the family, with whom she would be interacting on a continuing basis. ◎

[a]The author gratefully acknowledges Michael Petty, PhD, RN, APRN, CNS, for use of his direct care exemplar.

performing procedures (Becker et al., 2006; Verger et al., 2005). Verger and colleagues (2005) surveyed pediatric critical care NPs regarding their direct care activities, which included physical assessments, patient and family teaching, and performing procedures such as venipuncture, intravenous line insertions, lumbar punctures, feeding tube placements, endotracheal intubations, and central line placements. CNMs reported expansion of their direct care procedures to include first-assisting during cesarean sections and performing endometrial biopsies (Holland & Holland, 2007). CNSs and administrators need to have ongoing monitoring of the direct care components of the CNS role. With increasing complexity and diversity of the role, there is a propensity to have CNSs perform less and less expert direct care of patients, which is the main characteristic of APRN practice (Lewandowski & Adamle, 2009).

Regardless of the population being cared for, surveillance was a key direct care activity of APRNs identified in studies (Brooten, Youngblut, Deatrick, Naylor, & York, 2003; Brooten et al., 2007; Hughes et al., 2002). Surveillance is described as watching for physical and emotional signs and symptoms and monitoring dressing and wound care, laboratory results, medications, nutrition, response to treatment, and caregiving and parenting. Thus surveillance refers to an APRN's vigilant assessment of patient status, the rapid diagnosis of subtle or emergent conditions, and quick intervention to prevent or reverse a potentially negative outcome. Nursing surveillance can have a particularly important impact on the patient safety indicator of failure to rescue—situations in which providers fail to notice symptoms or respond adequately or swiftly to clinical signs, resulting in patient death from preventable complications. Failure to rescue has been linked to nursing surveillance; for example, the higher the nursing surveillance, as defined by staffing ratios, the lower the number of cases of failure to rescue (Aiken, Clarke, Sloane, Sochalski, & Silber, 2002; Clarke & Aiken, 2003). A study by Shever (2011) has also supported the concept that patients who receive higher surveillance, as documented by nursing in the electronic health record, are less likely to be involved in a failure-to-rescue situation.

In summary, direct care activities make up a large part of what most APRNs do, although there is considerable variation in which activities are performed and how much time is devoted to the direct care function across roles, settings, and patient populations.

Six Characteristics of Direct Clinical Care Provided by Advanced Practice Nurses

APRNs function in many roles and settings, and with different populations. Despite such variability in role implementation, there is a similarity in the components of direct care provided. Characteristics of advanced practice nursing care extend across advanced practice roles, health care settings, and populations of patients. These six characteristics are:

- Use of a holistic perspective
- Formation of therapeutic partnerships with patients
- Expert clinical performance
- Use of reflective practice
- Use of evidence as a guide to practice
- Use of diverse approaches to health and illness management

Accumulating evidence supports these features of APRN practice as having positive influences on patient outcomes. Throughout this chapter, the empirical evidence cited about APRN practice is illustrative and not based on a systematic review of research.

The six characteristics of APRN direct care practice have their roots in the traditional values of the nursing profession. These values are defined in nursing's social contract with society, as outlined by the American Nurses Association (ANA, 2010, p. 6):

- People manifest an essential unity of mind, body, and spirit.
- People's experiences are contextually and culturally defined.
- Health and illness are human experiences. The presence of illness does not preclude health, nor does optimal health preclude illness.
- The relationship between the nurse and patient occurs within the context of the values and beliefs of the patient and nurse.
- Public policy and the health care delivery system influence the health and well-being of society and professional nursing.
- Individual responsibility and interprofessional involvement are essential.

Nurses in advanced practice roles often have a deep commitment to the values on which these characteristics rest and are able to advocate persuasively and incorporate these values in daily practice. The expanded scope of practice of APRN roles often enables APRNs to fully enact these characteristics in their interactions with patients. An overview of strategies for enacting these characteristics is provided in Box 7.3.

BOX 7.3   Characteristics of Advanced Direct Care Practice and Strategies for Enacting Them

Use of a Holistic Perspective
- Take into account the complexity of human life.
- Recognize and address how social, organizational, and physical environments affect people.
- Consider the profound effects of illness, aging, hospitalization, and stress.
- Consider how symptoms, illness, and treatment affect quality of life.
- Focus on functional abilities and requirements.

Formation of Therapeutic Partnerships With Patients
- Use a conversational style to conduct health care encounters.
- Optimize therapeutic use of self.
- Encourage the patient, and family as appropriate, to actively engage in decision making.
- Look for cultural influences on health care discourse.
- Listen to the indirect voices of patients who are noncommunicative.
- Advocate the patient's perspective and concerns to others.

Expert Clinical Performance
- Acquire specialized knowledge.
- Seek out supervision when performing a new skill.
- Invest in deeply understanding the patient situations in which you are involved.
- Generate and test alternative lines of reasoning.
- Trust your hunches—check them out.
- Be aware of when you are time-pressured and likely to make thinking errors.
- Consider multiple aspects of the patient's situation when you are deciding how to treat.
- Make sure that you know how to use technical equipment safely.
- Make sure that you know how to interpret data produced by monitoring devices.
- Pay attention to how you move and touch patients during care.

- Anticipate ethical conflicts.
- Acquire technology-related skills for accessing and managing patient data and practice information.

Use of Reflective Practice
- Explore your personal values, belief systems, and behaviors.
- Identify your basic assumptions about health care, the advanced practice registered nurse role, and the rights and responsibilities of patients.
- Consider how your assumptions affect your judgments.
- Talk to colleagues and your teachers about your clinical experiences.
- Consider use of a journal to document experiences.
- Assess your current skill and comfort in reflection.

Use of Evidence as a Guide for Practice
- Learn how to search health care databases for studies related to specific clinical topics.
- Read research reports related to your field of practice.
- Seek out systematic revision of research and evidence-based clinical guidelines.
- Acquire skills in appraising the various forms of evidence.
- Work with colleagues to consider evidence-based improvements in care.

Diverse Approaches to and Interventions for Health and Illness Management
- Use interpersonal interventions to guide and coach patients.
- Acquire proficiency in new ways of treating and helping patients.
- Help patients maintain health and capitalize on their strengths and resources.
- Provide preventive services appropriate to your field of practice.
- Coordinate services among care sites and multiple providers.
- Acquire knowledge about complementary therapies.

Use of a Holistic Perspective

Holism Described

Holism has a variety of meanings. A broad view is that holism involves a deep understanding of each patient as a complex and unique person who is embedded in a temporally unfolding life. The holistic perspective recognizes the multiple dimensions of each person—physiologic, social, emotional, cognitive, and spiritual—and that the relationships among these dimensions result in a whole that is greater than the sum of the parts. People are in constant interaction with themselves, others, and the environment and universe and exhibit maximum well-being when all parts are balanced and in harmony (Erickson, 2007); this state of well-being can exist whether there are physical disorders or not. This comprehensive and integrated view of human life and health is considered in the health care encounter within the context of the full range of factors influencing patients' experiences (Box 7.4). Clearly, high-tech care environments with many health care providers, each focused on a particular aspect of a patient's condition and treatment, require coordinators who have a comprehensive and integrated appreciation of the patient and his or her experience of care as a whole. APRNs' capacity to keep the pieces together

and promote continuity of care in a way that focuses care on the unique individual is undoubtedly why many clinical programs have an APRN member or coordinator (see "Management of Complex Situations" later). Interprofessional team members caring for older adults view the APRN as a leader in facilitating holistic care (Cowley, Cooper, & Goldber, 2016). In addition, APRNs practicing in palliative care demonstrate practice at an advanced level by combining holistic care with treatment interventions to ameliorate symptoms, all while they are evaluating the care from a system context in terms of appropriate use of resources (George, 2016). The Shuler Nurse Practitioner Practice Model is based on a holistic understanding of human health and illness in older adults that integrates medical and nursing perspectives (Shuler, Huebscher, & Hallock, 2001; see Chapter 2).

Holism and Health Assessment

When working with a relatively healthy person, the APRN seeks to understand the person's life goals, functional interests, and health risks to preserve quality of life in the future. In contrast, when working with an ill patient, the APRN is interested in what the person views as problems, how he or she is responding to problems, and what the problems and responses mean to the individual in terms of daily living and life goals. In a study of 199 primary care clinical situations (Burman, Stepans, Jansa, & Steiner, 2002), NPs were found to engage in holistic assessment and ground their decision making within the context of the patient's life. In addition, NP faculty also engage students in and role-model provision of holistic care from a nursing perspective (Brykczynski, 2012).

The ability to function in daily activities and relationships is an important consideration for patients when they evaluate their health, so it is an appropriate and essential focus for holistic, person-centered assessment. Most functional assessment formats focus on the following: (1) how patients view their health or quality of life; (2) how they accomplish self-care and household or job responsibilities; (3) the social, physical, financial, environmental, and spiritual factors that augment or tax their functioning; and (4) the strategies that they and their families use to cope with the stresses and problems in their lives.

In pediatrics, measures of functional status have been developed, such as one for children with asthma (Centers for Disease Control and Prevention, 2013).

 BOX 7.4   **Factors to Consider When Helping the Patient Holistically**

- Patient's view of his or her health or illness
- Patterns of physical symptoms and amount of distress they cause
- Effect of physical symptoms on the patient's daily functioning and quality of life
- Symptom management approaches that are acceptable to the patient
- Life changes that could affect the patient's physical or psychological well-being (e.g., relationship changes, job change, intrafamily conflict, retirement, death of a loved one)
- Context of the patient's life, including the nuclear family unit, social support, job responsibilities, financial situation, health insurance coverage, responsibilities for the care of others (e.g., children, chronically ill spouse or partner, older parents)
- Spiritual and life values (e.g., independence, religion, beliefs about life, acceptance of fate)

In adults, APRNs may choose to use a disease- or problem-focused tool such as measurement of functional status in heart failure patients (Rector, Anand, & Cohn, 2006), of symptom distress in cancer patients (Chen & Lin, 2007; Cleeland et al., 2000), or of function and disability in geriatric patients (Denkinger et al., 2009), or a widely used general measure such as the Short Form-36 Health Survey (SF-36), which measures overall health, functional status, and well-being in adults and is available in several languages (Ware & Sherbourne, 1992).

Nursing Model or Medical Model

As APRNs have taken on responsibilities that were formerly in the purview of physicians, some have expressed concern that APRNs are being asked to function within a medical model of practice rather than within a holistic nursing model. This concern is raised when APRNs function as substitutes for physicians. However, there is evidence that a nursing orientation is an enduring component of APRN practice, even when medical management is part of the role (Brykczynski, 2012; Cowley, Cooper, & Goldberg, 2016; George, 2016; Mason, Jones, Roy, Sullivan, & Wood, 2015; Box 7.5). Activities described in these studies clearly reflect a nursing-focused practice.

Statements from professional organizations indicate that APRNs value both their nursing orientation and their medical functions. For example, the description of APRNs in the ANA's nursing social policy statement includes strong endorsement of specialized and expanded knowledge and skills within the context of holistic values (ANA, 2010). On the theoretical front, several models of advanced practice blend nursing and medical orientations (see "Shuler's

BOX 7.5 Nursing-Focused Advanced Practice Interventions

- Engagement of patients in their own care
- Patient education
- Guidance and coaching
- Care planning and care coordination
- Physical and occupational therapy referrals
- Use of communication skills
- Promotion of continuity of care
- Teaching of nursing staff
- Advance directive discussions
- Wellness and health promotion intiatives

Model of NP Practice" and "Dunphy and Winland-Brown's Circle of Caring: A Transformative, Collaborative Model" in Chapter 2).

Formation of Therapeutic Partnerships With Patients

The Institute of Medicine (IOM) has recommended patient-centered care as the foundation of safe, effective, and efficient health care (Committee on Quality Health Care in America, IOM, 2001). The person-centered, holistic perspective of APRNs serves as the foundation for the types of relationships that they cocreate with patients. APRNs are well prepared to develop therapeutic relationships as the cornerstone of patient-centered care (Esmaeili, Cheraghi, & Salsali, 2014; Kitson, Marshall, Bassett, & Keitz, 2012). The Gallup Poll has consistently reported that the public views nurses as the most trusted professionals (ANA, 2016). The skill of APRNs to develop therapeutic relationships with individual patients can influence broader public perceptions.

The development and maintenance of therapeutic relationships with patients and families is one of the key criteria in *The Essentials of Doctoral Education for Advanced Nursing Practice* (DNP Essentials), which is specific and foundational to advanced practice nursing (AACN, 2006). Studies have shown that APRNs form collaborative relationships with patients. In research of an APRN-directed transitional care model (Bradway et al., 2012), the authors found that a mutually trusting relationship between the APRN, the cognitively impaired patient, and the caregiver was key to providing the caregivers with the confidence and information they needed to optimally care for their loved one. This personal relationship and the availability of the APRN outside routine visits led to the avoidance of potentially negative outcomes. The APRNs utilized their advanced skills in tailoring information to improve caregiver skills and knowledge in these complex patient cases. Bissonette, Woodend, Davies, Stacey, and Knoll (2013) also found that an APRN-led collaborative team led to fewer emergency department visits and hospital admissions in kidney transplant recipients. In addition, Drennan et al. (2011) found that patients were satisfied with their relationships with nurses and midwives, including the consultation process, patient education, medication advice, and the patient's intent to comply with provider advice.

APRNs' therapeutic use of self contributes to the optimization of a therapeutic relationship with patient and family. Therapeutic use of self involves

APRN awareness of personal feelings, attitudes, and values and how that awareness influences the patient-provider relationship (Warner, 2006). This increased awareness on the part of the APRN helps increase empathy, allowing the APRN to engage more deeply with patients while maintaining appropriate boundaries to maintain objectivity (Warner, 2006). See Exemplar 7.2 for an example from a patient perspective when a therapeutic partnership is not established.

Shared Decision Making

In addition to eliciting information that increases understanding of the patient's illness experience, APRNs, in the studies cited, encourage patients to participate in decisions regarding how their diseases and illnesses should be managed. There is a continuum of patient involvement in making decisions for her or his own health care. At one end of the continuum are patients who want to be fully engaged

---

| EXEMPLAR 7.2 | A Cautionary Tale: The Founder of the First Nurse Practitioner (NP) Program on Disappointing NP Encounters |

Dr. Eileen O'Grady interviewed Dr. Loretta Ford, the founder of the NP role, on February 16, 2016. The following discussion captures a not-so-exemplary experience she had seeing a NP who did not meet her needs or appear to be practicing even the most basic nursing skills. This is presented as a cautionary tale about how patients can experience APRNs who do not embody the seven competencies.

Dr. O'Grady: I'd like to start with an incident you had a few years ago, seeing a NP who fell short of meeting your needs.

Dr. Ford: I ended up with a NP from the cardiologists' office. [The cardiologist] called himself the electrician of the cardiac team because he puts in the pacemakers. I began to have tachycardia attacks that were unusual, so I made an appointment but the cardiologist was busy, so they said I could see the NP.

So, I said "Fine!" That was good. I was on some medications and I felt they needed to be changed but when I checked them out, I was taking the maximum dose, so I didn't want to increase it until I had some information about it. So, I went to see the NP.

I hadn't seen her before and she came in and said her name; when I go to any health service I never tell them who I am or what my background is or anything. I'm careful not to use any technical language that might give me away. Right away there didn't seem to be any interest in me as a person, and so of course I didn't say anything. I didn't want to give it away, but I also didn't offer anything.

First of all, there was no history of any kind taken, not even a nursing history. There was no asking. She was looking at the computer more than at me and asking the computer "Now, is this unusual, this recent event?" or "What triggered it?" She never asked what I thought might trigger it. So from there on, it lacked human interaction. I could see no evidence of whether

she cared or not or whether or not there was any nursing presence at all. I didn't feel that there was any caring or compassion, it was purely technical.

As a matter of fact, the NP was not as caring as my primary care physician. There was no sense of coordination, and in the end she said "Well, I'll have to go and check with the cardiologist about new medication or different medication." And that ended the visit.

So, I didn't feel that nursing was there at all. I didn't think it was even good medicine myself, but I'm used to having a primary care physician who is an excellent clinician and a good teacher. So, I was disappointed, and I was never really sure if my primary care physician was consulted. I don't want any special treatment

Dr. O'Grady: So, the founder of the NP role has to do her own care coordination and sees an NP who does not appear to inhabit any of nursing's core values. What needs went unmet in that exchange?

Dr. Ford: Well, I'd like some human interaction, that the NP would indeed acknowledge that I was in the room instead of the computer. Now this is, in a way, an isolated incident, but it was repeated when my husband was in a rehabilitation center. The NP talked a little bit to me, but not much, and not to my husband, who didn't hear well anyway. So, it wasn't too different in that situation either. When I talk to my colleagues around the country, they have reported the same thing in terms of their experiences, so I don't know that this an isolated incident, but it seems to be the experience of nurses as patients around the country.

Secondly, my daughter has been cared for by another NP, and it's been phenomenally good. The coordination was excellent, the caring and communication for her worked out beautifully because she's finally had somebody to listen to her. So, you don't want to condemn all the NPs from my experience, but it's interesting

Continued

how variable it is and I don't know if its preparation or system problems. But certainly there's no legal restriction against practicing basic nursing care, the possibilities of nursing are so vast, in terms of patient care.

Dr. O'Grady: But this failure that you and your colleagues have experienced. What would you say is driving that? Where is the failure?

Dr. Ford: Well, I think there are failures in the systems controls. Some of the states are racing to the bottom as far as legal authorization for APRNs is concerned. But that shouldn't keep people from practicing basic nursing skills: caring, compassion, care coordination, teaching, and learning. After all, those nurses, many of them are practicing with specialists and know a great deal, and they ought to use that in teaching patients. None of us experienced that, those of us who haven't had a good experience seeing NPs as nurse patients.

On the other hand, I think the system has failed because in a sense the rewards are not there either. Rewards that they sometimes experience, is when they identify an unusual disease entity. It is a system that doesn't reward NPs with recognition, respect, or remuneration.

Then of course you have to ask about their preparation. A lot of people don't know the history of the NP; they're not interested in history, they're interested in what's going on today and tomorrow. And of course, once you take history out of the curriculum, you "integrate" it. Well, I say that integration means it's out of the curriculum. Because, all they know about is Florence Nightingale, but they don't know all of the things that Florence Nightingale encompassed as basic tenants of nursing.

Dr. O'Grady: So, given this disappointing NP experience, does your vision for the nurse practitioner future differ from what it was in the 1960s?

Dr. Ford: It does, because frankly the role has been increasingly medicalized. In that sense, the system is changing in prevention and promotion. We had four elements really: prevention, promotion, preservation, and protection. Henry [Silver] and I had many discussions about the language that we were using. We didn't call it physical exam; I insisted we call it physical assessment, because that is a nursing word. We have to keep nursing in the language and in concept, and to use the forward-looking concept of interdependence.

So that nurses were independent in nursing, but not independent in teams. Everyone was interdependent in the team care.

But the elements of nursing came right out of nursing. Because if you read the early literature, nursing was developing as a profession, and NPs needed to be independent in nursing, that it's health and wellness oriented and that the involvement of the patient as a member of the team is vital. That the nurse and the patient and others on the team were actually partners, and that's where many of the teaching elements came in.

So it was built on what the profession was saying at the time and we even used the nursing process; assessment, implementation, evaluation was part of what we were doing. And when we went to the state boards, we laid it out. That was the goal.

Dr. O'Grady: So how is your vision different today than it was in the 1960s for the future?

Dr. Ford: I think, for example, we're talking about nurses substituting for the primary care deficits of medicine. Well, I don't see that! I see them as being able to offer services to patients, regardless of their disease entity, with regards to health and wellness. How they cope with their illness, prevention. I mean, it was built on primary, secondary, and tertiary prevention of caring. And that could include adjusting medications; it has always involved medications, but not to the extent it does today. You know, we have made the cardinal error of developing legal authority by going after it task, by task, by task. It was the worst strategy and I never agreed with that because every time you turned around, we were running to the legislature to order equipment, to give certain scheduled drugs. Next thing you know, we'll be asking the legislature to allow us to pluck eyebrows, and that's ridiculous! So we've in some way painted ourselves into a corner by these efforts.

I've realized that creating one role (like the NP) was not going to change the system. The system was so strongly medically controlled. It's always one of these three things: power, control, and money. And you see them being played out every time, in every element, in every state: power, control, and money.

Dr. O'Grady: So, what could you say to a graduate student who's reading this book and doesn't want to become the NP who is not really assessing anything, not really being caring, not connecting. What would

EXEMPLAR **7.2**	**A Cautionary Tale: The Founder of the First Nurse Practitioner (NP) Program on Disappointing NP Encounters—cont'd**

you say to that NP when working in this metric-driven delivery system, that doesn't value these other things, these nursing things? What could the NP do?

Dr. Ford: Well, in the first place, I think the NP ought to select the place of employment very carefully, and negotiate ahead of time what she has to offer and find out what they don't have and say: "I cannot do what you don't have. You don't have physicians; you want physicians? Don't ask me. That's not what I do. Let me tell you what I do."

In that way, in Colorado by the way, there is a good example of this. I worked with a man who was a specialist and the best that ever happened is that I was a generalist in both pediatrics and family care (because I was a public health nurse). And we were a perfect match because he did what he did in medicine and I did all the family work and all kinds of things that made a difference in the outcome of the patients' wellness and health and living.

So, you don't need to be a specialist duplicate of what the specialist is. You need to be doing the thing that you can do best as a nurse. This doesn't mean that you shouldn't know a lot about what the specialist does and what the treatments are, and be able to adjust them to meet that patient's particular environment and experience. So it seems to me that you need to negotiate ahead of time, in terms of what you can and can't do and won't do—not because you can't do them, but because they're not where you want to spend your time.

Dr. O'Grady: So, it almost sounds like staying in your lane. Doing what you do really well.

Dr. Ford: Well, that will change. Because things change. For example, the technology is changing so rapidly today that we have to change with it, or we

have to invent it. We should not be flippant all the time of these inventions. And it doesn't need to be technology, but technology that we have at hand. Different ways and things to think about asking: "Why are we doing this? Do we really need to do it or does it matter?" I think we're in a time-warp in a sense.

Dr. O'Grady: So before we end, is there anything parting that you'd say about this whole incident or incidents that you've had with your husband and the NPs? Is there any parting advice or solution?

Dr Ford: Well, I think reflective practice has yet to come into being, so you must look at what you're doing every day and how you're spending the day. And it must include reflection on the interactions you are having with patients. Really know what a professional model of nursing is, and talk with others about it. Really talk with and listen to the patients. The listening has gone out the window you know.

Dr. O'Grady: Well, I'm writing the policy chapter and we are seeing the lay of the land and scope of practice for APRNs is moving at such a glacial place. The Affordable Care Act has largely decentralized decision-making and so the governance of delivery systems will dictate how APRNs get paid and how they're involved. So, there are just many more tables to be at. It's harder to influence because it's a one-by-one.

Dr. Ford: Well there's no doubt that there's going to be some changes in the air but as I say it's power, control, and money. But I'm sure that when I'd talk about independent practice, I'd sure talk about it in terms of the statutory authority. Because the states, anything in fact that raises such flags, and no one is independent, we're all interdependent. ◎

in a partnership with providers in making decisions, whereas at the other end of the continuum are patients who want to rely on family members or care providers to make all treatment decisions. This may include patients who are older, sicker, or cognitively impaired, or who have cultural beliefs that lead them to defer decisions to others. In general, patients express interest in wanting to be more involved in care planning and treatment decisions, and it is increasingly being demonstrated that with increased involvement, particularly in patients with chronic illness, there are improvements in individual care and outcomes and improved adherence to

recommended regimens (Houlihan, 2015; Kitson et al., 2012; Kullberg, Sharp, Johansson, & Bergermar, 2015; Robinson, Callista, Berry, & Dearing, 2008). No matter where the patient falls on this continuum, it is still incumbent on the provider to establish a collaborative partnership to ensure that regardless of whom the patient wants to make decisions, it is done in congruence with the patient's beliefs and values (Esmaeili et al., 2014).

APRNs should individually determine each patient's preference for participation in decision making and be sensitive to the fact that patients' preferences may change over time as they get to know the provider better and as different types of health problems arise. Once the patient's preference has been elicited, the provider should tailor his or her communication and decision-making style to the patient's preference. Many patients have not had prior health care experiences in which shared decision making was even a possibility but, when offered the opportunity, many choose it—tentatively in some cases, enthusiastically in others. Trying on a more active role may require some help from the provider, such as explaining how it would work and which responsibilities are the patient's and which are the provider's. Providers can encourage patients to bring up issues by asking open-ended questions such as "How have you been?" and focused but open questions such as "How are things going at home?" Patients can be encouraged to participate in decision making by offering them explicit opportunities in the form of questions such as "Does one of those approaches sound better to you than the other?" Gradually, patients approached in this way will learn that health care encounters will be organized around their concerns, not around a series of questions asked by the provider, and that they should feel safe to express their concerns and preferences.

Open and honest communication is foundational to a shared decision-making philosophy. APRNs have reported more advanced communication skills than those reported by basic RNs (Sivesind et al., 2003). The ability to adapt communication styles is a needed skill of APRNs (McCourt, 2006) and can result in patients reporting that they have more knowledge, confidence, and control of their own care (Esmaeili et al., 2014). It is a skill that is necessary for an APRN to maintain a therapeutic relationship with a patient while also supporting her or him in effective decision making. The APRN needs to use an approach that incorporates verbal and nonverbal behaviors exhibited by the patient while being careful to maintain professional boundaries (Elliott, 2010).

APRNs must be cognizant of their own personal beliefs and value systems in a partnership in which they are coaching patients in decision making (see Chapter 8). Although they are uniquely prepared to facilitate the holistic management of the physical, psychosocial, and spiritual aspects of care in these particular situations, APRNs may be involved in interactions in which it is difficult for them to help patients make decisions. If the APRN is unaware of or has unresolved issues of his or her own, he or she may risk exercising undue or unintentional influence on a patient's decision in emotionally charged situations. Bringing one's own beliefs and values to consciousness prior to a discussion focused on patient decision making, reflecting on one's own cognitive and affective responses to such discussions, and debriefing with a colleague can help APRNs maintain a therapeutic approach (or determine when it is appropriate for another clinician to become involved).

Cultural Influences on Partnerships

Another important factor affecting whether and how persons want to participate in health care decision making is their cultural background. It is easy to forget that not all cultures value individual autonomy as much as North Americans of Anglo-Saxon ancestry. Increasingly, recognizing and respecting the cultural identification of patients is being viewed as essential to building meaningful partnerships. Cultural groups form along lines of racial, national origin, religious, professional, organizational, sexual orientation, or age group identification. Some cultural groups are easier to identify than others. Physical differences in appearance may indicate to the provider that he or she is dealing with a person of a different cultural orientation. Other cultural identifications are less obvious—for example, people with religious beliefs about fate, God as healer, or treatment taboos. However, it is important to avoid making assumptions about cultural beliefs simply based on physical appearance or dress. In today's increasingly diverse society, many families have blended traditional beliefs and practices from a number of cultures. These beliefs are learned by asking the patient open-ended questions and responding in a way that makes the patient feel understood.

The DNP Essentials identifies the need for APRNs to synthesize and incorporate principles of cultural diversity into preventive and therapeutic interventions for individuals and populations (AACN, 2006). The preparation of APRNs in the area of cultural competence and culturally appropriate care is key because the demographics of nurses, including APRNs, do not match the overall demographics of the US population (Budden, Zhong, Moulton, & Cimiotti, 2013; Murray, Pole, Ciarlo, & Holmes, 2016). Interactions that are complicated by cultural misunderstandings can result in incomplete or inaccurate assessments and even in misdiagnoses and suboptimal outcomes (Barakzai, Gregory, & Fraser, 2007; Nokes, 2011; Sobralske & Katz, 2005). The APRN needs to individualize care based on an assessment of the cultural influences on the perception of illness and reporting of symptoms. Otherwise, differences in perceptions can cause confusion, misunderstandings, and even conflicts that disrupt the patient-provider relationship and discourse. Moreover, cultural influences often complicate attempts to resolve misunderstandings because different cultural groups approach conflict negotiation differently. Studies have shown that NPs can engender trust in a population such as African-Americans to an equal or greater extent than physicians (Benkert, Peters, Tate, & Dinando, 2008; Peters, Benkert, Templin, & Cassidy-Bushrow, 2014). In every encounter, the provider should expect that the patient may have values that are different in some ways from his or her own and must make a special effort to ensure that the care being given meets the patient's needs and is acceptable to him or her (Escallier & Fullerton, 2009). APRNs must always remain nonjudgmental and not impose their own beliefs or biases onto the patient.

Communication With Patients

A foundation of good communication with patients is essential to developing a therapeutic relationship. Research has shown that good communication between the APRN and patient can increase patient satisfaction, establish trust, increase adherence to a treatment plan, and improve patient outcomes (Bentley, Stirling, Robinson, & Minstrell, 2016; Burley, 2011; Charlton, Dearing, Berry, & Johnson, 2008; Gilbert & Hayes, 2009; Kinder, 2016; Persson, Hornsten, Wirkvist, & Mogren, 2011). Learning good communication skills takes ongoing practice throughout the APRN's career. Options for doing this include using standardized patients and simulation laboratories with feedback, which have been shown to improve APRN students' interpersonal and communication skills (Kesten, Brown, & Meeker, 2015; Lin, Chen, Chao, & Chen, 2013; Pittman, 2012; Rosenzweig et al., 2008).

One aspect of optimal communication is listening. Listening has been described as being fully present with the patient to garner patient details, increase the level of trust in the relationship, and improve patient compliance (Browning & Waite, 2010). Listening takes as much concerted effort to perform optimally as verbal communication. Key to good listening is the ability on the APRN's part to avoid being distracted by personal thoughts, forming instant judgments, and formulating a reply while the patient is still speaking and telling her or his story. In addition, the APRN must become aware of how individual expectations, experiences, and cultural paradigms can result in biases and misperceptions when working with patients (Browning & Waite, 2010). Reflective listening techniques can be useful when APRNs convey to patients that they have been heard and understood without judgment and can assist patients in exploring their personal situations more fully (Resnicow & McMaster, 2012). These techniques include taking patient statements and restating, rephrasing, reframing, and reflecting thoughts, feelings, and emotional undertones back to the patient (Miller, 2010).

Therapeutic Partnerships With Noncommunicative Patients

Some patients are not able to enter fully into partnership with APRNs because they are too young, have compromised cognitive capacity, or are unconscious. Examples of clinical populations who may be unable to participate fully in shared decision making are listed in Box 7.6. Unfortunately, staff nurses working with noncommunicative patients can become so focused on providing care that they forget about having meaningful interactions with the patient (Alasad & Ahmad, 2005). APRNs can role-model alternative forms of communication so that noncommunicative patients can receive optimal care.

Although these patients may have limited ability to speak for themselves, they are not entirely without opinion or voice. Situations in which patients will experience temporary alterations in cognition or verbal ability can often be anticipated. For example, in planned perioperative situations in which general

 BOX 7.6 Patient Populations Unable to Participate Fully in Partnership

- Infants and preverbal children
- Anesthetized patients
- Unconscious or comatose patients
- People in severe pain
- Patients receiving medications that impair cognition
- People with dementia
- People with psychiatric conditions that seriously impair rational thought
- People with conditions that render them incapable of speech and conversation
- People with congenital or acquired cognitive limitations
- People whose primary language is different from the provider's

anesthesia and intubation will be used, the CRNA has the opportunity to dialogue with the patient prior to the procedure. This creates a shared relationship in which the patient can feel comforted and confident about the upcoming procedure (Rudolfsson, von Post, & Eriksson, 2007). The CRNA can prepare patients for the period when communication will be a challenge and propose alternative methods for communication. In addition, the CRNA can discuss patients' preferences for handling possible events beforehand to elicit their wishes.

In the absence of this type of prior dialogue, experts who work with patients who cannot verbalize their concerns and preferences learn to pay close attention to how patients are responding to what happens to them; facial expressions, body movement, and physiologic parameters are used to ascertain what causes the patient discomfort and what helps alleviate it. In a study of persons who had experienced and recovered from unconsciousness (Lawrence, 1995), 27% of the patients reported being able to hear, understand, and respond emotionally while they were unconscious. These findings suggest that nurses should communicate with unconscious patients by providing them with interventions such as reassurance, bodily care, pain relief, explanations, and comforting touch.

There are tools that can be used for patients who are conscious but unable to communicate. Unfortunately, many nurses are not adequately educated in using alternative methods of communication and, if they are, may not be familiar or comfortable with the particular method required for an individual patient (Markor & Hazan, 2012; Thompson & McKeever, 2014). Other barriers include not having access to communication devices and time pressures that may not allow providers to engage adequately in a process that could take more time.

Other sources of information about patients who are unable to respond physically or to communicate should also be identified. For example, siblings visiting an adolescent male with a major head injury would be able to tell you what type of music he likes to listen to and could even bring you a playlist to play for the patient. His mother would know what has caused him to have skin reactions in the past. Responding to his father's offhand comment that he cannot stand to be without his glasses when he is not wearing his contact lenses would most likely help father and son. All of these are ways of building a partnership with an unconscious teenager in an intensive care unit. In adults and adolescents, advance directives, heath care proxy documents,

and organ donation cards are other sources of information regarding patients' wishes. Thus noncommunicative patients are not without voices, but hearing their voices does require presence and attentiveness, and establishing a relationship. Box 7.7 summarizes options for the APRN when engaging with noncommunicative patients.

Expert Clinical Performance

Few studies have clearly differentiated between the expert skills of the APRN and the practice of the basic RN. The expert performance of an APRN encompasses clinical thinking and skills. An expert's clinical judgment is characterized by the ability to make fine distinctions among features of a particular condition that were not possible during beginning practice. Benner's (1984) studies of expert clinical judgment, although not with APRN participants, inform this discussion of APRNs' clinical expertise. Tanner (2006) has reviewed the literature regarding clinical judgment and found that it requires three main categories of knowledge. The first is scientific and theoretical knowledge that is widely applicable. The second is knowledge based on experience that fills in gaps and assists in the prompt identification

 BOX 7.7   Techniques for Communicating With Noncommunicative Patients

- Maintain verbal interactions and eye contact with patient throughout care.
- Explain procedures.
- Monitor tone of voice to avoid inadvertently relaying emotional subcontext to the actual words used.
- Use appropriate touch for reassurance.
- Use other communication devices such as alphabet and word boards, writing, computers, and electronic communication devices.
- Use interpreters for foreign languages and sign language.
- Use other sources of information for patient's likes and dislikes—family, primary care providers, friends.
- Use physiologic cues—grimacing, frowning, turning away from touch, relaxing facial muscles, blood pressure and heart rate responses—as appropriate to evaluate patient responses to care and treatments.

of clinical issues. The final category is knowledge that is individualized to the patient, based on an interpersonal connection. Clinical judgment involves application of skills to the situation (Tanner, 2006; Victor-Chmil, 2013).

Clinical Thinking

APRNs' specialized knowledge accrues from a variety of sources, including graduate and continuing education, clinical experience, professional reading, reflection, mentoring, and exchange of information and ideas with colleagues within and outside nursing. The integration of knowledge from these sources provides a foundation for the expert clinical thinking that is associated with advanced direct care practice. Once an APRN has been in practice for a while, formalized knowledge and experiential knowledge become so mixed together that they may not be distinguishable to the outside observer. Illness trajectories and presentations of prior patients make an impression and come to mind when a patient with a similar problem is seen later (Benner, 1984). The expert also remembers which interventions worked and did not work in certain situations. Eventually, the expert's clinical knowledge consists of a complex network of memorable cases, prototypic images, research findings, thinking strategies, moral values, maxims, probabilities, behavioral responses, associations, illness trajectories and timetables, and therapeutic information. Thus experts have extensive, varied, and complex knowledge networks that can be activated to help them understand clinical situations and events. These networks are composed of internal and external resources. The APRN may mentally review internal resources such as educational knowledge, typical cases, and previously experienced cases when confronted with a complex or challenging patient. However, the APRN is also cognizant of when internal resources are no longer adequate and knows when to refer to external resources for consultation, more data, or guidance. Throughout the assessment, the APRN is using pattern recognition, deductive reasoning, and inductive reasoning to reach a differential diagnosis (Scordo, 2014).

Clinical reasoning brings together the clinical knowledge of the provider with specific observations, perceptions, events, and facts from the situation at hand to produce an understanding of what is occurring (Victor-Chmil, 2013). Sometimes, the understanding is arrived at by using cognitive processes to consider evidence and alternative explanations logically. At other times, the insight or understanding arrives intuitively—that is, through direct apprehension without recourse to deliberate reasoning (Benner, Tanner, & Chesla., 1996; Tanner, 2006). In these situations, APRNs can use reflective practice to sort through the intuition to understand the components better and identify new insights. With experience, they can then repackage these insights and incorporate them into their experiential learning to use the information in the next relevant case prospectively and deliberately. Clinical reasoning can be improved through use of tools such as external verbalization ("thinking aloud"), algorithms, and reflective journaling (Victor-Chmil, 2013).

APRN experts have the ability to scan a situation rapidly (e.g., past records, patient's appearance, the patient's unexpressed concern or discomfort) and identify salient and relevant information. The APRN is able to suspend judgment purposefully about personal strongly held beliefs that may be proposed by others, such as "he's a difficult patient" or "she's just drug seeking." The ability to do this ensures as much objectivity as possible when caring for patients. For example, research has shown that expert CNSs are able to transcend the labeling of a "difficult patient" to engage in problem resolution through the use of patient respect, communication skills, and increased self-efficacy (Wolf & Robinson-Smith, 2007). Relying heavily on their perceptions, observations, and assessment skills, APRNs quickly activate one or several lines of reasoning regarding what might be occurring. They then conduct a more focused assessment to determine which one best explains the situation at hand. These lines of reasoning can be informal personal theories about the specific patient situation; this formulation draws from personal knowledge of the particular patient, personal knowledge acquired from previous experiences, and formalized domain-specific knowledge (Tanner, 2006). In implementing the solutions, these lines of reasoning can be tested by performing a clinical intervention and noting how the patient responds. Throughout this process, the APRN may be teaching and role modeling with staff to assist in staff nurse self-awareness and reflection. A novice APRN may need to work through the situation in a formal logical way and be more deliberate about the use of formal educational knowledge, enriching it over time with experiential knowledge (Tanner, 2006).

It has been shown that the values and underlying knowledge a nurse brings to a situation also have a profound influence on his or her assessment of the patient. Results of one study demonstrated that a nurse's beliefs about older adults can affect how a nurse assesses the older confused patient and can affect prioritization of that patient's needs (Dahlke & Phinney, 2008). Another example is when a nurse's moral opinion of drug addiction and the interpretation of behavior as drug seeking may have more influence on the treatment of a patient's pain than does the actual assessment of the pain. If not self-aware, these potential values and perspectives may impede the APRN in making accurate diagnoses, impact determination of appropriate treatment plans, and alter the ability of the APRN to appropriately role model optimal care of patients for other interprofessional team members.

Most patient accounts unfold in a fairly predictable way, and the APRN arrives at a diagnosis and/or intervention with considerable confidence in her or his clinical inferences. At other times, however, there is uncertainty and lack of understanding regarding the situation. The uncertainty may pertain to information the patient provides, the diagnosis, the best approach to management, or how the patient is responding. When there is ambiguity, experts often break into conscious problem solving or "detective-like thinking and questioning" (Benner et al., 1996; Benner, Hooper-Kyriakidis, & Stannard, 1999) to try to determine what is going on.

Knowing the patient may be critical to perceptive and accurate clinical reasoning. Knowing the patient as an individual with certain patterns of responses enables experienced nurses to detect subtle changes in a patient's condition over time (Tanner, 2006; Tanner, Benner, Chesla, et al., 1993). The extent to which any nurse knows a patient may be associated with that nurse's ability to do the following:

- Recognize that risk factors are present.
- Detect early indicators of a problem (e.g., a subtle change in pattern).
- Take timely preventive action.
- Recognize nonfitting and atypical data.

Nonfitting data suggest to experts that they need to generate new or additional hypotheses because the current observations and parameters do not fully explain the clinical picture as it has been or as it should be. For example, when faced with a nonfitting sign or symptom, the nurse may generate alternative hypotheses pertaining to the onset of a complication or worsening of the disease process.

Thinking Errors

The clinical acumen of APRNs and the inferences, hypotheses, and lines of reasoning that they generate

are highly dependable. However, as practice becomes repetitive, APRNs may develop routine responses and then run the risk of making certain types of thinking errors (Scordo, 2014). Errors of expectancy occur when the correct diagnosis is not generated as a hypothesis because a set of circumstances, in the clinician's experience or patient's circumstances, predisposes the clinician to disregard it. For example, the NP who over several years has seen an older woman for problems associated with chronic pulmonary disease may fail to consider that the most recent onset of shortness of breath and fatigue could be related to worsening aortic stenosis; the NP has come to expect pulmonary disease, not cardiac disease. Or a patient presenting with nausea and vomiting during flu season may be treated for gastroenteritis, although appendicitis is the actual condition (Scordo, 2014).

Erroneous conclusions are also more likely when the situation is ambiguous—that is, when the meaning or reliability of the data is unclear, the interpretation of the data is not clear cut, the best approach to treatment is debatable, or one cannot say for sure whether the patient is responding well to treatment (Brykczynski, 1991). To avoid errors in these types of situations, experts often revert to the use of maxims (a succinct metaphor for a general truth) to guide their thinking (Brykczynski, 1989). One of the maxims that NPs use to deal with uncertain diagnoses is "When you hear hoofbeats in Kansas, think horses, not zebras." This reminds clinicians who are about to make a diagnosis that occurs infrequently to consider the incidence of the condition in the population. Thus an older adult with respiratory problems seen in a suburban office is unlikely to have tuberculosis; pneumonia is a more likely diagnosis. Because tuberculosis is rare in the older adult population, the clinical data for tuberculosis should be convincing if that diagnosis is proposed.

Poor judgment can also result from tunnel vision, overgeneralization, influence by a recent dramatic experience, premature closure (Croskerry, 2003), and fixation on certain problems to the exclusion of others (Benner et al., 1999). Faulty thinking is not the only source of error in clinical decision making. Others include inaccurate observations; misinterpretation of the meaning of data; a sketchy knowledge of the particular situation; and a faulty or outdated model of the disease, condition, or response.

It is important that APRNs recognize the potential for and avoid leaping to conclusions and making snap

BOX 7.8   Actions to Use to Avoid Thinking Errors

- Listen fully to patients' concerns and descriptions of their problems.
- Develop and utilize a systematic approach.
- Listen to input from other providers as to their assessments and perspectives.
- Use a diagnostic "time-out" to review the situation with fresh eyes.
- Pay attention to intuition that points to an incongruence in data; what cannot be explained?
- Avoid reliance on knowledge derived solely from rote memorization or repetition, but critically think through the source of knowing and how it relates to the individual patient.
- Remain constantly open to reevaluation of working diagnoses and treatments; avoid premature closure.
- Be aware of personal biases and assumptions.
- Continually evaluate what is "critical" data in each patient case.

judgments. It can become easy to allow biases to lead to premature diagnoses without fully listening to or assessing patients. The expert APRN has learned to scan data constantly and look for deviations. The ability to differentiate effectively between significant and insignificant data is needed to have safe practice. Box 7.8 presents actions that APRNs can take to prevent thinking errors.

Time Pressures

Regardless of setting, practitioners worry about the effect that time pressures have on the accuracy and completeness of their clinical thinking and decision making. A galvanizing report on errors and patient safety cited studies in which between 3% and 46% of hospitalized patients in the United States were harmed by error or negligence (Kohn, Corrigan, & Donaldson; Committee on Quality Health Care in America, IOM., 2000). It was estimated that more than 100,000 patients die from medical errors, and a more recent study suggested that little progress has been made in the decade following publication of the Kohn et al. report (Wachter, 2010). A heavy workload is associated with feelings of pressure, being rushed, cognitive overload, and fatigue adding to already burdened clinicians; these feelings clearly contribute to unsafe acts and omissions in care (Kohn et al., 2000). Time pressures have been shown to

lead to worsening diagnostic accuracy in physicians (Al Qahtani et al., 2016). Evidence also comes from studies of nurse staffing in hospitals in which fewer hours of nursing care per patient per day and less care provided by RNs were associated with poorer patient outcomes (Aiken et al., 2011; Blegen, Goode, Spetz, Vaughn, & Park, 2011; Needleman et al., 2011). Effectively addressing the issues of time pressures and insufficient hours of nursing care requires culture change, process redesign, and appropriate use of technology. The patient safety movement has led to a variety of efforts aimed at preventing errors—root cause analysis of sentinel events, improved work processes, redesign of delivery systems, use of technological aids, communication training, human factors analysis, and team building. All these factors can have significant direct and indirect effects on workload, fatigue, and time available for direct patient care.

The effects of a heavy workload on patient outcomes in nonhospital settings are less well understood; thus actions to address this issue have received less attention. However, as lengths of visits or contact times are decreased or the number of patients whom practitioners are expected to see in a day is increased, it is logical to assume that the number of errors in clinical thinking will increase. Each contact requires the practitioner to reset his or her clinical reasoning process by closing out one thinking project and starting on an entirely new one. This resetting, which is done back to back often during a day, is cognitively and physically demanding. How these performance expectations affect clinical reasoning accuracy is unknown.

Moreover, time pressures often get compounded by hassles, which come in the form of interruptions, noise in the environment, missing supplies, increasing time needed to interact with technology, and system glitches that make clinical data or even whole charts unavailable to providers. These hassles likely interfere with providers' ability to concentrate on what the patient is saying and disrupt their efforts to make clinical sense of a patient's account. In many settings, providers are required to multitask. They start a task but must attend to another before completing the original one. This clearly increases the risks of failure to obtain needed information, broken lines of thought, technological missteps, omissions in care, and failure to respond to patients' requests for service (Cornell, Riordan, Townsend-Gervis, & Mobley, 2011; Ebright, Patterson, Chalko, & Render, 2003).

Studies of emergency department physicians and NPs have demonstrated that their workflow patterns have frequent interruptions, which can result in shortcuts, failure to return to the original task, increased perceptions of stress, and a potential for commission of errors (Burley, 2011; Chisholm, Weaver, Whenmouth, & Giles, 2011; Westbrook, Woods, Rob, Dunsmuir, & Day, 2010). Admittedly, the emergency department may be an extreme example of a multitasking environment, but other settings also impose interruptions at a very high rate. An experienced APRN may be more skilled at focusing on and prioritizing tasks and quickly dismissing interruptions and extraneous information. The novice APRN, conversely, may take longer to perform tasks (allowing for more interruptions) and may need more assistance with consultations or accessing resources (Phillips, 2005). As time pressures for clinicians increase, organizational efforts to monitor for errors and potential errors and seek correction when there are system weaknesses are actions that APRNs owe patients and themselves as providers functioning in busy environments.

Many patients are sensitive to the pace with which staff and providers greet them, talk with them, and do things, particularly those activities that involve verbal interaction and physical contact. Some patients respond to the fast-paced talk and hurried movements of providers by not bringing up some of the questions that they had intended to ask. Others may just get flustered and forget to mention important information; still others may become hostile and withhold information. Thus errors in the form of information omission by the patient enter the clinical reasoning and decision-making process.

In summary, clinical thinking is a complex task. It involves drawing on knowledge in memory and attending to multiple sources of situational input, some of which are difficult to interpret. Often, multiple clinical issues must be addressed during a patient encounter. These complexities make clinical thinking a challenging task, even under the best of circumstances. Situational awareness—perceptions of the current environment in which the APRN is functioning—can make the APRN more cognizant of the potential for error and improve diligence to the thought process at critical junctures, such as when writing orders, when performing procedures, or during handoffs (Phillips, 2005).

Ethical Reasoning

Clinical reasoning is inextricably linked to ethical reasoning. Clinical reasoning generates possibilities of what *could* be done in a situation, whereas ethical reasoning adds the dimension of what *should* be done in the situation (see Chapter 13). Advances in health care and medical technology have increasingly resulted in gaps between care that is medically possible and care that is in the best interest of the patient. These gaps may be most notable when making decisions regarding withdrawing or withholding nutrition, hydration, or a treatment; when dealing with reproductive technology or human genetics; and when cost must figure into clinical treatment decisions. These situations are at high risk for becoming ethically problematic.

The literature regarding how to resolve ethical issues is extensive. One approach, incorporating preventive or prospective ethical considerations into clinical thinking and decision making, makes a great deal of sense (Epstein, 2012). Rather than waiting until a conflict arises, this approach places an emphasis on preventing ethical conflicts from developing by shaping the process of clinical care so that potential value conflicts are anticipated and discussed before outright conflict occurs. APRNs can use this approach with routine encounters with patients. For example, during an encounter with a healthy patient, an APRN may be able to say, "I'd like to discuss an important issue with you while you're well so I will know how to best help you if certain situations should come up in the future." Such issues could include pain management, advance directives, or organ donation. In addition to emphasizing early communication among the patient, significant others, and the health care provider(s) about values, preventive ethics requires explicit critical reflection on the institutional factors that lead to conflict (Epstein, 2012). An additional aspect of preventive ethics is an effort to create and preserve trust and understanding among providers, as well as between providers and patients (and their families). Thus the use of preventive ethics can be considered proactive in that it requires providers to consider how the routine processes of care foster or prevent conflicts from occurring or, at the very least, ensure that such issues are identified at an early stage. The preventive approach has the potential to avoid conflicts because clinicians integrate ethical reasoning into clinical reasoning at an earlier point in time than when a traditional, conflict-based ethics approach is used.

The concept of moral distress is being recognized increasingly as an issue for all nurses, including APRNs. Moral distress is defined as knowing what the ethically appropriate action should be but encountering barriers that discourage the provider from carrying out the action (American Association of Critical-Care Nurses, 2004; Rushton, Schoonover-Shoffner, & Kennedy, 2017). This results in internal conflict that is not resolved (see Chapter 13).

Laabs (2005) has found that among primary care NPs, distress is most frequently caused by patient refusal of appropriate treatment. This creates a conflict for the NPs between promoting patient autonomy and beneficence on the part of the NP, resulting in feelings of frustration and powerlessness. Some NPs changed jobs and others considered leaving advanced practice altogether.

The American Association of Critical-Care Nurses (2004) has developed a model to address moral distress. APRNs can use this "four As" model to understand and work toward the resolution of distressing situations; the "four As" are the following (American Association of Critical-Care Nurses, 2004):

- Ask—explore and understand where the distress is coming from.
- Affirm—confirm the distress and consider one's professional obligations.
- Assess—use self-awareness, reflection, and evaluation to assess barriers, opportunities, and potential consequences in preparation for action.
- Action—put into place actions that will initiate resolving the distress, anticipating setbacks and ways to cope with them.

Encountering these situations can feel overwhelming but can also be opportunities for an APRN to reassess her or his current beliefs and values. The APRN can use concurrent and retrospective reflection on these situations as a growth and development experience that can be used in positive proactive interventions with future patient encounters (Rushton, 2006).

Skillful Performance

Although the health care professions place high value on knowledge and expert clinical reasoning, it is important to keep in mind that the public values skillful performance in physical examinations, delivery of treatments, diagnostic procedures, and comfort care. Most graduate schools require students to perform a specific set of procedural skills recommended by a national specialty organization before they complete their program. However, little is known about how APRNs acquire competency in new or expanded procedural skills once they are in practice. Presumably, competency of APRNs to perform specific procedures and treatments is initially

ensured through the processes that agencies use to credential and grant privileges to APRNs. After that, the responsibility for acquiring new competencies lies with the individual APRN and employing agency. When an APRN or agency recognizes that patients would receive better care if the APRN could perform a new procedure, an agreement should be reached regarding exactly which new procedure the APRN will perform, the conditions under which the procedure will be done, how the APRN will acquire the necessary skill, and how supervision will be provided during the learning period. The APRN must also be aware that refinement of the technical component is only a piece of the procedure. He or she must also understand indications, contraindications, complications, and consequences of performing the procedures (Hravnak, Tuite, & Baldisseri, 2005). Documented evidence that formal training has occurred is required for regulatory purposes.

The types of skills nurses have performed have evolved over time. For example, it used to be within the physician's scope of practice (and outside the nurse's) to measure blood pressure and administer chemotherapy. With the advent of the APRN role, APRNs have acquired new performance skills when it made sense within their role and for the comfort, convenience, and satisfaction of patients. It is key for APRNs to be cognizant of the scope of their role, regulatory requirements of the states, and the reasonableness of acquiring the skill.

Advanced Physical Assessment

Discussion continues about what actually constitutes advanced physical assessment in the differentiation between the basic RN and APRN practice. In one survey, 99 APRNs, physician assistants (PAs), and their corresponding preceptor physicians were asked to rank the importance of 87 competencies as an advanced skill (Davidson, Bennett, Hamera, & Raines, 2004). All skills were ranked fairly high as being necessary for advanced practice care. Skills ranked highest as advanced skills were cardiac assessments, such as rhythm interpretation, and women's health skills, such as gynecologic and breast examinations. Competencies such as head, neck, and throat and skin assessment skills were rated lower on the advanced skill priority scale. The authors reported that higher rated skills appeared to need more use of clinical judgment to interpret or differentially diagnose when compared with lower rated skills, which tended to be more demonstration or technical skills.

Another component of advanced assessment is the use of evidence in assessing and formatting a diagnosis (Munro, 2004). APRNs should be skilled at understanding and using the concepts of sensitivity, specificity, and the kappa statistic to differentiate the likelihood of presence or absence of disease based on physical signs and the reliability of that finding. The increased use of technology does not preclude the importance of the physical assessment in reaching an accurate diagnosis (Munro, 2004). Using advanced practice nurses as specialized standardized patients in simulations can facilitate improved clinical reasoning in APRN students (Payne, 2015).

Patient Education

Patient education is a central and well-documented function of all nurses in any setting, and evidence of its effectiveness has been well established (Redman, 2004). Teaching and counseling are significant clinical activities in nurse-midwifery (Holland & Holland, 2007) and CNS practice (Parry, Kramer, & Coleman, 2006). There are several examples of the role of NPs in patient education to promote adherence to treatment regimens and provide health care information to improve outcomes and quality of life (Hahn, 2014; Lerret & Stendahl, 2011; Mao & Anastasi, 2010; McAfee, 2012; Whitehead, Zucker, & Stone, 2014). APRNs must understand the basic principles of patient education and the specific educational needs of their clinical populations. The teach-back method is especially helpful in ensuring understanding by the patient of the content the APRN is teaching (Agency for Healthcare Research and Quality [AHRQ], 2015). APRNs must be aware of the research in their specialties and be responsible for knowing the theoretical and scientific bases for patient teaching and coaching in their specialties and practice settings.

Students can develop competence by developing and implementing patient education. For example, a student could negotiate with a preceptor to co-lead a self-management group for patients with a chronic condition, using motivational interviewing and other chronic disease management strategies. Other activities could include developing limited literacy tools or evaluating existing patient education materials with regard to the appropriateness of content and health literacy level and evaluating the reliability and appropriateness of health information on the Internet. Consumers are increasingly using the Internet as a primary source of health care information. Students should know the health information resources likely to be used by their patient populations and be able to advise patients as to which websites are reliable and regularly updated.

BOX 7.9   Red Flags for Low Literacy

- Frequently missed appointments
- Incomplete registration forms
- Non-adherence with medication
- Unable to name medications, explain purpose or dosing
- Identifies pills by looking at them, not reading label
- Unable to give coherent, sequential history
- Asks fewer questions
- Lack of follow-through on tests or referrals

From Agency for Healthcare Research and Quality. (2015). Health literacy: Hidden barriers and practical strategies. Rockville, MD: Author. Retrieved from www.ahrq.gov/professionals/quality-patient-safety/quality-resources/tools/literacy-toolkit/tool3a/index.html.

In the United States, only 12% of adults have adequate health literacy to be able to navigate the health care system (AHRQ, 2016) (Box 7.9). Assessment of functional health literacy must be done sensitively. Years of education completed may not be an adequate indicator of reading and computational literacy. In addition, people with higher levels of education who experience a new diagnosis or other stresses may be unable to process complex information and consequently may benefit from the use of limited literacy materials (AHRQ, 2016). A variety of tools are available to assist clinicians in assessing patient literacy (Baker, Williams, Parker, Gazmararian, & Nurss, 1999; Davis et al., 1993; Sand-Jecklin & Coyle, 2013). APRNs involved in developing programmatic approaches to patient education must ascertain that materials are appropriate to the literacy level of participants in educational programs. Educational materials should use plain language—that is, text that exemplifies clear communication (National Institutes of Health, 2012; Stableford & Mettger, 2007). Plain language text is accessible, engaging, and reader friendly. Stableford and Mettger (2007) noted that reading levels alone are insufficient to determine whether text was prepared using plain language principles.

Numerous resources exist to help APRNs improve their abilities to assess health literacy and prepare useful, readable instructional materials. The Harvard T.H. Chan School of Public Health (2015) website is particularly useful; it includes slides documenting the problem of health literacy and its effects on health, as well as links to numerous resources. As APRNs work to improve the quality of educational materials for patients with limited literacy, they may encounter resistance to simplifying language and educational tools (Stableford & Mettger, 2007); therefore, slides and other resources that document the extent and impact of health illiteracy may be useful.

Adverse Events and Performance Errors

Since the publication of "To Err is Human" (Kohn et al., 2000), medical errors have been prominent in the public eye, as well as a focus of reform for health care institutions. Ideally, institutions and care providers should focus on improving the reliability of complicated systems to prevent failures or quickly identify, redesign, and rectify failures that do occur. Improving reliability ensures that care is consistently and appropriately provided. Traditionally, institutions and providers have been reluctant to be forthcoming with patients when errors or near misses have occurred. That stance is slowly changing with the movement toward increasing transparency in care and a focus on addressing system dysfunction to improve patient safety. In 2002 the National Quality Forum (NQF) first identified a list of adverse medical events that health care systems should work to prevent and publicly report when they occur to encourage public access to information about health care performance (NQF, 2008). This list was updated in 2006 and 2011. The 29 events are categorized into seven main areas: surgical or invasive procedure events, product or device events, patient protection events, care management events, environmental events, radiologic events, and potential criminal events (NQF, 2011). The Centers for Medicare and Medicaid Services is now denying payment for some of these publicly reported events, and it is anticipated that additional events will continue to be identified for denial of payment. There are increasing resources available in clinics and health care settings to try to prevent adverse events, including computer-generated alerts for ordering medications and laboratory tests; interdisciplinary colleagues, such as pharmacists and dietitians; electronic resources to access and verify recommendations and practice guidelines; appropriate steps in patient identification; and optimal team communication techniques (White, 2012). It is critical that APRNs consistently use them and be involved in decisions related to their development.

These changes are relevant to APRNs as the changes relate to their direct care role and the potential to be involved in "never," near miss, or medical error situations. It would be to the APRN's advantage to be cognizant of the institution's or practice group's policies related to appropriate actions when errors occur and what is required to be reported publicly based on federal and state regulations. APRNs may find themselves involved in these situations as a result of the many issues discussed, such as thinking errors and time pressures. APRNs involved as providers in these types of events should anticipate the need to readily inform the patient and family of the event. Honest open communication and sensitivity will help preserve trust and support ongoing care. When errors in care happen, patients expect to receive an explanation and an apology; doing so may help preserve a trusting relationship and at least ameliorate anxiety, fear, and confusion (Leape, 2012).

A consensus group of Harvard hospitals (Massachusetts Coalition for the Prevention of Medical Errors, 2006) has recommended four steps for communicating about adverse events:

1. Tell the patient what happened immediately, but leave details of how and why for later when a thorough review has occurred.
2. Take responsibility for the incident.
3. Apologize and communicate remorse.
4. Inform the patient and family what will be done to prevent similar events.

APRNs should take advantage of training and educational opportunities on how to communicate bad news and ways to promote safety. In addition, APRNs involved in incidents should anticipate the need for their own emotional support during this time.

Use of Reflective Practice

To continually grow and develop, APRNs must be reflective practitioners. APRNs may be familiar with multiple methods of learning—didactic, small group projects, clinical experiences with preceptors—but may be less familiar with this method of learning, which will be useful to them throughout their careers. Reflective practice is a way to take the experiences a practitioner has (positive or negative) and explore them for the purpose of eliciting meaning, critically analyzing, and synthesizing and using learning to improve practice (Atkins & Murphy, 1995; Kumar, 2011; Schön, 1992). The goal is to turn experience into personal knowledge by seeking insights that are not available with superficial recall (Atkins & Murphy, 1995; Kumar, 2011; Rolfe, 1997; Schön, 1992). Research findings have shown that reflective practice by APRN students is a valuable learning method, may increase self-confidence as a practitioner, and may improve clinical decision making (Raterink, 2016).

Forms of clinical supervision are frequently used in mental health nursing. Barron and White (2009) have described clinical supervision in this realm as a relationship between a more experienced and a more novice nurse in which the expected outcome is to assist the less-experienced nurse in the professional development of knowledge, skills, and autonomy. In these cases, clinical supervision may be used as a debriefing with a trusted and more experienced colleague of a situation that has been complex, intense, or characterized by uncertainty.

Reflection is not just a retrospective activity; it may occur prospectively or concurrently while providing care. Retrospective reflection occurs when an APRN takes the opportunity to consider how a situation could have been handled differently. Prospective reflection may occur when an APRN prepares to enter a difficult or uncertain clinical situation; one draws on experience and scientific knowledge to plan an approach and anticipates possible reactions or outcomes. Reflection can also occur concurrently. Concurrent reflection is termed *reflection-in-action* and can promote flexibility and adaptation of interventions to suit the situation. Reflection-in-action may be the goal of a more expert practitioner who has honed the skill of reflection (Benner et al., 1999). Although Benner's work was done with bedside staff nurses, it may be applicable to APRNs as well, as research by Fenton and Brykczynski (1993) suggested. Several models have been proposed to gain expertise in reflective practice (Atkins & Murphy, 1995; Brubakken, Grant, Johnson, & Kollauf, 2011; Johns, 2000; Kim, 1999), although they use similar processes to guide the practitioner through the reflective process. Deliberate self-reflection allows the APRN to anticipate alternative possibilities, remain flexible in challenging and changing situations, and strategically integrate the results of self-reflection with best practices to match interventions to patient and family needs.

Strengthening skills in self-reflection can be done in a number of ways for the APRN—through solitary self-evaluation, with a supervisor or teacher, or in small groups of supportive colleagues. With experience, the APRN may be asked to be the mentor in guiding others through a self-reflective process. Regardless of which model is used for reflection, the following guidelines can be considered:

- If reflection occurs in a small group, participants must feel safe to express thoughts, emotions, and thinking processes without fear of judgment.

- Practitioners need to gain self-awareness of personal values, beliefs, and behaviors.
- Practitioners need to develop the skills to articulate a situation with objective and subjective details.
- Critical debriefing and analysis are used to identify practitioner goals in the situation, extent of knowledge that was present or missing, feelings on the part of the practitioner and patient, consequences of actions, and which alternative options existed.
- Knowledge gained through this process can be integrated with current knowledge to change interventions in a current situation or improve approaches in future situations.
- Evaluation of this reflective process supports masterful practice and creates lasting improvements in practice.

There are several barriers to using reflection in daily practice. Lack of time may result in care and interventions becoming routine. The use of a reflective practice process will require dedicated time. If not thoughtfully arranged, it may seem to be extraneous and a "nice thing to do" rather than a necessary component to the APRN role. Acknowledging that one does not always know the right answer can be difficult for an APRN who is trying to establish a practice and role. In addition, reflection may elicit emotions that may be painful or difficult to deal with. It takes experience and skill to use reflection, which is particularly important when an APRN is very involved in a situation. Novice APRNs may need guidance in performing reflection to assist in ascertaining meaning and making connections that otherwise might be missed (Johns, 2000). Finally, some may see reflective practice discussions as official surveillance when supervisors are involved, and depending on the context (Clouder & Sellars, 2004). However, when reflective thinking is developed and incorporated into one's practice, it can be a means to demonstrate professional accountability for practice and a source of lifelong learning (Clouder & Sellars, 2004). Knowledge from reflection informs future clinical decision making, especially in those situations for which no benchmarks or best practice guidelines exist.

Use of Evidence as a Guide to Practice

An important form of knowledge that must be brought to bear on clinical decision making, for individuals and for populations, is the ever-increasing volume of evidence. For the nursing profession, the use of evidence as a basis for practice is more than the latest trend. (See Chapter 10) The profession has been intensively exploring and considering issues regarding the use of research since the early 1970s. Historically, CNSs have led efforts in many agencies to move toward research-based practice (DePalma, 2004; Hanson & Ashley, 1994; Hanson, 2015; Hickey, 1990; Mackay, 1998; Obrecht, Van Hull Vincent, & Ryan, 2014; Patterson, Mason, & Duncan, 2017; Stetler, Bautista, Vernale-Hannon, & Foster, 1995). They have brought research findings to the attention of the nursing staff and interprofessional teams and worked to develop the research appraisal skills of nursing staffs. With the advent of the DNP, evidence-based practice skills are seen as central to APRNs' role competency and a differentiating component to the PhD-prepared nurse, who is specifically prepared to conduct research (see Chapter 10).

Identifying and locating evidence and research findings is becoming easier with improved technology and categorization. However, clinicians often do not have sufficient experience in the use of various search engines available to retrieve information from databases. APRNs could benefit from education on simple tools that could greatly increase the efficiency of their searches. APRNs in all settings engaging in an evidence-based practice project would be well served by developing a relationship with a health sciences librarian who can assist with searches, save time, and prevent the omission of relevant evidence.

Evidence-Based Practice

It would be ideal to have all health care delivery based on research. However, in reality, there frequently may be no research on which to base decisions. Sackett (1998) has defined evidence-based practice as the explicit and judicious integration of best evidence with clinical expertise and patient values. Using only external evidence to make practice decisions is as unacceptable as using only individual clinical expertise.

Usually, when APRNs are involved in designing care for a population of patients, all forms of objective evidence should be used, including quality improvement data, data from internal databases, expert opinion panels, consensus statements, national guidelines data from benchmarking partners, and data from state and national databases (e.g., the Centers for Disease Control and Prevention). Agency-specific information, collected to pinpoint the nature of a problem, is particularly useful evidence that should be combined with the more general

knowledge gained from research evidence (see Chapter 10).

The process and extent of quality improvement (QI) has advanced significantly in the past few years with APRNs as QI leaders in their health care settings. Use of improved QI methods and tools and a national focus on the need to make significant changes in the care of patients provide nurses with the opportunity to identify patient care issues, evaluate the problem, and implement potential solutions in a more rapid fashion than ever before. APRNs can use QI methods such as the plan-do-study-act (PDSA) process and tools (Institute for Healthcare Improvement, 2011) and the lean principles (Lean Enterprise Institute, 2017) to lead and facilitate teams in improving care. Although QI data do not have broad generalizability and the rigor of official research, they can provide evidence for significant improvements that the APRN can implement on a daily local basis.

With the increasing bombardment of evidence available in the literature and via the Internet, APRNs must develop a plan to stay abreast of and manage the deluge of information. Examples of how an APRN can do this include: reading primary research reports and summaries of research findings on a regular basis; informally evaluating the soundness of the methods; and adjusting or fine-tuning his or her own practice on the basis of credible findings. This is the form of research use in which every professional nurse should engage. It is part of staying abreast of new knowledge in one's area of clinical practice.

Additionally, APRNs can subscribe to listservs, such as those from the AHRQ, that send timely summaries of emerging evidence and new national guidelines. Alternatively, an APRN could join or form an interprofessional group that meets monthly to discuss research reports on topics of mutual interest. Some APRNs keep a small notebook in which to jot down clinical issues and questions about which they are uncertain. Then they can make the most efficient use of library time to explore the evidence related to the questions of interest.

Evidence-based practice is a more systematic, rigorous, and precise way of translating research findings into practice. The evidence-based practice process is used in an organization to design a standard of care for a population of patients. This process is more formal because evidence-based care will be widely used as a guide to care; therefore the scientific conclusions on which it is based must be as free of bias and error as possible. In general terms, the process involves four steps: (1) locating, evaluating, and summarizing the science; (2) translating the science into clinical recommendations; (3) strategically implementing the recommendations; and (4) measuring and reporting their impact. The recommendations may take the form of a clinical practice guideline, decision algorithm, clinical protocol, or changes in policies or procedures.

Clinical Practice Guidelines

Evidence-based clinical practice guidelines can be useful decision-making and planning aids for clinicians. Many guidelines have been developed in close association with providers, are based on systematic and thorough reviews of research evidence, and have attained a balance between optimal care and economic reality. However, contractors also use clinical guidelines to ensure quality, limit variation of care, and control resource use. Guidelines should be based on research evidence that is evaluated and summarized by a credible panel, inside or outside the system, to ensure that the guidelines serve to incorporate science into practice and contain costs. Providers involved in the care of patients with the condition that the guideline addresses should have the opportunity to adapt guidelines produced by others. Ideally, clinicians should review proposed guidelines and negotiate problematic recommendations in advance to avoid situations in which the care of the individual becomes the focus of negotiation. In addition, clinicians should acknowledge that, although the guidelines may serve most patients well, some patients will require treatment and interventions not recommended in the guidelines. An explicit method for advocating for individual needs should be available to clinicians. Guidelines can be found through organizations such as the National Guideline Clearinghouse (www.guideline.gov) and AHRQ (www.ahrq.gov), and professional organizations such as the American Heart Association. Clinicians should review published guidelines carefully and be familiar with the criteria each organization uses to grade the strength of the evidence used to make care recommendations. It is important that APRNs be part of teams that are developing new guidelines for practice.

Theory-Based Practice

The preceding discussion of evidence-based practice recognizes how research evidence informs practice but ignores the role of theory. APRNs are becoming comfortable with the idea of research evidence as a guide to practice, yet the idea of theory-based practice is less familiar. It should not be because, contrary to common perception, theory can be a practical tool. Theory often brings together research findings in a way that helps practice be more purposeful, systematic, and comprehensive.

In the past, most discussions of theory-based practice addressed the use of conceptual models of nursing to guide care (Bonamy, Schultz, Graham, & Hampton, 1995; Hawkins, Thibodeau, Utley-Smith, Igou, & Johnson, 1993; Laschinger & Duff, 1991; Sappington & Kelley, 1996). However, more recently, emphasis has shifted to middle-range theories, which guide practice more specifically. Middle-range theories typically address a particular patient experience (e.g., living with rheumatoid arthritis) or problem (e.g., managing chronic pain); thus their range of applicability is relatively narrow. However, this narrow range allows them to be developed to address specific issues encountered in clinical practice. Schwartz-Barcott, Patterson, Lusardi, and Farmer (2002) have made a strong case for developing theories by using fieldwork so that the theories will be more closely aligned to the realities that practicing nurses encounter. Another approach to developing theories that are more specific to clinical situations is to generate a middle-range theory from one of the broader conceptual models. For example, Whittemore and Roy (2002) developed a middle-range theory describing adaptation to diabetes mellitus based on the concepts and theoretical statements of the broader Roy Adaptation Model. Middle-range theories have a structure of ideas and concepts that are more focused than general nursing theories and are more directly applicable to nursing practice (Smith, 2013).

Smith and Liehr (2013) have delineated middle-range theories that have the potential for impact on clinical nursing practice. The list in Box 7.10 provides

BOX 7.10 Middle-Range Theories

- Uncertainty in illness
- Theory of Meaning
- Self-transcendence
- Symptom management
- Unpleasant symptoms
- Self-efficacy
- Story theory
- Self-reliance
- Cultural marginality
- Caregiving dynamics
- Moral reckoning

From Smith, M. J., & Liehr, P. R. (Eds). (2013). *Middle range theory for nursing* (3rd ed.). New York: Springer.

a sampling of the middle-range theories currently available to practicing nurses, and the reader can see that the topics of the theories are substantively specific, although some are more specific than others. An APRN in a particular field may find that only one or two of these theories are applicable to her or his area of practice. However, as middle-range theories are developed for other topics, APRNs will be able to use several of these types of theories to guide different aspects of practice.

Diverse Approaches to Health and Illness Management

APRNs' holistic approach to care and their commitment to using evidence as a basis for care contribute to how they help patients. Generally, APRNs use a variety of interventions to effect change in the health status or quality of life of an individual or family and tailor their recommendations, approaches, and treatment to individual patients. Interpersonal interventions that are psychosocial in nature are frequently termed *support interventions.* Support interventions are somewhat distinct from educational interventions, which are informational in nature. Coaching uses a combination of support and educational strategies (see Chapter 8). There are also discrete physical actions, which are frequently categorized as nonpharmacologic and pharmacologic interventions. These distinctions are arbitrary because good clinicians craft interventions that are a combination of the various types as they seek to alleviate, prevent, or manage specific physical symptoms, conditions, or problems.

Interpersonal Interventions

Support is not a discrete intervention; it is a composite of interpersonal interventions based on the patient's unique psychological and informational needs. Supportive interpersonal interventions include providing reassurance, giving information, coaching, affirming, providing anticipatory guidance, guiding decision making, listening actively, expressing understanding, and being fully present. Each of these interventions can be described in terms of the circumstances for which it is indicated. For example, reassurance is indicated when a patient is experiencing uncertainty, distress, or lack of confidence; active listening is indicated when a patient has a strong need to tell his or her story. The actions that constitute these interventions are not mutually exclusive. For example, giving factual information can be

reassuring, instructional, guiding, or all of these things at the same time.

In practice, these interpersonal interventions are blended and APRNs may not be consciously aware of when they are doing one and when they are doing another. This is as it should be. APRNs have no need to think "Now I'm doing active listening; next I'm going to do anticipatory guidance." Instead, APRNs interact with patients in ways that intermingle the conceptually separate interventions. This crafting of support evolves as the APRN talks with patients; infers their worries, fears, and concerns; and, without a great deal of conscious thought, acts to alleviate their distress. A patient may experience the interaction as just a good talk with the APRN or as a feeling of being understood. However, support is a complex nursing intervention that is strategically crafted and purposefully administered, and that often makes a difference in how the patient feels and acts (Exemplar 7.3).

Therapeutic Interventions

The decision about whether or not to treat a particular condition can be difficult because the practitioner is faced with several probabilities that do not all lead to the same decision. Moreover, there is often pressure from patients to do something. When deciding whether and how to treat patients, clinicians consider the following five types of information:

- The degree of certainty about the diagnosis, condition, or symptom
- What is known about the effectiveness of the various treatment alternatives
- What is known about the risks of the treatment alternatives
- The clinician's comfort with a particular treatment or intervention
- The patient's preference for a certain type of treatment or management

In addition, there are resources available with recommendations on when not to provide an intervention because the intervention has no evidence to support that its use would positively impact the condition or outcome (American Board of Internal Medicine Foundation, 2017).

The most clear-cut situation is when the condition is definitely present, a particular treatment is known to be highly effective, the treatment can be expected to be low in risk for the particular patient, and the clinician and patient are comfortable with the treatment. Unfortunately, many (probably

J.E. is a certified nurse-midwife (CNM) in a joint CNM–obstetricians/gynecologists (OB/GYNs) practice model. The seven CNMs have an independent nurse-midwife patient panel. Consultants for the CNM practice are with the seven OB/GYNs in the shared clinical office space. Patients have access to both services at the initiation of care.

Patient care is coordinated and maintained in the respective patient panels. There is a formal process for patients to be seen by the alternative groups in the practice because patients are not allowed to alternate between CNM and OB/GYN provider patient panels. Transfers of care for patients who wish to have CNM care and are considered low risk are accepted in the same manner as transfers to the OB/GYNs of patients who develop high-risk complications outside the scope of the CNM practice.

J.E. has an appointment to see a couple in their early 30s who are expecting their first child. In this group CNM practice, he has met Jan and Steve once previously in this pregnancy. They are very excited about the upcoming birth because they are now 37 weeks and 5 days pregnant. Jan and Steve have prepared themselves with childbirth education classes and have hired a doula to assist them in the birthing process.

J.E. reviews the record and notes that Jan has had no complications during this pregnancy. Accurate dating has been established by the use of an early ultrasound, which corresponds with Jan's last menstrual period and estimated due date. Vital signs today are normal and the patient voiced no concerns to the medical assistant who did the initial intake for this routine, scheduled prenatal visit.

J.E. interviews Jan, who reports she feels well and has no concerns. Jan states that she has had more issues becoming comfortable—at night with increased hip pain, having to get up and urinate frequently, with the baby moving, and with itching. J.E. asks more about the itching and Jan relates that she has been noticing it more in the last few weeks but hadn't mentioned it before. She had looked up itching in pregnancy on the Internet and discussed it with her doula, who told her that this itching (pruritic urticarial papules and plaques of pregnancy [PUPPP]) seems pretty common in pregnancy. J.E. asks Jan more questions about the itching, and she states that it is primarily on the palms of her hands and soles of her feet and only scratching seems to help. Steve relates it is getting so bad lately it's like "watching a dog with an unrelenting scratch."

Jan states that she has tried Benadryl a couple of times but it didn't help.

J.E. performs a physical examination, which reveals some minor stretch marks but no notable trunk rash, as would be expected with PUPPP. There are some excoriated marks on Jan's palms because she has been rubbing her hands during the interview.

J.E. recognizes that this does not appear to be a typical PUPPP presentation and believes that the itching may be a symptom of intrahepatic cholestasis of pregnancy (ICP), a potentially serious complication. J.E. relays his thoughts to Jan and Steve and tells them that he is going to order additional blood tests. He orders a complete blood count (CBC), liver function tests, and total bile acid tests.

The laboratory results reveal a normal CBC but an elevated total bile acid level of 27.6 μmol/L (normal range, 0 to 7.0 μmol/L) and alanine aminotransferase level of 104 IU/L (normal range, 0 to 50 IU/L). These results confirm that the itching is related to ICP, which puts Jan at an increased risk of intrauterine fetal demise (IUFD). With confirmation laboratory data and a term pregnancy, J.E. calls Jan and informs her of the diagnosis and the need for induction of labor because of the increased risk of IUFD. She is upset and wants to have a direct conversation in the clinic to discuss if induction is really necessary.

J.E. sees Jan and Steve in the clinic and provides answers to their many questions about ICP. They want to discuss alternatives to induction because they had planned for a low-intervention, spontaneous labor and delivery. J.E. reviews with the couple that ICP is associated with a substantial risk of IUFD. This risk increases as a pregnancy approaches term. He explains that induction is considered the best option with a term pregnancy because routine antepartum testing such as ultrasound or electronic fetal monitoring (EFM) is used to evaluate for a placental insufficiency disease process and does not have the specificity to predict an increased risk of IUFD in ICP. J.E. also explains that the elevated bile acids in the amniotic fluid can cause the fetus to experience a sudden cardiac death because of effects on the umbilical artery and/or the electrical activity in the fetal heart. J.E. reviews other treatment options with the couple. Using ursodiol has been effective at decreasing the level of bile acids in the maternal system in preterm pregnancies, but its use to extend pregnancies to spontaneous labor is not recommended because the risk for IUFD still remains, even with decreased maternal bile acids at or beyond term. J.E. also informs Jan that the elevated levels of bile acid are caused by a genetic enzyme deficiency that she has and are not related to anything she did or did not do during her pregnancy.

Jan is crying out of fear and disappointment. J.E. reviews the couple's birth plan with them, pointing out that the desires they had expressed in their birth plan do not have to be revised at this time because of the need for induction. Although constant EFM with induction is required, the use of telemetry will not affect Jan's movement while she is in labor, nor will the use of hydrotherapy as an alternative to pharmaceutical pain management.

Jan and Steve agree with the plan of induction after this consultation and arrive at the hospital with their doula, Rita. After the initiation of induction, J.E. uses this early labor period to discuss and educate Rita privately on the rationale for induction and the

pathophysiology of ICP. J.E. recognizes that educating Rita is important so she can use this information with her future clients. J.E. also knows that as a member of a childbirth cooperative group, Rita is in a place to inform and instruct her doula peers that the subjective signs of increased itching of the palms of the hands and soles of the feet can be indicative of ICP, and they can advise future clients of doulas to notify their health care providers about these findings.

Emily is born to Jan and Steve at 7 pounds, 5 ounces, with an 8/9 Apgar score via normal spontaneous vaginal delivery after a 16-hour labor and delivery hospitalization for induction with prostaglandins and pitocin. Jan's maternal itching is resolved and total bile acid and liver function test results are returning to normal 48 hours postpartum. Baby and mother are discharged, with no additional follow-up needed for ICP, except for the increased risk of recurrence in future pregnancies. ◎

[a]The author gratefully acknowledges John Eads, MSN, APRN, CNM, for use of his exemplar.

most) therapeutic decisions are not so clear cut. In these cases, the weight of factors in support of a particular treatment and the weight of those against treatment or in support of another treatment are almost equal.

The treatment and management interventions that APRNs perform include a wide variety of self-care modalities and low-tech, nonpharmacologic modalities (Hahn, 2014; Hannon, 2013; Morilla-Herrera et al., 2016).When prescribing or recommending medications, APRNs consider the patient's financial status, the patient's previous experience with similar medications, ease of taking the medication, how many other medications the patient is taking, how often the medications must be taken, the side effect profiles of the drugs being considered, and potential drug and disease interactions. A systematic review of nurses as prescribers has shown that APRNs tend to prescribe similar or lower total numbers of medications overall compared with physicians, clinical parameters are the same or better for patients treated by prescribing APRNs, and quality of care is similar or better, with similar or improved patient satisfaction (Van Ruth, Mistiaen, & Francke, 2008).

As noted, considerable evidence indicates that APRNs use a broad range of interventions, with substantial reliance on self-care and low-tech

interventions. Surveillance, teaching, guidance, counseling, and case management are interventions used more often than procedural interventions (Brooten et al., 2003). The frequency with which the various categories of interventions are used varies moderately with patient populations. The repertoire of interventions used by individual APRNs clearly depends on the problems experienced by the population of patients with whom they work. Acute care NPs, CNMs, CRNAs, and CNSs working in inpatient settings, for example, use repertoires of therapeutic interventions different from those used by APRNs who provide primary care. The interventions that an individual APRN uses also depend on the customs of colleagues, practice setting, and reimbursement system. Nevertheless, APRNs must make an effort to extend and refine their repertoire constantly beyond the interventions learned during graduate education.

Individualized Interventions

One goal of treatment decision making is to choose from among several possible interventions and to use the one that will have the highest probability of achieving the outcomes the patient most desires. Usually, that probability is increased by particularizing the treatment or action to the individual patient

(Benner et al., 1996, p. 24). Particularizing requires that the recommendation or action take the following into account:

- Acceptability of the treatment to the patient
- What has worked for the patient in the past
- Patient's motivation and ability to use or follow the treatment (self-care)
- Likelihood that the patient will continue to use the treatment, even if side effects are experienced
- Financial burden of the treatment
- Health literacy of the patient

Nursing has always believed that individualizing nursing care—that is, tailoring care to the unique characteristics of the person and his or her situation—produces the best patient outcomes. In contrast, standardization of care and control of wide variation are important to quality control and cost containment. Clearly, a blending of the two perspectives is required to produce care that is effective for an individual and congruent with available resources. This can be accomplished by adopting evidence-based standards and guidelines to provide a framework for care while acknowledging that at the point of care (i.e., in the patient-provider interface), interventions and management may need to be tailored to reflect the patient's unique situation and needs.

Unfortunately, while individualized interventions have been shown to be effective in some cases (Janson, McGrath, Covington, Cheng, & Boushey, 2009; Richards et al., 2007), research support for the effectiveness of individualized interventions in general is not as strong as most APRNs would like. The extent to which the equivocal nature of the evidence is a function of methodologic difficulties in studying individualized interventions is unknown. Part of the difficulty stems from the various ways in which health messages may be customized—personalized, targeted, tailored, and individualized (Ryan & Lauver, 2002). An integrative research review of 20 studies in which interventions with varying degrees of customization to the individual were delivered has revealed that better patient outcomes were achieved with tailored interventions in only 50% of the studies as compared with standard interventions (Ryan & Lauver, 2002). The authors of the review proposed that another reason for the modest support for the efficacy of customized interventions is that patients with certain characteristics are more affected by these interventions than others; such uneven effects across subgroups would offset each other and present an appearance of little or no benefit. Even when a tailored intervention does not result in changed behavior or produce better patient outcomes, it may have other benefits. An example of this collateral gain was found in a study of 43 women with gynecologic cancer (Ward, Donovan, Owen, Grosen, & Serlin, 2000). The individualized sensory and coping message for pain management intervention had no demonstrable effect on analgesic use, pain intensity scores, or pain interference with life, but the women who received the individualized intervention reported that it contained useful information that helped them to feel more comfortable taking pain medication and to discuss pain more openly with a physician or nurse.

In today's technology-accessible world, many patients use the Internet to access information and educate themselves about their health and diseases. Patients may actually come to appointments knowing more about their disease than the APRN does. Although this can be disconcerting, it is important to recognize this as information-seeking behavior and capitalize on the opportunity to work with the patients to help them gain the information they need (Cutilli, 2006). Patients vary widely in terms of how much information they want and how they want it presented. Allowing them to make choices about how and what they learn should help prevent content overload and enhance the relevancy of the information given, resulting in better retention and application. Along similar lines, technology can be designed to allow patients to acquire information that is most important to them and to help them sort out their values, priorities, and preferences in their specific situation (Lin & Effken, 2010; Ryan, Pumilia, Henak, & Chang, 2009). It is apparent that technology-assisted learning and decision-making tools will become increasingly more acceptable.

It will be important for APRNs to help consumers differentiate among websites that are reputable and offer valid information and those that may not have solid evidence. The Internet is also now used for patients with similar or rare diseases to connect with each other as support in a way that might never have been possible before the advent and ease of use of the Internet. APRNs can also direct patients to state health department websites as excellent sites for accessing helpful information, such as immunization schedules, tobacco cessation tools, and information on diabetes care, sexually transmitted diseases, tuberculosis, and newborn screening.

Complementary Therapies

The extent of public use of complementary and alternative medicine (CAM) was well documented in the 1990s by Eisenberg and colleagues when they reported that approximately 33% of Americans were using at least one unconventional therapy (Eisenberg, et al., 1993; Eisenberg et al., 1998); this has been further supported in the most recent National Health Survey that included complementary therapy data (Blackwell, Lucas, & Clarke, 2014). Its use in certain ethnic groups is often higher than the national average. Many patients use complementary therapies (i.e., non-mainstream, non-Western therapies) in conjunction with conventional medical services; when complementary therapies are purposefully coordinated with conventional therapies in a treatment plan, the term *integrative therapies* is used.

The effectiveness and safety of complementary and alternative therapies vary widely. Some have been scientifically studied (e.g., relaxation, guided imagery, glucosamine and chondroitin for osteoarthritis), whereas others have not been studied at all. Of concern is that some may interact with other medications that the patient is receiving (National Center for Complementary and Integrative Health, 2016). Another issue specific to dietary supplements and herbal therapy is the lack of control over ingredients (National Center for Complementary and Integrative Health, 2016). Providers are caught between the desire of patients to use alternative therapies and reservations about their safety, often in the face of insufficient scientific evidence.

APRNs are incorporating complementary therapies into their practices in a variety of ways, albeit with some caution (Brykczynski, 2012; Maloni, 2013; Steefel, Hyatt & Heider, 2013; Yu, 2014). APRNs have expressed interest in being able to provide CAM for patients, even if it means expanding their scope of practice (Patterson, Kaczorowski, Arthur, Smith, & Mills, 2003). They are increasing their engagement in these therapies, are more willing to ask patients about complementary and alternative therapy practices, and are counseling patients on appropriate use. Many APRNs report a need to increase their own knowledge about complementary and alternative therapies to incorporate it fully into care. An interim solution to this situation may be for an APRN to consider developing a collaborative relationship with an expert CAM provider. In summary, because patients are using these therapies, APRNs seem to believe it is better that they do so with provider guidance and awareness.

Clinical Prevention

Population-Based Data to Inform Practice

The hallmark of the APRN role that differentiates it from other advanced nursing roles is the direct care that the APRN provides in the patient interface. Although this is a key component of the role, it is expected that APRNs also use a clinical prevention and population health focus (AACN, 2006). Clinical prevention refers to the health promotion and risk reduction components of individual health care that are learned as a result of population data. APRNs are considered to be nursing leaders in achieving national health goals for individuals and populations. Interventions outlined in the Healthy People 2020 campaign (Office of Disease Prevention and Health Promotion, 2017) can frequently be instituted or recommended by APRNs, regardless of their roles or settings. Monitoring for current vaccinations, advocating for tobacco cessation with patients, assisting in healthy diets, and identifying opportunities for increasing physical activity are all population-identified behaviors that can be implemented at the individual level. These interventions are key to addressing the increasing disease rates of diabetes, obesity, lung cancer, and asthma. The Healthy People 2020 website (http://www.healthypeople.gov/2020) is a great resource for APRNs and patients to access basic health care information. Work is currently underway to develop national health promotion and disease prevention objectives for Healthy People 2030 (Office of Disease Prevention and Health Promotion, 2017). In addition, APRNs should be cognizant of the ever-changing information related to infectious diseases and emergency preparedness based on today's global health care environment.

APRNs can use population trends to inform direct care and improve the assessments and interventions used at the direct care interface. Population data are frequently based on the diseases and conditions prevalent in the geographic setting in which the APRN practices, including the following:

- Monitoring for metabolic syndrome in the southeast United States
- Assessing for asthma in Virginia
- Surveillance for neurological disorders in Minnesota
- Cognizance of altitude-based disorders in mountain states
- High suspicion for tuberculosis in homeless patients with pulmonary symptoms who live in densely populated urban settings

Aggregated, individual clinical outcomes are also useful for the evaluation of program and practice effectiveness. By requiring that care be administered and individual outcomes be documented in standardized ways, the health care system can conduct programmatic evaluations of clinical outcomes. Population-based evaluations can also be used by APRNs to evaluate and improve the care they provide. Such evaluations can help answer questions such as the following:

- "Is the specific care I (we) provide patients the best way of managing their health or illness?"
- "Are my (our) patients doing as well as similar patients who are cared for by other providers?"

Conducting such an evaluation involves the following: (1) identifying groups of patients (i.e., populations) who have high costs of care, less than optimal outcomes, or both; (2) monitoring and analyzing variances in outcomes and costs; (3) examining processes of care to determine how management of the condition could be improved; and (4) incorporating management methods found to be effective in research or best practice networks. For example, population data in New Mexico have revealed a high mortality rate from alcoholism, prompting the state to invest more in alcoholism prevention programs and emphasize a sharper clinical focus on substance abuse.

Evaluation of the degree to which desirable outcomes are attained enables health care systems to compare their effectiveness with that of a comparable system or to evaluate the relative effectiveness of a new program or process of care. These types of evaluations and comparisons can lead to the identification of best practice methods at the health care system level. Use of services, readmission rates, complication rates, average total cost per case, and mortality rates are examples of population outcomes used in various types of evaluations and comparisons.

Preventive Services in Primary Care

Health promotion and disease prevention interventions are tools that APRNs in primary care regularly use to help people achieve and maintain a high quality of life. These preventive services include the following:

- Counseling regarding personal health practices that can protect a person from disease or promote screening for the presence of disease

- Immunization to prevent specific diseases
- Chemoprevention (e.g., use of aspirin for prevention of cardiovascular events)

Discernment is needed in the use of these interventions because time and effort can be wasted if their use is not based on current scientific knowledge and tailored to the individual person or community. Also, the public is confused regarding many of the preventive recommendations because new research evidence has been unseating long-established recommendations, such as the value of breast self-examination. The US Preventive Services Task Force (https://www.uspreventiveservicestaskforce.org) and the Canadian Task Force on Preventive Health Care (http://canadiantaskforce.ca) provide specific preventive guidelines for many health conditions. These include valuable summaries of the state of the science for each recommendation.

An important point made in the early document "Guide to Clinical Preventive Services" (US Preventive Services Task Force, 1996) is that primary prevention in the form of counseling aimed at changing health-related behavior may be more effective than diagnostic screening and testing. Many healthy people, as well as those who have had a recent health scare, are receptive to—even eager for—information and guidance about how to stay healthy and avoid age-related disabilities. However, other people who engage in one or several unhealthy behaviors can be defensive and resistant to talking about their risks and how behavior changes could reduce risks. Introducing behavior change issues with unreceptive people requires a high level of interpersonal skill and a good sense of timing. An APRN must consider that it is possible that no health care provider has previously attempted to discuss the problem (e.g., smoking, lack of exercise, alcohol abuse) with the person, even though signs of a problem have existed for a long time.

Talking about the risks of the current behavior and benefits of the behavior change is not enough. To be effective, counseling regarding these issues should also include a discussion of how the person perceives the burden of changing a personal behavior—that is, what would be lost and what would be required to make the change? The provider must first make the patient feel understood and must elicit how much effort will be required, what would give the individual the confidence to change, and which forms of self-help assistance are acceptable to the individual. Then and only then can a specific recommendation about a strategy or program be made. Theoretical models that can be useful in planning a behavior change program or protocol include the Transtheoretical Model (Cancer Prevention Research Center, University of Rhode Island, 2017) and the Health Belief Model (Resource Center for Adolescent Pregnancy Prevention, 2017). Both models include provider strategies for building a person's self-efficacy—confidence in one's ability to take action.

Clinicians also have at their disposal a wide array of screening tools, some of which are better with certain populations or age groups than others. For example, the US Preventive Services Task Force (2012) currently recommends against routinely screening women older than age 65 for cervical cancer if they have had an adequate recent screening with normal Papanicolaou (Pap) test results and are not otherwise at risk; they also recommend against performing routine Pap tests for women who have had a total hysterectomy as treatment for benign disease. Staying current with the latest screening recommendations in one's area of practice ensures that care is provided in a way that is scientific and cost-effective.

Preventive Services in Hospitals and Home Care

The preventive services provided in inpatient and home care settings are somewhat different from those provided in primary care. Many of the actions and assessments performed on behalf of acutely ill patients are aimed at early detection and prevention of problems related to treatment, disease progression, self-care deficits, or the hospital environment itself. Complications typically result from a complex set of factors, such as inadequate delivery systems or failure to assess patients for risk of complications common to their condition. Nurses assist patients by preventing adverse events and complications, including adverse medication reactions, unexpected physiologic decline, poor communication, pressure ulcers, and death. As noted earlier, this function is also termed *surveillance* or *rescuing* (as in rescuing from a bad course of events or death).

In the home setting, APRNs serve as advisors and partners. In addition to assessment and surveillance, guidance and coaching are particularly important. The patient may be new to the role of partner in this setting (Holman & Lorig, 2004). APRNs work with patients to prioritize measures that might prevent rehospitalizations. Interventions may include teaching about reportable signs and symptoms, guidance on how to communicate with their providers, and assistance in making connections between behaviors and situations in the home that directly affect health status.

Management of Complex Situations

APRNs' direct care often involves the management and coordination of complex situations. Many illustrations of this advanced practice nursing feature may be found in the chapters on specific advanced practice nursing roles (see Chapters 14 through 18). In some settings, APRNs have been designated as the providers responsible for coordination of complex follow-up care (Bradway et al., 2012; Looman et al., 2013; Morilla-Herrera et al., 2016). APRNs manage diverse and complex patient conditions and care requirements, which include the following:

- Confusion in older hospitalized patients and acute care of the elderly (ACE) units
- Frail older adults
- Pain in patients who are chronically or terminally ill
- Acute pain
- High-risk pregnant women
- Long-term mechanical ventilation
- Heart failure patients
- Neurosurgical patients
- Pediatric and adult palliative care
- Critically ill neonates

Many APRNs have been called in for consultation when there is a need for skilled communication, advocacy, or coordination of the various providers' plans—or some combination thereof (Exemplar 7.4). The patient's condition may not be improving because wound care, pain management, and physical therapy have not been well thought out and coordinated. Family members may be angry because plans keep changing and they are receiving conflicting information from various providers. Typically, the APRN talks with the patient and family to become familiar with their concerns and objectives and then brokers a new plan of care that reflects the patient's and family's needs and preferences, as well as the clinical objectives of the involved providers. The agreed-on plan must also be consistent with the care authorized by the third-party payers for the patient, or a special agreement must be negotiated. This brokering requires broad clinical knowledge regarding the objectives of various providers, interpersonal skill in dealing with the results of misunderstandings, diplomacy to encourage stakeholders to see each other's points of view, and a commitment to keeping the patient's needs at the center of what is being done.

| EXEMPLAR 7.4 | Management of Complex Patient Situations[a] |

C.M. is a diabetes clinical nurse specialist with 20 years of experience. She works in an 800-bed academic medical center, where she is accountable for overall outcomes of glycemic control in the inpatient setting. She is also responsible for evaluating, treating, and educating patients with complex diabetes needs.

C.M. has been asked to consult on and write treatment recommendations for a 30-year-old Somali woman. Before seeing the patient, C.M. reviewed the chart to ascertain patient history and information. The patient was diagnosed with type 2 diabetes mellitus (DM) 11 years ago and had been on oral hypoglycemic agents, although not well controlled. She has been managed by multiple providers over the years. The patient was not married and had two sons, 13 and 17 years of age; both have been diagnosed with type 1 DM.

Documentation in the chart indicated that the patient had been admitted to the hospital in diabetic ketoacidosis (DKA) caused by presumed nonadherence to her regimen. The health care team had initiated an insulin infusion but had not initiated the DKA protocol and had been having difficulty getting the patient's glucose level in the target range.

When C.M. entered the patient's room, she saw an African woman with truncal obesity, a puffy face, acne, and facial hair. The patient did not make eye contact and appeared standoffish. The patient was reluctant to answer questions. C.M. recognized the need to proceed thoughtfully in developing a relationship with the patient to establish trust. C.M. also realized that multiple visits would be required to fully ascertain the extent of needs for this complex patient. From C.M.'s experience and knowledge base, she knew that the symptomatology of DM in the African population is different from the typical presentation of DM in Caucasians. Type 1 DM symptoms in the African population may not be as severe on initial presentation and may not reflect ketosis; therefore this population can be misdiagnosed with type 2 DM and started on oral agents when they actually have type 1 DM and should be treated with insulin. C.M. suspected that this might have been the case with this patient. In addition, on first glance, C.M. immediately suspected that the patient had other endocrine issues (e.g., adrenal dysfunction or polycystic ovary syndrome) because of the presence of puffy face, acne, and facial hair.

C.M. decided the priority for this initial visit was to focus on the physical care aspects while clarifying the diagnosis and prescribing appropriate treatment to control the patient's glucose. She performed a physical examination and ordered the following diagnostic tests:

- C-peptide and antibodies (to differentiate between types 1 and 2 DM)
- Fasting cortisol
- Adrenocorticotropic hormone stimulation test
- Estradiol-androgen panel
- 24-hour urine
- Endocrinologist consult
- Initiation of standardized DKA protocol

C.M. returned the following day with the intent to explore knowledge and psychosocial areas with the patient. Again, the patient was wary in her interaction but started to have better eye contact. C.M. started by asking about the patient's psychosocial situation and determined that the patient was making ends meet financially. However, there were income issues, and C.M. determined that a social work referral was in order. The patient described having a good relationship with her sons and acknowledged an extensive family support system in the community. She identified herself as a Christian, not a Muslim, as most people assumed.

C.M. then started to inquire about the physical signs she had noticed on the previous visit by asking how long the patient had had acne and facial hair. At that point, the patient started to cry and stated that C.M. was the first person to have ever asked her about it. They were clearly distressing symptoms for the patient, and she relayed that she had tried multiple over-the-counter products to try to resolve the acne, but without success. C.M. shared with the patient what she suspected might be happening with other endocrine issues and reassured her that if that were the case, prescription dermatology creams and hormone therapies would help resolve the symptoms. It was at this point that the patient realized that C.M. was committed to helping her and a therapeutic relationship began to develop. The patient was now more receptive to allowing a full knowledge assessment.

C.M. discovered that the patient understood DM well and knew how to count carbohydrates and how to use that information when planning meals. Although the patient spoke English well, C.M. discovered that the patient could not read English and had some visual disturbances. What had been labeled as nonadherence was actually an inability to read and see health care instructions. When C.M. reviewed the diagnostic test results, it was determined that the patient had Cushing's syndrome, polycystic ovary syndrome, and type 1 DM, rather than type 2. Over the following days, in educational sessions with C.M., the patient quickly gained knowledge about insulin and how to administer it, and she became proficient at using a magnifier to read the insulin syringe. C.M. developed instructional tools that did not require the ability to read complicated English. Whenever the patient's sons were present, they were included in the teaching.

The patient was eventually discharged to home with new knowledge of insulin and type 1 DM management, as well as information about her new diagnoses and medications, ongoing support from external social services, and referral to a physician group that could manage the health needs of the entire family and provide continuity of care over time.

Highlights of Advanced Practice Nursing Care of a Complex Patient

This case exemplifies the role that an APRN can play in making accurate diagnoses and optimizing care for a complex patient. C.M. exhibited the following:

- Use of evidence and knowledge of unique population-based data applied to an individual patient, which resulted in prompt correction of a diabetes misdiagnosis
- Expert clinical assessment and intervention skills that identified new endocrine diagnoses and assisted in rapid correction of glycemic control
- Holistic approach to care, incorporating cultural assessment, psychosocial needs, and barriers to knowledge
- Individualized interventions to meet patient needs
- Interpersonal approach that allowed for rapid development of a trusting therapeutic relationship with a patient who was traditionally wary of health care providers who had consistently misidentified her as noncompliant ◎

[a]The author gratefully acknowledges Carol Manchester, MSN, APRN, CNS, BC-ADM, CDE, for the use of her exemplar.

Helping Patients Manage Chronic Illnesses

Another type of complex situation that APRNs manage effectively is chronic illness. Chronic diseases such as multiple sclerosis, cognitive degeneration, psoriasis, heart failure, chronic lung disease, cancer, acquired immunodeficiency syndrome (AIDS), and organ failure with subsequent transplantation affect individuals and families in profound ways. Most chronic illnesses are characterized by a great deal of uncertainty—uncertainty about the future life course, effectiveness of treatment, chances of leading a happy life, bodily functions, medical bills, and intimate relationships (Mast, 1995). The unique perceptions that the patient can experience with uncertainty in chronic illness has led to the proposal of a new model integrating the two concepts: the Health Change Trajectory Model (Christensen, 2015). For a variety of reasons related to the characteristics of advanced practice nursing, APRNs are successful in providing care in this complex situation to persons with chronic conditions and their families.

The US Department of Health and Human Services (HHS) has issued proposed rules for health care providers and systems based on the Patient Protection and Affordable Care Act (2010) to improve the coordination of patient care, particularly those with chronic or complex illnesses, through the establishment of accountable care organizations (HHS, 2011). Although the details of any specific legislative efforts will certainly change with time, the essential foundation of this accountable care organizations effort is to place patients at the center of their care, maintain quality standards of care, and lower health care costs.

APRNs who see chronically ill patients in a primary care or specialty setting improve care by coordinating the services patients receive from multiple providers. Chronic illnesses often affect several body systems or have numerous sequelae. Thus persons who are chronically ill often receive care from a primary care provider and several other clinicians, including physicians and APRN specialists, social workers, physical therapists, and dietitians. Without coordination, families coping with chronic illness can find themselves in an "agency maze" (Burton, 1995, p. 457). This vivid phrase captures the confusing experiences that ensue when the agencies and providers rendering care to a family do not communicate with one another. Families do not know where to go for help and, as a result, many resort to a trial-and-error approach to getting what they need. They often suffer the negative effects of misinformation, repetitive intake interviews, denial of service, conflicting approaches, and unsolved problems. A resource-savvy APRN can often assess these situations and intervene to reduce stress, improve communication, and benefit patients and families. By contacting other providers to develop a coordinated management plan and by linking patients with suitable agencies, the APRN can do much to relieve the burdens of chronic illness on a family.

Among the reasons that APRNs are successful in providing care to persons with chronic illness is their advocacy of patient self-care. It has been proposed that the key to self-care by patients with chronic illness is to provide self-management education and support in conjunction with traditional patient education (McGowan, 2012). Self-management education is aimed at promoting confidence to carry out new behaviors, teaching the identification and solving of problems, and setting patient-directed, short-term goals (Lorig, Ritter, & Gonzalez, 2003; McGowan, 2012). Many self-management educational interventions for those with chronic conditions are designed to bolster patients' sense of self-efficacy related to coping with their condition and gaining control over the impact of the disease on their lives. This can include engaging patients in shared decision making, promoting healthy lifestyles, and monitoring of symptoms (McGowan, 2012), all of which APRNs are skilled at providing and supporting. Although self-management education has had mixed results to date in physical and psychological health improvements, it is believed that it is a useful component of a comprehensive, chronic disease management program (Brady et al., 2013; McGowan, 2012).

Partnership in the management of a chronic illness requires a change in roles for patients and providers. Patients develop daily management skills, changes in behaviors, and accurate reporting of symptoms. Although providers continue as advisers and partners, they now also become teachers, a role that many are not adequately prepared to fulfill (Holman & Lorig, 2004). In this new partnership, patients develop more knowledge and experience over time and they know the most about the real consequences of chronic disease and their behaviors.

There are barriers to using a self-management education program in today's health care environment. These include lack of trained personnel in this intervention, patient dependence on the medical model that has been facilitated by paternalistic health care providers, and lack of reimbursement for these services (Bodenheimer & Grumbach, 2007).

Regardless, results of this model are compelling, with need for further research because the aging of the US population will only result in increasing numbers of patients living with chronic illness.

Through the use of diverse approaches and individualized, interpersonal, and therapeutic interventions, APRNs have the skills and resources to partner in managing populations throughout the care continuum, from preventive care to the most complex care required by patients with a chronic condition. This is important in view of the increasing complexity of patients' health problems in today's society.

Direct Care and Information Management

Health care is an information-rich environment. It has been said that health care encounters occur essentially for the exchange of information—between the patient and care provider and among care providers themselves (Committee on Quality Health Care in America, IOM, 2001). With the adoption of information technology (IT), health care information management has become increasingly complex. Inadequate resources and difficulty in accessing information at the time it is needed complicate the situation further (Committee on Quality Health Care in America, IOM, 2001). The IOM report recommended that government, health care leaders, and vendors work collaboratively to build an information infrastructure quickly to eliminate handwritten clinical data by the end of 2010. With the implementation of the Affordable Care Act, the HHS has made recommendations to encourage widespread implementation of electronic systems and databases to facilitate access to seamless and accessible health care information for everyone (HHS, 2010). Although there is still much to do, it is believed that appropriate use of these systems will decrease errors in prescribing and dosing, increase appropriate use of best practice guidelines, reduce redundancy, improve access to information for patients and providers, and improve quality of care. The direct care practice of APRNs is directly influenced by these changes as increasing numbers of health care systems and clinics implement electronic health records and databases.

The DNP Essentials task force recognized the increasing importance of information systems for APRN practice and education. Essential IV of the DNP Essentials requires that APRNs be prepared to participate in design, selection, and evaluation of systems used for outcomes and quality improvement; exhibit leadership in the area of legal and ethical issues related to information systems; and be knowledgeable about how to evaluate consumer sources of information available through technology (AACN, 2006). Borycki, Cummings, Kushniruk, and Saranto (2017) have outlined additional nursing informatics competencies required of multiple levels of nurses. With rapid changes in technology, it will be an ongoing challenge throughout an APRN's career to remain current in this area.

There is an expectation of increasing competence in the use of technology that can be a challenge for some APRNs. Wilbright et al. (2006) surveyed 454 nursing staff at all role levels in their self-reported skill in 11 key areas of computer use. Although the APRNs reported excellent to good skills at entering orders and accessing laboratory results, they rated their skills as fair or poor in 5 of 11 areas that were deemed essential to their role. APRNs may still struggle with optimal use of MEDLINE or CINAHL or skills such as use of Excel spreadsheets and project management programs, which may be essential to optimal functioning in their roles. If APRNs struggle with the need for increasingly complex technology skills, it will be difficult for them to use tools and their time optimally to care for their patients.

Well-functioning information systems can ease the workload of the APRN by optimizing the management of extensive data. However, meaningful IT needs more development to overcome challenges that APRNs may face on a daily basis in their use of IT, such as workflow disruptions, lack of interfaces between systems, work-arounds, in which providers subvert the IT to get the job done, and inappropriate use of order entry warning alerts (Magrabi, Ong, Runciman, & Coiera, 2010, 2012; Palojoki, Mäkelä, Lehtonen, & Saranto, 2016). Computer technology may actually require increased staff time when used for complex order entry and clinical documentation.

Health care institutions and private practices are rapidly implementing information systems across the country, so it is likely that APRNs will work in an environment in which a system is being implemented or upgraded. APRNs can have an impact on how these systems function to make them user-friendly and efficient at the direct care interface. Although APRNs may feel they have neither the time, inclination, nor expertise to participate in these implementations, user input is imperative and ultimately affects direct care.

As information systems are implemented, APRNs need to be cognizant of the potential for at least a temporary increase in errors, reduced charge capture, incomplete or difficult-to-access information, and increased time for routine tasks. Implementation of these systems is a major undertaking because it takes time to re-equilibrate workflow and organizational skills, regardless of APRN experience. When information systems are well implemented and used, the APRN will be able to use and view data in new ways to improve patient care.

The expansion of technology can lead to a corresponding increase in the number of tools and amount of data that are available for use—both within and external to the health care setting. Examples include: email or video communication with patients rather than telephone calls or office visits, patient use of "apps" to assist with dietary selections and recording intake when eating at restaurants, patient use of personal fitness devices that record activity levels and calories expended, data that can be downloaded and transmitted from mobile invasive technology to maintain life, the practice of telehealth for routine or specialty patient care, and the use of computers to assist in oncology protocol care decisions (e.g., Watson for Oncology: https://www.ibm.com/watson/health/oncology-and-genomics/oncology/). One commonality throughout these examples is the need to determine when and how to use these data to make patient care decisions (Harrington, 2017). There will be a need for robust analytics to obtain meaning from these data, and APRNs must partner with informaticists and be at the table when determining strategy regarding when and how to use analytics (Harrington, 2016a). The goal is to integrate technology with practice for value-added benefit (Harrington, 2016b). Although information systems and electronic resources can be great tools in the APRN's repertoire, the APRN must be constantly aware that these technologies bring with them their own pitfalls and unique potential for errors (Harrington, 2014). APRNs can play important roles in evaluating proposed technology and information management systems and the impact they have on APRN practice and patient care.

Conclusion

The central competency of advanced practice nursing is direct care, regardless of the specific role of the CNS, NP, CRNA, or CNM. APRNs are currently providing direct health care services that affect patients' health care outcomes positively and that are qualitatively different from those provided by other health care professionals. Of importance, these services are valued by the public and are cost-effective. APRNs can offer this essential care through the use of the six characteristics that comprise APRN direct care: use of a holistic perspective, formation of therapeutic partnerships with patients, expert clinical performance, use of reflective practice, use of evidence as a guide to practice, and use of diverse approaches to health and illness management. Their mastery accomplishes several goals, including differentiation of practice at an advanced level and context for the development of other competencies, such as consultation and collaboration. Together, these characteristics form a solid foundation for providing scientifically based, person-centered, and outcome-validated health care. Research evidence supports each of these claims and hence substantiates the nursing profession's and public's confidence in the care provided by APRNs. As APRNs continue to expand the scope and settings of their practice, it will be imperative that these six characteristics continue to be substantiated by solid research in each of the roles. In addition, research will be important in documenting the optimal so-called nurse dose of APRN intervention as we continue to face challenges in caring for culturally diverse, aging, and chronically ill populations.

Key Summary Points

- Direct care is the central APRN competency.
- The six characteristics of direct care are: use of a holistic perspective, formation of therapeutic

partnerships with patients, expert clinical performance, use of reflective practice, use of evidence as a guide to practice, and use of diverse approaches to health and illness management.
- While APRNs provide many strategic functions throughout and over the course of their role, time needs to continue to be spent in direct clinical care with patients in order to maintain differentiation between the APRN role and other DNP-prepared non-APRN roles.
- Mastery of these six characteristics of direct care delineates the differentiation of practice at an advanced level and sets the foundation for attaining skill in the other APRN competencies.

References

To access the references for this chapter, use your smartphone's QR code reader to scan the code below, or go to http://booksite.elsevier.com/ 9780323447751.

Guidance and Coaching

Eileen T. O'Grady • *Jean E. Johnson*

"You don't have to see the first staircase, just take the first step."
—*Martin Luther King, Jr.*

CHAPTER CONTENTS

This chapter defines guidance and coaching as distinct advanced practice registered nurse (APRN) competencies that are at the heart of nursing and are an effective means to engage patients in change leading to healthier lives. Since researchers first identified the teaching-coaching function of expert nurses and APRNs, guidance and coaching by APRNs have been researched, integrated into APRN competencies, and described through case studies and other writings about APRN practice (Benner, 1984; Benner, Hooper-Kyriakidis, & Stannard, 1999; Fenton & Brykczynski, 1993).

The American Association of Colleges of Nursing Essentials (Master's and doctoral knowledge, skills and competencies) have guidance and coaching integrated into nearly every competency, be it leadership, role development, or health promotion (American Association of Colleges of Nursing, 1996, 2006). Engaging others effectively to build rapport through deep listening is a key competency for all APRNs to build an authentic therapeutic exchange with patients. The core competencies of APRN guidance and coaching are explicated here within the context of theory and research. In addition, a description of which APRN situations are appropriate for guiding patients and which are appropriate for coaching patients is emphasized. Foundational skills of the coaching methodology are discussed, and guidance and coaching skills will be contrasted. Integrative health care, often linked with guidance and coaching, is not fully covered in this chapter; rather, a thorough discussion explores the relational skills needed across all four APRN roles. (See Chapter 7 for a discussion of integrative therapies in APRN practice.)

Why Guidance and Coaching?

Patient Engagement

In the United States, and around the world, people with serious illnesses or chronic conditions account for a disproportionate share of national health care spending. One of the main drivers of the Affordable Care Act (ACA) was to lower costs and reduce persistent racial disparities (Patient Protection and Affordable Care Act, 2010). Research shows that a multipronged approach is needed to reduce costs and health disparities and includes redesigning primary care, developing care teams that are accountable across sites of care, and managing transitions and medications (Schoen et al., 2011). Health providers working together with patients have the opportunity to design personalized interventions to sustain patients' involvement in their treatment and encourage patients to take an active role in their own health and health care.

Guiding and coaching patients requires activation and empowerment through placing the responsibility of the *pursuit* of health where it rightly belongs—with the patient. The ACA provided the structure to activate and empower patients by giving patients critical information about quality, enhancing patient-centered care through client-centered medical homes, and financing new models of care that empower patients. These elements of the ACA are designed to engage patients in their treatment, developing their abilities to manage their health and lower their modifiable risks, helping them express concerns and preferences regarding treatment, empowering them to ask questions about treatment options, and building strategic patient-provider partnerships through shared decision making (Chen, Mullins, Novak, & Thomas, 2016). Recognizing patients as the source of control for their health requires building confidence and empowerment and not having health care providers simply tell patients what they need to do.

This shift to a more patient-centered approach is a major component of improvement of population health.

Burden of Chronic Illness

The current biomedical model of care does not work for lifestyle-related diseases. Chronic diseases—including heart disease, stroke, type 2 diabetes, cancer, and chronic lung diseases—account for most deaths in the United States and globally and are costly, debilitating, and preventable (Centers for Disease Control and Prevention [CDC], 2016b). The World Health Organization (WHO) has identified four major risk factors responsible for the worldwide disease burden that now eclipses communicable diseases: (1) tobacco use, (2) poor diet, (3) alcohol abuse, and (4) physical inactivity. These four behaviors are responsible for 4 of every 5 deaths in the world and represent the most significant modifiable risk factors causing the chronic illness epidemic worldwide (WHO, 2014). Helping patients change these behaviors will greatly decrease untold suffering, early mortality, and disability. A startling statistic that represents opportunity for behavior change is that there are now more overweight people than undernourished people throughout the world (IFRC, 2011). This chronic illness epidemic is an impending disaster for worldwide health, for society, and for the global macroeconomy. Chronic noncommunicable diseases create a debilitating blow to economic development. They cause billions of dollars in losses of national income and push millions of people below the poverty line, each and every year (IFRC, 2011). In the United States alone, chronic diseases attributable to lifestyle factors are responsible for 7 of 10 deaths each year, and they account for 86% of our nation's health care costs, which in 2013 were $2.9 trillion (CDC, 2016b).

As every APRN knows, lifestyles associated with chronic illness can be prevented by choosing healthy behaviors. People can reduce their chances of getting a chronic disease or improve their health and quality of life if they already have a chronic disease by making healthy choices. The CDC (2016a) found that only 6.3% of US adults engaged in all five key health behaviors that can reduce their risk of chronic diseases: (1) avoiding alcohol consumption or only drinking in moderation; (2) exercising regularly; (3) getting enough sleep: (4) maintaining a healthy body weight; and (5) not smoking. These findings, based on nearly 400,000 adults aged 21 and older, showed that 1% failed to engage in any of the five health behaviors, while 24% engaged in four, 35% engaged in three, and 24% engaged in two. As APRNs bring a sharp focus to lifestyle change that can be addressed through guidance and coaching, their value in the health care marketplace will be more fully realized.

Context of Guidance and Coaching: Definition and Skills

There are relational approaches that focus on helping a person create change in his or her life to advance individual autonomy, well-being, and goal attainment. Although there is overlap among the approaches, several aspects differentiate them, such as length of time of engagement and the focus of the interaction. Understanding the characteristics of guidance versus coaching is a key APRN competency that is built on having trust and rapport with patients.

Guidance

Guidance is a broad term that means the provision of help, instruction, or assistance, and there are several forms of guidance. The distinguishing feature of guidance as compared to coaching is that guidance requires the provision of advice or education, whereas coaching is an inquiry, an excavation of answers from a person. To guide is to advise, or show the way to others, so guidance can be considered the act of providing expert counsel by leading, directing, or advising. To guide also means to assist a person to travel through or reach a destination in an unfamiliar area. Guidance is best used in situations when a person has a perceived knowledge deficit in an area for which expert APRN knowledge can fill the void. When providing guidance, the APRN is serving as a knowledge source for the patient. Guidance can include laying out, simplifying, or integrating the options for a patient to make a health care decision. It is imperative that the APRN determine the patient's level of knowledge before launching into guidance. Asking patients what they know about their condition is an important skill to respectfully build on what they know and make APRN guidance more powerful and effective. What follows are some common forms of guidance.

Anticipatory Guidance

Anticipatory guidance and teaching is a particular type of guidance aimed at helping patients and families know what to expect. Anticipating common problems or symptoms and what to do about them can go a long way in reducing unnecessary care and

promoting self-efficacy, as well as in reducing a patient's anxiety.

Anticipatory guidance is when the APRN informs the patient *a priori* about an expected health process that is likely to occur. For example when a patient sustains a cervical hyperextension injury (whiplash) after a car accident and a fracture has been ruled out, the APRN informs the patient that the muscles surrounding the neck will become far more painful within 48 hours. She or he may explain that torticollis may ensue and that this is normal, temporary, and to be expected. The APRN offers remedies and guidelines on when to seek more assessment. Another example of anticipatory guidance is when a woman experiences a miscarriage and the APRN lets the patient know to expect very heavy blood loss that may alarm her. The APRN provides guidelines about when to seek additional care, offers reassurance, and anticipates that the patient may experience intense feelings of loss and grief.

Patient Education

Patient empowerment can be achieved by teaching patients about their illnesses/conditions and by guiding them to be more involved in decisions related to ongoing care and treatment. The WHO defines patient education more broadly as any combination of learning experiences designed to help individuals and communities improve their health by increasing their knowledge or influencing their attitudes (WHO, 2016). The goal of patient education is to produce change and self-care. Clinicians have long thought that if the patient is provided with the right information, the patient will see the wisdom of making change in his or her life to be healthier and simply follow the recommendations.

For APRNs it is essential to determine what a person wants to learn before launching into a teaching or "telling" expert role. Patients often come with an array of information from available websites and other sources. As information has become so readily available, patients are looking for customized wisdom and a broker of information to cut through the large amount of confusing, often conflicting, sources of knowledge. They want to know what information applies to them and how should they use it. (See Chapter 7 for further discussion of patient education.)

Mentoring

There are many definitions of mentoring, but essentially it is a one-on-one relational process in which one person having more expertise or experience in a particular area provides guidance to another person. Mentors and mentees often have long-term relationships, sometimes for an entire career or lifetime. Although mentors help mentees move toward their goals, the goals of mentees are usually consistent with the career goals of the mentors. The similarity in interests is usually based on a shared knowledge area or achievement of a position. Mentors provide advice and support based on their experience to help their mentees attain their goals. The mentoring relationship can be highly structured, with set times for meetings and agendas, or very informal, with meetings at intervals as the mentee desires. These relationships are beneficial to both parties because the participants offer each other different perspectives and framing on modern APRN problems. The mentor is exposed to fresh thinking and to APRN problems that the mentee many be facing. Mentees are offered a longer view, wisdom, and perspective.

Counseling

In *20/20: A Vision for the Future of Counseling: The New Consensus Definition of Counseling,* the American Counseling Association defines counseling as the following:

> *Counseling is a professional relationship that empowers diverse individuals, families, and groups to accomplish mental health, wellness, education, and career goals.* (Kaplan, Tarvydas, & Gladding, 2014, p. 368)

Counseling can be a very long-term relationship that is focused on helping individuals address their problems. Counseling can take place within a work setting through programs such as employee assistance or with individuals on a personal basis. Counseling is generally focused on psychological, social, or performance issues. The key distinction is that counseling is intended to "fix" a problem through gaining insight and advice from the counselor. Counseling as a technique operates from a problem-based approach as opposed to building on a person's strengths.

Coaching

Coaching is a broad umbrella term that encompasses different approaches, philosophies, techniques, and disciplines. Coaching is defined by the International Coach Federation (ICF) as "partnering with clients in a thought-provoking and creative process that inspires them to maximize their personal and professional potential" (ICF, 2016a). For APRNs this definition also extends to a health potential. The ICF (2016a) identified four main components of a coach's responsibility:

- Discover, clarify, and align with what the client wants to achieve
- Encourage client self-discovery
- Elicit client-generated solutions and strategies
- Hold the client responsible and accountable

The ICF definition and components of coaching provide significant leeway in the development of different philosophical approaches to coaching. Although there are common principles, there are different philosophies and schools of thought in the coaching sphere. One example is motivational coaching, based on a focused approach to explore and ignite motivation for change and address ambivalence. Another is integrative coaching, developed by Duke University to help patients make changes to lead healthier lives (Duke Integrative Health, 2016). Integrative coaching is intended to address the gap between medical recommendations and the patient's success in implementing the recommendations. Each of these approaches has commonalities, including working toward change that is defined by a patient. In addition, there are different foci of coaching, such as health and wellness, executive, life transition, end of life, and attention-deficit/hyperactivity coaching, to name a few. A meta-analysis on coaching by Sonesh et al. (2015) found wide-ranging impacts of coaching, including that coaching is an effective way to change patient behaviors and improve leadership skills, job performance, and skill development. Specific findings included that coaching:

- Improves personal and work attitudes, including self-efficacy, commitment to the organization, and reducing stress.
- Can elicit a strong bond, which in turn facilitates joint goal setting, and may be the mechanism through which goals are reached.

Coaching is based on a relationship in which the *individual identifies his or her goals*. It is founded on the recognition that the person seeking coaching is mentally healthy and has internal resources to deploy toward attaining her or his goals. The role of the coach is to work with that person in accomplishing those goals. The coach helps individuals clarify, define, reflect, and move forward. Coaching can be thought of as leading change from behind as well as walking with the patient (McLean, 2012). This concept clearly puts the individual in charge while the coach fully engages with the patient. Coaching can last from a "spot" coaching session of one time to several years in length. Many coaching relationships last about 6 to 10 interactions to move a person forward far enough so that he or she can self-coach to continue to attain and sustain her goals.

There is considerable discussion within coaching as to how much advice giving should be offered. Because coaching is usually considered a partnership with an individual requiring the asking of powerful questions, the APRN must trust that the person has her or his own answers that are true and right for him or her. However, working with patients to make change is different in that providers have specific health-related information that patients need and want. Providing that information is providing guidance within a coaching context. Combining coaching with guidance is essential to a complete provider-patient relationship. Table 8.1 differentiates guidance and coaching.

Nurse Coaching

Nurse coaching is aimed at working with individuals to promote their maximal health potential by integrating the skills of nursing and coaching. The relatively new International Nurse Coach Association supports the concept of integrative nurse coaching. Hess and colleagues (2012) have created momentum to integrate coaching into all registered nurse programs. Professional nurse coaching is defined as "a skilled, purposeful, results-oriented, and structured relationship-centered interaction with clients provided by a registered nurse for the purpose of promoting achievement of client goals" (Dossey, Luck, Schaub, 2015, p. 3). Although this definition is specific to nursing and nursing care, it is consistent with the intent of the ICF definition. The International

Nurse Coach Association offers certification as a nurse coach through their text *The Art and Science of Nursing Coaching: The Providers Guide to the Nursing Scope and Competencies* (Dossey et al., 2013), published by the American Nurses Association (ANA), as well as *Nurse Coaching: Integrative Approaches for Health and Wellbeing* (Dossey, Luck, & Schaub, 2015). These works have been endorsed by the American Holistic Nurses Association.

Coaching has been explicitly integrated into several APRN practices, although the extent is unknown. Hayes and Kalmakis (2007) have asserted that coaching is a critical component of a holistic care approach for nurse practitioners. Most midwives might say that their practice incorporates coaching throughout the mother's pregnancy and delivery (Exemplar 8.1). There has long been the concept of being a labor coach within midwifery. Clinical nurse specialists have worked within the spheres of both consultant and coach. As coaches, they have worked with patients and family members to manage multiple chronic illnesses or a specific disease. Many clinical nurse specialists have roles that incorporate coaching when working with nurses to develop skills. A certified registered nurse anesthetist uses coaching to customize and personalize pain management or anesthesia to meet the patient's stated goals and needs.

Theories and Research Supporting APRN Guidance and Coaching

There are numerous evidence-based theories and frameworks that inform the APRN guidance and coaching competency. These are deeply rooted in Florence Nightingale's environmental theory as well as the science of human caring, which broadens and deepens the therapeutic use of self. In fact, the importance of the APRN-patient therapeutic relationship is foundational to the APRN guidance and coaching competency. Although there are many theories and models, we will note those that are important to informing and developing the APRN guidance and coaching competency.

Nightingale's Environmental Theory

Florence Nightingale's *Notes on Nursing: What It Is and What It Is Not* (1860), makes a strong link between a person's environment and her or his health. Working with a person to manage his or her environment is the fundamental role of nursing, and as we experience a chronic illness epidemic in

TABLE 8.1	Elements of Guidance and Coaching Competencies
Guidance	**Coaching**
Expert APRN has higher authority gradient	Power is shared
APRN is the expert	Patient is the expert/has the answers
Provides advice	Seeks understanding
Fixes problems	Builds on strengths
Expertise is valued	Curiosity is valued
Telling	Asking
Teaching	Inquiring
Anticipates	Explores
APRN leads/sets agenda	Patient leads/sets agenda

EXEMPLAR 8.1   **Being a Midwife and Family Nurse Practitioner Is Being a Coach**

Dawn Lovelace, DNP, CNM, FNP

Dawn Lovelace, DNP, RN, CNM, FNP, is both a certified nurse-midwife (CNM) of 22 years and a family nurse practitioner (FNP) of 17 years who believes coaching is integral to her practice. She lives in Grand Coulee, Washington, an area with approximately 1000 people in the town and about 10,000 people in the 20-square-mile service area surrounding the town. She and several colleagues worked to build a full-scope health service with her focus on developing maternity care services that did not exist. She was on call 24/7 for births, saw patients 4 days a week in clinic, and provided emergency room coverage. She saw patients in the hospital and nursing home. The practice has added more clinicians and is now a medical home.

Dr. Lovelace says that coaching has always been part of "being" a midwife and FNP, and she has a strong commitment to helping people be as healthy as possible. As a midwife, she helps a woman prepare for and meet her goals for the birth as well as helping her become a parent. The beauty of coaching pregnant women is that she has 9 months and often much longer to engage in a coaching relationship. Coaching has been part of the very deep and long value she has had. It is integral to her personal belief system. She starts where the person is, helps her evolve based on her reproductive life plan, and determines how to help get her there. For Dr. Lovelace, it is difficult to tease out what is coaching because it is so embedded within the role. She describes how being with women outside the hospital setting helps one truly be present with them. She knows she is present when she loses track of time

and is in the "zone" or "flow." She has used the transformative power of pregnancy and birth knowing that this is a time of life when people want to grow and that tapping into that desire is easy.

When asked what she likes best about coaching, Dr. Lovelace says she has seen so many amazing outcomes of coaching. She described working with a 14-year-old pregnant girl who was heavily involved in drugs. Dr. Lovelace's coaching went beyond the birthing process as she worked with the young woman to get her life together. In spite of every roadblock conceivable, that young woman is now in college and is an effective parent. She also described another young girl who came for birth control and who was going from house to house sleeping on sofas. This young woman is now a nurse practitioner, and when she recently saw Dr. Lovelace, she said that it was really important in how she saw herself that Dr. Lovelace treated her like a human being and saw the potential in her.

When asked what she would say to her students about integrating coaching into their practice, Dr. Lovelace quickly said, "Start where the person is. Accept them where they are. We all have people we don't like, but we need to accept them and don't ever write anyone off." In asking how she would advise students to be able to be present with patients, Dr. Lovelace said, "It takes work and self-evaluation, you need to know your prejudices and beliefs. We have off days in which we don't listen but we need to keep working at deep listening. Helping people figure out how to change their lives—that is what matters. You have to be committed to having coaching being part of your practice and value it." ◎

---

modern times, this observation still holds true. In fact, Nightingale built the foundation of nursing as a distinct profession on her observation that external factors associated with patients' surroundings greatly affect their lives, their development, and their biologic and physiologic processes (Nightingale, 1860). This seminal conceptual thinking lies at the heart of modern APRN guidance and coaching.

Midrange Theory of Integrative Nurse Coaching

A theoretical framework for nurse coaching has been developed by Dossey and colleagues (2015). They defined an integrative nurse coaching framework as

"a distinct nursing role that places clients/patients at the center and assists them in establishing health goals, creating change in lifestyle behaviors for health promotion and disease management, and implementing integrative modalities as appropriate" (p. 29). The authors identified five components of this model: (1) self-reflection, self-assessment, self-evaluation, and self-care; (2) integral perspectives and change; (3) integrative lifestyle health and well-being; (4) awareness and choice; and (5) listening with HEART (healing, energy, awareness, resiliency, and transformation) (Dossey et al., 2015, p. 29). Based on this theoretical framework, the ANA published a guide to nurse coaching competencies (Dossey et al., 2013) (Exemplar 8.2).

The Story of a Nurse Coach Champion

Barbara Dossey, PhD, RN, AHN-BC, FAAN, HWNC-BC

Barbara Dossey is changing the practice of nursing. She has been building on 50+ years of nursing experience, including a 23-year focus in critical care and cardiovascular nursing. As she cared for critically ill patients, she realized that many of her patients could have prevented their serious health issues if they had changed their lifestyles. That was the beginning of her focus on holistic nursing, healing rituals, and health and wellness through coaching.

In 2010 a seminal experience for Dr. Dossey occurred after an interprofessional coaching conference with over 1000 people, where not a single nurse presented on a topic that is the foundation of nursing. She asked herself, "Where are the nurses in this health and wellness coaching conversation, what can I do, and how can I do it?" Her answer was to look at the power of coaching as an integral role and part of nursing practice.

Dr. Dossey then moved quickly—knowing how to create change. She invited five like-minded holistic nursing colleagues engaged in health and wellness coaching to craft a roadmap to move the philosophy and role of coaching into mainstream nursing. Strategically, she and her colleagues obtained permission to use the American Nurses Association template of nursing specialties scope and standards and developed a template for coaching applicable to all levels and disciplines within nursing. As a result, she and her colleagues published *The Art and Science of Nurse Coaching: A Provider's Guide to Scope and Competencies* (Dossey et al., 2013). This is the study guide for the American Holistic Nurses Credentialing Corporation Nurse Coach certification examination. She and two colleagues also developed the Theory of Integrative Nurse Coaching, a midrange theoretical model for nurse coaching, and published the first Nurse Coach textbook, *Nurse Coaching: Integrative Approaches for Health and Wellbeing* (Dossey, Luck, & Schaub, 2015).

Dr. Dossey speaks eloquently about the "heart" of nursing being coaching. As she considers advanced practice registered nurse (APRN) work, she describes APRN clinical expertise as necessary but not sufficient and says that coaching brings the "heart" of nursing back to the APRN-patient relationship. It is the integration that fulfills Florence Nightingale's vision of nursing as focused on the health of humanity and a healthy world—local to global.

Her philosophy is firmly based on the richness of the integrative nurse coaching model. She is clear that the requisite to being an effective nurse coach is to know yourself and to continuously develop oneself through self-awareness, self-reflection, self-evaluation, and self-care. As we go to a deeper level of our own story, we can listen at a deeper level to patient stories to more effectively help them to create healthy change—often with baby steps leading to sustained change and healing on many levels.

Dr. Dossey speaks passionately about the beauty of hearing the stories of patients and how important that is to understanding who each patient is and what patients' hopes are for their health in order to help them understand their own strengths and resilience. She believes that APRNs have deep capacity to bear witness—to let go of their agenda and to be aware of the qualities of stillness and be open to the present moment. The critical component of an APRN working effectively with a patient is to work with the patient to identify his or her goals, strengths, and actions for change, and to be present and listen with HEART (*h*ealing, *e*nergy, *a*wareness, *r*esilience, and *t*ransformation).

Dr. Dossey believes that positive psychology is key to coaching by believing in the strengths that patients have and recognizing that everybody has resilience. When APRNs increase the self-awareness of patients, those patients make better choices and have power to make life changes. She knows this can be done because she has a personal nurse practitioner care provider who has integrated coaching into her practice and begins each visit with a joyful greeting of "I am very glad to see you and I want to hear what you have being doing since I last saw you," setting the stage for deep listening and hearing Dr. Dossey's story. The focus is on her as a patient and a person, not on a routine physical examination or a symptom. ◎

Transtheoretical Model

The transtheoretical model is an integration of several hundred psychotherapy and behavior change theories, hence the term *trans* (Prochaska, Redding, & Evers, 2002). Using smokers as research subjects, Prochaska et al. learned that behavior change unfolds through a series of sequenced stages of change, which were not delineated in any of the existing multitude of theories. The transtheoretical model has been used successfully in a number of maladaptive lifestyle behaviors such as alcohol and substance abuse, eating disorders, anxiety/panic disorders, obesity, sedentary lifestyles, high-risk sexual behavior, and nonadherent medication use. This model is highly relevant to the APRN who can tailor the intervention to the patient's specific stage of change to maximize the likelihood that the patient will proceed through a needed change process. Providing specific knowledge about disease trajectories or prevention strategies and advice is overused and often counterproductive when it comes to motivating patients toward sustained lifestyle change. A thorough discussion on readiness for change and application of this theory is provided later in this chapter.

Watson's Model of Caring

The theoretical framework for Watson's model of caring is based on loving kindness. Her work has focused on the science of caring and moving from carative to caratas (love), that is, the process of relating to others in an authentically present way, going beyond the ego (Watson, 2017). The APRN would go beyond self-interest and ego to fully and spiritually integrate body, mind, and spirit. This model provides a strong feelings-based approach to coaching, recognizing the openness of spirit to another person as essential in a therapeutic relationship. Honoring and respecting the patient's values, history, beliefs, autonomy, goals, and being is foundational in this model. It also requires self-reflection for the APRN to reach deep love and respect in a relationship. This includes, for example, being present to and supportive of the expression of positive and negative feelings, the creative use of self and using *all* ways of knowing, and assisting with basic needs with intentional caring consciousness (Watson, 2017).

Positive Psychology

Seligman (2011) found five dimensions that lead to a flourishing life or a high degree of well-being (Fig. 8.1). These dimensions can be cultivated to build one's capacity to flourish. The five dimensions of positive psychology are directly applicable to the APRN interacting with a wide range of people. In looking at the dimension of positive emotions as an example, Fredrickson (2001) proposed that feeling positive emotions broadens people's momentary thought-action choices, which builds their enduring personal resources. Broadening and building suggest that the capacity to experience positive emotions may be a fundamental human strength central to human well-being. The APRN can facilitate a person's positive psychology, especially in a guidance and

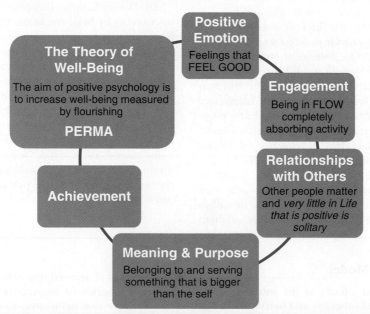

FIG 8.1 The theory of well-being. *(From Seligman, M. E. P. [2011]. Flourish: A visionary new understanding of happiness and well-being. New York, NY: Free Press.)*

coaching interaction, by promoting any or all of the five dimensions of well-being.

Growth Mindset

Dweck (2006), in her study of mindset and its impact on achievement, found that there are two types of belief systems. One is a *growth mindset* in which the individual believes she or he can learn and practice and achieve success. In addition, there is the belief that hard effort can remedy setbacks and that people with a growth mindset have a high degree of resilience. *Fixed mindset* people believe they are endowed with talents that are fixed; they focus on documenting and defending their talent rather than developing skills. People with fixed mindsets de-link talent from effort, acting on the belief that talent is a fixed, immutable entity. Fostering a growth mindset in the clinical space can create motivation and productivity, leading to improved outcomes. Guiding patients to shift from a hunger for approval (fixed mindset) to a passion for learning (growth mindset) by the tiniest degree can have profound impact on nearly every aspect of life (Dweck, 2006).

Self-Determination Theory

Ryan and Deci (2006) provide a framework for the understanding of human motivation and conditions that promote it and thwart it. The theory purports that there are two forms of motivation, intrinsic and extrinsic, and that all humans are motivated both by rewards (outside of ourselves) and by our interests, curiosity, and abiding values (inside). This framework offers three conditions that are associated with the level of a person's motivation for engagement (Fig. 8.2). These three psychological needs have a robust impact on wellness (Ryan & Deci, 2006).

This framework is directly applicable to the APRN guidance and coaching competency because the APRN can promote the environment that supports competence, autonomy, and human relatedness (Exemplar 8.3). When these three needs are satisfied, it leads to enhanced self-motivation and health, and when thwarted, diminishes motivation and well-being. Placing high value on positive regard, warmth, and giving patients as much psychological freedom as possible will lead to more engaged patients and better health outcomes (Ryan & Deci, 2000).

Transitions in Health and Illness

The emerging importance of guidance and coaching is also related to a better understanding of the importance of assisting patients with a variety of life experiences in order to reduce health care costs and increase quality of care (Naylor, Aiken, Kurtzman, Olds, & Hirschman, 2011). Early work by Schumacher

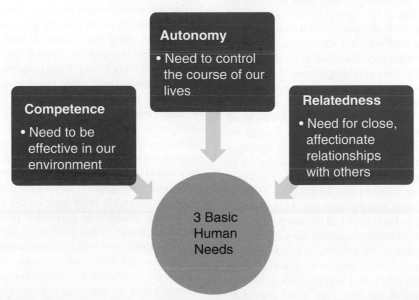

FIG 8.2 Self-determination theory posits that all humans have three central areas of motivation: competence, autonomy, and relatedness.

My Journey From the ICU to Wellness

Eva Schmidt, APRN, FNP-BC, CHWC

Starting my nursing career as an ICU nurse, I witnessed first-hand the unnecessary devastation of poor lifestyle choices and very often poorly informed choices. Almost from the very beginning, I found myself questioning how such patients had ended up there. Who had failed them? What could have been different for them? I started asking questions and quickly learned that it wasn't about a lack of desire to change. Most of the patients had tried. Many had even been through disease education programs. So, what was missing? My deep desire to answer that question is, in part, what led me to become a nurse practitioner.

I knew I needed to act "upstream," before an illness appeared, and that maybe I could help more people from that vantage point. I also knew that the foundation of the nurse practitioner role is based on health promotion and disease prevention. I intended to build on that concept to help people improve their health, not just treat disease and illness.

When I finished my NP program, I went to work for a 10-physician family practice. I had high hopes and stars in my eyes about how I would practice. They, however, had a different idea. I was seeing nearly 30 patients a day, never getting to really know any of them. I always felt as if I had my hand on the door, watching the clock, knowing the next patient had already been waiting too long. I was not only exhausted, I was sad. It became clear to me how those ICU patients had been failed. I finally had to ask myself, "Now what?"

I took a leap of faith and partnered with a physician in that practice to start our own MD-NP practice. Being the owner of my own practice seemed to be the answer. It was going to provide a new opportunity for me to finally deliver care in the way I knew it should be. We offered 30-minute appointments and were committed to delivering a different experience. At least I was. Word got out! We were very successful. Within 5 years we had built a practice of over 5000 patients. Having a business background, it made perfect sense for me to act as the practice administrator as well as a full-time provider. However, it didn't take long to see the signs. We were slowly falling into the same trap. I found myself working 24/7 just to keep up. I had no time for the very thing I set out to accomplish—putting the patients first!

As that environment became more toxic, with my partner and I having more and more disagreements about how I would practice, I began ignoring my own health. By the end of the fifth year, I had gained 40 pounds and was in the worst shape of my life. I started to feel like an imposter. I was supposed to be helping people improve their health and I certainly wasn't "walking the talk." I was spending so much time trying to prove myself as an equal to my physician partner that I had lost sight of the very foundation I started out on. I was failing my own patients and knew the only way to gain integrity with them was to gain integrity with myself and my own health. It was time to let the physician do his work and to focus on applying my NP skills where it would be most impactful.

I had one particular patient at that time who I had been seeing for several months. She was 150 pounds overweight, with all of the comorbidities one would expect. She was on several medications, and it seemed that despite her apparent desire to lose weight, each visit was spent adjusting those medications as the number on the scale continued to climb. I would give her a list of "good foods" and "bad foods." I'd advise her on how to cook, how to shop, and how to exercise. Yet every visit she would sit in my exam room and cry, saying things like "I don't know why I can't seem to stay on a diet" or "I was so bad this week." I knew we needed a new approach. I finally started asking her why losing the weight was important to her. She admitted that she didn't want to follow in her mother's footsteps; her mother had a heart attack before the age of 55 and died at 60. Once I took off the expert hat and we started focusing on her own motivation for change, the weight started coming off. She was able to set small goals for herself at each visit that led to lasting behavior changes. Within 6 months, she had lost over 70 pounds and is now off all of her medications.

I started using that approach with more patients. I would use the time scheduled for "follow up" or "medication checks" to have powerful conversations about wellness. I saw more improvements in the next 12 months than I had in 5 years with some of them. It became clear to me that coaching patients by putting them in the driver's seat was leading to much better outcomes. It felt right, stepping back and empowering the patients to make decisions about why, what, and how they would change. I was also building warmth and trust with them, making the visits very positive for both of us.

As my work life improved, so did my own health. I made the decision to leave that practice and toxic business partner. It has reinforced for me that health coaching, combined with foundational nursing concepts, is what our society needs. I know that through the coaching competency, I'm impacting people's lives and blazing a trail to better health outcomes. It has also established that when I'm taking care of myself, I'm a stronger advocate and role model for my patients. ◎

and Meleis (1994) remains relevant to the APRN guidance and coaching competency and contemporary interventions, often delivered by APRNs, designed to ensure smooth transitions for patients as they move across settings (e.g., Aging and Disability Resource Centers, 2011; Coleman & Berenson, 2004; Coleman & Boult, 2003).

Schumacher and Meleis (1994) defined the term *transition* as a passage from one life phase, condition, or status to another: "Transition refers to both the process and outcome of complex person-environment interactions. It may involve more than one person and is embedded in the context and the situation" (Chick & Meleis, 1986, pp. 239-240).

Transitions have been characterized according to type, conditions, and universal properties. Schumacher and Meleis (1994) have proposed four types of transitions—developmental, health and illness, situational, and organizational. Developmental transitions are those that reflect life cycle transitions, such as adolescence, parenthood, and aging. Health and illness transitions require not only adapting to an illness but more broadly reducing risk factors to prevent illness, changing unhealthy lifestyle behaviors, and numerous other clinical phenomena. Situational transitions are most likely to include changes in educational, work, and family roles. These can also result from changes in intangible or tangible structures or resources (e.g., loss of a relationship or financial reversals) (Schumacher & Meleis, 1994). Organizational transitions are those that occur in the environment: within agencies, between agencies, or in society. They reflect changes in structures and resources at a system level.

Developmental, health and illness, and situational transitions are the most likely to lead to clinical encounters requiring guidance and coaching. Successful outcomes of guidance and coaching related to transitions include subjective well-being, role mastery, and well-being of relationships, all components of quality of life (Schumacher & Meleis, 1994).

This description of transitions as a focus for APRNs underscores the need for and the importance of incorporating guidance and coaching into the APRN-patient therapeutic partnerships.

APRN Guidance and Coaching Skills

There are several important skills that must be in place to establish effective relationships. Chapter 7 presents a thorough discussion on communication with patients and with those who are unable to fully participate in verbal communication. These skills are necessary to be an effective APRN. Even though the skills noted in this section are part of basic nursing care, the following discussion of skills is described within the context of APRN guidance and coaching. Note that there is considerable interaction among the skills—they are interdependent and should be part of every APRN toolbox.

Listen

We listen every day. It is part of our ability as human beings (as long as our hearing is anatomically and physiologically intact). However, how often are we thinking of other things when someone is talking to us? We intend to give our attention to the patients we serve—but there is so much work to do and so many patients to see. Every aspect of patient care has to do with highly skilled listening: listening for energy, what the person wants or needs, resistance, choices made, and how choices move toward or away from goals. Coaching in particular requires that patients do most of the talking, with the APRN doing most of the listening. We could not adequately guide patients or do anticipatory teaching without knowing what the person already understands.

Rachel Naomi Remen (2006) is a pioneer of relationship-centered care and has noted, "The most basic and powerful way to connect with another person is to listen. Just listen. Perhaps the most important thing we give to each other is our attention" (p. 34). Listening is a foundational skill to both guidance and coaching and in any relationship. Listening is the process of understanding others and establishing trust in the relationship. Trust is the foundation of the APRN–patient therapeutic relationship.

There are several different taxonomies of listening. A useful classification described by Whitworth and colleagues (2007) includes three levels of listening (Fig. 8.3). The level 1 listener is tuned out, either ignoring the person talking or pretending to listen. This level is also referred to as internal listening, where the listening is all about the listener. Level 2 listening is selective, with the listener sometimes focusing but at times being distracted by his own inner dialogue. Level 2 listening has a sharper focus on the other person than level 1. In level 3, the APRN becomes a mirror in which the information is reflected back. This listening is collaborative, empathic, and clarifying. The APRN is unattached to his agenda and his own interests. Level 3 is empathic listening, representing the highest level, in which the listener gives time and attention to listening and gives her

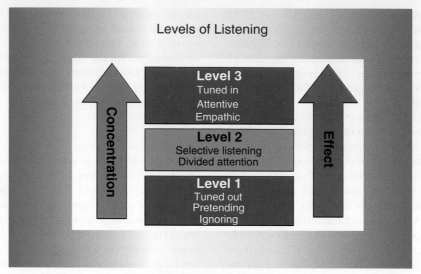

FIG 8.3 Levels of listening.

or his full self. Empathic listening is not only hearing what is said but also understanding the words, emotion, and meaning. It is considered "deep" listening or listening with the heart. Deep listening is hearing what is *not* said and includes tone of voice and nonverbal expressions. It is a global form of listening, in which one is using all the senses to listen, noticing gestures, the action, inaction, and interaction. It requires the APRN to be very open and softly focused without an agenda or judgment of any kind. Level 3 listening is often described as a force field with invisible radio waves in which only the skilled listener can receive the information, often unobservable to the untrained listener (Whitworth et al., 2007). Guiding and coaching require Level 3 listening in order to fully engage with the patient's baseline knowledge, goals, actions, and emotions. Suggestions for level 2 and 3 listening are:

- Stop talking!
- Relax for a minute prior to engaging with a patient by deep breathing, visualizing a pleasant memory that triggers relaxation.
- Review the health record prior to beginning a dialogue.
- Remove distractions and potential interruptions, and clear your head of intruding thoughts.
- Listen for the tone of the conversation as well as the words.
- Acknowledge what is said by reflecting and probing further.
- Ask powerful questions.

Literature reflecting the benefits of listening includes patient satisfaction with care, enhanced patient engagement in care planning, and improved health outcomes (Wentlandt et al., 2016). Listening is the most critical of skills for APRNs, as discussed in Chapter 7. There is no guidance or coaching without deep listening.

Build Strengths

There is an increasing recognition that building on patient strengths is a way for patients to gain confidence in their ability to change. The tendency in the past has been to focus on what is broken, not working, or what an individual does not do well. This is likely based on the medical model paradigm, that the health issues that a patient has are the result of not doing something or not doing something correctly, and that gap needs to be addressed. Rather than fixing what is broken, building on strengths can make the broken parts desiccate and shrink. For example, if a person has a great *appreciation for excellence* in their profession, that inherent skill can be applied to a weight loss journey by raising the quality of food they are ingesting or using *love of learning* to experiment with different strategies to manage their stress. A recent interprofessional summit was convened to identify that a major change that must occur in care delivery is to build on patient strengths to assist patients to achieve their goals (Swartwout, Drenkard, McGuinn, Grant, & El-Zein, 2016).

The recent focus on building strengths is based on seminal research by Peterson and Seligman (2004), who demonstrated the benefit of assessing and using people's strengths in making and sustaining change in a person's life. There are years of research showing the benefits of building on strengths (Values in Action [VIA] Institute on Character, 2016). The Classification of Strengths is an important tool that has been used in a growing body of evidence since the mid-1990s (Peterson & Park, 2009). This classification has six "virtues"—wisdom and knowledge, courage, humanity, justice, temperance, and transcendence. In addition, there are 24 characteristics within the overall classification (Table 8.2). Although the research has not been specific to health care, there are clearly applications to health promotion by assessing and then building on patients' strengths for a healthier future.

Building on strengths has become an approach broadly used in health coaching (Exemplar 8.4). Confidence gained from building on strengths helps individuals to not only deploy those strengths toward achieving their goals but to also work on areas to be developed. Often people do not recognize their strengths, and the initial work of the APRN is to help the patient identify her strengths. There are strengths assessments available online that have strong validity profiles. One example is the VIA Survey of Character Strengths, which can be found at http://www.viacharacter.org/www/Character-Strengths-Survey. If there is no formal VIA assessment, the APRN can help the patient recognize his or her strengths to build on by asking:

- "Tell me about a challenge that you feel you successfully managed."
- "What would your friends and family say were the best parts about you?"
- "What strengths helped you be successful?"
- "How would you describe your strengths to create the change you want to make?"

APRNs can incorporate strength finding into any visit. Identifying strengths could take place during the history or physical examination. APRNs already respect, value, and engage with each patient, and identifying and building on their strengths will help in the APRN efforts to build capacity to relate well to patients.

Cultivate Unconditional Positive Regard

At times we may be frustrated with a patient because she or he does not follow advice or adhere to a care plan. There are patients whose political philosophy may be different, who may be racist, who like to smoke, and who are highly resistant to change. There may be patients who are difficult to relate to. Having unconditional positive regard (UPR) for all people does not mean we have to like every patient. Mearns (1994) noted that liking someone is based on shared values and complimentary needs and is therefore conditional. However, it is especially important to have UPR for all patients and particularly for those we find most frustrating. UPR is essential to building a trusting and effective relationship.

Being completely accepting toward another person, without reservations (UPR), is a concept developed by the psychologist Carl Rogers. He proposed that each individual has vast resources to marshal for self-understanding and self-directed behavior but an interpersonal climate of positive regard was necessary to facilitate this (Rogers, 1961). Joseph (2012) defined UPR as "valuing the person as doing their best to move forward in their lives constructively and respecting the person's right to self-determination no matter what they choose to do" (p. 1 on website). It is about accepting a person as he or she is and without judgment. It has been the basis for patient-centered therapy. It is important to note that UPR also includes setting boundaries by creating clarity of expectations in the relationship. Examples of boundaries linked to UPR include not supporting hurtful behaviors or being treated disrespectfully as an APRN. Each APRN needs to establish her or his own set of boundaries and clarify and maintain them with her or his patients.

TABLE 8.2	The Classification of Human Strengths
Values in Action Classification of Strengths	
6 Virtues	**24 Characteristics**
1. Wisdom and Knowledge	creativity, curiosity, judgment, love of learning, perspective
2. Courage	bravery, perseverance, honesty, zest
3. Humanity	love, kindness, social intelligence
4. Justice	teamwork, fairness, leadership
5. Temperance	forgiveness, humility, prudence, self-regulation
6. Transcendence	appreciation of beauty and excellence, gratitude, hope, humor, spirituality

From Peterson, C., & Seligman, M. (2004). *Character strengths and virtues: A handbook and classification.* Washington, DC: APA Press/Oxford, England: Oxford University Press.

Deborah McElligott, DNP, HWNC-BC

Setting: Nurse practitioner (NP) private coaching practice.

Issue: Marie's Narrative: Marie is a 35-year-old female who comes to the office to see what a "coaching session" entails. She has a history of migraines, obesity, prediabetes, and fatigue. She is married, works full time, and has two children under the age of 7. Her migraine pain ranges from 5 to 8 (scale of 1 to 10), with nausea and occasional vomiting; the symptoms are worse with stress and relieved by her "additional migraine medication" and lying down, but followed by a day of fatigue and dull 2- to 4-level pain. The frequency ranges from three times a week to once a month, with no identifiable pattern. Marie has seen multiple specialists over the last 20 years, including her primary care physician, neurologist, pain specialist, allergist, and chiropractor. Her laboratory values are normal with the exception of an elevated hemoglobin A_{1c} (5.7%). Her body mass index was 30 and her body fat was 42%.

Session 1

Marie scheduled a 1-hour appointment with the NP for a coaching session after reading an article linking lifestyle to migraines. The NP prepared for the appointment by reviewing the questionnaires Marie completed online and then doing a brief centering exercise before Marie entered the room. During the introductions, the NP described the coaching process and asked Marie what she was hoping for (eliciting the agenda). She described her need to lose weight in order to have the energy to care for her family and complete her responsibilities at work. She was fearful of "diabetes" because she has a family history (personal motivators). Although she has had migraines for 15 years, her increased responsibilities have made coping with them more difficult (awareness raised about the link to stress). The NP reflected that Marie did have a lot on her plate. Marie was clearly ready to make changes but didn't know where to begin (moving from contemplation to preparation).

The NP asked if she could share what others in her situation have done and Marie was interested. The NP shared that some patients have found a relationship between food, stress, and headaches, receiving some relief by following an elimination food plan. Marie said she tried everything—she had been to an allergist,

nutritionist, Weight Watchers. She did lose some weight, but her headaches didn't improve (resistance emerging).

The NP recognized the success Marie had in the past and focused on her strengths. Marie acknowledged that she did feel lighter and had more energy with the weight loss. But her most recent attempt at Weight Watchers failed and her migraines didn't decrease. She was willing to try anything.

The NP asked if she could review the elimination food plan (a chart of healthy foods to eat while eliminating dairy and gluten) and a food log planner (chart to log food, activity, migraine, sleep, bowel movement, and stress) with her and Marie agreed. The NP identified that the purpose for the tracking was for Marie to be able to identify any patterns that existed. Marie said she had done all these things in the past but not together. She said she would do this, she was ready to try and would "complete the log sheet each day and eat only the foods on the chart for 2 weeks."

The NP asked how confident she was that she could do this (on a scale of 1 to 10) and Marie replied 5. She felt it was easy enough but that stress either at work or at home may trigger her to eat the wrong food. The NP asked what would make it a 7. Marie replied that if she could control her stress, she would be more confident in her plan. On questioning, Marie preferred to run to reduce stress, but identified that running is not an option at work or when caring for the kids, so she eats. The NP asked if Marie wanted to try a short meditation and she agreed. After a 5-minute practice, Marie replied that she felt relaxed and was confident that she could incorporate this into her plan—she said she almost felt like she had had a nap. At the end of the session, Marie agreed to log her food, eliminate dairy and gluten (for 1 week), and do 5 minutes of meditation 4 days a week (actions/goal setting). She was going to be accountable to the NP and come back in 1 week to review the plan and see if patterns emerged. Her new confidence level rose to a 7 of 10.

Sessions 2–7

Marie returned for weekly visits. On week 2 she had only one migraine, improved sleep, and success with her meditation—she logged everything on her weekly log sheet and noted an extremely busy day prior to her migraine. Over the next 3 weeks she continued on the elimination plan as her energy increased and her cravings for sugar decreased. The NP explored her next goals and Marie wanted to decrease her migraine

Patient Seeking Coaching for Obesity, Prediabetes, and Migraine Pain—cont'd

medications. The NP asked her to speak to her neurologist before she made any medication changes. Marie also wanted to begin an exercise plan—she already belonged to a gym, and set a goal to exercise 3 times a week for 30 minutes prior to going to work. The NP asked if she would begin to reintroduce dairy or gluten but Marie did not want to. She continued on the elimination plan with an occasional "cheat day."

Session 8
By week 8 Marie had been successful in meeting her activity goal, food goal, meditation, and food log. She decreased her migraine medication to half the dose, had an average of two migraines a month, and didn't

need any additional medication to control them. She felt better, her clothes were looser, and people noticed a difference in her appearance, even though she had only lost 1 pound. She became aware that she was building muscle. The NP summarized all the changes she had made as they compared her initial evaluations to the most recent one, seeing a dramatic decrease in symptoms. Her A_{1c} was 5.6%. She was less stressed and had more energy. She was determined to stay on her routine and was comfortable introducing small amounts of gluten on special occasions. Marie continues to follow up with her medical team, feeling empowered by her efforts. ◎

Cultivate a Culture of Empathy

Carl Rogers built on Maslow's hierarchy of needs by adding that in order for a person to "grow," she or he needs acceptance, genuineness, and empathy. Rogers believed that each person can achieve his or her deepest desires in life and achieve self-actualization, but that empathy helps foster that growth, just the way that a seed needs soil and water. His greatest contribution was in his study of accurate empathy and its role in the growth of humans. He described empathy as an underappreciated way of being and posited that accurate empathy is "being one with the patient in the here and now, being highly sensitive to their experience and their world" (p. 34). He stressed that listening is not a passive endeavor because active listening can bring about changes in people's attitudes toward themselves. People who experience accurate empathy and are listened to in this way become more emotionally mature, more open, and less defensive (Rogers, 1961). There is increasing recognition and evidence that provider–patient relationships, the quality of their communications, and accurate empathy influence quality, safety, and health outcomes (Price, Elliott, Zaslavsky, et al., 2014).

The upcoming section in this chapter on "Self-Knowledge as an APRN" focuses on the skills essential to cultivating a culture of empathy.

Create a Safe Environment

Creating a safe environment includes deep listening, unconditional positive regard, and other elements of presence. A patient must feel physically and

psychologically safe in order to fully engage in a relationship. We often take for granted that people seek health care and trust APRNs to do the best for them simply because we are credentialed health care providers. However, they often feel that they must "please us" rather than be honest about their concerns. Pleasing a provider is deeply rooted in patient behavior. Patients want their APRN to like them. They may be afraid that the APRN will be angry or judgmental of them if they are challenging or have not adhered to a treatment plan, so they may tell APRNs what they think we want to hear.

Patients' desire to please is ultimately derived from a fear that if the provider does not like them, they will not get good care. There are reasons for patients wanting APRNs to like them based on a vast literature related to prejudice and bias. Currently, more attention is being paid to implicit (unconscious) bias as a contributing factor in health disparities in the United States. One definition of implicit bias is "attitudes or stereotypes that affect our understanding, actions, and decisions in an unconscious manner" (Kirwan Institute, 2015). Everyone has implicit biases. Kahneman (2011) included a summary of research that has taken place on bias in his book *Thinking Fast and Slow*. Biases are not only based on race, ethnicity, or religion but may be based on manner of dress, weight, gender, political views, and other issues. And they may be based on how we perceive the behavior of a patient as a patient. Is the patient deferential? Is he or she personable? Is she or he a complainer?

We often give subtle messages of greater acceptance when patients are "compliant" and of nonacceptance if they are not. That message can be conveyed simply through a smile or frown. APRNs in a coaching mode need to invite open conversation and let patients know that it is safe for them to challenge and to be honest about their issues. Creating the safe environment will support having a truthful conversation with the APRN far above any kind of approval-seeking by the patient.

In addition to establishing safety within a relationship, there are considerations about establishing safety in the environment. A room with "thin walls" that is sterile and unpleasant may inhibit a patient from feeling safe. Creating an inviting and accepting environment can be a challenge but one that is worth the time. Having pictures on the wall, freshly painted rooms with privacy, and places to comfortably sit are critical to establishing an environment of safety. Some health care services have to manage the potential of physical violence in creating safe places. Accomplishing this in any clinical space will require engaging many different people in order to invest in creating a safe physical environment. Paying attention to the environment tells patients that you care about them. The space in which we engage patients needs to match the eloquence of the conversations we are having with them on a daily basis.

Self-Knowledge as an APRN

An important element of integrating guidance and coaching into APRN clinical practice is knowing yourself as a person (see Chapter 7). This differentiates coaching from mentoring, consulting and advising, and motivational interviewing. Although we want to form relationships with our patients that lead to highly important, impactful, and meaningful outcomes, each of us has a unique understanding of others and of ourselves. Being an effective APRN requires staying open and teachable to new learning and self-reflection to continue to grow. Learning not only includes staying current with emerging health care evidence but, perhaps most importantly, knowing ourselves and growing personally and professionally.

McLean (2012) has formulated a model of self that applies to the APRN. She identifies six areas of self-knowledge that are useful in optimizing the role as coach: presence, empathetic stance, boundary awareness, somatic awareness, range of feelings, and courage to challenge.

Presence

How well honed is your ability to be present? Thich Nhat Hah (2015), a Buddhist philosopher, has said, "The most precious gift we can give others is our presence." In a guiding or coaching relationship, presence is not only a gift but a prerequisite to being a full partner. The International Coach Federation defines coaching presence as the "ability to be fully conscious and create [a] spontaneous relationship with the client, employing a style that is open, flexible and confident" (ICF, 2016b). This definition uses the word "fully conscious"; others may use the words "fully aware" or "mindful." Some people equate the words "mindful" and "presence." A definition of mindfulness is noted by Bazarko (2013), a nurse working in the area of mindfulness. She writes, "Mindfulness means to purposefully pay attention in the present moment with a sense of acceptance and nonjudgment" (p. 109). The commonality of both definitions is paying attention and being fully conscious. Presence requires mindfulness and mindfulness requires presence.

Being present is foundational to building a trusting relationship with the patient (see Chapter 7). McLean (2012) points out that a useful way to think about presence and coaching is being alert to "what's being said, what's not being said, what's being acted out, what's observable somatically and what's a pattern you have observed before" (p. 26). In other words, being present means coming to the relationship with listening at levels 2 and 3 as described earlier in the "Listen" section.

There are two common pitfalls to being present that relate to APRNs: external distractions and the well-honed ability to try and anticipate what the patient needs. We are often physically present, but our minds tend to jump from one thought to another. When you are with a patient, you may be thinking about the patient you just saw, your frustration with one of your colleagues, or getting your child to basketball practice. When you take the time to be aware of what you think during a patient visit, you may be astounded by how many thoughts unrelated to the patient enter your mind.

In addition to the challenges of our work environment, we have deeply rooted ways of thinking as APRNs to anticipate patient problems. (See Chapter 7 for a discussion on thinking errors in practice.) We have been taught that we need to have answers for problems so we can fix a problem and thereby fix a patient. We think ahead of what we hear from the patient. Once we start anticipating, we have stopped being present. We need to slow our thinking and follow what the patient is saying. This is a fundamental challenge to the APRN coach. The art of nurse coaching is to develop the ability to set aside distractions—including jumping ahead in problem solving, which often leads to misdiagnosis and care that is not patient centered—and engage fully in the moment with the patient.

Presence can be enhanced through practice, which can take place at any time. It may be useful to start the day with 5 minutes of doing nothing or to spend 1 minute doing nothing before seeing each patient. Practice being aware of when you are not present and bring yourself back to being present. When you find you are not present, do not consider that a failure, just bring yourself back to being present. Practice at home and at work. The more you practice being present, the easier it will be to achieve. Both you and your patients will benefit.

Empathic Stance

To what extent are you able to be empathic? Empathy has been described as being able to walk in another person's shoes and is foundational to nursing and coaching. It is the ability to understand and share the feelings of another. This requires knowing the boundaries of your empathy, which can range from one extreme of accepting a patient's emotions as your emotions to the other extreme of failing to recognize a patient's emotional status altogether. Although empathy is woven into basic nursing, as we get pressed for time and get frustrated by demands of patients, exhibiting empathy requires constant vigilance.

Although we accept empathy as an emotional state, there is increasing understanding of the neurophysiology of empathy. Research beginning in the mid-1990s has led to identifying neural networks of "mirror neurons" that may explain the capacity for empathy (Rizzolatti & Craighero, 2004). Mirror neurons are activated by both the action of an individual and the observation of a similar action performed by another (Lamm & Majdandzic, 2015; Preston & de Waal, 2002). It appears that mirror neural pathways extend to multiple structures in the brain based on the stimuli producing the effect. A possible explanation for empathy is that when we are listening to and looking at a patient, our mirror neurons are activated as if we are experiencing what the patient is doing or experiencing. With ongoing research into mirror neurons, there is great promise to better understand the neural activation that forms and supports relationships and how feelings are experienced.

One way of expanding empathy is to record a visit with a patient and reflect on the content of the visit. Ask yourself if you were listening and able to reflect back to the patient your understanding of the feelings the patient was experiencing. Were you able to walk in that patient's shoes? The more experiences that we personally have in a variety of situations, particularly with illness and encounters with the health care system, enables us to better understand patient experiences.

Boundary Awareness

Do you know your boundaries with your patients? The concept of boundary awareness in coaching is founded on the initial work of Kerr and Bowen (1988) on self-differentiation within the context of family. The concept of self-differentiation can be extended to any unit of people and is explained by Kerr and Bowen (1988), who state, "The more differentiated a self, the more a person can be an individual while in emotional contact with the group" (p. 235). The important concept in Bowen's theory is centered on differentiation with the extreme of emotional fusion in which a coach would become part of the patient's system, experiencing the patient's feelings and needs. In an APRN coaching relationship, there is a fine line between boundaries that are too tight and those that are too loose, and it can be a significant challenge to maintain a coaching balance. To be more aware of boundaries, pay attention to situations in which you feel stressed. Reflect on the sources of stress related to how you are establishing boundaries. Another exercise in clarifying boundaries is to be aware of feelings of resentment, discomfort, and/ or guilt (Gionta & Guerra, 2015). If you experience these feelings within a patient relationship, it is time to reset boundaries.

Somatic Awareness

Can you identify the physical expression of your emotional discomfort? Somatic awareness refers to the physical feelings and behaviors experienced while working with a patient, such as tightening of stomach muscles, pulling at strands of hair, or crossing of the arms. Silsbee (2008, p. 154) offers the insight that "sensation provides an early warning system of our habits." There may be times when you are feeling very "relaxed" and you may need to draw your attention to your level of listening and presence. You also have physical manifestations when you are feeling like you are getting into uncomfortable emotional territory. Some people may feel a physical tenseness, while others may clench their teeth or cross their arms. Whatever the reaction may be, it is important to be aware of the somatic feeling in order to make adjustments, such as taking deep breaths or mentally calming yourself for effective APRN guidance and coaching. A technique that may be useful to enhance somatic awareness is using Silsbee's (2008) "body scan" approach. Starting with the feet and, moving up your body, scan for physical responses to a situation. This can be done quickly—in a few seconds.

Range of Feelings

Are you aware of your comfort level with a wide range of feelings for both yourself and the patient? Being comfortable with the breadth (e.g., anxiety, anger, fear, happiness, sadness) and intensity of your feelings in relation to those of patients is essential to give patients the opportunity to talk about their feelings. If a patient senses your discomfort with anxiety, she will not talk about it. Transformational change for patients occurs at the emotional level, and the APRN coach will only be able to support this by recognizing and accepting his or her own feelings in order to accept those of the patient. A patient with newly diagnosed breast cancer or who is having unexpected triplets will have a range of feelings, and if the APRN is not comfortable with the patient's feelings, the patient will feel inhibited to share those feelings.

To get a better understanding of one's own feelings when interacting with a patient, use root cause analysis applied to the exploration. Create some mental space (between patients) and keep asking yourself why you were experiencing your feelings. This can take you to a deep level toward understanding your feelings. It is also useful to pay attention to triggers. When you note a particular feeling while guiding or coaching, reflect on what might have contributed to that feeling.

Courage to Challenge

Are you comfortable challenging a patient? The APRN coach must be willing to challenge a patient in order to help move the patient forward. While it is important to maintain a good working relationship, wanting to be liked may interfere with the effectiveness of challenging a patient's view or with interpretation of situations, beliefs, or values. Patients often get "stuck," and respectfully challenging them to think differently or see themselves or their situation differently can get them "unstuck" (Moore & Tschannen-Moran, 2010). Challenging patients is a way of deepening awareness and forwarding action by making a request or suspending a belief. For example, a challenge might be, "Could I challenge you to 30 days with no sugar?" or "What would it be like to approach this situation without any fear or anxiety,

instead cultivating calm confidence?" One useful way of maintaining an effective APRN therapeutic relationship while challenging the patient is to inquire about feedback. Ask the patient if the conversation was useful, what part was most helpful, and what created discomfort. In challenging, make sure patients know that you are fully with them on their journey and that the point of the journey is to create change.

APRN Proficiencies Specific to Coaching

Ask Permission

Although nursing is a wonderful blend of science, technology, and caring, nurses have a strong drive to make people better, whatever the specific situation. APRNs have embraced the idea of holistic health care and are empathic with patients, but there continues to be an attitude that providers know what is best for patients. Integrating coaching into practice requires a culture shift and a change in personal philosophy and approach to caring for patients. To effectively integrate coaching into personal beliefs as well as the practice culture, there are many small actions that can support stronger APRN encounters.

A crucial first step is asking permission from each person prior to initiating a coaching conversation. Asking permission, such as "May I coach you on this?" or "Is it okay for me to explore this with you further?," is a way of respecting boundaries. Asking permission also demonstrates to the person that he or she has a choice and power in the relationship (Kimsey-House, et al, 2011) . If the patient decides against coaching, the APRN should move to providing guidance as part of basic care.

Support Small Changes

Although big change is often desired, small changes are what create forward movement. Nearly everyone at some time has intentions to lead a healthier life by making adjustments in lifestyle. Each New Year millions of resolutions fall by the wayside because we try to take big leaps to change behaviors and then realize a big leap is too difficult.

When coaching a patient, there is a tendency by both APRN and patient to jump to big interventions. Well-intentioned patients may want to initiate major interventions to manage their health but they overestimate the change they can realistically make in their lives. Overestimating the ability to make lifestyle changes can then be demoralizing when the changes are not successful. Often, a patient will commit to making a change in order to please the APRN but cannot follow through.

Having patients consider small changes may produce bigger and more lasting results. According to Seligman (2011), humans are more likely to achieve their goals if they have early success. Success breeds success, with small changes being easier to integrate into a lifestyle. A person trying to lose a few pounds may believe that a strict diet is mandatory, requiring considerable changes, such as how food is purchased and prepared, who does the preparation, limiting food intake, and changing social patterns to adhere to the diet. However, as a coach you can work with your patient to make a small change, such as taking a walk to add exercise or decreasing the amount of liquid low-nutrient calories. Small changes are part of a larger process of change. Patients can be coached to do one intervention, and once that is integrated into their lives, additional small changes can be added. These small changes can add up to major lifestyle changes.

Although small changes can have a big impact and are a useful start for lifestyle change, there may be patients who need to decide on a big change in their lives, such as having bariatric surgery to achieve weight loss, or leaving a toxic relationship.

Be Curious

Perhaps one of the most useful coaching tools is to be curious (Moore & Tschannen-Moran, 2010). Being curious will provide the foundation for asking questions—and likely the right questions. Patients nearly always give clues as to what is on their minds—but may not be direct. One should follow with up with questions such as "I wonder what … means to you?" or "I am curious about what you just said that …." These very simple questions based on curiosity often net a rich conversation and help bring out issues that are important to patients. In a time-constrained environment, APRNs may feel inhibited from opening any doors to topics that they may not be able to pursue with patients. However, not opening the door deprives patients of being able to talk about what is really important to them, and opportunities to positively impact their life are missed.

Getting to the Feelings

Change happens when people understand and incorporate the need for change at an emotional level. Although knowledge of data is helpful, it is usually only a starting point because the knowledge

alone usually does not create transformative change. In coaching patients, it is important to get to the emotional meaning of their issues (Stober & Grant, 2006). Naming emotional feelings is a driver for motivation to change. Exploring feelings related to change links mindfulness and contemplation to taking action.

A universal response to change—even change we believe we should make—is resistance. We create reasons for or exceptions to why we cannot change, such as, "It's too hard," "I don't really like/need/want to do this," or "I've tried before and failed." A major reason for resistance to change is simply fear—fear of not being successful, fear of what other people may think, and many other types of fears. As an APRN, having a trusting relationship with your patients can help them name and understand their fears and other feelings about change.

Getting to the feelings has boundaries. This does not mean getting to feelings that relate to psychopathology or feelings related to issues that require counseling. Naming/identifying feelings should not be focused on the past, such as on past relationships with family members, but on the present and future. It is about getting to the feelings related to the present circumstances creating the need for change, the change process itself, and the potential outcome. The following statements can be used to get to feelings:

- "Tell me about how you feel when you think about (or talk about)…."
- "Knowing how you feel about … is important to me."

APRN Coaching Process

Although the skills noted in the previous section are critical to being an effective APRN coach, bringing the coaching process into practice is the foundation of coaching. The process includes assessing the readiness of the patient to engage in change, preparation to make the change, taking action, and finally maintaining the change (Fig. 8.4).

Patient Readiness

In order to be coached, the patient must be functionally able, creative, and resourceful. Therefore most people in the general population are appropriate to receive/participate in coaching. If an APRN is considering using coaching, the patient must first be deemed well enough to imagine a better future for herself. Consequently, coaching will not be productive

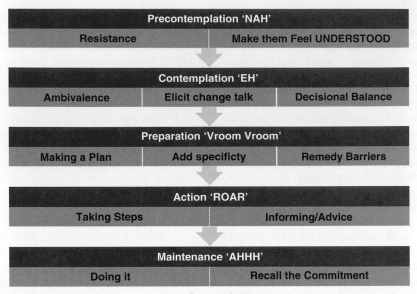

Precontemplation 'NAH'	
Resistance	Make them Feel UNDERSTOOD

Contemplation 'EH'		
Ambivalence	Elicit change talk	Decisional Balance

Preparation 'Vroom Vroom'		
Making a Plan	Add specificty	Remedy Barriers

Action 'ROAR'	
Taking Steps	Informing/Advice

Maintenance 'AHHH'	
Doing it	Recall the Commitment

FIG 8.4 Stages of change.

with people who cannot envision a different future. Explicitly, those who are severely mentally ill, psychotic, manic, severely depressed, suicidal, inebriated, obtunded, demented, or high or who are in a severe emotional state such as acute grief or trauma are not appropriate to engage in a coaching partnership. People with mental illness or in an acute intense emotional state are best engaged with empathy and guidance. A simple way to determine if a person is coachable is to ask the individual to describe his or her life in the future, if everything went as well as it possibly could for her or him. If the person cannot articulate an answer, the APRN should not enter into a coaching dialogue, but instead work with him or her to be able to envision a future, healthier life.

After rapport has been developed and some degree of empathy expressed, the APRN must determine the person's readiness for change. The person's stage of change in any given self-defeating lifestyle must be documented in the health record for the entire health care team to use and build on, measure progress, and guide interventions. According to Norcross (2013), only about 30% of the general population seen in health care is in the "Action (making changes)" stage (Fig. 8.5). Staging people is a necessary first step to any coaching encounter because it drives the skilled conversation. Taking the time to assess where the person is in the change process sets the stage for a deeper, more meaningful, and more effective encounter.

Resistance

When people are resistant, they are saying they will not change, they have no plans to change in the near future, or they are wholly not interested in changing. The main task for the APRN in working with people who are resistant to change is to help them *feel understood.* These interactions need not take a great deal of time, and the patient should leave the APRN with the feeling of being understood, that the APRN "gets me." The challenge for the APRN is to see how the self-defeating patient activity serves a larger purpose in the patient's life and to offer a partnership statement for the future, such as "I can see how smoking makes you feel like you are making your own decisions in your life and how important that is to you. If you ever want to quit, come back and we can work together for you to stop smoking." Specific advice at this stage can drive resisters deeper into resistance. If a patient is not interested in being coached, guidance can be offered as a more passive way for the patient to be engaged.

Contemplation

APRNs most often see patients when they are in the contemplation phase. It is the place of ambivalence, where they both want to change but do not want to. Advice at this stage can be harmful. Instead, the APRN should determine personal motivators and bring forth the emotional conflict the person is experiencing. The APRN should approach the person

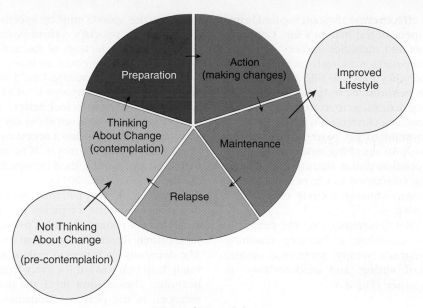

FIG 8.5 Stages of change.

in ambivalence with a neutral stance, without pushing. To determine his readiness for change, using questions such as "Why is this important? Why now? What if you did nothing and stay on this course—what is your future like in 10 years?" can move the person to identify personal motivators. The key task in this stage is to arouse emotions and encourage people to start talking about their ambivalence.

Preparation

Once a patient moves to the preparation phase, the task of the APRN is to identify barriers and develop remedies for these obstacles in partnership with the patient. With many life changes, it is important to set a start date and prepare the environment for change, such as finding an exercise partner or identifying impulse control techniques. Suggestions, gently offered, can be helpful in this stage as long as the APRN has no strong ownership in the person's willingness to adopt a specific suggestion.

Action

Action is when the patient is actively engaged in making a lifestyle change. This stage is one in which direct advice and guidance is most helpful. Brainstorming on strategies to overcome obstacles and what to do in the event of a short-term lapse (a one-time re-emergence of an unwanted behavior)

or relapse (fully reverting back to prior behavior) are important conversations. A common technique is to create "if, … then" scenarios. For example, if a patient was working to reverse her or his type 2 diabetes and was excluding sugar from his or her diet, she or he could plan that *if* he or she ingests sugar, *then* she or he gets right back to avoiding sugar at the next meal. Anticipating setbacks and having remedies planned for lapses and relapses are crucial during the action stage (Norcross, 2013).

Maintenance

Maintenance often requires the APRN to acknowledge the patient's success, and to ask about how the patient holds himself or herself accountable, how he or she manages lapses, and what he or she would do if a relapse occurred. When a patient experiences a full relapse, she or he reverts to consistently exhibiting old behaviors. The APRN must determine where the patient is in the cycle of change again (e.g., are they in resistance vs. contemplation, or are they back in action?). It is important for the APRN to approach change as a process and to be aware that having setbacks can be common for some people.

The "Four *A*s" of the Coaching Process

According to Rogers (2012), coaching is a partnership of equals whose aim is to achieve speedy, increased, and sustainable effectiveness through focused learning on some aspect of the patient's life. Coaching raises awareness and identifies choices, with the APRN coach and patient working from the patient's agenda. Together they have the sole aim of closing the gap between performance and potential. A crucial first step is asking permission from each person prior to initiating a coaching conversation. As noted previously, it is important to get permission from the patient to move into coaching mode. Initiating a coaching conversation differs sharply from shared decision making (discussed in Chapter 7), in that APRNs hand control almost entirely over to the patient in coaching.

Once the APRN determines that the person is appropriate for coaching, a four-step coaching methodology—agenda setting, awareness raising, actions and goal setting, and accountability—is followed in sequence (Fig. 8.6).

Agenda Setting

Agenda setting, and the broader coaching methodology, requires handing over control and the choice of topic to the patient. The APRN elicits the agenda (the topic the patient wants to discuss) from the patient and the APRN and patient work together to address the patient's agenda. For example, the APRN may say, "You have a lot of things going on with you and we have 15 minutes together today. What would be most useful for you to have accomplished when our time together is done?" *Allow for silence* because this is a powerful question in and of itself. The patient may struggle with that question, and the APRN may need to ask more probing questions;

however, the agenda must be specific, measurable, and within the patient's control. Agendas cannot be centered around feelings or the actions of others. Acceptable agendas could include, "I need a plan for managing sugar cravings" or "I want to be able to manage the colostomy myself," while unacceptable agendas are "I want to feel better" or "I want my wife to have more concern about my pain." Eliciting and clarifying the agenda is a necessary and important step in the coaching process. If no agenda is determined by the patient, then no coaching can occur (Kimsey-House et al., 2011).

Focusing on the patient's agenda is a sharp departure from what is typically provided by APRNs in the form of patient education because the encounter is entirely directed toward what the patient wants. The decisions each person makes, no matter how small, lead him toward (or away from) a life that is healthier. Thus at some level, the patient agenda is wrapped in the person's fundamental values and truth.

Awareness Raising

Awareness raising requires challenging the patient's mindset and assumptions about an issue with which she is struggling. It requires skillful inquiry in which the APRN adopts a highly curious approach to understand what and how the patient thinks about an issue. Awareness is raised by asking powerful questions (Table 8.3) that have likely never been asked of the patient and require deep reflection. This phase of coaching generally is the most time consuming. As the APRN builds coaching skills, it can be helpful to have five powerful questions that are used regularly to begin an inquiry. During the awareness phase, the APRN is using deep listening skills, watching for nonverbal messages. The APRN may become aware of the moment in which the patient has a major insight or makes new connections. The APRN can identify when awareness has been raised because there may be more silence and the patient will begin to identify changes he or she wants to make.

Actions and Goal Setting

The APRN asks the patient what she or he wants to do and when he or she wants to do it. Goals flow directly from the awareness raised, which arouses emotions, and the patient has a higher degree of self-efficacy in pursuing the goal(s). If the patient seems stuck on developing a solution, the APRN

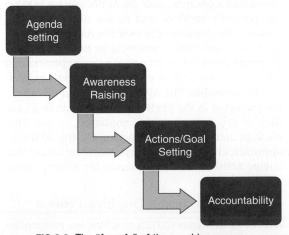

FIG 8.6 The "four *A*s" of the coaching process.

TABLE 8.3	Coaching Phases, APRN Skills, and Examples of Questions for Patients	
Coaching Phase	**APRN Skill**	**Examples**
Agenda elicited	Excavate what is most meaningful	What is most important/meaningful/helpful to you at this time?
	Clarify needs	What do you need from our time together?
Awareness raised	Ask powerful questions	What are you **not** willing give up?
	Shift consciousness	If you say "YES" to *X*, what do you say "NO" to?
	Let the person do most of the talking	What's working well in this situation?
	Explore assumptions with curiosity	Who do you need to become to make it happen?
	Promote "generative moments"	What do you want to see happen?
		What do you want to be held accountable for?
		What do you most value about yourself?
		What would your life be like if you were not *(name limitation)*?
		What is your deepest desire for yourself?
Actions/Goal setting	Link raised awareness to specific goals to forward into action	What do you want to do and when do you want to do it?
		On a scale of 1 to 10, how successful do you think you will be?
	Brainstorm	What is going to get in your way?
	Determine self-efficacy	What is the remedy to that obstacle?
	Challenge if the person could do more (gently and once)	Can I challenge you to … (do more)?
Accountability	Help person use resources, not pursue goals alone	How do you want to be accountable?
	Partner with supportive others	What will you do if you go off your plan?
	Use technology	What is your "when-then" plan?
	Confirm agenda met	Did you get what you needed today?

can set up a brainstorming exercise in which the patient and APRN take turns coming up with a list of ideas/solutions. The key competency in brainstorming is to not allow the patient to judge the ideas until they are all laid out. Once the goals or actions are determined, the APRN must determine *self-efficacy* (the belief a person has in herself or himself to complete a task). The APRN asks, "On a scale of 1 to 10, how successful are you likely to be in doing this (10 = success)?" If the chosen number is less than 7, the goal must be modified. Success breeds success, so as any adult embarks on a change process, it is important to have early successes. During this phase of the coaching, the APRN is letting the patient talk. The APRN may need to ask clarifying questions to make the patient's goal more specific. If the APRN has a sense the patient could do more, he or she can *challenge* the patient. This skill is only used during the goal-setting phase and when the APRN thinks the patient could do more. For example, if the patient commits to ambulating down the hall once a day, the APRN can challenge him or her to do so 3 times a day. The patient will respond to the challenge in one of three ways: (1) agree to it, (2) reject it, or (3) modify it. It is crucial that the APRN accepts fully however the patient responds and challenges the patient no further.

Accountability

The final step in the coaching method is determined by the APRN asking, "How do you want to hold yourself accountable?" Ideally, it is best to use the patient's own resources to achieve accountability, such as relatives, coworkers, or apps. The APRN could offer himself or herself as a way to hold a patient accountable, but it must not present *any* burden to the APRN. Accountability could be in the form of an email, text, or follow-up visit. It is important in this phase to have the patient outline a plan if the goals are not being met; this may include developing "when-then" strategies such as "When a week goes by and I haven't done what I said I would, I will reschedule with you" (Rogers, 2012).

The Dilemma of Guiding or Leading From Behind

Shifting into APRN coaching practice will require the APRN to learn when coaching will be useful and when patient education is most appropriate. Health care information is now easily accessible, and social networks such as PatientsLikeMe (www.patientslikeme.com) significantly alter the needs of patients. An increase in customization, translation, and wisdom is needed for patients who have difficulty seeing their way forward. Applying the right intervention at the right time for patients receptivity to change is critical. The right intervention may likely be a combination of guidance and coaching.

Building Coaching Into Practice

Although building coaching into APRN practice is largely based on integrating the skills and mindset of coaching as a way of relating to patients, there are small things that the APRN can do to integrate coaching into practice. Some examples of building coaching into the structure and process of care include:

- Collecting information from patients while they are in the waiting room or waiting in the examination room that is related to their goals for the visit. Questions on an intake form could include:
  - What are your current goals for maintaining or managing your health?
  - Do you feel you are committed to pursuing these goals?
  - What makes these goals important to you now?
- Focusing on the patient's goals and ask what would be useful from the APRN to move toward achieving those goals.
- Establishing a section in the medical record that summarizes the patient's goals, actions, and follow-up plan. If using an electronic health record, there may need to be negotiation with the service provider to integrate this information into the record.
- Creating a safe and welcoming environment in the examination rooms using pictures, soft colors, and other visuals that are comforting.

There are several useful resources that include sample coaching contracts, exercises to practice skills, and other useful materials (Donna & Wheeler, 2009; Dossey et al., 2015; Hudson Institute, 2016).

Conclusion

Guidance and coaching are effective, rewarding, and critical skills to bring to patient care. APRNs are providers who have already integrated the value of patient-centered care, and guidance and coaching brings the focus of care to the patient's goals,

preferences, and abilities. Guidance is different from coaching in that it is directive and values patient education. Guidance relies on the APRN as the expert. Coaching is focused on goals established by the patient and assists the patient to understand and use his or her capacity to achieve those goals. Although many APRNs have built guidance and coaching into their practice, there is a need to have all APRNs examine their mental model of interacting with patients to build on the guidance and coaching processes and skills and partner with patients to help them create healthy change. Guidance and coaching are necessary skills for all APRNs.

Key Summary Points

- Guidance and coaching require deep listening and strong empathic skills.
- All patients must be assessed for appropriateness of guidance and/or coaching.
- Guidance requires exploring what the patient already knows.
- Patients must be assessed for readiness to change before the coaching methodology is used.
- Integrating guidance and coaching is integral to patient-centered care.
- Although there is broad agreement that patient-centered care is important, developing ways to support it has been challenging.
- Integrating coaching with guidance establishes the patient as the center of care and as the full source of control.

References

To access the references for this chapter, use your smartphone's QR code reader to scan the code below, or go to http://booksite.elsevier.com/ 9780323447751.

Consultation

Geraldine S. Pearson

> *Let us never consider ourselves finished nurses... we must be*
> *learning all of our lives.*
> — *Florence Nightingale*

CHAPTER CONTENTS

The author wishes to thank the following authors of previous chapters used in the writing of this edition: Anne-Marie Barron, PhD, RN, PMHCNS-BC, FNAP; Patricia A. White, PhD, ANP-BC; Julie Vosit-Steller, DNP, FNP-BC, AOCN; and Allison B. Morse, ScM, ANP-BC, WHNP, AOCNP.

Consultation is an essential part of the advanced practice registered nurse (APRN) role. It is both a skill and an art and requires knowledge, experience, and an integration of the essential aspects of the APRN role that are brought into clinical practice. The evolution of the APRN role, supported by the Institute of Medicine report, *The Future of Nursing* (2011), has resulted in parallel development of consultation as a required competency for APRNs. This has increased professional attention toward the specific competencies required to provide consultation.

Historically the nursing literature on consultation focused most on the clinical nurse specialist (CNS) role. As advanced practice nursing has evolved, the consultation competency has received more attention and is explicitly addressed as a role expectation for all four APRN roles. The American Association of Colleges of Nursing (AACN, 2006, 2011) has highlighted consultation as an essential component of master's and Doctor of Nursing Practice (DNP) programs. In defining the essentials of DNP education, the AACN emphasizes the need for explicit skills in the areas of collaboration and consultation for DNP-prepared advanced practice nurses. While acknowledging that the roles in any specialty nursing practice have overlap and differences, consultation activities for all are essentially the same process with varying specialty content emphasis. The complexities of today's health care settings require that all APRNs offer and receive consultation and understand, clinically and legally, the differences between consultation and collaboration.

At this time in nursing history, with advanced practice nursing skill development and political support, APRNs are poised to provide consultation to patient populations and systems with the power to change the quality of health care. The Institute of Medicine's landmark report, *The Future of Nursing: Leading Change, Advancing Health* (2011), cemented the role of nursing in transforming the health care system in the United States. This report, along with the Patient Protection and Affordable Care Act (2010; Carthon, Barnes, & Sarik, 2015), focus attention on new health care delivery and payment models that emphasize teamwork, care coordination, prevention, and value. Nurses are contributors to the health care system at all these levels of health care. The process of consultation is integrated into each.

The purpose of this chapter is to define consultation in APRN practice, explore theoretical models that have defined this activity, and distinguish the process of consultation from other APRN activities, including supervision, collaboration, and co-management. These activities have different meanings, outcomes, and responsibilities. The specific definitions of consultation originally posed by Caplan (1970) and later by Lipowski (1974, 1981, 1983) and Barron and White (2009) form the theoretical underpinnings for this chapter. The author of this chapter has been a psychiatric APRN for over 35 years in many capacities—as a practitioner, educator, journal editor, and consultant. This chapter reflects this experience and lessons learned from errors and mistakes. Theoretical models have endured, adapted to more current practice, and positively guided the interprofessional practice of consultation.

Consultation and Advanced Practice Nursing

Consultation has been a key part of the APRN role since the role was first conceptualized. The 1960s marked an increase in graduate training for specialty advanced practice roles. In the United States this was facilitated by increased federal funding for graduate nursing education (Hoeffer & Murphy, 1984). By 1980 the American Nurses Association had developed a social policy statement that defined and supported specialization of advanced nursing practice (American Nurses Association, 1980). When the predominant advanced practice role was the CNS designation, the course content around consultation was "embedded in the clinical practice aspect of educational preparation" (Pearson, 2014, p. 270).

This embedded clinical role was furthered by increasing visibility of role models and more defined actions encompassed in the consultation process. Benner's model of expert nursing practice (1984) formed the basis of Fenton's work (1985) that defined the CNS consultation role as a specific practice domain. This was characterized by patient care consultation to nursing staff, interpreting the role of nursing to other professional staff, and providing patient advocacy by consulting to staff treating complex patients and families. Fenton was one of the first nurses to describe advocacy as a fundamental aspect of consultation. By embracing this, APRNs are able to differentiate their consultation role from that of other health professionals. The overarching principle of consultation has to be the element of caring, essential to all nursing practice. From this comes the specific process providing expert information about a particular situation, health issue, or patient or staff issue.

State laws and regulations may mandate a "consultative" or "collaborative" role with a physician for advanced practice and prescriptive privileges; awareness of statutes and norms that regulate practice is essential for each APRN. The wording of these regulations may imply a hierarchical relationship between the APRN and physician. APRN consultation, as it is described here, is not dependent upon a physician and comprises an independent activity.

The goals and outcomes of consultation are relevant to ongoing efforts to reform health care. APRNs can help bring about the national goal of high-quality, cost-effective health care for every American. Consultation creates networks with other APRNs, physicians, and other colleagues, offering and receiving advice and information that can improve patient care and APRNs' own clinical knowledge and skills. Interacting with colleagues in other disciplines can enhance interprofessional collaboration while shaping and developing the practices of consultees and protégés. This indirectly and significantly shapes the quality, depth, and comprehensiveness of care available to patient populations and their families. Consultation offers the APRN the opportunity to positively influence health care outcomes beyond the direct patient care encounter.

Defining Consultation

The term *consultation* is used in many ways. It is sometimes used to describe direct care—the practitioner is in consultation directly with the patient. It may be used interchangeably with the terms *referral* and *collaboration,* which are actually different activities. Thus, how the term is being used in a given situation may be unclear, and it may be difficult to determine exactly what is being requested and what is expected. A lack of clarity about the specific process being used for clinical problem solving leads to confusion about roles and clinical accountability. The more precisely the word *consultation* is defined, the more likely consultation will be used for its intended purposes of enhancing patient care and promoting positive professional relationships that result in true collaboration and optimal patient outcomes. Because consultation is a core competency of advanced practice nursing, this precision is needed for communication within (intraprofessionally) and outside of nursing with other professionals (interprofessionally). It is extremely important to understand the differences between consultation and other types of professional interactions. Table 9.1 summarizes these differences, which are further described in the remainder of this section.

Caplan's Definition of Consultation

The term *consultation* has many definitions for APRNs working in a variety of clinical specialties. Although Caplan originally defined consultation as it applied to mental health, his interdisciplinary tenets about the types and process of consultation have endured and have applicability to all APRN specialties.

At a broad level, consultation is defined as "any professional activity carried out by a specialist" (Caplan & Caplan, 1993, p. 11). At the other end of the definition continuum, consultation has very specific and strictly applied parameters. Consultation was specifically defined by Caplan as an indirect service model that involves "a process of interaction between two professionals—the consultant, who is a specialist, and the consultee, who invokes the consultant's help in a current work problem that he believes is within the consultant's area of specialized competence. The work problem involves managing or treating one or more clients of the consultee, or

---

TABLE 9.1 Clarifying Definitions of Clinical Consultation, Co-Management, Referral, Supervision, and Collaboration

Type of Interaction	Goals	Focus	Responsibility for Clinical Outcomes
Clinical consultation	To enhance patient care and/or improve skills and confidence of consultee	Consultant may or may not see patient directly Degree of focus on consultee's skill is negotiated with consultee	Remains with consultee, who is free to accept or reject the advice of consultant
Co-management	To enhance patient care through availability of expertise of two (or more) professionals working together to optimize outcomes	Both professionals see patient directly and coordinate their care with one another (e.g., physician may monitor complex medication regimen while APRN focuses on adaptation and human response)	Shared
Referral	To enhance patient care by relinquishing care (or aspects of care) to another professional whose expertise is perceived to be more essential to care than that of the professional making the referral	Establish connection between patient and professional who is accepting referral Negotiate responsibilities for outcomes	Negotiated, but responsibility is often assumed (at least for aspects of care by professional accepting referral)
Supervision	To foster a supportive and educational process between a more senior, expert clinician and a less senior, novice clinician	Establish a supportive relationship that enhances the clinician's care of the patient	May be shared, but usually rests with the supervisor, who is ultimately responsible for the delivery of care
Collaboration	To foster a dynamic, interpersonal process in which two or more individuals make a commitment to each other to interact authentically and constructively solve problems	Establish the collaborative relationship between professionals or professionals and patients to accomplish established goals, purposes, or outcomes	May be shared between professionals, but responsibility rests with the provider(s) responsible for the patient

Adapted from Barron, A. M., & White, P. (2009). Consultation. In A. B. Hamric, J. A. Spross, & C. M. Hanson (Eds.), *Advanced practice nursing: An integrative approach* (4th ed., pp. 191–216). Philadelphia: WB Saunders.

planning or implementing a program to cater to the clients" (Caplan, Caplan, & Erchul, 1995, p. 11).

Other principles of consultation include:

1. The client is the layperson who is the focus of the consultation.
2. The consultant is not responsible for implementing interventions or remedial actions.
3. The consultee continues to have professional responsibility for any corrective action.
4. The consultee is free to accept or reject any of the consultant suggestions.

For purposes of this discussion, the "layperson" defined by Caplan could be any individual for whom the consultee requests consultation. This could be a patient, a client, another nurse, or other health care providers.

Realistically APRNs are often asked to consult in situations in which the parameters of their influence and authority are less clear when compared to physicians or other health care professionals. Real-life consultations are rarely neatly compartmentalized.

The principle of maintaining boundaries around identified responsibilities and roles has merit, and the consultation might be clearer for all involved in the process if there is adherence to guiding principles.

Additionally, Caplan (1970) has identified four major types of consultation: client-centered and consultee-centered case consultation and program-centered and consultee-centered administrative consultation. They are discussed here from a nursing perspective.

Client-centered case consultation is a traditional type of consultation typically occurring when a generalist asks a specialist for an expert opinion about a particular case or patient. An additional unspoken goal can also be to further the knowledge of the generalist about a particular clinical dilemma that can be generalized to other patient populations or cases. APRNs frequently receive these types of consultation requests in all settings. They tend to be uncomplicated and rely on the nurse's expert clinical knowledge. Exemplar 9.1 represents a client-centered case consultation.

EXEMPLAR 9.1   **CNS-to-ICU Staff Consultation on a Young Man With an Overdose**

A young man was admitted to the intensive care unit (ICU) after ingesting acetaminophen as part of an overdose. He had been drunk the night before and had revealed to his mother that he had overdosed on the acetaminophen but his mother had not believed him and told him to go to bed and "sleep it off." When he became violently ill the next day, she rushed him to the emergency department. He was later transferred to the ICU. This was nearly 12 hours after the overdose. Immediately the psychiatric service and liaison clinical nurse specialist (CNS) were consulted to assess his current suicidal risk and to make treatment recommendations.

The young man's mother was distraught and upset that she had not believed him when he told her he had taken the bottle of acetaminophen. The gastroenterologist was not optimistic that liver failure could be prevented given the length of time from ingestion to hospitalization. The psychiatrists assessed the patient to no longer be at imminent risk of suicide. Everyone involved was deeply distressed by the tragedy. The nurses requested that the liaison CNS be available for additional supportive care for the patient, support and referral for the family, and assistance in planning nursing care for the patient.

Within 36 hours of admission the patient had slipped into a coma and appeared to be dying. His mother accepted referral to a local mental health center. This was arranged by the consultation liaison nurse. A day

later the mother, who had been a constant presence in the ICU and had been verbal about her guilt, regret, and pain, stopped coming to the unit. She said it was too painful to see him in a coma. His friends and other family members were with him constantly as he slipped farther and farther into a coma. All talked continually with the nursing staff and consultation liaison CNS. When Friday evening came the CNS invited the nursing staff to call her if they needed her over the weekend. They called her later that night and said they were concerned about his mother, who had come to the unit to say goodbye to her son.

The CNS came in and was present with the family and friends as he died. His mother left, and as the young man passed away, his friends and family were with him. They sang songs and held his hands during the vigil. The CNS and nursing staff remained nearby and ensured that the death was peaceful.

This client-centered consultation focused primarily on the needs of the patient and family. The consultant and staff regularly shared their own feelings of impotence and despair with one another as they discussed the care of the patient. That sharing and planning helped shape the nursing perspective in the situation and clarify the goal of promoting a peaceful and comfortable death, once cure was no longer a viable goal. The consultation contributed to an active and compassionate nursing presence in the midst of tragedy and pain. ◎

Consultee-centered case consultation also involves focus on improving patient care, but the emphasis is focused directly on the consultee's difficulty in handling the situation. The focus of the consultant is on better understanding the consultee's difficulties and helping that person clarify and correct the problem in a particular case. The goal is education of the consultee, using questions as a springboard for teaching and improved understanding of the patient and the situation. The focus is on the task and on knowledge development. Thus the consultant may educate the consultee further on the issues presented by the patient or may suggest alternative strategies for dealing with the problem. This is probably the most common type of consultation sought by APRNs. The consultant may seek to bolster the confidence of the consultee in handling the problem if, in the opinion of the consultant, the consultee has the ability and potential to do so. If the problem presented by the consultee is a lack of professional objectivity, the consultant can help the consultee identify the factors interfering with the consultee's ability to see the patient realistically.

The consultee may hold a stereotyped view of the patient, or perhaps the patient's difficulties in some way mirror or symbolize the consultee's personal difficulties and cloud the consultee's ability to see the reality of the situation. This type of consultation has been an important aspect of traditional CNS practice (Exemplar 9.2).

Program-centered administrative consultation focuses on a work problem that requires planning and administration and an expert opinion about the development of a new clinical system to provide care. The goal, similar to the first type of consultation, is to provide expert consultation around a program administrative question (Exemplar 9.3).

Consultee-centered administrative consultation is similar to case consultation but involves a focus on the consultee's difficulties with programming and/or organizational objectives rather than a particular patient. The primary concern of the consultant is to correct difficulties of a consultee or among a group of consultees that interfere with program development and organization. These difficulties could be related to group functioning, leadership

---

EXEMPLAR 9.2 NP-to-CNS Consultation for a Disabled Man Living in the Community

Mr. P is a 49-year-old man residing in a group home. He is considered intellectually challenged with an IQ in the mild range of disability. He also has a seizure disorder requiring daily medications and frequent laboratory monitoring. He attends a sheltered workshop 5 days a week and manages his activities of daily living but needs supervision for cooking, shopping, and managing money. The staff at the group home have noticed that over the past few months he has become agitated and less cooperative. Referred to his primary care provider, a physical assessment ruled out a physical cause to his irritability. The primary care nurse practitioner (NP) sought the consultation of a clinical nurse specialist (CNS) expert in the care of the older intellectually challenged population. The consultant shared clinical experiences in caring for this population and noted the lack of research in the area of behavioral changes in this population. He also recommended a physician colleague whose subspecialty is assessing and treating psychiatric issues in this specific population. In this case, the consultant reinforced appropriate interventions by the primary care NP, offered new ideas for potential interventions, and shared resources for ongoing support, including a physician resource for future needs. ◎

EXEMPLAR 9.3 Program-Centered Administrative Consultation

A federally qualified health center (FQHC) is getting ready to open a new outpatient pavilion in conjunction with an established community hospital. This FQHC interfaces closely with the community hospital and hopes to continue this process with the new outpatient pavilion. A consultation is requested from an APRN with extensive experience in both types of care settings to best plan how to provide optimal continuum of care for a patient population that will receive treatment in both settings. Models of community care, reimbursement, and specific nursing roles are part of the consultation. The APRN has not worked specifically in either of these settings and has no personal investment in the outcome of the consultation other than improved care delivery to an underserved population. ◎

Consultee-Centered Administrative Consultation

Administration is recommending a patient education program for teaching breast health in an inner-city, underserved medical-surgical unit. To assist in the development of this program, the certified nurse-midwife is asked to consult with the nursing leader of the unit and offer perspective on how the program might be implemented considering the patient population and the ability of nursing staff to facilitate this within the boundaries of their current workload. ◎

issues, authority issues, or role confusion. The goal is to help the consultee develop and implement adaptive behaviors to work within administrative boundaries (Exemplar 9.4).

Differences Between Consultation, Co-Management, Referral, Supervision, and Collaboration

It is easy for APRNs to become confused about the subtle differences between consultation, co-management, referral, supervision, and collaboration. Each term suggests specific roles and responsibilities and the process for each is different.

Consultation activities can be interprofessional between different professional groups (such as physicians, APRNs, social workers, and physical therapists) or intraprofessional between nurses (such as APRN, staff nurse, or nurse leader). Consultation is also used by APRNs to offer clinical expertise to other colleagues and expertise in program development. Given APRNs' advanced knowledge and assessment skills, and in some cases expansion of the APRN role into areas of specialization, consultation between APRNs can foster improved accessibility, consultation, and timely and potentially improved care for patients without relying on another professional group to provide specialty consultation.

In contrast, *co-management* is the process by which one professional manages some aspects of a patient's care while another professional manages other aspects of the same patient's care. Co-management is not a simple process, especially because it involves a commitment to ongoing, clear, and explicit communication with the other provider; awareness and acknowledgment of differing professional styles; and shared responsibility of clinical care.

Referral occurs when the APRN directs the patient to another provider or APRN for specialized care, especially when it is beyond the expertise or scope of the APRN. In a referral the clinician temporarily or permanently relinquishes responsibility for care (or aspects of care) to another clinician, who is likely a specialist, for an opinion or management of part of a patient's care. Referral implies a responsibility to facilitate care to the referrant and ensuring that there is a seamless transfer of care from the APRN to another provider. This transfer could be temporary or a permanent transfer of care, which should be clarified prior to the transfer. In most cases, once the care associated with the referral is complete, the patient will return to the full-time care of the referring clinician. An example involves the pediatric APRN recommending a referral to a psychiatric provider for assessment of complex psychotropic medication needs.

The term *clinical supervision,* as used in mental health practices, describes an ongoing supportive and educational process between a more senior, expert clinician and a less senior, novice clinician. The goals of clinical supervision are to develop the knowledge, skills, self-esteem, and autonomy of the supervisee (Caplan & Caplan, 1993). Unlike the consultant, the supervisor is generally responsible for safeguarding the care of the supervisee's patients and is accountable for the care provided to these patients.

Supervision is different from consultation. A consultant is often an outsider of the organization or unit in which the consultation occurs. The supervisor and supervisee are generally in hierarchical positions, whereas the consultant should be neutral in this hierarchy. Although the ultimate goal of clinical supervision and consultation is likely the same (assisting another professional to enhance knowledge, skills, and abilities in patient care), the processes, relationships, and responsibilities are different.

APRNs are often confused in practice between consultation and *collaboration.* Chapter 12 provides a thoughtful definition of collaboration that was first offered by Hanson and Spross (1996):

Collaboration is a dynamic, interpersonal process in which two or more individuals make a commitment to each other to interact authentically and constructively to solve problems and to learn from each other in order to accomplish identified goals, purposes, or outcomes. The individuals recognize and articulate the shared values that make this commitment possible. (p. 232)

Collaboration is a process that underlies the professional interactions involved in consultation, co-management, and referral. Whatever the nature of the consulting relationship, the APRN keeps the patient at the center of her or his actions; therefore consultation requires collaboration on some level when two professionals come together to meet patient-centered goals. Recruiting other professionals for collaboration organizes support of an interprofessional group, thereby increasing the impact on the patient or problem through the synergy of multiple experts. An example of collaboration may involve a geriatric CNS and palliative care nurse practitioner (NP) participating in a family meeting to discuss goals of care with a frail older patient and his or her family regarding end-of-life wishes, including code status and hospice. It is important to note that the American College of Nurse-Midwives (2011) used the term *collaboration* to describe the process whereby the certified nurse-midwife (CNM) and physician jointly manage the care of the woman or newborn; that is, the terms *co-management* and *collaboration* were used synonymously.

This definition of collaboration suggests a process that underlies the professional interactions involved in consultation, co-management, referral, and supervision. Therefore in the discussion of consultation, collaboration is assumed to be essential to the process.

Model of APRN Consultation

Barron (1989) proposed a model of consultation for CNSs that was based on the nursing process and incorporated principles from the work of Caplan (1970) and Lipowski (1974, 1981, 1983). This model, expanded by Barron and White (1996), has evolved into a model of APRN consultation (Fig. 9.1) Box 9.1 presents the principles of consultation derived from the field of mental health (Caplan, 1970; Caplan & Caplan, 1993; Lipowski, 1981) on which this model is based.

Ecologic Field of the Consultation Process

APRNs tend to have a holistic orientation and understanding of systems theory that enables them to apply this consultation model in practice. At the center of Barron and White's (1996) proposed model are the purposes and outcomes of consultation.

BOX 9.1 **Principles for the Model of Advanced Practice Nursing Consultation**

- The consultation is usually initiated by the consultee.
- The relationship between the consultant and consultee is nonhierarchical and collaborative.
- The consultant always considers contextual factors when responding to the request for consultation.
- The consultant has no direct authority for managing patient care.
- The consultant does not prescribe, but makes recommendations.
- The consultee is free to accept or reject the recommendations of the consultant.
- The consultation should be documented.

Surrounding the center is the ecologic field of the consultation. Consultations are embedded in the context of the specific circumstances surrounding the consultation request, so the ecologic field in which the consultation takes place must be understood in order to provide effective consultation (Caplan & Caplan, 1993). This involves an appreciation of the interconnection and interrelatedness of the systems and contexts influencing the consultation problem and process. Thus the consultation process is an integral part of the ecologic field. The process—in which the consultant evaluates the request, performs an assessment, determines the skills required to address the problem, intervenes, and evaluates the outcome—is expanded in Fig. 9.2, as described later. Other elements of the ecologic field include the characteristics of the consultant, consultee, patient and family, and situational factors. It is assumed that there are reciprocal influences among the purposes, process, and contextual factors that can affect consultation processes and outcomes. Each component of the model is elaborated in the following sections.

Purposes and Outcomes

The purpose of a consultation may be to improve care delivery processes and patient outcomes, enhance health care delivery systems, extend the knowledge available to solve clinical problems, foster the ongoing professional development of the consultee, or a combination of these goals. Consultants should be aware that the purposes for which they

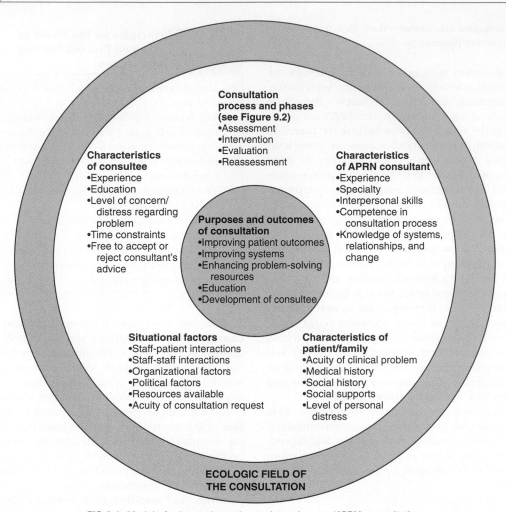

Consultation process and phases (see Figure 9.2)
•Assessment
•Intervention
•Evaluation
•Reassessment

Characteristics of consultee
•Experience
•Education
•Level of concern/ distress regarding problem
•Time constraints
•Free to accept or reject consultant's advice

Characteristics of APRN consultant
•Experience
•Specialty
•Interpersonal skills
•Competence in consultation process
•Knowledge of systems, relationships, and change

Purposes and outcomes of consultation
•Improving patient outcomes
•Improving systems
•Enhancing problem-solving resources
•Education
•Development of consultee

Situational factors
•Staff-patient interactions
•Staff-staff interactions
•Organizational factors
•Political factors
•Resources available
•Acuity of consultation request

Characteristics of patient/family
•Acuity of clinical problem
•Medical history
•Social history
•Social supports
•Level of personal distress

ECOLOGIC FIELD OF THE CONSULTATION

FIG 9.1 Model of advanced practice registered nurse (APRN) consultation.

have been consulted may contract or expand during the process of consulting. Often, APRN consultants accomplish several purposes at once. If additional purposes and possible outcomes are uncovered during consultation, these should be made clear to the consultee. The consultee may want the consultant's assistance with a patient but does not have the time or interest to focus on his or her own development, which could inform the consultee's problem solving in similar patient situations. Patients may also reveal information that requires a shift in the consultation's focus, purpose, and outcome. Over the course of the consultation, being explicit about the goal or outcome of the consultation is essential if APRNs are to evaluate the impact of consultation on practice.

Process for Formal Consultation

The algorithm for the consultation process presented in Fig. 9.2 defines the process of assessment and intervention in consultation (Barron & White, 2005). It follows the nursing process of assessment, planning, intervention, and evaluation. The process detailed in this figure suggests a continuous loop through the consultation process conducted by the APRN with continual reassessment and evaluation of outcome. This best reflects the reality of consultation in an APRN practice. Rarely is it a neatly executed, clear process with a definite beginning and ending. Rather, as the APRN role develops and deepens, the consultation process builds on itself to establish credibility, effectiveness, and clarity in the APRN role regardless of nursing specialty. However, with

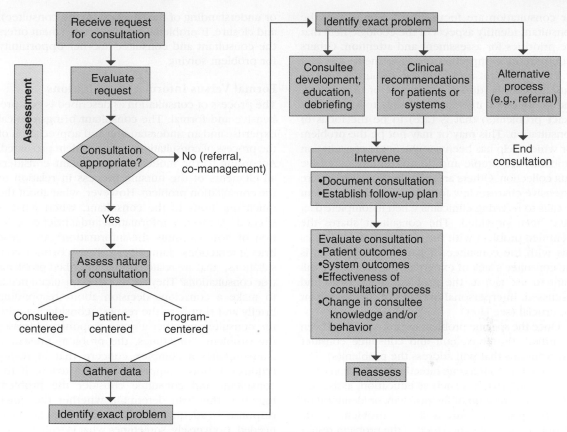

FIG 9.2 Algorithm for the consultation process.

experience and expertise, the process may occur fairly rapidly so that the expert consultant may not be consciously aware of using these steps. In addition, in some situations, the problem for which help is sought is clear cut and the consultation is brief. These types of consultations are discussed later in the chapter.

Once a request for consultation has been received, assessment of the consultation problem begins with evaluation of the request itself. An important component of assessment is confirming with the consultee that consultation is, in fact, the appropriate strategy for addressing the problem. At this stage, the consultant and consultee may decide that an alternative process is needed (e.g., a shift to co-management or referral). The consultant confirms that the problem has been accurately identified and falls within the realm of the consultant's expertise and clarifies the nonhierarchical nature of the relationship between the consultant and consultee. The consultant also confirms that the consultee will remain clinically

responsible for the patient who is the focus of the consultation. The consultant must remember that the consultee is ultimately free to accept or reject the consultant's recommendations. Once the request itself has been considered, the consultant gathers information from the consultee about the specific nature of the problem. The consultant tries to determine whether the patient has unusually difficult and complex problems (patient-centered consultation) or whether the problem results from the consultee's lack of knowledge, skill, confidence, or objectivity (consultee-centered consultation). Once the request, the nature of the relationship, and the appropriateness of consultation have been established, the consultant focuses on gathering data related to the consultation problem. This may include direct assessment of the patient. The consultant considers the ecologic field of the consultation, which includes the systems and contexts that may influence the patient and family, consultee and staff, and setting in which the consultation takes place. Some requests for consultation are focused and require that the consultant identify aspects of the ecologic field that are priorities for assessment and attention. Others require more comprehensive assessment.

The consultant uses available resources such as patient records, direct assessment of the patient, and interviews with staff and family to identify the exact problem(s) that is (are) to be the focus of consultation. This may or may not be the problem for which help has been sought. Some consultation problems are simple and do not require extensive data collection. Others are complex and may require extensive chart review for a long-standing problem or calls to referring clinicians when incomplete data have been provided. The consultant shares the identified problem with the consultee and validates this with the consultee. If part of the problem is the consultee's lack of expertise, the consultant will want to use tact as the problem is identified and discussed. Interpersonal qualities of the consultant are crucial (see later).

Once the specific problem or problems have been identified, the consultant and consultee consider interventions that will address the problem(s). The consultant may intervene directly with the consultee by using approaches such as education, assistance with reinterpretation of the problem, or identification of appropriate resources if the problem is the consultee's lack of experience. If the problem results from a particularly difficult patient situation, the consultant may assist with the process of clinical decision making by providing alternative perspectives on the problem and recommending specific interventions. More data may be needed to analyze the situation further, and a decision may need to be made about whether the consultee or consultant will gather more data. If the consultee accepts the recommendations of the consultant, together they negotiate how the interventions will be carried out, and by whom. If the consultant is to intervene directly with the patient, the consultee must understand his or her ongoing responsibility for the patient and agree to the consultant's interventions. Together, they identify additional resources and determine the time frame for the consultation (one time or ongoing).

After the intervention, the consultant and consultee engage in evaluation. Evaluation of the success or lack of success of the intervention and overall consultation is essential to the consultation process. If the problem is resolved, evaluation offers an opportunity for review, confirmation of the enhanced effectiveness of the consultee in managing the problem (underscoring the new skills and abilities

or understanding of the situation by the consultee), and closure. If problems remain, reassessment offers the consultant and consultee another opportunity for problem solving.

Formal Versus Informal Consultations

The process of consultation as described is comprehensive and formal. The consultant brings clinical expertise and an understanding and appreciation of the process of consultation to the problem presented. According to the model, the consultant considers all elements of the nursing process in relation to the consultation problem. However, what about the quick questions to the consultant, when what is needed is a piece of information and a brief description of how to apply the information? Are these brief interactions, sometimes called "corridor consultations," that are related to circumscribed problems true consultations? They are, but the consultant needs to make a conscious decision about responding briefly and simply to the request, considering with the consultee whether a quick response addresses the problem. Sometimes, the problem presented oversimplifies a complex concern that in reality requires a more comprehensive approach. If the consultant and consultee consider the problem together, they can determine whether the quick response is adequate or whether consultation is needed. Conversely, sometimes what is truly needed is a short answer to a clinical question or validation that the approach to the problem is appropriate.

Barron and White (2005) offered a cohesive description of the differences between formal and informal consultation. Informal consultations occur spontaneously and can involve a quick question about a patient care or system issue. APRNs provide these types of consultations regularly but need to be cautious and able to decide when a quick answer is not appropriate for a complex problem or when a more planned approach to the problem is warranted. As APRNs move into expert status in their practice setting, they get more requests for consultations. They also become increasingly adept and proficient at quickly responding to consultation requests. The art of the process is being able to quickly differentiate when a simple answer is sufficient or when such an answer only worsens the problem.

Informal consultations, which can occur frequently in an APRN's practice, require additional considerations. Guidelines for informal consultations are described in Box 9.2. An example of an informal consultation would be an unplanned discussion of a patient with nursing care questions that occurs

BOX 9.2 Guidelines for Informal Consultation

- Include a disclaimer to emphasize that the consultation is not a formal consultation.
- Keep conversations short.
- Frame responses in general terms.
- Suggest several possible answers, and note that all depend on the specifics of the case.
- Be cautious of evaluating any test results and rendering a specific diagnosis.
- Keep communications about a particular patient to a minimum.
- Advanced practice registered nurses (APRNs) should document all informal consultations, if not in the medical record, then in their own files. This would include their assessments and recommendations in relation to the informal consultation problem. APRNs need to make well-considered judgments about where and what to document about informal consultations.

Adapted from Barron, A-M., & White, P. A. (2005). Consultation. In A. B. Hamric, J. A. Spross, & C. M. Hanson (Eds.). *Advanced practice nursing: An integrative approach* (3rd ed., pp. 225-255). St. Louis: Elsevier Saunders.

during a staff meeting. The meeting is attended by the APRN on the unit, and guidelines are given for planning a more focused and formal consultation for the unit staff.

Staff nurses sometimes equate this brief type of consultation with consultation in general because they have experienced only this type of consultation with physicians, who quickly impart information and are then off to the next patient. The idea of the roving clinical expert dropping by with tidbits of expert advice is the concept that non-APRNs can have of a consultant. This is another reason why it is important to make a conscious decision about responding in a brief way to the consultation request. In the informal situation the consultee may not realize that a more comprehensive and thorough investigation of the problem and solutions with the consultant is possible. Also, some clinical situations require a more formal approach to the consultation problem. APRNs should consider the types of problems in practice that require a formal approach and develop a system for integrating nurse-nurse and interprofessional consultations, which make advanced practice nursing skills more visible and extend their knowledge and skills.

Characteristics of the APRN Consultant

In addition to theoretical understanding, self-awareness and interpersonal skills are essential for the consultant. For a model of consultative practice to be implemented, it is critical that APRNs first value themselves and the specialized expertise that they have developed. One must appreciate one's own skills and knowledge before the possibilities for consultation can be envisioned. The knowledge and skills acquired by APRNs could serve to inform and expand the practices of staff nurses, other APRNs, and health care professionals of various disciplines involved in the care of these patient populations. However, APRNs must first appreciate that they have valuable understanding and knowledge to share.

APRNs with expert status can carry large amounts of informal authority and power. This may extend beyond the formal boundaries of their role and make them more apt to be approached for consultation. APRNs have to be knowledgeable about systems, relationships, and change (Barron & White, 2005). In addition, ideally, consultants know themselves well—they are aware of their own personal issues, strengths, weaknesses, areas of expertise and motives. A good consultant must be able to suspend judgment and avoid stereotyping and incorporate the core concept of caring in all communications in their nursing practice. When consultation is sought, a fresh perspective is often needed. Self-understanding allows the consultant to see consultation issues realistically, without prejudice. It is not uncommon for a consultant to step into a highly emotionally charged situation and use self-awareness, understanding, and self-possession to remain objective, clear, and effective. It can be meaningful and helpful for the consultant to have a trusted colleague or supervisor with whom to share and review consultation situations. These discussions can offer support and enhance the consultant's understanding of personal and interpersonal responses to the consultation material.

The consultant should also be able to establish warm, respectful, and accepting relationships with consultees (Carter & Berlin, 2007; Perry, 2011). The initiation of a consultation request is often associated with a sense of vulnerability on the part of the consultee, who recognizes that assistance is required to help manage the situation at hand. The consultant must communicate (and sincerely believe) that the problem and consultee are important and worthy of consideration. The consultant must also communicate confidence in the consultee's ability to overcome the difficulties resulting in the consultation request. When the consultant creates a climate of trust and acceptance, the consultee can then be willing to risk vulnerability and genuineness with the consultant. A respectful, trusting connection between the consultant and consultee allows a deep examination of the problem, implications, solutions, and ultimately resolution and learning.

An APRN may be the consultee, requesting consultation from a physician or another APRN. As a consultee, the APRN should be able to identify and articulate the nature of the problem for which help is being sought. It may be necessary to clarify the collegial, nonhierarchical nature of the consultation relationship. Before consulting with an APRN colleague or physician, APRNs have likely tried alternative plans or directions based on knowledge of the patient or clinical situation. It is important to relay this information to the consultant planning the approach because it can be useful to the consultation. Dialogue with APRN colleagues and physicians can improve the effectiveness and efficiency of the consultation and can strengthen collaboration among colleagues. In addition to their intrapersonal knowledge and interpersonal skills, APRNs must be competent in the consultative process. Although skill in consultation develops over time, the attributes of the consultant and consultation process described here can help novice APRNs learn to consult with confidence (Carter & Berlin, 2007).

Characteristics of the Consultee Requesting the Consultation

The consultee identifies a problem that exists in a clinical situation because of uncertainty, complexity, or a lack of knowledge on his or her part and believes that increased knowledge and assistance with clinical decision making would enhance practice and patient care. Characteristics of the consultee may need to be considered. Education, experience, the consultee's level of distress regarding the clinical problem for which help is sought, organizational skills, and availability to solve problems with the consultant are factors that can influence the consultation. What prompted the consultation, and how is the request related to specific consultee characteristics? Who is asking for the consultation, and is this person in a position to implement consultant recommendations?

Understanding the ecologic field of the consultation involves knowing the APRN role in the situation, identifying the person requesting the consultation, and understanding involved patient/family factors as well as the situational factors that influence the process (Barron & White, 2005).

Patient and Family Factors

Among factors to consider are the acuity and complexity of the clinical problem, the patient's medical history, social history, social supports, and other resources. Depending on the nature of the problem, it may be important to consider concurrent stresses being experienced by the patient and family. An acute problem may demand the consultant's immediate assistance, requiring a shift in the consultant's priorities. A complex or unusual problem may take more time to solve. Asking the following questions may help guide the process of the consultation:

- What is the patient's medical history?
- What are the acute and chronic issues affecting the patient's current status?
- What family issues are influencing the patient's status currently and historically?

Situational Factors

Perhaps the most important of all considerations, situational factors are those issues within the organization and staff that influence the consultation process. In this model, the term *situational factors* refer to those inherent factors in the organization and staff caring for the patient. Numerous situational factors can affect the consultation process. For example, the mood or atmosphere of the care environment, the power differential between different levels of leadership or nursing staff, and professional differentiations between various professional groups all influence the situation (Barron & White, 2005). The quality of relationships and interactions between staff and patients or among staff members themselves may be important issues. For example, a patient perceived as being nonadherent to some therapy may be responding to conflicts among team members that the patient has inferred from clinicians' behaviors. A clinician may seek validation from a consultant as a way of getting support for an unpopular but potentially productive approach to a clinical problem. Time pressures and lack of adequate resources can affect consultation. Organizational factors include legal factors, regulatory considerations, and credentialing mechanisms for a specialty practice. Organizational politics, power imbalances, and rapid or frequent system changes also are to be considered. All these factors can affect the consultee's view of the importance of the request.

For APRNs, the status of advanced practice nursing and APRNs in a particular agency or state may influence consultation. For example, organizational policies and procedures regarding consultation and nursing practice, statutes regarding APRN-physician consulting relationships (e.g., required collaborative/consultation agreements versus independent practice), protocol agreements, reimbursement policies, malpractice, and degree of prescriptive authority may all affect the consultation process.

Other Models of Consultation

Other nurse experts have defined nursing consultation. In psychiatric–mental health nursing, the psychiatric consultation liaison nurse (PCLN) role was implemented as a way to have psychiatric–mental health nurses involved in medical-surgical environments, identifying comorbid psychiatric disorders and the ways that they manifest in patients on the medical-surgical unit. PCLNs traditionally consulted directly with staff, but also with managers in health care systems, around organizational issues and administrative concerns. The PCLN role has been in existence for nearly 50 years to offer:

> immediate, short-term, crisis-oriented mental health intervention and education to individuals in medical-surgical settings, to bridge the gap often found between psychiatric and medical-surgical nursing care, and to facilitate clients' transition to additional health services of both a physical and psychosocial nature. (Yakimo, Kurlowicz, & Murray, 2004, p. 215)

Similarly, the CNS role has historically had a strong consultation component. Benner's model of expert nursing practice (1984) further informed the CNS role in consultation. This included:

- Providing patient care consultation to the nursing staff through direct patient intervention and follow-up
- Interpreting the role of nursing in specific clinical patient care situations to nursing and other professional staff
- Providing patient advocacy by sensitizing staff to the dilemmas faced by patients and families seeking health care

These concepts, while linked more specifically to CNS functioning, have applicability to all APRN roles. Barron and White (2009) evaluated the differences between consultation and other APRN practices. Few APRN staff function only as consultants because this competency is most likely combined with other aspects of APRN practice. Acknowledging and defining the role activity at the time it is being performed is the responsibility of the APRN.

Standards of Practice

The *Consensus Model for APRN Regulation* (APRN Joint Dialogue Group, 2008) was an effort aimed at unifying the different types of advanced practice nurses that were practicing throughout the United States. Standards have been set forth by the National Council of State Boards of Nursing in conjunction with the Advanced Practice Nursing Consensus Work Group. The APRN regulatory model emphasizes consultation activities as part of the APRN's role function (National Council of State Boards of Nursing, 2008). In addition, *The Essentials of Doctoral Education for Advanced Nursing Practice* (AACN, 2006) sets the practice stage for DNP-prepared APRNs to engage in consultation activities as part of their indirect and direct care management of complex health care situations and patient populations.

In a similar manner, the National Association of Clinical Nurse Specialists (2004) organizes CNS practice into three domains: patient, nurses and nursing practice, and organizations and systems. This integrated model of CNS practice is referred to as the Spheres of Influence model (Fulton, 2014). The Association identified the consultation competency as a required skill in a CNS role. Historically, consultation in these spheres was the hallmark of a CNS role. Yet the influence of third-party reimbursement and fiscal restraints on the CNS consultation role cannot be underestimated because the demand for third-party reimbursement has escalated and requires justification of a consultation role. Many CNSs have woven consultation into their reimbursement, citing that this work is highly impactful on the health care environment (Pearson, 2014). Many hospitals and clinics eliminated CNS positions prior to fully understanding that consultation could and should be billed. All systems that utilize third-party reimbursement need to ascertain a way to formally bill for consultative services provided by nurses.

NP core competencies were updated by the National Organization of Nurse Practitioner Faculties in 2017. Although not formally listed as an NP core competency, the concept of consultation can be indirectly ascertained within each competency. This is in contrast to the CNS competencies, which clearly delineate the consultative aspects of this role.

Applicability of Benner's Concept of Expert Practice to Consultation

Benner noted that nursing practice undergoes a shift from competent to proficient to expert in the course of experiential role development. Proficient practice is described as:

> an increased capacity for recognizing whole patterns and a budding sense of salience where relevant aspects of the situation simply stand out without recourse to calculative reasoning. Proficient practitioners can read a situation, recognize changing relevance, and accordingly, shift their perspective on the whole situation. (Benner, Tanner, & Chesla, 2009, p. 137)

This proficiency leads to expert practice, which is characterized by the ability of nurses to intuitively understand and respond to the pertinent issues in a situation. Engaging in expert practice makes the process of consultation more effective and easier. Expert nursing practice encourages a broader view of the situation, using engaged practical reasoning. This reasoning relies on a mature understanding and perceptual grasp of the nuances of a particular situation. APRNs at the level of expert practice have embedded knowledge of nursing practice, are engaged in the process, and are able to understand their role definition in the larger health care system while confident they can make a difference in the system to which they are consulting.

This is not to suggest that APRNs at earlier stages in their practice are unable to provide expert consultation. It means that as APRNs become more expert in their chosen specialty area, their ability to provide consultation becomes easier and more seamless. The clinical expertise gained from experience translates into increasing levels of confidence in the ability to provide consultation that is thoughtful, intelligent, and clear about professional boundaries, and that ultimately, in many situations, can improve patient care or system functioning.

Common APRN Consultation Situations

APRN-Physician Consultation

Consultation and collaboration with the physician and patient care team remain integral components of APRN interprofessional development. When consulting with other nurses or physicians, an APRN is likely to be far along in the problem-solving process. The need for consultation is often related to the consultee's level of diagnostic uncertainty or complex management issues. Experienced APRNs often have a clear definition of the problem and a preliminary plan to address it that they wish to

validate or reformulate, depending on the consultant's advice. Truly collaborative relationships between physicians and APRNs ensure consultation that is bidirectional. Physicians in primary care often consult APRNs regarding issues such as assisting patients in making lifestyle changes or in coping with the effects of chronic illness. Many APRNs in primary care have specialty expertise in women's health care and are sought out by physicians for consultation on such issues. Physicians might then choose to comanage patients with APRNs so that patients benefit from the expertise of both professionals. An APRN, in turn, might consult a physician regarding a patient in a medically unstable condition, which evolves into co-management by the physician and APRN, with each assuming responsibility for the outcomes of decision making.

The American College of Nurse-Midwives (2011) was deliberate in describing the various types of interactions that CNMs have with physicians. Unfortunately, APRN-physician consulting relationships have often been structured by laws and regulations that mandate or imply supervisory oversight, which can reinforce stereotypical nurse-physician relationships. Many organizational cultures reinforce traditional nurse-physician relationships and the behavioral norms associated with them. One of the major challenges facing advanced practice nursing educators is to fully delineate/explore the APRN-physician relationship to ensure that students understand the autonomous expression of advanced practice nursing. This is key to developing collegial relationships, including use of consultation that is not hierarchical in nature. When a hierarchical relationship exists between an APRN and a physician, the APRN who consults may defer to the physician's decisions, downplaying or ignoring first-hand knowledge of the patient. However, interactions between physicians and APRNs can be extremely successful, and these practices embrace the collaborative relationships that are key to effective consultation (see Chapter 12).

Consultation between APRNs and physicians can highlight the strengths of each—that is, the APRN's deep appreciation for the human responses related to health and illness and the physician's deep understanding of disease and treatment. When both areas of expertise are available to patients and their families, truly holistic, comprehensive, and individualized care is offered. As APRN knowledge evolves and deepens, an emerging issue in relation to APRN-physician consultation is the crossing of traditional nurse-physician boundaries. As APRNs become more and more specialized, the knowledge embedded in practice may be more closely related to what is generally thought of as medical practice. For example, a certified registered nurse anesthetist may have highly developed skills in the area of pain management and the requisite skills to perform procedures to address complex pain issues. In women's health practices, APRNs may specialize in using complementary therapies for menopausal symptoms. Physicians often refer interested patients to the collaborating women's health APRN in the practice for consultation about using complementary therapies. Tact and understanding of the long-standing boundaries that are being crossed can elevate the consultation relationship to a new level.

APRN–Staff Nurse Consultation

Early on, as CNSs implemented their consultative roles, it became apparent that the culture of nursing had not adopted consultation as an important strategy in providing patient care. Staff nurses were expected to take care of the patients by themselves. A novice nurse might consult a head nurse or more senior nurse, but staff members were expected to know how to solve problems and use the policy and procedure manual. An important component of implementing consultation means teaching staff members how and when to consult. Early on, CNSs often engaged in active case finding to identify patients who needed the knowledge and skills they had because CNSs were not actually assigned to patients and staff nurses. By building this type of clinical caseload, they demonstrated to nursing staff how intraprofessional consultation might be helpful. This process may still occur when an APRN is new to a unit or program, when trust needs to be established with staff nurses, or when an APRN role is entirely new to a unit or organization and staff nurses are unclear what to expect of the new role. Of note, CNSs tended to carry out direct consultation with patients and to consult with other professionals to assist the staff with problem solving and enhancing patient care. For example, staff nurses might call the Adult-Gero CNS regarding a patient with Guillain-Barré syndrome because they have no experience caring for patients with this disorder. The CNS may have had little or no experience as well but can mobilize the resources needed, such as arranging an in-service consultation by the neuroscience or rehabilitation CNS or NP, providing articles, being available to staff on all shifts as they implement

unfamiliar assessments, and assisting with care plan development. The APRN initiates processes (including additional consultation) and provides knowledge directly.

Once relationships are established and staff members perceive that the APRN consultant is approachable, respectful, and helpful, staff will initiate contact with the consultant when complex clinical issues arise. Exemplar 9.1 presents an example of a consultation resulting from staff nurse identification of care needs. This example demonstrates evolution of the consultation process. The APRN has specific clinical expertise and is called on to support the ICU nursing staff in managing a complex overdose patient. Nursing staff are provided with evidence-based practice knowledge around mental health issues, including suicide risks, death and dying, and family care.

Consultation in the International Community

The APRN role as a consultant has applicability internationally as evidenced by literature from Switzerland (Bryant-Lukosius et al., 2016), Taiwan (Lu et al., 2016), and Australia (Fry et al., 2013). The increasing recognition of the APRN role as key in health care prevention and provision is prominent around the world. Consultation is one of numerous competencies required in all APRN roles.

Within the past 15 years, there has been increased success in establishing international consultative relationships in nursing. The role and use of consultation internationally has expanded, especially in the areas of midwifery (Vosit-Steller, Morse, & Mitrea, 2011) and palliative care. Vosit-Steller and coworkers (2011) reported that with the support of agencies such as Sigma Theta Tau International and the International Council of Nurses, cross-cultural consultation has grown to provide more advanced nursing care to many developing areas of the world.

International consultation is challenging and rewarding. The creation of sustainable international collaborations that attend to consultation is congruent with the mission and values of nursing and the philosophy of nursing education (Vosit-Steller et al., 2011). Consultative relationships must initially be built on trust and a common mission, with a commitment to establishing a relationship. Once rapport and appreciation for cultural differences have been established, effective communication in international consultation can be achieved by personal visits,

---

EXEMPLAR 9.5   **American APRN–Romanian Registered Nurse International Consultation[a]**

Mrs. P is a 60-year-old widow who has lived all of her life in Romania. She is Christian Orthodox but does not practice her religion. She receives a modest pension from the government, which meets her financial needs. Her past medical history includes cardiovascular disease. Mrs. P was diagnosed with breast cancer this year and was treated surgically. Following her mastectomy, she refused chemotherapy and radiation therapy. Several months after the mastectomy, she presented with metastatic disease and a fungating breast lesion. The major concerns of the Romanian nurses were related to ineffective control of the drainage and foul odor and the patient's perception of her body image. As they changed the patient's dressing at her home, the Romanian nurse described the current approach to Mrs. P's management to the American advanced practice registered nurse (APRN).

The nurse irrigated the area with povidone-iodine (Betadine) and saline and applied a wet gauze dressing. Then petroleum jelly (Vaseline) and crushed metronidazole tablets were applied to reduce odor and prevent infection. Calcium alginate was applied to the edges of the wound to assist with hemostasis.

The APRN consultant prepared for the consultation by considering the following questions:

1. How would we manage this type of lesion in the United States?
2. What type of dressings are used in Romania, and why?
3. What solutions are used for irrigating?

4. How can our (US) practice suggestions translate to resources available in Romania, and are there cultural implications?
5. How can nurses communicate with patients with poor body image and compromised sexuality?
6. How do you extend care to family members to inform them about the challenges?

The management issues that were raised for input from the APRN consultant included the fact that the wound soaks through the dressing, requiring dressing changes twice daily and resulting in maceration of the wound edges. This then required large amounts of absorbent material and diapers to assist with the drainage. The APRN offered several recommendations regarding how to optimize use of dressings considering the materials and medication solutions at hand in Romania.

There was an interactive discussion at the bedside and debriefing following the visit regarding the exploration of which interventions would be useful. The Romanian nurse noted that it was difficult to obtain some of the materials on a consistent basis, such as zinc oxide or alternative dressing materials. Recognizing the limitations in accessing materials for symptom management allowed the consultant to identify areas of creative management, which provided care that was redirected and evidence-based. The eventual outcome was equivalent to using materials that were suggested and available in the United States. ◎

---

[a]The author is grateful to Julie Vosit-Steller, DNP, FNP-BC, AOCN, and Allison B. Morse, ScM, ANP-BC, WHNP, AOCNP, for this exemplar.

---

telecommunication, video conferencing, and written vehicles for collaboration. Consultation is a dynamic process that benefits both parties when they understand one another's needs (Exemplar 9.5). There is a current need to expand consultation in the areas of training resources in primary care and specialty areas, to expand education traditionally and through telehealth, and to offer support in utilizing research and writing for publication (Vosit-Steller et al., 2011). Soeren, Hurlock-Chorostecki, and Reeves (2011) noted that the international expansion of the NP role has contributed positively to both intraprofessional and interprofessional utilization of the expertise provided by APRNs. They noted that the capacity to perform holistic care for patients is not limited by traditional role boundaries.

Issues in APRN Consultation

Developing Consultation Skills in APRN Students

For APRNs to learn the theoretical and practical issues involved in the development of consultative abilities, relevant content must be included in graduate education curricula. In highlighting consultation as an essential aspect of DNP education, the AACN (2006) recognized consultation as a central competency for all APRN practice. In addition to faculty-initiated experiences with consultation, APRN students have much to offer each other as they move through DNP programs. Consulting with peers on challenging clinical issues offers students experience with the consultation process as they begin to think of themselves as consultants.

Learning how to evaluate and consider the implications of consultation related to the outcomes of care can be valuable for students. Focusing on the impact of APRN consultation illuminates documentation issues, cost-effectiveness, and related curricular needs. These findings could translate to insurers and policymakers who determine policy and payment for health care services.

Developing comfort and skill with seeking, providing, and evaluating consultation is an important goal for DNP education. APRNs are expected to influence patients, other providers, and the systems in which they work. Therefore, when APRNs graduate, they should be equipped with knowledge, skill, and confidence in the consultation process. Effective consultation, whether it is sought or provided, enables APRNs to establish credibility, build collaborative relationships with other members of the health care team, and influence the processes and outcomes of care.

Using Technology to Provide Consultation

The use of new technologies to enhance care delivery has affected every aspect of the health care delivery system. Consultation is now not limited to the physical setting. Teleconferencing has been used successfully in consultation, medical education, supervision, and simulation (Flodgren, Rachas, Farmer, Inzitari, & Shepperd, 2015). In addition, educational models are teaching nursing students how to implement and utilize telehealth models to connect, collaborate, and consult with nurses and other health care specialties providing care (Gray & Rutledge, 2014). The use of technologies in these models of care and consultation are challenging reimbursement, liability, and the definitions of technology-enhanced interprofessional collaboration. This requires clarity about the definition of precise telehealth activities and an understanding of legal and ethical issues related to access, privacy, confidentiality, security, jurisdiction, and licensure standards for APRNs. These differ by state and by practice institution and have to be clarified depending on the geographic location of the practice.

Several programs have been implemented using APRN consultation and telehealth. Miller and colleagues (2008) assessed consults completed in the emergency department by APRNs over a 1-year period. The APRNs tended to minor injuries with the assistance of a telemedicine network, if necessary. Of these consults, 60% were found to be appropriate for APRNs (Miller et al., 2008). This figure increased to 84% if children younger than 14 years and those with shoulder injuries were excluded.

Schweickert and colleagues (2011) provided a rural, high-risk population access to telehealth stroke education. The program was found to be equivalent to in-person stroke education with regards to satisfaction, knowledge, and making health behavior changes to reduce vascular risk.

A team of CNSs has been gathering clinical data from the electronic health record (EHR) about falls, delirium, and the use of restraints prior to consultation with geriatric patients (Purvis & Brenny-Fitzpatrick, 2010). They are using these computer-generated, high-risk indicators to facilitate nursing practice guidelines, nursing plans of care, and real-time indicators prior to consultation (Purvis & Brenny-Fitzpatrick, 2010).

Some of the care provided by APRNs in retail clinics, minor emergency areas, and rural health clinics can be carried out within the digital arena (Lee, 2011). APRNs have branched out beyond triaging patients in call centers. In a California study, nurses used interactive audio and visual systems to collect and transmit vital signs and provided "palliative care, rehabilitation, and chronic disease management" to patients suffering from HIV/AIDS (Lee, 2011). During a 4-month period, telehealth monitors were placed in patients' homes and, at the end of the trial, patients reported being satisfied with their care.

Midwestern Veterans Affairs Medical Centers have created a link through teleconference and electronic medical records. The collective bariatric surgery departments conducted initial consultations through this system for patients who resided at distances of more than 300 miles away (Sudan, Salter, Lynch, & Jacobs, 2011). The satisfaction rate for patients who used the system was 82%; the rate of surgical outcomes and satisfaction was 96.6% (Sudan et al., 2011).

Wright and Honey (2016) described a teleconsultation process in New Zealand that sustains the coordination, advocacy, and support of patients and caregivers on the health care team. It was especially useful for distance consultation by specialty nurses. This qualitative research found that teleconsultation provided for more timely care for patients by increasing the access to specialist expertise. The program represents a shift to a technological model that allows patients to remain in their community.

Telehealth has also been used in transcultural consultation on palliative care between APRNs in an established collaborative relationship among Brasov, Romania; the University of Rhode Island; and Simmons College (Gerzevitz et al., 2009). Once collegial and trusting relationships were established, teleconferencing was used among the three sites to consult on difficult cases from a hospice in Romania. Electronic communication presented the opportunity to advance practice methods and provide validation for nursing actions (Gerzevitz et al., 2009).

Privacy, security, and access to telehealth create unique, additional ongoing concerns in the world of telehealth and consultation. Documentation parameters for security and privacy and the need for security related to the online sharing of private medical information must be delineated by the system where care is being provided. Providing information through telecommunication across state lines raises concerns about liability and differences in state nurse practice acts regarding scope of practice. Documentation guidelines and protocols should be established for the application of any telecommunication considering confidentiality and security issues in telehealth practice.

Reimbursement for telehealth and telehealth consultation regularly occurs in most states. The Patient Protection and Affordable Care Act, signed into law on March 23, 2010, addresses the use of telehealth as a means of delivering efficient and effective health care in the United States (Lee & Harada, 2012). Telehealth has become more mainstream as a care model as increasingly there is reimbursement available for the service. States have a variety of implemented reimbursement strategies for telehealth; not all states incorporate these policies into their Medicaid programs. In spite of this, the Center for Connected Health Policy (cchpca.org) noted that 48 states and the District of Columbia have some form of reimbursement for telehealth in their public programs. Notably, no states are alike in definitions of law or policy (CCHPA, 2017).

APRNs are currently leaders in telenursing practice and should be aware of important policy issues to advance the use of telehealth further (Schlachta-Fairchild, Varghese, Deickman, & Castelli, 2010), including consultation. Issues such as technology selection and implementation principles, interstate licensure, malpractice, and telehealth reimbursement are important to advancing telenursing further. In addition, evidence-based strategies for demonstrating caring using technology in patient interactions are key for advancing telenursing in APRN practice.

Finally, APRNs should be aware of how telenursing can affect the nursing shortage in the United States, providing access to care irrespective of geographic location of provider and patients (Schlachta-Fairchild et al., 2010).

The application of technology in delivering health-related information continues to be studied in terms of process and outcomes. APRNs should consider the potential opportunities that exist to enhance consultation activities with these modalities but should exercise caution regarding their implementation until legislative and policy initiatives related to access, security, and mutual recognition of APRN practice across state lines are more fully developed and future research elucidates specific processes, outcomes, and concerns related to telehealth strategies and practices.

Documentation and Legal Considerations

Although it has been stressed that the consultee remains clinically responsible for the patient who is the focus of the consultation, it is critical to appreciate that APRN consultants are accountable for their practices relative to the consultation problem. Once a consultant-consultee relationship has been established, scope of practice is implied and responsibility is assumed. This is initiated once the patient has been seen, recommendations have been rendered, and documentation has been entered into the patient chart. The duty of care and the legal responsibility to follow up on the consultation is of principal importance. The initial consultation should end with a summary communication to the consultee. This communication should ideally echo the documented recommendations but should be presented in person to the consultee or by telecommunication. Whether the consultee adopts the recommendations is entirely optional, according to professional skill and standard in the specialty.

APRN consultation is influenced by factors such as professional standards of practice within the specialty, state and certification regulations, nurse practice acts, and institutional and group policies (Christensen, 2009). If malpractice were to be questioned involving consultation, it would be these specific documents and regulations that would be used to determine duty of care, standard of care, and/or damages, and with which type of provider the consultation is most appropriate.

Inherent in the consultation process is the ability to communicate effectively, but little emphasis is placed on written communication through consultation notes. The art of writing a consultation note is learned primarily through trial and error or through mentorship with a senior practitioner (Stichler, 2002). Documentation is the best defense for the APRN consultant, whether the patient is seen or not. If the consultation is on the telephone, sidebar questions have been answered, or medical information interpreted about a patient, an event note should be entered into the chart. The EHR has become a convenient tool for documenting consultations and outcomes (McElwaine et al., 2014). Establishing a formal consultation relationship is protective to the APRN consultant and the consultee. The EHR has shifted legal trends to a more formal level. Legal action has been taken against APRNs and APRN consultants for informal consultation, and the establishment of a relationship between the consultant and patient should be delineated to avoid later legal risk due to lack of role clarity. The current trend for APRN consultation is more formal than informal.

As the role of APRN consultant has expanded, it brings with it greater risk of professional liability in a litigious society. It is advisable that APRNs be aware of their malpractice coverage and, if employed in a high-risk area, be aware of the elements that constitute malpractice and plan for the management of risks involved. NPs often work with other health care professionals in collaborative settings. The laws governing the degree of supervision and protocol vary by state. These agreements address the level of physician oversight and consultation allowed independently by the APRN. In the most constructive settings, collaborative practice results in optimal patient care. Collaborative practice may create a lack of cooperation among physicians, NPs, health care entities, and pharmacies in the course of defending themselves against allegations of malpractice. These consultative situations raise complex issues in the event of a professional liability claim.

In addition, evidence to substantiate claims regarding prescribing practices may be difficult to obtain. Because the APRN has the ability to examine, diagnose, and establish treatment plans for patients, friction may develop among the various health care professionals. Should these professionals become codefendants in professional liability litigation, an adversarial situation may result. In some jurisdictions, physicians may carry lower limits of professional liability coverage than an NP. In such cases, the NP may become the focus of the defendant's claim in an effort to collect from the NP's additional liability insurance coverage (Burroughs et al., 2007).

Some APRNs prefer to purchase additional liability insurance. When obtaining insurance, the APRN consultant must consider the following: the practice setting, types of policies, components of the policy, costs, and the means to obtain adequate coverage (Scott & Beare, 1993). The best protection during a consultation includes good client communication and individualized client contracts. A well-written contract serves as a legal document to delineate responsibilities and outcomes, provide a professional image, and protect against possible negative developments.

Discontinuing the Consultation Process

There are circumstances in which an APRN has initiated the consultative process and recognition of safety or necessity warrants the closure of a consult. If the APRN has become aware that she or he or the patient is in a dangerous situation, and the consultee is not willing to intervene, the consultant would need to assume responsibility for ensuring safety needs and step out of the consultation role (Barron, 1983, 1989).

Developing the Practice of Other Nurses

Consultation from an APRN can enhance the clinical knowledge and practice of nurses requesting consultation. An outcome of APRN consultation, especially over time, is to encourage the professional development and practice of nurse consultees (Barron & White, 2009). One of the most rewarding aspects of the consultative process is to observe the growth in consultees and the mastering of new skills (Gray & Rutledge, 2014). The increasing number of DNPs in practice has significantly supported the confidence of engaging and effective consultation as a critical part of practice (Christensen, 2009).

Christensen (2009) has emphasized the importance of self-evaluation following consultation. The approach and process of APRN consultation largely follows a medical model, focused on symptoms, at times excluding the fact that nurses possess the best traits of empathy, compassion, and holism. As consultants, APRNs are in a position to use the reflection skills they develop as graduate students and contribute to the consultation as a whole, being mindful of identifying the awareness of a therapeutic interpersonal relationship with patients. This process can enhance the learning of the consultee and the consultant, contributing in a meaningful way to the process (Barron & White, 2009). It is through critical reflection of the consultative process that nursing practice is advanced. The reflective nature of this element of advanced practice work promotes the development of future APRNs (Christensen, 2009).

APRN Consultation and Research

There is a decided gap around research evaluating the evidence-based impact of consultation on health care systems. In 2006 Yakimo wrote that there was a lack of outcome measurement, particularly in psychiatric consultation liaison nursing. In 2004, Yakimo, Kurlowicz, and Murray had systematically reviewed PCLN studies that looked at outcome in practice. They recommended that there be a mechanism for measuring change in patients or system using an established tool for measuring outcome. They stated that outcomes should be based on the particular interest/specialty group and that the measurement tool chosen should be specific enough to measure the intent of the intervention (Yakimo et al., 2004). While their study was applicable specifically to psychiatric consultation liaison nursing, it has merit for other subspecialties of APRN practice. Measuring outcome might involve using a tool but might also be viewed from a patient care perspective or improvement in functioning. The differences will involve who has requested the consultation, who the target group is for the intervention, and how the consultation is being used to improve patient care.

The body of national and international research about the role of the APRN is growing. In each, consultation is cited as essential to the practice (Bryant-Lukosius et al., 2016; Fabrellas et al., 2015; Kutzleb et al., 2015; Perrin & Kazanowski, 2015). This reflects consultation as a core aspect of functioning in a broad picture of the APRN role as it is currently conceptualized. This is especially applicable in this era of shrinking resources, too few providers for the medical needs of the population, and a growing need for nursing expertise. Consultation, delivered in any manner, can expand the influence of the APRN and allow this expertise to reach a larger population of patients.

Billing for Consultation

Payment for consultation services is improving in some APRN roles, but APRNs need a clear understanding of the requirements for payment. Traditionally, the CNS, CNM, and certified registered nurse anesthetist were considered essential consultants and collaborators within the teams of specialty units.

BOX 9.3   Centers for Medicare and Medicaid Services Criteria to Bill for Consultation

1. Specifically, a consultation service is distinguished from other evaluation and management visits because it is provided by a physician or qualified nonphysician practitioner (advanced practice registered nurse [APRN]) whose opinion or advice regarding evaluation and/or management of a specific problem is requested by another physician or other appropriate source.
2. The qualified APRN may perform consultation services within the scope of practice and licensure requirements for APRNs in the state in which he or she practices. Applicable collaboration and general supervision rules (by state) apply, as well as billing rules.
3. A request for a consultation from an appropriate source and the need for consultation (i.e., the reason for consultation services) shall be documented by the consultant in the patient's medical record and included in the requesting physician or qualified APRN's plan of care in the patient's medical record.
4. After the consultation is provided, the consultant shall prepare a written report of her or his findings and recommendations, which shall be provided to the referring physician. There are five levels of current procedural terminology code for consultation.

Adapted from Buppert, C. (2012). Update on consultation billing: Legal limits. *Journal for Nurse Practitioners, 5,* 730-732; and Burroughs, R., Dmytrow, B., & Lewis, H. (2007). Trends in nurse practitioner professional liability: An analysis of claims with risk management recommendations. *Journal of Nursing Law, 11,* 53-60.

Yet these APRNs did not bill or were not reimbursed for their services (Buppert, 2012). In 2005 the Centers for Medicare and Medicaid Services decided that the shared visit rules for billing were not applicable to consultation (Buppert, 2012). Specifically, consultations cannot be billed "incident to." There are specific Centers for Medicare and Medicaid Services criteria that must be met for APRNs to bill individually (Box 9.3).

Consultations may be billed based on time if the counseling and coordination of care constitute more than 50% of the face-to-face encounter between the physician or qualified APRN and the patient. The preceding requirements (request, evaluation or counseling and coordination, and written report) shall also be met when the consultation is based on time for counseling and coordination (Buppert, 2012).

When billing a consultation, the APRN must select the current procedural terminology code that is supported by documentation under Medicare's documentation guidelines. These guidelines can be found at www.cms.gov/. Also, Medicare administrative contractors have published their audit score sheets for evaluation/management on their websites. The most current information about billing is found on the website of the local contractor or agency billing representative.

Evaluation of the Consultation Competency

Ongoing evaluation of an APRN's skill in consultation is a requirement of the role. This involves overall evaluation of the consultative process and effective use of skills. APRNs should consider strategies that will assist them in determining their overall and specific effectiveness in relation to consultation. Data may be obtained from consultees, peers, administrators, review of the APRN's documentation of consultation, and the APRN's self-evaluation.

Guidelines for consultation may vary by areas of specialty, which will dictate an individual APRN's practice. This variation in consultation practice also leads to variability in the appropriate questions and criteria used to evaluate the consultation skill. Examples of questions that may help with the evaluation of consultation skills include:

- Are the consultant recommendations appropriate for the patient situation and do they result in improved patient outcomes?
- Is the consultant contacted again after the initial consultation?
- Are consultation requests for the APRN becoming more sophisticated over time?
- Was the APRN able to respond to all requests for consultation?
- Do glaring issues or needs seem to be going unaddressed?
- Do there seem to be patterns in terms of the theme, number, or location of consultations?
- Are there delays in doing consultation triage?

The subjective experiences of the APRN consultant should be considered. Were the consultees open and comfortable with the consultant? Were consultees anxious or resistant? These data are subjective but important in evaluating the overall success of the consultation.

Clinical competency, competency in applying the consultation process, interpersonal skills, and professionalism are all areas to be considered in evaluation. Identifying the individuals involved in the evaluation and developing a systematic approach to data collection regarding the consultation of the APRN practice are important and validate the need for the APRN consultant. Over time, assessment of change in the consultees or consultee system is the best evaluation of the competency.

Obstacles to Successful Consultation

Many obstacles can be identified for the APRN engaging in consultation. They include a lack of education about consultation models and the nuanced complexities of the process. Students are encouraged to read extensively about the process of consultation, the various types, and the ways nurse consultation can be implemented. Approaching a complex consultation without the knowledge of the system, the question being asked, or the aspects of the consultee that influence the process sets the consultant up to potentially fail in positively completing the consultation. Being set up by the broader system to fail with the consultation is a risk best avoided by knowledge and planning. When the consultation process is not about the consultation at all but about roles and expertise of the APRN, it can be indicative of larger problematic issues within the system. Students are encouraged to study the consultation process and to proceed thoughtfully when asked to provide a consultation. Knowledge and awareness of all the influencing factors provide the power that helps ensure successful consultation.

Conclusion

APRNs have a long tradition of involvement in various aspects of direct and indirect patient care activities, including consultation. APRNs use their consultation skills to improve care processes and patient outcomes. The power of consultative activities to inform and advance practice compels all APRNs to consider consultation as an integral aspect of role performance. Consultation offers APRNs the opportunity to both acquire and share the clinical expertise necessary to meet the increasingly challenging and diverse demands of patient care in a changing health care environment.

APRN consultation contributes to positive patient outcomes and may promote more appropriate use of scarce health care resources. These assumptions require testing through quality improvement studies, cost-benefit studies, and research that examines the processes and outcomes of care. This procedure can result in effective measurement of consultation activities and resulting care outcomes. Consultation can facilitate having comprehensive and specialty-related knowledge directly and indirectly available to all patients who might need it and should be an expected and integral aspect of APRN role performance.

In summary, this chapter has examined the art of consultation as it pertains to the APRN. As the sphere of nursing influence expands, APRNs are likely to have increased requests and demand for the consultation part of their specialty nursing practice.

Key Summary Points

- Consultation is an essential part of APRN practice regardless of role or specialty.
- Consultation differs from co-management, referral, supervision, and collaboration.
- Consultation, as described in this chapter, is an independent, autonomous nursing function,

though APRNs must be aware of specific state regulations that impact APRN consultation activity.
- It is important for the consultant and consultee to define expectations and responsibilities of the consultation, and there should be closed-loop communication to ensure successful closure of the consult.

References

To access the references for this chapter, use your smartphone's QR code reader to scan the code below, or go to http://booksite.elsevier.com/ 9780323447751.

Evidence-Based Practice

Mikel Gray

> *"Efficiency is doing the things right, effectiveness is doing the right things."*
>
> **—Peter Drucker**

Evidence-based practice (EBP) is the dominant approach for clinical decision making in the 21st century and a core competency of advanced practice registered nurse (APRN) practice (American Association of Colleges of Nursing [AACN], 2006, 2011). The primary purpose of this chapter is to review principles of EBP and how the APRN incorporates these principles into practice. It also describes the four steps of the evidence-based process and identifies resources that the APRN can use when making clinical decisions.

EBP is defined as the conscientious, explicit, and judicious use of current best research-based evidence when making decisions about the care of individual patients (Sackett, Rosenberg, Gray, Haynes, & Richardson, 1996). Current best evidence is drawn from *research* produced by nurses or a variety of other members of the interprofessional team providing care to individual patients, groups of patients, or communities. *Nursing research* is defined as systematic inquiry that generates new knowledge about issues of importance to the nursing profession; individual studies may focus on clinical practice, education,

administration, and informatics (Polit & Beck, 2016). Although all such research contributes to the nursing profession, *current best evidence* entails the application of research findings from studies that evaluate interventions or assessments used by nurses and other care providers to improve patient outcomes. For the APRN, much of this research will be generated by nurses. Nevertheless, the APRN will also draw upon research produced by multiple members of the interprofessional team who deliver modern health care and apply these findings to evidence-based clinical decision making as an individual provider or as a mentor or consultant to front-line nurses, physicians, and other care providers.

Advanced practice nursing has evolved significantly since its inception in the 20th century. Entry into APRN practice now occurs following completion of a master's or doctoral degree. All APRNs are educated to seek out and apply current best evidence, which is the core component of EBP. In addition, the master's-prepared APRN may be involved with generation of original research, acting as a data collector or a member of a multisite clinical trial (AACN, 2011). The master's-prepared APRN also may participate in and lead quality improvement projects that collect and analyze data from a specific unit, facility, or multisite health system in order to evaluate and improve care processes in the unit, facility, or health system.

The APRN who wishes to play a more active or lead role in generating original research may complete a doctoral program with a research focus. Most research-based doctoral programs in the United States lead to a Doctor of Philosophy (PhD) degree (AACN, 2011). These PhD programs prepare nurses for a research-intensive career; extensive coursework focuses on theory and metatheory, research methodology, and statistical analysis of findings needed to produce new knowledge for the advancement of nursing. Having completed a research doctorate, the PhD-prepared APRN may act as principal investigator or coinvestigator of studies with other nurse researchers. In addition, the PhD-prepared nurse may act as a member of an interprofessional team designing a research project, overseeing data collection, analyzing findings, and disseminating these findings via the professional literature. Many PhD-prepared nurses will function primarily in a faculty role, while others will engage in clinical practice based on their knowledge and training as an APRN.

More recently, many APRN students are electing to complete a practice-focused doctorate degree, the Doctor of Nursing Practice (DNP). The DNP-prepared APRN is ideally prepared to synthesize existing research findings essential for EBP, to use data from increasingly sophisticated databases linked to Electronic Medical Record systems and national databases, and to participate in the formation of policies and procedures on a facility-wide or health system–wide basis. In addition, this individual may participate in the generation of original research as a data collector or clinical consultant to a research team charged with designing a particular study. The DNP-prepared APRN is also prepared to design and participate in quality improvement projects that analyze practice and processes within a specific facility or health system. Quality improvement projects are the evaluation of practice processes within a specific unit, clinic, facility, service, or community in order to change (improve) patient-centered outcomes, while a formal research study is designed to generate new knowledge. The DNP- prepared APRN also may synthesize findings from multiple studies via a systematic or scoping literature review resulting in ranking of levels of evidence, differentiate evidence-based from best practice–based assessments or interventions, and identify gaps in research.

Whereas the role of the APRN in EBP is well established, the role of the master's- or DNP-prepared APRN in generating original research continues to evolve. Education programs provide essential knowledge and skills needed to enter into practice as a master's-prepared, DNP-prepared, or PhD-prepared APRN. As DNP-prepared APRNs move into practice and gain greater expertise and knowledge through continuing education or individualized teaching from clinician or academic mentors, the individual's role in the generation of original research may evolve. Such evolution is especially likely for the first generation of DNP-prepared APRNs, who are just now entering practice in significant numbers. As these individuals move through their careers and gain expertise, they are likely to form strategic and productive alliances with PhD-prepared nurse researchers, physician researchers, and others who are likely to strengthen current best evidence and enhance current methodologic approaches via real-work clinical trials or use of metadata in order to more fully understand the processes of nursing and interprofessional clinical practice. The AACN (2015) has published a white paper concerning the role of the DNP in generation of new knowledge that provides initial expert opinion concerning this new level of APRN education and practice, but additional time is needed to determine the DNP's optimal involvement in the generation and synthesis of evidence.

Evidence-Based Practice and the APRN

EBP is the dominant approach for clinical decision making and a core competency for APRNs who hold a master's in nursing or a DNP (AANC, 2006, 2011; Stiffler & Cullen, 2010; see Chapter 3). The AACN has defined essentials of master's and doctoral education in nursing (AACN, 2006, 2011). All APRNs are expected to translate current best evidence into practice. The master's-prepared APRN is expected to integrate policies and seek evidence for every aspect of practice; this skill requires application of principles of EBP to clinical decision making and professional practice. Education within a DNP program builds on these skills by further developing the student's competencies to use analytic methods to appraise existing literature and other forms of evidence (such as abstracts or other forms of grey literature[a]) into determining best practices; designing

---

[a]Grey literature are document types that are protected by intellectual property rights and of sufficient quality to be collected and preserved by libraries and institutional repositories, but they are not controlled by commercial publishers.

and implementing processes to evaluate practice outcomes; developing practice patterns that influence these outcomes; and comparing practice within an individual unit, facility, or health system against national benchmarks. The DNP-prepared APRN is also able to use information technologies in order to collect data related to current nursing practice patterns and outcomes, analyze these data, and play a leadership role in designing and implementing quality improvement initiatives and projects essential for application of current best evidence to the local unit, facility, or regional or national health system.

Although components tend to overlap, three levels of this core competency for APRN practice can be identified: (1) interpretation and use of EBP principles in individual clinical decision making; (2) interpretation and use of EBP principles to determine policies, standards, and procedures for patient care; and (3) use of EBP to evaluate clinical practice.

A formal, four-step process for identifying and determining EBP has been defined; it consists of: (1) formulation of a clinical question; (2) identification and retrieval of pertinent research findings based on literature review; (3) extraction and critical appraisal of data from pertinent studies; and (4) clinical decision making based on results of this process (Sackett, Strauss, Richardson, Rosenberg, & Haynes, 2000). This process was originally developed as a teaching strategy for medical students, and it remains the central process for creating current best evidence. Given the growing number of clinical practice guidelines and related EBP resources, this four-step process acts as a template for incorporating current best evidence in practice.

Principles of EBP are used to guide clinical decision making for individual patients, for creating policies and procedures that influence current practice on a facility-wide or health system–wide level, and for determining policies for delivering care to large groups (Gerrish et al., 2011; Stiffler & Cullen, 2010). Despite widespread acceptance of the concept of EBP, adoption of current best evidence into daily practice remains limited. For example, analysis of mammogram use by the Behavioral Risk Factor Surveillance System found no significant change in rates of mammography screening among women less than 50 years of age despite a 2009 change advising against routine screening mammography in younger women (Dehkordy et al., 2015). Similarly, a random sample of 850 children from 28 school-based health centers in six states found that, despite recommendations from a multidisciplinary expert panel of physicians, nurses, nutritionists, psychologists, and epidemiologists, body

mass index was not calculated on 27% of children's health records and blood pressure was not documented on 68.5% of records (Gance-Cleveland et al., 2015). Additional analysis revealed that slightly more than half of obese children (51.7%) were identified based on recommended screening procedures. A number of factors are thought to influence clinician acceptance and application of this problem-solving approach to direct patient care, including a lack of knowledge of the principles of EBP. This chapter defines EBP, differentiates it from concepts of research and quality improvement, and defines three levels of advanced practice nurse competency related to EBP (Table 10.1):

Level I: use of evidence in individual APRN practice
Level II: use of evidence to change practice
Level III: use of evidence to evaluate practice

Exemplars 10.1, 10.2, and 10.3 provide examples of each of these EBP-related competencies.

The term *evidence-based practice* represents a blending of several related concepts, including evidence-based nursing and evidence-based medicine. The original term, *evidence-based medicine,* traces its historical roots to a strategy for educating medical students developed by the faculty at McMaster Medical School in Hamilton, Ontario (Rosenberg & Donald, 1995). Evidence-based nursing is defined as the process that nurses use to make clinical decisions using the best available research evidence, their clinical expertise, and patient preferences (DiCenso, Cullum, & Ciliska, 2002). The explicit inclusion of patient preference and clinical expertise is significant for APRNs because they reflect the holistic approach central to nursing practice while maintaining the focus on current, research-based evidence.

EBP offers several advantages when compared with previous models of clinical decision-making. For example, tradition-based practice is based on clinical and anecdotal experience, combined with received wisdom, often provided by instructors or clinical preceptors and expert opinion from those perceived as experts or expert clinicians in a given area of care. By substituting a standard of current best evidence for received wisdom or expert opinion, EBP encourages the advanced practice nurse to update and refine clinical practice continually as newer evidence is generated and published. EBP also offers distinctive advantages when compared with rationale-based clinical decision making.

Rationale-based clinical decision making relies on identifying a rational explanation for an intervention

TABLE 10.1   Overview of Evidence-Based Practice Competencies and Levels

Competency	Fundamental Level	Expanded Level
Level I: Interpretation and use of research and other evidence in clinical decision making	Incorporate evidence-based practice (EBP) principles and processes into individual clinical practice.	Create and incorporate EBP practices and principles on a unit, clinic, department, facility, health care system, national, or international level. The advanced practice registered nurse (APRN) may serve as member of interprofessional team formulating policies and procedures on a unit-wide, facility-wide, or health system–wide level. The APRN may function as member of an expert panel that formulates best practice, evidence-based, or blended practice guidelines intended for use on a national or global level.
Level II: Use of EBP to change practice	Incorporate best practice changes according to EBP principles into own practice or act as mentor to front-line staff incorporating change.	Design and implement a process for changing practice beyond the scope of individual practice on a unit, clinic, facility, health care system, or national basis.
Level III: Use of EBP to evaluate practice	Identify benchmarks for evaluating own practice or participate in evaluation of practice among front-line nursing and other clinical staff.	Design and implement a process to evaluate pertinent outcomes of practice beyond the scope of individual practice (e.g., generic nursing practice, group APRN practice, interprofessional team practice, facility-wide or health care system–wide practice).

EXEMPLAR 10.1   Level I: Interpretation and Use of Evidence-Based Practice in Individual Clinical Decision Making

The most basic level of evidence-based practice (EBP) competency is the application of the four steps for clinical decision making in an individual patient. This proficiency requires more than formulation of a clinical question and identification of pertinent studies needed to determine best available evidence. The advanced practice registered nurse (APRN) must combine knowledge of best evidence with an assessment of individual patient factors likely to affect treatment effects, such as the presence of comorbid conditions, psychosocial and cultural factors such as locus of control, preference and impact on quality of life, and cost considerations.

Example: As an APRN in a urology department, I am often asked by patients and physician colleagues whether cranberry juice or supplements (including cranberry capsules) should be prescribed to prevent urinary tract infection (UTI). This persistent query led me to formulate a clinical question, "Are cranberry juice or cranberry products effective in the prevention or management of urinary tract infection?" A systematic literature review based on current best evidence available in 2002 suggested that regular consumption of cranberry juice reduces the incidence of UTIs in community-dwelling women and residents of long-term facilities but does not reduce the risk in patients who undergo intermittent or indwelling catheterization (M. Gray, 2002). The findings of this systematic review

were further supported by a recent randomized controlled trial (RCT) that evaluated a 6-week course of cranberry juice versus placebo capsules in 106 women following gynecologic surgery. Analysis revealed a lower incidence of UTI in women allocated to active cranberry tablets; this difference persisted after adjusting for likely confounding variables, including intermittent self-catheterization (Foxman, Cronenwett, Spino, Berger, & Morgan, 2015).

However, additional evidence has emerged that influences these conclusions. Specifically, two RCTs published in 2011 and 2012 found that cranberry juice was no more effective than antimicrobial therapy or cranberry-flavored placebo drink for preventing UTI (Barbosa-Cesnik et al., 2011; Stapleton et al., 2012). On initial consideration, this evidence appeared to support discontinuing recommendations of consumption of cranberry for women seeking to prevent recurrent UTIs. However, additional evaluation of findings from one of the studies, a study using a placebo group (Barbosa-Cesnik et al., 2011), revealed that both groups experienced a considerably lower incidence of UTIs than anticipated. In a subsequent interview with one of the investigators, the researchers acknowledged a possibility that the placebo-flavored drink might have contained some of the ingredients hypothesized to exert an antimicrobial effect in the urine (Larson, 2010). In addition, I considered the fact that consumption of

Level I: Interpretation and Use of Evidence-Based Practice in Individual Clinical Decision Making—cont'd

cranberry juice twice daily is not associated with any known harmful side effects. I also considered the fact that cranberry juice is relatively inexpensive compared with dietary supplement cranberry capsules. As a consequence of all these factors, cranberry juice is preferred as a natural means for preventing UTIs among many women in my practice.

This example of basing individual clinical decisions on an EBP process illustrates several important points. It points out the importance of remaining abreast of emerging evidence and the real possibility that newer evidence may significantly alter our understanding of the benefits or harmful effects associated with a specific intervention. In addition, this case illustrates the role of patient preference in clinical decision making. Clinical experience strongly suggests that a significant proportion of women prefer nonpharmacologic interventions for preventing UTIs, and regular consumption of cranberry juice tends to increase overall fluid intake and provide possibly beneficial effects without associated adverse side effects. Therefore, given the absence of harm, low direct cost, and mixed evidence concerning efficacy of this preventive intervention, I discuss consumption of cranberry juice with women as a possibly effective intervention that is free from harmful side effects. I also counsel women to consider engaging in other behavioral interventions for the prevention of UTIs, including adequate daily fluid intake based on recent recommendations from the Institute of Medicine, daily consumption of a dietary source of the probiotic lactobacillus, and consideration of avoiding use of a diaphragm and vaginal spermicide as birth control strategies (Salvatore et al., 2011).

This case also illustrates the time-consuming and rigorous demands of basing individual clinical decisions on the EBP process. Fortunately, APRNs have access to various evidence-based resources such as the *Cochrane Database of Systematic Reviews* and the systematic reviews available at the U.S. Preventive Services Task Force web page.

In addition to these resources, a growing number of professional societies have generated evidence-based clinical practice guidelines that address measurable clinical questions with thorough and extensive systematic reviews of existing evidence to formulate clinical recommendations covering comparatively broad topics such as heart failure, diabetes mellitus, chronic obstructive pulmonary disease, breast cancer, end-stage renal disease, osteoporosis, and other topics of special interest to APRN practice. In addition to searching the resources of the appropriate professional association's web page, the National Clearinghouse of Practice Guidelines, operated by the Agency for Healthcare Research and Quality, houses a large collection of evidence-based clinical practice guidelines that can be accessed at http://www.guideline.gov. ◎

Level II: Interpretation and Use of Evidence-Based Practice to Create Policies for Patient Care

For many advanced practice registered nurses, the growing demand to formulate evidence-based policies and protocols needed to prevent the growing list of "never events" provides an opportunity to master the second competency level, interpretation and use of evidence-based practice (EBP) to create policies for patient care.

Example: Fineout-Overholt, Melnyk, Stillwell, and Williamson (2010a, 2010b, 2010c) have described the EBP process needed to answer a clinical question about whether a rapid response team affects the number of cardiac arrests and unplanned intensive care unit admissions in hospitalized adults. Based on this question, the authors described the process used to search the evidence for pertinent studies, code and extract data from these studies using a standardized protocol, and synthesize data to implement policies needed to launch a rapid response team at their facility. Based on this process, the team concluded that there is sufficient evidence to justify developing policies and committing the resources needed to form a rapid response team at their facility. In addition to providing an example of the EBP described in this chapter, this series of articles describes the processes required to implement such a program. Although a detailed discussion of this translation from research-based evidence to clinical practice is beyond the scope of this chapter, the authors identified and briefly reviewed essential components of this step in the implementation process, including engaging stakeholders in their facility; securing administrative support; preparing a campaign to launch the rapid response team, including staff education and changes in care protocols; and measuring outcomes following implementation of the practice change. ◎

Level III: Evaluation of Evidence-Based Practice to Determine Standards of Care

Participation in an interprofessional team to evaluate and determine standards of care using evidence-based practice (EBP) is the third and most advanced level of the EBP competency for advanced practice registered nurse (APRN) practice. Generation of an evidence-based clinical practice guideline entails identification of a number of clinically measurable questions required for establishing and evaluating clinical practice in a broad area of patient care, along with an extensive systematic review of pertinent studies. This often encompasses major assessment strategies related to the management of a particular disorder and first-line and alternative interventions for management.

Example: A professional nursing society charged a task force of three APRNs with clinical expertise in chronic wound care with development and validation of an evidence-based algorithm for use of compression for prevention and treatment of chronic venous insufficiency (CVI) and venous leg ulcers (VLUs) (Ratliff, Yates, McNichol, Gray, 2016). The task force began this task by identifying pertinent clinical questions, an appropriate theoretical framework for clinical decision making in patients with CVI and/or VLUs, and an exploratory literature review. The nursing society committee selected a PhD-prepared APRN with experience in literature review and generation of evidence-based guidelines for clinical practice, including algorithms. Patient population/Problem, Intervention, Comparison, and Outcome (PICO)–formatted questions were generated by the three-member task force and a literature review was initiated. It soon became apparent that the algorithm must combine evidence-based decisional nodes with clinical decision points that lack sufficient evidence to be deemed evidence based. Based on this initial review, the task force elected to complete a scoping review that focused on current clinical practice guidelines and research specifically focusing on a single aspect of CVI and VLU prevention and treatment: compression. This search revealed eight clinical practice guidelines; each recommended compression as part of a bundle of interventions for prevention and management of CVI and VLUs, but none provided adequate guidance concerning when to select a specific type of compression (stockings, bandages, intermittent pneumatic compression devices) or best practices for donning and removing compression devices. Based on these initial findings, a second phase of the literature review was completed that included studies in adult patients that compared one or more types of compression, or evaluated techniques for aiding patients or lay caregivers in donning or removing compression devices. This two-step scoping literature review was used to develop a draft algorithm that incorporated evidence-based interventions and interventions lacking adequate clinical evidence, along with evidence-based statements supporting the algorithm and best practice statements linked to clinical decisions not supported by adequate research-based evidence.

A multidisciplinary team that represented all regions of the United States was assembled that reviewed and critiqued the algorithm and reached consensus on best practice statements supporting the algorithm. This panel comprised APRNs, specialty practice nurses in wound, ostomy and continence vascular care, physical therapists, physicians, and basic science researchers in the area of compression devices. Under the direction of this multidisciplinary group, the algorithm was modified, including addition of supplemental materials deemed necessary for adaptation of the algorithm by clinicians with limited experience and knowledge in management of CVI and VLUs. It was also adapted into an electronic format for ease of use in multiple care settings. This second draft of the algorithm was submitted to content validation by a second and separate multidisciplinary group that was composed of APRNs, specialty practice nurses, physicians, and physical therapists. The resulting guideline has been downloaded by more than 7000 providers in North America, including APRNs, specialty practice nurses, vascular surgeons, and physicians and physical therapists specializing in chronic wound care. The construction and validation of this algorithm demonstrates how a small task force of APRNs consulted with a PhD-prepared APRN to design PICO-based questions and complete a scoping literature review that combined evidence-based decisions with best practice decisions essential to construction of a clinically relevant and pragmatic algorithm guiding APRNs, specialty practice and front-line nurses, physicians, and physical therapists in selecting, applying, and reapplying compression for prevention and management of VLUs in adult patients with CVI. Research concerning the influence of this algorithm in two settings, long-term care and home care, is ongoing. ◎

(Gray et al., 2002). This form of clinical decision making relies on findings from a wide variety of studies, including pathophysiologic research designed to identify the principal action of an intervention or the main reason it exerts a particular effect, and in vitro or in vivo research models that measure outcomes in animals, tissues, or individual cell lines. Although these types of studies are enormously valuable to our overall understanding of health, disease, and the reasons that interventions exert a particular effect, EBP limits its search for evidence to studies that directly measure the efficacy or effectiveness of a particular intervention, the predictive power of diagnostic studies, and the presence and severity of adverse side effects.

Evidence-Based Practice, Research, and Quality Improvement

The process and outcome of EBP should be differentiated from the process of generating a research study or completing a quality improvement (QI) project (Shirey et al., 2011; Table 10.2). Research is a systematic investigation designed to generate or contribute generalizable new knowledge to health care or advanced practice nursing (Arndt & Netsch, 2012). In contrast, EBP combines findings from multiple research studies that focus on the efficacy of a particular intervention or the accuracy of a specific diagnostic procedure. EBP has been described as the study of studies; its goal is the synthesis of existing knowledge generated from multiple research studies, whereas the goal of an individual research study is to generate new knowledge about an intervention or assessment technique (Gray et al., 2002). QI is defined as a systematic activity that generates outcome data in order to achieve rapid improvements in health care delivery in a specific setting (Arndt & Netsch, 2012; US Department of Health and Human Services, Health Resources and Services Administration, 2011). The data generated during a QI project is designed to improve specific outcomes within a local facility, clinic, or community. Unlike the data generated by a research study, the results of a QI project can only be generalized to the specific patient population that comprised the project setting.

Despite these differences, the APRN should remember that research, EPB, and QI projects share a common goal—improvement of patient care. Further, research, EBP, and QI should be viewed as complementary and combined in a manner that improves individual clinical decision making and

care processes affecting an entire facility, health care system, or larger community. For example, an acute care APRN may observe that the ventilator-associated pneumonia (VAP) incidence in his or her facility's critical care unit is higher than published benchmarks. As a result, the APRN elects to complete a QI project designed at reducing the incidence of VAP. Initially, the APRN should review the unit's current prevention protocol to determine whether it is based on current best evidence, such as routine oral hygiene, regular evaluation for readiness to extubate, elevation of the head of the bed, and prophylaxis for peptic ulcer disease and deep vein thrombosis (Eom et al., 2014). This review may incorporate principles of EBP and findings from individual research studies to answer two questions:

- Are the preventive interventions used by local staff based on current best evidence?
- Does existing research suggest that combining these interventions into a prevention bundle actually reduces the incidence of VAP?

In reference to the first question, a review of current best evidence suggests that bundled interventions are effective for reducing the incidence of VAP (Eom et al., 2014; Ramirez, Bassi, & Torres, 2012). When examining individual interventions, the acute care APRN may note that current best evidence supports regular oral hygiene that incorporates chlorhexidine as effective for preventing VAP (Vilela, Ferreira, Santos, & Rezende, 2015). In contrast, limited evidence suggests that ongoing elevation of the head of the bed may not affect VAP incidence, even though it is associated with an increased likelihood of sacral pressure ulcer formation (Edsberg, Langemo, Baherastani, Posthauer, & Goldberg, 2014; Leng, Song, Yao, & Zhu, 2012;). Finally, the APRN also may identify findings from an individual study, the NASCENT randomized clinical trial. This study demonstrated that a silver-coated endotracheal tube reduced the incidence of VAP (Kollef et al., 2008) in 9417 critically ill adults from 54 facilities in North America.

Thus the APRN has synthesized essential research-based knowledge using principles of EBP to provide a platform for a QI project. Depending on existing policies in the local critical care unit, the APRN may collaborate with others to create a modified or novel prevention bundle and measure VAP incidence before and following implementation of this bundle. Findings of this process comprise a QI project; although these results cannot be generalized to every critical care unit, they can be used to evaluate care processes in the local critical care unit.

TABLE 10.2   Evidence-Based Practice, Research, and Quality Improvement: Understanding the Similarities and Differences

	Evidence-Based Practice	Research Study	Quality Improvement Project
Overall Goal	Apply current best evidence to clinical decision making for individual patient, facility, or large group	Produce generalizable new knowledge	Enhance quality of care delivery by evaluating the effect of specific action plan on local unit, clinic, facility, or health system
Methodology for Generating Results	Systematic review with ordinal ranking of strength of evidence and/or meta-analysis Scoping literature review (study) may be combined with consensus-based expert opinion for identifying best practice documents when evidence is lacking	Various methods employed: • randomized controlled trial • comparison cohort study • prospective cohort study • retrospective comparison control study • qualitative	Various models used; most common include: • CHRONIC CARE model (Problem solving, Decision Making, Resource utilization, Taking Action, Counseling, Community Resources) • LEAN model • PDSA (Plan-Do-Study-Act) model (also referred to as Model for Improvement) • Focus-Analyze-Develop-Execute-Evaluate (FADE) model • Six Sigma model (DMAIC: Define, Measure, Analyze, Improve, Control)
Unit of Study	Individual studies, systematic review with pooled analysis of multiple studies	Varies, typically aggregate (sample) of individual patients, families, communities	Varies, typically one or more units within facility, individual facility, or individual health system
Does involvement of human subjects require Institutional Review Board review and approval?	Not indicated; evidence-based practice is the study of studies and application in daily practice	Always indicated when study has any involvement of human subjects	May be indicated if project involves evaluation of novel or nonstandard care (intervention) of patients
Tangible Product (may or may not be published or made available to public)	Individual clinical judgment Policy for care on individual unit/clinic, facility wide or health system wide Protocol for care delivery Clinical practice guideline	Research report, may be initially presented as abstract or poster at scientific meeting; ultimate goal is to publish as research report in peer-reviewed scholarly journal	Internal report to health system leadership and/or administration; may be published as quality improvement report in peer-reviewed scholarly journal

Evidence and Current Best Evidence: Historical Perspective

Although the concept of "best evidence" may appear transparent on initial consideration, a more careful analysis of the historical roots of evidence generation in health care is needed. The Oxford English Dictionary Online (2016) defines evidence as an object or document that serves as proof. The objects or documents acceptable for use as evidence vary for each discipline or profession; historians seek out original documents or artifacts, and lawyers have developed a complex system for identifying evidence codified with federal, state, or other rules of evidence documents. Within the context of EBP, clinicians seek studies to establish evidence for the efficacy and safety of an intervention, or the predictive power of a diagnostic procedure. Although the search for evidence can be traced back more than 2000 years, definitions for what constitutes sufficient evidence to reach these conclusions have evolved significantly over time.

Despite a growing number of study designs used to evaluate the effectiveness of various interventions, diagnostic procedures, and intervention bundles, the randomized controlled trial (RCT) remains the gold standard research design for generating evidence (Sackett, 2015; Turner, 2012). The RCT is based on three critical elements: (1) manipulation of an experimental intervention; (2) comparison of the group receiving the experimental intervention to a control or comparison group that receives a placebo, sham device, or standard intervention, depending on ethical considerations; and (3) random allocation of subjects to the intervention or comparison/control group. Random allocation, advocated since the early 1930s, is an essential element of an RCT because it is the most effective technique for spreading potentially confounding factors evenly among treatment and control groups (Hill, 1937). A well-known RCT that compared streptomycin with standard care at the time (bed rest) is usually cited as the world's first, large-scale, controlled trial (Streptomycin treatment, 1948). Randomization was achieved using a closed envelope system and subjects were blinded to treatment group. However, at least one trial was completed and published before this landmark study. Amberson, McMahon, and Pinner (1931) compared the antibiotic sanocrysin for treatment of pulmonary tuberculosis with a placebo. In addition to random allocation of subjects by flipping a coin, they also blinded physician data collectors to group assignment to minimize bias, another important design feature of the modern RCT.

Based on this historical legacy and guided by the pioneering efforts of Archibald Cochrane, current best evidence is now defined as the best available studies evaluating the efficacy and safety of an active or preventive intervention or the predictive accuracy of an assessment (Gray et al., 2004; van Rijswijk & Gray, 2012). These studies must directly evaluate the effect of an intervention; compare the intervention with a placebo, standard care, or a sham device; and document adverse side effects associated with the intervention. Studies used to establish current best evidence must be executed in human (rather than animal) subjects and must measure the most direct outcome of treatment, rather than relying on interim outcomes based on convenience. For example, a study of the efficacy of a topical wound therapy should measure wound closure rather than concluding efficacy based on the percentage of wound closure completed at a convenient or arbitrary point after the initiation of treatment (van Rijswijk & Gray, 2012).

This definition of current best evidence raises a corollary question: What criteria must be fulfilled to define an intervention as "evidence-based?" At least two major regulatory groups, the U.S. Food

and Drug Administration (FDA) and the European Medicines Agency (EMA), have established specific criteria for labeling an intervention as evidence based (Cormier, 2011). For a drug to receive an indication for clinical use, the FDA requires results from two well-designed RCTs with consistent results, both of which must compare the agent with a placebo- or sham-based control group; the EMA criteria are similar (EMA, 2000).

Although these groups provide well-defined criteria for defining an intervention (administration of a drug) as evidence based, achieving this level of evidence is complex and enormously costly. For example, the total cost of achieving a new drug indication has risen sharply over the past decade and may be as high as $2.5 billion (Mullin, 2014). Based on these rigid criteria, only a minority of interventions that APRNs use to manage their patients would qualify as evidence based, and limited research in this area has suggested that 40% of clinical decisions used in daily practice are unsupported by evidence (G. E. Gray, 2002; Greenhalgh, 2001). As a result, APRNs often must search the literature and identify relevant evidence to support clinical decision making in a particular case or group of patients, or retrieve this information from EBP resources, such as clinical practice guidelines or best practice documents.

Steps of the Evidence-Based Process

Step 1: Formulate a Measurable Clinical Question

Clinical decision making using the EBP process begins with the formulation of a measurable clinical question. Questions arise from various sources. For example, many APRNs will formulate their first clinical questions as part of an EBP process when planning their final scholarly project as part of a DNP degree. Individual clinical APRN or staff nurse practice provides another rich source for clinical questions. Queries may arise when the APRN is faced with a questionably effective intervention or when managing an uncommon or rare disorder that is not addressed in major clinical practice guidelines. APRNs often serve on multidisciplinary committees that may be charged with developing a policy or protocol for presenting or managing a particular clinical challenge. For example, the growing list of "never events" (National Quality Forum, 2016) presents an ongoing challenge to APRNs practicing in the acute and critical care settings, who are often charged with designing facility-wide prevention programs for conditions such as catheter-associated urinary tract infections, surgical site infections, and central line–associated bloodstream infections.

After identifying the general topic to be scrutinized, the APRN must formulate a measurable question that can be meaningfully addressed using evidence-based clinical decision strategies. Results of several studies have suggested that application of the PICO model aids nurses in formulating clinically relevant and measurable questions as well as assisting in efficiently searching the literature for available evidence (Balakas & Sparks, 2010; Hastings & Fisher, 2014; LaRue, Draus, & Klem, 2009; Smith-Strøm & Nortvedt, 2008; Table 10.3).

The *P* in PICO indicates patient or population (Hastings & Fisher, 2014), although the P is sometimes expanded to include the primary problem (Balakas & Sparks, 2010). This element of the formula alerts the APRN to define the population to be studied and the nature of the problem to be scrutinized carefully. The population may comprise a subgroup of patients in a facility, such as critically ill patients receiving mechanical ventilation or all patients with an indwelling urinary catheter, but it often incorporates much larger populations, such as any individual with a wound or any patient recently diagnosed with diabetes mellitus. As these examples illustrate, identification of the primary problem is closely tied to the population under scrutiny. Examples of primary problems may be a disease such as sinusitis, a disorder such as chronic osteoarthritis, or a

predisposition to a potentially preventable condition such as a pressure ulcer.

The *I* in the PICO model represents the main intervention to be considered. In many cases, an APRN will examine a single intervention such as using a follow-up telephone intervention for reducing fasting blood glucose levels in patients with diabetes mellitus (Evans, 2010). In contrast, the combined effect of more than one intervention used to prevent or treat a specific disorder can be evaluated. For example, the APRN can identify a protocol or bundle of interventions and analyze their effect on a given outcome. Searching for evidence that evaluates the combined effect of multiple interventions is clinically useful, but it presents unique challenges. For example, Hagiwara, Henricson, Jonsson, and Suserud (2011) studied whether decision support tools decrease the time to receive definitive care in acutely ill or trauma patients prior to hospital admission. They operationally defined "decision support tools" as active knowledge systems that use two or more items to generate case-specific advice. They further classified these tools as electronic or nonelectronic. However, their literature search retrieved only 2 of 33 studies that specifically addressed this clinically relevant question. Despite the use of a well-accepted definition for decision support tools, the authors observed that a number of studies were excluded because it was not possible to classify the study intervention as a decision support tool.

Nayan, Gupta, and Sommer (2011) faced a similar challenge when studying whether smoking cessation rates were higher in oncology patients who receive smoking cessation interventions as compared with usual care. Their initial search identified a meta-analysis of data from eight RCTs that detected no differences in self-reported cessation rates when these interventions were compared with usual care. However, subclassifying smoking interventions into pharmacologic, behavioral, and combined interventions suggested that cessation protocols that combine pharmacologic and behavioral interventions appeared to increase cessation rates when compared with usual care or single-intervention protocols.

The *C* in the PICO model represents the approach used as a basis for comparison to the intervention undergoing scrutiny. This approach is frequently described in research reports as standard care or usual care. Although these terms are descriptive, it is essential that the APRN specifically define the intervention(s) that comprise standard care and ensure that the studies retrieved enable adequate differentiation of this standard care from the

---

◎ **TABLE 10.3**   **PICO(T) Model for Generating EBP Clinical Questions**

Component	Definition
P	*P*atient/*P*opulation—identify the population of interest *P*roblem—identify the primary problem
I	*I*ntervention—identify the intervention(s) to be considered
C	*C*omparison—identify to what the intervention will be compared
O	*O*utcome—identify the goal of the intervention(s)
T*	*T*ime—time frame for measuring outcomes

*Optional.

Adapted from Smith-Strøm, H., & Nortvedt, M. W. (2008). Evaluation of evidence-based methods used to teach nursing students to critically appraise evidence. *Journal of Nursing Education, 47*, 372–375; and Sackett, D. L., Strauss, S. E., Richardson, W. S., Rosenberg, W., & Haynes, R. B. (2000). *Evidence-based medicine: How to practice and teach EBM* (2nd ed.). London: Churchill-Livingstone.

intervention under scrutiny, especially when evaluating the effect of a bundled intervention or protocol.

The *O* in PICO represents the outcome, or intended goal of the intervention. When determining the outcome, it is important to identify and evaluate the most direct result indicating clinical efficacy and avoid reliance on indirect outcomes that are more easily measured. Careful consideration of the most direct and clinically relevant outcome is essential when constructing a clinically relevant question. For prevention studies, the most direct outcome is generally a reduction in the incidence of the disease or disorder under scrutiny. For example, an APRN evaluating the effect of a prevention protocol on surgical site infection rates should base conclusions of efficacy on incidence rates, rather than on interim outcomes such as differences in a nurse's knowledge after education on prevention or self-reported changes in practice following in-service training. The APRN should also measure process outcomes that may influence whether the intended goal or outcome is met.

A final element, *T,* indicating time, may be added to the PICO conceptual framework. The time frame is meant to indicate the relevant observation period for outcomes; it may be short, such as the first 24 to 48 hours following surgery, or long, such as years to decades following the onset of a chronic condition such as dementia or diabetes mellitus (Balakas & Sparks, 2010; Hastings & Fisher, 2014; Milnes, Gonzalez, & Amos, 2015).

Step 2: Search the Literature for Relevant Studies

Evidence-based clinical decision making relies on identifying research-based evidence. Therefore, it is essential for the APRN to develop expertise in searching the literature to identify and retrieve appropriate studies. Fortunately, the development of modern electronic databases has revolutionized our ability to search the published literature rapidly and access pertinent research reports. A number of electronic databases are now available to the APRN (Table 10.4). Although full access to these databases usually requires a paid subscription, APRNs may access these electronic databases via a facility-based subscription. Specifically, the vast majority of health system, university, or college libraries maintain institutional subscriptions to Ovid, ensuring access to multiple electronic databases such as MEDLINE or CINAHL. In addition, access to PubMed, a service of the MEDLINE database, is available without charge on the Internet.

MEDLINE and PubMed

Administered by the US National Library of Medicine, MEDLINE is the world's largest electronic database of health-related research and literature (US National Library of Medicine, 2016). There are articles from a number of professions, including medicine, nursing, dentistry, veterinary medicine, and associated disciplines such as physiology, pharmacology, and molecular biology. Approximately 5600 journals are

---

TABLE 10.4   **Examples of Electronic Databases for Identifying and Retrieving Pertinent Research**

Name	Description	URL
MEDLINE	Largest online database for nursing, medical, and allied health journals	https://www.nlm.nih.gov/bsd/pmresources.html
PubMed	Freely accessible online version of MEDLINE database; lacks the robust Boolean features of MEDLINE	http://www.ncbi.nlm.nih.gov/sites/entrez?db=PubMed
Cumulative Index to Nursing and Allied Health Literature (CINAHL)	Largest database for nursing and allied health literature; includes multiple nursing journals not indexed in the MEDLINE database	http://www.ebscohost.com/biomedical-libraries/the-cinahl-database
Education Resource Information Center (ERIC)	Linked to more than 320,000 articles from 1966 to the present; focuses on educational literature, including undergraduate and graduate nursing	http://www.eric.ed.gov/
PsycINFO	Contains more than 3 million resources dating back to 1888; excellent resource for the APRN who specializes in providing mental health care	http://www.apa.org/pubs/databases/psycinfo/index.aspx
Web of Science	Includes journals in the basic and clinical sciences drawn from approximately 9300 journals with impact factors; administered by Clarivate Analytics	https://apps.webofknowledge.com/WOS_GeneralSearch_input.do?product=WOS&search_mode=GeneralSearch&SID=1At DcGoWCHV3rnpT4ub&preferencesSaved=

indexed. The MEDLINE database is primarily organized around MESH (*me*dical *s*ubject *h*eadings) terms. Entering a MESH term, such as "coronary artery disease" or "osteoporosis," will trigger a number of subheads that are potentially useful to identify evidence for answering a clinical question, such as "diagnosis," "drug therapy," "diet therapy," and "nursing." The MEDLINE database may also be searched using various keywords that are not official MESH terms; these searches retrieve articles that include the keyword in its title, abstract, or in a list of identifying keywords, but they will not provide the subheads available when a MESH term is accessed. The MEDLINE database includes articles published in 39 languages; 91% are printed in English and 83% of those published in other languages have English language abstracts, greatly increasing access for English-speaking searchers.

MEDLINE has robust Boolean functions, allowing the APRN to focus or narrow a search by combining two or more MESH terms or keywords using the functions "AND," "OR," and "NOT" (U.S. National Library of Medicine, 2016). For example, an APRN might pose a question about the effectiveness of administering an angiotensin-converting enzyme inhibitor for the prevention of mortality and disease progression in patients with heart failure. In this case the APRN might initially select the MESH term "heart failure" along with the MESH term "angiotensin-converting enzyme inhibitors." By using the "AND" Boolean function, the database will retrieve articles that merge the intervention (angiotensin-converting enzyme inhibitor agents) with the primary patient problem under scrutiny (heart failure).

A second Boolean function, "OR," allows the searcher to retrieve articles that contain either of two keywords or MESH terms. This function is useful when terms that are recently coined or historically relevant differ from the corresponding MESH term. For example, an APRN may be seeking information about patients who experience chronic lower urinary tract pain not associated with bacterial infection. The MESH term for this condition is "interstitial cystitis." However, a more recent term (bladder pain syndrome) has been increasingly used to describe this condition (Hanno et al., 2014); combining the MESH term "interstitial cystitis" with the keyword "bladder pain syndrome" retrieves more citations that entering either term alone.

A third Boolean function, "NOT," allows the APRN to limit a search by eliminating articles that do not address the intervention, assessment, or patient population under scrutiny. For example, an APRN interested in prevention of central line infections might enter the MESH term "indwelling catheters," which will retrieve studies focusing on infections associated with multiple types of catheters, including urinary and peritoneal dialysis catheters. Use of the "NOT" Boolean function will enable the APRN to eliminate articles about various types of catheters not pertinent to a clinical question focusing on hospital-acquired central line infections.

The MEDLINE database allows searches via multiple alternative fields, including author, journal, publication type (e.g., review article), language, experimental approach (human, in vivo, or in vitro), gender, age range, and publication year. These options are useful for focusing searches based on the parameters specified in the clinical question.

The PubMed webpage (http://www.ncbi.nlm.nih.gov/pubmed) provides free access to the MEDLINE database. The basic search engine will retrieve articles based on keywords. Clinicians searching PubMed can click on an advanced search icon and access a site that allows a combination of keywords or keyword and author or journal using the Boolean function "AND." However, the PubMed database does not have the robust search functions characteristic of MEDLINE. In addition, although a limited number of articles can be downloaded directly from the PubMed site, access to most articles is restricted to the complete citation and abstract.

Cumulative Index for Nursing and Allied Health Literature

The Cumulative Index for Nursing and Allied Health Literature (CINAHL) is an electronic database containing more than 2.6 million elements from approximately 3000 nursing and allied health journals and books. Similar to MEDLINE, the CINAHL database is available online as a subscription service typically accessed as part of an EBSCO Information Services subscription maintained by larger health care facilities and universities. Articles can be searched using keywords; the CINAHL database also contains the Boolean features "AND," "OR," and "NOT" and multiple search fields similar to those described for MEDLINE. CINAHL also indexes doctoral dissertations, an important source for gray literature (unpublished documents) in the field of nursing.

Online Evidence-Based Resources

In addition to retrieving individual research reports from electronic databases such as MEDLINE and

CINAHL, the APRN should also search online evidence-based documents such as the Cochrane Library and PubMed Health. The Cochrane Library is part of the Cochrane Collaboration; it is administered by a nonprofit organization, and reviews are generated by more than 28,000 volunteers from across the globe (Cochrane Collaboration, 2016). The Cochrane Library contains multiple resources for identifying current best evidence, including the Cochrane Database of Systematic Reviews and the Cochrane Central Register of Controlled Trials. The Database of Systematic Reviews contains more than 5000 systematic literature reviews based on clinical questions covering almost every specialty practice area in contemporary health care. Whenever possible, these reviews include a meta-analysis of data pooled from comparable studies. The systematic reviews can be accessed by multiple search fields, including keywords found in the title or abstract and author. Systematic reviews can be retrieved as a summary, standard report, or full report. A plain language summary provides a brief synopsis of the review's main findings. A standard report provides more detailed information, including a structured abstract of the review, plain language summary, background, objectives, methods, results, and discussion, along with reference lists for included and excluded studies. Systematic reviews are also available as a full report that incorporates all the elements of the standard report plus a detailed summary of all analyses generated for the review.

The plain language summary is useful as a quick reference when the APRN is only interested in a succinct summary of the main findings of a systematic review; this document may also be shared with a patient or family with a college-level education who may wish to know more about evidence supporting a particular intervention or assessment strategy. The full summary provides the more detailed information necessary when the APRN is evaluating current best evidence for individual decision making or generation of recommendations for practice. The detailed report also may be used for this purpose; study of this longer version is especially recommended for the novice APRN who is learning to synthesize evidence for clinical decision making or generating evidence-based documents such as a plan for a scholarly project.

Other online resources include the Joanna Briggs Institute, Essential Evidence Plus, and PubMed Health. The Joanna Briggs Institute is an international collaboration of nurses and other allied health care professionals, including the Cochrane Nursing Care Field and Cochrane Qualitative Research Methods Group, that provides evidence-based resources for nursing (Joanna Briggs Institute, 2016). Essential Evidence Plus is a subscription service administered by Wiley-Blackwell Publishers (Essential Evidence Plus, 2016) that enables users to access multiple electronic databases, including the Cochrane Library, to obtain evidence-based resources and information. An individual or institutional subscription to Essential Evidence Plus also provides access to POEMS (*Patient-Oriented Evidence that Matters*). POEMS are regularly updated synopses of evidence from individual studies and an archive of more than 3000 previously posted summaries. They may be downloaded online, downloaded to a smartphone, or viewed via podcast.

PubMed Health is an electronic database for evidence-based resources administered by the National Center for Biotechnology Information, US National Library of Medicine (http://www.ncbi.nlm.nih.gov/pubmedhealth). This electronic database includes reviews of clinical effectiveness research; reviews are available in brief reports designed for use by consumers, along with full reports designed for use by clinicians such as APRNs. In addition to its link to the extensive MEDLINE/PubMed database, PubMed Health is linked to evidence-based resources from the Cochrane Library, the Agency for Healthcare Research and Quality (AHRQ), the National Cancer Institute, the National Institute for Health and Clinical Excellence (NICE) guidelines program, and the National Institute for Health Research, Health Technology Assessment Program. Table 10.5 summarizes additional online resources for EBP.

Clinical Practice Guidelines

Searches of electronic databases should also incorporate the identification and retrieval of existing clinical practice guidelines or best practice documents. Clinical practice guidelines may be enormously helpful to the APRN because they represent a systematic review of existing evidence based on measurable clinical questions and recommendations for management of the disease, disorder, or condition (Fletcher, 2008). Identification and incorporation of appropriate guidelines is also important to APRNs because these documents are increasingly being viewed as a standard of care among clinicians, especially given the widespread acceptance of EBP principles. In addition to increasing scrutiny by clinicians, courts within the United States have also begun to grapple with the issue of clinical practice guidelines and their relationship to the *legal* definition of a standard of care. The current legal definition

TABLE 10.5   **Additional Online Resources for Evidence-Based Practice**

Name	Description	URL
Clinical Practice Guidelines		
Agency for Healthcare Research and Quality (AHRQ)	Evidence report topics, technical reviews, and clinical guidelines	https://www.ahrq.gov/
National Guideline Clearinghouse (NGC)	Evidence-based clinical practice guidelines and measurement tools	https://www.guideline.gov/
Institute for Healthcare Improvement	List of published articles about developing and using evidence-based protocols	http://www.ihi.org/
General Sites With Links to Other EBP Sites		
Star Model Research	Comprehensive list of EBP resources	http://nursing.uthscsa.edu/onrs/starmodel/star-model.asp
Centre for Evidence-Based Healthcare	Lists of reviews and evidence research reports	https://nottingham.ac.uk/research/groups/cebhc/index.aspx
Centre for Evidence-Based Medicine (CEBM)	Links to evidence-based resources, tools, continuing education, and discussion groups	http://www.cebm.net/
Joanna Briggs Institute	Privately owned EBP site with some free resources and subscription pages	http://joannabriggs.org/
Essential Evidence Plus	Subscription service administered by Wiley-Blackwell Publishers	https://www.essentialevidenceplus.com/
Advanced Practice Nursing	Subscription site for evidence-based resources	http://www.enursescribe.com/evidencebased.html
Registered Nurses Association of Ontario	Repository of best practice guidelines focusing on front-line nursing practice	http://rnao.ca/bpg/

for standard of care for physicians is "that which a minimally competent physician in the same field would do under similar circumstances" (Moffett & Moore, 2011, p. 111). Legal precedents concerning use of these documents continues to evolve; nevertheless, multiple courts have ruled that guidelines may be used as learned treatises to lend credence to or impeach an expert witness, to defend a clinician for using recommendations with the document as a standard of care, and to suggest that the clinician failed to deliver standard of care by not following guideline recommendations (Moffett & Moore, 2011; Taylor, 2014). The evolving use of practice guidelines provides another powerful rationale for the inclusion of EBP principles as a core competency for APRNs.

The National Guideline Clearinghouse is the largest online resource for clinical practice guidelines (http://guideline.gov/help-and-about). Administered by the AHRQ, this database houses more than 3000 clinical practice guidelines formulated within the past 5 years. The APRN should also search the webpage of the appropriate nursing and medical societies for relevant clinical practice guidelines. The number of professional societies producing clinical practice guidelines has grown from a few pioneers, including the American Academy of Pediatrics and

Oncology Nursing Society, to the vast majority of societies and organizations, including many smaller subspecialty groups.

The APRN should also search for best practice documents pertaining to the clinical question under scrutiny. Best practice guidelines are a synthesis of expert and clinical opinions when higher levels of evidence are not available to guide clinical decision making (Triano, 2008). Although these documents do not provide the systematic review and evidence-based recommendations of care incorporated into a clinical practice guideline, they can provide an excellent source of current knowledge of a specific intervention or assessment technique. In addition to housing clinical practice guidelines, the National Guideline Clearinghouse also indexes best practice documents produced within the past 5 years. The Registered Nurses' Association of Ontario (RNAO) is another excellent resource for best practice guidelines that affect multiple areas of nursing care, including many areas pertinent to advanced practice nursing (http://rnao.ca/bpg/).

Strategies for Searching Electronic Databases
Because of their robust size and ability to identify potential resources in a matter of seconds to minutes,

any hunt for best current evidence begins with a search of more than one electronic database. Searching multiple databases is strongly suggested because limited evidence has shown that searching a single database is likely to miss meaningful research identified when a search is expanded to more than one database (Bramer, Giustini, & Kramer, 2016). Studies further suggest that even a competent search using appropriate databases fails to identify all of the studies pertaining to a clinical question (Bramer et al., 2016; Helmer, Savoie, Green, & Kazanjian, 2001). An RCT found that the efficiency of identification and retrieval of studies is significantly improved when a medical librarian is consulted (Gardois et al., 2011). Several factors probably contribute to the incomplete retrieval of pertinent studies when relying solely on searches of electronic databases. Challenges related to keywords are postulated to be a primary cause of incomplete retrieval. Many conditions and interventions are referred to by multiple names and these terms evolve over time. For example, the chronic wound currently referred to as a "pressure ulcer" was historically labeled a "bedsore," a term that was later changed to "decubitus ulcer" or "pressure sore" before the current term was popularized and added to the MESH term taxonomy. In addition to this limitation, electronic databases typically identify keywords for search purposes from the title, abstract, and a short list of key terms provided by the author and/or publisher. Although authors and publishers share the goal of maximizing the number of times an article is read and cited in subsequent peer-reviewed publications, even subtle changes in narrative or selection of less widely used terms limit the likelihood that a particular study report will be identified in subsequent searches.

Although the lag time between publication and indexing in the major databases has decreased dramatically over the past decade, the significant growth in production of clinical studies by scholars from a number of health care fields means that newer research pertinent to a clinical question typically appears within a matter of months to 1 year of a focused search. In addition, electronic databases are heavily weighted toward published documents. Publication bias is defined as the tendency for studies with provocative results to achieve favorable peer review and acceptance for publication as compared with research reporting negative results (Smith, 1956). In the current era of blended print, electronic, and open access sources of health care research, publication bias arises from multiple sources; specifically, articles are more likely to be published if they report statistically significant findings, or provocative findings that challenge current thinking or are perceived as novel, or if they are likely to attract lay media attention (Song, Hooper, & Loke, 2013). The magnitude of this effect is hypothesized to be substantial (Guyatt et al., 2011). For example, Sutton, Duvall, Tweedie, Abrams, and Jones (2000) carried out meta-analyses of 48 systematic reviews and reported that 20% were found to have omitted or missed studies reporting negative results. Electronic databases are also limited by the relative paucity of gray literature, which is especially significant in nursing research. The term *gray literature* is defined as unpublished results of studies available as abstracts or short reports in conference proceedings or journal supplements. Sparse research has suggested that the magnitude of nursing studies that remain unpublished despite completion is substantial. For example, Hicks (1995) reported that only 16 of a group of 161 British nurses who completed a study and presented results at a professional conference submitted their findings for publication in a peer-reviewed journal, and only 14 (9%) were ultimately published.

Several strategies can be used to increase the proportion of pertinent studies identified during a literature search for current best evidence. They include doing ancestry searches, searching gray literature sources, consulting experts in the field, and using Internet-based search engines. Ancestry searches are completed by reviewing the reference list of individual research reports, review articles, or systematic reviews identified during a literature search (Melnyk & Fineout-Overholt, 2010). Weak evidence suggests that ancestry searches may reveal multiple studies that are missed during electronic database searches (Horsley, Dingwall, & Sampson, 2011). Identifying pertinent gray literature sources remains a challenge. Hand searches of one or more peer-reviewed journals that publish research abstracts in a supplement to or regular issue of the society's official journal, or abstracts made available to conference attendees as a proceedings booklet or in an electronic format, may serve as a rich source of pertinent studies. Although these sources may identify multiple potentially pertinent studies, they typically contain limited details of the study design and analyses of findings, thus limiting their value as evidence-based resources. In contrast, the CINAHL, PsycINFO, and ERIC databases index doctoral theses and dissertations that provide intensely reviewed and detailed reports of graduate students' supervised research.

Internet-based search engines, such as Google or Google Scholar, are an increasingly robust source of published and unpublished studies. They are particularly useful when attempting to retrieve full reprints of older articles not yet incorporated into the major electronic databases. Nevertheless, considerable caution must be used when relying on unpublished information from the Internet, especially if the source material has not undergone peer review. An evaluation of the coverage, recall, and precision of search strategies used in 120 systematic reviews found that Google Scholar lacked the full coverage needed for performing a systematic review (Bramer et al., 2016; Gehanno, Rollin, & Darmoni, 2013). Consulting with an experienced researcher or clinical experts in a particular field can also lead to identification of pertinent studies (Godin et al., 2015).

Step 3: Critically Appraise and Extract Evidence

Although a careful search of the literature using the strategies described will recover pertinent studies, it will also retrieve much information that does not comprise evidence of effectiveness, predictive accuracy, or safety. Therefore, the APRN must critically appraise the various documents for their contribution to current best evidence, extract pertinent data, and set aside findings that do not address the clinical question under scrutiny. This process begins with separation of individual research reports and systematic reviews summarizing research findings from secondary sources, such as integrative review articles or editorials, via a title search. An integrative review is a comprehensive discussion of research, expert opinion, and theoretical knowledge about a topic (Gray & Bliss, 2005). Although the integrative review typically includes studies that may provide valuable sources of evidence when subjected to an ancestry search, it is ultimately a synthesis of knowledge about a given topic, rather than an evidence-based review of studies intended to establish efficacy or predictive accuracy. Similarly, opinion-based articles such as editorials are eliminated because they report expert opinion rather than original research data.

Evidence Pyramid

After eliminating articles that do not report or systematically review original data, the remaining studies are evaluated based on a pyramid of evidence (Bracke, Howse, & Keim, 2008; Fig. 10.1). The pyramid provides a taxonomy for ranking a study's potential

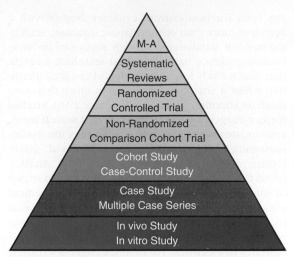

FIG 10.1 Pyramid illustrating levels of evidence used to evaluate efficacy of an intervention. *M-A,* Meta-analysis.

contribution to evidence based on its design. The base of this pyramid comprises laboratory-based studies using animals (in vivo model), tissue samples, cell lines, or chemical media (in vitro models). Although these studies are typically well designed and apply much more rigid controls than those used in clinical research, they are nevertheless eliminated because their findings do not yield evidence about efficacy, safety, or predictive value when an intervention is applied to human subjects in a clinical setting.

The second rung up from the base of the evidence pyramid is typically occupied by individual or multiple case series. A case study is a detailed description of results when an individual patient, family, inpatient care unit, long-term care facility, health care system, or community is subjected to an intervention or intervention bundle (Crowe et al., 2011; Polit & Beck, 2016). Multiple case series summarize results from more than one patient with a similar condition when exposed to a common intervention or intervention bundle. The results of case studies or multiple case series can be used as evidence that an intervention is feasible, offers an attractive alternative to usual care, can be applied safely in a selected patient or patients, and merits further investigation to determine clinical effectiveness. However, individual case studies or multiple case series do not compare the intervention of interest with a control or standard care, and their results cannot be used to reach conclusions about efficacy, effectiveness, or predictive power. The APRN must remain aware that findings from these designs tend to favor positive effects of the intervention and often imply evidence of efficacy or effectiveness. In addition, results of individual case studies (sometimes labeled testimonials) are frequently used in marketing campaigns to imply a positive effect when a particular product is used. Nevertheless, case studies and multiple case series do not compare the intervention under scrutiny to a placebo or to standard (usual) care, and their results cannot be used to establish efficacy or predictive power.

The higher rungs of the evidence pyramid are occupied by the RCT, nonrandomized comparison cohort trials, and cohort or case-control studies. Depending on the nature of the clinical question and availability of research-based evidence, results of one or more studies employing these designs will be used to determine current best evidence. The nonrandomized comparison cohort trial shares certain similarities with the RCT; it compares outcomes from at least two groups, including one cohort that is exposed to an experimental intervention and a second group exposed to usual care, a sham device, or placebo (Polit & Beck, 2016). However, this study design uses non–randomly selected groups because of ethical, financial, or other considerations. Because the nonrandomized comparison cohort trial lacks random assignment, the potential for bias in group membership is high and the likelihood that these differences will influence study findings is significant.

A cohort study is an observational design in which a large sample is identified and followed over time to determine which participants will develop a disease or disorder under scrutiny (Polit & Beck, 2016). During this prolonged observation period, the incidence of the disease or disorder is measured prospectively. A cohort study allows researchers to identify new (incident) cases, and temporal relationships between preventive interventions or constitutional factors and incidence can be analyzed. Although the cohort study provides valuable results, data collection requires an extended observation period, resulting in a comparatively high likelihood of subject dropout and significant cost.

The case-control study, sometimes called the nested case-control design, provides a less expensive but less robust alternative to the cohort study. It requires comparison of two groups, one with the condition under study and the other free from the condition at a single point in time. The cohort study prospectively identifies cases from persons who remain free of the disorder of interest, and the nonrandomized comparison cohort study relies on identification of two groups, those with a condition

(cases) and a second group without the condition (controls). Selection of this second group (controls) is especially difficult and often acts as a source of bias within this retrospective design (Polit & Beck, 2016). The nested case-control study uses retrospective analysis of data from a sample population participating in a parallel group or factorial RCT (Polit & Beck, 2016). These study designs differ from that of the RCT because they are observational rather than interventional in nature. Study findings can be used to identify relationships between the presence of a given factor and the likelihood of the condition being studied, but they cannot be used to establish a cause-and-effect relationship between the associated factor and disease or disorder that is needed to determine efficacy.

The most powerful research design is the RCT, which is considered the gold standard for measuring the efficacy of an intervention or the predictive power of an assessment strategy (Sackett, 2015; Turner, 2012). Efficacy is defined as the likelihood that an intervention will achieve the desired outcome in a group of subjects based on evaluation in a research setting that controls for random effects produced by extrinsic factors. The concept of efficacy must be differentiated from effectiveness, which is defined as the effect of a specific intervention when administered to a particular patient at a given point during the course of an illness or condition.

Several types of RCTs are commonly reported in the health care literature (Chow & Liu, 2014). The parallel design RCT assigns subjects randomly to an experimental group exposed to the intervention under scrutiny or to a control group exposed to a placebo, sham device, or standard intervention based on ethical considerations. A crossover RCT is characterized by random assignment of subjects to an experimental or control group, followed by crossing the subject over to the alternative group after a washout period designed to remove (wash away) initial exposure effect. Although the crossover RCT potentially needs to enroll fewer total subjects and may incur less cost than the parallel group design, it is performed less often because of the potential for contamination of findings caused by residual effects when subjects are crossed over. The factorial RCT compares two or more experimental interventions with a control group treated with a placebo or sham versus a group receiving usual care or some alternative intervention. Because the RCT is the most powerful study design, it should be routinely included when reviewing the literature for current best evidence; it is generally considered to be of higher quality than designs that do not involve randomization of subjects, such as the cohort or case-control study.

Systematic Reviews and Meta-Analyses

Even though the RCT is considered the most powerful individual research design, the highest rungs of the evidence pyramid are occupied by systematic reviews and meta-analyses (see Fig. 10.1). These designs form the apex of the evidence pyramid because they combine the results of multiple studies to determine the effect created by a specific intervention. A systematic review uses a structured methodology to comprehensively seek out, select, appraise, and analyze studies based on a measurable clinical question (Engberg, 2008; Holly, Salmond, & Saimbert, 2017). The methods used for generating a systematic review are comparable to those used to identify current best evidence for clinical decision making, and the rise of EBP closely parallels the recent explosion of systematic review articles published in the professional literature. Combining results from multiple studies is more powerful than consideration of a single RCT because it allows for the qualitative analysis of results produced by multiple researchers in various study settings to determine whether the effects of the intervention are beneficial (greater than placebo or standard care), mixed (no more effective than placebo in some studies versus more effective than control group findings in others), or ineffective (less effective than placebo or standard care or associated with adverse side effects that exceed its beneficial effects).

The meta-analysis is the highest rung of the level-of-evidence pyramid because it provides a quantitative technique for pooling and analyzing results from more than one study to determine the direction and magnitude of an intervention's effect (Engberg, 2008). Although the benefits of meta-analysis are apparent, studies must be carefully analyzed before completing this type of statistical analysis. This evaluation is based on data extraction and consideration of the sample populations of the various studies, experimental intervention, study methods, and outcome variables used to determine treatment effect. The outcomes of a meta-analysis based on a dichotomous (nominal) outcome measure are usually expressed as an odds ratio, relative risk, or absolute risk reduction, depending on the nature of the clinical question. The results of a meta-analysis based on a continuous outcome variable will be based on the weighted mean difference and standardized mean difference, sometimes referred to as effect size. The precision of the magnitude of the effect size is expressed by the accompanying confidence interval.

The level of the evidence pyramid is useful for the APRN engaging in EBP because it provides a taxonomy for categorizing studies based on underlying design for their potential contribution to current best evidence needed to answer a clinical question. Nevertheless, research design alone cannot be used to judge the quality of individual studies or their contribution to current best evidence (Holly et al., 2017). Although RCTs provide excellent designs for minimizing bias in the evaluation of some forms of interventions—a medication designed to improve hemodynamic instability; physical manipulation, such as insertion of a catheter for parenteral fluid replacement; or positioning to prevent ventilator-associated pneumonia—it may not be feasible or desirable to limit a systematic review seeking current best evidence to RCTs alone. In many cases, the APRN will find that there are insufficient RCTs to define current best evidence. As a result, nonrandomized trials or observation epidemiologic studies examining the association between preventive or interventional measures and the outcome of interest may be included because they provide the best available evidence. In other cases, the quality of one or more RCTs may be compromised, limiting the APRN's ability to extract data and reach meaningful conclusions about efficacy from these studies. Ogilvie, Egan, Hamilton, and Petticrew (2005) evaluated systematic reviews of evidence related to the efficacy of psychosocial interventions and observed that the inclusion of RCTs alone might miss most pertinent evidence because these interventions tend to be embedded or applied along with physical interventions in many RCTs. In this case, measuring only direct outcomes produced in an RCT may paradoxically miss results from alternative studies that examine the effect of the psychosocial interventions that comprise an essential component of APRN practice.

Critical Appraisal
Individual Studies

After eliminating studies that do not contribute to determining current best evidence, the APRN must evaluate the quality of individual studies by seeking out sources of potential bias in order to determine the magnitude of their contribution to current best evidence for a given topic (Higgins & Green, 2011). In selected circumstances, this evaluation may be used to eliminate studies that do not meet criteria for meta-analysis or contain sufficient flaws that

TABLE 10.6	Critical Appraisal Guide for Quantitative Studies
Question	**Evaluation Criteria**
Why was the study done?	Does the study include clearly stated research questions, aims, hypotheses, or purpose statements?
What is the sample size?	Did the study enroll enough subjects to allow statistical analysis so that results did not occur by chance?
Are the instruments used to measure major variables valid and reliable?	Were the outcome measures of the study clearly defined? Were instruments used to measure these outcomes valid and reliable?
How were data analyzed?	What statistical tests were used to determine whether the study purpose was achieved?
Were there any untoward events during the study?	Did subjects withdraw before completing the study; if so, why did they withdraw?
How do results fit with previous research in this area?	Did the researchers base their work on a thorough literature review?
What does this research mean for clinical practice?	Is the study purpose an important clinical issue?

Adapted from Melnyk, B. M., & Fineout-Overholt, E. (2010). *Evidence-based practice in nursing and healthcare: A guide to best practice.* Philadelphia, PA: Wolters-Kluwer.

severely compromise the generalizability of findings. However, studies must not be eliminated because they report negative findings or the study is not an RCT. Although no standardized form for evaluating study quality exists, several models have been developed that provide a useful framework for evaluating the quality of individual studies. Melnyk and Fineout-Overholt (2010) have advocated a Critical Appraisal Guide for Quantitative Studies (Table 10.6). Alternatively, the CONSORT (Consolidated Standards of Reporting Trials) criteria for improving reporting the results of RCTs and the STROBE (Strengthening Reporting of Observational Studies in Epidemiology) criteria for reporting the results of observational studies in epidemiology can be adapted to enable systematic assessment of the quality of individual studies and their contribution to evidence-based clinical decision making (Moher, Schulz, & Altman for the CONSORT Group [Consolidated Standards of Reporting Trials], 2001; von Elm et al. for the STROBE Initiative, 2007). Fig. 10.2 is the individual study form used by the Cochrane Collaboration for evaluating individual studies as part of their production of a systematic review of current best evidence. It is based on a three-level ranking—0 to 2—in which a score of 2 indicates that the criterion was clearly met, a score of 1 indicates that it was partially met, and a score of 0 indicates that it was not met. Tables 10.7 and 10.8 summarize criteria for an initial evaluation of study quality adapted from the CONSORT and STROBE statements, respectively (Moher et al., 2001; von Elm et al., 2007). These statements are designed to serve as a guide when publishing individual study results in a peer-reviewed scholarly journal; they can be easily adapted as a guide for

evaluating individual study quality as part of an EBP process.

Systematic Reviews and Meta-Analyses

Because systematic review and meta-analytic techniques are much newer than the design techniques used to generate RCTs, nonrandomized comparison cohort trials, or observational epidemiologic studies, few instruments have been developed and validated for the evaluation of potential bias in systematic reviews with or without meta-analysis of pooled data. A technical report prepared for the AHRQ identified more than 20 guidelines for evaluating the quality of systematic reviews, but only 2 were considered high quality (West et al., 2002). Nevertheless, this report identified common factors that should be incorporated into any evaluation of the quality of these documents, including a clinical question, methods for searching the literature and extracting data, and recommendations for practice or policy based on evidence identified (Table 10.9).

The APRN should evaluate the systematic review for sources of potential bias associated with study retrieval. Common sources of bias include time-, language-, and geography-related bias, as well as publication bias (discussed earlier) (Campbell et al., 2015).

Time-related bias is created when systematic reviews limit the time frame for study inclusion. Although systematic reviewers are understandably concerned with limiting their reviews to the best current evidence, searches must use original research reports rather than summaries of studies contained in integrative or systematic reviews. Therefore, decisions about time frames in systematic reviews

Review:
Quality Assessment Tool
Study ID #__   Raters initials: __   Date__

	Scoring	Score	Query	A/B/C
A: Was the assigned treatment adequately concealed prior to allocation?	2 = Method did not allow disclosure of assignment 1 = Small but possible chance of disclosure of assignment or unclear 0 = quasirandomized or open list/tables Clearly yes = A Not sure = B Clearly no = C			
B: Were the outcomes of patients who withdrew described and included in the analysis (intention to treat)?	2 = withdrawals well described and accounted for in analysis 1 = withdrawals described and analysis not possible 0 = no mention, inadequate mention or obvious differences and no adjustment			
C: Were the outcome assessors blinded to treatment status?	2 = effective action taken to blind assessors 1 = small or moderate chance of unblinding of assessors 0 = not mentioned or not possible			
D: Were the treatment and control group comparable at entry?	2 = good comparability of groups, or confounding adjusted for in analysis 1 = confounding small; mentioned but not adjusted for 0 = large potential for confounding, or not discussed			
E. Were the subjects blind to the assignment status after allocation?	2 = effective action taken to blind subjects 1 = Small or moderate chance of unblinding of subjects 0 = not possible, or not mentioned (unless double-blind) or possible but not done			
F. Were the treatment providers blind to assignment status?	2 = effective action taken to blind treatment providers 1 = Small or moderate chance of unblinding of treatment providers			

FIG 10.2 Individual study quality assessment tool. *(From the Cochrane Collaboration. [2013]. Study quality guide: Guide for review authors on assessing study quality. Retrieved from https://cccrg.cochrane.org/sites/ cccrg.cochrane.org/files/public/uploads/StudyQualityGuide_May%202013.pdf.)*

	0 = not possible, or not mentioned (unless double-blind) or possible but not done		
G: Were care programmes, other than the trial options, identical?	2 = Care programmes clearly identical 1 = Clear but trivial differences 0 = Not mentioned, or clear and important differences in care programmes		
H. Were the inclusion and exclusion criteria clearly defined?	2 = clearly defined 1 = inadequately defined 0 = not defined		
I. Were the interventions clearly defined?	2 = clearly defined 1 = inadequately defined 0 = not defined		
J. Were the outcome measures used clearly defined?	2 = clearly defined 1 = inadequately defined 0 = not defined		
	Outcome 1:		
	Outcome 2:		
	Outcome 3:		
	Outcome 4:		
	Outcome 5:		
K. Were diagnostic tests used in outcome assessment clinically useful?	2 = optimal 1 = adequate 0 = not defined, not adequate		
	Outcome 1:		
	Outcome 2:		
	Outcome 3:		
	Outcome 4:		
	Outcome 5:		
L. Was the surveillance active, and of clinically appropriate duration?	2 = optimal 1 = adequate 0 = not defined, not adequate		
	Outcome 1:		
	Outcome 2:		
	Outcome 3:		
	Outcome 4:		
	Outcome 5:		

FIG 10.2—cont'd

should include the latest publications at the time the review was conducted and extend backward to a meaningful point in time. This time frame may be based on a landmark event, such as passage of legislation, development of an intervention or diagnostic technology, or publication of a Phase 3 RCT and approval of a drug for clinical use. Gaps in the timeline for searches should not be present.

Language-related bias is common in systematic reviews. Although English is the predominant language of science (Meneghini & Packer, 2007), and most articles in MEDLINE and CINAHL are published in English, many studies are only published in other languages. The potential for language-related bias associated with the use of English language–only sources should be acknowledged in the methods section or discussion of a systematic review.

The Risk of Bias in Systematic Studies (ROBIS) instrument is a validated instrument that was specifically developed for assessment of bias in systematic reviews; it was intentionally designed to reflect the domain-based structure of the instrument used by the Cochrane Collaboration for identifying possible bias in individual studies (Whiting et al. for the Robis

TABLE 10.7   **Evaluating Quality of the Randomized Controlled Trial and Nonrandomized Comparison Cohort Trial**

Criterion Section of the Research Report	Evidence That Criterion Was Met
Study purpose (introduction and background)	The purpose of the study is clearly stated. A rationale for the study is clearly stated and supported by appropriate literature.
Study participants (methods)	Inclusion and exclusion criteria for study participants are described, along with the study setting.
Study aims (methods)	Measurable research aims, questions, or hypotheses. These statements include measurable study outcomes consistent with the stated purpose of the study.
Sample size (methods)	The authors describe how the sample size was determined. Ideally, sample size is based on a power analysis to determine the number of subjects needed to determine group differences. The sample size recruited may be slightly larger than the minimum group size suggested by the power analysis to account for subjects who withdraw prior to completion of data collection.
Random allocation (methods)	Methods used to achieve random allocation are described, the success of randomization may be illustrated in a table comparing demographic and key clinical characteristics between experimental and control groups, and inferential analysis should identify no significant differences between groups. Procedures for group selection in the nonrandomized comparison cohort trial are described. Absence of randomization in group assignment is clearly acknowledged, and a table comparing demographic and key clinical characteristics of intervention and comparison group is provided.
Blinding (methods)	Study participants and data collectors are blinded to group assignment whenever feasible; blinding is not feasible for multiple nursing interventions, such as education or counseling.
Statistical methods (methods)	Appropriate statistical methods are used to compare primary and secondary outcomes. Descriptive statistics and inferential statistical analyses are based on considerations of level of measurement (nominal, ordinal, or continuous) and distribution of data. Multivariate analyses are used when multiple outcome measures are analyzed. Intention to treat analysis is used, when indicated.
Participant flow (methods and results)	Study procedures are thoroughly described in the methods section; a diagram of participant flow may be placed in the results section. The number of subjects who do not complete data collection is stated, and reasons for early study withdrawal are clearly stated. Ideally, the proportion of patients who do not complete the study is ≤15%.
Outcomes (results)	Outcomes based on research questions or aims are stated for each group and the precision of the outcomes is measured using a 95% confidence interval.
Adverse events	Adverse events are reported, along with their impact on study completion.
Generalizability	Results are interpreted in the context of current evidence along with limitations of the study, including potential sources of bias. Limitations associated with multiple analyses are discussed.

Adapted from Moher, D., Schulz, K. F., & Altman, D., & CONSORT Group (Consolidated Standards of Reporting Trials). (2001). The CONSORT statement: Revised recommendations for improving the quality of reports of parallel-group randomized trials. *JAMA, 285,* 1987–1991.

group, 2016). The instrument is divided into three phases. In the first phase, the user is prompted to evaluate whether the systematic review adequately adhered to the stated inclusion and exclusion criteria; whether these criteria were clearly stated, mutually exclusive, and unambiguous; and whether these criteria appeared appropriate for the clinical question(s) or aim(s) of the systematic review. The second phase of the instrument includes an evaluation of the techniques used to identify and retrieve studies, such as use of more than one electronic database, selection of search terms, restrictions based on language or publication format, and efforts to minimize errors in study selection. It also prompts users to evaluate the methods used to synthesize findings, extract data, and present findings using appropriate quantitative or semiquantitative criteria such as sensitivity analyses or funnel plots. Phase 3 prompts users to evaluate the methods used to detect sources of potential bias within individuals studies, the relevance of studies based on stated PICO question or review aims, and avoidance of summarizing findings exclusively based on statistical significance. Access to this instrument, along with guidance for

TABLE 10.8	Evaluating Quality of Observational Studies: Adapted From the STROBE Statement
Criterion Section of the Research Report	**Evidence That Criterion Was Met**
Study purpose (introduction and background)	The purpose of the study is clearly stated. A rationale for the study is clearly stated and supported by appropriate literature.
Study participants (methods)	Eligibility criteria for study participation and follow-up criteria are clearly described for the cohort study. Criteria for cases and controls are described for the case-control study; criteria used to match cases and controls are clearly described.
Study outcomes (methods)	Outcome variables are clearly defined, along with confounding factors and potential associated (predictive) factors. Diagnostic criteria for differentiating cases and controls are clearly described for cohort and case control studies.
Bias (methods)	Potential sources of bias are acknowledged.
Statistical methods (methods)	Appropriate statistical methods are used to analyze primary and secondary outcome measures. Descriptive statistics and inferential statistical analyses are based on considerations of level of measurement (nominal, ordinal, or continuous) and distribution of data. Multivariate analyses are used when multiple outcome measures are analyzed. An explanation of methods used to control for confounding factors and how missing data were managed is provided.
Participants (results)	Demographic and pertinent clinical characteristics of cases and controls are described.
Outcome data (results)	For the cohort study, a report of incidence or summary measures over time should be reported. For the case-control study, outcomes of variables potentially associated with likelihood of status as a case or control subject are reported. Association between outcome as a case or control should be based on multivariate analysis when multiple factors are analyzed.
Generalizability (discussion)	Key findings are presented based on study questions or aims. Limitations of the study are clearly acknowledged, including sources of bias and inability to determine cause and effect based on the presence of statistically significant associations. Limitations associated with multiple inferential analyses are acknowledged.

Adapted from von Elm, E., et al. & STROBE Initiative. (2007). Strengthening the Reporting of Observational Studies in Epidemiology (STROBE) statement: Guidelines for reporting observational studies. *BMJ, 335,* 806–808.

its use, is available at http://www.bristol.ac.uk/social-community-medicine/projects/robis/.

Data Extraction

The decision-making process associated with EBP relies on more than simply retrieving studies and basing a clinical decision on a generalized impression of reported findings. Instead, the APRN should use a consistent process to extract only pertinent outcomes based on criteria determined in the clinical question posed in Step 1. To ensure consistency, study review and data extraction should follow a predetermined protocol, just as original research adheres to established study procedures, regardless of whether results will be used for writing a formal systematic review, evaluating existing evidence for the purposes of a QI project, or formulating new policies in a local facility. The process used to extract data varies based on the nature of the clinical question. For example, the protocol used to

extract data from a group of RCTs—possibly combined with results of one or more nonrandomized trials—to determine the efficacy of a given intervention will differ from data coded and extracted for a review of the predictive accuracy of a diagnostic examination. The Cochrane Collaboration (http://bjmt.cochrane.org/resources-developing-review) provides excellent resources for coding forms enabling a standardized protocol for data extraction. Fig. 10.3 is a data extraction form used for coding data from an individual study evaluating the efficacy of a single experimental intervention. This form can be used when measuring outcomes of trials comparing two groups, one of which was exposed to the intervention of interest and the other exposed to a placebo, sham device, or standard care. The webpage also provides a standardized form designed to aid the clinician when extracting data from RCTs comparing the effects of multiple interventions.

TABLE 10.9	Criteria for Evaluation of a Systematic Review, With or Without a Meta-Analysis
Criterion	**Evidence That Criterion Was Met**
Study question	A clearly defined clinical question is provided; the question should define the patient population and problem, intervention or assessment strategy under scrutiny, comparison treatment, and outcomes indicating intervention effect or predictive power of the assessment strategy.
Inclusion or exclusion criteria	Search methods are clearly described. Techniques used to identify studies include electronic database searches along with techniques to increase the efficiency of the search, such as ancestry search, consultation with experts in the field of inquiry, web engine searches, trial registries, and conference proceedings.
	Inclusion and exclusion criteria for studies are clearly stated. Potential sources of bias in selection criteria (time-, language-, and geography-related) are acknowledged and minimized.
Data extraction	The process for data extraction from individual studies is clearly described.
	A standardized protocol for data extraction is included in the methods section of the systematic review. This protocol specifies persons involved in data extraction and procedures for coding data, ranking study quality, building consensus about data extraction, and resolving conflicts in individual study coding.
	Incorporation of an independent coder is used to measure reliability (interrater agreement rates) similar to that used for reporting original data when multiple data collectors participate in a research protocol. Interrater agreement rates should vary from 75% to 100%.
	A persuasive rationale for excluding studies based on methodologic quality is provided and excluded studies are clearly identified.
	The process used to weight evidence (e.g., results of meta-analysis, ranking of evidence) is clearly defined.
	The process for determining study quality, including weighting of the study for purposes of evidence ranking or meta-analysis, is clearly explained. Evidence ranking is based on consensus among authors and a process for resolving disagreements concerning quality rankings via consensus is clearly described.
Recommendations for clinical practice	Recommendations for clinical practice are supported by evidence extracted from the systematic review. The strength of recommendations should be specified and the process for determining strength of recommendation clearly explained. Ideally, evidence ranking and determination of strength of recommendations for clinical practice are based on validated and published ranking systems.

Adapted from Schlosser, R. W. (2007). Appraising the quality of systematic reviews. FOCUS Technical Brief No. 17. Retrieved from http://ktdrr.org/ktlibrary/articles_pubs/ncddrwork/focus/focus17/Focus17.pdf; and West, S., King V., Carey, T. S., Lohr, K. N., McKoy, N., Sutton, S. F., et al. (2002). Systems to rate the strength of scientific evidence. Evidence Report–Technology Assessment No. 47. AHRQ Publication 02-E016. Rockville, MD: Agency for Healthcare Research and Quality.

Step 4: Implement Useful Findings in Clinical Decision Making

Implementing useful findings is a deceptively complex process that goes beyond simply combining study results to create a protocol for implementation of a given intervention or assessment strategy. This process occurs on multiple levels, including clinical decision making when caring for an individual patient, creation and implementation of policies on a facility- or community-wide level, and creation of evidence-based clinical practice guidelines designed to set standards of care on a national or global level. Implementing EBP when caring for individual patients, establishing local policies for clinical practice, or establishing guidelines for practice on a national or global basis requires a synthesis of knowledge of the intervention's predictive power or efficacy, consideration of individualized physical and psychosocial factors likely to have an impact on effectiveness when applied to an individual patient, and knowledge of its direct cost or economic impact (van Rijswijk & Gray, 2012). For example, whereas a new drug may be shown to be effective in an RCT when compared with a placebo, its adaptation into an evidence-based clinical practice guideline must also address its comparative effectiveness to existing agents with similar pharmacologic actions, the frequency and nature of the adverse side effects associated with the drug, and its cost. The increased cost associated with a new drug may be justified if it proves more effective than existing agents in the same class or is associated with a lower risk of adverse side effects. In contrast, the novelty of a drug does not provide justification for inclusion in evidence-based clinical practice guidelines or protocols if it does not offer clinically relevant advantages in terms of the efficacy or safety needed to justify the increased patient cost likely to be associated with a newer agent.

The process of implementing findings from an EBP process begins with the generation of recommendations for clinical practice, which are derived

{Review name}- Basic information for study ID: ....

Method

Randomisation	Blinding	Intention to treat - Loss to Follow-up

Participants

N	Age	Sex	Type of injury:
Country	Hospital	Period of Study	Other participants (not review?)

Inclusion criteria		Exclusion Criteria	

Interventions

Intervention (including description, when started, frequency, duration & when stopped etc)

Outcomes

Overall length of follow-up:

Outcomes	Tick if available	How measured	When done

Notes - see over   **Reviewer:**

FIG 10.3 Data extraction form of individual studies comparing two groups. *(From the Cochrane Collaboration. [2013]. Study quality guide: Guide for review authors on assessing study quality. Retrieved from https:// cccrg.cochrane.org/sites/cccrg.cochrane.org/files/public/uploads/StudyQualityGuide_May%202013.pdf.)*

from the data extracted from pertinent studies. However, just as the strength of individual evidence underlying assessment strategies or interventions varies, so must the strength or associated recommendations for clinical practice. Similar to the various systems used to grade evidence, a review of the literature reveals that more than 60 different taxonomies for grading the strength of practice recommendations have been incorporated into various clinical practice guidelines and best practice documents (Garcia, Alvarado, & Gaxiola, 2010). Widely used systems include the Strength of Recommendation for Treatment taxonomy (SORT) scale, Grading of Recommendations Assessment, Development and Evaluation (GRADE) scales, NICE scale, Center for Preventive Medicine scale (developed in Oxford), and Scottish Intercollegiate Guideline Network (SIGN) taxonomy. Garcia et al. (2010) have compared the effect of evidence-based clinical decision making for a child with diarrhea using four scales (NICE, GRADE, Centre for Evidence-Based Medicine [CEBM], and SIGN scales) in a group of 216 novice physicians (pediatric residents). A significant number of physicians changed their recommendation for management of the index case based on review of the various clinical recommendations. Of the four scales recommended, the GRADE scale was found to exert the greatest influence on clinical decision making.

The GRADE scale was developed by a group of clinicians to rank the strength of clinical recommendations based on current best evidence (Atkins et al. for the GRADE Working Group, 2004; Brozek et al., 2009). The GRADE Working Group has recommended evaluating the quality of evidence based on a four-point ordinal scale:

1. High evidence indicates that additional research is unlikely to change confidence of the direction or magnitude of the effect size associated with a specific intervention.
2. Moderate evidence indicates that additional research may significantly influence the magnitude of treatment effect.
3. Low evidence indicates that new research may affect the direction and magnitude of treatment effect.
4. Very low evidence indicates insufficient evidence to determine treatment effect.

Using this underlying scale for grading evidence, the GRADE Working Group advocated a scale for recommendations for clinical practice in which the highest grade indicates benefits that clearly outweigh potential for harm, the second level indicates that benefits of treatment must be carefully weighed against potential adverse sides effects, the third level indicates that balance between benefit and harm cannot be clearly distinguished based on best available evidence, and the lowest grade level indicates that the best available evidence suggests the intervention is likely to produce more harm than benefit.

A second ranking system will be familiar to many APRNs practicing in North America. The US Preventive Services Task Force uses an ordinal scale with grades ranging from A to D and a fifth category labeled I (Trinite, Cherry, & Marion, 2009). Similar to the rankings advocated by the GRADE Working Group, recommendations for practice are linked to the direction, magnitude, and balance between benefit and harm. Table 10.10 summarizes the Task Force scale for recommendations for clinical practice.

From Policy to Practice: Tips for Achieving Meaningful Changes in Practice Based on Current Best Evidence

Although the EBP process is effective for identifying current best evidence, completion of the process does not guarantee meaningful changes in practice needed to achieve desired clinical outcomes. In contrast, evidence strongly suggests that merely introducing a new policy or directing clinicians to alter their current practice is unlikely to lead to meaningful or sustained changes in practice (West, 2001). Many EBP innovations introduced through the efforts of one or more clinician advocates tend to result in short-term adoption by a limited number of clinicians that is not likely to be sustained over time (Stetler, 2003). To overcome this problem, the APRN must be aware of successful strategies to design and implement a structured program for translating practice innovations into meaningful and sustained changes.

Rogers' Diffusion of Innovation Theory provides a useful framework for the APRN seeking to implement successful and sustained changes in practice based on EBP processes (Rogers, 2003). This theoretical framework describes four stages that an individual clinician or group will experience when evaluating and deciding to adopt or reject a practice innovation. The first phase, described as the knowledge stage, occurs when clinicians are made aware of the innovation and its potential impact on practice and patient outcomes. For many clinicians, knowledge may be introduced through continuing education activities, announcement of a practice innovation, or informal communication from colleagues or informal clinical

⊙ TABLE 10.10	US Preventive Services Task Force Scale for Strength of Recommendations for Clinical Practice	

Rank	Description	Recommendation for Practice
A	The service* is recommended and supported by evidence of substantial benefit.	The APRN should offer or provide this service when indicated.
B	The action is recommended and supported by strong evidence of moderate benefit associated with the service, or moderate-level evidence suggesting moderate to substantial benefit from the service.	The APRN should offer or provide this service when indicated.
C	Evidence suggests that the service provides only a small benefit.	The APRN should offer or provide this service only when other considerations support offering or providing this service.
D	Evidence demonstrates no benefit from the service or potential harm outweighs the service.	The APRN should discourage use of the service.
I	Current evidence is insufficient to assess the balance between harm and benefit of the service.	The APRN should counsel patients about the uncertainty of the balance between benefit and harm before offering or providing this service.

*Service is defined as an intervention, intervention bundle, or assessment strategy.
From Trinite, T., Cherry, C. L., & Marion, L. (2009). The U.S. Preventive Services Task Force: An evidence-based prevention resource for nurse practitioners. *Journal of the American Academy of Nurse Practitioners, 21,* 301–306.

leaders. Historically, many clinicians have believed that simply introducing a practice innovation is sufficient to ensure a sustained practice change, but research utilization studies have repeatedly proven this assumption false (Rogers, 2003; Stetler, 2003).

The second stage is characterized by a process of persuasion. During this stage, clinicians will form a favorable or unfavorable attitude toward a practice innovation. Although the decision-making process is highly individualized, formation of a positive attitude toward a practice innovation is primarily determined by two major factors—the perceived benefit of the practice change on patient outcomes and the perceived investment associated with the practice change as compared with current practice. Outcomes of research studies tend to focus on benefits to patients, but the APRN must also carefully consider the impact of a proposed practice innovation on existing practice. Such considerations are particularly relevant when an EBP innovation comprises a bundle of interventions. For example, current best evidence reveals that prevention of facility-acquired pressure ulcers is based on a number of preventive interventions, including regular skin assessment, pressure ulcer risk assessment, selective use of support surfaces, and regular patient turning and repositioning (National Pressure Ulcer Advisory Panel, European Pressure Ulcer Advisory Panel, and Pan Pacific Pressure Injury Alliance, 2014). Research has also demonstrated that pressure ulcer risk assessment is more effective when based on a validated

instrument as compared with an individual clinician's judgment. Various pressure ulcer risk instruments have been validated, but the Braden Scale for Pressure Sore Risk has emerged as being predominant in North America (Bolton, 2007). This is not based on its predictive power alone; a number of scales have been shown to exert robust predictive power in evaluating pressure ulcer risk. Rather, clinical experience overwhelmingly suggests that the parsimony of the Braden scale profoundly influences it predominance in clinical practice, especially when compared with other scales that require far longer to complete.

The third phase (decision stage) occurs when individual clinicians reach a decision about the proposed practice innovation (Rogers, 2003). At this point, the clinician will elect to support (accept) the practice innovation as valuable and worthy of implementation or oppose (reject) the innovation as offering insufficient benefit for the patient or being too costly when compared with outcomes achieved using current practice patterns. Historically, the decision to accept or oppose a practice innovation when reached by a key decision maker, such as a physician or nurse administrator, was thought to be the same as adopting or rejecting it, but the rise of EBP and interprofessional care teams has led to a more transparent separation of individual decision making from adoption of a practice innovation.

The final stage of innovation diffusion is adoption into daily clinical practice. Similar to the other stages of innovation diffusion, successful adoption requires more than assent to integrate the innovation into practice. It also requires varying levels of adapting or restructuring the practice environment in a manner that enables clinicians to engage in the behavior changes needed to adopt an innovation. When planning to introduce an EBP innovation, the APRN should consider the following factors: (1) its relative advantage; (2) its compatibility with current practice patterns; (3) the degree to which the innovation can be adapted on a trial basis; and (4) the degree to which results of the innovation can be observed (Rogers, 2003). Judging the relative advantage of a practice innovation requires comparing the time required to execute its various assessments and innovations as compared with the time and effort committed to existing practice patterns. Demonstrating the relative advantage of an EBP innovation is particularly challenging when it requires a greater time investment than current practice patterns. In this case, the APRN should clearly communicate and emphasize advantages to patient outcomes. Additional factors that favor adoption of an EBP include support from organizational administration, clinical leadership at the inpatient unit or clinic level, and manipulation of the practice environment to enhance adoption of new practices.

The degree to which a practice innovation can be adopted on a trial basis can also enhance the likelihood of its successful and sustained adoption (Rogers, 2003). For example, implementation of a facility-acquired pressure ulcer prevention program might include risk assessment using the Braden Scale for Predicting Pressure Sore Risk. In this case, integration of the Braden scale into the hospital's electronic medical record, combined with an online training program, allows nurses to familiarize themselves with use of the instrument prior to officially adopting this assessment into routine practice (Magnan & Maklebust, 2008, 2009).

Adoption of an EBP innovation is also enhanced by the degree to which results are observable. Meaningful feedback has traditionally been reserved for administrators or selected clinical leaders. However, front-line clinicians must be included in this feedback loop if they are to adopt practice changes on a sustained basis.

The process of implementing EBP in the APRN's local facility must be individualized based on existing practice patterns, staffing and resources of the facility, and organizational culture of the facility (Carlson, Rapp, & Eichler, 2012). Nevertheless, experience and existing research provide insights into key elements needed for achieving a successful and sustained change in practice patterns: (1) identification of an interprofessional team of stakeholders needed to plan and implement the practice innovation; (2) support from the organization's administration; (3) a clinical leadership structure that supports EBP principles; and (4) feedback data for monitoring improvement and rewarding clinician stakeholders.

Stakeholder Engagement

Formation of an interprofessional team of key stakeholders is essential to the implementation of a successful and sustained EBP innovation (Gallagher-Ford, Fineout-Overholt, Melnyk, & Stillwell, 2011; Powell, Doig, Hackley, Leslie, & Tillman, 2012). This group should include key clinical leaders who will be affected by the proposed practice innovation, such as clinical nursing leaders, physicians, and other clinicians (e.g., physical or occupational therapists, case managers). This group will be most directly responsible for completing the initial EBP process to identify current best evidence or using available resources, such as clinical practice guidelines, to aid with this determination. This group should also take primary responsibility for determining how the practice innovation should be incorporated into existing practice patterns. The key stakeholder group must consider a number of factors when designing an implementation strategy, including potential facilitators and barriers to implementation. Although evidence is limited, Weiner, Amick, and Lee (2008) have provided a detailed description of strategies that have proven effective for assessing organizational culture and barriers or facilitators likely to influence introduction of an EBP innovation. The core group should also design strategies to gain administrative support and support from key clinical leaders essential to the implementation of an EBP innovation. An APRN is often the coordinator or leader of this interprofessional team.

Organizational Support

In some cases, administrative personnel may approach the APRN concerning the need for a practice innovation based on regulatory changes, such as the introduction of "never events" by the National Quality Forum and Centers for Medicare and Medicaid Services in 2008 (Drake-Land, 2008). However, clinical experience strongly suggests that most EBP innovations are initiated by a clinician seeking to improve patient care outcomes. Ensuring administrative support involves more than merely informing administrative personnel of an intention to change organizational practice based on EBP principles (Brindle, Creehan, Black, & Zimmerman, 2015). Instead, the APRN must work with other key stakeholders to formulate a proposal that provides key administrative personnel with knowledge of the rationale for the recommended practice innovation, its anticipated impact on patient outcomes and associated costs, and the extent of needed resources, which will vary depending on the practice innovation proposed. Essential resources usually include a commitment to clinical leaders and staff education about the proposed practice innovation, alterations to the electronic health record needed to facilitate the innovation, disposable supplies or durable medical equipment needed to implement the practice change, and a system for measuring outcomes and providing staff and stakeholders with meaningful feedback about outcomes.

Clinical Leadership Support

The presence of a corporate culture and clinical leadership structure that supports EBP principles may be the single most important factor influencing the adoption of EBP innovations (Creehan et al., 2016; Rapp et al., 2010). Rapp et al. (2010) evaluated barriers to the implementation of EBP initiatives and observed that the behavior of clinical supervisors forms a substantial barrier to statewide EBP innovation projects. Specifically, they found that although clinical leaders did not oppose the use of EBP principles for clinical decision making, they did not set expectations among front-line clinicians, relying instead on informal methods of practice adoption. Although this approach may not act as a barrier to select clinicians who share an inherent interest in EBP and practice innovation, it ultimately favors maintenance of the status quo rather than organizational adoption of EBP principles and associated practice innovations.

Fortunately, several strategies have been identified to avoid this potential barrier to the adoption of EBP innovations. Obtaining Magnet status is a strategy for promoting an organizational environment that promotes EBP in nursing practice. Magnet status from the American Nurses Credentialing Center requires the integration of EBP principles into nursing care (Reigle et al., 2008). Although obtaining Magnet status is a major undertaking that goes well beyond the implementation of a single EBP innovation, it has been shown to aid facilities when transforming an organizational culture to one that promotes the principles of EBP among clinical nursing leaders and front-line clinicians.

Involvement of clinical leadership facilitates unit- or facility-based adoption of EBP practice innovations. Clinical leaders, such as the clinical nurse specialist, may act as facility-wide leaders for EBP changes by working with an interprofessional team evaluating facility-wide or health system–wide policies and procedures for care delivery. The clinical nurse specialist also may act as mentor and educator for unit- or clinic-based champions, which has been shown to facilitate adoption of EBP innovations in multiple health care settings (Taggart, McKenna, Stoelting, Kirkbride, & Mottar, 2012; Yevchak et al., 2014). The unit- or clinic-based champion is a clinician who practices on the unit in question and agrees to act as a mentor to front-line staff nurses and others to implement the EBP innovation. Selection of the proper individual as a champion is critical; Rogers (2003) noted that group adoption of innovation occurs in a stepwise manner, with some individuals acting as early adopters, followed by most group members who adopt the innovation based on positive results and feedback from early adopters, followed by a second minority of individuals (late adopters) who change practice only after it becomes apparent that the innovation is inevitable. Clinicians who are early adopters, and who are recognized on their units as influential practitioners, are preferred to the appointment of clinicians who are not persuaded that the innovation is advantageous when compared with current practice patterns.

Beyond careful selection and adequate administrative support, limited research allows identification of some fundamental strategies that enhance the effectiveness of unit-based champions (Taggart et al., 2012; Yevchak et al., 2014). These include scheduling time for unit-based champions to receive essential education for their enhanced role and to meet with clinical experts and unit managers as their role is delineated. Production and distribution of easily accessible educational materials for staff, including online information, pocket cards, and traditional education sessions tailored to staff with varying work hours, have been shown to enhance the effectiveness of unit-based champions on daily practice. Specific strategies such as rounding or case presentations are also perceived as valuable, as is quick access to specialty practice nursing or interprofessional staff.

Evidence-Based Practice Innovation: Feedback

As noted earlier, generating objective and meaningful outcomes when engaging in an EBP change is essential to determine its impact on clinical outcomes and cost. Feedback should be easily interpretable to all stakeholders and provided on a regular basis to promote sustained changes. For example, feedback may include regular reporting of facility-wide pertinent clinical outcomes, such as reduction in surgical site infections or indwelling catheter days, or it may include individual provider or unit outcomes. While the concept of providing feedback as a means of engaging clinical staff in an EBP innovation seems attractive, evidence concerning its impact is mixed. For example, a study of a structured monthly feedback program on a ventilator care prevention bundle in two urban critical care units found no effect on adherence after 1 year (Lawrence & Fulbrook, 2012). Similarly, researchers conducted an RCT that analyzed the impact of a monthly, multifaceted feedback strategy on nursing shifts (the unit of analysis for this cluster RCT) in 24 Dutch intensive care units limited to quarterly feedback (de Vos et al., 2015). No differences in adherence to evidence-based guideline standards were found when the structured feedback intervention was compared to standard feedback. Whether these results reflect the lack of efficacy of any structured feedback program versus lack of effect owing to the nature of the feedback is not clear. Additional research is needed before recommendations concerning routine feedback for front-line clinicians participating in an EBP innovation can be made.

Future Perspectives

The identification and evaluation of studies to identify current best evidence is currently based on a hierarchy that identifies the RCT as the most powerful study design for generating evidence, along with systematic reviews and meta-analytic techniques that combine data from multiple RCTs to reach conclusions about the strength of evidence. Although the RCT remains the best research design for evaluating the efficacy of an intervention, it does not necessarily follow that determination of efficacy indicates that an intervention will prove effective when applied in daily clinical practice as opposed to the rigidly controlled clinical trial setting (van Rijswijk & Gray, 2012). In addition, evaluations of current best evidence do not incorporate other real-world factors that influence treatment effectiveness when applied to the management of individual patients, including patient preference and the impact of cost. In order to address these gaps, clinicians, researchers, and policy makers are working together to look at sources of real-world data as complementary to data generated from traditional research designs, including the RCT. For example, in 2010, Congress allocated funds for development and generation of comparative effectiveness studies that seek to measure clinical effectiveness based on considerations of treatment effect, patient preference, and resource allocation (2010; U.S. Department of Health and Human Services, Health Resources and Services Administration, 2011). At the same time, the National Institutes of Health formed the Patient-Centered Outcomes Research Institute (PCORI), which was charged with generating research to help patients and providers make more informed decisions about their own care. The Institute continues to fund comparative effectiveness studies. This approach differs from traditional EBP processes because it relies on data collected under daily clinical practice and outside the controlled environment of the RCT (AHRQ, 2016). Other sources of real-world data include real-world clinical trials and health sciences research. The essential components of a well-designed, real-world trial continue to evolve, but basic principles include comparison of existing options for treatment; enrolling participants with few inclusion and exclusion criteria; minimal or no manipulation of treatment interventions outside individual clinical judgment; and consideration of treatment effect, cost, and patient preference (Lurie & Morgan, 2013). Health services research is generated by an interprofessional or transdisciplinary research team that investigates how social factors, financing systems, organizational structures, technologies, and individual behaviors affect access to health care (Lohr & Steinwachs, 2002). In addition, large electronic databases provide an increasingly rich source of real-world data that extends knowledge of how interventions perform beyond that provided by the RCT.

Conclusion

EBP involves the generation of a clinically measurable question, identification of pertinent research findings, coding and extraction of essential data, and implementation of findings. Intimate knowledge of this process is critical for the APRN to master three core levels of the EBP competency: application to individual clinical decision making, formulating policies for patient care in a local facility, and evaluating evidence in order to establish standards of care via clinical practice guidelines. These competencies are increasingly essential as the APRN functions as a team member, leader, and decision maker within an interprofessional health care team.

Key Summary Points

- Evidence-based practice is a central competency of advanced practice nursing.
- Evidence-based clinical decision making arises from a four-step process beginning with identification of a pertinent clinical question, systematic literature review, extraction of pertinent data, and implementation of findings into clinical practice.
- The APRN is well prepared to synthesize existing research findings needed to translate current best evidence into clinical practice on an individual, unit-wide, facility-wide, or health system–wide basis.
- Translating current best evidence into clinical practice requires more than simply introducing new policies or procedures in order to achieve

meaningful or sustained changes in clinical practice.
- Formation of an interprofessional team of key stakeholders, clinical support, and clinical leadership on a facility-wide level from an APRN and others, along with unit-based support from clinical champions, is essential for achieving sustained changes in clinical practice.

References

To access the references for this chapter, use your smartphone's QR code reader to scan the code below, or go to http://booksite.elsevier.com/ 9780323447751.

Leadership

Michael Carter • *Laura Reed*

"Anyone can hold the helm when the sea is calm."

—Pubilius Syrus

CHAPTER CONTENTS

The purposes of this chapter are to describe the advanced practice registered nurse (APRN) leadership competency, provide useful literature and resources on leadership and change, describe characteristics of effective leaders, identify obstacles to effective leadership, and discuss strategies for developing leadership skills. This chapter will help APRNs define their need for leadership abilities and develop a plan for acquiring the necessary skills appropriate to their particular positions and professional goals.

The Importance of Leadership for APRNs

Leadership is a core competency of APRNs. This competency may come as a surprise to some new

The authors acknowledge Charlene Hanson and Mary Fran Tracy for their contributions to earlier editions of this chapter.

APRNs in that they are often focused so much on understanding and applying the art and science of clinical practice that leadership seems like a distant concern. Yet APRNs quickly learn in clinical practice that care is provided in complex systems and these systems require leadership to function effectively. APRNs have unique knowledge and clinical legitimacy that provide a strong basis for their leadership.

Health care systems are under constant redesign and transformation (Gilman, Chokshi, Bowen, Rugen, & Cox, 2014; Institute for Healthcare Improvement [IHI], 2011; Institute of Medicine [IOM], 2000, 2001, 2011; Leape et al., 2009; Reynolds et al., 2015), and there is continuing evolution in health professional education as well (American Association of Colleges of Nursing [AACN], 2006; Dreher, Clinton, & Sperhac, 2014). Interprofessional care among a variety of different clinicians has become more important to ensure quality outcomes, and leading these teams is very complex (Canadian Interprofessional Health Collaborative, 2010; Farrell, Payne, & Heye, 2015; Greiner & Knebel, 2003; Interprofessional Education Collaborative, 2011). The unique leadership provided by APRNs takes place in the systems where they provide care. Clinical care is usually delivered at the individual, patient level but is embedded within larger organizations. These larger care delivery organizations rely on leaders to improve safety, quality, and reliability and to evaluate the results of care. In short, systems leaders must be able to identify the need for innovation and change and implement strategies to achieve them. In partnership with others, APRNs craft approaches to evaluate, reassess, and implement systems redesign and innovation.

APRNs provide leadership in several areas. Their activities range from taking a stand on behalf of an individual patient to advocating for a change in national health policy. Competency in leadership does not stand alone but interacts with other APRN competencies. In the United States, the movement of APRN education to the Doctor of Nursing Practice (DNP) has implications for the APRN's leadership competency (AACN, 2004). For example, one of the essentials of DNP education is expertise in systems leadership (AACN, 2006).

Constantly Evolving Health Care Systems

The World Health Organization (2013) has reasoned that everyone in the world should have access to the health services they need without being forced into poverty when paying for these services. This goal requires substantial changes in the health systems of many countries, including the United States. The passage of the Patient Protection and Affordable Care Act (2010) and the subsequent enactment of the Act's many provisions moved the United States much closer to universal coverage, but the United States remains the only developed country in the world without universal coverage. Other nations are experiencing similar evolution of their systems of care, and these changes are often related to the new types of health care problems seen in these countries, the organization of their health care systems, and the ways in which these countries pay for care.

The IOM released their groundbreaking *The Future of Nursing* report in the United States in 2011, and the subsequent work in monitoring these changes highlights the important goals for APRNs to lead change and advance health. This report contends that it is essential for nurses to be full partners and leaders in the transformation of health care.

The IOM has issued a number of reports over the years calling for radical redesign and transformation of the American health care system. Such changes do not occur quickly in part because they require a significant rethinking of how care is delivered, the roles of patients and education of providers, effective channels for diffusing innovation, how health care is financed, where and how care is delivered, and which provider activities are valued and paid for (Hunter, Nelson, & Birmingham, 2013). These IOM reports calling for transformation of the health care system are predicated on six national quality aims—safety, effectiveness, patient-centeredness, timeliness, efficiency, and equity (IOM, 2001). The IOM has long noted that patients throughout the health system are at high risk for the occurrence of adverse events, yet numerous institutional barriers to reporting these events still exist. One barrier has been the long-standing tendency toward naming and blaming individuals rather than exploring gaps in systems of care and organizational culture (Wagner, Capezuti, & Ouslander, 2006). Leaders have come to realize that errors occur because of a continuum of reasons. APRN leaders can use the six quality aims to facilitate the evaluation of errors, near misses, and questionable behavior to determine root causes of situations in which employee behavior does not match organizational values. Causes for these situations can range from organizational culture to defective systems and processes to bad choices on the part of employees.

The IHI launched a campaign in 2001 to save 100,000 lives from medical errors (Berwick, Caulkins, McCannon, & Hackbarth, 2006; Patient Safety and

Quality Health Care, 2005). This campaign was so successful, with an estimated 122,000 lives saved between January 2005 and June 2006, that a new goal was created to decrease mortality and morbidity in 5 million lives (IHI, 2012). Yet with all these efforts, medical errors remain the third leading cause of death in the United States per year, estimated to total 251,454 deaths (Makary & Daniel, 2016). Many health care systems are participating in efforts to improve safety and quality, such as Magnet hospital recognition or participation in the IHI campaign. APRNs not only have a stake in these efforts but also have the clinical expertise and leadership that can ensure success.

Evolving Health Professional Education

Just as health care has been evolving throughout the world, so too has health professional education. Part of these educational changes reflect the new or expanded competencies health professionals must have for future practice based on changes in the type of health care conditions being treated and new emphasis being placed on patient quality, costs, access, and patient-centered care. The Josiah Macy Jr. Foundation makes recommendations on how health care providers need to be trained to meet the needs of primary health care and has been providing yearly updates on interprofessional education (Cronenwett & Dzau, 2010; Kahaleh, Danielson, Franson, Nuffer, & Umland, 2015; Pohl, Hanson, Newland, & Cronenwett, 2010). There continues to be substantial interest in expanding and improving interprofessional education. This approach to education is very complex in that health professionals come from different theoretical perspectives, educational programs may not be co-located, academic calendars are seldom synchronized, and faculty obligations often preclude working with other professions. Measuring the impact of interprofessional education on provider practice and the outcomes for patients has been very difficult. This may be attributed to the substantial length of time from when the professionals were in education until actual changes in patient outcomes could be measured. In addition, the system of care delivery is changing the way it is financed, and this can compound the measurement of outcomes from education alone.

APRN Competencies

In the AACN's *The Essentials of Doctoral Education for Advanced Nursing Practice* (2006), several specific competencies relate to leadership for all DNP graduates, including APRNs. Of the eight essentials, four inform the leadership competency—organizational and system leadership for quality improvement and systems thinking, clinical scholarship and analytic methods, information systems and patient care technology for the improvement and transformation of health care, and clinical prevention and population health for improving the nation's health. Core competencies developed by the National Association of Clinical Nurse Specialists (NACNS, 2010) address leadership requirements of clinical nurse specialists (CNSs), and those developed by the National Organization of Nurse Practitioner Faculties (NONPF, 2017) address nurse practitioners (NPs). Nurse practitioner leadership competencies are also in place for Canada (Canadian Nurses Association, 2010) and Australia (Nursing and Midwifery Board of Australia, 2014).

Earlier APRN education programs focused a good deal on learning to provide expert clinical care. This focus was necessary but is no longer sufficient for future practice. Health care has changed in many ways. Practice today and for the future means that APRNs must possess knowledge, skills, and abilities to address larger system issues in a way not expected in the past. APRNs have a social covenant with the society that they serve. New issues concerning the social determinants of health have emerged and must be understood by APRNs. Patients are living longer and some of this extension of life includes periods of active dying. Many health conditions have no cure or hope of cure. Learning to diagnose and treat patients with acute and chronic health conditions is central for much of APRN practice, but the work does not stop there. Understanding the evolving structures, regulations, and ethos of care is mandatory for APRNs to deliver high-quality care with the greatest access for those in need and at the lowest costs. These changes in focus of care mean that APRNs must be able to seamlessly move from the individual recipient of the service to the much larger system context and then back.

In summary, numerous contextual and educational factors that require APRN leadership have been identified in calls for the redesign and transformation of the health care system. Certain themes are apparent—in particular, patient-centeredness (see Chapter 7), teamwork (see Chapter 12), quality improvement, the use of information technology, and complexity. These factors are an appropriate part of graduate and continuing education so that APRNs acquire the knowledge and skills they need to lead effectively (Cronenwett et al., 2009; Scott & Miles, 2013; Sherwood, 2010).

Leadership: Definitions, Models, and Concepts

APRNs can draw on numerous models of leadership and change processes to inform their leadership development. Most leadership models are predicated on leaders having an ability to understand themselves. Leadership grows out of personal characteristics that can be learned and are associated with successful leadership. One model of self-awareness is the emotional awareness model of Goleman (2005). This model proposes that there are four core skills that lead to improved leadership effectiveness. These are self-awareness, self-management, social awareness, and relationship management. Most important is that successful leaders understand the importance of self-regulation in their relationships.

Definitions of Leadership Useful for APRNs

Contemporary definitions of leadership generally fit into one of two categories: transformational leadership (Carlton, Holsinger, Riddell, & Bush, 2015; Vance & Larson, 2002) or situational leadership (Carlton et al., 2015; Grohar-Murray & DiCroce, 1992). Both categories are built on attributes of the leader that are learned and can be taught.

Leadership Models That Lead to Transformation

Vernon (2015) asserted that transformational leaders constantly ask themselves and their team questions about what the goal is, how to try things differently, and what are the costs of maintaining the status quo. This form of leadership transforms the team by leading to changes in values, attitudes, perceptions, and/or behaviors on the part of the leader and the follower and lays the groundwork for further positive change. Thus, transformational leadership occurs when people interact in ways that inspire higher levels of motivation and morality among participants. How do leaders do this? Transformational leaders analyze a situation to understand the particular leadership needs and goals; they use this information, together with their interpersonal skills, to motivate, stimulate, share with, conciliate, and satisfy their followers in an interdependent interactional exchange. DePree (2011) defined leadership as an art form in which the leader does what is required in the most effective and humane way.

This definition proposes that contemporary leadership may be viewed as a process of moving the self and others toward a shared vision that becomes a shared reality. Successful transformational leadership is relational, driven by a common goal or purpose, and satisfies the needs of leader and followers. It is the leadership style often associated with effective change agents. Schwartz, Spencer, Wilson, and Wood (2011) have studied the effects of transformational leadership on the Magnet designation for hospitals and report that transformational leadership brought about the change needed to obtain and maintain Magnet status. Other authors who have described a transformational approach to leadership include Wang, Chontawan, and Nantsupawat (2012), who studied transformational leadership with Chinese nurses. Transformational leadership was associated with job satisfaction in nurses.

Many different models of leadership are available (Table 11.1). One model that is frequently used is the work of Stephen Covey, begun in 1989.

The Eight Habits of Highly Effective People

Stephen Covey (1989) presented personal and interdependent characteristics that foster acquisition of leadership skills (Box 11.1). In creating a personal view of leadership, Covey suggested that the most effective way to "keep the end in mind" is to create a personal mission statement that becomes a standard to live by as one progresses from independence to interdependence. In Covey's model, interdependence is achieved only after one has defined and integrated this personal mission or standard into one's practice.

 BOX 11.1 **Covey's Eight Habits of Highly Successful People**

- Be proactive.
- Begin with the end in mind.
- Put first things first.
- Think win-win.
- Seek first to understand, then to be understood.
- Synergize.
- Sharpen the saw.
- Find your voice and inspire others to find theirs.

Adapted from Covey, S. (1989). *The seven habits of highly effective people: Powerful lessons in personal change.* New York, NY: Simon & Schuster; Covey, S. (2004). *The 8th habit. From effectiveness to greatness.* New York, NY: Free Press; and Covey, S. (2006). Leading in the knowledge worker age. *Leader to Leader Journal, 41,* 11–15.

⊚ TABLE 11.1	Useful Models of Transformational Leadership and Change		
Author	**Title**	**Relevant Concepts**	**APRN Use**
Senge	*The Fifth Discipline* (1990, 2006)	Describes five actions or processes that characterize effective teams and organizations that manage change well: • Personal mastery • Awareness of mental models • Shared vision • Team learning • Systems thinking	APRNs can use these concepts to identify: • Personal leadership goals • Strengths and needs of the teams and organizations with whom they work • Strategies to enhance team development and collaboration
Covey	*The Seven Habits of Highly Effective People* (1989) *The 8th Habit* (2004) "Leading in the Knowledge Worker Age" (2006)	Development of a personal mission statement to live by as one develops independence and interdependence. The eight habits that foster acquisition of leadership skills are: • Be proactive. Take the initiative, choose your response. • Begin with the end in mind. Define success. • Put first things first; personally manage yourself. • Think win-win, with a willingness to cooperate. • Seek first to understand and then to be understood. • Synergize; the whole is greater than the sum of its parts. • Sharpen the saw; renew your physical, mental, spiritual, and social dimensions. • Find your voice and inspire others to find theirs	APRNs can use these characteristics to: • Acquire leadership skills • Attain interdependence by fully incorporating one's personal mission statement into practice • Use influence and inspiration as a creative catalyst for change
Nelson et al.	"Microsystems in Health Care: Learning from High-Performing Front-Line Clinical Units" (2002)	Studied 20 varied microsystems; identified nine common success characteristics associated with delivery of high-quality, cost-efficient care: • Leadership • Culture • Organizational support • Patient focus • Staff focus • Interdependence of care team • Information and information technology • Process improvement • Performance patterns	APRNs can use these characteristics to assess one's system and identify gaps in and opportunities for leadership.
Massoud, Nielsen, Nolan, Schall, and Sevin	"A Framework for Spread" (2006)	Model evolved by the Institute for Healthcare Improvement to understand phases of successful system change. Key elements: • Prepare for spread. • Establish aim for spread. • Develop an initial spread plan. • Execute and refine plan.	APRNs can use ideas for each phase of spread. Also useful for: • Understanding the importance of leadership in planning for spread • Detailing elements of the aim and initial plan for spread (addresses the who, what, when, where)
Cooperrider Whitney, and Stavros	*Appreciative Inquiry Handbook* (2008)	Uses a 4D cycle to seek positive attributes to build on through conversations and relationship building rather than focusing on problem areas: • Discovery • Dream • Design • Destiny	APRNs can use these concepts to: • Motivate and inspire colleagues to excellence in practice • Develop partnerships to capitalize on positive attributes of individual team members to solve complex problems in health care

Covey described attributes of those who lead from a philosophy of interdependence: listening twice as much as you speak, remaining trustworthy by never compromising honesty, maintaining a positive attitude, and keeping a sense of humor. Interdependence allows one to hear and understand the other person's viewpoint, leading to a synergistic or win-win level of communication. In 2004, Covey expanded on this leadership model by proposing an eighth habit—leaders need to find their voice and help others to find theirs. He noted that leaders at any level can use their inspiration and influence to overcome negativity and use creativity to move the organization to greatness; this type of leader can be a catalyst for change. Covey (2006) also developed leadership ideas in light of managing people in the information age. A key concept in this update is that leaders must be aware that the ways they lead will influence the choices that followers make.

Situational Leadership

The term *situational leadership* is defined as the interaction between an individual's leadership style and the features of the environment or situation in which he or she is operating. Leadership styles are not fixed and may vary based on the issues being addressed or on the environment. Situational leadership depends on particular circumstances, with leaders and followers assuming interchangeable roles according to environmental demands (Huber, 2014). The role of follower is important because APRNs will find themselves in both roles from time to time. Leaders must have followers and followers must have leaders. It is important for leaders to learn to follow and allow others to lead. DePree (2011) expanded on this idea and used the term *roving leadership* to describe a participatory process in which leadership in a particular situation may shift among the team members. This notion of leadership is relevant because APRNs' work in collaborative health care teams requires the roles of leader and follower to be interchangeable depending on the complex needs of the patient.

Leadership Models That Address System Change and Innovation

Change is a constant in today's clinical environments. Efforts to transform the health care system are generally focused in three areas: diffusion of innovation, clinician behavior change, and patient behavior change. The reality is that change is often messy and not always welcome even when it seems straightforward. An integrative review of diffusion and dissemination of innovations reveals why redesign and transformation are messy—they are exceedingly complex (Greenhalgh, Robert, MacFarlane, Bate, & Kyriakidou, 2004; Kwamie, 2015). For example, an NP was very concerned about how long it was taking patients to schedule return visits. The booking system was controlled by the larger health care organization and was not easily adapted to a specific purpose. In addition, all the providers wanted to keep all slots filled for the next 2 weeks so double booking was common, resulting in some clinic times being overloaded. Office staff had no authority to override the system and billing staff could not determine if a particular insurance plan would pay for more frequent visits. Making any change in scheduling involved the information technology staff, the office staff, the billing staff, and the clinicians—any one of whom could stop the change.

Nelson et al. (2002) argued that clinical microsystems are the front-line units in which patients and providers interface and are the foundation for providing safe and high-quality care within large organizations. Thus transforming care at the front-line unit is essential to optimizing care throughout the continuum. They studied the processes and methods of 20 high-performing sites and identified the characteristics that were related to high performance: leadership, organizational culture, macro-organizational support of microsystems, patient focus, staff focus, interdependence of the care team, information and information technology, performance improvement, and performance patterns.

APRNs practice at the patient-provider interface, and their leadership can contribute greatly to the optimization of other successful characteristics. APRNs are skilled at creating cohesive teams, identifying and advocating patient and staff needs, leading performance-improvement efforts at the front-line interface, and contributing to a positive organizational culture.

One helpful model for understanding leadership in complex organizations is complexity theory. Henry (2014) contends that complexity theory is focused on understanding the ways in which individuals are free to act in interconnected but not predictable ways. This means that one person's actions lead to changes in the context for others in the organization. Some theories of leadership and management are built on the assumption that individuals and organizations are logical and predictable in the way they function. Complexity theory holds that some actions are not predictable in a linear manner and evolve more organically.

APRNs who are learning to lead change may find the use of complexity theory helpful. Clancy, Effkin, and Presut (2008) provide insights when there are multiple providers, new technology competition, and complex information systems involved.

Spread of Innovation

Massoud and colleagues (2006) developed a model to address the difficulty in spreading effective, evidence-based innovation beyond the immediate environment. Diffusion within and among health care organizations is key with today's goal of implementing best practices throughout health care. Founded on Rogers' (2003) definition of diffusion, this framework for spread is based on four main components—preparing for spread, establishing an aim for spread, developing an initial spread plan, and executing or refining the spread plan. Leadership is essential in preparing a plan to spread innovation. As leaders, APRNs must take an active role in ensuring the innovation is evidence based throughout all aspects of the spread plan. During the development of the spread plan, the leader oversees the project and may take an active role in developing the plan. Finally, the APRN leader needs to ensure collection and use of information about the effectiveness of the plan, supporting course correction as needed.

Several common themes emerge when considering models of leadership and change. Effective leadership requires sound knowledge of oneself and one's organization with regard to values, strengths, and weaknesses, as well as expert communication and relationship-building skills and the ability to think and act strategically.

Appreciative Inquiry

Appreciative inquiry (AI) is a leadership model that seeks to find positives through appreciative conversations and relationship building (Cooperrider, Whitney, & Stavros, 2008). Rather than focusing on a problem, this model encourages a focus on what is working well and what the organization does well, and then broadens and builds on the strengths. This model is predicated on the belief that when we expand what we do best, problems seem to fall away or are outgrown. Leading through positive interactions results in people working together toward a shared vision and preferred future without the burden of being weighed down by problems. Leaders using this leadership model are open to inquiry without having a preconceived outcome in mind; rather, they facilitate a search for shared meaning and build and expand on what is working well. For example, faculty in an APRN graduate program wanted to create a DNP program, but there were quality concerns about some of their existing Master of Science in Nursing options. Through an AI process, the faculty decided to build a DNP program based solely on the certified registered nurse anesthetist (CRNA) role because that was their strongest offering at the time. Moreover, through this process they decided to phase out two of their Master of Science in Nursing options because they were not up to the same level of quality. Over time, the CRNA program was recognized as one of the nation's top programs. So, rather than investing solely in "fixing what's broken," the AI model directs resources and visioning to an organization's greatest strengths. This leadership model uses a 4D cycle:

- *D*iscovery—an exploration of what is; finding organizational strengths and processes that work well
- *D*ream—imagining what could be; envisioning innovations that would work even better for the organization's future
- *D*esign—determining what should be; planning and prioritizing those processes
- *D*estiny—creating what should be; implementing the design

AI uses a positive perspective that can be motivational and inspirational for employees with the goal of increasing exceptional performance. This model can work well for APRNs who are skilled in developing partnerships. Although evidence for the effectiveness of this leadership model is limited, there is enough evidence to support further rigorous research (Jones, 2010). The consequences of leading with an emphasis on defects are that the process lacks vision, places attention on yesterday's causes, and can lead to narrow and fragmented solutions. The AI model shifts from asking "What is the biggest problem?" to "What possibilities exist that we have not yet considered?" This approach quickly leads individuals to a shared purpose and vision.

Concepts Related to Change

Change refers to the various types of initiatives aimed at improving the quality and safety of practice, whether by revising policies or helping clinicians master new knowledge and change behavior. In other words, change is seen as any clinical or systems effort to encourage the adoption and diffusion of innovation, including quality improvement, product rollouts, clinician education, and skill development. Change is viewed as a process so that it does not have a discrete beginning and end but, instead, appears to be a series of continuous transitions that overlap one another. This means that the ability to bring about change must be woven into the fabric of the everyday life and work of APRNs. As with patient assessment to effect individual behavior change, APRNs must be skilled at assessing and reassessing their organizations and the complex forces that drive the health care system to be effective change agents. Systems innovation requires leadership that is continuous and flexible and demands ongoing attention to and redefinition of appropriate strategies (Greenhalgh et al., 2004; Klein, Gabelnick, & Herr, 1998; Kwamie, 2015; Massoud et al., 2006; Shirey, 2015; Thompson & Nelson-Martin, 2011).

Opinion Leadership

One way that change can be initiated is through the use of opinion leadership (Anderson & Titler, 2014). Opinion leaders are clinicians who are identified by their colleagues as likeable, trustworthy, and influential (Flodgren et al., 2007). Clinicians are likely to listen to the opinion leader and make a change in practice based on what has been learned from the opinion leader. One study of opinion leaders in several different clinical settings has indicated that contextual factors influence the ability of an opinion leader to promote guideline adoption by colleagues (Locock, Dopson, Chambers, & Gabbay, 2001). Shirey (2008) pointed out that there are several elements of being the opinion leader, including being knowledgeable, respected, trusted, and well connected within the organization; in addition, opinion leaders must also be generous with their time and advice. APRNs become opinion leaders as they are recognized for their astute clinical decision making and influence of others. They are sought out by others and, when APRN opinion leaders speak, others listen. Thus a staff nurse may ask a CNS wound care specialist to examine a wound and provide treatment advice. Colleagues are eager to try the new information when an NP returns from a conference and shares what was learned. CRNAs are consulted for their opinion on airway management. These examples suggest the importance of attending to environmental cues when change is planned. Unfortunately, there is very limited evidence on the effectiveness of opinion leaders concerning change. This may be because there have been few studies of this model of leadership.

Driving and Restraining Forces

Driving and restraining forces are useful concepts for APRNs planning for change, including managing the intended and unintended consequences of change. For example, the movement toward multistate licensure has gained momentum as APRNs extend their practices across state lines (Young et al., 2012; see Chapter 12, Fig. 12.1, for an illustration of driving and restraining forces). These forces can serve as driving or restraining influences for APRNs depending on different policies and procedures for reimbursement and prescriptive authority within states. As multistate licensure for APRNs evolves, telehealth may be considered a driving force and states' rights may be a restraining force. For example, a psychiatric/mental health NP in one state may wish to use telehealth methods to treat patients in an adjoining state to save patients the time and expense of driving to therapy sessions. The states allow for this under the RN license but do not allow for this under the APRN approval. The APRN would have to seek and obtain recognition from the board of nursing in the state where the patient is located. There may be very different rules in the two states about physician collaboration or supervision, scope of practice, and prescription rules, and these could be a restraining force for extending this practice. The unintended consequence of these rules and regulations could be to restrict care by APRNs to rural residents.

Understanding driving and restraining forces helps in analyzing the organizational settings in which APRNs work. For example, an organizational assessment of these various forces is useful in determining an institution's level of commitment to diversity.

At times, physicians have been both driving and restraining forces for change. Experienced APRNs know that one of the challenges in system redesign and transformation has been engaging physicians in the work of improving quality as a team member. Berwick (2016) has argued that there is now a new era in health care that calls for an end to the protectionism seen earlier. He points out that better care, better health, and lower costs can be brought about by working with others to improve care in a transparent way. APRNs and physicians are players who can lead together to offset professional prerogative and greed while listening to the voices of the people served.

Pace of Change

A major concern is the rapidity with which change occurs in the health care industry. Even when one develops detailed plans for a change, events may occur that reshape the process and progress so that what gets implemented may not be the same as the original proposal. As the rapidity of change increases, the time frame to accomplish change strategies shortens. This phenomenon makes change more difficult for individuals and organizations to manage. As a consequence, many of the traditional models still being used to implement change will not be successful.

Planned versus unplanned change is based predominantly on issues of time—time to plan for and think through the desired change, time to orient and allow stakeholders to become comfortable with the proposed change, and time to educate and allow the change process to occur. Many required changes in health care do not have sufficient time to allow the proposed change to naturally evolve. Transitional leadership may offer the best hope for survival in rapid change situations.

Whether health care organizations can sustain fast-paced change is not clear unless there is a commitment to the culture of change. This commitment assists and supports adaptation to new systems and ways of knowing and doing. A culture of change requires several components, including learning about change and change strategies, encouraging dialogue, valuing collaboration and differences, and being committed to enacting change. In a classic work, O'Connell (1999) proposed strategies for promoting a culture of change within an organization (Box 11.2).

APRNs can use one or more of the models of leadership described here to assess their systems. Knowing where one's system is in terms of readiness for change and identifying the forces that will support or restrain adoption of an innovation can help the APRN design strategies that will work. It is also helpful to consider the techniques used for implementing change, such as building alliances, creating a shared vision, being assertive, negotiating conflict, and managing transitions as they relate to providing a positive culture for change. As leaders, APRNs can use their skills to translate the need for and perspectives on change among clinicians, patients, families, and administrators. In addition, APRN leaders need to be prepared to identify when it is not in an organization's best interest to pursue a change based on context, environment, inadequate problem solving, or unresolved barriers. Repetitive, rapid change can take a toll on engagement and productivity and potentially on patient safety, particularly if implications and consequences are not thoroughly considered. Most importantly, leaders need to understand the personal implications of change if a culture of change is to be realized. Box 11.3 provides a useful set of strategies for APRN leaders who are helping their organizations and colleagues work through change transitions.

Types of Leadership for APRNs

Some APRNs are not comfortable with the idea of being leaders. This may be because they see leadership as outside of their goal of caring for their

---

◎ BOX 11.2 O'Connell's Strategies That Promote a Culture of Change

- Maintain momentum toward change.
- Emphasize managerial support in the process of changing workflow and practice patterns.
- Encourage the question "why" and exercise tolerance for the results.
- Emphasize the importance of personal concerns and address them.
- Find new and different ways to demonstrate administrative support.

Adapted from O'Connell, C. (1999). A culture of change or a change of culture. *Nursing Administration Quarterly, 23,* 65–68.

◎ BOX 11.3 Leadership Strategies for Moving Through Change

- Spark a passion; believe in what you are doing; shine a light on activities that inspire and excite.
- Understand the organizational culture.
- Create a vision.
- Get the right people involved.
- Hand the work over to the champions of change.
- Let values serve as the compass for where you are headed.
- Change people first; organizations evolve.
- Seek and provide opportunities for professional renewal and regeneration.
- Maintain a healthy balance.

Adapted from Kerfoot, K., & Chaffee, M. W. (2007). Ten keys to unlock policy change in the workplace. In D. J. Mason, J. K. Leavitt, & M. W. Chaffee (Eds.), *Policy and politics in nursing and health care* (pp. 482–484). Philadelphia: Saunders; and Kerfoot, K. (2005). On leadership: Building confident organizations by filling buckets, building infrastructures, and shining the flashlight. *Dermatology Nursing, 17,* 154–156.

patients. However, upon a more careful view, leadership is understood to be necessary to bring about the kinds of things that ensure good patient care. APRN leadership competency can be conceptualized as occurring in four primary areas: in clinical practice with patients and staff, within professional organizations, within health care systems, and in health policymaking arenas. The extent to which individual APRNs choose to lead in each of these areas depends on patients' needs; personal characteristics, interests, and commitments of the APRN; institutional or organizational priorities and opportunities; and priority health policy issues in nursing as a whole and within one's specialty. These four areas have substantial overlap. For example, developing clinical leadership skills will enable the APRN to be more effective at the policy level as clinical expertise informs policymaking.

Clinical Leadership

Clinical leadership focuses on the needs and goals of the patient and family and ensures that quality patient care is achieved. Clinical leadership is a foundational component to attaining and maintaining a productive environment in which safe and excellent care employing best practices is provided (Murphy, Quillinan, & Carolan, 2009). This leadership occurs when APRNs acquire and apply knowledge about how to build appropriate working relationships with health care team members, how to instill confidence in patients and colleagues, and how to problem-solve as part of a team (Bally, 2007). APRN leaders propose and implement change strategies that improve patient care. Some clinical leadership skills are part of the competencies of consultation (see Chapter 9) and collaboration (see Chapter 12). The most common clinical leadership roles APRNs fulfill are those of advocate (for patient, family, staff, or colleagues), group leader, and systems leader. APRNs may advocate for a particular patient or family, as when an acute care nurse practitioner (ACNP) discusses with the attending surgeon the need for the patient to have a clear understanding of the potential adverse effects of an elective surgery. The surgeon may have concluded that the patient and family fully understood the potential outcomes of the surgery but the ACNP discovered that there was broad misunderstanding by the patient and family. Presenting talks or writing articles on clinical topics are other ways of expressing clinical leadership and influencing others. The important aspect of clinical leadership is that the APRN steps up,

assuring the best clinical outcome for any particular patient.

Group leadership may be informal, as when an APRN agrees to coordinate multiple referrals for a patient with complex care needs or has expertise in a particular clinical problem such as pain management, skin care, or screening for cervical cancer and assumes a team leadership role reflecting this expertise. APRNs may also have more formal leadership responsibilities; for example, an APRN may lead a weekly team meeting or agree to convene a group and lead the development of a new practice protocol to bring care into line with newly released standards of care. One function of the APRN leader is to motivate colleagues and facilitate their use of new knowledge and/or the adoption of new practices with the goal of improved patient outcomes.

APRNs often exercise leadership to ensure that clinical problems are addressed by administrative leaders at a systems level. This type of leadership requires that APRNs move between the clinical and administrative arenas, interpreting the needs of one to the other. Advancing clinical excellence requires financial, creative, and political skills to promote innovative care with others (Murphy et al., 2009). Having these additional skills improves the success of this form of clinical leadership and the compelling translation of ideas between distinct, sometimes competing perspectives. APRNs recognize the clinical problems related to their specialty that require attention or intervention from the larger (macro) system of which they are a part. For example, when a CNS called a patient to learn why he had not kept his appointment at the heart failure clinic, she learned that the patient could not find parking nearby because of hospital construction, did not know that a shuttle would take him from the satellite lot to the clinic, and did not have the energy to walk from the satellite lot. The CNS knew that this could be a problem for other clinic patients and worked with administrators to make sure patients had knowledge of and access to the resources that were needed and available. The CNS understood the clinical implications (patients might experience more complications requiring readmission) and systems implications (e.g., lower care quality, increased risks for patients, higher costs, missed appointments) of construction-related missed appointments for her patient population.

APRNs who lead patient care teams effectively find that their interprofessional leadership skills are in demand. For example, an APRN who was successful in leading a quality improvement initiative to improve care of patients with asthma who were admitted to the hospital was invited to chair a national task force of health care professionals developing practice guidelines for the treatment of asthma. The ability to provide clinical interprofessional leadership requires a firm grasp of clinical and professional issues while responding to the challenges of other disciplines and the larger society. It necessitates a deep respect for other clinicians and the creation of a safe and welcoming place for all voices to be heard. APRNs develop the attributes needed to lead in other domains as they build on a solid foundation of strong clinical leadership.

Professional Leadership

Active participation and leadership are particularly important and exercised in professional organizations. Novice APRNs may begin by seeking membership on a committee of a local, state, or national nursing or interprofessional organization. These organizations are built on the voluntary contributions of their members and rely on members to achieve the organization's goals. As APRNs become more experienced, they may seek opportunities to apply the leadership skills that they have learned in their work to their professional organizations. Most APRNs are members of one or more nursing and interprofessional organizations. These memberships provide a myriad of leadership opportunities, including organizing continuing education offerings, presenting at national conferences, chairing a committee, and running for the board of directors. In these situations, APRNs exercise more choice as to whether and when they will participate in leadership activities than they do in their usual work roles.

Professional leadership often begins locally and proceeds to state, national, and international levels. Novice APRNs can acquire leadership skills and experience by becoming involved in the leadership and committee work of local advanced practice nursing coalitions and organizations and progressing into state and regional leadership roles as they develop their style, strengths, and network as APRN leaders. The ability to place APRN leaders in key local, state, and national positions is critical to the visibility and credibility of APRNs and to the establishment of their place within nursing and the larger health care community. In addition to informal leadership development opportunities, there are also formal programs in which APRNs can develop the skills to lead in positions such as board membership (Carlson et al., 2011).

Systems Leadership

Systems leadership means leading at the organizational or delivery system level—a skill that requires a multidimensional understanding of systems. Systems leadership often requires a "big picture" view and understanding elements in care delivery far beyond nursing. Within health care organizations, APRNs may lead clinical teams, chair committees, chair or serve as members of boards, manage projects, and direct other initiatives aimed at improving patient care as well as the clinical practice of nurses and other professionals. Systems leadership overlaps professional situations in which leaders are elected or appointed to positions within defined organizations and groups. For example, APRNs may identify an increase in the rate of patient falls and lead a task force to evaluate the problem and design corrective interventions. A critical care CNS or ACNP may initiate interprofessional rounds to monitor patients on mechanical ventilation and gather data on clinical variables such as complication rate and time to weaning. APRNs may be asked to participate in or lead standing or ad hoc interprofessional committees such as credentialing, ethics, institutional review board, or pharmacy and therapeutics committees. APRNs may be asked by administrators to participate in organizational reengineering or other activities aimed at improving the environment in which others practice.

APRNs need to be aware that the characteristics of successful entrepreneurs are desirable and valued in systems leaders. The term *entrepreneurial leadership* refers to leaders who go outside of traditional employment systems to create new opportunities to exercise their unique abilities (Shirey, 2004). When these leaders use the entrepreneurial skills of innovation and risk taking and assume responsibility for achieving specific targets in an organization, they are termed *intrapreneurs*. Because this leadership style is consistent with the call for health care system redesign, it is worth reviewing characteristics associated with entrepreneurial leadership. Shirey (2007b) has stated that nurse entrepreneurs have a desire to make a difference and see opportunities in situations in which others see barriers or challenges. Blanchard, Hutson, and Willis (2007) have developed tools for leaders to assess their entrepreneurial strengths and have identified attributes of entrepreneurs, including being resourceful, purposeful, a risk taker, a problem solver, innovative, communicative, and determined. Universities that prepare APRNs are offering coursework on innovation, entrepreneurship, and innovative thinking to prepare entrepreneurial and intrapreneurial APRN leaders (Shirey, 2007a). APRNs frequently underestimate their transferable skills, which can be used in entrepreneurial or intrapreneurial opportunities (Shirey, 2009). Recognition of these skills will assist intrapreneurial APRNs to build a case for how their services can assist the organization in achieving innovative clinical excellence (Shirey, 2007b). Entrepreneurial leadership skills are illustrated in Exemplar 11.1, which also illustrates the evolving nature of advanced practice nursing leadership and how it can expand in breadth over time to lead national and international policy. Dr. Bednash moved from staff nurse to NP to leader of one of the premier national organizations in nursing education. She credits her NP education with providing her the basis for her international leadership.

Willingness to Name Difficult Organizational Problems

A common human characteristic in organizations is to operate around the periphery of problems and not in the heart of them. Rare is the leader who directly acknowledges and names dysfunctional activities that are deeply embedded in organizations. A key role of APRNs is to name the problem without implying blame. This approach to leadership brings a problem into the light without the burden of having to solve it. In this way, the APRN is inviting others into the conversation for a better understanding of barriers to collaborative practice and state-of-the-art, patient-centered care. For example, if office staff think that they do not have the authority to make scheduling and patient flow work better, the APRN can name this problem and invite members of the organization to explore it further. The willingness for APRNs to enter into these courageous conversations is a key skill set to effective collaboration. When there are high-stakes issues with high emotions, it is tempting to focus instead on peripheral issues.

In another example, a primary care practice had for some time had a significant number of patient and staff complaints about waiting times to see a physician who was excellent but slow. She was always behind in her appointment times and could not keep pace with the demands of primary care. This created conflict in the waiting room and with support staff as patients frequently waited more than 2 hours to be seen for a scheduled appointment. Sometimes patients left without being treated after they had been checked in. The APRN who recently joined the practice was able to name the problem and the impact on the entire system, including paying overtime for medical assistants to work late. This naming of a problem that had been going on for years greatly relieved the organization. Once the problem and its dimensions were defined, the physician became aware of the impact that these long waits had on the entire office, as well as on her patients. The team came up with an approach that allowed this particular physician to have longer appointments and booked some vacant slots to allow for catch up. The manner in which the APRN raised the quality concerns made it safe because it was always in the context of patient care.

APRNs can enter these conversations by naming troubling dynamics or environmental threats. A patient's problem cannot be resolved without having its dimensions clearly defined. The same holds true for organizational leadership and the need to foster more collaboration and unity at the systems level. This type of acknowledgment of issues and willingness to name problems without having to solve them is a powerful way for APRNs to model true leadership.

Health Policy Leadership

Some APRNs may not see themselves as being particularly interested in or talented at political advocacy. However, all APRNs have a vested interest in policymaking that affects their patients' care, health care funding, national priorities in health, and state and local policies related to the health of the community they serve. Understanding and leading in health policy has become increasingly important as more laws and regulations are enacted with implications for APRN practice (see Chapters 19 and 22). APRNs should be aware of and must often respond to local, state, and national policymaking efforts likely to affect these laws and regulations. Organizations that define competencies for APRNs also have competencies related to health policy. Leadership in health policy requires an ability to analyze health care systems, an understanding of the personal qualities associated with effective leadership, and the skill to use this knowledge strategically.

Across these four domains of leadership, APRNs use their clinical expertise, team building, and collaborative skills to build community around shared values such as patient-centeredness and commitment to quality. To exert leadership in health policy, APRNs will be expected to remain informed about current and emerging issues in health care such as changes in federal and state regulations concerning scope of practice and nursing education funding proposals.

Geraldine (Polly) Bednash, PhD, RN, FAAN, Nurse Practitioner

Dr. Geraldine "Polly" Bednash attributes much of her rise to national and international leadership to her preparation as a nurse practitioner. Her childhood was spent in San Antonio, Texas, which was primarily a small military town at the time with strong Latin American roots. She fondly recalls making tamales with family and going to market with her grandmother to acquire the needed ingredients to help treat family illnesses. She did not grow up with the idea of becoming a nurse but selected this when she entered university. Money was tight so she worked throughout her time in school. She enrolled in the Army Nurse Corps for the last 2 years of school and immediately entered service after graduation. She met her husband while serving as a Nurse Corp officer in Vietnam. She and her husband moved to New York after her Army service, and she assumed a position as a faculty member at a diploma nursing school in the New York area.

Later, her husband's company moved them to the Washington, DC, area, but there she quickly discovered that her baccalaureate degree would not garner her a faculty position. She obtained her master's degree in medical-surgical nursing at Catholic University and again assumed a faculty position in nursing education.

She was accepted into the Robert Wood Johnson Foundation program to prepare nursing faculty to become nurse practitioners. She describes becoming a nurse practitioner in the early 1980s as "eye opening" and "ground breaking." In this new role she was expected to be a risk taker, to be on top of her game, and to have good working relationships with physicians and other health care professionals. She credits this education with forming the foundation for much of her future success as a national and international leader in nursing. Nurse practitioners diagnosed and treated patients but also considered the cultural and economic issues related to their care. As an independent practitioner she was required to understand the needs of the individual within the context of the larger system. This was not a part of traditional hospital nursing practice at the time. She went on to complete her PhD at the University of Maryland and transitioned her career to policy leadership.

For 3 years, Dr. Bednash was Director of Government Affairs of the American Association of Colleges of Nursing (AACN), and she was then selected to be Executive Director. She led that organization through its dramatic evolution as one of the nation's most important voices for nursing education, practice, and research. Her leadership at the AACN is credited with establishing the Association as the national voice for baccalaureate and graduate nursing education. Dr. Bednash was the driving force behind expanding the AACN's reach and influence in all health care and higher education circles as well as in the US Congress and with the Administration. She mobilized support for the AACN's signature initiatives, including the creation and ongoing revision of the *Essentials* documents, the establishment of the Commission on Collegiate Nursing Education, the advancement of the practice doctorate, and the development of the clinical nurse leader role and the Commission on Nurse Certification. In addition, Dr. Bednash spearheaded dozens of grant-funded initiatives, including the End-of-Life Nursing Consortium and the New Careers in Nursing Program.

Like many leaders, Dr. Bednash credits a number of individuals who helped her along the way. These include internationally renowned leaders in nursing and health care who provided support, words of wisdom, and encouragement at important times in her life. For example, when a patient experienced an adverse effect from a medication Dr. Bednash had prescribed, it was a physician colleague who helped her to understand that sometimes the work of nurse practitioners may place patients in harm's way and that she must learn from this event to help other patients.

She has devoted a good deal of her leadership experience to mentoring, coaching, and assisting others who aspire to leadership. The unique nature of her work as the head of a nursing organization that served many nursing schools meant that she had to be judicious in the selection of individuals to assist. Most of the people for whom she has served as a mentor are in professions other than nursing.

Her suggestions for advance practice registered nurses (APRNs) who are building competence in leadership is to always be open to the advice of those around you, even if you are not sure at the time you want to hear that advice. She also encourages APRNs to cultivate colleagues who will tell it like it is rather than rapidly agreeing with your position. And, always strive for transparency in your leadership work. ◎

APRNs are expected to understand the broad elements of government so that there can be timely and effective contact with policymakers to ensure that the APRNs' patients will be well represented in any proposed changes in laws or regulation. The APRN may not passively allow changes to happen but is expected to actively participate in discussion and actions for policy change. This policy work can combine leadership in clinical care, professional activities, and systems leadership. The defining characteristics of APRN leadership—mentoring, innovation, change agency, and activism—may be apparent in all four domains, but the emphasis accorded to each one depends on the particular leadership demands.

Characteristics of APRN Leadership Competency

The three defining characteristics of APRN leadership—mentoring, empowering others, and innovation—are listed, along with their core elements, in Table 11.2. These are discussed separately here to assist in understanding the differences among them. However, there is considerable overlap in the knowledge and skills needed for each characteristic. Experienced APRNs can demonstrate these characteristics in all four domains of leadership. APRNs often focus on developing clinical leadership first because the new clinical work can be time consuming. As APRNs gain more confidence in their advanced clinical abilities, they tend to expand their leadership in additional domains such as mentoring and empowering others.

Mentoring

A key element of APRN leadership competency is mentoring others. The ability to help others grow and encourage them toward developing their full potential requires competent, caring leaders who are interested in the success and well-being of others. Mentoring also ensures the development of future nurse leaders (McCloughen, O'Brien, & Jackson, 2010). Mentoring bridges the gap between professional education and the experiences of the subsequent working world (Barker, 2006). Guiding and coaching, leading by example, and role modeling with awareness and attentiveness to the needs and concerns of followers are basic characteristics of successful leaders. The ideas behind the colloquial statements of "taking someone under your wing" or "giving a colleague a leg up" are grounded in the

TABLE 11.2	Characteristics and Core Elements of the Leadership Competency
Defining Characteristic	**Core Elements (Knowledge and Skills)**
Mentoring	• Shared vision • Seeks mentors and serves as a mentor • Willing to share power • Empowering self and others • Self-reflection
Empowering Others	• Educate to empower through increasing the individual's knowledge base. • Use inspiration, motivation, and encouragement. • Provide structure that offers protection and security as one moves into new territory. • Provide resources to support others' growth and development. • Give the support and direction necessary for change toward empowerment. • Foster actualization, empowering others to evoke change.
Innovation	• Knowledge of models of leadership and change • Systems thinking • Systems assessment skills • Flexibility • Risk taking • Expert communication • Credibility • Change agent

mentoring process. Mentors are competent and self-confident, having qualities that epitomize success in their own careers and having the ability and desire to help others succeed. Other characteristics of successful mentors include inspiring, confident, committed to the development of others, and being willing to share. Mentors take on responsibility for the development of protégé skills, such as flexibility, adaptability, judgment, and creativity (McCloughen et al., 2010). Protégés are viewed as individuals who express a desire to learn, are committed to the long course of events, and are open to the process of trial and error. Successful protégés have high self-esteem, can self-monitor, and are resilient risk takers (Tourigny & Pulich, 2005). The reward for the mentor is to step back and enjoy the success and achievements of the protégé. APRNs who have had the benefit of mentoring report that it affected the progression of their career and enriched their leadership development (McCloughen, O'Brien, & Jackson, 2009).

Two types of mentoring are described in the literature. The first, termed *formal mentoring,* has the approval and support of an organization with objectives, a selection process, and a mentoring contract. Mentors are chosen from the ranks of experienced clinicians and provide exposure to clinical situations that offer opportunities to demonstrate competence, coaching, and role modeling and afford protection in controversial situations (Tourigny & Pulich, 2005). Many professional organizations, such as Sigma Theta Tau International and the National Organization of Nurse Practitioner Faculties, offer formal mentoring programs, and information is usually available on the organizations' websites. The term *informal mentoring* is a relationship that is unstructured and mutually beneficial; the experiences usually last longer and are self-selected (Tourigny & Pulich, 2005). Good mentors foster growth rather than dependency and instill the internal strengths to enable protégés to traverse rough spots in their career development. Mentors lead protégés on a journey of self-discovery and help them find the value they bring to the role and to nursing leadership (Vos, 2009). As mentoring relationships progress, the protégé takes on more freedom to try new behaviors and develops confidence in trying new skills, always with the knowledge that someone is behind him or her.

Mentoring relationships can be developed based on specific needs of the APRN protégé, such as writing for publication or developing professional presentation skills, or on the general development of career and leadership skills. Harrington (2011) has reported that mentoring new NPs will accelerate their development as primary care providers. Finding a mentor in one's geographic location may not be feasible, depending on the skill to be developed. In today's technological world, however, APRN leaders can establish mentoring relationships at a distance that can be a rewarding experience as well. Use of conference calls, videoconferencing, social media, and networking at professional conferences can all be feasible means to support a distance mentoring relationship.

There are two parts to the APRN mentorship equation: APRNs who are seeking to be mentored by those they aspire to emulate and APRNs who can serve as mentors. Some APRN leaders are reluctant to serve as a mentor for a variety of reasons. However, Vance (2002) has asserted that a chaotic health care environment makes mentoring support more important than ever. She suggested that mentors and protégés adopt a mentoring philosophy that encourages collaboration with others, not competition. Novice APRNs are fortunate if they can find a mentoring relationship that lasts over time. The APRN mentor creates a safety net in which the protégé can expose vulnerabilities and be coached to develop confidence in new skills. Mentoring is a gift that allows new APRN leaders to emerge. Today, APRNs taking on large leadership roles engage executive coaches, and more often paid executive coaches. There is a cadre of nurses who do executive coaching, and these relationships can be highly valuable because the mentor is safely outside of the organization. APRNs who take on new executive leadership positions can negotiate in their employment package for the organization to pay for executive coaching.

An interrelationship exists among the concepts of mentoring, organizational culture, and leadership. Watkins (2013) described organizational culture as the patterns of behavior of an organization, and these patterns are dynamic, changing over time. A positive organizational culture offers social support and a sense of well-being and empowerment that fosters the mentoring process (Harrington, 2011). Thus APRNs should seek opportunities to mentor or be mentored and articulate the benefits of mentoring activities to their organization.

Empowering Others

The term *empowerment* is best understood as giving power to others, and this is often done by encouraging others and giving them authority. APRNs operationalize empowerment by sharing power with others, including patients, as well as by enabling them to access or assert their own power. Empowerment as a leadership strategy is guided by the shared vision of the leader and follower and a willingness of the leader to delegate authority to others. Leaders who empower their followers greatly increase the influence of APRNs within nursing and beyond nursing's boundaries. In some ways, empowerment shares some characteristics with mentoring. There is a continuously developing reciprocal relationship between the two key players.

Empowerment requires more than just giving others permission to act on their own. It is a developmental process that a good leader fosters over time; it encourages constituents to feel competent, responsible, independent, and authorized to act. Quast (2011) provided six ways to empower others to succeed (Box 11.4).

For example, certified nurse-midwifes (CNMs) empower pregnant women by putting them in control of the birthing process through education,

BOX 11.4 Six Ways to Empower Others to Succeed

- Share information.
- Create clear goals and objectives.
- Teach that it is OK to make mistakes.
- Create an environment that celebrates both successes and failures.
- Support a learning environment.
- Let teams become the hierarchy.

Courtesy of Lisa Quast. Adapted from Quast, L. (2011). 6 ways to empower others to succeed. *Forbes.* Retrieved from http://www.forbes.com/sites/lisaquast/2011/02/28/6-ways-to-empower-others-to-succeed/#18b792493cc8.

mentoring, and providing resources for parenting that nurture self-esteem and enhance family structure. CNMs are quick to let others know that they do not deliver babies—mothers deliver babies and midwives assist. This changes the power gradient in such a way that the mother is no longer dependent or passive in the birthing process. Instead, she is the decision maker and in control. This is very different from the paternalistic and hierarchical relationships seen in many obstetric medical practices.

Innovation

As the prior discussion suggests, initiating and sustaining innovation are critical elements of the APRN leadership competency. Covey's work (1989) with interprofessional groups is instructive to APRNs who are learning innovation skills. Innovation requires the capacity of the person to envision a world that can be and not just a world that is. This can be difficult for some because such a vision requires stepping over boundaries, cultures, politics, personal likes, and other elements that we hold very closely. Change occurs at the system and personal levels, and one must deal with core values to change or to serve as an agent for change successfully. Covey contended that people have a changeless core inside them that they need if they themselves are to be able to change. Thus one key to the ability of people to change is a strong sense of who they are and what they value. Lasting change comes from the inside out. This observation is relevant to APRNs. First, APRNs need to identify their own core values to become effective in leading change. Second, Covey's insight can help APRNs who encounter resistance to change initiatives, especially when it persists. The resistance may come from the sense that a core value is being threatened.

There is an affective dimension to change. Although many people express an excitement at the prospect of change, some changes are difficult and painful, and any change contains an element of loss. Mastering emotional tension during change requires perseverance, patience, and compassion. At best, change can be described as challenging and invigorating. Lazarus and Fell (2011) have suggested that it is important to close the gap in creativity and use innovation as a process to induce change in health care. To understand change in today's health care environment, APRNs must explore the dynamics of change and the culture in which it occurs.

APRNs generally consider several factors when they are proposing an innovation—the relevance of power and influence, stakeholders' concerns and interests, contextual factors, individuals' values, and the affective dimensions of change. Understanding these important factors is integral to the APRN leadership competency.

Political Activism

Political activism and advocacy will become even more important as APRNs hone their skills for systems leadership and change. Many of the skills needed to navigate successfully in political waters are closely associated with good leadership. The core elements that define contemporary leadership, such as shared vision, systems thinking, and the ability to engage in high-level communication within the context of a changing environment, are all basic to political effectiveness. Again, change leading to care improvement is the common element that drives APRNs to advocate for advanced practice and patient issues. There is little room for discussion about whether APRNs need to take on the mantles of policymaker and patient advocate as part of their leadership role (see Chapter 19). For many, this falls within the context of a moral imperative: "Nurses practice at the intersection of public policy and the personal lives (of their patients); they are, therefore, ideally situated and morally obligated to include sociopolitical advocacy in their practice" (Falk-Rafael, 2005, p. 222). Working for social justice is seen as part of the ethical decision-making competency of APRNs (see Chapter 13). APRNs must position themselves strategically at the policy table to advocate for access to care and appropriate interventions for everyone. Great strides have been made in developing nurses' skill and acuity as policymakers (see Chapter 19). Rapidly evolving policy situations mean that APRNs are often faced with trial-by-fire learning when it comes to activism and advocacy. However, policy issues tend to wax and wane so that APRNs do not always have to be highly engaged and can at times monitor the situation. Identifying trusted mentors with whom to debrief and developing a plan of action can help APRNs develop the poise and skills needed to respond effectively in unexpected, chaotic, and tense political situations.

Although activism is frequently associated with advocacy in the political realm, activism can occur in the clinical and system environments as well. The same leadership skills apply in those settings when advocating for issues such as access to care, ethical decision making, and resolving injustice.

Attributes of Effective APRN Leaders

Several personal attributes are deemed necessary for successful leadership (Box 11.5). Effective leaders demonstrate these broad qualities because they are needed in the interprofessional context of today's health care. Nurses are called to exert their leadership expertise far beyond nursing circles. The history of advanced practice registered nursing (see Chapter 1) demonstrates that nurse leaders have always led outside the realm of organized nursing education and practice.

Timing

A good sense of timing may come easily to some, but for most people it requires painstaking development and practice. APRN leaders know when to act and when to hold back. They recognize the need for urgency at times as, for example, during an unexpected legislative vote in Congress; they also know to take the time to develop a carefully thought-out plan with deliberate strategy when a change in scope of practice is being considered. The notion of timing is apparent when APRNs use mandated change as an opportunity to introduce other changes. For example, institutions applying for accreditation by The Joint Commission (TJC) are expected to demonstrate compliance with TJC's current evidence-based standards for specific health care problems (TJC, 2016). Many institutions use these mandated changes to launch a variety of initiatives aimed at improving care management.

An example of timing took place during a legislative session in Tennessee. APRNs were seeking to have a joint Senate and House committee remove regulations that restricted NP practices to limited locations. During the committee meetings, an NP

BOX 11.5 Attributes of APRN Leaders

Expert Communication Skills
- Articulate in speech and in writing
- Able to get own point across
- Uses excellent listening skills
- Desires to hear and understand another's point of view
- Stays connected to other people

Commitment
- Gives of self personally and professionally
- Listens to own inner voice
- Balances professional and private life
- Plans ahead; makes change happen
- Engages in self-reflection

Developing One's Own Style
- Gets and stays involved
- Sets priorities
- Manages boundaries
- Uses technology
- Engages in lifelong learning
- Maintains a good sense of humor

Risk Taking
- Gets involved at any level
- Demonstrates self-confidence and assertiveness
- Uses creative and big picture thinking
- Willing to fail and begin again
- Has an astute sense of timing
- Copes with change

Willingness to Collaborate
- Respects cultural diversity
- Desires to build teams and alliances
- Shares power
- Willing to mentor

Adapted from Hanson, C., Boyle, J., Hatmaker, D., & Murray, J. (1999). *Finding your voice as a leader.* Washington DC: American Academy of Nursing.

---

testified about the many challenges the restrictive language imposed on NPs in providing good care in rural and underserved communities. The chairman of the committee stated that, if the NPs were "unshackled" from their communities, they would leave and that the existing rules kept the NP tied to the community. Clearly, this language offended nurses, patients, and communities, but this committee meeting was not the time to call the chairman out. Following the committee hearing, the press got wind of the statement with the help of some very astute nurses in the audience, and the public outrage over these insensitive comments was explosive. The news media reported that the chairman, who happened to be African American, should have recognized the inappropriateness of his statements, particularly in a former southern slave state. The chairman subsequently met with the NP who testified before the committee, apologized for the language, and sponsored a new bill to revoke the restrictive language during the next session. The timing of the release of the chairman's comments by the media made all the difference in this situation.

Self-Confidence and Risk Taking

Taking risks is inherent in the leadership process and is tied inextricably to self-confidence. The willingness to take a chance, try, and occasionally fail is the mark of a true leader. Risk-taking behaviors differentiate APRNs who will be recognized as leaders and change drivers from other capable nurses. By learning to take risks, APRNs enhance their leadership repertoire, allowing for more spontaneity and flexibility in response to conflict, resistance, anger, and other reactions to change and high-risk situations. Motivation is the desire to move forward and can also be viewed as a component of risk taking. Wheatley (2005) has affirmed that another component of risk taking is the willingness to be disturbed. Certainty is more comfortable. Staying put is rarely as risky as taking the chance to move ahead. Risk taking should be differentiated from risky leadership behaviors. Taking good risks involves evaluating all types of evidence available at the time and making educated decisions based on that information. It also involves trying to anticipate consequences of actions, having a plan in place to evaluate the implementation, being willing to accept that the risk was not successful, and learning from the experience. Risky behavior, on the other hand, involves making decisions impulsively without fully exploring available information or having a strategy to address unintended consequences.

Several of the key attributes in Box 11.5 incorporate some form of the word *willingness*. The abilities to be open, to learn, to change one's mind, to be willing to take what comes, and to work through differences are key to all levels of leadership. Leadership is about negotiation and interactions with others to reach common goals. To do this may mean failing and trying again and again to reach the desired outcome. This quality of personal hardiness—the ability to pick oneself up and start again—is seen repeatedly in biographies of successful leaders who have made change happen in difficult times.

Communication and Relationship Building

The relevance of communication skills and collegial relationships to quality health care has received attention (Castledine, 2008). APRNs who lead must be able to communicate effectively with others (see Chapter 12) and participate in the identification and resolution of clinical and ethical conflicts among team members (see Chapter 13). The successful leader must have the requisite communication skills to build the trust and cooperation necessary to negotiate difficult intraprofessional and interprofessional issues. The ability to understand another's viewpoint and respect opposing views is key to effective communication and ultimately to reaching a mutually satisfactory outcome. Covey (1989) has suggested that leaders will need to understand and be understood by others. Good leaders listen and understand the other person's viewpoint before they speak. The charisma that is associated with many leaders is often simply outstanding listening and communication skills. The ability to influence a key power strategy used to gain the cooperation of others is an outcome of excellent communication. A second part of expert communication is relationship building. The art of building strong alliances and coalitions with others and staying connected with colleagues and groups is basic to the sense of community needed to lead effectively. Building relationships within the work environment can minimize the impact of organizational structures that hinder one's ability to collaborate and solve problems (Wheatley, 2005). These alliances are important, whether at the highest levels of international policymaking or at the local level when building a coalition to address a recurring patient issue. Building relationships is central to the effectiveness of a team who cares for patients. Not only must APRNs establish effective relationships with their coworkers, but they are often in a position to strengthen relationships among other members of the team through role modeling and mediation.

Thought leaders use conversational leadership as a way to bring key groups together to raise critical questions and issues and gain collective intelligence leading to innovation and wise actions. Open conversations are one way in which leaders share what they know with colleagues and create new ways of knowing and doing. This type of open conversation may lead to having the courageous conversations that are sometimes needed to name a problem so that the communication can move forward. Building relationships is also central to another APRN communication skill, conflict negotiation (see Chapter 12). APRN students may come to their educational programs having been socialized to be silent or suppress their opinion in situations of conflict. Specific approaches to identifying conflicts and resolving them successfully have been identified and used successfully in business (Fisher, Ury, & Patton, 2011) and in health care (Longo & Sherman, 2007). The website for the Conflict Resolution Network (www.crnhq.org) is a resource on conflict negotiation.

Boundary Management: Balancing Professional and Personal Life

Managing boundaries refers to how APRNs deal with various aspects of advanced practice nursing within the professional and personal components of their lives. Sometimes, APRNs are in the position of guarding the boundary, such as when they are approached to undertake a task that is not within their scope of practice. Productivity requirements mean that APRNs must be clear about the numbers and types of patients that they can care for on a given day. Often, managing boundaries means extending them—building a bridge that enables the APRN to partner with other groups or expanding a boundary as other patient or health care needs are identified. For example, although CRNAs may not need prescriptive authority in a given state, they assist other APRN colleagues in their quest for state prescriptive authority. Extending a boundary may also mean expanding one's scope of practice at an agency level so that patient needs can be better met. Boundaries in practice tend to be fluid and often situation dependent. For example, in some practices, family NPs treat patients in the emergency department of the hospital, whereas in others only ACNPs treat patients there. Pushing boundaries in practice is usually based on education and experience in a particular area. That may mean that the APRN will have to acquire new training or credentialing in an area or technique and then be supervised in performing this new skill before expanding the boundary in autonomous practice.

As boundary managers, APRNs recognize communications and behaviors that breach or enhance interpersonal relationships. APRN leaders also teach others how to collaborate with colleagues in other disciplines, build coalitions, and set limits while maintaining their own boundaries—a fine distinction, but strategically important. For example, a CNM may negotiate the boundaries or responsibilities among the neonatologist, obstetrician, and nurse-midwifery staff. Clinical leadership and professional leadership require the negotiation of boundaries, regardless of whether the borders are drawn around professional roles, patient populations, or organizations.

Important to this discussion is the issue that APRNs are people with lives outside their work. They are often spouses, parents, grandparents, members of their religious communities, and members of their broader community. Each of these components of their lives will carry boundary requirements in addition to their professional boundaries. There are no easy answers as to how to manage boundary issues that arise between personal and professional demands. APRN leaders will find an almost constant interplay between personal and professional boundaries. Grant (2013) pointed out that asking for help results in a cascade of important assistance from family and colleagues. The successful APRN leader is quick to ask for help and use that help to achieve goals.

Self-Management/Emotional Intelligence

Most people know when they have overextended themselves; their bodies give clues such as fatigue, stress signals, feelings of frustration, and even physical illness. One of the challenging aspects of being a good leader is the provocative realization that one is being asked to play many important cutting edge roles at the same time. These invitations are exciting and seductive because they open new opportunities and speak to the high regard that others have for the leader. For these reasons, it is easy for good leaders to overextend their activities well beyond manageable, realistic boundaries. The skills of being able to delegate tasks; say no and mentor others to take on some of the load; and enlarge the circle of leaders, strategists, and followers are integral to effective leadership. Unfortunately, the inability to set realistic personal boundaries can lead to stress, frustration, and burnout. Being a leader and competent APRN provider at the same time is not easy, but it can be done. This skill requires APRNs to decline a request when competing responsibilities make it not possible to accept the request. Skillful practice with saying "no" uses the sandwich technique. It begins with saying the larger "yes"—what the APRN is currently reaching for in the practice or trying to accomplish—followed by a firm "no," and ends with a hopeful statement such as "Perhaps I can help you find somebody else" or "Maybe I can help in the future." The goal is to leave the requester with a sense of respect and a better understanding of the APRN. The following is an example: "I am really trying to build the prenatal care outreach service to underserved women. So, I cannot serve on the hospital CEO search committee. Perhaps I can help you find another qualified CNM to serve."

The process of self-reflection is useful for APRNs to determine which personal and work characteristics seem to set off imbalances. Three strategies are useful and simple in concept but can be complicated in execution. First, expecting perfection is often a setup for imbalance. Keeping in mind the axiom, "Perfect is the enemy of good," may help APRNs establish realistic expectations. Reframing the notion to "good enough for now" allows the leader to move along. Another strategy is for APRNs to examine what makes them say "yes" or "no." It is easy to think, "If I just do this one more thing, everything will be fine." One APRN kept a note on her phone reminding her either to decline something that would tip the scales to overcommitment or to buy time by asking, "Can I think about it and call you tomorrow?" One colleague avoids commitments that are large but far into the future; these are invitations for activities months or even years in the future. Such activities may not appear to threaten one's usual commitments and deadlines but, as the time to fulfill the commitment approaches, these commitments can become very threatening. The challenge for the APRN is to ensure that adequate time to plan for, develop, and organize the work is budgeted well in advance of the due date. The third strategy is to make appointments with oneself for important personal and professional activities. By putting these appointments into a calendar, APRNs can lessen the risk of giving away time that they need to maintain balance. Using "the three things rule" may be helpful; identify the three most important things that must be done before any new commitments are made or started.

Respect for Cultural and Gender Diversity

Successful APRN leaders strive for cultural competence and value diversity in their work. These attributes require awareness of one's own biases, attitudes, and behaviors that surface at all levels of interaction and in all settings. An APRN leader needs to serve as a role model by demonstrating respect for the cultural differences of individuals and constituencies in any given situation. When a systems framework is used for understanding a complex concept such as culturally competent leadership, four levels can be identified—societal, professional,

organizational, and individual. For the APRN, the responsibility for culturally competent care includes all four of these levels. A useful aid for developing a sound respect for cultural diversity can be found in the Interprofessional Education Collaborative competencies developed in 2011 (see Chapter 12, Box 12.1, for this resource). Culturally competent care is delivered with knowledge, sensitivity, and respect for the patient's and family's cultural background and practices. Cultural competence is an ongoing process that involves accepting and respecting differences (Giger et al., 2007). This definition is built on the assumption that care providers are aware of and sensitized to their own cultural backgrounds and that they are able to integrate this sensitivity into their delivery of care. The interactive nature of caregiving requires the authentic engagement of the provider with the patient to appreciate and respond to differences that may affect giving or receiving care. A good example of the challenge that culturally competent care presents has been provided by Wheatley (2005). In this example, a group practice offered free car seats and training in their use to a group of parents, but no one took advantage of the gift. On debriefing, the providers learned that for this group of parents, using a car seat was an invitation to God to cause a car accident. Differences are issues for every person, and they become even more important when one becomes a leader and role model. Working with colleagues who are different provides APRNs with opportunities for soliciting information about others' experiences. Box 11.6 presents strategies for enhancing cultural awareness.

Gender can play an important component in leadership. Gender stereotypes can exert a strong influence similar to cultural stereotypes and affect the way a leader is viewed and how the leader actually performs (Burgess, Joseph, van Ryn, & Carnes, 2012). As with culture, successful leaders understand their own biases about gender, the role gender may play in the provision of care, and gender issues in team functioning.

Global Awareness

The world is highly interconnected and interdependent; this affects APRN leaders because issues such as access to care, patient safety, and quality care are global issues that are not confined to any particular geographic region. There are workforce challenges throughout the world, natural and human catastrophes occur with regularity, and there are fewer barriers to interactions among countries (Abbott &

BOX 11.6   Strategies to Achieve Cultural Competence

- Explore and learn about your own racial and ethnic culture and background.
- Explore and learn about the different racial and ethnic cultures most frequently encountered in your practice.
- Read ethnic newspapers, magazines, and books.
- Listen to the music from a different culture.
- Learn the language of a different culture. Become bilingual with the verbal and nonverbal behavior of the culture.
- Take advantage of training opportunities to increase your cultural awareness and sensitivity.
- Be able to identify personal biases and develop strategies to manage, eliminate, or sublimate those potentially damaging attitudes and behaviors.
- When faced with a patient difficulties, consider whether unconscious biases may be operating for you or your colleagues.

Adapted from Hanson, C. M., & Malone, B. (2000). Leadership: Empowerment, change agency, and activism. In A. B. Hamric, J. A. Spross, & C. M. Hanson (Eds.), *Advanced nursing practice: An integrative approach* (2nd ed., pp. 279–313). Philadelphia: Saunders.

 BOX 11.7   Global Competencies for Nurse Leaders

Develop global mind-set and worldview:
- Global environmental awareness
- Cultural adaptation
- Awareness of social, political, and economic trends

Understand needs of technology:
- Enhanced ability of communication and technology
- Create global networks
- Individuals can now drive change just as businesses used to drive change

Respect diversity and cultivate cross-cultural competencies:
- Institutional mergers and growth
- Multicultural work force
- Multicultural patient populations

Adapted from Nichols, B., Shaffer, F., & Porter, C. (2011). Global nursing leadership: A practical guide. *Nursing Administration Quarterly, 35,* 354–359.

Coenen, 2008; Carter, Owen-Williams, & Della, 2015). APRN leaders interface with a multicultural workforce in their immediate setting or through professional organizations, and they are asked to lead multicultural teams (Nichols, Shaffer, & Porter, 2011). APRNs may look to other countries for problem-solving ideas or may be asked for consultation in person or via technology from health care providers across the globe.

The sharing of new techniques, therapies, and knowledge resources is important as we work together to address global issues such as the global chronic illness epidemic, infectious diseases, and common health crises (Abbott & Coenen, 2008; World Health Organization, 2008). Nichols et al. (2011) have identified global competencies for nurse leaders as outlined in Box 11.7. In addition, they have outlined areas for nurse leaders to consider in development of a worldview that includes sense of self and space, cultural dress, family relationships and decision making, values and beliefs, nutrition habits, and religious preferences (Nichols et al., 2011). Friedman (2006) has termed this view *global*

citizenship and suggested that individuals and groups in leadership positions have a responsibility to think and act as global citizens. There are several organizations that have a global perspective of their mission, which can be accessed for resources:

- International Council of Nurses
- World Health Organization
- Sigma Theta Tau International
- Pan American Health Organization

Developing Skills as APRN Leaders

There are formal and informal strategies that are useful when considering a leadership development plan. Students will need to have experiences in their educational program to help them develop leadership skills. These can occur in the classroom, clinical practice, and student leadership and health-related service projects. In general, lessons learned in one domain will apply to leadership situations in other domains. Health policy leadership is discussed separately because it has specific features that are somewhat different from the APRN's everyday leadership activities.

Factors Influencing Leadership Development

There may be a misconception that leadership is a trait that one is born with rather than a skill that can be learned. There are a number of resources that new APRNs can access to help them learn to be leaders. These resources include many of the attributes described in this chapter, such as education, experience, expert communication, networking, assertiveness, and collaboration. Zaccaro (2007) has argued that with increases in conceptual and methodologic resources, learned attributes are more likely to predict leadership than once was believed. Leadership represents complex patterns of behavior explained in part by multiple leader attributes (Zaccaro, 2007). In this section, we explore leadership traits and attributes of leadership-competent APRNs.

Personal Characteristics and Experiences

Allen (1998) explored the primary factors and individual characteristics that influenced leadership development in nurse leaders. Self-confidence, traced to childhood and subsequent risk-taking behaviors, was reported as a critical factor. Feedback from significant others led to enhanced self-confidence over time. The nurse leaders also spoke about having innate qualities and tendencies of leaders, such as being extroverted or bossy and wanting to take charge, and about having roles as team captains and officers in organizations. They saw themselves as people who rise to the occasion. A third important factor was a progression of experiences and successes that were pivotal in moving them forward. Being at the right place at the right time and taking advantage of opportunities presented in those situations allowed them to grow as leaders. Closely aligned with this factor was the influence of people important to them, such as mentors, role models, faculty, and parents, who had the ability to encourage and provide opportunities for advancement. Personal life factors, such as time, family, health, and work schedules, influenced leadership development. For example, supportive spouses and relatives who assisted with family and home responsibilities and employers who were flexible were important to the leadership development process. Upon close examination, one can see that the leadership abilities grew out of a combination of education and learning opportunities and depended on the support of others. These same characteristics can be used by aspiring APRN leaders.

Zaccaro, Kemp, and Bader (2004) have developed a model that describes distal attributes, including personality, cognitive abilities, motives, and values, along with proximal attributes, including social appraisal skills, problem-solving skills, expertise, and tacit knowledge. In this model, the leader's operating environment influences the trajectory toward success, which supports the importance of organizational culture described by Watkins (2013) (see "Mentoring" section earlier). Carroll (2005) identified six factors that were present in women leaders and nurse executives: personal integrity; strategic vision and action orientation; team-building and communication skills; management and technical competencies; people skills (collaboration, empowering others, valuing diversity); and personal survival skills. These factors share similarity with the attributes in Box 11.5.

Strategies for Acquiring Competency as a Leader

Formal educational opportunities in leadership are an expected part of APRN education. Opportunities to work with faculty and other mentors help students acquire leadership skills and further reinforce self-confidence as a leader. Running for office while a student or for local leadership positions in professional organizations and serving on local and national coalitions are other good strategies for developing this competency (Sandrick, 2006). Also, leadership conferences that foster effective communication and interaction are beneficial. Exemplar 11.2 shows how students can practice their leadership development while in school.

Leadership skills are developed and enhanced over time and in many ways. Communication is one of the strengths often attributed to nurses; it is a skill that can be strengthened through practice. Staying connected is important for busy APRNs and can be achieved in a variety of ways, from social media and shared projects to attending conferences that allow for time to interact and problem-solve with colleagues about similar professional issues. A community of APRN leaders is important for faculty and students involved with raising the visibility of advanced practice nursing roles in their institutions and communities.

Developing Leadership in the Health Policy Arena

Health policy issues affecting APRNs and their patients, including strategies for political advocacy, are explored in Chapter 19. The following section describes how APRNs can develop skills to influence health policy through creative leadership and political advocacy, whether by means of local grassroots endeavors or directly through top government

| EXEMPLAR 11.2 | Mentoring an Advanced Practice Nurse Student in Community Leadership |

John was required to complete a course in the family nurse practitioner program focused on health care leadership. John was not too sure just why this was required since his primary goal was to graduate and open a practice in northeast Alaska, where he would be providing care to Alaska Native people in a small village. This had been a long-term dream, and he had selected a very strong clinical program and an experienced Alaskan Native preceptor so he would be ready to begin providing care upon graduation. He was unclear about what leadership activities would be expected of him as a primary care provider. One of the assignments he had in the leadership course was to complete a community assessment of his future site of practice to determine areas in which he could lead change. John learned many things about his future practice site during this assignment.

The community where he would be in practice did not have a potable water supply. Untreated water was taken from a nearby stream during the summer months, but the stream was frozen during the long and very harsh winter. Ice could be melted for water but there was no assurance that the water would be clean enough for drinking. John also learned that the sewage system was a "honey bucket" self-haul system that is nearly impossible for the elderly to use and exposed children to raw sewage.

Working under the mentorship of his preceptor, who lived in the village, John began to grasp the scope of the problem and quickly learned that substantial leadership would be required to bring an acceptable and affordable solution to the problems of potable water and sewage management. Solutions suitable for other climates just would not work in this community. Previous plans had failed because they did not fit the culture of the community, could not survive the harsh winter climate or spring floods from ice dams on the river, and were far too expensive for the small community to afford. John also learned that what he thought was a simple issue was a very large problem and would likely take many years to remedy. He was able to engage community elders to begin the process of finding long-term solutions. He had skills in grant writing that were very useful in securing funds to help with the planning. Most of his success was a result of the excellent mentorship he received from both his faculty member and his Alaskan Native preceptor. They gently guided him through the many complex areas related to this problem.

Following graduation and after beginning practice in the village, John has continued his leadership. A new drinking/washing water system is in place but work continues on the community sewage system. His project in his leadership class has led to a longer-term role in leading his village to build other needed infrastructure. ◎

involvement. The term *advocacy* can be defined as the act of pleading another person's cause and is multifaceted with diverse activities (Halpern, 2002; Kendig, 2006): "the endpoint of advocacy is the health and welfare of the public" (Leavitt, Chaffee, & Vance, 2007, p. 37). APRNs are being called on, both collectively and individually, to make their voices heard as governments struggle with budget constraints and difficult decisions about health policies, organization, and the funding of health care programs.

In the political arena, developing power and influence uses a number of leadership skills. Leadership strategies used by APRNs in the political arena include developing influence with policymakers, motivating colleagues to stay informed of current issues, and providing bridges to other leaders who have access to important resources. The policy arena is made of a variety of rules, regulations, laws, court opinions, funding strategies, and other interrelated areas. There is often no one simple approach to this area. Mentoring APRNs to understand their power and influence in the health policy arena is a key role for the APRN leader. The developmental process for becoming a political activist begins early in life with an understanding of how government and the political systems work. Focused understanding often begins when health policy is introduced in the nursing curriculum (see Exemplar 11.2). These students are usually coached to understand the power inherent in policymaking, the power of politics to influence practice, and the ways that they can influence the system, individually and collectively, to better their own practice and be high-level patient advocates. Faculty members keep students informed about key legislative issues and introduce them, through role modeling, to the role of political advocacy. Inviting APRN students to accompany faculty who are giving testimony at a legislative hearing is one way to model the advocacy role. Faculty may also be members of committees or boards that focus on policy issues, and students can accompany the faculty member in this work. Many professional organizations also offer tools about how to engage in the political process, such as the NACNS (2011) and the American Association of Nurse Anesthetists (2016; Zenti, 1998).

There is no question that influencing policy takes substantial commitment, time, and energy. Timing is an important consideration. APRNs ask themselves several personal and professional questions to determine the degree of involvement and level of sophistication at which advocacy is to be undertaken, including the following:

- What are my personal responsibilities related to wage earning, small children, dependent parents, single parenthood, health issues, school, and gaining initial competence as an APRN?
- How can I best serve the APRN community at this time?
- What data sources can I access that keep me informed and up-to-date?
- What learning opportunities will help me be an effective APRN advocate?
- How can I develop short-term and long-term plans for becoming a more politically astute advocate for myself, my patients, and nursing?
- What do I care deeply about?
- What am I able to commit to, based on the responses to these questions?

APRNs will need to find an appropriate mentor once they have made a decision about the depth of involvement to which they can commit. There are numerous effective nurse leaders and advocates who are willing and able to move new advocates into positions to make positive changes in health policy. Opportunities for input and influence exist at various levels of the legislative process (Larson, 2004; Park & Jex, 2011; Winterfeldt, 2001; see Chapter 22).

Using Professional Organizations to the Best Advantage

For APRNs, close contact with their professional organizations is an important link for staying current of national and state policy agendas, finding a support network of like-minded colleagues, and accessing information about changes in credentialing and practice issues. This means being an active member of more than one affiliate organization to stay on the cutting edge of pertinent issues. Most APRNs are aligned with at least one nursing organization; those who aspire to an active role in influencing policy will need to have memberships in several.

As new graduates move into diverse practice settings, they must align with the advanced practice nursing organizations that best meet their needs and offer the strongest support, choosing to engage actively in some and remaining on the periphery in others. Choosing the "right" organizations to belong to is based on particular needs, comfort level, specialty, and experience.

Internships and Fellowships

One excellent way to develop enhanced skills as an advanced practice nursing policy advocate is to apply for a national or state policy internship or fellowship. These appointments, which last from several days to 1 or 2 years, offer a wide range of health policy and political experiences that are targeted to novice and expert APRNs. For example, the Nurse in Washington Internship (NIWI), sponsored by the Nursing Organizations Alliance, is a 4-day internship that introduces nurses to policymaking in Washington, DC. This internship serves as an excellent beginning step in learning the APRN policy role. Federal fellowships and internships that link nurses to legislators or to the various branches of federal and state government are invaluable in assisting APRNs to understand how leaders are developed and how the system for setting health policy operates.

New Modes of Communication

The ability to communicate with others accurately, efficiently, and in a timely manner is a driving force in making effective change. There is substantial opportunity to share information and to engage with others at a distance (Wakefield, 2003). Time and distance are no longer serious obstacles to communication. The multiple modes of Internet access make virtual communication a reality.

Obstacles to Leadership Development and Effective Leadership

There are a number of areas in which leaders encounter obstacles to developing effective leadership. Some of these have been touched on earlier but there are other areas in which obstacles can arise in unanticipated ways.

Clinical Leadership Issues

APRNs can find that exerting clinical leadership can be challenging at times. Some health systems have archaic rules and regulations that can infect professional staff privileges and the ability for APRNs to lead. For example, some health systems do not credential APRNs as independent practitioners but rather as dependent practitioners. This means that records must be signed by another professional; admissions, transitions of care, and discharges are a challenge; and procedures or scope of practice can be restricted. The world of health care is changing and the astute APRN will keep pushing the boundaries in this area. Sometimes these issues can be resolved by creativity. For example, in one state there was a statewide regulation governing all hospitals that there must be a physician appointed to be the chief of the medical staff. The particular hospital wanted to appoint a CNM to be in charge of all clinical services offered by the hospital. This was done by appointing the CNM to the title of Chief Clinical Officer and having the Chief of the Medical Staff report to this position. This approach allowed the hospital to achieve its goal and to conform to state regulations.

Many rules and regulations that limit practice will fall away as new APRNs join the team and their unique expertise is valued. Some hospitals that claim that they do not credential APRNs do credential CRNAs to practice. They would have to close their surgical services if they did not do so. The day will come when the rest of the APRNs will be viewed as similarly valuable.

Professional and System Obstacles

There are several obstacles to achieving recognition as an APRN leader. Most of the obstacles result from conflict or competition among individuals, groups, or organizations. These obstacles can develop as the scopes of practice of various professionals overlap in clinical practice. A lack of legal empowerment to practice to the fullest extent of knowledge and skills has been a dominant barrier to the optimal practice of APRNs in recent years. CNMs and CRNAs have the longest track record in America of dealing with these issues and have earned many successes. Competition can be intraprofessional, as among APRN groups, and interprofessional, as among pharmacists, optometrists, physicians, and nurses. One approach to good leadership is to focus on bringing dignity to self and others rather than being liked; for most people, this is difficult because being accepted and liked by others is important. Trying to do it all rather than delegating to others is a common challenge for busy leaders. As noted, a good leader can encourage a shared workload that recognizes the talents and abilities of followers.

Dysfunctional Leadership Styles

Leadership can be a lonely place, and successful leadership requires careful nurturing. Although good leaders are sought after and desired, we have all experienced the other side of the coin—a dysfunctional leader. There are a multitude of traits and styles that can be attributed to a dysfunctional leader, such as micromanager, passive-aggressive, narcissistic personality, conflict avoidant, a quest for personal power, and a game player. The dictatorial leader or the leader who is most interested in empire building is easily recognized. Dysfunctional leaders often have poor self-control, have no time for others, or fail to accept responsibility for their own actions. At its worst, dysfunctional leadership moves into the realm of horizontal violence.

Horizontal Violence

Horizontal violence is described as an aggressive act carried out by one colleague toward another (Longo & Sherman, 2007). This type of behavior is often seen among oppressed groups as a way for individuals to achieve a sense of power. Some of these behaviors are being overly critical, intentionally undermining another's actions, fighting among colleagues, and wrongfully blaming others. These behaviors leave one feeling humiliated and overwhelmed and unsupported. Although there are many barriers to leading effectively and creating community, several constellations of behaviors that are particularly destructive have been identified. Nurses may be vulnerable to these destructive behaviors because of the profession's historical marginalization as being female and a relatively powerless group in health care. The culture of an organization as described earlier is also a factor in the development of these dysfunctional styles. These behaviors undermine successful APRN leadership. APRNs must avoid engaging in such behaviors and intervene assertively when they do occur. Four manifestations of horizontal violence in workplace culture limit the ability of APRNs to lead: the *star complex*, the *queen bee syndrome, failure to mentor* ("eating one's young"), and *bullying*. These behaviors are of particular concern because the profession needs to recruit and develop new nurses to help them have satisfying careers and pass on the legacy of a satisfying career to future generations of nurses. Faculty and preceptors need to be alert to the appearance of such toxic behaviors and assure that they are not tolerated. Readers are referred to the articles by Anderson (2011), Longo and Smith (2011), King (2002), Rider (2002), Longo and Sherman (2007), and Bally (2007) for specific suggestions on strategies for communicating with students and colleagues who demonstrate these negative interpersonal styles.

Abandoning One's Nursing Identity: Star Complex

Effective APRN leaders are proud of their identity as a nurse. Those with a star complex deny or minimizing their nursing identity when being identified as a nurse might diminish their influence. The star complex is a condition that is seen in some experienced APRNs or in APRNs who have not been well socialized into nursing as a profession. Individuals with a star complex are those whose sense of self and identity depend a great deal on the opinions of powerful others. Acknowledging or promoting their identity as nurses is seen to diminish their power or the opinions that powerful others hold about them. As an example, consider Janice, an expert APRN who provides superior patient-focused care. Physician colleagues consider her to be a partner in the delivery of care, but staff and other APRNs gave up consulting with her because her self-promotion often interfered with patient and colleague interactions. In a recent conversation, a well-respected physician colleague told her how impressed he was with her practice. "In fact," he stated, "you're really not a nurse. You're different from all the other nurses I know." Janice graciously accepted this compliment, knowing that stardom, although overdue, had finally arrived. She had ascended to the heights of provider status and crashed through the nursing ceiling into a zone beyond nursing. Clearly, Janice's understanding of herself as an APRN was dormant.

APRNs are particularly vulnerable to being seduced into believing that they are something other (more) than a nurse. Advanced practice nursing specialties that have expanded roles may seek the status of medicine. This vulnerability stems from the historical lack of recognition of nursing by physicians, other disciplines, and even other nurses; the need for approval; and a lack of personal mastery.

A primary strategy for the management of this obstacle is effective mentoring by a powerful APRN with a strong nursing identity. An additional essential strategy is to use clear and concise communication skills to provide an appropriate response to a colleague who believes that it is a compliment to be identified as other than a nurse. An appropriate response for Janice to have made would have been, "Thank you, but I'm proud to be an APRN. It is good that we can work together to help our patients." The existence of a star complex may represent a more fundamental problem for the APRN than good communication skills can address. The issue is whether the APRN truly desires to be identified as a nurse, performing at the boundaries of nursing practice and being accepted by other nurses as a valued member of the nursing profession. As APRNs are increasingly recognized as valued members of the health care team and as mentoring and empowerment become understood as core elements of leadership, star complex behavior will become less tolerated, unnecessary, and less frequent.

Hoarding or Misusing Power: Queen Bee Syndrome

An effective leader is generous, looking for opportunities to lift colleagues up by sharing opportunities, knowledge, and expertise and acknowledging the contributions of others. Queen bee syndrome refers to individuals who believe they have achieved a level of prominence by their own individual hard work, with little or no assistance from others, and that everyone else should do the same. These people hoard all the visible leadership tasks for themselves. Like those with a star complex, the effort to garner power is a theme. In this case, power derives not from powerful others but from the queen bee's own knowledge and expertise. Such APRNs are threatened by strong individuals and tend to denigrate them instead of sharing power. This type of leader prefers to be surrounded by servile individuals who will not challenge personal authority. For example, Rita, an experienced wound and ostomy APRN, makes sure that she sees every patient and that patients know she is the authority on wounds and ostomies. Staff nurses who are competent in these skills report that Rita undermines them with patients by saying that the care should have been done a certain way. Rita was not happy when the staff on a surgical unit, who had tried unsuccessfully to involve her in a unit project, conducted a quality improvement project during which both physicians and patients identified some service delivery issues relative to ostomy care. These staff members changed the way wound and ostomy services were managed.

The antidote to a queen bee syndrome is to use knowledge and expertise to move away from hoarding power toward collaborative, empowered leadership. Queen bee behavior is the antithesis of good leadership. Queen bees will have more difficulty remaining as leaders and keeping positions of power as APRN become more confident in their leadership abilities and join the circle of leaders. All effective leaders empower others.

Failure to Mentor

A distressing form of horizontal violence is common. "Nurses eat their young" is an epithet that characterizes the experience of many novice nurses and APRNs, as well as of some older, more experienced nurses (Baltimore, 2006). Nurses who advance in their profession may forget their roots and leave novice nurses behind or, worse, actively undermine their advancement. For example, nurses are often criticized by other nurses for continuing their education and moving into APRN roles. This denigration of important values and goals by colleagues is dispiriting and discouraging; it can hamper nurses from moving forward in their careers. In another example, the orientation process for a new position may become a survival test to see whether the new APRN can survive without mentoring or a supportive network. Because perceived powerlessness is at the root of this behavior, an important antidote is empowerment. The common practice of mentoring, taking an active interest in another's career, apprenticing, and "giving a leg up" to the least experienced is not as common in nursing as it is in many other professions. Box 11.8 lists the behaviors that provide evidence that there has been a failure in mentorship (Baltimore, 2006; Longo & Sherman, 2007; Longo & Smith, 2011).

Bullying

Bullying is a severe form of horizontal violence attributed to oppressed group behavior. Plonien (2016) and the American Nurses Association (2015) have suggested that horizontal violence is a more complex phenomenon and includes those external to nursing who make up the organization's culture and add to stress in the work setting. Curran (2006) reported that there will be more career nurses vying for leadership positions and that forms of horizontal violence such as bullying will worsen. Bullying is not a one-time event but instead is a subtle, deliberate, and ongoing behavior that accumulates over time and leaves the victim feeling hurt, vulnerable, and powerless (Anderson, 2011; Hutchinson, Vickers, Jackson, & Wilkes, 2005; Longo & Sherman, 2007).

Strategies to Overcome Horizontal Violence

Personal and organizational symptoms of horizontal violence are job dissatisfaction, increased stress levels, and physical and psychological illness. If the broader cause is a negative organizational culture, then the most effective leadership strategy to prevent its occurrence is to adopt a zero tolerance policy and a shared set of values with the staff (Longo & Sherman, 2007; Longo & Smith, 2011) that support positive behaviors. For example, fostering mentoring opportunities and enhancing the transition of colleagues into new positions of leadership can create a positive culture that does not tolerate horizontal violence. Box 11.9 presents suggested leadership strategies to eliminate horizontal violence.

Negative behaviors that are expressed as failure to mentor, bullying, and disenfranchising others may

---

BOX 11.8 Failure in Mentorship Behaviors

- Gossiping or bad-mouthing
- Criticizing
- Failure to give assistance when needed
- Setting up roadblocks by withholding information
- Bullying
- Scapegoating
- Undermining performance

BOX 11.9 Leadership Strategies to Stop Horizontal Violence

- Examine the organizational culture for symptoms of horizontal violence.
- Name the problem as horizontal violence when you see it.
- Educate staff to break the silence.
- Allow victims of horizontal violence to tell their stories.
- Enact a process for dealing with issues that occur.
- Provide training for conflict and anger management skills.
- Empower victims to defend themselves.
- Engage in self-reflection to ensure that your leadership style does not support horizontal violence.
- Encourage a culture of zero tolerance for horizontal violence.

Adapted from Longo, J., & Sherman, R. O. (2007). Leveling horizontal violence. *Nursing Management, 38,* 34–37, 50–51.

continue to be present in an increasingly stressful health care environment (McAvoy & Murtagh, 2003; Thomas, 2003). It is not an overstatement to claim that the future health of the profession depends on overcoming this barrier and relegating it to history. APRN leaders as role models create a more empowering and humane work environment for their colleagues and those who follow them.

Strategies for Implementing the Leadership Competency

Developing a Leadership Portfolio

Throughout this chapter, definitions, attributes, and components of leadership and key strategies for developing competency in APRN leadership have been presented. These approaches will help new APRNs acquire leadership skills and can assist faculty in teaching these skills. Developing a leadership component as part of a professional portfolio is helpful to novice APRNs who desire to individualize continuing development of the leadership competency consistent with their personal vision, goals, timeline, and APRN role in the practice setting. An Australian study reported increased knowledge, skill sets, and outcomes in clinicians and leaders who used portfolios to enhance their effectiveness (Dadich, 2010). Falter (2003) has suggested the use of a strategy map that includes vision, goals, and objectives that outline steps to achieve a particular strategy. Portfolios are designed to meet the needs of individual APRNs and should be consistent with clinical and personal interests and professional goals and provide a timeline that allows for personal and professional balance and boundary setting. Chapter 20 provides the elements of a marketing portfolio.

Promoting Collaboration Among APRN Groups

At different times, each subgroup of APRNs in America has emerged as a leader for the nursing profession. Psychiatric CNSs were early APRNs to enter private practice, despite the litigious climate in which they could be threatened with lawsuits for "practicing medicine." CNMs and CRNAs have led the way in using data effectively to justify their practice and attain appropriate scopes of practice. Early in their history, both groups began to record the results of their practices, showing the quality and suitability of their care (see Chapter 1). In the 1990s, NPs, with their flexible, community-based primary care practices, stood at the forefront of the changing health care delivery system. Although these subgroups of APRNs have made impressive strides, an obstacle to effective leadership is the tendency for APRN specialty groups to separate and establish rigid boundaries that distinguish them from one another, thereby fragmenting APRN groups and blocking opportunities for the increased power that unity would bring.

The tension and fragmentation created by rigid boundaries require leaders who can transcend APRN roles and specialties. Consensus groups have developed at the national level to discuss policy issues in which the power of the collective numbers of all APRN groups speaking with one voice cannot be overemphasized (see Chapters 2, 12, and 22). An excellent example of professional collaboration among nurse leaders is the Consensus Model work (Chapter 22). APRN organizations have joined to speak out collaboratively about state regulations regarding reimbursement, prescriptive authority, and managed care empanelment.

Each APRN, regardless of specialty, has the responsibility of moving toward an integrative and unified understanding of advanced practice nursing. Creating community in the current health care environment is particularly challenging because of the realignment of clinical decision making, changing scopes of practice for APRNs, and new roles that blur boundaries between and among providers.

An understanding of change, effective communication, coalition building, shared vision, and collaborative practice leads to the development of structures on which unity is built. These five building blocks form the foundation of interprofessional leadership and practice.

Networking

Networking is a valuable technique used by leaders to stay informed and connected regarding APRN issues. Networking is not a new strategy for APRN leaders. Formal networks take the form of committees, coalitions, and consortia of people who come together to share information, collaborate, and plan strategy regarding mutual issues. Formal networks open doors to new opportunities and provide shared resources that ensure a competitive edge in the organization (Carroll, 2005). Informal networking is a strategy that takes place behind the scenes and allows for contact with APRNs and others who speak similar language, share viewpoints, and offer support and feedback at critical times. The ability of APRNs to stay connected to important practice and education issues through networking is key to leadership competency. The most effective strategy for becoming an insider is networking with colleagues within the circle of APRN peers and with other health care providers who have a stake in the outcomes of a particular issue.

Effectively Working With Other Leaders to Advance Health Care

Other strategies also assist in the process of planning and implementing change. It is important to analyze the situation and explore the need for change. If change is warranted, one must craft an implementation plan that involves the key players. Box 11.3 lists leadership strategies that are useful for moving through these transitions. Bonalumi and Fisher (1999) have suggested that an important component of leadership during times of change is the ability to foster and encourage resilience in change recipients. O'Connell (1999) and Grafton, Gillespie, and Henderson (2010) have defined resilient people as being positive and self-assured in the face of life's complexities; having a focused, clear vision of what they want to achieve; and having the ability to be organized but flexible and proactive rather than reactive. Helping colleagues and followers develop resilience should be a major focus for APRN leaders who seek to facilitate the growth of their followers.

Institutional Assessment Regarding Readiness for Change

With the emphasis on evidence-based practice and the knowledge that evidence-based guidelines and therapies are underused (IOM, 2001; McGlynn et al., 2003), overused, or misused (IOM, 2001), APRNs have an important systems leadership role in improving care. This can be accomplished by leading and collaborating with nurses and interprofessional colleagues to ensure the adoption of best practices (Duffy, 2002; Spencer & Jordan, 2001; Spross & Heaney, 2000; Weaver, Salas, & King, 2011). An institutional assessment of specific factors will help the APRN identify facilitators of and barriers to change. These data can then be used to design a plan for change in collaboration with others. Box 11.10 lists key assessment questions to consider.

BOX 11.10   Assessment Questions to Evaluate Readiness for Change

- What is the nature of the change (e.g., policy, procedure, new skill, behavior)?
- Is the issue significant? For all stakeholders or just one group?
- Is a national policy, guideline, or standard the focus of the change? Is it a mandate with which the agency must be in compliance?
- Is the change simple or complex? Will different stakeholders perceive its simplicity or complexity differently?
- Do you foresee major problems associated with change, such as an increase in errors or resistance on the part of a group?
- Will it be possible to address these major problems?
- Are there vested interests—who is likely to gain from the change, who will view the change as a loss (e.g., of power)?
- Are there opinion leaders who will promote the change? Do you anticipate strong opposition?
- Have you observed a gap between public statements and private actions (e.g., a colleague agrees to serve on a committee but never shows up or participates in the committee's work)?
- Are there resource implications? What are the costs (e.g., staffing, materials, lost revenue)?

Adapted from the University of York National Health Centre for Reviews and Dissemination. (1999). Getting evidence into practice. *Effective Health Care Bulletin, 5,* 1–16.

Followship

As APRNs focus on developing their leadership skills, they discover the importance of being a good follower. Skill is necessary to recognize when one should be a follower rather than a leader—when another is more skilled or more appropriate to lead a particular situation, or when it is appropriate to let others who are developing leadership skills take the lead on a project. Successful collaboration and teamwork require not just leadership but skilled followers as well. Expert followers know how to accept direction, be forthcoming with pertinent information that is valuable to the team, seek clarification, and provide appropriate constructive feedback.

Conclusion

The health care system is constantly evolving and while this evolution can appear rather chaotic at times, most of the changes seen are the results of leadership. This means that the future is bright for APRNs as clinical, professional, health policy, and systems leaders. APRNs can exert their leadership influence in far-reaching ways, from the bedside and clinic to the highest political office. APRNs are also constantly evolving in all the various roles, and these changes have had substantial influence on the health care system, as well as on the nursing profession itself. APRNs exercise leadership when they present ideas or dilemmas and offer solutions to colleagues or communities, whether through social media or at a national meeting. Small changes often lead to much larger changes, so APRNs should not underestimate the impact of leadership exercised with patients, colleagues, and administrators. APRNs can consider how they can lead, make a difference, and commit to doing so, knowing that they can redefine the scope of their leadership influence in response to opportunities or changing life circumstances. The dynamic, ever-changing environment of health care sets the stage for ceaseless opportunities for APRNs to innovate and lead.

Nursing practice is based on an interactive style that empowers patients and colleagues. This foundation holds APRN leaders in good stead as they move into the emerging interprofessional practices that are developing. APRNs can work toward identifying, clarifying, and demystifying the health care system of today, for within today's reality lies the basis of tomorrow's change. APRNs are poised to lead change as they operate at the boundary between today's health care system and that of tomorrow. The attributes, goals, and vision of APRN leaders put them at the forefront of the health care frontier.

Key Summary Points

- Leadership is a core APRN competency, requiring deep knowledge of the art and science and an emphasis on interpersonal skills.
- The health care system is evolving continuously, requiring APRNs to create mastery around change management.
- Effective leaders use mentors, mentor others, network, and learn how to follow.

References

To access the references for this chapter, use your smartphone's QR code reader to scan the code below, or go to http://booksite.elsevier.com/ 9780323447751.

Collaboration

Michael Carter • Cindi Dabney • Charlene M. Hanson

"For the strength of the pack is the Wolf, and the strength of the Wolf is the pack."

—*Rudyard Kipling*

CHAPTER CONTENTS

Advanced practice nursing is highly complex and requires that the advanced practice registered nurse (APRN) be competent in collaboration. Collaboration takes place in a number of reciprocal relationships and includes the APRN, the patient, families, other health care providers, and a number of others who are a part of the treatment experience. Patients assume that their health care providers communicate and collaborate effectively and become concerned when this does not occur. Patient dissatisfaction with care, unsatisfactory clinical outcomes, and clinician frustration can often be traced to a failure to collaborate among those caring for the patient. Collaboration depends on

clinical and interpersonal expertise and is built on strong collegial relationships. The primary focus of this chapter is on collaboration among individuals and work groups. The goal is to make explicit the values, behaviors, and processes that facilitate collaboration and thus improve patient care.

Definition of Collaboration

Collaboration: What It Is

The term *collaboration* is often used in health care and is associated with teamwork and partnership.

These are necessary components of collaboration but are not sufficient. The American Nurses Association's (ANA's) *Nursing's Social Policy Statement* (ANA, 2010) clarifies that collaboration for nurses, including APRNs, means a true partnership in which there is a valuing of expertise, power, and respect for all members. Collaboration also means recognizing and accepting each participant's sphere of activity and responsibility.

The Essentials of Doctoral Education for Advanced Nursing Practice, released by the American Association of Colleges of Nursing (AACN) in 2006, specifies that APRNs are expected to provide interprofessional collaboration for improving patient and population health outcomes. APRNs are expected to establish, participate, and lead collaborative teams when appropriate.

Hanson and Spross' (1996) earlier definition of collaboration is still appropriate today:

> Collaboration is a dynamic, interpersonal process in which two or more individuals make a commitment to each other to interact authentically and constructively to solve problems and to learn from each other to accomplish identified goals, purposes, or outcomes. The individuals recognize and articulate the shared values that make this commitment possible. (p. 232)

Characterizing collaboration as an interaction conveys the communicative and behavioral aspects of this competency. This definition implies partnership, shared values, commitment, and goals yet allows for differences in opinions and approaches. Including the notions of shared values and commitment makes it clear that collaboration is a process that evolves over time.

The Interprofessional Education Collaborative (IPEC) (2011) has developed four core competencies of collaborative practice for health professionals. These focus on values and ethics, roles and responsibilities, communication, and teamwork across the full spectrum of care. Additionally, the Institute of Healthcare Improvement (2017a) has developed a Triple Aim framework dealing with improving the patient experience of care, including quality and satisfaction with care; improving the health of populations; and reducing the per capita cost of health care. These aims can only be achieved through collaborative practice for health professionals.

The ability to commit to interprofessional interaction over time requires that participants bring a set of characteristics and qualities to the encounter. To interact authentically means partners share the emotional satisfactions and frustrations of clinical work and develop ways of supporting each other. Successful collaboration can lead to an intimacy that arises from working closely together over time. A collaborative practice may include the challenge of dealing with the same person(s) daily over clinically important matters that are large or small. Managing conflict and engaging in crucial conversations are key to success and require the skills found in the definition of collaboration.

Collaboration requires relationships that are productive for professionals, patients, and communities. There is room for disagreement in collaborative relationships; partners and teams develop strategies for dealing with disagreements that are mutually satisfactory and enhance the process. Collaboration demands a sophisticated level of communication; collaboration cannot be mandated, legislated, or regulated.

Collaboration: What It Is Not

Several forms of interaction occur among clinicians, patients, families, and administrators in the complex processes that occur in care delivery. Collaboration is likely the most sophisticated and complicated among these forms. At times there can be confusion as to what collaboration is and what other forms of communication exist. These other forms listed below do not meet the definition of collaboration used by the nursing profession.

With the exceptions of parallel communication, the processes described here require some level of interaction among providers but may not involve collaboration. Information exchange, coordination, consultation, co-management, and referral may be sufficient to achieve clinical goals in particular situations. Effective and timely communication is required among clinicians for these processes to work to benefit patients, minimize errors, and enhance quality.

Parallel Communication. Parallel communication occurs when clinicians interact with a patient separately. They do not talk together before seeing a patient nor do they see the patient together; there is no expectation of joint interactions. For example, the staff registered nurse, medical student, attending physician, acute care nurse practitioner (NP) and the certified registered nurse anesthetist (CRNA) all ask the patient the same questions about medications. In this example, multiple interactions are burdensome and frustrating for the patient. The patient is inconvenienced, and fragmented information has been gathered from multiple sources that may lead to errors in clinical decision making. This practice of asking the same question is often perceived as a safety issue, requiring different providers to ask the same questions, especially regarding medication review and reconciliation. The patient expects that, at the minimum, the information is captured in the medical record and all those involved with care will read and understand this information. Repeated questioning over the same topic can be interpreted as either the information was not recorded or the clinician failed to read the record.

One-Sided Compromise. Communication that demonstrates a one-sided compromise occurs when the APRN is overly agreeable, consistently yields to the other health care providers, and senses a personal lack of integrity in the care. This yielding results in compromised care and occurs when the APRN lacks the will or skill to engage in a collaborative negotiation.

Faux Collaboration. Faux collaboration occurs when persons in a position of authority believe that they are being collaborative because those around them are agreeing with the authority figure but not engaging in meaningful dialogue. This form of communication can be rather subtle and difficult for others to understand.

Parallel Functioning. Parallel functioning occurs when providers care for patients, addressing the same clinical problem, but do not engage in any joint or collaborative planning. For example, nurses, physical therapists, and physicians document their interventions for pain in separate parts of the patient record but do not communicate about the case. The effect of such interactions is the same as for parallel communication.

Information Exchange. Informing may be one-sided or two-sided and may or may not require action or decision making. If action is needed, the decision is unilateral, not a result of joint planning. Information exchange may be sufficient and exert a neutral or beneficial effect on care processes and outcomes. There is a risk of a negative outcome if the situation actually requires joint planning and decision making.

Coordination. This form of communication lends structure to the encounter and may include actions to minimize duplication of effort but not interaction.

Calling the supplier to assure that the patient receives the durable medical equipment needed following an office visit is one way that the APRN may engage in coordination. This form of communication is usually one-sided and direct and may achieve the goal, but this is not collaboration.

Consultation. The clinician who is caring for a patient seeks advice regarding a patient's concern but retains primary responsibility for care delivery (see Chapter 9). For example. the certified nurse-midwife (CNM) may believe that there is a need for an evaluation and recommendation for treatment of a mother who is experiencing symptoms of depression and asks for a consultation by the psychiatric/mental health nurse practitioner. The result is a recommendation to the CNM for treatment of the mother, but the CNM retains the responsibility of actually prescribing the intervention if the recommendation is determined to be appropriate.

Co-Management. Two or more clinicians provide care and each professional retains accountability and responsibility for defined aspects of care. This process usually arises from consultation in which a problem requires management that is outside the scope of practice of the referring clinician and the treatment will be continuing (see Chapter 9). Providers must be explicit with each other about their responsibilities. Co-management may also be a process used by interprofessional teams, such as palliative care. There is the possibility that co-management can become parallel functioning, and this should be avoided.

Referral. A referral occurs when the APRN directs the patient to another clinician for the management of a particular problem or aspect of the patient's care when the problem is beyond the APRN's expertise (see Chapter 9). For example, the APRN may determine that a patient could benefit from a course of physical therapy and a referral is initiated, or the APRN decides that the patient has appendicitis and requires surgery, so a referral to a surgeon is initiated.

Supervision. Some clinicians may confuse collaboration with supervision. Supervision occurs when one clinician delegates aspects of care to another clinician but retains full authority for the care. Authority and accountability for all aspects of the care are retained by the supervisor and billing for the care is done by the supervisor. All APRNs are autonomous practitioners and supervision of them by other disciplines is not appropriate. APRNs may supervise other nursing personnel for aspects of nursing care they provide but are not appropriate to supervise other disciplines.

Domains of Collaboration in Advanced Practice Nursing

APRNs execute the collaboration competency in several domains—among individuals, work groups, and organizations. Competency in collaboration is often executed at the same time as other competencies, and it is dynamic, shifting as the particulars of a situation change.

Collaboration With Individuals

Collaboration with patients, families, and colleagues in the delivery of direct care is the primary domain in which collaboration is practiced. For example, in forming partnerships with patients (see Chapter 8), APRNs aim to understand how the patient wants to interact, and in turn collaborate with patients and families when they mutually set and revise goals and determine barriers for outcomes; these activities are aimed at uncovering a common purpose, a hallmark of collaboration. APRNs also collaborate with individual clinicians. For example, the diabetes clinical nurse specialist (CNS) may collaborate with the cardiac CNS and a staff nurse to determine who will carry out which aspects of patient education for a patient. The collaborative process may include determining the order and timing of content to be taught. In this case, the APRN is also executing the direct care (interacting with the patient to assess learning needs) and guidance (guiding patients in lifestyle changes) competencies.

Collaboration With Teams and Groups

Another common domain in which APRNs implement collaboration is in their work with clinical teams and on departmental and institutional committees. These groups may be composed of individuals from multiple disciplines. A key function of the collaborative competency is the facilitation of teamwork to ensure the delivery of effective, safe, high-quality care leading to positive outcomes. APRNs play key roles in facilitating and leading interprofessional teams, which ultimately requires integrated collaboration of leadership competencies. As APRNs become more experienced, their skill in facilitating collaboration in groups grows.

Collaboration in the Organizational and Policy Arenas

In this domain, the focus of collaboration extends beyond the delivery of care to individuals and groups. The organizational and policy forces shaping advanced practice nursing and clinical care require that even novice APRNs cultivate collaboration. Initiatives aimed at clarifying credentialing requirements, making it easier to practice across state lines, and improving reimbursement for APRNs require them to use their status as clinicians, citizens, and members of professional organizations to collaborate with organizational leaders and policymakers.

Collaboration in Global Arenas

Global or international collaboration is becoming an essential domain for APRNs, as noted by the AACN (2006), the Institute of Medicine (IOM, 2011; IOM, Committee on Quality Health Care in America, 2001), and the National Organization of Nurse Practitioner Faculties (NONPF, 2012; see also Chapter 6). Friedman (2005) has argued that global communication and collaboration will be the keys to successful living, working, and economic success over the next century, and we believe that this is true for health care. There is evidence that globalization is already affecting practice; the APRN covering the emergency room at night may be communicating with a radiologist in Australia about a diagnostic image that was sent electronically to be interpreted in real time. In addition, APRNs' experiences with volunteerism in other countries (e.g., Doctors Without Borders, mission trips to Haiti and Africa) are shaping their goals and opportunities.

Terms of Collaboration

The terms *multidisciplinary, interdisciplinary, transdisciplinary,* and, most currently, *interprofessional collaboration* are often used interchangeably. There are differences among these terms; the prefix actually indicates the level and depth of interactions to which the term refers. Choi and Pak (2006) provided a review of the key differences among the terms. Multidisciplinary teams use the knowledge from different disciplines, but these teams stay within their own boundaries. Interdisciplinary teams blend the various disciplines into a single whole. Transdisciplinary teams integrate the sciences with the humanities and move beyond usual boundaries. This clearly defined idea of interprofessional collaboration moves beyond these traditional forms of teamwork and takes these types of collaboration a bit further in an attempt to eliminate traditionally prescribed boundaries through negotiation and interaction (Alberto & Herth, 2009; Bainbridge, Nasmith, Orchard, & Wood, 2010; IPEC, 2011).

Interprofessional collaboration occurs when more than one professional works together to focus on a particular health problem or concern. Interprofessional collaboration requires that there be mutual respect and commitment for the sake of a response to a problem. Petri (2010) has suggested that it is an interpersonal process characterized by health care professionals with shared objectives, decision-making responsibility, and power working together to solve patient care problems. The Interprofessional Collaborative Initiative (IPEC, 2011; Schmitt, 2011) is a partnership made up of the AACN, American Association of Colleges of Osteopathic Medicine, American Association of Colleges of Pharmacy, American Dental Education Association, Association of American Medical Colleges, and Association of Schools of Public Health. This group takes this definition further with their goal of preparing all health professions students to work together deliberatively to build a safer and better patient- and community-centered health care system in the United States. IPEC has developed a framework for interprofessional collaborative practice based on four domains, described in Box 12.1. Each IPEC domain has several behaviors that further define the competency (IPEC, 2011).

The move to reintroduce team approaches to care is evident across the spectrum of health care today (Clausen et al., 2012; IOM, 2011; Patient Protection and Affordable Care Act [ACA], 2010; Young et al., 2012). Interprofessional and transdisciplinary work foster the development of new approaches to clinical care. This level of interaction leads to new insights in the interpretation of assessments and creative and effective clinical problem solving, leading to successful outcomes.

Interprofessional Collaboration

The need for collaboration among health care professionals has been a serious concern over many years (Bainbridge et al., 2010; Dumez, 2011; Petri, 2010; World Health Organization, 1978). Efforts to transform health care systems around the world to improve the reliability of care, safety, quality, efficiency, and cost-effectiveness will not be successful unless clinicians, teams, and administrators undertake the important collaborative work leading to transformation.

Several phenomena have coalesced to bring the struggles to attain interprofessional collaboration to a critical point. The IOM report on quality and safety in the late 1990s (IOM, Committee on Quality Health Care in America, 2001) identified shortages of providers, especially in primary care, and the need for team approaches through community-based care, accountable care organizations, and nurse-managed clinics. In addition, the 2011 IOM report *The Future of Nursing* urged teamwork among health care providers. These initiatives have all led to a continuing focus on the need to foster interpersonal and interprofessional competency for all health care providers. The pressing need for collaboration among health care professionals led to the development of specific interprofessional competencies in 2011 (ACA, 2010; Canadian Interprofessional Health Collaborative [CIHC], 2010; IPEC, 2011).

A paradox of the contemporary health care systems of several countries is that there are incentives and disincentives for members of different disciplines, work groups, and organizations to collaborate. Incentives and disincentives may be equally powerful so that motivation to collaborate can be diminished or eliminated by a compelling counterforce (Fig. 12.1) (Young et al., 2012). An understanding of this paradox can help APRNs and their colleagues approach opportunities for collaboration strategically and build and sustain clinical environments that support collaboration. Numerous clinical initiatives aimed at improving quality and safety, the need to eliminate health care disparities, and an increasing proportion of health care professionals other than physicians underscore that interprofessional collaboration at the educational, clinical, and institutional levels is essential in the current health care marketplace (IOM, 2011; Pohl, Hanson, Newland, & Cronenwett, 2010; Schmitt, 2011). The ability to collaborate is essential for APRNs to implement interprofessional practice models and analyze complex health problems in an interactive environment (Cronenwett & Dzau, 2010; IOM, 2011; Pohl et al., 2010).

Characteristics of Effective Collaboration

The definition of collaboration invites exploration of the characteristics that make up a successful collaborative relationship. Personal and setting-specific attributes are pivotal to successful collaborations.

BOX 12.1   Interprofessional Collaborative Initiative Domains and Competencies

Competency Domain 1: Values and Ethics for Interprofessional Collaboration
- Place patients and populations at center of care.
- Respect dignity and privacy of patients and confidentiality of team members.
- Embrace cultural diversity.
- Respect unique cultures, values, and roles.
- Work in cooperation with patients and providers and those who support care.
- Develop trusting relationships with patients, families, and team members.
- Demonstrate ethical conduct and quality care as a member of the team.
- Manage ethical dilemmas in interprofessional care situations.
- Act with honesty and integrity.
- Maintain personal and professional competence.

Competency 2: Roles and Responsibilities for Collaboration
- Communicate role and responsibilities clearly to patients and professionals.
- Recognize skill, knowledge, and ability limitations.
- Engage with professionals who complement one's practice.
- Explain roles and responsibilities of other team members.
- Use the full scope of the knowledge, skills, and abilities of all team members.
- Communicate with the team to clarify roles and responsibilities.
- Forge interdependent relationships.
- Engage in continuous interprofessional development.
- Use unique and complementary abilities of all members to optimize care.

Competency 3: Interprofessional Communication
- Choose effective communication tools to enhance team function.
- Communicate information to patients and team members, avoiding discipline-specific terminology.
- Express knowledge and opinions to team with confidence, respect, and clarity to ensure common understanding.

- Listen actively and encourage ideas and opinions of other team members.
- Give timely, sensitive, and instructive feedback to team members about their performance and respond respectively to feedback from others.
- Use respectful language in difficult situations or interprofessional conflict.
- Recognize one's own uniqueness and contributions to effective communication, conflict resolution, and positive working relationships.
- Consistently communicate the importance of patient-centered care.

Competency 4: Interprofessional Teamwork and Team-Based Care
- Describe the process of team and role development and the role and practice of effective teams.
- Develop consensus on ethical principles to guide all aspects of patient care and teamwork.
- Engage other health professionals in shared, patient-centered problem solving.
- Integrate knowledge and experience of other professionals to inform care decisions while respecting patient and community values and priorities.
- Apply leadership practices that support collaborative practice.
- Engage self and others to manage constructively any disagreements about values, roles, and goals of care.
- Share accountability with other professionals, patients, and communities for relevant health care outcomes.
- Reflect on individual and team performance to improve individual and team performance.
- Use process improvement strategies to improve the effectiveness of interprofessional teamwork and practice.
- Use available evidence to inform effective teamwork and team-based practice.
- Perform effectively on teams and in different team roles in a variety of settings.

Adapted from Interprofessional Education Collaborative. (2011). Core competencies for interprofessional collaborative practice: Report of an expert panel. Retrieved from http://www.aacn.nche.edu/education/pdf/IPECreport.pdf.

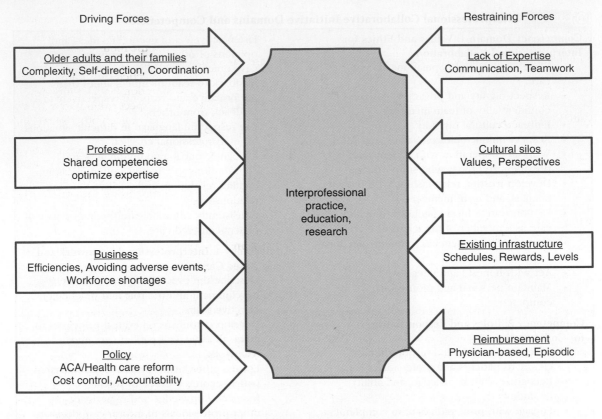

FIG 12.1 Driving and restraining forces for interprofessional practice, research, and education. *(From Young, H. M., Siegel, E. O., McCormick, W. C., Fulmer, T., Harootyan, L. K., & Dorr, D. A. [2012]. Interdisciplinary collaboration in geriatrics: Advancing health for older adults.* Nursing Outlook, 59, *243–250.)*

Some characteristics of collaboration have long been recognized, but clinicians and organizations have often resisted adopting the necessary philosophy, commitment, and behaviors. Steele's early analysis (1986) of collaboration among NPs and physicians revealed several characteristics—mutual trust and respect, an understanding and acceptance of each other's disciplines, positive self-image, equivalent professional maturity arising from education and experience, recognition that the partners are not substitutes for each other, and a willingness to negotiate. Petri (2010) and Hughes and Mackenzie (1990) have outlined four characteristics of NP-physician collaboration: collegiality, communication, goal sharing, and task interdependence. Spross (1989) described three essential elements of collaboration: a common purpose, diverse and complementary professional knowledge and skills, and effective communication processes. These early works highlight the core elements necessary for collaboration that are listed in Box 12.2.

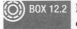 **BOX 12.2 Essential Characteristics of Collaboration**

- Clinical competence and accountability
- Common purpose
- Interpersonal competence and effective communication
- Trust
- Mutual respect
- Recognition and valuing of diverse, complementary knowledge and skills
- Humor

Collaboration requires clinical competence, common purpose, and effective interpersonal and communication skills or, at a minimum, a willingness to learn them. Trust, mutual respect, and valuing each other's knowledge and skills are equally important but develop over time. For these characteristics to develop, prospective partners must approach encounters with a willingness to trust, a commitment to respect each other, and the assumption that the other's knowledge and skills are valuable. In one sense, these characteristics are prerequisites; however, they are fully realized only after many constructive and productive interactions. Finally, a sense of humor among team members often serves many functions in helping team members stay committed to each other's collaborative practice.

Clinical Competence and Accountability

Clinical competence is perhaps the most fundamental characteristic underlying a successful collaborative experience among clinicians; without it, the trust and desire needed to work together are not possible. Trust and respect are built on the assurance that each member is able to carry out his or her role, function in a competent manner, and be accountable for practice. Clinical competence is a critical element of collaboration and has been supported by research (Bosque, 2011), yet stereotyped views of nursing and medical practice may interfere with collaborative efforts. These stereotypes may include physicians as having ultimate responsibility and nurses as having little responsibility.

Mutual trust and respect develop when collaborating clinicians can rely on each other's clinical competency. Partners share decision-making power because they recognize that leadership is problem based, not team or role based. Contemporary leadership shifts among partners in a departure from the traditional "captain of the team" approach. Thus the person with the most expertise, interest, talent, or willingness to lead can respond to the particular demands of the situation or problem. The accountable care organization and medical home concepts are excellent examples of how this approach works. The trust and respect among collaborators are such that they can count on the satisfactory resolution of the problem, even when they know as individuals that they might have approached the issue differently. This openness to shared leadership and alternative solutions allows partners to learn from each other. Collaboration offers APRNs and physicians opportunities to model their varied assessment and intervention strategies, which fosters mutual learning and appreciation for the contributions of each to the care of patients and families.

However, the environments in which APRN students and new graduates work must support them as they learn and mature clinically. Trust and assertiveness seem to act reciprocally in collaboration; as trust grows, so does the ability to communicate in difficult situations. Responding assertively in situations of risk and keeping the focus on the patient's welfare can enhance trust.

Respect for others' practice and knowledge is key to successful collaboration because it enhances shared decision making. Respect extends to acknowledgment and appreciation for each other's time and competing commitments.

Being accountable for practice enhances collaboration. APRNs model full partnership on caregiving teams when they share planning, decision making, problem solving, and goal setting for patient care (Clausen et al., 2012; IPEC, 2011).

Common Purpose

Collaboration is predicated on the notion of having a common purpose (Murray-Davis, Marshall, Gordon, 2011; Petri, 2010). Even if partners have not discussed the purposes and goals of their interactions, the organizations in which they work usually have an explicit mission and goals. Goals can be the starting point for identifying the purposes of clinical collaboration. Common purposes may range from ensuring that an underserved patient gains access to preventive services, such as mammography, to a more ambitious quality improvement agenda to improve the management of heart failure patients across settings.

One of the paradoxes of collaboration is that the partners are autonomous (self-governing, accountable) but interdependent, reflecting a reciprocal reliance on each other for support in carrying out their responsibilities. Recognizing their interdependence, team members can combine their individual skills to synthesize care plans that are more complex and comprehensive than what they could have created working alone. Like other characteristics, the common purpose that initially brought partners together may change over time. The situation that brought two clinicians together may become secondary to the deep personal commitment to work together in ways that improve patient care and are interpersonally and professionally satisfying. In addition to a common purpose, partners who are guided by a shared vision of the possibilities inherent in collaboration, believe in the value of collaboration, and are committed to achieving the relationship's potential (Young et al., 2012) will be most able to develop transdisciplinary and interprofessional collaboration. Developing a shared vision permits partners to value each other's ideas, opinions, and actions.

Interpersonal Competence and Effective Communication

Interpersonal competence is the ability to communicate effectively with colleagues in a variety of situations, including uncomplicated routine interactions, disagreements, unique cultural value conflicts, and stressful situations. The key to demonstrating interpersonal competence is the ability to communicate openly, clearly, and convincingly. Oral and written communications share some commonalities but require different abilities.

The concept of transparency is important. The IOM's *Crossing the Quality Chasm* lists transparency as one of the rules for the 21st century health care system (IOM, Committee on Quality Health Care in America, 2001). The term *transparency* can be defined as the honest and open sharing of information and ideas. It includes open communication among parties and not pretending everything is fine when it is not. Transparent communications are closely linked to accountability; transparency engenders trust and thus is an underlying requisite for collaboration. After clinical competence, interpersonal competence and effective communication may be the most important characteristics needed for APRNs to establish collaborative relationships.

Assertiveness is a key element of interpersonal competence needed by all APRNs. Assertiveness may be a challenge for women in some cultures and will have to be carefully exhibited. A range of qualities may be required for APRNs to be able to do the following: take risks; discuss disagreements in clinical judgment and agree to criteria for resolving such conflicts; be able to avoid a near-miss clinical situation, such as an error in prescribing or interpretation of clinical data; and admit that a mistake, miscommunication, or oversight has happened. Assertiveness is not sufficient in certain situations and environments and, in these cases, courage will be required to confront the problem.

Recognizing and Valuing Diverse, Complementary Culture, Knowledge, and Skills

High-quality patient care requires an interpersonal belief that the complementary knowledge other team members have will enhance one's own personal plan for patient care. Appreciation for the diverse and complementary knowledge each party brings to the work, commitment to quality and patient-centeredness, and willingness to invest in the partnership or team are all necessary for collaboration to become the normative process in team interactions.

A lack of knowledge about another's discipline is a barrier to developing effective teamwork (Dumez, 2011). Team members must recognize and value the overlapping and diverse skills and knowledge that each discipline brings to the team (CIHC, 2010; IPEC, 2011) so that mutual trust and respect can develop and deepen over time. Partners observe that patients benefit from their combined talents and efforts. They come to depend on each other to use good clinical judgment and to take appropriate actions.

Initially, collaborators have limited knowledge of each other as individuals and as professionals; collaboration is a conscious, learned behavior that improves as team members learn to value and respect one another's practice and expertise (IPEC, 2011). The first step is to recognize these differing contributions. For example, medicine and nursing, although overlapping disciplines, are culturally distinct and have diverse goals for patient care. In many cases, they complement each other. These complementarities also extend to other disciplines. Collaboration is built on the respect and valuing of the contributions of each profession to the common goal of optimal health care delivery.

Humor

Humor can serve as an important aspect of the collaborative process. Despite the serious nature of nurses' work, there's always room for levity somewhere. And, perhaps, serious work is where humor is needed the most (Rosenblatt & Davis, 2009). In collaborative practice, humor serves to decrease defensiveness, invite openness, relieve tension, and deflect anger. Humor helps individuals keep perspective and acknowledge the lack of perfection, and it sets the tone for trust and acceptance among colleagues so that difficult situations can be reframed. Ciesielka, Conway, Penrose, and Risco (2005) suggested that humor is essential to successful collaboration because it is a bridge to different backgrounds. The use of humor helps defuse the need for persons to argue their own point of view and allows them to refocus on how they can work together to meet common goals. APRN students can be encouraged to observe how humor is used by preceptors and colleagues and identify those uses that seem effective for improving communication and defusing conflict situations. Humor can be a challenge at times, however. Humor is a complex cognitive experience usually designed to cause laughter, but these experiences are often very contextual. This means some attempts at humor can be misinterpreted and invoke a negative response. Care will need to be exercised in using humor to have the desired outcome.

Although this list of characteristics of effective collaboration may seem daunting to the novice, a consistent commitment to and practice of collaboration can develop this competency over time in an APRN's practice. Exemplar 12.1 showcases the elements of collaboration in an individual practice. All health professionals need to recognize that investing the time and energy to build these relationships is an important component of clinical practice. The high levels of exchange of ideas and expertise that become possible when all of these characteristics come together is one of the great satisfactions of collaborative practice.

Impact of Collaboration on Patients and Clinicians

There is common agreement that collaboration is an important part of clinical practice as an APRN (Bosque, 2011; Young et al., 2012), but some clinicians struggle to be adept at collaboration. Common barriers to interprofessional communication and collaboration include personal values and expectations, personality differences, hierarchy, culture and ethnicity, generational differences, and gender (O'Daniel & Rosenstein, 2008).

Patient and provider benefits of collaboration have been documented. Patients are sensitive to the relationships among caregivers and are quick to recognize the lack of respect or trust among their providers. Collaborative relationships with interdisciplinary health care providers can ameliorate some of these negative effects (Remonder, Koch, Link, &

EXEMPLAR 12.1 | **Elements of Collaboration in One Advanced Practice Nurse's Practice**

Caesar M. is a family nurse practitioner who has a nursing home practice. He also volunteers one evening per week at a free clinic serving people living in poverty and without insurance. Donna is a 35-year-old patient with Crohn's disease; she is married to a welder and they have two children under 10 years of age. Donna had previously worked as a home health aide but had to stop because of her illness. She applied for disability coverage but was denied. The staff at the University Medical Center 75 miles away had initiated intravenous (IV) immune system suppression therapy. Donna was charged $6000 for each treatment, which occurred every 6 weeks. Donna's family income was $22,000 per year.

The company that produced the drug approved the free clinic to receive the medication without charge given Donna's family income. This medication had to be reconstituted by a pharmacist under a laminar-flow hood and administered IV over a 2-hour period. Once constituted, the medication was only viable for 4 hours. An additional complicating condition was that Donna had a history of extreme difficulty with IV access via peripheral veins.

Caesar knew that only through multiple collaborative arrangements would he be able to assure that Donna would repeatedly receive this needed treatment. The free clinic lacked the necessary supplies or equipment to administer the medication. Caesar's nursing home did have this ability. The administration and the director of nursing at the nursing home were approached and

both agreed that this could be done in their facility at no charge to Donna.

The next issue was to collaborate on developing a plan to mix the medication. The director of pharmacy at the local critical-access hospital agreed to mix the medications when needed as long as the clinic provided the medication. What was left was obtaining the free services of a surgeon to place an access port through which the IV medication could be administered. One of the volunteer ministers at the free clinic was married to a woman who was the clinic manager for a local surgeon. The surgeon was reluctant to offer the surgical placement for free but he placed the port after substantial pressures from Caesar and the minister's wife/office manager.

Now the medication administration dance began. On the day of administration, Donna stopped by the clinic and obtained the medication vial. She took it to the hospital, where the pharmacist reconstituted the drug under the hood and gave the IV bag to Donna. She brought this to the nursing home, where Caesar obtained an IV pump and administered the medication through her port over 2 hours.

One year later, the state approved the Medicaid expansion under the Patient Protection and Affordable Care Act. Donna received full insurance to cover her existing condition and she was able to be treated at a facility that could take over all aspects of this care. This is an example of multiple collaborations that might be required to assure treatment. ◎

Graham, 2010). Successful collaborative practices facilitate patients easily moving among providers as situations dictate. Collaboration requires an ability to transform competitive situations into opportunities for working together that are mutually beneficial and in which all parties can imagine the possibility of creating a win-win situation. In the past, this movement among providers was hampered by a lack of ability for the patient's information to flow with the patient. This is becoming easier with the migration to electronic record systems with patient portals.

The impact of APRNs on disease management and care transition interventions indicates that there are positive outcomes for patients. Table 12.1 illustrates the types of patient and provider benefits that have been ascribed to collaboration. Collaboration competencies have been in place for APRNs for several years in the United States, Canada, and Australia (AACN, 2006; Canadian Nurses Association, 2010; NONPF, 2012; Nursing and Midwifery Board of Australia, 2014).

Evidence That Collaboration Works

The United States has been undergoing a number of transitions in health care, and one of these changes has been the introduction of a patient-centered medical home for primary care. This model of care has several elements, but the critical element is collaboration among the health professionals treating the patient (Agency for Healthcare Research and Quality [AHRQ], n.d.). Research on medical homes shows reductions in cost measures and a decrease in overall utilization (Bosque, 2011; Nielsen, Buelt, Patel, & Nichols, 2016).

Additional literature, especially from Canada, shows similar findings (CIHC, 2010; Dumont, Briere, Morin, Houle, & Hoko-Fundi, 2010; Rice et al., 2010). Of note, publications that address interdisciplinary collaboration (particularly with physicians) and APRNs specifically have increased with the IPEC development of interprofessional competencies. Important ideas about collaboration from leaders in other disciplines have informed this discussion of collaboration (Bainbridge et al., 2010; Dumez, 2011; Palinkas, Ell, Hansen, Cabassa, & Wells, 2011). One goal of collaboration is to improve the quality of care. Exemplar 12.2 provides an example of one way in which collaboration can accomplish this goal.

Research Supporting Interprofessional Collaboration

Impact on Health Outcomes

NPs have been shown to be effective in managing health conditions in primary care and have been shown to be cost-effective in prior research (Newhouse et al., 2011). The outcomes of NP and CNM care were found to be equal to or in some cases better than outcomes for care provided by physicians alone. CNS care was found to help reduce hospital costs and length of hospital stay. There were insufficient data to evaluate CRNA practices. Competency in collaboration is a part of the clinical requirement for APRN practice and is likely a part of the reason for these findings.

Concern has been expressed by some groups that APRNs should not be provided full practice authority as autonomous practitioners. The opposition for APRN autonomy reasons that APRNs will not collaborate if not mandated by regulations. Evidence does not support this contention. Oliver, Pennington, Revelle, and Rantz (2014) reported that NPs who had full practice authority had better health outcomes and decreased hospitalization rates for Medicare and Medicaid beneficiaries compared to those in states that mandated collaboration.

TABLE 12.1	Benefits of Collaboration
Who Benefits?	Benefits
Patients	Improved quality of care
	Increased patient satisfaction
	Lower mortality rate
	Improved patient outcomes
	Patients feel more secure, cared for, closer to health care providers
	Empowers patients and family to become team members
Providers	Improved trust and respect for caregivers
	Improved communication and clarity of message
	Increased sharing of responsibility
	Increased sharing of expertise
	Mutually satisfying problem solving
	Improved communications
	Increased personal satisfaction
	Increased quality of professional life
	Enhanced mutual trust and respect
	Bridges care-cure dichotomy
	Expands horizons of providers
	Avoids redundant care and ensures coverage
	Empowers providers to influence health policy

Adapted from Sullivan, T. J. (1998). *Collaboration: A health care imperative* (pp. 26–27). New York, NY: McGraw-Hill Health Professionals Division.

EXEMPLAR 12.2   **Collaboration Works for Patients and Clinicians**

Dr. C. is a psychiatric clinical nurse specialist at a large tertiary hospital that is part of a rapidly expanding health system. This system includes hospitals, clinics, rehabilitation centers, and home health services and has been participating in new demonstration projects with the US Centers for Medicare and Medicaid Services. These projects are designed to improve the quality of care and to decrease the overall costs of care. New for this health system is changing from a fee-for-service payment system to a global payment for the care received by the patient across settings. In the past, each element of care was paid for as the service was provided and there was little linkage among the various aspects of care. Dr. C has reviewed the past 3 months' data on readmission following discharge from the acute care hospital because this is one of the key quality improvement measures. The new single electronic health record allows providers to follow the patient's care across different sites of care. What Dr. C. determined was that about 70% of the patients who were readmitted to the hospital had depression or anxiety identified during their acute care admission, yet no evidence-based plan of care was provided to deal with these problems. Based on this analysis, Dr. C. decided to build a collaborative pathway to assure that patients who experience depression or anxiety during acute care hospitalization were identified and provided with appropriate treatment.

Dr. C. quickly discovered that many providers would be involved in creating and delivering this plan. The first requirement was to assure that all patients received appropriate screening for depression and anxiety. Dr. C. engaged the assistance of social work in helping select the screening tools that were best suited to this situation. Next, Dr. C. met with the manager of the hospitalist program. In this particular hospital, acute care nurse practitioners and internal medicine physicians provide hospitalist services. The nurse manager for critical care was also included because the decision had to be made as to whether the screening would be done by nursing staff or by the hospitalists. The screening tools selected were such that they could be completed easily and accurately by the staff nurse who performs the admission assessment and included in the electronic record. Scores indicating the potential for depression or anxiety in the patient were automatically flagged by the record so that the hospitalists could request a consult by the psychiatric team for further analysis and recommendations for treatment. Evidence-based plans of care were then prescribed as appropriate by either the consultant or the hospitalist.

Dr. C. led a formative evaluation as this new approach to screening, diagnosis, and treatment unfolded and was able to make modifications in the plan based on the information provided by all concerned, including the patients and families. Three months after implementation, Dr. C. then conducted a summative evaluation of the program. What was found was that almost all patients had been screened. Those who scored as being at risk for depression or anxiety were placed into a treatment pathway that continued across sites of care, and readmissions to the hospital following discharge were reduced by 50%. Dr. C. continues to monitor the system and to provide written reports to the key collaborators in a timely manner. ◎

Effects of Physician and APRN Collaboration on Costs

Burke and O'Grady (2012) reported that group visits carried out by transdisciplinary health care teams are efficacious and hold promise for improved outcomes and better cost containment. Similarly, an integrative review of the impact of transdisciplinary teams on the care of the underserved demonstrated other benefits such as better primary care access and quality for underserved populations (Ruddy & Rhee, 2005).

Brooten et al. (2005) have reported the positive effects of APRN and physician collaboration on caring for women with high-risk pregnancies. Jackson et al. (2003) reported that fewer fiscal resources were required when obstetricians and CNMs worked within a collaborative care birth center model.

One of the challenges of evaluating cost-effectiveness with respect to clinical collaboration is the ability to measure change over an appropriate time horizon. As the Litaker et al. (2003) study suggested, a 1-year collaborative intervention was enough to change patient behaviors in ways that reduced important clinical markers but was not sufficient to assess and measure the impact of complications and disease-related comorbidities on the disease trajectory over time. The fact that the 1-year intervention was insufficient to sustain the behavior changes that led to the reduced clinical markers supports our conceptualization of collaboration as a process that evolves over time. It is also suggested that our understanding of long-term changes in patient behavior and clinical outcomes may depend on a complete empirical understanding of collaborative processes. Even so, there is evidence that organizationally supported teams, such as rapid response teams, can improve patient outcomes (Scherr, Wilson, Wagner, & Haughian, 2012).

In 2010, the Robert Wood Johnson Foundation (RWJF) reported examples of increased quality of life and safety in patients who were cared for by health care professionals who had overcome professional boundaries to work together. Results from such studies will continue to shape our understanding of collaboration and guidance and coaching competencies of APRNs (see Chapter 8).

There are many fine examples of collaboration initiatives leading to positive changes in health care and collaborative interactions among the health care disciplines. In 2007, boards of nursing, pharmacy, medicine, occupational therapy, physical therapy, and social work joined in a collaborative effort to assist regulatory bodies and legislators (National Council of State Boards of Nursing [NCSBN], Association of Social Work Boards, Federation of State Boards of Physical Therapy, Federation of State Medical Boards of the United States, National Association of Boards of Pharmacy, and National Board for Certification in Occupational Therapy, 2006). New competencies for education and practice that include collaboration and team work have been developed (IPEC, 2011; NONPF, 2012). Both the IOM Committee on the Robert Wood Johnson Foundation Initiative on the Future of Nursing (IOM, 2011) and the Josiah Macy Jr. Foundation recommendations for training primary care providers (Cronenwett & Dzau, 2010) include strong recommendations for collaboration among health care professionals. These efforts are encouraging; new positive strides in preparing health professions students for collaborative practice will be fulfilled.

Effects of Failure to Collaborate

Concerns about the quality of health care began to take on new importance in the United States and elsewhere during the latter part of the 20th century. Some time ago, the Committee on Quality Health Care in America of the IOM (2001) highlighted that patients were not receiving the best care possible and that thousands were dying each year by errors in care delivery. The Institute for Healthcare Improvement (IHI) (2017b) launched their work during this time as well. The problems continue in spite of substantial effort. In 2016 medical error was reported as the third leading cause of death in the United States (Makary & Daniel, 2016).

The emerging approaches for improving the quality of health care traced to the work of W. Edwards Deming (1982), who argued that organizations can increase quality and simultaneously reduce costs. The basic assumption of these new approaches to improving health care was that problems were not the fault of any particular individual clinician but were better understood as problems with systems of care delivery. The new idea to decrease errors and improve quality was that collaboration among providers, administrators, and patients would lead to improved quality, decrease injury, decrease costs, and save lives. Failures of collaboration often resulted in harm to patients, including morbidity and mortality. This means that failure to collaborate not only results in less than optimal working conditions for the professionals but also results in serious harm and increased costs of care for the patients (Makary & Daniel, 2016).

Balik and colleagues (2011) provide an in-depth analysis of research, studied organizations, and interviewed experts in hospital care to better understand how to improve care to patients and their families during hospitalization. One of the key drivers of quality care was respectful partnerships among providers and administrators. Respectful partnership is one of the critical elements of quality collaboration. These researchers reported that quality care did not occur without respectful partnership. Failure to collaborate results in poor-quality care, increased costs often associated with high staff turnover, and harm to patients.

Imperatives for Collaboration

Failure to collaborate in health care can result in harm to patients. Therefore, organizations and clinicians have an obligation to collaborate under the moral requirement to do no harm. The effects of collaboration or its failure can be seen in the way that ethical and institutional dilemmas are resolved and how research is conducted. A substantial driving force for collaboration came about as a part of the adoption of the ACA in 2010. There were key elements of this act that required improvements in quality that could only be achieved by interprofessional collaboration.

Based on the reality that medical and diagnostic error is a major concern in health care, research and planning are underway at both the AHRQ and through the 2016 Culture of Safety project at the ANA to find a way to provide a culture of safety to undergird patient care (ANA, 2016; Weaver, Dy, Lubomski, & Wilson, 2013). Interventions to promote safety are not easily defined, but safety cultures are described as those in which there is shared commitment to safety and effective teamwork as the highest priority.

Although many studies and plans do not attribute lack of collaboration and communication as a direct cause of medical error, collaboration and relationships among caregivers are seen as major forces in alleviating the problem (Manojlovich et al., 2014). Mutual respect, an important component of successful collaboration, ranked high as a predictor of a safe patient environment.

Ethical Imperative to Collaborate

Collaboration is required to minimize harm from care. Logically, that means that failure to collaborate is an ethical issue. The clinical imperative of APRN roles to collaborate is embedded within the ethical imperative. The IPEC (2011) proposed that all future health professionals assert the values and ethics of interprofessional practice by placing the needs and dignity of patients at the center of health care delivery and included a specific ethics domain and competencies (see Box 12.1). Compassionate and ethical patient care that provides a healing environment requires collaborative working relationships among all the providers, including APRNs (Petri, 2010; Schmitt, 2011). Environments that foster collaboration may also create a more supportive context for addressing ethical issues.

Quality patient care requires collaboration because it reinforces commitment to a common goal and reaffirms the central goal of patient welfare. Collaboration enhances shared knowledge because all health care providers repeatedly educate each other about the patient. Collaboration also demonstrates that how care is delivered is as important as who delivers the care. Collaboration is a moral imperative; good patient care requires it.

Institutional Imperative to Collaborate

The evidence that collaboration works has suggested that there are structural and interpersonal dimensions to collaboration; that is, although institutional policies or standards do not guarantee collaboration, they can establish expectations for collaboration. These institutional expectations can provide a structure that facilitates interpersonal communication and relationship building (ACA, 2010; IOM, 2011). The mutual goals of quality patient care and the ethical imperative to collaborate are at the center of interprofessional efforts to provide care or resolve conflicts in approaches to care for patients. For example, institutions that apply for Magnet status are expected to have a structure in place for interprofessional collaboration as one of the key characteristics (American Nurses' Credentialing Center, 2016). The incentive for hospitals to move to Magnet status has never been higher, with the current emphases on nurse retention, quality, costs, and safety. Institutions that have applied for the American Nurses' Credentialing Center (2016) Magnet credential must demonstrate that they meet five characteristics. These criteria have been associated with the ability to attract and retain nurses. APRNs are usually intimately involved in efforts to seek Magnet status, such as leading quality improvement initiatives, facilitating professional development of staff, and contributing to the establishment of policies and procedures that shape an environment in which effective collaboration can occur.

Finally, reducing error and increasing the reliability of care by adopting evidence-based practices constitute another significant institutional imperative to foster collaboration. Improvements that result from such initiatives are often tied to payment for the organization.

An example of the institutional imperative to collaborate has been the progression of the Doctor of Nursing Practice (DNP). The national concerns about the quality and safety of health care have informed the development of the DNP and helped form consensus among schools, faculty, and other stakeholders (AACN, 2004). The DNP Essentials (AACN, 2006) set collaboration as a core competency for this degree for APRNs. The document includes numerous mentions of the terms *collaboration* and *collaborative* in the competencies required for DNP graduates. Examples that require collaborative competencies include the ability to create change in health care delivery systems, the need to collaborate across settings to enhance population-based health care, and the need for interprofessional collaboration to implement practice guidelines and peer review processes (AACN, 2006). Current competencies for all APRN groups include competencies based on high-level communication and interprofessional practice skills.

Research Imperative to Study Collaboration

Schmitt (2011) suggested that collaboration be examined as an intermediate outcome when health care is evaluated. In a review of the literature, Schmitt cited a number of challenges faced by health services researchers in trying to understand collaboration and its impact on outcomes. Methodologic challenges include the need for more robust, well-designed studies, including clinical trials, to provide more conclusive evidence about the impact of collaboration on patient outcomes. In addition, sample selection, measurement of collaboration, and outcome measurement pose dilemmas for those interested in studying the phenomenon. A major limitation of existing knowledge is that much of it comes from hospital-based practice and, according to Schmitt, studies of collaboration and its outcomes are underdeveloped.

Institutional imperatives to collaborate and the research imperative to study collaboration are becoming more closely aligned. For example, the AHRQ has become an important resource for funding and disseminating the results of research on quality improvement, patient safety, adoption of evidence-based practices (EBPs), and other issues associated with the delivery of safe and reliable health care. Manojlovich et al. (2014) stressed the need to build a better safety climate through improved interprofessional collaboration.

In addition, the National Institutes of Health Common Fund continues to expect collaboration among clinical investigators. Drenning (2006) has urged collaboration among nurses, APRNs, and nurse researchers to understand and implement EBP changes likely to improve patient care.

The National Center for Interprofessional Practice and Education (2017) reports that it supports over 80 research projects across the United States to focus on interprofessional practice and education. The projects are evaluating how interprofessional practice can be used effectively in different clinical and learning environments. The focus is on clinical practice and community engagement through onsite training and classroom learning.

Collaboration among providers with different perspectives results in a creative and multidimensional intelligence that is emotionally rewarding because patients do better and clinicians derive personal and professional gratification from this work. This has implications for APRNs, administrators, clinicians, researchers, and others. APRNs and administrative and clinical colleagues need to assess the collaborative climate, determine facilitators and barriers, and work together to strengthen relationships while building an organizational culture that values collaboration. Researchers must help APRNs and administrators understand the structures and processes associated with collaboration and the extent to which collaboration affects patient and utilization outcomes.

Context of Collaboration in Contemporary Health Care

The pressures on APRNs and others to improve quality, work more efficiently, and allow others to be involved in decisions about patient care could be expected to foster collaboration among clinicians. Paradoxically, these same factors may undermine collaboration. As APRNs practice autonomously and collaboratively, other clinicians have experienced concerns including the increasing supply of APRN providers, which can encroach on the autonomy of others and their willingness to collaborate. Pressures on some physicians may generate concern about relinquishing authority and power and fears that may cause individuals to withdraw from or sabotage efforts to collaborate. Moreover, collaboration can also take more up front time, which may appear to decrease efficiency but improves outcomes and saves time in the long run. Thus the transition to a presumably more effective, accessible, and efficient health care system may actually undermine collaboration

In addition, confusion about scope of practice can be damaging to collaboration for all involved. Other independent practitioners may ask themselves the following (Safriet, 2002):

- What's in it for me to collaborate?
- What areas of my work do I get to expand because other providers can do things that I have traditionally done?

APRNs may be uncertain about how to proceed with collaboration, for example, when they are asked to assume responsibility for a new skill such as performing an invasive procedure. The reality is that regulatory initiatives and payment structures are rearranging collaborative relationships frequently. These changes are often at the heart of the tension associated with collaboration among players as the roles and boundaries of disciplines have blurred and expanded.

Incentives and Opportunities for Collaboration

Efforts to reduce costs and improve quality of health care provide APRNs, other clinicians, and administrators with common goals toward which to work and with opportunities for learning from each other. National interdisciplinary guidelines and standards of care are intended to reduce unwarranted and often expensive variations in health care. Many guidelines specify interdisciplinary collaboration as a critical component of effective care. Standards and guidelines developed and agreed on by interdisciplinary groups, whether at the local (office or institution), national, or international level, offer a sound starting point for jointly determining patient care goals, processes, and outcomes. Accreditation activities offer another opportunity to build collaborative relationships. The Joint Commission requires documentation that demonstrates collaborative, interdisciplinary practice to help providers develop stronger interdisciplinary approaches to care. The need for a highly coordinated system of chronic care management led the Health Sciences Institute to promulgate interdisciplinary competencies. The goals for chronic illness care, which include promoting health and preventing disease, managing disease and disease impacts, and promoting consumer independence and life quality, are centered on a model in which all players are valued for their contributions and collaborative effort.

The move toward a more community-based, health promotion and disease prevention model of care has also been creating new opportunities for collaborative practice in primary care (Bodenheimer & Grumbach, 2012). The use of telehealth and electronic health records also offers creative opportunities for interaction. For these systems to work, APRNs and other clinicians need to be involved in selecting, piloting, modifying, and implementing new technologies. From the selection of vendors to full deployment of the technology, the adoption of new technologies offers opportunities for clinicians to develop collaborative learning communities. In the current global market, innovative new alliances among advanced practice nursing groups and physician groups need to be developed and nurtured (McCaffrey et al., 2010; Young et al., 2012).

Barriers to Collaboration

Implementing effective collaborative professional relationships in the workplace can be challenging. Barriers to collaboration exist and can be characterized as professional, sociocultural, organizational, and regulatory. Part of the challenge is that team members see themselves primarily as representatives of their own discipline rather than as members of a collaborative team.

Disciplinary Barriers

The way health professional education is conducted in the United States has long been a barrier to successful collaboration. Each profession is a culture with its own values, knowledge, rules, and norms, and education programs reflect this culture. Additionally, education programs are frequently conducted at different types of colleges and universities where there may be little opportunity for shared learning. The basic epistemology that underlies each type of profession may be unique and, at times, may conflict with that of other professions. This leads to differences in understanding what constitutes truth, goals of practice, and expected outcomes even when there is joint practice. One profession may firmly believe that it is the only one that has the whole picture for the patient, as evidenced by the continuing efforts to place CRNAs under physician supervision (see Chapter 18). Similar issues are seen at times for NPs and CNMs. Pharmacists may believe that they are the single authority for questions concerning medication. In an evaluation of the Hartford Foundation initiative to strengthen interdisciplinary team training in geriatrics (Reuben et al., 2004), faculty and students in advanced practice nursing, medicine, and social work were found to be influenced by disciplinary attitudes and cultural factors that were obstacles to teamwork, a phenomenon the authors termed *disciplinary split*. They observed that disciplinary heritage and a differential willingness to participate in teamwork characterized disciplinary split and constituted an obstacle to implementing effective interdisciplinary teamwork in geriatrics training.

There are few opportunities for interdisciplinary education as health care providers learn their professions. The RWJF Partnerships for Training initiative (Rice et al., 2010; RWJF, 2003; Young et al., 2012) identified many of the stresses inherent in building and sustaining interprofessional academic-community partnerships. Stresses encountered by participants as they developed partnerships centered on money, differing agendas, systems that were not integrated, varying philosophies, and long-held beliefs about how things should be done.

Collaboration is often easier to implement and maintain at the community grassroots level than at the professional organizational level. Although collaboration happens daily among practicing clinicians, collaboration may not exist at the national level, impeding efforts to move toward a coordinated health care system. The dated positions espoused by some policymakers from all disciplines may be based on stereotyped beliefs about disciplinary roles and responsibilities, rather than reflecting consideration of the issues or what is best for patients. These factors make it increasingly important for APRNs and other clinicians practicing at local levels who have learned the art of collaboration to take an active role in bringing their perspectives and experiences to policymaking at institutional, community, state, and national levels to foster collaboration. A broader statutory definition of professional autonomy for APRNs than what is found in many states is necessary if the more complex autonomy of interdependent collaborators is to be exercised effectively (Lugo, O'Grady, Hodnicki, & Hanson, 2007; Safriet, 2002).

Despite these existing challenges to collaboration, there is evidence of progress. The US Preventive Services Task Force, which is part of the federal AHRQ, is made up of an interdisciplinary group of providers and researchers who develop, disperse, and revise evidence-based recommendations on screening and prevention for a variety of health care concerns (US Preventive Services Task Force, 2012).

Ineffective Communication and Team Dysfunction

Communication styles may also be a barrier to collaboration. Dysfunctional styles of interactions among health care professionals that particularly undermine collaboration include being difficult, bullying, or abusive (Anderson, 2011). The term *disruptive behavior* has been used to include these and other intimidating behaviors. Clinicians whose behavior is disruptive display arrogance, rudeness, and poor communication (Longo & Smith, 2011; Saxton, Hines, & Enriquez, 2009). APRNs have a responsibility to recognize disruptive behaviors as risks to collaboration and safe patient care and to develop a repertoire of interpersonal and system strategies with which to address these behaviors directly and promptly.

Lencioni (2005), a business consultant on team effectiveness, has proposed a model of team dysfunction that has a practical use by APRNs. In this model, the first four of the five dysfunctions reflect the absence of key components of our definition of collaboration: absence of trust, fear of conflict, lack of commitment, and avoidance of accountability. The fifth dysfunction, inattention to results, is consistent with the observation that efforts within health care to improve safety, reliability, and quality represent an opportunity to foster teamwork and collaboration by examining the processes and outcomes of care, attending to results.

Sociocultural Issues

Tradition, role, and gender stereotypes are obstacles to collaboration (Rafferty, Ball, & Aiken, 2001). Safriet (1992) has suggested that the field of medicine staked out broad professional territory early on and considers any movement into this turf by other clinicians, at any level, to be unacceptable. This bias can lead to challenges to successful collaboration.

Nursing remains a predominantly female profession and, despite the influx of women into medicine, pharmacy, and dentistry, gender role stereotypes still exist and affect collaboration. Gender stereotypes dominate images of staff nurses in the media and how APRNs are commonly portrayed on television. However, the rules are changing as all of health care becomes increasingly female.

Stereotypical images of APRNs influence how they are viewed by consumers, and this can be positive. Australia has only had very limited experience with NPs in primary care. Parker et al. (2012) asked consumers in five Australian states their thoughts about receiving their primary care from NPs. Almost none of the consumers had any knowledge about what NPs were. The consumers indicated that they highly valued registered nurses and that NPs would be very acceptable for their primary care since they were registered nurses who could also prescribe drugs and authorize referrals.

Organizational Barriers

Competitive situations arise that can interfere with collaboration. The patchwork of US federal and state policies, rules, and regulations along with organizational rules and policies concerning APRN practice can make collaboration difficult. This set of rules can also lead to unproductive competition among clinicians. For example, the intent of Medicare billing requirements was to foster cooperation among clinicians, but they also discourage collaborative relations between health care providers and may actually serve as disincentives. "Incident-to" billing (see Chapter 21) requires that patient care services provided by APRNs be directly supervised by physicians and offers reimbursement inequities, severely hampering a collaborative environment (Centers for Medicare and Medicaid Services, 2016).

Regulatory Barriers

Legislation and regulations pose a number of barriers to the implementation of collaborative roles. In the early days of advanced practice nursing, the overlap in APRNs' and physicians' scopes of practice was often addressed by requiring physician supervision of aspects of APRN practice. An outcome of this early requirement was that physician supervision often appeared in advanced practice nursing literature on collaboration and in state practice acts and regulations. In the past 30 years, there has been a slow but steady movement away from references to protocols and language requiring physician supervision toward emphasizing consultation, collaboration, peer review, and use of referral (Lugo et al., 2007).

APRN practice based on joint purposes and the public interest is more likely to foster collaboration between the professions (ACA, 2010; IOM, 2011; Safriet, 2002). A supervision requirement precludes the development of a collaborative relationship and physicians cannot supervise advanced practice nurses.

Eliminating regulatory barriers to full practice authority has been one of the pillars of the IOM work in *The Future of Nursing* (2011). Substantial work continues to remove these and other barriers for APRNs throughout the United States. Similar efforts are taking place in other countries as they discover that creating artificial barriers to full practice is counter to national goals of access to high-quality care for their people (Carter, Owen-Williams, & Della, 2015).

Adopting a multistate licensure compact for APRNs has become important to ensure that collaboration and continuity of care can occur (NCSBN, 2017). Consumers are consulting quality scorecards, licensing boards, websites, blogs, and other Internet resources to identify agencies and individual clinicians who provide the best health care.

Opportunities to create collaborative relationships can be lost during rapid changes in health care (Remonder et al., 2010; Young et al., 2012). Furthermore, nurses and other clinicians who are confronting their own professional concerns may not fully appreciate the stresses that others experience in today's volatile market. This factor is a serious deterrent to collaborative relationships.

Collaboration within the APRN nursing community is also problematic at times. Overall, there are four dimensions of APRN regulation—licensure, accreditation, certification, and education. Often, language and policy barriers make it difficult for the groups responsible for each of these to collaborate. These groups have created a collaborative network that allows them to match their individual organizational priorities to the priorities for APRNs overall. Exemplar 12.3 describes this effort and illustrates how an initial

---

EXEMPLAR 12.3 **A Long-Term Collaboration for the Education and Regulation of Advanced Practice Registered Nurses (APRNs)**

The implementation of the Consensus Model for APRN Regulation is an exemplary illustration of how collaboration works to accomplish a challenging component of advanced practice nursing.

In the United States, the board of nursing in each state has the responsibility and authority to regulate nursing at the beginning and advanced levels. In the 1990s there was a rapid proliferation of educational programs and certification processes for postgraduate education, particularly for nurse practitioners. The National Council of State Boards of Nursing was confronted with an array of different and potentially confusing sets of credentials that varied from state to state. There had been a long history of practice by nurse anesthetists and nurse-midwives but these roles were regulated by the nursing board in some states and by the medical board in others. Multiple new nurse practitioner programs were developing and often in narrow areas such as pediatric oncology or palliative care. Emerging from what had become confusing regulation was the creation of the Consensus Model for APRN Regulation: Licensure, Accreditation, Certification and Education.

Over 70 nursing organizations engaged in high-level collaboration to bring the consensus process for APRN regulation into successful implementation. Currently, interacting through a social media entity entitled LACE, nursing legislators, accreditors, certifiers, and educators accomplish the difficult and challenging work of implementing the Consensus Model for APRN Regulation across all states. As implementation of this model evolves, a more seamless practice environment for APRNs exists across all states. In most cases, the state legislatures and the governors must pass legislation to meet the new standards for education and certification as well as recognize independent practice and independent prescribing by all four roles of APRNs. Progress is being made each year to achieve this goal of common recognition.

Prior to this work, there were very few examples of nationwide collaboration among APRN nurse associations, educators, certifiers, accreditors, and the member boards of nursing. Through this important collaboration, this work continues today with regularly scheduled meetings and recognition of the consensus process. ◎

failure to collaborate can turn into a win-win situation for all involved.

Processes Associated With Effective Collaboration

Recurring Interactions

A trusting and collaborative relationship develops over time and depends on recurring, meaningful interactions (Alberto & Herth, 2009). Development of trust particularly takes place over time. This means that collaborative relationships are difficult to develop in organizations in which there is a high staff turnover or frequent rotation of clinicians, such as with house staff physicians. A series of less-complicated interactions that have been clinical or personal will contribute to the development of trust in collaborative relationships. Team members need recurring interactions to acquire an understanding of each other's backgrounds, roles, and functions and develop patterns of interaction that are constructive, productive, and supportive. Projects focused on quality and outcomes of care that involve joint collection and analysis of data build collegiality and foster collaboration. Membership on interdisciplinary committees, such as pharmacy and therapeutics, performance improvement, institutional review boards, ethics, and others with a patient care focus, also foster communication and collegiality.

Effective Conflict Negotiation and Resolution Skills

Conflict will arise as individuals, teams, and organizations work more closely together on their shared goals. APRNs need to have some general approaches to conflict negotiation and resolution. Box 12.3 lists some key conflict resolution skills (Conflict Resolution Network, 2016).

Partnering and Team Building

Health care leaders are examining ways to improve the functioning of teams (Bosque, 2011; IPEC, 2011). Effective models of teamwork have been used in subspecialties in psychology and health care. APRNs can draw on the lessons learned in these fields to improve team functioning. Some of the processes that have been associated with effective team building and conflict negotiation are listed in Box 12.3. Partnering is often a long-term process over several years with different partners, as illustrated in Exemplar 12.3.

BOX 12.3   Conflict Resolution Network's 12 Skills Summary

- Win-win approach (How can we solve this as partners rather than opponents?)
- Creative response (Transform problems into creative opportunities.)
- Empathy (Develop communication tools to build rapport; use listening to clarify understanding.)
- Appropriate assertiveness (Apply strategies to attack the problem, not the person.)
- Cooperative power (Eliminate "power over" to build "power with" others.)
- Managing emotions (Express fear, anger, hurt, and frustration wisely to effect change.)
- Willingness to resolve (Name personal issues that cloud the picture.)
- Mapping the conflict (Define the issues needed to chart common needs and concerns.)
- Development of options (Design creative solutions together.)
- Introduction to negotiation (Plan and apply effective strategies to reach agreement.)
- Introduction to mediation (Help conflicting parties to move toward solutions.)
- Broadening perspectives (Evaluate the problem in the broader context.)

Adapted from Conflict Resolution Network. (2016). 12 Skills summary: Conflict resolution skills. Retrieved from http://www.crnhq.org/12-Skills-Summary.aspx?rw=c.

Implementing Collaboration

There are times when APRNs may feel as though they are the only ones with an active commitment to collaboration. Collaboration may be the most difficult competency to accomplish because it is mediated by social processes such as attitudinal and cultural factors that are ingrained in their professions or in society. Efforts to change the environment to one that is more collaborative involve proving oneself over and over and challenging colleagues' behaviors that restrain attempts to work together. These intrapersonal demands, along with clinical demands, can be exhausting. Therefore APRNs need to evaluate the potential for collaboration when seeking career opportunities. Questions about how clinicians work together, the degree of hierarchy, the interpersonal climate, and organizational structures that support collaboration should be a high priority. A realistic appraisal of collaboration is needed to determine whether APRNs can provide the standards and quality of care that are characteristic of advanced practice nursing and whether they can expect a reasonable level of job satisfaction.

Assessment of Personal and Environmental Factors

APRNs bring many personal attributes to a professional partnership. Assessment of their current attributes compared to the characteristics of collaboration listed in Box 12.4 can help beginning APRNs to determine the areas most in need of development.

Covey (1989) offered a perspective on moving toward a higher level of interdependence with colleagues. He portrayed interdependence as a higher level of performance than independence. Only individuals who have gained competence and confidence in their own expertise are able to move beyond autonomy and independence toward the higher synergistic level of collaboration. Collaboration appears to have the same meaning as interdependence in Covey's work. This view is provocative when one considers the hierarchical context that often frames clinical collaboration. The notion that interdependence is the higher level of performance is supported in the evolution of advanced practice nursing. A number of clinical specialties are evolving to such a stage as disciplines mature and identify a shared interprofessional component to their work. For example, in the specialty of diabetes, advanced diabetes management involves

interprofessional collaboration (Gucciardi, Espin, Morganti, & Dorado, 2016) and is recognized by a certification examination open to a number of disciplines (see Chapter 5).

Teams are expected to collaborate with patients and their families in addition to each other. This collaborative relationship can be problematic for clinicians and/or patients. Saxton et al. (2009) suggested that when patients are abrasive or ill-equipped to deal with conflict, clinicians should remember to treat these patients with dignity and respect, even when disagreeing with them, and remember that a patient is more than his or her illness. In addition, illness can interfere with or diminish a patient's normal or effective communication skills. Crocker and Johnson (2006) found that patients may assert themselves by honoring their body's wisdom and firing caregivers whom they view as not compassionate. Self-assessment is one important component to consider when embarking on a new professional relationship or evaluating the success or failure of current or potential collaborative relationships. The self-directed questions in Box 12.4 may help individuals identify personal strengths and weaknesses. APRNs should also consider contextual factors in the systems in which they practice.

Administrative leadership plays a key role in the development of collaborative relationships among organizational members. Administrators who support team and interprofessional administrative models, and who are themselves good communicators, can do a great deal to increase the momentum of new collaborations. The common vision of quality patient care and provider satisfaction makes collaboration a worthy goal for APRNs and nursing administrators.

Global interactions require high levels of individual and organizational collaboration beyond what can be envisioned. APRNs who recognize the need for global participation and collaboration at the personal, organizational, and systems levels are more likely to be successful.

Strategies for Successful Collaboration

Individual Strategies

Box 12.5 lists strategies that promote collaboration (Rider, 2002). APRNs can examine their interactions for opportunities to implement these ideas and strengthen their interpersonal competence.

One strategy is for APRNs to promote their exemplary nursing practices to help other health

---

 BOX 12.4   **Personal Strengths and Weaknesses Strategies**

- Am I clear about my role in the partnership?
- What values do I bring to the relationship?
- What do I expect to gain or lose by collaborating?
- What do others expect of me?
- Do I feel good about my contribution to the team?
- Do I feel self-confident and competent in the collaborative relationship?
- Are there anxieties causing repeated friction that have not been addressed?
- Has serious thought been given to the boundaries of the collaborative relationship?

Adapted from Rider, E. (2002). Twelve strategies for effective communication and collaboration in medical teams. *BMJ Clinical Research, 325,* S45.

BOX 12.5 **Strategies to Promote Effective Communication and Collaboration**

- Be respectful and professional.
- Listen intently.
- Understand the other person's viewpoint before expressing your opinion.
- Model an attitude of collaboration, and expect it.
- Identify the bottom line.
- Decide what is negotiable and non-negotiable.
- Acknowledge the other person's thoughts and feelings.
- Pay attention to your own ideas and what you have to offer to the group.
- Be cooperative without losing integrity.
- Be direct.
- Identify common, shared goals, and concerns.
- State your feelings using "I" statements.
- Do not take things personally.
- Learn to say "I was wrong" or "You could be right."
- Do not feel pressure to agree instantly.
- Think about possible solutions before meeting and be willing to adapt if a more creative alternative is presented.
- Think of conflict negotiation and resolution as a helical process, not a linear one; recognize that negotiation may occur over several interactions.

Adapted from Rider, E. (2002). Twelve strategies for effective communication and collaboration in medical teams. *BMJ Clinical Research, 325*, S45.

professionals and consumers better understand the strengths of APRNs as health care providers (Pohl et al., 2010). Participating in interdisciplinary quality improvement initiatives and developing and evaluating EBP guidelines (see Chapter 10) are other ways to engage with colleagues within and across disciplines. One way to share excellence in practice in grand rounds or a team conference is to include the opportunity for each care team member to describe her or his own decision making about patients and suggest new strategies for care to the team.

Team Strategies

The development of effective teams was one of the IOM's recommendations for improving health care quality (ACA, 2010). Lencioni's field guide (2005) provides activities aimed at helping team members overcome the team dysfunctions described earlier,

noting that there are two important questions team members must ask themselves:

- Are we really a team?
- Are we ready to do the heavy lifting that will be required to become a team?

A group of collaborators will be able to use the field guide to their advantage if they can respond affirmatively to both questions. The activities are aimed at helping teams address each of the five dysfunctions by helping them build trust, master conflict, achieve commitment, embrace accountability, and focus on results.

One serious challenge to collaboration is team members who are not interested in developing collaborative teams. In this type of situation, APRNs must step up and operate from a stance and expectation of collaboration; that is, APRNs should model collaboration in all interactions and expect the same from all other members of the team. Building a group of like-minded colleagues can also increase the momentum toward collaboration as the expected style of interaction within a team. APRNs should understand that collaboration is only beginning to be taught in health professions schools. Consequently, they must be prepared to teach this process to others.

A recent concept is the idea of a group visit by a collaborative group of providers. The group visit can be understood as an extended office visit during which not just physical and medical needs are met, but educational, psychological, and social concerns are also addressed by a collaborative group of caregivers invested in caring for the patient (Burke & O'Grady, 2012; Young et al., 2012). A suggested starting point might include consideration of ways to plan ahead before starting collaborative group visits, how to let patients know about the new change, who needs to be part of the collaborative provider group, who does what, and an agenda for the visit (Bodenheimer & Grumbach, 2012). An example of a group visit practice that includes an NP, a CNS, and a CNM is "Centering Pregnancy: A New Program for Adolescent Prenatal Care" (Moeller, Vezeau, & Carr, 2007). The great significance of the group visit is the inclusion of the patient as part of the group and the cost-effective use of resources to address multiple aspects of the patient's care.

Working together on joint projects is an excellent way to facilitate collaboration. Collaborative research and scholarly writing projects, as well as community service projects that tap into the strengths of various members, demonstrate the benefits of collaboration. These strategies move across lines from personal life to organizational settings and from education to practice arenas. New models that foster team care are needed in primary care and within specialty practice in all settings. More importantly, collaboratively developed practice guidelines improve communication and clarify clinicians' roles in patient treatment (Cooper, 2007; US Preventive Services Task Force, 2012).

Organizational Strategies

The numerous initiatives to improve safety and quality that have evolved from the IOM reports can help health administrators and leaders create organizational structures that facilitate collaboration while attending to important quality and safety goals. The IHI's white papers, The Joint Commission and Magnet requirements for evidence of interdisciplinary collaboration in patient care, toolkits for interdisciplinary education, and clinical and organizational toolkits to facilitate the adoption of EBP guidelines (e.g., from the Registered Nurses Association of Ontario [http://rnao.ca/bpg]) are available. These toolkits often include assessments that can be done to identify the location of the barriers and the opportunities for improvement. APRNs and other clinical colleagues and leaders can use these assessments to develop strategic plans for improving the collaborative environment. Clinicians may need professional development to enable them to collaborate depending on the results of the assessment.

Organizational leaders must take seriously reports of disruptive behavior and take action to eliminate this behavior. Kinnaman and Bleich (2004) have observed that collaboration requires more resources and suggested that the type of problem-solving behavior should be matched to the degree of complexity and uncertainty inherent in the problem. APRNs will find it useful to pay attention to the costs in time, money, resources, and patient outcomes of collaborating and not collaborating. Documenting positive and negative patient and institutional outcomes of collaboration or its absence can contribute to identifying which clinical resources are needed to achieve clinical and institutional goals.

One strategy that fosters successful collaboration is a move toward interdisciplinary education programs that allow for face-to-face interaction and joint problem solving among health science students (Alberto & Herth, 2009; Bainbridge et al., 2010; Petri, 2010). Definitive changes in the structure of clinical education and sequencing of content will be required. This will be a difficult task given the entrenched bureaucracies involved and will require stronger interactions among education programs. Health care providers need to be learning about health policy issues from a perspective that offers broad solutions. Faculty across programs need to be evaluating and treating patients and supervising students together. Joint appointments among the faculty of different professions provide the opportunities to model advanced practice nursing care and build rapport.

Health professional organizations have endorsed the shift toward a collaborative model (IHI, 2017a; NCSBN et al., 2006). As noted, there are some successful models of consensus building in some sectors of health care. These models, across disciplines, must be replicated more widely in health care if barriers to successful interprofessional collaboration are to be reduced.

Exemplar 12.4 is an example of how APRNs from different specialties can work together to alter a hospital policy. They pooled the expertise in their particular specialty and their knowledge of the political issues that often surround hospital-based work. They knew that if they wanted to make this change, the key players in the decision-making process would have to buy into the idea. The usual pattern is not to change because past policy and procedures have been in place and there is substantial pressure not to change something that is viewed as working. The pull of the familiar was in place, yet it was not working for the mothers who wanted different options available to them.

These APRNs all knew that in their facility, policy approval was the purview of the medical staff. They would have to be included to make this change. Also, the hospital was governed by strong department chairs in medicine and they would also have to agree. These APRNs well understood that science, although critically important, was not sufficient to bring about this change. All the stakeholders had to be included. The APRNs knew which parts of the policy were open for negotiation and which were not, and crafted their proposal cleverly. This change did not happen quickly; several months were required to gain the support of all the key players. However, in the end, the women who used the birthing center were greatly advantaged by the collaborative efforts of all involved.

Conclusion

Many of the barriers to successful collaboration occur because of values, beliefs, and behaviors that have until recently gone unchallenged in society and in the organizations in which nurses practice. Radical change is needed if the conditions conducive to

Ms. Smith is a certified nurse-midwife (CNM) who provides full-scope midwifery services to women who choose this approach for pregnancy and delivery. The birthing center at which Ms. Smith attends the delivery by her patients has a policy that women must choose no analgesia during labor and delivery or they must have an epidural. Many of the women were not happy with having only two choices. Some women believed that they might need some help with the pain of delivery but did not want to be confined to labor in a bed by use of the traditional epidural anesthesia. Ms. Smith investigated this issue and found that the policy seemed to have been developed in the past by a committee that consisted of obstetrics and gynecology (OB-GYN) physicians and anesthesiologists. The policy was approved by the medical staff. No mothers, CNMs, or certified registered nurse anesthetists (CRNAs) were part of the policy making. There have been a number of advances in care since this policy was developed, and Ms. Smith wished to bring about a change to improve care to the mothers and their families.

In this particular facility, only anesthesia providers (physician or CRNA) were credentialed to administer any analgesic or anesthetic agents, a practice touted as necessary for the quality of care for recipients of these agents. Ms. Smith did not believe that she would be able to alter this policy, nor did she really wish to do so. However, she wanted to provide an expanded set of options for her mothers. Although many of the mothers did not choose to receive any analgesia for labor or delivery, they wanted to have the option available prior to needing it.

Ms. Smith consulted with a CRNA colleague who specialized in obstetric anesthesia. They met and discussed a number of options and decided that there were types of epidural approaches that could allow the mother to continue to walk while in labor and thereby improve the likelihood of a normal vaginal birth. Also, additional approaches were added to the list of available agents. One was a handheld device that delivered inhaled nitrous oxide when the mother thought she needed it. The services of a pediatric nurse practitioner were requested because the advanced practice registered nurses (APRNs) believed that the substantial literature on the topic indicated that newborns have better outcomes if the mother does not receive a standard epidural and that normal vaginal birth could be encouraged.

This trio of APRNs crafted the new policy proposal; engaged support from the Chair of OB-GYN, Chair of Pediatrics, Chair of Anesthesiology, and nursing supervisor; and advanced the change in policy to the medical staff committee. After a great deal of argument, discussion, and negotiation, the policy was changed and approved by the hospital board. Now, women could choose from a wide range of approaches that best met their wishes and particular situations. This group of APRNs knew that there were some parts of the policy that would not change, including the administration of anesthetics by anesthesia providers only. Also, all the anesthesiologists and CRNAs who provided obstetric anesthesia were not equally adept at all the new approaches, so the CRNA provided in-service education for them. The nursing staff of the birthing center needed additional training and the CNM provided this education, along with the CRNA. Although the change in policy was created to accommodate the wishes of the patients in the midwifery practice, the outcome was that all women who delivered in the facility now had options that improved their satisfaction and quality of care. In addition, all the APRN caregivers believed that they had enhanced the labor experience of their maternity patients. ◎

collaboration are to become the norm. Collaborative relationships not only are professionally satisfying but also improve access to care and patient outcomes. Although APRNs collaborate successfully with many individuals within and outside of nursing, they may find that one of their most important collaborative relationships—with physicians—may also be the most challenging. Despite the fact that there are many successful individual APRN-physician collaborative practices, including many with evidence demonstrating their beneficial effects on health care, tradition and stereotypes are often powerful negative influences on policymaking and in health care and professional organizations.

To meet the demands for cost-effectiveness and quality, clinicians from all disciplines have been meeting together to discuss the care they provide and to define ways to deliver it to maximize quality and minimize duplication of effort. These interactions foster the trust and respect required for mature collaboration. They enable collaborators to recognize their interdependence and value the input of others, thus creating a synergy that improves the quality of clinical decision making. Systems citizenship starts with seeing the systems we have shaped and that in turn shape us (Friedman, 2005). Collaboration becomes a priority as global interconnectedness enters our everyday interactions in the complex health care arena in which APRNs practice. In today's health care environment, collaboration may flourish, regardless of the barriers identified in this chapter.

Key Summary Points

- There is a need for a better understanding of the organizational structures, communication processes, and interactive styles that enable clinicians to collaborate in ways that benefit clinical processes and outcomes.
- APRNs can contribute to this understanding in several ways:
  - By documenting and analyzing their experiences with collaboration in published case studies;

- By serving as preceptors for students and helping them develop the skills essential for collaboration; and
- By working with researchers who are studying the characteristics and clinical implications of collaboration.
- Effective collaboration must be at the heart of any redesign of the health care delivery system whether that redesign occurs in a unit, in a clinic, within and between organizations, or globally.

References

To access the references for this chapter, use your smartphone's QR code reader to scan the code below, or go to http://booksite.elsevier.com/9780323447751.

Ethical Decision Making

Lucia Wocial

> *"The very first requirement in a hospital is that it should do the sick no harm."*
>
> *—Florence Nightingale*

CHAPTER CONTENTS

Nurses in all areas of health care routinely encounter disturbing moral issues, yet the success with which these dilemmas are resolved varies significantly. Because nurses have a unique relationship with the patient and family, the moral position of nursing in the health care arena is distinct. As the complexity of issues intensifies, the role of the advanced practice registered nurse (APRN) becomes particularly important in the identification, deliberation, and resolution of complicated and difficult moral problems. Although all nurses are moral agents, APRNs are expected to be not just leaders in recognizing and resolving moral problems, but role models, creating ethical practice environments and promoting social justice in the larger health care system. They are expected to exercise their moral agency; that is, fulfill their obligation to act to do good work. It is a basic tenet of the central

definition of advanced practice nursing (see Chapter 3) that skill in ethical decision making is one of the core competencies of all APRNs. In addition, the Doctor of Nursing Practice (DNP) essential competencies emphasize leadership in developing and evaluating strategies to manage ethical dilemmas in patient care and organizational arenas (American Association of Colleges of Nursing [AACN], 2006). This chapter explores the distinctive ethical decision-making competency of advanced practice nursing, the process of developing and evaluating this competency, and barriers to ethical practice that APRNs can expect to confront.

Foundations of Ethical Practice

Perhaps one of the biggest challenges for APRNs in attaining competence in ethical decision making is the path taken to become an APRN. Some individuals will pursue APRN education after years of clinical practice and others will begin practice as an APRN

The author would like to acknowledge Ann B. Hamric and Sarah A. Delgado for their work on previous editions of this chapter.

with no experience in nursing. As a profession, we expect nurses to demonstrate everyday ethical comportment, to integrate a strong moral competence into every aspect of nursing practice (Benner, Sutphen, Leonard, & Day, 2010). This requires at the very least cultivating one's moral sensitivity, which is an individual's capacity, acquired through experience, to sense the moral significance of a situation (Lützén, Dahlqvist, Eriksson, & Norberg, 2006). This necessitates a capacity to distinguish between feelings, facts, and values and reflect on these with the ability to articulate what is good, recognizing that defining what is good can be fraught with pitfalls if one has not engaged in rigorous self-reflection of personal values and potential biases (Feister, 2015).

Evidence suggests that when people face ethical decisions, they engage in mental processes outside their conscious awareness (may rely on intuition) and their decisions may be affected by their emotional state (Guzak, 2015). Ethically challenging situations often evoke strong emotions. Guarding against emotional responses in ethically challenging situations requires APRNs to rigorously and continuously practice self-awareness, becoming exquisitely sensitive to their own hidden biases, which in turn helps them develop strong moral agency. The Code of Ethics for Nurses includes a provision calling attention to the duties nurses owe to themselves, including preservation of wholeness of character and integrity (ANA, 2015). This attention to the self enables nurses to hold themselves and others accountable even and especially in emotionally charged situations.

One often overlooked element of ethical practice is a deep understanding of dignity and the role it plays in fostering positive relationships. While each of us desires to be treated with dignity, we have an innate talent for lashing out when we feel our dignity is violated. Our default is to attack, which contributes to a cycle of psychologic warfare against others, effectively destroying relationships and poisoning the environment (Hicks, 2003). When we learn to embrace the essential elements of dignity (Table 13.1), we can overcome our autopilot and promote healthy human relationships, which are essential for an ethical environment. Exemplar 13.1 is a brief but powerful example of how an APRN demonstrates how to honor dignity through everyday ethical comportment.

Characteristics of Ethical Challenges in Nursing

In this chapter, the terms *ethics* and *morality* or *morals* are used interchangeably (see Beauchamp

⊚ TABLE 13.1	**Ten Essential Elements of Dignity**
1. Acceptance of Identity	Approach people as neither inferior nor superior to you; give others the freedom to express their authentic selves without fear of being negatively judged; interact without prejudice or bias, accepting how race, religion, gender, class, sexual orientation, age, disability, and so on are at the core of their identities; assume they have integrity.
2. Recognition	Validate others for their talents, hard work, thoughtfulness, and help; be generous with praise; give credit to others for their contributions, ideas, and experience.
3. Acknowledgement	Give people your full attention by listening, hearing, validating, and responding to their concerns and what they have been through.
4. Inclusion	Make others feel that they belong at all levels of relationship (family, community, organization, nation).
5. Safety	Put people at ease on two levels: physically, where they feel free of bodily harm; and psychologically, where they feel free of concern about being shamed or humiliated and feel free to speak without fear of retribution.
6. Fairness	Treat people justly, with equality, and in an evenhanded way according to agreed upon laws and rules.
7. Independence	Empower people to act on their own behalf so that they feel in control of their lives and experience a sense of hope and possibility.
8. Understanding	Believe that what others think matters; give them the chance to explain their perspectives and express their points of view; actively listen in order to understand them.
9. Benefit of the Doubt	Treat people as trustworthy; start with the premise that others have good motives and are acting with integrity.
10. Accountability	Take responsibility for your actions; if you have violated the dignity of another, apologize; make a commitment to change hurtful behaviors.

Adapted from Hicks, D. (2011). The dignity model. Retrieved from http://www.pyeglobal.org/wp-content/uploads/2013/09/Summary_of_Dignity_Model.pdf.

EXEMPLAR 13.1	Clinical Situation Demonstrating Everyday Ethical Comportment: Honoring Dignity[a]

Lori is a clinical nurse specialist who is eager to promote evidence-based practice changes. Armed with the latest research demonstrating the effectiveness of simple interventions to reduce urinary catheter–related infections, she encounters Kathy, a busy direct care nurse. Following Hicks' (2003) essential elements of dignity (see Table 13.1), Lori approaches Kathy as a colleague, not one who has superior knowledge. Lori knows Kathy has not attended her in-service program outlining the new protocol and, rather than mention that, Lori acknowledges the heavy patient assignment Kathy is managing and complements her on her organization. When Kathy mentions that there is an order for a routine culture of the urinary catheter, Lori takes the opportunity to explain key points from the new protocol. Lori cheerfully offers to contact the physician, giving him the benefit of the doubt that he did not realize there was a new nurse-led protocol to guide appropriate removal of urinary catheters and check cultures only when a patient is symptomatic. Despite Lori's best efforts, Kathy feels that Lori has not been responsive to the workload she faces and lashes out at Lori, suggesting she is pushing this new protocol simply because it will save money. Lori does not respond to Kathy's heated comments. She instead helps Kathy focus on the primary goal, reducing the risk of infection for the patient. Lori offers to help Kathy remove the catheter, and makes several suggestions to assure the patient has assistance to void, including returning in an hour to help Kathy monitor the patient to make sure he has assistance to void. ◎

[a]Thanks to Lori Alesia, MN, CNS, RN, for her assistance with this exemplar.

& Childress, 2012, for a discussion of the distinctions between these terms). A problem becomes an ethical or moral problem when issues of core values or fundamental obligations are present. An *ethical* or *moral dilemma* occurs when obligations require or appear to require that a person adopt two (or more) alternative actions, but the person cannot carry out all the required alternatives. The agent experiences tension because of the moral obligations resulting from the dilemma of differing and opposing demands (Beauchamp & Childress, 2012; Doherty & Purtilo, 2016). In some moral dilemmas, the agent must choose between equally unacceptable alternatives; that is, both may have elements that are morally unsatisfactory. For example, based on her evaluation, a family nurse practitioner (FNP) may suspect that a patient is a victim of domestic violence, although the patient denies it. The FNP is faced with two options that are both ethically troubling: connect the patient with existing social services, possibly straining the family and jeopardizing the FNP-patient relationship, or avoid intervention and potentially allow the violence to continue. As described by Silva and Ludwick (2002), honoring the FNP's desire to prevent harm (the principle of nonmaleficence) justifies reporting the suspicion, whereas respect for the patient's autonomy justifies the opposite course of action.

Jameton (1984, 1993) has distinguished two additional types of moral problems from the classic moral dilemma, which he termed *moral uncertainty* and *moral distress*. In situations of moral uncertainty, the nurse experiences unease and questions the right course of action. When nurses experience moral distress, they believe that they know the ethically appropriate action but feel constrained from carrying out that action because of institutional obstacles (e.g., lack of time or supervisory support, physician power, institutional policies, legal constraints). There is growing recognition that moral distress is a complex construct with considerable debate over an exact definition (Fourie, 2015; Hamric, 2012; Musto et al., 2015). Noting that nurses and others often take varied actions in response to moral distress, Varcoe, Pauly, Webster, and Storch (2012) have proposed a revision to Jameton's definition:

> [M]oral distress is the experience of being seriously compromised as a moral agent in practicing in accordance with accepted professional values and standards. It is a relational experience shaped by multiple contexts, including the socio-political and cultural context of the workplace environment. (p. 60)

The phenomenon of moral distress has received increasing national and international attention in nursing and medical literature. There is growing recognition that failing to address moral distress may have negative consequences for clinicians and patients. Moral distress occurs when conscientious persons are practicing in challenging contexts and is not due to moral weakness of the person experiencing it (Garros, Austin, & Carnevale, 2015; Halpern, 2011). Studies have reported that moral distress is significantly related to unit-level ethical climate and to health care professionals' decisions to leave clinical practice (Corley, Minick, Elswick, & Jacobs, 2005; Epstein & Hamric, 2009; Hamric, Borchers, & Epstein, 2012; Hamric, Davis, & Childress, 2006; Lamiani, Borghi, & Argentero, 2015; Pauly, Varcoe, Storch, & Newton, 2009; Schluter, Winch, Holzhauser, & Henderson, 2008; Varcoe et al., 2012; Whitehead, Herbertson, Hamric, Epstein, & Fisher, 2015). APRNs work to decrease the incidence of moral uncertainty and moral distress for themselves and their colleagues through honest self-reflection, education, empowerment, and problem solving.

Although the scope and nature of moral problems experienced by nurses, and more specifically APRNs, reflect the varied clinical settings in which they practice, three general themes emerge when ethical issues in nursing practice are examined. These are problems with communication, the presence of interprofessional conflict, and nurses' difficulties with managing multiple commitments and obligations.

Communication Problems

The first theme encountered in many ethical dilemmas is the erosion of open and honest communication. The erosion begins when clinicians fail to speak up in crucial situations. Research suggests that even when patient safety is at risk, fewer than 2 in 10 clinicians will speak up (Maxfield, Grenny, McMillan, Patterson, & Switzler, 2005; Maxfield, Grenny, Lavandero, & Groah, 2010). With medical error now listed as one of the leading causes of death in the United States (Makary & Daniel, 2016), it is essential that we focus on stopping the silent erosion of communication. APRNs must be willing and able not only to speak up in high stakes situations but to coach nurses in how to break the silence and create an atmosphere in which open communication is the rule rather than the exception.

Clear communication is an essential prerequisite for informed and responsible decision making. Some ethical disputes reflect inadequate communication rather than a difference in values (Hamric & Blackhall, 2007; Ulrich, 2012). The APRN's communication skills are applied in several arenas. Within the health care team, discussions are most effective when members are accountable for presenting information in a precise and succinct manner. In patient encounters, disagreements between the patient and a family member or within the family can be rooted in faulty communication, which then leads to ethical conflict. The skill of listening is just as crucial in effective communication as having proficient verbal skills. Listening involves recognizing and appreciating various perspectives and showing respect to individuals with differing ideas. To listen well is to allow others the necessary time to form and present their thoughts and ideas.

Understanding the language used in ethical deliberations (e.g., terms such as beneficence, autonomy, and utilitarian justice) helps the APRN frame the concern in rational terms. This can help those involved to see the components of the ethical problem rather than be mired in their own emotional responses. When ethical dilemmas arise, effective communication is the first key to negotiating and facilitating a resolution. For example, Jameson (2003) found that when certified registered nurse anesthetists (CRNAs) and anesthesiologists focused on the common goal of patient care (shared values) rather than on the conflicting opinions about supervision and autonomous practice, they were able to transcend role-based conflict and promote effective communication.

Interprofessional Conflict

The second theme encountered is that most ethical dilemmas that occur in the health care setting are multidisciplinary in nature. Issues such as refusal of treatment, end-of-life decision making, cost containment, and confidentiality all have interprofessional elements interwoven in the dilemmas, so an interprofessional approach is necessary for successful resolution of the issue. Health care professionals bring varied viewpoints and perspectives into discussions of ethical issues (Hamric & Blackhall, 2007; Piers et al., 2011; Shannon, Mitchell, & Cain, 2002). These differing positions can lead to creative and collaborative decision making or to a breakdown in communication and lack of problem solving. Thus an interprofessional theme is necessary in the presentation and resolution of ethical problems.

For example, a clinical nurse specialist (CNS) is facilitating a discharge plan for an older woman who is terminally ill with heart failure. The plan of care, agreed on by the interprofessional team, patient, and family, is to continue oral medications but discontinue intravenous inotropic support and all other aggressive measures. Just prior to discharge, the social worker laments to the CNS that medical coverage for the patient's care in the skilled nursing facility will be covered by the insurer only if the patient has an intravenous line in place. The patient's daughter wishes to take her mother home and provide care. The attending cardiologist determines that the patient can be discharged to her daughter's home because she no longer requires skilled care; however, the bedside nurse is concerned that the patient's need for physical assistance will overwhelm her daughter and believes that the patient is better off returning to the skilled nursing facility. The CNS engages the patient in a careful conversation about her condition and her preferences. Although each team member shares responsibility to ensure that the plan of care is consistent with the patient's wishes and minimizes the cost burden to the patient, they differ in perspective and approach for how to achieve these goals. Such legitimate but differing perspectives from various team members can lead to ethical conflict.

Multiple Commitments

The third theme that frequently arises when ethical issues in nursing practice are examined is the issue of balancing commitments to multiple parties. Nurses have numerous and, at times, competing fidelity obligations to various stakeholders in the health care and legal systems (Chambliss, 1996; Hamric, 2001). Fidelity is an ethical concept that requires persons to be faithful to their commitments and promises. For the APRN, these obligations start with the patient and family but also include physicians and other colleagues, the institution or employer, the larger profession, and oneself. Ethical deliberation involves analyzing and dealing with the differing and opposing demands that occur as a result of these commitments. An APRN may face a dilemma if encouraged by a specialist consultant to pursue a costly intervention on behalf of a patient, whereas the APRNS's hiring organization has established cost containment as a key objective and does not support use of this intervention (Donagrandi & Eddy, 2000). In this and other situations, APRNs are faced with an ethical dilemma created by multiple commitments and the need to balance obligations to all parties.

Another significant threat to ethical practice is the failure of APRNs to practice self-care. As noted in the *Code of Ethics for Nurses* (American Nurses Association [ANA], 2015), nurses owe the same duty to themselves that they do to their patients. For example, an APRN may receive a referral to see a patient late in the day. She will feel compelled to

stay late and meet the patient's needs, even if she has already worked well beyond a "normal" day. As a one-time event, this is laudable. When it becomes a pattern, particularly when the APRN is sacrificing personal time or family time, she puts herself at risk for long-term health consequences (Fox, Dwyer, & Ganster, 1993). Something as commonplace as interrupted sleep or lack of sleep contributes to a negative emotional state (Tempesta et al., 2010), which in turn may deplete self-control and lead to unethical behavior (Barnes, Schaubroeck, Huth, & Ghumman, 2011; Gino, Schweitzer, Mead, & Ariely, 2011).

The general themes of communication, interprofessional conflict, and balancing multiple commitments are prevalent in most ethical dilemmas. Specific ethical issues may be unique to the specialty area and clinical setting in which the APRN practices.

Ethical Issues Affecting APRNs

Primary Care Issues

Situations in which personal values contradict professional responsibilities often confront nurse practitioners (NPs) in a primary care setting. Issues such as abortion, teen pregnancy, patient nonadherence to treatment, childhood immunizations, regulations and laws, and financial constraints that interfere with care were cited in one older study as frequently encountered ethical issues (Turner, Marquis, & Burman, 1996). Ethical problems related to insurance reimbursement, such as when implementation of a desired plan of care is delayed by the insurance authorization process or restrictive prescription plans, are an issue for APRNs. NPs practicing within a managed care environment often feel the necessity to balance the needs of patients against the organization's interests (Ulrich, Soeken, & Miller, 2003). The problem of inadequate reimbursement can also arise when there is a lack of transparency regarding the specifics of services covered by an insurance plan. For example, a patient who has undergone diagnostic testing during an inpatient stay may later be informed that the test is not covered by insurance because it was done on the day of discharge. Had the patient and NP known of this policy, the testing could have been scheduled on an outpatient basis with prior authorization from the insurance company and thus have been a covered expense.

Viens (1994) found that primary care NPs interpret their moral responsibilities as balancing obligations to the patient, family, colleagues, employer, and society. More recently, Laabs (2005) has found that the three issues most often noted by NPs as causing moral dilemmas are (1) being required to follow policies and procedures that infringe on personal values, (2) wanting to bend the rules to ensure appropriate patient care, and (3) dealing with patients who have refused appropriate care. Issues leading to moral distress in NPs included pressure to see an excessive number of patients, clinical decisions being made by others, and a lack of power to effect change (Laabs, 2005). Increasing expectations to care for more patients in less time are routine in all types of health care settings as pressures to contain costs escalate. APRNs in rural or ambulatory care settings often have fewer resources than their colleagues working in or near academic centers in which ethics committees, ethics consultants, and educational opportunities are more accessible.

Issues of quality of life and symptom management traverse primary and acute health care settings. Pain relief and symptom management can be problematic for nurses and physicians (Oberle & Hughes, 2001). APRNs must confront the various and sometimes conflicting goals of the patient, family, and other health care providers regarding the plans for treatment, symptom management, and quality of life. The APRN is often the individual who coordinates the plan of care and thus is faced with clinical and ethical concerns when participants' goals are not consistent or appropriate.

Acute and Chronic Care Issues

In the acute care setting, APRNs struggle with dilemmas involving pain management, end-of-life decision making, advance directives, assisted suicide, and medical errors (Shannon, Foglia, Hardy, & Gallagher, 2009). Rajput and Bekes (2002) identified ethical issues faced by hospital-based physicians, including obtaining informed consent, establishing a patient's competence to make decisions, maintaining confidentiality, and transmitting health information electronically. APRNs in acute care settings may experience similar ethical dilemmas. Recent studies of moral distress have revealed that feeling pressured to continue aggressive treatments that respondents thought were not in the patients' best interest or in situations in which the patient was dying, working with physicians or nurses who were not fully competent, giving false hope to patients and families, poor team communication, and lack of provider continuity were all issues that engendered moral distress (Hamric & Blackhall, 2007; Hamric et al.,

2012). Emergency department NPs experience moral distress with poor patient care results related to inadequate staff communication and working with incompetent coworkers in their practice (Trautmann, Epstein, Rovnyak, & Snyder, 2015).

APRNs bring a distinct perspective to collaborative decision making and often find themselves bridging communication between the medical team and patient or family. For example, the neonatal nurse practitioner (NNP) is responsible for the day-to-day medical management of the critically ill neonate and may be the first provider to respond in emergency situations (Juretschke, 2001). The NNP establishes a trusting relationship with the family and becomes aware of the values, beliefs, and attitudes that shape the family's decisions. Thus the NNP has insight into the perspectives of the health care team and family. This "in-the-middle" position, however, can be accompanied by moral distress (Hamric, 2001), particularly when the team's treatment decision carried out by the NNP is not congruent with the NNP's professional judgment or values. Botwinski (2010) conducted a needs assessment of NNPs and found that most had not received formal ethics content in their education and desired more education on the management of end-of-life situations, such as delivery room resuscitation of a child on the edge of viability. Knowing the best interests of the infant and balancing those obligations to the infant with the emotional, cognitive, financial, and moral concerns that face the family struggling with a critically ill neonate is a complex undertaking. Care must be guided by an NNP and health care team who understand the ethical principles and decision making related to issues confronted in neonatal intensive care unit practice.

Societal Issues

Ongoing cost containment pressures in the health care sector have significantly changed the traditional practice of delivering health care. Goals of reduced expenditures and increased efficiency, although important, may compete with enhanced quality of life for patients and improved treatment and care, creating tension between providers and administrators, particularly as reimbursement changes from a procedure-based to a quality/value-based system. Studies suggest that changes in payment systems can lead to ethical challenges for providers.

Ulrich and associates (2006) surveyed NPs and physician assistants to identify their ethical concerns in relation to cost containment efforts, including managed care. They found that 72% of respondents reported ethical concerns related to limited access to appropriate care and more than 50% reported concerns related to the quality of care. An earlier study of 254 NPs revealed that 80% of the sample perceived that to help patients, it was sometimes necessary to bend practice or institutional policies to provide appropriate care (Ulrich et al., 2003). Most respondents in this study reported being moderately to extremely ethically concerned with cost containment; more than 50% said that they were concerned that business decisions took priority over patient welfare and more than 75% stated that their primary obligation was shifting from the patient to the insurance plan. Although many hoped the passage of the Patient Protection and Affordable Care Act (ACA, 2010) would help with these concerns to some extent, the ethical tensions that underlie cost containment pressures and the business model orientation of health care delivery no doubt will continue. Changes in government leadership bring shifts in health care policy, and the 2016 election is a prime example. Ongoing attempts to repeal and replace the ACA have highlighted the complexity of the healthcare system and vividly underscore the ongoing debate about what constitutes "fair" distribution of resources, different conceptions of what is good, and a predisposition to seek power and advantage (Obama, 2017; Sorrell, 2012). Even as lawmakers debate how to address healthcare delivery, real life challenges such as the opiate epidemic will stress the system and pose more ethical challenges for advanced practice nurses ((Friedmann, Andrews & Humphreys, 2017).

A survey of primary care providers—physicians, NPs, and physician assistants—indicates that overall, providers are more negative about the increased reliance on quality metrics and financial penalties to promote high performance (Commonwealth Fund and Henry J. Kaiser Family Foundation, 2015). It may be too soon to know for sure; however, history suggests ethical challenges will continue as the system of health care delivery evolves. While a number of myths surround the impact of patient satisfaction scores on reimbursement, the data suggest that patients are good discriminators of the care they receive. Ultimately, it is about communication and relationships, not simply acquiescing to what a patient says he or she wants (Siegrist, 2013).

An example of how cost containment goals can create conflict is a situation in which an NP wishes to order a computed tomography scan to evaluate a patient complaining of abdominal pain. The NP knows that the patient has a history of diverticulosis resulting in abscess formation, and the current presentation with fever and abdominal tenderness justifies this testing; however, the insurance approval process takes a minimum of 24 hours. By sending the patient to the emergency room, the test can be done more quickly, but the patient will also face a long wait and a high co-pay if she does not require subsequent hospital admission. Limiting access to computed tomography scans is based on containing costs and avoiding unnecessary testing, which are two laudable goals. In this situation, the lengthy approval process means that the NP must make decisions about the treatment plan without important information. The pressure to alleviate the patient's suffering in a timely manner may tempt the NP to advise the patient to go to the emergency room, which may result in a greater financial burden on the patient and may ultimately prove more expensive to the system. The availability of modern technology forces difficult choices, especially challenging providers to redefine "timely," urgent, and emergent, and may cause providers to feel as though they are choosing between what is best for patients and what is best for organizations.

Technologic advances, such as the rapidly expanding field of genetics, are also challenging APRNs (Caulfield, 2012; Harris, Winship, & Spriggs, 2005; Horner, 2004; Pullman & Hodgkinson, 2006). As Hopkinson and Mackay (2002) have noted, although the potential impact of mapping the human genome is immense, the challenge of how to translate genetic data rapidly into improvements in the prevention, diagnosis, and treatment of disease remains. To counsel patients effectively on the risks and benefits of genetic testing, APRNs need to stay current in this rapidly changing field. A helpful resource for this and other issues is the text by Steinbock, Arras, and London (2012) and a more recent article by Seibert (2014). As one example, genetic testing poses a unique challenge to the informed consent process. Direct-to-consumer marketing, with phrases such as "Your DNA has an incredible story!" by companies that provide genetic testing, projects an image of a cutting-edge, risk-free opportunity (https:// www.23andme.com). Patients may feel pressured by family members to undergo or refuse testing, and they may require intensive counseling to understand the complex implications of such testing (Erlen, 2006). APRNs may be involved in posttest counseling, helping patients navigate such thorny issues as disclosure of test results to family members or potential future family members and what to do if the information makes its way to an employer or insurance company. Because genetic information is crucially linked to the concepts of privacy and confidentiality, and the availability of this information is increasing, it is inevitable that APRNs will encounter legal issues and ethical dilemmas related to the use of genetic data. The cost of genomic testing may effectively put this technology out of reach for disadvantaged populations. It will be important for the health care system to create a model that will ensure the sustainability of funding for genomic-guided interventions, their adoption and coverage by health insurance, and prioritization of genomic medicine research, development, and innovation (Fragoulakis, Mitropoulou, van Schaik, Maniadakis, & Patrinos, 2016).

APRNs may engage in research as principal investigators, coinvestigators, or data collectors for clinical studies and trials. In addition, leading quality improvement initiatives is a key expectation of the DNP-prepared APRN (AACN, 2006). Ethical issues abound in clinical research, including recruiting and retaining patients in studies, protecting vulnerable populations from undue risk, and ensuring informed consent, fair access to research, and study subjects' privacy. As APRNs move into quality improvement and research initiatives, they may experience the conflict between the clinician role, in which the focus is on the best interests of an individual patient, and that of the researcher, in which the focus is on ensuring the integrity of the study (Edwards & Chalmers, 2002).

Access to Resources and Issues of Justice

Issues of access to and distribution of resources create powerful dilemmas for APRNs, many of whom care for underserved populations. Issues of social justice and equitable access to resources present formidable challenges in clinical practice. Trotochard (2006) noted that a growing number of uninsured individuals lack access to routine health care; they experience worse outcomes from acute and chronic diseases and face higher mortality rates than those with insurance. McWilliams, Meara, Zaslavsky, and Ayanian (2007) found that previously uninsured Medicare beneficiaries require significantly more hospitalizations and office visits when compared with those with similar health problems who, prior to Medicare eligibility, had private insurance. The ACA has improved access to quality care and decreased the incidence of these circumstances. Regardless of patients' insurance status, the costs of health care will

continue to present ethical dilemmas for providers. The shift in payment structure to a value-based system adds to the complexity of health care reform. A report of projects funded by the Robert Wood Johnson Foundation concluded that achieving the objectives of reduced cost and improved quality will require a trusted, widely respected "honest broker" that can convene and maintain the ongoing commitment of health plans, providers, and purchasers (Conrad, Grembowski, Hernandez, Lau, & Marcus-Smith, 2014). The allocation of scarce health care resources also creates ethical conflicts for providers; regardless of payment mechanisms, there are insufficient resources to meet all societal needs (Bodenheimer & Grumbach, 2012; Trotochard, 2006). Scarcity of resources is more severe in developing areas of the world, and justice issues of fair and equitable distribution of health care services present serious ethical dilemmas for nurses in these regions (Harrowing & Mill, 2010). A further international issue is the "brain drain" of nurses and other health professionals who leave underdeveloped countries to take jobs in developed countries (Chaguturu & Vallabhaneni, 2007; Dwyer, 2007).

Allocation issues have been described in the area of organ transplantation, but dilemmas related to scarce resources also arise in regard to daily decision making, for example, with a CNS guiding the assignment of patients in a staffing shortage or an FNP finding that a specialty consultation for a patient is not available for several months. Whether in community or acute care settings, APRNs must, on a daily basis, balance their obligation to provide holistic, evidence-based care with the necessity to contain costs and the reality that some patients will not receive needed health care. As Bodenheimer and Grumbach (2012) have noted, "Perhaps no tension within the U.S. health care system is as far from reaching a satisfactory equilibrium as the achievement of a basic level of fairness in the distribution of health care services and the burden of paying for those services" (p. 215).

One of the value-added components that APRNs bring to any practice setting is creativity and a wide range of patient management strategies, which are crucial in caring for large numbers of uninsured and underinsured persons. It is not uncommon for an APRN to encounter a patient who has been forced to stop taking certain medications for financial reasons. Although many practitioners prescribe generic forms of medications, if available, some patients still have to pay an exorbitant price for their medications. For example, an acute care nurse practitioner (ACNP) managing an underinsured patient with chronic lung disease and heart failure discovers that the patient is unable to pay for all the medications prescribed and has elected to forego the diuretic and an angiotensin-converting enzyme inhibitor. Because the ACNP knows that angiotensin-converting enzyme inhibitors are associated with reduced morbidity and mortality rates, and that diuretics control symptoms and prevent rehospitalization, these changes are discouraged. Instead, the ACNP helps the patient make more suitable choices when altering medications, such as dosing some medications on an every-other-day basis. The ACNP has helped the patient cope with the situation but must face the morally unsettling fact that this plan of care is medically inferior.

Finally, as APRNs broaden their perspectives to encompass population health and increased policy activities, both essential competencies of the DNP-prepared APRN (AACN, 2006), they will experience the tension between caring for the individual patient and the larger population (Emanuel, 2002). Caregivers are increasingly being asked to incorporate population-based cost considerations into individualized clinical decision making (Bodenheimer & Grumbach, 2012). Population-based considerations present a challenge to APRNs, who have been educated to privilege the individual clinical decision.

Legal Issues

Over the last 30 years, the complexity of ethical issues in the health care environment and the inability to reach agreement among parties has resulted in participants turning to the legal system for resolution. A body of legal precedent has emerged, reflecting changes in society's moral consensus. Ideally, moral rights are upheld or protected by the law. For example, the culturally and linguistically appropriate services standards mandate that health care institutions receiving federal funds provide services that are accessible to patients regardless of their cultural background (US Department of Health and Human Services, Office of Minority Health, 2001). These standards provide a legislative voice for the ethical obligation to respect all persons, regardless of their cultural background and primary language. In a different voice, the ACA (2010) has mandated that persons who can afford health insurance purchase it or pay a penalty. According to this law, societal beneficence, in the form of limiting high expenditures on the care of uninsured persons, is preferred over individual autonomy (Trautman, 2011).

APRNs must use caution and not conflate legal perspectives with ethical decision making. In many cases, there is no relevant law to guide decision making. Thoughtful deliberation of the ethical issues rather than searching for a legal answer to avoid litigation offers the best hope of resolution. In addition, looking to the judicial system for guidance in ethical decision making is troubling because the judicial aim is to interpret the law, not to satisfy the ethical concerns of all parties involved. In addition, clinical understanding may be absent from the judicial perspective. Involvement of the media may further confuse the situation, as was evident in the Schiavo case (Gostin, 2005).

At age 26, Terri Schiavo was in a persistent vegetative state following cardiac arrest and severe anoxic brain damage. Ms. Schiavo had no advance directive, and her husband was appointed her guardian. Her parents did not contest this until a lawsuit resulted in a financial settlement with money put in trust to provide care for her. Mr. Schiavo wished to remove his wife's feeding tube and her parents wished to keep her alive. The legal guidelines in that case were clear; the Florida court system repeatedly upheld the right of Ms. Schiavo's spouse to refuse nutrition and hydration on her behalf. However, advocacy groups, politicians, and Ms. Schiavo's parents used the media to offer a variety of interpretations of the case and wielded political power to prevent removal of the feeding tube and to have it replaced twice after it was removed. Clearly, the legal perspective did not satisfy the moral concerns of all involved. Unfortunately, much of the publicity about the case focused on the emotional experience of the parents fearing the loss of their daughter and not on the medical facts of the case or careful consideration of the ethical elements.

Sometimes, the law not only falls short of resolving ethical concerns but contributes to the creation of new dilemmas. Changes in the Medicare hospice benefit under the ACA (2010) offer a clear example. Designed to prevent hospice agencies from enrolling and reenrolling patients who do not meet criteria, the new regulations require a face-to-face assessment by a health care provider to recertify hospice eligibility at set intervals after the initial enrollment (Kennedy, 2012). Often, patients with dementia or another slowly progressive disease who enroll in hospice experience an initial period of stability, likely because they have improved symptom management and access to comprehensive services. If this stability extends to the next certification period, the patient may face disenrollment. For the practitioner conducting the assessment, this creates the ethical dilemma of wanting to be truthful regarding the patient's status and at the same time avoiding removing a service that is benefiting the patient and family.

Ethical Decision-Making Competency of APRNs

There are a number of reasons why ethical decision making is a core competency of advanced practice nursing. As noted, clinical practice gives rise to numerous ethical concerns and APRNs must be able to address these concerns. Also, ethical involvement follows and evolves from clinical expertise (Benner, Tanner, & Chesla, 2009). Another reason why ethical decision making is a core competency can be seen in the expanded collaborative skills that APRNs develop (see Chapter 12). APRNs practice in a variety of settings and positions but, in most cases, the APRN is part of an interprofessional team of caregivers. The team may be loosely defined and structured, as in a rural setting, or more definitive, as in the acute care setting. The recent reemergence of an interprofessional care model is changing practice for all providers (Interprofessional Education Collaborative [IPEC], 2016). Regardless of the structure, APRNs need the knowledge and skills to avoid power struggles, broker and lead interprofessional communication, and facilitate consensus among team members in ethically difficult situations.

Elements of Core Competency Development

The core competency of ethical decision making for APRNs can be organized into four elements (Fig. 13.1). Each element is enhanced by the acquisition of the knowledge and skills embedded in other areas. The competency of ethical decision making is understood as an evolutionary process in an APRN's development. APRNs should be exposed to all elements in graduate school; however, particular attention should be paid to knowledge acquisition and developing moral sensitivity. The other elements of the ethical decision-making competency evolve as APRNs mature in their roles and develop clinical expertise, becoming comfortable in the practice setting. Creating an ethical work environment and promoting social justice represent leadership behavior and the full enactment of the ethical decision-making competency. Although this is an expectation of the practice doctorate, all APRNs should develop

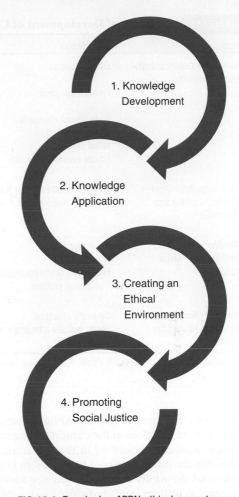

FIG 13.1 Developing APRN ethical competency.

their ethical knowledge and skills to include all four elements of this competency. The essential components of each element are described in Table 13.2 (Hamric & Delgado, 2014).

Element 1: Knowledge Development

The first element in the ethical decision-making competency is developing core knowledge and terminology in ethical theories and principles and the ethical issues common to specific patient populations or clinical settings. This dual knowledge enables the APRN student to integrate philosophical concepts with contemporary clinical issues. The emphasis in this initial stage is on learning the language of ethical discourse and achieving cognitive mastery. The APRN learns the theories, principles, codes, paradigm cases, and relevant laws that influence ethical decision

TABLE 13.2   Elements of Development of Core Competency for Ethical Decision Making

Element	Knowledge	Skill or Behavior
1. Knowledge Development— Moral Sensitivity	Ethical theories	Sensitivity to ethical dimensions of clinical practice
		Identify alternate perspectives through reframing
	Professional code	Values clarification: self-reflection
		Tempered emotion (through insight and experience)
	Professional standards	Sensitivity to fidelity conflicts
	Legal precedent	Gather relevant literature related to problems identified
	Moral distress	Interpret reactions and emotions of others
	Ethical issues in specialty	Identify ethical issues in the practice setting and bring to the attention of other team members
2. Knowledge Application— Ethical Judgment and Motivation	Ethical decision-making frameworks	Apply ethical decision-making models to clinical problems
	Mediation and facilitation strategies	Use skilled communication regarding ethical issues
		Facilitate decision making by using select strategies
		Recognize and manage moral distress in self and others
3. Creating an Ethical Environment—Moral Action	Preventive ethics	Use preventive ethics to decrease unit-level moral distress
		Identify "at risk" for ethical conflict situations
	Awareness of environmental barriers to ethical practice	Mentor others to develop ethical practice
		Address barriers to ethical practice through system changes
		Role model collaborative problem solving
4. Promoting Social Justice Within the Health Care System	Concepts of justice	Ability to analyze the policy process
	Health policies affecting a specialty population	Advocacy, communication, and leadership skills
		Involvement in health policy initiatives supporting social justice

Modified from Hamric, A. B., and Delgado, S. (2014). Ethical decision making. In *Advanced practice nursing: An integrative approach* (5th ed., p. 334). St. Louis, MO: Elsevier.

making. With this knowledge, the APRN begins to compare current practices in the clinical setting with the ethical standards described in the literature.

Mastering the components of this element is the beginning of the APRN's personal journey toward developing a distinct and individualized ethical framework. Initially the APRN must work to develop sensitivity to the moral dimensions of clinical practice (Weaver, 2007). A helpful initial step in building moral sensitivity involves exploring one's values, intentionally clarifying the personal and professional values that inform one's practice (Feister, 2015; Fry & Johnstone, 2008). Engaging in this work uncovers personal values that may have been internalized and not openly acknowledged and is particularly important in today's multicultural world.

Another key aspect of this element is developing the ability to distinguish a true ethical dilemma from a situation of moral distress or other clinically problematic situation. This requires a general understanding of ethical theories, principles, and standards that help the APRNs define and discern the essential elements of an ethical dilemma. Novice APRNs should be able to recognize a moral problem and seek clarification and illumination of the concern. Once an APRN can identify ethical issues and name the concerns about which others are uneasy, the APRN will gain self-confidence and begin to earn credibility with others. If the issue remains a moral concern after clarification, the APRN should pursue resolution, seeking additional help if needed.

Although some beginning graduate students will have had significant exposure to ethical issues in their undergraduate programs, most have not. A 2008 US survey of nurses and social workers found that only 51% of the nurse respondents had formal ethics education in their undergraduate or graduate education; 23% had no ethics training at all (Grady et al., 2008). APRN students with no ethics education or clinical experience will be at a disadvantage in developing this competency because graduate education builds on the ethical foundation of professional practice. The current master's essentials (AACN, 2011) do not address ethics education directly but include competencies in the use of ethical theories and principles. *The Essentials of Doctoral Education for Advanced Nursing Practice* (AACN, 2006) contains explicit ethical content in five of the eight major categories (Box 13.1). Even categories that do not explicitly list necessary ethical content imply it in referring to issues such as improving access to health care, addressing gaps in care, and

BOX 13.1 **Ethical Competencies in the DNP Essentials[a]**

- Integrate nursing science with knowledge from ethics and biophysical, psychosocial, analytic, and organizational sciences as the basis for the highest level of nursing practice. (I)
- Develop and/or evaluate effective strategies for managing the ethical dilemmas inherent in patient care, the health care organization, and research. (II)
- Design, direct, and evaluate quality improvement methodologies to promote safe, timely, effective, efficient, *equitable* [emphasis added], and patient-centered care. (III)
- Provide leadership in the evaluation and resolution of ethical and legal issues within health care systems relating to the use of information, information technology, communication networks, and patient care technology. (IV)
- Advocate for social justice, equity, and ethical policies within all health care arenas. (V)

[a]Essential number in parentheses.
From American Association of Colleges of Nursing. (2006). *The essentials of doctoral education for advanced nursing practice.* Washington, DC: Author.

using conceptual and analytic skills to address links between practice and organizational and policy issues.

Exposure to ethical theories, principles, and concepts is not enough. Processes that accommodate and value the unique nature of each ethical problem, incorporating personal values and ethical theories, are gaining influence (Cooper, 2012). Knowledge development must extend beyond classroom discussions to include discussion of ethical dimensions of clinical practicum experiences. In one study, Laabs (2005) noted that 67% of NP respondents claimed that they never or rarely encountered ethical issues. Some respondents showed confusion regarding the language of ethics and related principles. In a later study, Laabs (2012) found that APRN graduates, most of whom had had an ethics course in their graduate curriculum, indicated a fairly high level of confidence in their ability to manage ethical problems, but their overall ethics knowledge was low. These studies provide compelling commentary on the need for ethics knowledge development in graduate curricula.

The core knowledge of ethical theories should be supplemented with an understanding of issues central to the patient populations with whom the APRN works. As APRNs assume positions in specific clinical areas or with particular patient populations, it is incumbent upon them to gain an understanding of the applicable laws, standards, and regulations in their specialty, as well as relevant paradigm cases. This information may be garnered from current literature in the field, continuing education programs, or discussions with colleagues. Information on legal and policy guidelines should be offered during graduate practicum experiences in the area of clinical concentration.

Knowledge development is an ongoing process. APRNs will gain core knowledge in graduate education but, as societal issues change and new technologies emerge, new dilemmas and ethical problems arise. The ability to be a leader in creating ethical environments involves a commitment to lifelong learning about ethical issues, of which professional education is just the beginning. At least one study suggests it is continuing education in ethics beyond basic training that can have the largest impact on moral action (Grady et al., 2008).

Developing an Educational Foundation

Because the APRN will apply theories, principles, rules, and moral concepts in actual encounters with patients, it is imperative that consideration of the context in specific situations be strengthened. Simulation has been shown to be an effective environment for students to learn and practice skills necessary to navigate complex environments involving ethical conflict (Buxton, Phillippi, & Collins, 2015). Howard and Steinberg (2002) maintained that graduate curricula need to go beyond traditional ethical issues to encompass building trust in the APRN-patient relationship, professionalism and patient advocacy, resource allocation decisions, individual versus population-based responsibilities, and managing tensions between business ethics and professional ethics. As technology changes and new dilemmas confront practitioners, the APRN must be prepared to anticipate conditions that erode an ethical environment. Knowledge and skills in all phases of this competency depend on the application of current ethical knowledge in the clinical setting; ethical reasoning and clinical judgment share a common process and each serves to teach and inform the other (Dreyfus, Dreyfus, & Benner, 2009). Therefore the importance of clinical practice cannot be overemphasized.

BOX 13.2 | **Principles and Rules Important to Professional Nursing Practice**

- Principle of respect for autonomy: The duty to respect others' personal liberty and individual values, beliefs, and choices
- Principle of nonmaleficence: The duty not to inflict harm or evil
- Principle of beneficence: The duty to do good and prevent or remove harm
- Principle of formal justice: The duty to treat equals equally and treat those who are unequal according to their needs
- Rule of veracity: The duty to tell the truth and not to deceive others
- Rule of fidelity: The duty to honor commitments
- Rule of confidentiality: The duty not to disclose information shared in an intimate and trusted manner
- Rule of privacy: The duty to respect limited access to a person

Adapted from Beauchamp, T. L., & Childress, J. F. (2009). *Principles of biomedical ethics* (6th ed.). New York: Oxford University Press.

Overview of Ethical Approaches

Principle-Based. Although ethical decision making in health care is extensively discussed in the bioethics literature, two dominant models are most often applied in the clinical setting. The first model of decision making is a principle-based model (Box 13.2), in which ethical decision making is guided by principles and rules (Beauchamp & Childress, 2012). In cases of conflict, the principles or rules in contention are balanced and interpreted with the contextual elements of the situation. However, the final decision and moral justification for actions are based on principles. In this way, the principles are binding and tolerant of the particularities of specific cases (Beauchamp & Childress, 2012). The principles of respect for persons, autonomy, beneficence, nonmaleficence, and justice are commonly applied in the analysis of ethical issues in nursing. The ANA *Code of Ethics for Nurses* (2015) has endorsed the principle of respect for persons and underscores the profession's commitment to serving individuals, families, and groups or communities. The emphasis on respect for persons throughout the code implies that it is not only a philosophical value of nursing but also a binding principle within the profession.

Although ethical principles and rules are the cornerstone of most ethical decisions, the principle-based approach has been criticized as being too formalistic for many clinicians and lacking in moral substance (Gert, Culver, & Clouser, 2006). Other critics have argued that a principle-based approach conceals the particular person and relationships and reduces the resolution of a clinical case simply to balancing principles (Rushton & Penticuff, 2007). Because all the principles are considered of equal moral weight, this approach has been seen as inadequate to provide guidance for moral action (Gert et al., 2006; Strong, 2007). Another significant challenge to the principled approach is a shallow understanding of autonomy. Honoring a person's autonomy does not mean that that person should get whatever they want. Respect for persons (the broader understanding of autonomy) requires a more nuanced understanding of how to balance what a person may want with the responsibility to avoid harm and promote a person's well-being. This is especially important when, for example, APRNs face pressure from patients to prescribe medication they do not need or (worse) may cause them harm. In spite of these critiques, bioethical principles remain the most common ethical language used in clinical practice settings.

Casuistry. The second common approach to ethical decision making is the casuistic model (Box 13.3), in which current cases are compared with precedent-setting cases (Beauchamp & Childress, 2012; Jonsen & Toulmin, 1988; Toulmin, 1994). The strength of this approach is that a dilemma is examined in a context-specific manner and then compared with an analogous earlier case. The fundamental philosophical assumption of this model is that ethics emerges from human moral experiences. Casuists approach dilemmas from an inductive position and work from the specific case to generalizations, rather than from generalizations to specific cases (Beauchamp & Childress, 2012).

Concerns have also been raised regarding the use of a casuistic model for ethical decision making. As a moral dilemma arises, the selection of the paradigm case may differ among the decision makers and thus the interpretation of the appropriate course of action will vary. In nursing, there are few paradigm cases of ethical issues on which to construct a decision-making process. Furthermore, other than the reliance on previous cases, casuists have no mechanisms to justify their actions. The possibility that previous cases were reasoned in a faulty or inaccurate manner

BOX 13.3   Alternative Ethical Approaches

Casuistry

- Direct analysis of particular cases
- Uses previous paradigm cases to infer ethical action in a current case
- Analogues in common law and case law
- Values practical knowledge rather than theory (pretheoretical)
- Privileges experience

Narrative Ethics

- Supplements principles by emphasizing importance of full context
- Gathers views of all parties to provide more complete basis for moral justification
- Story and narrator substitute for ethical justification, which emerges naturally
- Privileges stories

Virtue-Based Ethics

- Emphasizes the moral agent, not the situation or the action
- Right motives and character reveal more about moral worth than right actions
- Character more important than conformity to rules
- Right motives make for right actions
- Privileges actor's values and motives

Feminist Ethics

- Views women as embodied, fully rational, and having experiences relevant to moral reasoning
- Emphasizes view of the disadvantaged—women and other underrepresented groups
- Emphasizes importance and value of openness to different perspectives
- Concerned with power differentials that create oppression
- Emphasizes importance of attention to the vulnerable and to resulting inequalities
- Privileges power imbalances

Care-Based Ethics

- Emphasizes creating and sustaining responsive connection with others
- Emphasizes importance of context and subjectivity in discerning ethical action
- Sees individuals as interdependent rather than independent; focuses on parties in a relationship
- Privileges relationships

may not be fully considered or evaluated (Beauchamp & Childress, 2012). In spite of these concerns, the case-based moral reasoning used in casuistry appeals to clinicians because it mimics clinical reasoning, in which providers often appeal to earlier similar cases to make clinical judgments. Artnak and Dimmit (1996) applied the casuistic model to an analysis of a complex case, concluding that the use of this approach allows fuller consideration of the contextual particulars of the case and provides a systematic approach for organizing and analyzing the facts of the case. An adaptation of this approach, sometimes referred to as the "four box" approach, has been developed by Jonsen, Siegler, and Winslade (2010). These authors have advocated clustering patient information according to four key topics—medical indications, patient preferences, quality of life, and contextual features—and then using that information to resolve a dilemma.

Narrative Ethics. Because neither of these theoretical approaches has been seen as fully satisfactory, alternatives have emerged (see Box 13.3). Narrative approaches to ethical deliberation have evoked considerable interest (Charon & Montello, 2002; Nelson, 2004; Rorty, Werhane, & Mills, 2004). Narrative ethics emphasizes the particulars of a case or story as a vehicle for discerning the meaning and values embedded in ethical decision making. The argument is that all knowing is bound up in a narrative tradition and that all participants in ethical deliberations need the coherence and singular meaning given to a particular situation that only narrative knowledge can provide. Narrative ethics begins with a patient's story and has some similarities with casuistry in its inductive particularistic approach. Critics of this approach have argued that although narrative is a necessary element in ethical analysis, it cannot supplant principle- or theory-based ethics (Arras, 1997; Childress, 1997). There is, however, recognition that careful consideration of a patient's stories can enlarge and enrich ethical deliberations. In commenting on narrative versus principle-based approaches, Childress (1997) noted that "We need both in any adequate ethics" (p. 268). As with casuistry, narrative-based approaches appeal to nurses, who find much of the meaning in their work through entering into the stories of their patient's lives.

Care-Based Ethics. Other approaches, such as virtue-based ethics, feminist ethics, and care-based ethics, provide alternative processes for moral reflection and argument (Beauchamp & Childress, 2012; Wolf, 1996). Historically, nursing ethics was virtue based, with an emphasis on qualities necessary to be a virtuous nurse. Although this is no longer a dominant theme in nursing literature, it can still be seen. For example, Gallagher and Tschudin (2010) based their understanding of ethical leadership in professional values and virtues.

The ethics of care has emerged as relevant to nursing (Cooper, 1991; Edwards, 2009; Lachman, 2012). The care perspective constructs the moral problem as sustaining responsive relationships with important others, and consequently focuses on issues surrounding the needs and responsibilities that occur in relationships (Gilligan, 1982; Little, 1998). In this approach, moral reasoning requires empathy and emphasizes responsibilities rather than rights. The

response of an individual to a moral dilemma emerges from important relationship considerations and the norms of friendship, care, and love. Viens (1995) reported that NPs she interviewed used a moral reasoning process that mirrored Gilligan's model in the major themes of caring and responsibility.

Although every ethical theory has some limitations and problems, an understanding of contemporary approaches to bioethics enables the APRN to appeal to a variety of perspectives in achieving a moral resolution. In the clinical setting, ethical decision making most often reflects a blend of the various approaches rather than the application of a single approach. Although there is some danger in over-simplifying these rich and complex approaches, Exemplar 13.2 shows how they can be reflected in ethical decision making. A more thorough discussion

---

EXEMPLAR 13.2   **Clinical Situation Demonstrating Differing Ethical Approaches**

To illustrate the different ethical approaches, consider the case of a 64-year-old female, M.H. She presented to the emergency department with jaw pain and was admitted to the hospital. Her medical history is significant for stage IV glioblastoma multiforme and multifocal stroke. The neurosurgeon has no more curative therapy options for M.H. She underwent a palliative surgery in an attempt to relieve pain and pressure from an abscess. On a previous hospitalization M.H. completed an advance directive specifying a preference to forgo resuscitation if her condition is not curable. Currently M.H. is not able to communicate beyond tracking with her eyes. Her daughter K.J. is concerned that M.H.'s inability to communicate is due to the high level of pain medication she is receiving. The neurosurgeon believes it is a manifestation of her progressing tumor. The daughter expresses doubts about her mother's wishes to be on do-not-resuscitate (DNR) status and has asked the team to lighten up on pain medication so she can communicate more with her mother and escalate support, including intubation if necessary. The team caring for the patient, including a staff nurse, resident, attending physician, chaplain, social worker, and clinical nurse specialist (CNS), apply different ethical theories when they approach this case.

The staff nurse believes that K.J.'s inability to support her mother's advance directive and lack of concern for her mother's suffering renders her an inappropriate decision maker. The nurse believes the harm of allowing M.H. to suffer more pain with no real benefit is unethical. The nurse believes her first obligation is to M.H. alleviating her pain, and not to K.J.'s need for closure.

The attending physician adopts a principle-based approach, favoring patient autonomy and respect for persons. He recognizes the daughter's distress but believes that K.J.'s desire to lighten up on pain medication comes from her fear of losing her mother and is not based on her knowledge of her mother's wishes. Because M.H. should be respected as a person, reducing her pain medication to alleviate her daughter's fears is unethical. He sees no reason to put M.H. on a ventilator and favors institution of comfort measures only.

The resident had a case a year ago, when she was an intern, in which a patient's illness was thought to be terminal but his family insisted on aggressive interventions and the patient recovered from the acute episode, lived another 3 months, and was able to attend his daughter's wedding. This case, occurring early in her career, profoundly influences her to pursue at least a trial at intubation and aggressive interventions for M.H. Applying a casuistry-based approach, the resident supports the daughter's request. She writes orders to reduce pain medication and agrees to speak to the attending physician about aggressive interventions. She asks the CNS to help the nurses implement this new medication plan for the patient.

The social worker adopts a care-based approach, privileging the relationships within the patient's family. He himself has a long-standing relationship with the neurosurgeon and he trusts that the prognosis is correct. He has worked with this patient and her family on previous hospitalizations. He believes if K.J. has a chance to see that less medication will not change M.H.'s ability to communicate, she will be able to accept the terminal nature of her mother's condition. He helps K.J. to agree to a DNR order and closes the discussion by encouraging her and the rest of the family to stay with the patient and to "be together at this crucial time." He also asks the staff nurse to relax the regulations regarding family visitation so that the daughter and her children can spend more time at M.H.'s bedside.

The chaplain is able to spend quiet time with K.J. and her children while they are at M.H.'s bedside. He learns that the family has limited financial resources and that K.J. has a 10th-grade education. Prior to M.H.'s diagnosis, the daughter's only interactions with the health care system were the births of her two children. Her mother has assisted her in the care of her children, making it possible for her to work. The chaplain hears one of the intensive care unit nurses describe K.J. as "totally clueless." Interpreting the case from a feminist viewpoint, she worries that the family's socioeconomic status and the daughter's educational background are creating a bias against K.J. The chaplain is determined to advocate for the patient's daughter to correct this power imbalance.

The CNS's involvement in the case begins when the staff nurse consults her because his appeals to the resident and attending physician have failed to result in what he believes is the right course of action—maintenance of the current medication schedule. The CNS listens to the staff nurse's story and attends carefully to the details he gives. She then seeks out the resident, attending physician, chaplain, and social worker to hear their perspectives. She adopts a narrative-based approach and wants to hear all the contextual features of the case before deciding about the best course of action to address the conflict. When she speaks to M.H.'s daughter, she learns about the conversation that K.J. had with her mother shortly before M.H. became unresponsive, in which M.H. expressed a desire to plan her grandson's birthday party. It is this conversation that led the patient's daughter to request a change in

medication and a plea for aggressive interventions: "I know she wants to be here for my kids," she weeps; "she wouldn't give up without telling me."

Resolution of the Case
The CNS organizes a team meeting. She has discerned that personal biases may be influencing different perspectives of team members. She asks the members to work toward a consistent message that can be given to M.H.'s daughter because the contrasting views are clearly creating confusion. This request results in careful review of the clinical aspects of the case, including the most recent magnetic resonance imaging scan, and brings the team to an agreement that the patient's condition is most likely unrecoverable and she is dying. The chaplain has an opportunity to ask questions and share what she overheard. She is reassured that the team was unaware of the daughter's educational background and economic status and that they are not basing their care treatment plan on these factors. She is further reassured that what she heard was not intended as disrespect toward the daughter but rather a reflection of frustration at the situation. The CNS then moves forward to establish a mutually acceptable plan of care.

In a subsequent family meeting, the team explains the patient's prognosis to the patient's daughter using layperson's terms and simple pictures to clarify the growth of the tumor and its position. After addressing K.J.'s questions, the CNS explains that the team has met separately to consider carefully her request for a change in medication and that the potential harm of such a plan outweighs potential benefits. The CNS ends the meeting with the family by offering them additional time to discuss their options and ask any further questions. After several hours the daughter asks to speak with someone from hospice. The CNS's impact in this case is through influencing the flow of communication, not controlling the discussion. ◎

---

of ethical theory is beyond the scope of this chapter, but the reader is referred to the references cited for more detail.

Professional Codes and Guidelines
The ANA's *Code of Ethics for Nurses* (2015) describes the profession's philosophy and general ethical obligations of the professional nurse. It describes broad guidelines that more reflect the profession's conscience than provides specific directions for

particular clinical situations. It provides a framework that delineates the nurse's overriding moral obligations to the patient, family, community, and profession.

Professional organizations delineate standards of performance that reflect the responsibilities, obligations, duties, and rights of the members. These standards also can serve as guidelines for professional behavior and define desired conduct. Although the general principles are relatively stable, professional organizations often reflect on specific or contemporary issues and take a proactive position on pivotal concerns. For example, the American Association of Critical-Care Nurses (2008) has issued a position paper on moral distress, acknowledging that it negatively affects quality of care and influences nurses who are considering leaving the profession. The paper then lists the responsibilities of nurses to address moral distress, some resources that can be helpful to them, and the obligations of nurses' employers to offer support, such as employee assistance programs and ethics committees, to assist with managing moral distress. An additional example is the International Association of Forensic Nurses' position paper (2009) supporting the use of emergency contraception for victims of sexual assault. This document provides ethical and clinical rationales for policies that permit dispensing of these medications.

Personal and Professional Values

Individuals' interpretations and positions on issues are a reflection of their underlying value system. Value systems are enduring beliefs that guide life choices and decisions in conflict resolution (Ludwick & Silva, 2000). Viens (1995) found that values were an essential feature of the everyday practice of the 10 primary care NPs she interviewed. Values of caring, responsibility, trust, justice, honesty, sanctity and quality of life, empathy, and religious beliefs were articulated by the study participants, often as ideals that motivated their actions. An awareness of personal values generates more consistent choices and behaviors; it can also assist APRNs to be aware of the boundaries of their personal and professional values so that they can recognize when their own positions may be unduly influencing patient and family decision making.

Values awareness should include an understanding of the complex interplay between cultural values and ethical decision making (Buryska, 2001; Ludwick & Silva, 2000). When patient and family decisions contradict traditional Western medical practice, health care providers may inadvertently resort to coercive or paternalistic measures to influence patients' choices to be more consistent with the provider's values. APRNs and other health care providers must understand that their recommendations for particular treatments may be unduly influenced by their own cultural values. Providers must intentionally explore factors that guide a patient's decisions so that the treatment plan is consistent with the patient's value preferences. For example, a patient from a Southeast Asian culture may show respect to authority figures by obeying the APRN's treatment suggestions, even if he or she disagrees with the plan. In this situation, the APRN could assure the patient that questions about the plan of care are welcomed and are not disrespectful.

By the same token, claims made in the name of religious and cultural beliefs are not absolute. Buryska (2001) offered helpful guidelines for clinicians to assess the defensibility of patient and family claims made in the name of cultural or religious considerations. For example, he maintained that spiritual or cultural claims grounded in an identifiable and established community are more defensible than those that are idiosyncratic to the person making the claim. Although it is critical for caregivers to respond with respectful dialogue, support, and compassionate care, patient and family demands for treatment must be considered in relation to other claims that also have ethical weight—the professional integrity of providers, legal considerations, economic realities, and issues of distributive justice.

Professional Boundaries

In their professional capacity, APRNs often develop long-term therapeutic relationships with many of their patients. The intimate nature of the relationship, coupled with the compassionate nature of nurses, may make them vulnerable to boundary violations. A violation may be the result of a well-intentioned provider who rationalizes crossing lines for the benefit of the patient (Holder & Schenthal, 2007). For example, the APRN forms a close relationship with a terminally ill patient and his spouse. When the patient dies, the APRN feels compelled to offer support to his wife and agrees to go to lunch with her. The death of her patient is the catalyst that causes the APRN to drift across a boundary, profoundly altering the expectations and therapeutic nature of the relationship. The obligation to maintain professional boundaries within a therapeutic relationship is shared with all nurses (ANA, 2015), and APRNs are also in a position to observe for boundary violations by others and to intervene when they occur.

APRN boundary crossings may lead to transgressions and ultimately violations. This is known as boundary drift (Holder & Schenthal, 2007). A frequent opportunity for transgression occurs when patients and families express gratitude for a provider's care. Gifts such as boxes of candy or flowers are routine. When the gifts become excessive or have significant financial worth (e.g., expensive tickets to a sporting event), providers are challenged to acknowledge the gratitude and redirect it, for example, by suggesting a charitable donation to the facility. When the transgression is initiated by the provider, regardless of the magnitude, the behavior must be addressed immediately and the culpable individual must be removed from interaction with the patient. Other members of the health care team will need to step in and reestablish therapeutic boundaries (National Council of State Boards of Nursing, 2009).

Element 2: Knowledge Application

The second element of the core competency is applying the knowledge developed in the first level to the clinical practice arena. Because skill in ethical decision making cannot be developed in a moral vacuum, APRNs must actively seek out positions different from their own so that they can develop new perspectives to approaching an ethical dilemma (Robichaux, 2012). As APRNs acquire core ethical decision-making knowledge, the responsibility to take moral action to address ethical dilemmas becomes more compelling. Action is more successful if the APRN learns to identify situations that are at risk for ethical conflict (Pavlish, Brown-Saltzman, Hersh, Shirk, & Nudelman, 2011). When the APRN is proactive in identifying ethical issues and can mount a timely response to an identified ethical conflict, he or she can change the course in present and future situations. Therefore moral action should not be underestimated as a core APRN skill and should be recognized, fostered, and valued by others. *Once an advanced nursing role is assumed, the APRN accepts the responsibility to be a full participant in the resolution of moral dilemmas rather than simply an interested observer or one of many parties in conflict.*

When APRNs apply core knowledge of ethical concepts, they begin to develop the practical wisdom of moral reasoning. Learning how to approach crucial conversations is a necessary skill for APRNs to master because it will enable them to be leaders in resolving conflicts that arise (Maxfield et al., 2005, 2010). The success and speed with which the APRN gains these behavioral skills is related to the presence of mentors in the clinical setting and the willingness of the APRN to become immersed in ethical discussions.

Institutional resources, such as ethics committees and institutional review boards, provide valuable opportunities for APRNs to participate in the discussion of ethical issues. Typically, hospital ethics committees serve three functions: policy formation, case review, and education. As a member of the ethics committee, the APRN exchanges ideas with colleagues and gains an understanding of ethical dilemmas from a variety of perspectives. In addition, the APRN is informed of current legislation, regulations, and hospital policies that have ethical implications. This is an extremely valuable experience that can accelerate the development of ethical decision-making skills.

Unfortunately, most APRNs do not have the opportunity to serve on interprofessional ethics committees and, in some cases, may have few resources or professional colleagues available to mentor and develop the skills of ethical decision making. Thus the APRNs must advance their ethical decision making competency by actively seeking opportunities to read about and apply ethical knowledge and, more importantly, engaging in ethical dialogue with professional colleagues. Professional organizations offer materials such as *The 4 A's to Rise Above Moral Distress* (American Association of Critical-Care Nurses, 2004) and workshops in which case studies are discussed and analyzed. This format is helpful to the inexperienced APRN, who needs guidance in applying knowledge to clinical cases.

Ethical Decision-Making Frameworks

Several authors have proposed a stepwise approach to ethical decision making (Doherty & Purtilo, 2016; McCormick-Gendzel & Jurchak, 2006; Rushton & Penticuff, 2007; Spencer, 2005; Wueste, 2005). In Box 13.4, the steps suggested by Doherty and Purtilo (2016) are listed as an example. The reader will note that this framework uses many elements of the various ethical approaches discussed earlier in considering contextual factors, seeking full information on a case, and specifying a step that explicitly appeals to ethical theory. This framework for ethical decision making is intended for all health professionals and therefore is applicable to a wide variety of situations. Regardless of the model chosen, there are a number of common mistakes or fallacies that NPs should avoid when justifying their ethical position. Some examples include giving undue weight to someone in authority, focusing on the characteristics of the people involved in the conflict rather than on their positions, and providing only a basic rationale for their positions (a necessary but not sufficient step) without exploring broader features in the situation (Cooper, 2012).

Most frameworks for ethical decision making include information gathering as a key step. Generally, information about the clinical situation, the parties involved, their obligations and values, and

BOX 13.4 **Sample Ethical Decision-Making Framework**

1. **Gather information:**
   - Clarify the additional information needed.
   - Categories of information to consider include clinical indications, patient preferences, quality of life, and contextual factors.
   - Caution is advised not to make this step an end in itself.

2. **Determine that the problem is an ethical one and identify the type:**
   - Locus of authority—conflict involves determining who should make a decision.
   - Ethical dilemma—conflict in which two opposing courses of action are both ethically justifiable but cannot both be satisfied.
   - Moral distress—conflict in which the ethical course of action seems clear but the agent feels unable to carry it out.

3. **Use ethical theories or approaches to analyze the problem:**
   - A utilitarian approach would focus on the consequences of potential actions.
   - A deontologic approach would focus on the duties of involved parties.
   - Various ethical theories provide additional perspectives (see "Overview of Ethical Approaches" and the references cited).

4. **Explore the practical alternatives:**
   - Imagination is required to ensure that a wide range of alternatives are identified.
   - Diligence in assessing the feasibility of identified actions is also essential.

5. **Complete the action:**
   - Once determined, motivation to carry out the ethical action is essential.
   - Not to act at this point is a conscious choice, with consequences.

6. **Evaluate the process and outcome:**
   - What went well, and why?
   - To what other situations might this experience apply?
   - What do the patient, family, and other providers say about the course of action taken?

Adapted from Doherty, R. F., & Purtilo, R. B. (2016). *Ethical dimensions in the health professions* (6th ed.). Philadelphia, PA: Saunders.

legal, cultural, and religious factors are needed. However, this factual information is not sufficient unless tempered with the contextual features of each case. Identifying the cause of the problem and determining why, where, and when it occurred, and who or what was affected, will help clarify the nature of the problem.

Problem identification is also a common step in most frameworks. Strong emotional responses to a situation can be the first signal that ethical conflict exists. However, many conflicts that arise in the clinical setting generate powerful emotional responses but may not be ethical issues. Ethical issues are those that involve some form of controversy about conflicting moral values and/or fundamental duties or obligations. The APRN must distinguish and separate moral dilemmas from other issues, such as administrative concerns, communication problems, and lack of clinical knowledge. For example, a communication problem between a staff nurse and physician may be resolved if an APRN acts as a facilitator, ensuring that each understands the perspective of the other. In this case, ethical decision making may not be needed; the conflict does not result from a difference in values but rather a failure to communicate. As noted, effective and compassionate communication skills undergird this competency.

Although a framework provides structure and suggests a method of examining and studying the ethical issues, the essential component of resolution of ethical dilemmas is moral action. Simply knowing the right course of action does not guarantee that a person has the motivation or courage to act (LaSala & Bjarnason, 2010; Rest, 1986; Rushton & Penticuff, 2007).

Strategies for Resolution of Ethical Conflict

Conflict in any workplace is a daily occurrence. Learning to manage conflict of any kind will make it less likely that individuals will engage in behaviors that are destructive to teams (The Foundation Coalition, n.d.). The challenge in most cases of ethical disputes is to have all involved parties listen to each other's perspectives to understand the basis of the disagreement and work together to create a collaborative solution. In cases in which conflict is intense and resolution seems difficult, it may be helpful to solicit help from a member of the institution's ethics committee or another professional colleague not involved in the case. However, in many cases the APRN must serve as a facilitator for the parties in dispute. The objective of successful facilitation in ethical disputes is to achieve an integrity-preserving solution that is satisfactory to all parties. In reality, however, that is not always possible. The issues of time, cost, available resources, level of moral conviction, prognostic uncertainty, and perceived value of the relationship play important roles in the strategy used and likelihood of reaching a desired outcome (Spielman, 1993).

Spielman (1993) applied Thomas' (1992) five strategies for managing conflict to resolving ethical conflicts, of which collaboration is the preferred approach. Her typology is useful for evaluating ethical conflict resolution. As described in Chapter 12, collaboration is a core competency of advanced practice nursing. Recent attention to interprofessional competencies has also emphasized the importance of collaboration (Canadian Interprofessional Health Collaborative, 2010; IPEC, 2011). In ethical conflicts, a collaborative approach is the most likely to result in a solution that preserves the integrity of all involved parties.

Collaboration, however, is not always possible in resolving ethical disputes. The other four approaches include the following:

1. *Compromise* is an appropriate approach to ethical decision making when the parties involved are committed to preserving their relationship and each possesses a high moral certainty about their position.

2. Alternatively, *accommodation* occurs when one party is more committed than the other to preserving the relationship; the committed party defers to the other, with the result that only one perspective directs the outcome. Accommodation is unlikely to promote the integrity of all involved parties and should be used only when time is limited or the issue is trivial.

3. *Coercion* is also a strategy unlikely to result in an integrity-preserving outcome. In this approach, the more powerful party, who has a strong commitment to a particular position, determines the outcome of the conflict through an aggressive stance.

4. *Avoidance* is the most dangerous of the strategies considered by Spielman (1993) because the less powerful party does not articulate his or her ethical concerns.

Exemplar 13.3 provides examples of each of these strategies in a situation that evoked considerable ethical conflict.

There is an additional dynamic that may be operating in environments in which avoidance is the norm in dealing with ethical conflict. In a series of observational qualitative studies of hospital-based nurses, Chambliss (1996) documented a phenomenon he called "routinization" of the moral world (p. 38).

EXEMPLAR 13.3 **Strategies Used in Resolving Ethical Conflict**

An acute care nurse practitioner (ACNP) in an ambulatory clinic provides comprehensive care to patients with narcotics addiction. J.S., a 36-year-old male patient, also has a history of asthma, cigarette smoking, alcohol use, and an anxiety disorder. He arrives at the clinic and is disruptive in the waiting room. He is pacing back and forth and loudly stating he needs his methadone. In the interval since his last visit, he has wrecked his car and has no easy form of transportation. He has missed multiple days of work and is worried about losing his job.

At this visit, J.S. reports that he has not taken medications for his anxiety because he ran out of pills and had no mechanism for refilling them. He is not carrying an inhaler and is wheezing mildly. He denies any recreational drug use. The ACNP wants to see him for follow-up regarding his asthma and anxiety in 1 week and gives him prescriptions for an anxiolytic and an inhaler.

The following day, J.S. shows up for his methadone. He states that he lost the prescriptions and asks if he could get new ones. The clinic nurse expresses frustration and concern that the patient is "working the system." She claims in exasperation, "He does this all the time!!" She feels the patient may be selling his prescriptions and wants to report him to the police. She suggests that the ACNP tell the patient that if he continues to be irresponsible and disrupt the clinic, the clinic will no longer provide treatment.

The social worker, whose ongoing contact with the patient was instrumental in getting him to attend clinic regularly and stay out of trouble, advises the ACNP that there is no evidence of a crime. He states his belief that using coercion will raise the patient's anxiety and likely result in him not following up on treatment for his asthma and will likely not change his disruptive behavior.

The ACNP notes the emotional responses of the interprofessional team members, which signal an ethical conflict. Her initial thought is to provide the new prescriptions and say nothing. This strategy is an

Continued

EXEMPLAR 13.3   **Strategies Used in Resolving Ethical Conflict—cont'd**

example of avoidance. Another avoidance option would be to send the patient to another provider for his medications. For example, a pulmonologist could be consulted for the asthma medication. The ACNP considers but does not select either of these courses of action.

In communications with the clinic nurse, the ACNP uses accommodation as a strategy for managing ethical conflict. She validates the nurse's concern about the negative impact of the patient's behavior on the other clinic patients and agrees that the behavior is inappropriate and needs to be addressed. The strategy favored by the social worker is also an example of accommodation. He believes that the obligation of the clinic staff is the delivery of patient care and that they should be able to overlook "minor" inconveniences for this patient, who clearly has limited resources. He suggests not providing prescriptions to J.S. again but adopting a policy of calling or faxing all prescriptions for him directly to a pharmacy.

The clinic nurse's strategy is an example of coercion. In coercive strategies, the ethical decision maker resolves the conflict by exerting a controlling influence on another party whose actions or values are fueling the conflict. Suggesting to J.S. that his actions may affect his access to the care he needs exerts power over this patient. The disadvantage of this type of strategy is the powerlessness it imposes.

When J.S. arrives for his follow-up appointment the next week, the ACNP informs him that the staff in the clinic are concerned about his disruptive behavior. She tells the patient, "I do not want you to be in trouble. Being disruptive in clinic is not fair to other patients or the staff who are working to provide care. In addition, losing prescriptions is frustrating and causes others to be suspicious about what happened to the first prescription. I want to work with you to help you stay well." When she invites the patient to help her understand what happened, the patient reveals some important information. J.S. explains that being in the clinic is hard because it makes him more anxious, especially when there are lots of other patients in the waiting room. He accepts his minor wheezing as "normal" and does not see his asthma as a big problem.

The ACNP offers to help J.S. identify strategies to lower his anxiety when he has to wait and offers the suggestion that the clinic fax prescriptions directly to the pharmacy in the future. J.S. agrees to these changes and states he will work harder to be less disruptive in the future.

Another conflict evident in this case is between the clinic nurse and the social worker. Compromise is needed to maintain an effective working relationship because the two provide care to the same patient population. Compromise can be achieved if the two parties focus on a common goal and relinquish control of some elements of the final decision. In this case, the ACNP meets with both parties and they identify that their common goal is efficient delivery of quality health care. Through compromise, the clinic nurse recognized the value that the social worker placed on keeping the patient in care and relinquished her desire to coerce the patient to get him to change his behavior. Similarly, the social worker recognized that the nurse wanted to avoid disruptive behavior that upsets other clinic patients. He agreed to relinquish his accommodating approach to the patient's behavior if it negatively affected the clinic's operation in the future. ◎

In routinization, nurses became enmeshed in the tasks and routines of care delivery and, over time, became accustomed and desensitized to the ethical conflicts around them. The routine blunted the nurses' moral sensitivity and moral agency so that moral difficulties were not recognized; nurses commented, "You just get used to it." Chambliss (1996) also noted that nurses were aware of problems but often did not see them as "ethics problems," and neither did those in authority. The great ethical danger in such environments is not that nurses would make the wrong choice when faced with an important decision, but that they would never realize that they are facing a decision at all. APRNs must be alert for signs of routinization of the moral dimension of practice in the environments in which they care for patients. Identifying and addressing features of the system that blunt or dismiss the moral sensitivity of any care provider is a critical part of APRN leadership.

Element 3: Creating an Ethical Environment

As the APRN becomes more skilled in the application of ethical knowledge, she or he is better positioned to help create and sustain ethical environments. The ethical health of the work environment is a critical factor in whether ethical problems are productively addressed. The foundation of an ethical work environment includes respectful, productive interpersonal relationships and skilled communication (American

Association of Critical-Care Nurses, 2015). APRNs must demonstrate what it means to be respectful to colleagues in all disciplines. Multiple studies show that poor relationships between physicians and nurses can contribute to moral distress, a sign of ethical conflict (Bruce, Miller, & Zimmerman, 2015; Gutierrez, 2005; Hamric & Blackhall, 2007; Kälvemark, Höglund, Hansson, Westerholm, & Arnetz, 2004; Piers et al., 2011). Without respect, healthy relationships are doomed, communication is ineffective, and not only can this be unethical, it can be harmful (The Joint Commission, 2008).

In one study of NPs, the participants' perception of the ethical environment was the strongest predictor of ethical conflict in practice; the more ethical the environment, the lower was the ethical conflict (Ulrich et al., 2003). Too often, other nurses and members of the health care team remain silent about ethical issues (Gordon & Hamric, 2006; Maxfield et al., 2005). When APRNs demonstrate effective ethical decision making, they can lead the way in the creation of a climate in which ethical concerns are routinely addressed.

Once the APRN transforms ethical knowledge into moral action, he or she can emerge as a mentor for others who are grappling with ethical dilemmas. In a mentoring capacity, the APRN helps colleagues deal with moral uncertainty and develop the ability to voice ethical concerns. In this way, the APRN supports and empowers other team members to develop confidence and fosters an environment in which diverse views are expressed and problems are moved toward resolution. APRNs can broaden their influence by intentionally engaging colleagues in thoughtful reflection of moral issues by leading ethics rounds and case reviews. CNSs in particular have abundant opportunities to foster nurses' everyday ethical comportment through the seemingly mundane details of patient care.

In a classic article, Shannon noted that the roots of interprofessional conflict in the clinical setting are often based on preconceived stereotypes of the moral viewpoints of other disciplines and perceptions of the moral superiority of one's own discipline (Shannon, 1997). APRNs can help professionals from other disciplines understand the perspectives and socialization of nurses. Teaching and mentoring activities of the mature APRN often focus on other professional colleagues to prepare them proactively to communicate openly with patients about ethical concerns.

Creating an ethical environment encompasses aspects of coaching and teaching patients and families in ethical decision making. It is not sufficient for the APRN simply to provide information to patients and families facing difficult moral choices and expect them to arrive at a comfortable decision. The ethical competency is linked closely with the ability to mobilize patients and the APRN's colleagues so that those who need help move through the necessary steps to reach resolution.

APRNs should strive to develop environments that encourage patients and caregivers to express diverse views and raise questions. Thoughtful ethical decision making arises from an environment that supports and values the critical exchange of ideas and promotes collaboration among members of the health care team, patients, and families. A collaborative practice environment, in turn, supports shared decision making, shared accountability, and group participation, fostering relationships based on equality and mutuality. The APRN is integral to the development and preservation of a collaborative culture that inspires and empowers individuals to respond to moral dilemmas.

The current nature of health care delivery across and through care settings creates a climate in which many workers feel overwhelmed, stressed, and discouraged by the lack of time to care for patients and their increased acuity levels. Combined with a sense of powerlessness and routinization (Chambliss, 1996), these factors can result in nurses retreating from a stance of moral agency. An ethically sensitive environment is one in which providers are encouraged to acknowledge when they feel overwhelmed and seek help when they need it (Hamric, Epstein, & White, 2013). The *Code of Ethics for Nurses* (ANA, 2015) has affirmed the importance of nurses contributing to an ethically sensitive health care environment, as well as preserving personal integrity. One provision states that "The nurse owes the same duties to self as to others, including the responsibility to preserve integrity and safety" (p. 4). Only when care providers recognize and attend to their personal needs will they be better able to detect and nurture the needs of others.

Preventive Ethics

An additional important role of the APRNs in Element 3 is to extend the concept of ethical decision making beyond problem solving and to move toward a paradigm of preventive ethics. The term *preventive ethics* is derived from the model of preventive medicine; the term was coined by Forrow, Arnold, and Parker (1993). It emphasizes developing effective organizational policies and practices that prevent ethical problems from developing (McCullough, 2005). The ability to predict areas of conflict and develop plans in a proactive rather than reactive manner will avert some potentially difficult dilemmas and can lead to more ethically responsive environments (Forrow et al., 1993; Fox, Bottrell, Foglia, & Stoeckle, 2007; McCullough, 2005; Nelson, Gardent, Shulman, & Splaine, 2010).

When value conflicts arise, resolution becomes more difficult because one value must be chosen over another. Preventive ethics emphasizes that all important values should be reviewed and examined prior to the conflict so that situations in which values may conflict can be anticipated. In other words, the goals of the health care team should be articulated as clearly as possible to avoid potential misinterpretations. For example, a CRNA should have an understanding of a terminally ill patient's values regarding aggressive treatment in case a cardiopulmonary arrest occurs during surgery. However, the CRNA's moral and legal obligations should be openly discussed so that the patient and professional appreciate and recognize each other's values and moral and legal positions. Modeling this preventive approach in ethical deliberations encourages the early identification of values and beliefs that may influence treatment decisions and allows time to resolve impending issues before problems arise. In much the same way, early anticipation of potential complications in patients can lead to proactive discussions of ethical issues and restructuring of the care environment to anticipate and avoid ethical conflict.

A conscientious inspection of other factors that influence the evolution of moral dilemmas reveals a number of environmental factors that can become barriers to ethical practice. Chambliss (1996) made the important point that features of the work setting and their role as employees often create moral problems for nurses. Examining roles and responsibilities of all parties may expose power imbalances. Issues related to powerlessness are an area in which the APRNs can influence change. By providing knowledge, promoting a positive self-image, and preparing others for participation in decision making, the APRN empowers individuals. APRNs must avoid the trap of trying to fix problems for others. When faced with a dilemma, the APRN is not responsible for identifying the "one right answer." The skill of the APRN is used not to resolve moral dilemmas single-handedly, but rather to mentor others to assume a position of moral accountability and engage in shared decision making. Enhancing others' autonomy and providing opportunities for involvement in reaching resolution

is a key concept in preventive ethics (Forrow et al., 1993).

Ethically responsive environments are enhanced by a process of ongoing, rather than episodic, ethical inquiry. Throughout this process, the APRN incorporates his or her skills, ethical expertise, and clinical background on issues necessary to facilitate dialogue, mediate disputes, analyze options, and design optimal solutions. The ethical decision-making skills of the APRN move the resolution of moral dilemmas beyond individual cases toward the cultivation of an environment in which the moral integrity of individuals is respected. Development and preservation of this ethical environment is the key contribution of the APRN. Although ethical issues may develop with little warning, the practice of preventive ethics greatly improves a team's ability to handle these issues in a morally responsible and innovative manner.

Exemplar 13.4 provides an example of preventive ethics in addressing staff moral distress. This case highlights how the ethical decision-making competency of APRNs can lessen the reoccurrence of moral problems. In this situation, Dea's actions went beyond resolving a single case of moral distress and focused on the features of the system that were contributing to the distress of the staff. As this exemplar shows, recurring ethical problems, particularly moral distress, are sometimes a result of the structure of care delivery systems in an institution. Dea's case demonstrates that applying a preventive ethics approach to the system requires perseverance and ongoing identification of new strategies to change complex and interrelated system features.

Element 4: Promoting Social Justice Within the Health Care System

Nursing as a profession plays a pivotal role in society, focusing specialized knowledge, skills, and caring on improving the health of the public (ANA, 2010). The final element in the ethical decision-making competency is seen in mature APRNs who have expanded their focus of concern to incorporate the needs of their larger specialty population. This element builds on the previous ones as APRNs expand their sphere of involvement beyond their institution into the societal sector. Moving into the arena of social justice is an historic legacy and a current imperative. Falk-Raphael (2005) has noted that Florence Nightingale's work bequeathed to professional nursing "a legacy of justice-making as an expression of caring and compassion" (p. 212). Increasing attention to social justice has been seen in nursing literature in the United States and

Dea, a clinical nurse specialist (CNS) in a neuroscience intensive care unit (ICU), seeks to change the management of patients with traumatic brain injury (TBI). She and other members of the staff have noted that the care of this population is inconsistent, and many staff have a fatalistic attitude about these patients' hope of recovery. She is also aware of recent research on the use of a new technology, brain tissue oxygen monitoring, that has shown promise in improving outcomes for these patients. As an initial step, she invites a CNS from another state, an expert in the management of TBI whom she knows to be an inspiring speaker, to give a presentation on brain tissue oxygen monitoring. Dea arranges for staff coverage so that all neuroscience ICU registered nurses can attend the presentation, in which the speaker describes how the technology is used to prevent progressive injury in patients with TBI. Members of the respiratory therapy team, staff in the emergency room, and nurses from the trauma ICU are also invited to the presentation, which is highly successful. Dea then collaborates with the nurse manager and administration to implement brain tissue oxygen monitoring in the neuroscience ICU. She obtains key physician support, provides training sessions, supports the staff when the technology is introduced into patient care, and develops algorithms for acting on the information this technology provides. Dea also creates a Wall of Fame, highlighting all unit patients who have recovered, to help staff celebrate successes in caring for this challenging patient population.

As staff develop skills and knowledge related to the management of TBI patients, they notice the improved outcomes in monitored patients as the technology detects changes in cerebral oxygen level; these data promote early aggressive intervention. However, Dea begins to realize that this success itself is creating a new source of moral distress. Although patients with TBI are often managed in the neuroscience ICU, they are also admitted to other ICUs where this technology is not available. In addition, the application of the technology varies depending on the preferences of the attending physician and residents assigned to manage TBI patients. Although some of the medical staff are open to the use of the brain tissue oxygen monitor, others do not agree that it is a valid tool. Because the nurses see the better than expected outcomes of monitored patients as compared with those who do not receive monitoring, they believe that all patients should receive this technology. The staff's moral distress heightens after a particularly troubling case of a young TBI patient who was never monitored with the new technology and subsequently died.

Recognizing an ethical conflict with the potential to recur with increasing frequency, Dea takes action using a preventive ethics approach. She consults a nurse with expertise in ethics to meet with the staff. During that meeting, their moral distress is articulated. The nurses value their growing expertise in brain tissue oxygen monitoring and note that this new technology has served as the impetus for improving the care of TBI patients. However, the nurses are not empowered to maximize its application because decisions about the admission of patients with TBI to an ICU are made without nursing input and because the medical staff, not the nursing staff, makes the final decision to make use of the brain tissue oxygen monitor.

During the meeting, the staff identify a number of strategies for decreasing their moral distress. One is directing admission of TBI patients to the neuroscience ICU, recognizing at the same time that patients with thoracic and abdominal trauma as well as TBI would still be admitted to the trauma ICU; in addition, many TBI patients are first admitted to the trauma ICU while these other problems are ruled out. Better communication between ICU charge nurses was considered as a means to improve nursing input into bed assignment. Another strategy discussed in the meeting was advocacy for patients' needs on the part of the neuroscience nurses with the medical staff. The staff is encouraged to use Dea as a resource when they encounter resistance from their medical colleagues. A final strategy identified at this meeting was to track the outcomes of patients who have received brain tissue oxygen monitoring and thus develop a database to support the value of this tool. Dea agrees to collect the data, review each case, and follow up on quality-of-care issues.

Dea then works with a colleague in the trauma ICU to improve communication among the neuroscience ICU, trauma ICU, and neurosurgical team. They arrange a meeting with nurses from both ICUs and surgeons from the neurosurgery and trauma teams. At that meeting, the use of aggressive measures in TBI patients, including brain tissue oxygen monitoring, are discussed. In follow-up, Dea and her physician colleagues in neurosurgery and neurocritical care develop algorithms for the management of TBI, identifying patients who may benefit from brain tissue oxygen monitoring and facilitating their admission to the neuroscience ICU.

Continued

| EXEMPLAR 13.4 | Addressing Staff Moral Distress Through Preventive Ethics[a]—cont'd |

These algorithms are reviewed by the trauma service for incorporation into the trauma manual, a document used by all trauma residents.

Dea also continues to encourage and support her staff to be proactive advocates. She coaches the nurses toward effective advocacy and role-models collaboration and information sharing in her own communications with residents and attending physicians. Over time, Dea begins to see an increased acceptance of the new technology and of an aggressive approach to managing TBI among the neurosurgery teams.

Two members of the nursing staff, with Dea's encouragement and guidance, developed a poster about their moral distress and steps to address it. The poster was accepted and presented at a national conference (Pracher, Moss, & Mahanes, 2006). The nurses attending the conference to present the poster learned that their situation is not unique; other conference attendees noted similar conflicts in their own units and validated the distress experienced as a result.

Although a closer connection between the neuroscience and trauma ICUs is a secondary benefit, concerns about inconsistencies in care continue. Patients with TBI continue to be admitted to the neuroscience and trauma ICUs and are not always transferred quickly if they need monitoring. Through a collaborative process with the CNS in the trauma ICU, a new approach to standardizing the care of TBI patients is identified and plans are made to incorporate brain tissue oxygen monitoring in the trauma ICU. The database that Dea has maintained demonstrates positive patient outcomes that support this change. Dea lends support to the CNS in that unit as she begins to train the staff in the use of the technology and the algorithms for responding to the information it provides. Two years after the initial education session on this technology, Dea notes that "there is still work to do to optimize the care of these patients." However, because of her proactive response to the staff's distress, champions for this technology now exist on both units, and an environment for effecting positive change has been created. ◎

[a]We gratefully acknowledge Dea Mahanes, MSN, RN, Charlottesville, VA, for sharing this exemplar.

internationally (Bell & Hulbert, 2008; Buettner-Schmidt & Lobo, 2011; Grace & Willis, 2012; Tarlier & Browne, 2011). Although APRNs prepared at the master's level may develop social justice practices over time, the AACN's *The Essentials of Doctoral Education for Advanced Nursing Practice* (2006) strongly supports APRNs moving into a larger arena of ethical decision making, with explicit preparation in DNP programs. The need for nursing to speak to mounting concerns regarding the quality of patient care delivery, resource allocation, and outcomes in policy and public forums is one justification for doctoral-level education for APRNs. Most of the DNP Essentials address the need for systems leadership in these larger forums; one in particular, "Health Care Policy for Advocacy in Health Care," advocates for DNP graduates to "design, implement and advocate for health care policy that addresses issues of social justice and equity in health care. The powerful practice experiences of the DNP graduate can become potent influencers in policy formation" (p. 13).

In a number of hallmark reports, the Institute of Medicine (2000, 2001, 2003) has highlighted the fragmentation and systems failures in health care and called for restructuring efforts to achieve safe, effective, and equitable care. Equity is primarily an issue of justice; as noted, concerns about access to and distribution of health care resources are key justice concerns of APRNs.

Nurses in many roles have been increasingly concerned by the current health care system and the gaps in care provision to many of the neediest members of society. Some have asserted that all nurses should include sociopolitical advocacy in their practice if the profession is to fulfill its social mandate (Falk-Raphael, 2005). This is a tall order because many formal education programs, undergraduate and graduate, may not include such content, so the APRN must commit to continued skill development and involvement in national organizations to achieve competence at this level. The clinical expertise and an APRN's cutting-edge understanding of the clinical needs of her or his patient population provide the platform from which the APRN speaks to social justice issues. Nurses in policy, research, or other non-APRNs roles often call on APRNs to provide expert information on the policy and larger system issues that confront their specialty populations.

To enact this level of the ethical decision-making competency requires sophisticated use of all of the core competencies of advanced practice nursing. In particular, advocacy, communication, collaboration (see Chapter 12), and leadership (see Chapter 11) are required. APRNs active at this level are often consultants to policymakers or serve on expert panels crafting policies for specialty groups. Essential knowledge needed for this element includes an understanding of the concepts of justice, particularly distributive justice (the equitable allocation of scarce resources) and restorative justice (the duty owed to those who have been systematically disadvantaged through no fault of their own). In addition, knowledge of the health policy process in general (see Chapter 19) and specific health policies affecting their specialty population are needed by APRNs to move into this level of activity.

Exemplar 13.5 describes one APRN's development through the different elements of the ethical decision-making competency, including beginning activity in promoting social justice. Chapter 19 also provides examples of actions by nurses who have expanded their concerns about individual patients into working for social justice in the policy arena.

Although this element of the ethical decision-making competency may sound daunting to the novice, beginning activities in this arena, such as involvement in institutional or community policymaking groups and sustained efforts to build ethical knowledge, can establish the foundation for larger policy involvement. Many graduate programs and almost all DNP programs have courses dedicated to the development of policy skills. It is often the case that the experience of moral outrage over the unethical treatment of patients propels the APRN into the policy arena as the APRN sees the consequences of the gaps in the current health care system.

Evaluation of the Ethical Decision-Making Competency

The evaluation of ethical decision making should focus on two areas—the process and the outcome. Process evaluation is important because it provides an overview of the moral disagreement, interpersonal skills used, interactions between both parties in conflict, and problems encountered during the phases of resolution. Whether the APRN is the facilitator or a party in conflict, there must be a deliberate and reflective evaluation of the process of resolution that includes assessing the type of ethical issue, interrelational and situational variables, ethical shifts that occurred during the process, and strategies used by all parties during the negotiation phase. Mediation, a process in which a neutral third party negotiates a resolution between parties who are in conflict, helping them find solutions consistent with their values, can be a very useful process (Dubler & Liebman, 2011). As the APRN reflects on the process, attention should be given to how similar situations could be anticipated and resolved in the future. Debriefing situations with the affected parties are also an important process evaluation strategy. To avoid the debriefing session becoming simply a venting of emotions, the APRN must keep the focus on preventive ethics and what needs to change in the environment to avoid or minimize future problems.

Deliberate and consistent review of the process will help the APRN assess various approaches to the resolution of ethical dilemmas and identify the onset of moral conflict earlier. This ongoing evaluation of process is particularly important in issues of social justice because it takes years for changes in system-wide health policies that support social justice to be implemented. Evaluating grassroots and legislative efforts as they occur will help identify strategies likely to be successful versus those that ought to be abandoned.

Evaluation of the outcome is also critical because it acknowledges creative solutions and celebrates moral action. Components of the outcome evaluation include the short- and long-term consequences of the action taken and the satisfaction of all parties with the chosen solution. Unfortunately, a successful process does not always result in a satisfactory outcome. Occasionally, the outcome reveals the need for changes in the institution or health care system. The APRN may need to become involved in advancing these desired changes or identifying appropriate resources to pursue them. The goal of outcome evaluation is to minimize the risks of a similar event by identifying predictable patterns and thereby averting recurrent and future dilemmas. The questions "What do we want to happen differently if we are confronted with a similar situation?" and "What first steps can we take to achieve this change?" can be helpful in framing the discussion.

Although evaluation of the ethical problem is an important step for preventing future dilemmas and building ethically sensitive environments, tension and uneasiness will remain in some situations. In true ethical dilemmas, even the best process may still result in a course of action that is not seen positively by all participants. It is important for APRNs to acknowledge that many issues leave a "moral

EXEMPLAR 13.5	Putting It All Together: Development of the Elements of the Ethical Decision-Making Competency[a]

R.T. is a family nurse practitioner (NP) who is completing a DNP program. Her experience with providing health care to Hispanic migrant farm workers in rural Virginia has given her many opportunities to use her ethical decision-making skills. This exemplar portrays her journey through the ethical decision-making competency including social justice as she has developed her APRN practice.

One fall evening, R.T. accompanies a team of outreach workers into a migrant farm camp to screen workers for diabetes and heart disease. Three older men approach her with concerns regarding Antonio, one of the new younger workers. They report that he has been losing weight, sweating all the time, and shaking and that he appears ill. They are scared for him and a little frightened that he could be contagious. R.T. encourages the men to have him schedule an appointment with her the following night because she would be staffing a mobile clinic in the community. The men are concerned that Antonio would be unwilling to give his information to anyone because he lacks legal documentation to be in the United States. The men promise that they will encourage Antonio to make an appointment and reassure him that R.T. will not report him to the authorities.

The next night, R.T. waits for someone to come to her with these concerns. When this does not happen, she walks outside the mobile clinic and luckily sees Antonio. He is easy to identify because he is sweating profusely and his hands are trembling. R.T. asks her community health worker to ask him to join her in the mobile clinic and, to her surprise, he agrees. Antonio looks much older than his reported age of 19. He is frail, anxious-appearing, and sweaty. After taking a history and doing an examination, R.T. suspects that he might have hyperthyroidism. She convinces Antonio to allow her to check some laboratory values.

The laboratory results confirm R.T.'s suspicions. Normally, she could refer a patient with hyperthyroidism to endocrinology for urgent treatment because she is concerned that he or she could go into a coma or die. Instead, she is faced with many barriers to accessing care for him. He is in this country illegally and uninsured. Although he lives well below the poverty line, he does not qualify for Medicaid. He might qualify for financial assistance but he would be leery of providing any identification or pay stubs. Furthermore, Antonio does not want to see any doctors in the United States, preferring to wait until he returns to Mexico in 6 months to have the issue addressed. He does not want to miss time from work because he thinks he might get fired. In addition, he has transportation and language barriers, which would make it difficult to see a specialist. R.T. struggles to determine whether the principle of beneficence or the principle of respect for autonomy should carry the most weight in her decision making.

Stories such as this are common when working with migrant Hispanic farm workers. Early on in her emerging in ethical decision making, R.T. would have thought only about the individual situation. Knowledge regarding professional obligations and ethical theories can help her deal with this situation by providing a solid foundation in her thinking about the ethical nature of this situation. As R.T.'s ethical competency developed, she began to look at the bigger problem, the system. The existing referral system placed most of the burden on patients to obtain appointments with specialists. The referral staff was not allotted the needed time to assist non-English speaking or illiterate patients, such as Antonio, with obtaining financial assistance at the local academic hospital. R.T. realized that ethical dialogue would need to occur among staff and administration for the health care center's culture to change. Antonio's case helped shape a new system. The outreach coordinator now assists migrant farm workers with the financial screening process, interpretation, and transportation. Antonio's case was the first success. Although it took three times as long to get him the care he needed, he finally underwent thyroid ablation and is now a healthy 20-year-old.

As R.T. is developing her practice as a DNP-prepared NP, she is looking for ways to promote social justice within the health care system. She knows that making changes in the ethical practice of one health care center is not enough to make changes across the system. To have a voice in the larger political arena, R.T. joined the leadership committee of her region's NP organization. She has taken on the role of governmental affairs chairperson. This allows her to be involved in health care legislation that affects APRNs and patients. Her hope is that this will become an avenue for addressing the ethical problems associated with caring for undocumented Hispanic migrant farm workers. ◎

[a]We thank Reagan Thompson Holland, MSN, RN, NP, for her assistance with this exemplar.

residue" that continues to trouble participants involved in the conflict (Epstein & Hamric, 2009). Part of the outcome evaluation must address the reality of these lingering feelings and the related tensions that they create.

Barriers to Ethical Practice and Potential Solutions

A number of factors influence how moral issues are addressed and resolved in the clinical setting. Some barriers are easily corrected, but others may require attention at institutional, state, or even national levels. Regardless of type, the APRN must identify and respond to the barriers that inhibit the development of morally responsive practice environments.

Barriers Internal to the APRN

Lack of knowledge about ethics; lack of confidence in one's own ability to name, define, and resolve ethical conflicts; lack of skill in communicating in high-stakes situations; and a sense of powerlessness are potent barriers to the APRN achieving competence in ethical decision making. To address these barriers, APRNs need to seek out opportunities for ethics education through schools of nursing and professional organizations. Engaging in periodic values clarification exercises can be helpful for APRNs and all members of the health care team who experience conflict. Once personal values are realized, the APRN can more easily anticipate situations in which these conflicts will arise and develop strategies for managing them. For example, an emergency department NP may be faced with providing care for a criminal injured in a gunfight that killed innocent bystanders. The *Code of Ethics for Nurses* (ANA, 2015) emphasizes that all individuals be treated with dignity and respect; however, it can be disturbing and difficult to provide care for an individual who has caused harm to others, particularly if the NP has not examined her or his own personal views. The process of values clarification is helpful when preparing for this type of situation.

APRNs can empower themselves by role-modeling ethical decision making within their team. For example, in the primary care setting, a clinic nurse mentions to the APRN a concern about how a patient situation was handled. In addition to reflective listening and emotional support, the APRN can encourage the nurse to gather all the necessary information and guide the nurse in an analysis of the ethical elements and consideration of practical solutions.

This process demonstrates the process of ethical decision making for the clinic nurse and empowers the APRN in the development of this core competency. Including ethical aspects of a patient's case in interprofessional rounds, scheduling debriefing sessions after a particularly difficult case, reading and discussing ethics articles specific to the specialty patient group in a journal club, and/or using simulation activities in which caregivers role-play different scenarios are additional strategies that APRNs can use to empower themselves and other nurses to examine ethical issues.

Lack of time is often a barrier faced by APRNs seeking to enact this competency. In some cases, the APRN may need to resolve a presenting dilemma in stages, with the most central issue addressed first. The APRN also needs to enlist the aid of administrative and physician colleagues in recognizing the ongoing consequences of lack of time for team deliberations. For example, if a patient is not receiving adequate pain management because the bedside nurse is concerned about hastening death and is unaware of the full treatment plan, the CNS should first focus on relieving the patient's pain. Once the immediate need is addressed, the CNS can help the bedside nurse identify nonpharmacologic interventions to promote comfort and educate the nurse about the dosage and timing of medications to prevent wide fluctuations in pain management. At this point, the administrative leadership should be approached about supporting ongoing staff education. An additional strategy, such as arranging for the nurse to rotate to a hospice unit or attend End-of-Life Nursing Education Consortium training (http://www.aacn.nche.edu/elnec/about/fact-sheet), represents a preventive approach to help avert similar dilemmas in the future.

Interprofessional Barriers

Different approaches among health care team members can pose a barrier to ethical practice. For example, nurses and physicians often define, perceive, analyze, and reason through ethical problems from distinct and sometimes opposing perspectives (Curtis & Shannon, 2006; Hamric & Blackhall, 2007; Shannon, 1997). Although the roles are complementary, these differing approaches may create conflict between a nurse and physician, further separating and isolating their perspectives. A physician may be unaware of the nurse's differing opinion or may not recognize this difference as a conflict (Hamric & Blackhall, 2007; Shannon et al., 2002). One study has indicated that physicians and nurses deal with the same ethical problems and use similar moral reasoning but that differences are related to professional roles, the types of responsibilities each group had in the situation, and the resulting different questions each group raised (Oberle & Hughes, 2001). Similar to an optical illusion, the nurse and physician may look at the same ethically troubling clinical situation but, because of differences in their perspectives, they focus on opposing features and arrive at different conclusions about the appropriate course of action. In such situations, the APRN first seeks to understand alternative interpretations of the situation and establish respectful and open communication before seeking resolution of ethical problems.

Physicians, nurses, and APRNs need to engage in moral discourse to understand and support the ethical burden that each professional carries (Curtis & Shannon, 2006; Hamric & Blackhall, 2007; Oberle & Hughes, 2001). Encouraging examples of interprofessional collaboration include the European MURINET (Multidisciplinary Research Network on Health and Disability) project (Ajovalasit et al., 2012), a joint policy statement on requests for inappropriate treatment (Bosslet et al., 2015), and the National Consensus Project, composed of nursing and medical professional organizations that appointed a team of physicians and nurses to revise the *Clinical Practice Guidelines for Quality Palliative Care* (National Consensus Project for Quality Palliative Care, 2009).

A third robust initiative including multiple professions has been the establishment of the Interprofessional Education Collaborative, whose mission is to advance interprofessional education so that students entering the health care professions not only seek collaborative relationships with other providers but also view collaboration as the norm and not the exception (IPEC, 2016). An expert panel developed core competencies for interprofessional education; one of the four domains focuses on values and ethics (IPEC, 2016). The emphasis of this domain is developing climates of mutual respect and shared values. Box 13.5 lists the 10 competencies identified.

These statements focus on values shared by all health care disciplines and can serve as a basis for building collaborative interprofessional teams that emphasize preventive ethics. As noted, collaboration is the key strategy for eliminating interprofessional barriers.

Patient-Provider Barriers

Additional barriers to ethical practice arise from issues in the patient-provider relationship. Health

---

BOX 13.5   Values and Ethics Competencies[a]

1. Place the interests of patients and populations at the center of interprofessional health care delivery.
2. Respect the dignity and privacy of patients while maintaining confidentiality in the delivery of team-based care.
3. Embrace the cultural diversity and individual differences that characterize patients, populations, and the health care team.
4. Respect the unique cultures, values, roles and responsibilities, and expertise of other health professions.
5. Work in cooperation with those who receive care, those who provide care, and others who contribute to or support the delivery of prevention and health services.
6. Develop a trusting relationship with patients, families, and other team members.
7. Demonstrate high standards of ethical conduct and quality of care in one's contributions to team-based care.
8. Manage ethical dilemmas specific to interprofessional patient/population-centered care situations.
9. Act with honesty and integrity in relationships with patients, families, and other team members.
10. Maintain competence in one's own profession appropriate to scope of practice.

[a]Competencies as identified by the Interprofessional Education Collaborative. From Interprofessional Education Collaborative. (2011). *Core competencies for interprofessional collaborative practice: Report of an expert panel.* (p.18). Washington, DC: Author.

---

care providers, employees of the health care institution, and patients and families all contribute to the settings in which most APRNs practice, offering opportunities for both personal enrichment and cultural conflict (Linnard-Palmer & Kools, 2004). For example, parents may inform an NP in a pediatric outpatient setting that for cultural and religious reasons, they do not want their child immunized. In this case, the NP is faced with a belief that places the child and community at risk. The NP wants to preserve the parent's rights and preferences but is concerned about the child's best interests and the potential harm to other children if they are exposed to an illness from a nonimmunized child (Fernbach, 2011). Issues that result from cultural diversity are difficult to resolve without help from others who are more familiar with the specific cultural practices and beliefs. Occasionally, hospital chaplains, local clergy, or individuals from the patient's culture who may teach in the language department in a local university can assist with obtaining an expanded understanding of specific belief systems. Internet-based resources such as "The Provider's Guide to Quality and Culture" (Overman, 2006) also provide specific information about cultural groups.

Ensuring appropriate care for patients at the end of life is an additional challenge to ethical practice. Although some patients use advance directives to convey their wishes, these forms are not always applicable to specific clinical situations and the appointed decision maker may never have discussed end-of-life care with the patient. APRNs in primary care settings should encourage such conversations or guide patients, particularly those with life-limiting conditions, through the process of making their wishes known if they become incapacitated. The POLST (Physician Orders for Life-Sustaining Treatment) approach to end-of-life planning (Center for Ethics, Oregon Health and Science University, 2017) provides an effective strategy to discuss and document patient wishes for patients with serious illness or frailty. In states that have adopted this practice, patient wishes addressing resuscitation, additional medical interventions, food and fluids, and antibiotics are documented on a form that translates decisions into actionable medical orders. In acute care settings, particularly intensive care units (ICUs), APRNs can broker conversations with families who are facing difficult decisions and ensure that the choices in care are based on what the patient would want and not on the desires of family members who are in a state of anticipatory grief, focused on the pending death of the patient rather than on what is in his or her best interest. In a study of families of ICU patients, Ahrens, Yancey, and Kollef (2003) found that 42 of 43 families receiving support and enhanced communication from a CNS-physician team were able to make decisions to withhold or withdraw care at the end of life. The authors noted that "This finding underscores the importance of intentional and well-designed communication and support systems for families making medical and moral decisions" (p. 322). More recently, Curtis et al. (2012) reported an evidence-based intervention involving "communication facilitators" to improve interprofessional team and family communications in the ICU.

Another barrier to ethical practice that challenges many APRNs is the issue of patient nonadherence. Patients and families may choose not to be actively involved in their care or resist an APRN's attempts to improve their well-being, which raises clinical and ethical questions. Managing nonadherent patients is ethically troubling because they consume a disproportionate amount of health care resources, including the APRN's time, redirecting these resources from patients who are more amenable to the established plan of care. There are no easy solutions to managing the nonadherent patient (Resnick, 2005); however, full consideration of this issue is beyond the scope of this chapter (see Chapter 8 for effective strategies for those patients in resistance). In many cases, other factors, such as impaired thinking and concentration, knowledge deficits, financial issues, and emotional disorders, can conflict with the patient's ability to follow the prescribed treatment plan (Bishop & Brodkey, 2006). APRNs should seek additional support from resources such as social workers or home health nurses to discover the underlying causes and find solutions.

Organizational and Environmental Barriers

Lack of support for nurses who speak up regarding ethical problems in work settings is a potent barrier to ethical practice. Unfortunately, early research and recent literature have revealed disturbing examples of environments in which nurses' concerns were minimized or ignored by physicians, administrators, and even other nurses (Ceci, 2004; Gordon & Hamric, 2006; Klaidman, 2007; Ulrich, 2012); such environments can lead to moral distress. Recent studies have revealed significant correlations between the level of moral distress and turnover of nurses and physicians (Hamric et al., 2012; see Schluter et al. [2008] for a review of other studies). These findings lend urgency to the need for APRNs to provide leadership in building ethical practice environments. APRNs need to assess the level of support that nurses receive from others and work to create environments that are "morally habitable places" (Austin, 2007, p. 86). Consideration should be given to organizational ethics programs that focus on building structures and processes to deal with conflicts of roles and expectations (Hamric et al., 2013; Rorty et al., 2004). APRNs need to develop skills in collaborative conflict resolution and preventive ethics to build ethical practice environments in which moral distress is minimized and the moral integrity of all caregivers is respected and protected.

APRNs should identify resources within and outside the institution to assist with the resolution of ethical problems. Internal resources may include chaplain staff, liaison psychiatrists, patient representatives, social work staff, ethics committees and their members, and ethics consultation services. Resources outside the institution include the ANA's Center on Ethics and Human Rights (www.nursingworld.org/ethics), the Veterans Administration's National Center for Ethics in Health Care (www.ethics.va.gov), ethics groups in national specialty organizations, and ethics centers in universities or large health care institutions. The recognition of a moral dilemma does not commit the APRN to conducting and managing the process of resolution individually. APRNs should engage appropriate resources to address the identified needs and work toward agreement.

As noted, nursing's ethical obligations to patients and their families can also be challenged when organizations implement cost containment practices. Continuity of care and knowing the patient and family are significant issues for APRNs in acute and primary care settings. In outpatient settings, pressures to see more patients in less time can decrease the APRN's opportunity for individualized problem solving for patients and families. Thomas, Finch, Schoenhofer, and Green (2004) noted that NPs' interpersonal skills can enhance the patient's "personhood," an essential part of the caring relationship and the provision of holistic care. Whittemore (2000) has argued that resolving ethical dilemmas requires knowing the patient as a person to be able to recognize the salient aspects of a situation that are important for resolution. However, in time-pressured settings, the emphasis is on efficiency and not on the patient-provider relationship or the provision of holistic care. APRNs struggle in these types of environments to balance the needs of individuals with generalized treatment approaches and productivity targets.

However, it is also the case that the costs of the US health care system are unsustainably high and growing (Emanuel et al., 2012). Improving the efficiency and effectiveness of care delivery at a reduced cost can itself be seen as a moral good, one that requires clinicians to work together with administrators to achieve cost-effective goals. Also, there are times when cost-conscious care can enhance accessibility and quality. APRNs can bridge clinical and administrative perspectives and collaborate with administrators to help achieve quality patient outcomes at reduced cost to the system. One proposal for decreasing costs involves removing scope of practice barriers to increase the use of APRNs in the United States (Emanuel et al., 2012; Institute of Medicine, 2011). APRNs can be instrumental in decreasing the adversarial view between clinicians and administrators that hampers decision making in many settings.

Many institutions are willing to make changes in the delivery of patient care if there are clear outcome data that support a change in practice. APRNs can successfully navigate the cost-conscious health care environment if they effectively demonstrate how their unique contributions to patient care, although more time intensive, ultimately reduce health care expenditures (see Chapter 23). Because patients have shorter hospital stays, open communication and collaboration with the health care team, patients, and families are essential behaviors for optimal planning. APRNs also should maintain and affirm patient's rights and articulate strong ethical reasons for interventions. It may be necessary to question and challenge features in the health care system that negatively affect the quality of care delivered. Finally, there is a need to review patient outcomes consistently and the quality of nursing care provided (see Chapters 23 and 24) because these data can be powerful in building the case for quality changes to promote ethically responsive environments. With its emphasis on cost-effectiveness research and incentives for achieving positive patient outcomes, together with sanctions for underachievement (e.g., charging hospitals for high levels of readmissions), the ACA is accelerating reliance on outcome data as a guide to practice and payment.

Box 13.6 lists websites that contain valuable ethics resources for clinicians. Many specialty organizations issue policy statements related to ethical issues or publish guidelines for their members' use in responding to ethical problems. Box 13.6 also contains sites useful for gathering current literature on legal and ethical issues.

Conclusion

The changing health care environment has placed extraordinary demands on nurses in all care settings. Many forces conflict with nursing's moral imperatives of involvement, connection, and commitment. The ethical decision-making competency involves four elements, including complex knowledge and skill development necessary to move individual patient care, promoting ethical caregiving environments, and moving the larger system toward ethical practices. As a core competency for the APRN, ethical decision making reflects the art and science of nursing. The APRN is in a key position to assume a more decisive role in managing the resolution of moral issues and helping create ethically responsive

BOX 13.6 Organizations With Electronically Available Ethics Resources

Ethics Policy Statements or Guidelines

ABCD Caring (Americans for Better Care of the Dying): http://www.abcd-caring.org

American Academy of Neurology, Practice Guidelines: https://www.aan.com/Guidelines

American Academy of Pediatrics, Policy Statements: http://www.aap.org/en-us/advocacy-and-policy/Pages/Advocacy-and-Policy.aspx

American Association of Nurse Anesthestists: http://www.aana.com

American College of Medical Genetics, Policy Statements: http://www.acmg.net/ACMG/Publications/Policy_Statements/ACMG/Publications/Policy_Statements.aspx

American College of Nurse-Midwives: http://www.acnm.org

American College of Physicians, Center for Ethics and Professionalism: http://www.acponline.org/ethics

American College of Surgeons: http://www.facs.org

American Medical Association, Council on Ethical and Judicial Affairs: https://www.ama-assn.org/about-us/council-ethical-judicial-affairs-ceja

American Nurses Association, Center for Ethics and Human Rights: http://www.nursingworld.org/MainMenuCategories/EthicsStandards/About

American Society for Reproductive Medicine: http://www.asrm.org/?vs=1

American Society of Anesthesiologists, Ethical Guidelines and Statements: http://www.asahq.org/resources/ethics-and-professionalism

American Society of Law, Medicine and Ethics: http://www.aslme.org

American Society of Transplantation, Key Position Statements: https://www.myast.org/public-policy/key-position-statements/key-position-statements

Canadian Resource for Nursing Ethics: http://www.NursingEthics.ca

Center for Jewish Ethics, Academic Coalition for Jewish Bioethics: http://www.rrc.edu/ethics-center/sje-bioethics-group

Center for Practical Bioethics: https://www.practicalbioethics.org

The Hastings Center: http://www.thehastingscenter.org

International Care Ethics (ICE) Observatory: http://www.surrey.ac.uk/fhms/research/centres/ICE/

International Council of Nurses: http://www.icn.ch

The National Academies of Sciences, Engineering, and Medicine, Health and Medicine Division: https://www.nationalacademies.org/hmd

National Catholic Bioethics Center: http://www.ncbcenter.org

National Hospice and Palliative Care Organization: https://www.nhpco.org

National Human Genome Research Institute: http://www.nhgri.nih.gov

National Institutes of Health Resources on Bioethics Interest Group: https://sigs.nih.gov/bioethics/Pages/default.aspx

Office for Human Research Protections: http://www.hhs.gov/ohrp

Organ Procurement and Transplantation Network: https://optn.transplant.hrsa.gov

Presidential Commission for the Study of Bioethical Issues: https://bioethicsarchive.georgetown.edu/pcsbi

Society of Critical Care Medicine: http://www.sccm.org/Pages/default.aspx

United Network for Organ Sharing: http://www.unos.org

University of Pennsylvania Department of Medical Ethics & Health Policy: http://medicalethicshealthpolicy.med.upenn.edu

Veterans Administration's National Center for Ethics in Health Care: www.ethics.va.gov

Yeshiva University Center for Bioethics: http://www.yu.edu/ethics/bioethics

Ethics and Legal Search Sites

American Bar Association Public Resources: http://www.americanbar.org/portals/public_resources.html

Bioethics Information Resources, U.S. National Library of Medicine, National Institutes of Health (bioethics online literature search): https://www.nlm.nih.gov/bsd/bioethics.html

Bioethics Research Library at Georgetown University: https://bioethics.georgetown.edu/

Legal Information Institute: http://www.law.cornell.edu

Medical College of Wisconsin, Center for Bioethics and Medical Humanities: http://www.mcw.edu/Center-for-Bioethics-and-Medical-Humanities.htm

health care environments. The identification of patterns in the presentation of moral issues enables the APRN to engage in preventive strategies to improve the ethical climate in patient care environments. Ethical decision-making skills, together with clinical expertise and leadership, empower the APRN to assume leadership roles in public policy processes that promote social justice within the larger health care arena. Preparation for this competency begins in graduate education but continues throughout the APRN's career.

Key Summary Points

- APRNs face a variety of moral problems typically centered around three themes: problems with communication, the presence of interprofessional conflict, and managing competing commitments and obligations.
- APRNs must be careful not to conflate following laws and rules to avoid litigation with a thoughtful deliberation to determine an ethical path.
- APRNs must rigorously and continuously practice self-awareness, becoming exquisitely sensitive to

their own hidden biases, which in turn helps develop strong moral agency.
- As a core competency for the APRN, ethical decision making reflects the art and science of nursing.

References

To access the references for this chapter, use your smartphone's QR code reader to scan the code below, or go to http://booksite.elsevier.com/ 9780323447751.

The Clinical Nurse Specialist

Mary Fran Tracy • Sue Sendelbach

"If you obey all the rules, you miss all the fun."
—Katharine Hepburn

CHAPTER CONTENTS

Overview and Definitions of the Clinical Nurse Specialist

The clinical nurse specialist (CNS) role was created: (1) to provide direct care to patients with complex diseases or conditions; (2) to improve patient

The authors would like to acknowledge Patricia S.A. Sparacino, PhD, RN, FAAN; Garrett K. Chan, PhD, APRN, FAEN, FPCN, FAAN; and Cathy Cartwright, MSN, RN, PCNS, FAAN for their excellent work in previous editions.

outcomes by developing the clinical skills and judgment of staff nurses; and (3) to retain nurses who were experts in clinical practice, particularly in emerging specialty areas at that time, such as psychiatry, oncology, and critical care (Cockerham & Keeling, 2014). Expert clinical practice is the essence, the core value, of the CNS role. Historically, the role has been versatile, evolving, flexing, responsive, and adaptable to patient populations and health care environments, notably the same characteristics that have led to concerns regarding role confusion and ambiguity because of variability in implementation. However, the core strength of the CNS in providing complex specialty care while improving the quality of care delivery has remained central to the understanding of this advanced practice registered nurse (APRN) role. The American Nurses Association (ANA) has defined APRNs as nurses who "practice from both expanded and specialized knowledge and skills" (ANA, 2003, p. 9). An expanded knowledge base and skill set refers to the "acquisition of new practice knowledge and skills, including the knowledge and skills that authorize role autonomy within areas of practice that may overlap traditional boundaries of medical practice" (ANA, 2003, p. 9; see Chapter 3). The ANA defines the primary role of the CNS as working to continually improve the nursing care of patients and patient outcomes (ANA, 2010).

In its *Statement on Clinical Nurse Specialist Practice and Education,* the National Association of Clinical Nurse Specialists (NACNS) defined the CNS as an APRN who manages the care of complex and vulnerable populations, educates and supports nursing and nursing staff, and provides the clinical expertise to facilitate change and innovation in health care systems (NACNS, 2004). NACNS describes CNSs as practicing in the three interrelated spheres of patient direct care, nurses and nursing practice, and organizations and systems. As noted earlier in this text, direct care of patients is the primary distinguishing feature of CNS practice (see Chapter 7).

Interventions in the other two spheres of influence are intended ultimately to affect the care of patients to improve outcomes. Examples of interventions in these two spheres include guiding and educating staff nurses in the nursing practice sphere and leading quality improvement projects and redesigning the delivery of care in the organizations and systems sphere. In the NACNS model, therefore, the patient direct care sphere encompasses the interventions of the other two spheres to depict the centrality of the patient care focus. In this chapter, the NACNS spheres of influence and the Hamric model of competencies are used to illustrate the unique contributions of the role of the CNS and how the CNS role differs from other APRN roles.

A foundation of expert practice and competencies undergirds the CNS role; however, the activities of CNSs are as varied as their individual specialty practices. The diversity of CNS specialties, differences in their individual practices, practice differences seen among CNSs in the same institution, and required variation of an individual CNS' practice

over time has created confusion about what CNSs do. Unlike other APRNs, whose primary role is to deliver direct patient care, the multifaceted CNS delivers direct patient care specifically to complex and vulnerable populations, educates and supports nurses and nursing staff, provides leadership to specialty practice program development, and facilitates change and innovation in health care systems (Lewandowski & Adamle, 2009). This variability in CNS practice, even within the same institution, has characterized the role since its creation. The definition of the CNS role has remained deliberately broad so that CNSs can respond to changing health care environments.

A hallmark of the role is the ability of the CNS to adapt to changing needs of patients, nurses, and health care systems (Kilpatrick, Tchouaket, Carter, Bryant-Lukosius, & DiCenso, 2016). For example, a unit- or population-based critical care CNS with an experienced, certified specialty staff may balance his or her time equally among direct patient care activities, educating nursing staff, and system-wide improvements. However, if there was an acute increase in staff turnover and the unit had predominantly inexperienced staff, the CNS focus would likely shift to primarily support, education, and role modeling for the new staff. Conversely, if a preventive cardiology CNS works in an outpatient clinic in the same institution and sees a panel of patients as a provider of expert specialty care, that CNS practice may focus more on direct patient care and less on education and system-wide improvements. Several clinical, staff, and system variables must be weighed when planning for CNS positions and implementing the role, including the number, type, and background of nurses and other clinical staff; clinical, educational, or institutional resources; and patient population, acuity, and outcomes.

The versatility of the role is what attracts nurses to become CNSs—the ability to impact patient care on many levels. However, this versatility in CNS practice has continued to challenge the CNS role definition and understanding of the impact of CNSs on clinical outcomes and costs of care. Role confusion and variability, regulatory drivers, and fiscal retrenchment in the last 25 years have resulted in the loss of CNS positions in many parts of the country to save hospitals money without jeopardizing direct care registered nurse (RN) positions. The most recent numbers from 2004 estimate approximately 70,000 nurses prepared to practice as CNSs and more than 14,000 prepared as both a CNS and a nurse practitioner (NP) (NACNS, 2017a). It is difficult to know the exact number of CNSs in the United States because the Bureau of Labor Statistics collects APRN data for NPs, certified registered nurse anesthetists (CRNA), and certified nurse-midwives (CNM) only. CNS clinical practices are shaped by many factors, such as health care agency needs, community needs, payor and other regulatory agency mandates, statutory limitations, supervisor requests, and individual CNS interests. Over the past few decades, CNSs have been able to change their practices in response to these influential forces.

Clarifying the work and core competencies of all CNSs, regardless of specialty, has been complicated because specialty organizations have historically established varying educational, competency, and practice standards for CNSs (e.g., critical care, oncology, and neuroscience specialties). NACNS was not established until 1995 (see Chapter 1; www.nacns.org). The NACNS itself has acknowledged that advanced practice organizations for the other three APRN roles had a significant head start in defining competencies and influencing health policies related to advanced practice nursing (NACNS, 2004). The ANA, many specialty organizations, and APRN leaders have worked diligently to define CNS practice, standards, and competencies and to develop CNS curricula (see Chapter 1; NACNS, 2004; NACNS, National CNS Competency Task Force, 2010). More work, however, is required to educate colleagues, administrators, and the public about the role of the CNS. With the increasing emphasis on patient outcomes, efficiencies, patient safety, and appropriate use of technology, the CNS is uniquely prepared to address the nation's health care needs (American Association of Colleges of Nursing [AACN], 2006a; NACNS, 2012b; NACNS, Validation Panel, 2011). According to the *Consensus Model for APRN Regulation,* a defining factor for all APRNs is that a significant component of the education and practice be focused on direct care of individuals (APRN Joint Dialogue Group, 2008). If CNSs want to be recognized nationally or statewide as APRNs, they must have direct care of individuals in their role. If the focus is mainly on educating nurses or process improvement without direct care of individuals, the clinician is not practicing in the role of a CNS (Cronenwett, 1995). For the purposes of clinical practice and licensure, accreditation, credentialing, and education, the work and contributions of CNSs as APRNs must be made unambiguously clear.

New opportunities for CNS practice have presented themselves with the introduction of the Patient Protection and Affordable Care Act (ACA; 2010).

CNSs have consistently delivered direct and indirect care that improves patient care quality and outcomes, patient safety, and nursing practice and that ensures efficient use of resources, cost efficiency, cost savings, and revenue generation (NACNS, 2004; Newhouse et al., 2011; see Chapter 23). This is in complete alignment with the purpose of the ACA and the public's and health care's interests in improving the overall quality of health care. CNSs' clinical acumen and expertise are not limited to their patients' physiologic and psychologic needs. Their clinical expertise permeates the other elements of their multifaceted responsibilities—education, evidence-based practice (EBP), health policy, organizational and system factors, and political change—and they are highly qualified to lead interprofessional teams in health care reform. The purpose of this chapter is to describe the core competencies, current marketplace challenges, and future directions for CNSs.

Clinical Nurse Specialist Practice: Competencies Within the Spheres of Influence

Although other models of APRN practice have been described (see Chapter 2), the NACNS's three spheres of influence and Hamric's seven competencies (see Chapter 3 and Chapters 7 through 13) will primarily be used to organize and explain CNS practice in this chapter. CNS students are encouraged to familiarize themselves with the *Statement on Clinical Nurse Specialist Practice and Education*[a] (NACNS, 2004) and with specialty-specific standards (e.g., American Association of Critical-Care Nurses, 2014; Emergency Nurses Association, 2011) to understand the discussion of spheres and competencies better. To be successful, a CNS must understand and apply the seven competencies of advanced practice nursing across the three spheres of influence, regardless of setting or specialty (Chan & Cartwright, 2014). The NACNS, along with other nursing organizations, has endorsed and defined entry-level competencies to be used by graduate programs in the preparation of CNSs (NACNS, National CNS Competency Task Force, 2010) (Table 14.1).

Advanced practice competencies are categories of expected proficient performance and include specific knowledge and skill sets. The direct care

---

[a]As of the writing of this chapter, NACNS is in the process of revising the *Statement on Clinical Nurse Specialist Practice and Education* as well as the entry-level core competencies. Please check the website at nacns.org for the updated statement and competencies

TABLE 14.1   National Association of Clinical Nurse Specialist Core Competencies

Core Competencies	Behavioral Statement
A. Direct Care Competency	Direct interaction with patients, families, and groups of patients to promote health or well-being and improve quality of life Characterized by a holistic perspective in the advanced nursing management of health, illness, and disease state
B. Consultation Competency	Patient-, staff-, or system-focused interaction among professionals in which the consultant is recognized as having specialized expertise and assists consultee with problem solving
C. Systems Leadership Competency	Ability to manage change and empower others to influence clinical practice and political processes within and across systems
D. Collaboration Competency	Working jointly with others to optimize clinical outcomes Clinical nurse specialist collaborates at an advanced level by committing to authentic engagement and constructive patient-, family-, system-, and population-focused problem solving
E. Coaching Competency	Skillful guidance and teaching to advance the care of patients, families, groups of patients, and the profession of nursing

F. Research Competency
  F.I. *Interpretation, Translation, and Use of Evidence*
  F.II. *Evaluation of Clinical Practice*
  F.III. *Conduct of Research*
	The work of thorough and systematic inquiry
	Includes the search for, interpretation of, and use of evidence in clinical practice and quality improvement, as well as active participation in the conduct of research

G. Ethical Decision Making, Moral Agency, and Advocacy Competency	Identifying, articulating, and taking action on ethical concerns at the patient, family, health care provider, system, community, and public policy levels

Adapted from the National Association of Clinical Nurse Specialists, National CNS Competency Task Force. (2010). Clinical nurse specialist core competencies: Executive summary 2006–2008. Retrieved from http://www.nacns.org/wp-content/uploads/2017/01/CNSCoreCompetenciesBroch.pdf.

of patients and families is the central competency in Hamric's model (see Fig. 2.4) and links every other competency. According to the NACNS model, the impact and influence of CNSs are felt within three spheres of influence—direct care of patients,[b] nurses and nursing practice, and organizations and systems (NACNS, 2004; see Fig. 2.2).

The NACNS model also emphasizes the importance of direct care; clinical expertise and direct care are basic to CNS practice. For this reason, the direct care of patients sphere is the largest sphere in the NACNS model and encompasses the other two spheres. Box 14.1 presents examples of activities in this sphere.

CNSs often execute some competencies simultaneously. They exert influence in the nurses and nursing practice sphere by caring for patients directly and by serving as coaches, educators, guides, and role models for nursing staff and other caregivers. They provide consultation. They demonstrate EBP competencies by working with staff to develop, implement, and evaluate EBP changes. They may collaborate

in clinical research, an activity likely to affect all three spheres of influence. Similarly, they collaborate and facilitate team development, assess and intervene to alleviate the moral distress inherent in clinical care, and create environments that support clinicians' ethical decision making. Box 14.2 lists examples of CNS interventions in the nurses and nursing practice sphere. CNSs exert influence in the organizations and systems sphere by providing clinical and systems leadership through articulating nursing issues to team members, advocating for patients or nurses, or evaluating the quality and cost-effectiveness of technologies and care processes. Box 14.3 lists example activities in this sphere.

Throughout all three spheres, CNSs apply the nursing process; assessment, planning, implementation, and evaluation activities. These are designed to improve the care of patients, develop nurses, and improve the systems in which nurses work and care is delivered. Experienced CNSs understand that activities in each sphere of influence and their advanced practice competencies exert reciprocal influences on each other. Implementing competencies across the three spheres can result in improvements in clinical outcomes, patient safety, patient/

[b]In the NACNS document, this sphere is termed *client direct care*. For clarity in this chapter, this sphere is termed *direct care of patients*.

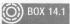 **BOX 14.1** **Examples of Clinical Nurse Specialist (CNS) Interventions in the Care of Complex and/or Vulnerable Patients**

Direct Care

1. Provide expert, specialized assessment of complex patients.
2. Provide evidence-based treatment and care of illness, symptoms, and responses to illness using advanced concepts related to the nursing process.
3. Provide coaching and guidance to patients and families regarding illness management, health maintenance, and health behavior goals.
4. Monitor and prescribe pharmacologic and nonpharmacologic therapies.
5. Order and interpret laboratory and diagnostic tests.
6. Perform advanced procedures.

Collaboration and Ethical Decision Making

1. Facilitate movement of patients and families through and across health care settings.
2. Facilitate health care system access.
   a. Provide outcomes management.
   b. Provide discharge planning, providing and/or ensuring ambulatory and community follow-up.

3. Advocate for patient and family.
   a. Promote collaboration between the patient and family and the nurse and interprofessional team.
   b. Provide leadership in interprofessional ethical situations.
   c. Utilize sound ethical principles when partnering with patients and families to determine therapeutic options and plans of care.
   d. Facilitate patient/family and/or health care team conferences.
4. Facilitate communication among interprofessional team members.

Consultation

1. Appropriately order consults for expertise needed outside of the CNS's skill competencies.
2. Provide consultations when requested for patients within the CNS's specialty expertise.
3. Provide consultation to nurses on complex patients.
4. Comanage complex patients with health care colleagues within CNS's specialty expertise.

---

family satisfaction, resource allocation, professional nursing staff knowledge and skills, advancement of clinical nursing practice, health care team collaboration, and organizational efficiency (Adams et al., 2015; Fabbruzzo-Cota et al., 2016; Soltis, 2015).

The variety of activities, the challenge of in-the-moment problem solving that characterizes clinical work, and intermediate- and long-range planning efforts to improve the care of patients attract CNSs to this work. Throughout the history of CNS practice, and despite the changes in health care, reimbursement, and credentialing that have affected advanced practice nursing, CNSs have remained focused on championing excellence in nursing practice and on improving clinical care and the systems in which the care is delivered.

Without sustained engagement in direct care (direct care of patients sphere), it would be difficult, if not impossible, to continue to be effective in the other two spheres because the effectiveness of CNSs depends on their clinical credibility. However, because CNSs provide more than just direct care, maintaining their commitment to patient care is often challenged as organizational priorities change.

In the following sections, the ways in which CNSs implement the seven competencies across three spheres of influence are described.

Direct Clinical Practice

Specialization was the genesis of the CNS role, but expert clinical practice—and direct patient care—is its heart. The central competency of direct clinical practice is explicitly linked to the patient sphere of influence; the insights and outcomes of providing direct care influence the CNS's work in the other two spheres of nursing practice and systems. It is direct practice that is core to the CNS role; otherwise the CNS can be replaced with experts in project management, policy revision, quality improvement, and nursing education. The direct care expertise at the APRN level adds perspective not provided by others.

CNS practice includes advanced assessment skills and the integration of "biophysical, psychosocial, behavioral, sociopolitical, cultural, economic, and nursing science" (AACN, 2006b, p. 16) into specialized, expert nursing practice. Many authors have described strategies for successfully implementing the

BOX 14.2   Examples of Clinical Nurse Specialist (CNS) Interventions in the Nurses and Nursing Practice Sphere

Guidance and Coaching
1. Educate nurses and interprofessional staff.
   a. Provide formal classes.
   b. Provide informal, bedside teaching.
   c. Develop skills of experienced staff nurses to perform as consultants on basic nursing care for colleagues so the CNS can focus on consultations for complex and vulnerable patients.
2. Provide role modeling, preceptorship, and mentoring.
3. Ensure professional growth opportunities for both novice and experienced nurses.
4. Disseminate knowledge through publication and conference presentations.

Consultation
1. Provide case consultation to nursing staff on complex and vulnerable patients.

Collaboration
1. Collaborate with nurse manager.
   a. Assist with financial planning for units.
   b. Assist in recruiting and retaining staff.
   c. Contribute to formal and informal evaluation of nursing staff.
2. Collaborate with researchers on clinical research projects.

Leadership
1. Provide unit leadership.
   a. Develop and contribute to staff communication forums.
   b. Assist in conflict resolution among staff.
   c. Inform staff of organizational changes.
2. Evaluate and introduce new technology.

Evidence-Based Practice (EBP)
1. Role-model use of EBP when developing guidelines, developing new procedures, and evaluating new technology.
2. Educate and mentor nurses and interprofessional staff in the process of evaluating and implementing new evidence.

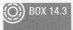

BOX 14.3   Examples of Clinical Nurse Specialist Interventions in the Organizations and Systems Sphere

1. Assess needs of patients, families, communities, nurses, and organizations.
2. Develop evidence-based protocols, policies/procedures, clinical pathways, and standards of care.
3. Cultivate unit culture that values research utilization and evidence-based practice.
4. Lead quality improvement efforts.
   a. Identify and prioritize quality improvement issues.
   b. Develop indicators, methods, and metrics to measure patient outcomes.
   c. Perform unit-based quality improvement projects.
5. Develop innovative models of care.
6. Develop, implement, and evaluate programs.
7. Participate on advisory and policymaking boards and committees.

health care environment. It is easy for the direct care component of the role to be overemphasized or underemphasized because of institutional priorities and competition for CNS expertise. The unique skill set of CNSs may result in them being continually pulled away from direct care to lead projects that are of high priority for the institution. Conversely, if an institution recognizes value only in the revenue generation component of direct care, the CNS may be required to focus exclusively on that component of the role. The CNS role is optimally enacted when CNSs have the opportunity to use what they learn from direct clinical practice to improve care for individual patients, families, and patient populations, whether that occurs at the patient-CNS interface, through nursing personnel, or through organizational improvements.

Providing regular and consistent direct patient care is essential for the CNS to do the following:

- Evaluate the quality, effectiveness, efficiency, and safety of patient care and determine whether inadequacies are the result of a lack or ineffective use of nursing resources, insufficient equipment and supplies, or systems inefficiencies (see Chapter 7).
- Demonstrate one's clinical competency and maintain clinical expertise, thereby role-modeling clinical behaviors, establishing credibility, and maintaining team relationships and collegial trust.

expert clinician dimension (Duffy, Dresser, & Fulton, 2016; Fulton, Lyon, & Goudreau, 2014; Zuzelo, 2010). Each strategy is highly dependent on the individual CNS and her or his practice setting and can fluctuate from year to year in relation to the prevailing

- Identify nursing staff learning needs, including knowledge and skill development.
- Refine one's clinical expertise and reflective abilities.
- Maintain CNS credentials and certification.

Direct care, or direct clinical practice, refers to CNS activities and responsibilities that occur within the patient-nurse interface (see Chapter 7). For many years, a CNS's direct clinical practice was not clearly linked to measureable goals, such as patient outcomes or resource use. Thus few data were available to justify the role and correlate its expense with the cost avoidance and quality improvement aspects of the role when health care institutions were restructuring their operating systems. However, most patients requiring the expertise of a CNS are sicker, more frail, and in need of specialized expert care. CNS care of high-risk patients with complex conditions has consistently shown improved patient outcomes and reduced health care costs when CNSs and other APRNs were directly involved with patient care, including assessing, teaching, counseling, and negotiating systems (Avery & Schnell-Hoehn, 2010; Newhouse et al., 2011; Schmidt & Ulch, 2012).

A CNS is most likely to care directly for a patient whose diagnosis or care is complex, unique, or problematic. Examples of complex patients include a very–low-birth-weight infant, a frail older person with multiple chronic conditions, a child with complex congenital heart disease, a young pregnant woman with a transplanted organ, or a man diagnosed with bipolar disorder who has survived a suicide attempt but who requires prolonged physical rehabilitation. Examples of unique situations include the care of a child with a rigid external distraction device for midface advancement; evaluation and implementation of a new intervention, such as teletechnology to assess the efficacy of preventive interventions for pressure ulcers; and introduction of an experimental chemotherapeutic agent. CNSs have the advanced skills to care for these complex patients by incorporating a holistic perspective, forming therapeutic partnerships, and using expert clinical thinking and skillful performance to optimize outcomes. The CNS has the access and ability to evaluate the latest evidence and apply it in diverse ways to manage complex cases.

Direct care also affords a CNS the opportunity to assess the quality of care for a specific patient population. This qualitative assessment enhances the interpretation of quantitative data and directs changes in care processes. For example, a CNS might notice a pattern of frequently missed clinic appointments for a heart failure patient. Through the therapeutic partnership, the CNS may determine that a lack of clinic parking results in a barrier for this patient to keep appointments. The outcome is not one of a nonadherent patient but of a logistical failure that requires immediate resolution for the benefit of all clients with heart failure. When a home care nurse notes that an older patient is not taking medications consistently, a CNS's engagement with that patient can provide a more detailed and complex assessment. The result of such an assessment may be that this older patients is cognitively impaired and forgets to take his medications; that the medication regimen is too complex, causing the patient to miss doses; or that the medication is too expensive and not covered by supplemental insurance or Medicaid, causing the patient to halve or skip doses and let prescriptions go unfilled. The CNS's evaluation might integrate advanced assessment skills, such as cognitive screening, into the admission assessment of all older patients; might identify therapeutic alternatives, such as a simpler or more economical medication regimen to improve adherence; or might introduce other creative interventions to promote health and quality of life.

A CNS's clinical practice interventions may be continuous, in which the CNS carries a consistent caseload, or time-limited, regular, or episodic, in which the CNS cares for complex cases as they arise. Examples of regular ongoing care include: providing care for high-risk newborns in a pediatric special care clinic; providing psychotherapy, medication management, and other specialized nursing care for patients requiring mental health care; delivering total patient care to the first patients in an innovative surgery program; or providing yearly comprehensive neurologic care for children with spina bifida in a hospital-based clinic. Episodic care helps a CNS assess and intervene in a particular problem. Examples of episodic care include planning and coordinating a patient's complex hospital discharge, facilitating a support group for families of children with hydrocephalus, and working with a patient and family who are disagreeing about the plan of care in order to facilitate decision making. Involvement in either regular or episodic care enables CNSs to identify nursing or systems problems that interfere with care and require CNS intervention, such as lack of staff knowledge, the need for clinical policies or procedures, or the need for a streamlined process for ethics consults to address ethical dilemmas. For each clinical situation, a CNS takes a comprehensive approach, using discriminative judgment, advanced knowledge, and expert skills, including expertise in the technical, humanistic, and organizational aspects of care. In these situations, CNSs are particularly skilled at the use of surveillance, quickly identifying patient and system issues and intervening to avoid further complications. A CNS intervention may be as simple as assisting a patient and family to navigate a hospital's bureaucracy. A CNS knows how and when to bend the rules and when to bypass organizational or philosophical roadblocks, thus ensuring the focus on the patient and family and a successful outcome.

If clinical skills—particularly psychomotor ones, such as administering chemotherapy and troubleshooting external ventricular drains—are not used periodically, CNSs become less proficient. Regular clinical practice helps a CNS maintain the expertise and clinical competence needed to practice and develop the skills of other nurses. In addition to maintaining and refining clinical skills, direct clinical practice is imperative at two pivotal points: during a CNS's orientation to establish credibility and before and occasionally throughout the implementation of organizational change to assess the impact of the change on patient care. CNSs must weigh the benefits and costs of different ways to implement direct care. Advantages, such as developing credibility with staff or maintaining one's skills, are evaluated against potential disadvantages, such as competing demands or time pressures.

Indirect Practice

Clinical practice can also occur indirectly. For example, a CNS can guide the direct care being performed by a novice staff nurse with the goal to improve the direct care skills and knowledge of nurses. A CNS may select a patient population in which there are recurrent problems or poor outcomes and collaborate with members of the health care team to develop and implement standards of care, clinical pathways, clinical procedures, and/or quality or performance improvement plans.

Implementation of and adherence to recommended practice changes should be evaluated to assess the impact of the change on outcomes, refine algorithms or guidelines, improve clinical management, and promote consistent adherence. Algorithms and guidelines are rarely self-sustaining and require a champion who continuously facilitates their implementation, constantly evaluating new evidence that may result in the need for revisions. This role is imperative if the algorithm or guideline is to be successful and achieve its intended outcome. A CNS is often the person to fulfill the champion role.

System responsibilities for evaluating technology and its impact on patients and resources are another facet of the CNS's indirect clinical practice. Technologic advances have accelerated changes in health care delivery. These advances, however, coupled with the pressure of cost containment, increased competition, heightened consumer expectations, and capped budgets, create conflicting demands and priorities. Technologic advances have provided the objective data necessary to make clinical judgments (e.g., medication titration based on hemodynamic indices), devices to remotely assess a patient (e.g., telemonitoring of vital signs and weights), and interventional alternatives to treat disease (e.g., fiberoptic, robotic, and virtual reality surgery). However, technology warrants close scrutiny because with it comes responsibility to evaluate its impact on budgets, quality of care, the environment, risk-benefit ratios, staff, and patients as well as anticipation and evaluation of new types of errors that can occur with new technology.

Patient Safety

Patient safety is integral to all aspects of direct and indirect clinical practice, including CNS availability to and support of novice nurses (Altmiller, 2011; Barton & Makic, 2015; Makic, 2015). The CNS's familiarity with The Joint Commission's National Patient Safety Goals (2016), the Agency for Healthcare Research and Quality's (AHRQ's) Patient Safety Network (PSNet: https://psnet.ahrq.gov), teaching strategies from Quality and Safety Education in Nursing (QSEN Institute, 2014), and the Open School at the Institute for Healthcare Improvement (IHI, 2016) are resources that can help the CNS keep abreast of patient safety issues. It is this direct clinical practice that empowers a CNS to assume a leadership role in evaluating patient safety, exploring root cause analyses, and preventing adverse events. A CNS can build an atmosphere of trust in situations in which adverse events are investigated, bring systems and individual patient–level thinking to the discussion, and then facilitate implementation of changes that are needed to prevent recurrence of those adverse events.

Although providing direct care to patients is a core competency, how CNSs provide direct care varies across CNS specialties and practice settings; it is determined by population needs, influenced by the expertise of other nursing personnel, and affected by regulatory designations of CNSs as APRNs and their scopes of practice. When, how, for whom, and with whom direct care is given are fluid and are negotiated and renegotiated with professional nursing staff and organizational leadership based on patients' needs and the knowledge and clinical skill of nursing personnel.

Exemplar 14.1 illustrates how a pediatric CNS uses her professional competencies to provide expert care to a specific patient population and demonstrates the importance of direct care to execution of the other CNS competencies and how the care impacts functioning across the three spheres of influence.

Guidance and Coaching

One of the essential components of the CNS role is that of expert coach. This role of guide or coach is used during teaching and mentoring to facilitate transition from one situation to another and depends on the interaction of technical, clinical, and interpersonal competencies and self-reflection (see Chapter 8). CNSs use formal and informal coaching and teaching strategies with patients and families, nurses and nursing personnel, graduate

---

EXEMPLAR 14.1   **Direct Clinical Practice and Core Competencies of the Clinical Nurse Specialist[a]**

CC, a pediatric neurology clinical nurse specialist (CNS), performs preoperative history and physical examinations in the pediatric neurology clinic; orders appropriate radiographs, laboratory tests, and consultations; and obtains cephalometric measurements and photographs for patients undergoing surgery for craniosynostosis. On the day of surgery, CC notifies the staff nurses who will be caring for the patient about pertinent findings and specific needs. Postoperatively, CC assesses the patient for adequate pain control, dietary needs, vital sign changes, incision status, swelling, and neurologic function. She facilitates discussions about these findings, staff nurses' concerns, parents' concerns, and the plan of care among care team members. She adapts standing orders for each patient in collaboration with the neurosurgeon.

Consultation
CC is frequently consulted by staff nurses, referring physicians, or other advanced practice registered nurses to assess misshapen heads by physical assessment or reviewing radiographs. These consultations provide opportunities to teach health care professionals how to recognize the differences between positional plagiocephaly and craniosynostosis, leading to earlier referrals for improved outcomes.

Guidance and Coaching
The Internet can be an excellent resource for families seeking health care information about medical conditions and treatment options. To help families learn more about craniosynostosis, CC created a website that describes the various types of craniosynostosis and treatment options, including a new, less invasive technique. As a result, she receives many inquiries from families seeking information about this new technique for their babies. Providing accurate information on the website is critical so that families can make informed decisions

about surgery. Much of the preoperative teaching is done by telephone or in the clinic because parents and other family members have many questions.

CC has educated nurses about the early recognition of craniosynostosis, surgical options, and positional plagiocephaly through professional journal articles, a book chapter, presentations at national nursing conferences, teaching at the local school of nursing, and in-service education programs for the staff nurses. Mentoring graduate students has provided additional opportunities for role modeling.

Evidence-Based Practice
Collaboration on research with the pediatric neurosurgeon has yielded data demonstrating that the new surgical technique decreases patients' hospital stays, lowers costs, and improves patient outcomes. When parents noticed a sharp decrease in fussiness in their baby immediately after surgery, CC developed a questionnaire to survey parents' perceptions of fussiness and irritability in their baby before and after surgery. Statistically significant decreases in fussiness and irritability were found postoperatively, suggesting that babies with craniosynostosis experience increases in intracranial pressure.

Leadership
In this unique role, CC can provide care throughout the continuum, using clinical pathways to help families navigate the hospital system in an efficient manner. Bringing a baby to an unfamiliar city for surgery by surgeons that they have never met is a daunting experience for most parents. CC's leadership skills are put to the test coordinating preoperative directed donor blood; arranging lodging at the Ronald McDonald House; scheduling preoperative workups and follow-up appointments with the neurosurgeon, plastic surgeon, ophthalmologist, and anesthesiologist; and coordinating the postoperative molding helmet.

Continued

EXEMPLAR 14.1	Direct Clinical Practice and Core Competencies of the Clinical Nurse Specialist[a]—cont'd

Collaboration

Collaboration occurs at many levels. First, CC collaborates with the pediatric neurosurgeon to provide for and coordinate optimal patient and family care. She collaborates with the staff nurses who care for the babies with craniosynostosis, providing in-service educational programs about the disorder and conducting rounds with them on the postoperative patients. Collaboration also occurs with other members of the craniofacial team, such as ophthalmologists, genetics counselors, plastic surgeons, and orthotic designers. CC confers with referring health care providers to provide continuity after the patient leaves the hospital and between follow-up visits.

Ethical Decision Making

Although this new surgical treatment for craniosynostosis results in minimal blood loss, an infant will occasionally present with a low hemoglobin level or experience excessive intraoperative blood loss. Some families refuse blood transfusions for religious reasons, requiring more intensive preoperative preparation to minimize the need for a blood transfusion. Being present for the conversations that the neurosurgeon has with the family who refuses blood transfusion assists in understanding the reasons for refusal and allows the CNS to reinforce the plan of care should the child need blood during or after surgery. A protocol for preoperative erythropoietin injections can be sent to the patient's pediatrician in an attempt to increase the hemoglobin level.

A great deal of preparation is required for a family to bring their baby to the hospital for this type of surgery. The CNS is instrumental in facilitating this process, using the core competencies and spheres of influence. ◎

[a]The authors thank Cathy Cartwright, MSN, RN, PCNS, FAAN, for this exemplar.

nursing students, other CNSs, health professionals, consumer groups, and organizations or systems (see Chapter 8).

Patients and Families

A CNS's expert guidance and coaching are pivotal in providing or influencing patient and family education and behavior. CNSs may use coaching and teaching skills in educating patients and families with complex situations to complement the care given by other nurses and health professionals. CNSs continually seek better ways to coach patients and families using combinations of cognitive, educational, and behavioral strategies to improve patient education and adherence to interventions. However, a CNS cannot teach every patient and family and so must assess and prioritize whom to teach. For example, a CNS could mentor a case manager or presurgical program educator to provide routine preoperative teaching for cardiac surgical patients. A CNS could then allocate more time to coach high-risk, complex, unusual, or challenging patients, such as a teenage girl with congenital heart defects with a history of an eating disorder who is afraid she will die if she undergoes another cardiac surgery, or a patient with multiple comorbidities who neither speaks nor reads English and who will be going home after surgery to housing with no running water.

A CNS may demonstrate to nurses how to facilitate difficult conversations with patients and their families by supporting the parents of a newborn who has died, working with a patient and family on end-of-life decisions, or "translating" a physician's technical explanation into lay terms.

As health care systems are restructured, there is increasing emphasis on patients' accountability for their own health. This means that in addition to coaching individuals, CNSs are even more likely to be involved in education program planning and implementation aimed at helping groups of patients manage chronic illnesses and associated symptoms. A study of rheumatoid arthritis patients in the United Kingdom showed that the patients had positive relationships with their CNSs—viewing the CNSs as their main source of information, providing guidance on how to manage their arthritis, and providing them reassurance and self-confidence in knowing how to manage their chronic condition (Hardware, Johnson, Hale, Ndosi, & Adebajo, 2014). Many patients know that they need to be better informed and educated about health risk determinants, preventive self-care, treatment options, and risks and benefits of treatments, but their health care behaviors are influenced by many personal, psychologic, and sociocultural factors. Because a patient is not always able or willing to change his or her lifestyle or to adhere to health care recommendations, a CNS must determine which patient or patient population is most appropriate for the advanced coaching requiring a CNS, such as a patient with early-onset dementia who has poor social support living in an economically depressed community.

Nurses and Nursing Personnel

A CNS is a role model for nurses, demonstrating the practical integration of theory and EBP into nursing practice. Whereas NPs and CNMs primarily coach patients and families, a CNS strives continuously to improve clinical practice and integrate new knowledge into the practice of nurses as well. A CNS's time can often be better spent by teaching others the why, what, and how of common patient care interventions rather than repeatedly personally providing those same interventions. For example, a wound, ostomy, and continence CNS can guide and coach unit skin champions to assist their peers to use standards in assessing and intervening for patients with simple types of wounds. The CNS is then appropriately consulted for complex wounds. By providing guidance and coaching, optimal patient outcomes and cost avoidance can be realized (Boyd et al., 2014; Clements, Moore, Tribble, & Blake, 2014). Bedside coaching can reinforce EBP and new skills through real-time feedback to the staff RN (Clements et al., 2014). Developing standards for patient education and providing resources to ensure consistent information across populations are equally important CNS educational activities. As a nurse applies the new knowledge and skills taught by a CNS, the CNS can attend to new or more complex responsibilities. The nurse can then become the role model for the skill mastered or the knowledge gained, and so a CNS's influence will continue to impact patient care. CNSs may also guide and coach RNs in professional development areas as well, such as advancing their skills in education, publishing, and presenting (Hoke & Papa, 2014). The professional development of nurses in clinical practice settings is a key distinguishing feature of the CNS. CNSs' abilities to guide and mentor nurses toward stronger specialty practice can reduce turnover, improve patient safety, and support enhanced patient outcomes (Muller, Hujcs, Dubendorf, & Harrington, 2010).

This notion of extending the reach of the CNS through professional RN expertise can be considered a defining characteristic of the guidance and coaching competency of CNS practice. The cycle of enrichment and professional development is never complete. Whenever major staff turnover occurs or a CNS enters a new practice setting, the cycle of guiding and coaching nurses must begin anew.

Students

A CNS has a professional responsibility to educate, guide, and coach graduate nursing students and, when the opportunity arises, to be their mentor. In working with graduate nursing students in the classroom or clinical setting, a CNS, models the integration of practical and scientific knowledge into expert clinical practice, and demonstrates the level of advanced practice nursing to which a student can aspire. A CNS can provide opportunities for a graduate nursing student to do a clinical practicum or residency; the reward of working with an excellent student is being able to do more, extend one's influence more broadly, and make advanced practice expertise more widely available. In addition to providing patient care, the CNS guides students to complete projects (e.g., writing patient education materials or clinical procedures) or tasks (e.g., a literature review to support proposed changes in clinical practice) that also benefit the practice setting.

Consultation

The nursing literature offers classic descriptions of the essential components of consultation and strategies for ensuring the success of a CNS as a consultant (Barron, 1989; Hamric,1983; Sneed, 1991). Consultation is an expected CNS competency, though each CNS's consultative proficiency and the need to use this competency varies. The CNS can provide consultation to others in the care of a patient; however, consultation also occurs when the CNS requests advice from another member of the health care team yet retains primary responsibility for that patient's care (see Chapter 9).

As a content expert, a CNS can suggest a wide range of alternative approaches or solutions to clinical or systems problems, whether internal or external to the practice setting. As a consultant, the CNS often directs staff to other resources (e.g., other colleagues, community resources, practice guidelines) that enable nurses and others to make decisions based on relevant and appropriate alternatives. A CNS is a process consultant and facilitates change so that decisions can be made for immediate and future situations. Process activities and outcome achievement are two critical and measurable elements of the CNS consultation competency. Documenting consultations and linking them to outcomes is essential. An example of this connection has been described by Gurka (1991), who used four consultative process activities (the fact finder, educator, informational expert, and advocate modes) from Lippitt and Lippitt's consultation model (1978) and measured three major outcomes (prevention of complications, maintenance or development of standards of care, and improvement in nurses' clinical judgment skills).

A CNS is both an internal and an external consultant. Because consultation is an increasingly important role for the CNS, care must be taken to optimize opportunities to develop resources and guide and coach RNs to advance their skills with basic care situations so CNS consultations are more appropriately focused on complex patient cases.

Internal Consultation

Internal consultation includes assisting staff and facilitating organizational development in one's own practice setting, especially through the creative use of resources and alternative strategies to overcome or eliminate perceived system obstacles. A CNS may determine that a request for internal consultation requires the collaboration of a number of consultants, including other CNSs and members of other disciplines. A CNS often initiates the plan, mobilizes the resources, convenes team meetings, defuses the politics, and facilitates the resolution. Box 14.4 presents examples of CNS internal consultation.

External Consultation

External consultation occurs apart from the CNS's practice or employment setting. External consultation offers approaches or solutions to specific problems to assist the nursing profession, a specialty organization, other health care providers, and health systems. Box 14.5 presents examples of external consultation.

Unless internal or external consultation is a CNS's primary responsibility (e.g., as part of a consult team or service), problems may arise if a CNS's time is used more for consultations than for direct care. The impact on patient care is less visible unless the content and process of consultations are well documented and the outcomes are measured. Chapter 9 contains further discussion of the consultation competency.

Evidence-Based Practice

In implementing the EBP competency, CNS involvement in the evaluation and improvement of nursing

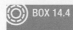 **BOX 14.4   Examples of Clinical Nurse Specialist (CNS) Internal Consultation**

- A rheumatology CNS consults on follow-up visits with patients with inflammatory arthritides, resulting in higher patient satisfaction and no difference in outcomes compared to physician follow-up (Koksvik et al., 2013).
- A pediatric CNS (neurosurgery) consults with a pediatric CNS (endocrine) about hormone replacement for a 13-year-old girl who recently underwent resection of a pituitary tumor and now has panhypopituitarism.
- Initiation of a night-shift CNS to be available as a resource and consultant throughout an acute care hospital results in increased registered nurse (RN) satisfaction, increased RN engagement, and earlier intervention for decompensating patients (Becker, 2013).
- A CNS joins a newly formed palliative care consult team at a large facility with long-term care, post–acute care, and long-term acute care hospital patients. The CNS performs all assessments on initial team consult and triages to other team members as appropriate while also consulting with RNs to increase palliative care knowledge (Mahler, 2010).
- An oncology CNS who rarely cares for patients with brain tumors consults a neurology or neurosurgery CNS when brain tumor patients are admitted for assistance in developing a care plan that addresses neurologic deficits and ensures the effective monitoring of potential complications.
- A neurologist consults with a cardiovascular surgery CNS for assistance in preparing a patient admitted with a brain abscess and a previously undiagnosed congenital cardiac anomaly for urgent cardiac surgery.

practice and activities may range from scholarly inquiry to formal scientific investigation. The Doctor of Nursing Practice (DNP) degree adds to the knowledge base of traditional master's programs for CNSs by expanding depth in EBP and quality improvement knowledge and skills (AACN, 2012). DNP-prepared CNSs can implement the science developed by nurse researchers, such as those with a Doctor of Philosophy (PhD) or Doctor of Nursing Science

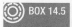 **BOX 14.5** **Examples of Clinical Nurse Specialist (CNS) External Consultation**

- An oncology CNS provides consultation to Romanian nurses on complex wound care for a breast cancer patient to discuss care options based on supplies available in Romania (Vosit-Steller & Morse, 2014).
- A pediatric CNS (neurosurgery) in a children's hospital provides consultation for the medical-surgical CNS in an adult clinic about transitioning care of an 18-year-old spina bifida patient with shunted hydrocephalus.
- Two oncology CNSs study telephone consults they received related to patients with metastatic breast cancer. Of received calls, 63% came from patients while 21% came from other health care professionals to provide information, provide symptom management, and address psychosocial and other issues (Warren, Mackie, & Leary, 2012).

(DNS) degree (AACN, 2012). There has been increasing collaboration between PhD-prepared nursing faculty and CNSs in the clinical setting, in which the CNS lends clinical expertise to the research component and supports EBP in the practice setting (Fulton, 2011). Specific EBP competencies, each of which has basic and advanced levels of activity, include interpretation and use of research findings (evidence- or research-based practice) and participation in collaborative research (see Chapter 10).

CNSs have the knowledge, skills, and clinical expertise to use EBP to advance clinical practice and improve patient outcomes. Nurse-sensitive indicators have been defined that capture nursing's unique contributions to patient outcomes. Assuming responsibility for identifying nursing-sensitive and interprofessional quality indicators and using outcomes data to improve patient care are prime opportunities for a CNS to assess patient care strategies and community systems, analyze interprofessional communication and collaboration, coordinate care, and monitor patient and system progress. Much work has yet to be done, however, to develop the science linking nursing, health care processes, available measures, and quality outcomes (Naylor, 2007). All CNSs must demonstrate the EBP competency and have ongoing accountability for monitoring and improving their practice and the practice of other

nurses (NACNS, 2004). CNSs implement this competency in a variety of ways, depending on experience, expertise, circumstances, setting, and resources.

Interpretation and Use of Evidence in Practice

Evidence-based practice has become an umbrella term for research utilization, research-based practice, and outcomes research (see Chapter 10). Integration of new scientific findings and science-based knowledge influences the development and evaluation of new approaches to clinical practice (AACN, 2006b).

For CNSs, the interpretation and use of research and other evidence often begins with a clinical question identified by the CNS or staff with whom he or she works. Knowledge is the basis for practice but, too frequently, routine practice may not be based on sound evidence. The foundation of improved quality of care and patient outcomes is the analysis of research-based evidence and expert consensus-dependent practice changes to ensure best practice and achieve quality patient care. Inherent in the CNS role is the evaluation of the appropriateness of evidence and the application of its findings to clinical practice. A CNS is the ideal clinician to assess factors that are barriers and facilitators to change and to develop, implement, and evaluate EBP. EBP is integrated into clinical procedures, administrative policies, educational materials for patients and staff, and care guidelines. A CNS's involvement in developing policies and procedures means that evidence informs clinical practices and standards.

A CNS who develops an evidence-based guideline of care for a patient population promotes improved patient outcomes throughout the three spheres of influence. Ideally, nursing practice improves, the patient's physical or mental function improves, care is as consistent as possible accounting for individual preferences/variances, treatment is safer and with fewer complications, and there is continuity of care across the health care continuum (McCabe, 2005). Multiple examples of CNS-led EBP improvements can be found in the literature. CNS contributions to improving patient outcomes by providing evidence-based care include the following: CNS-led implementation of innovative strategies that led to a decrease in central line–associated blood stream infections (Richardson & Tjoelker, 2012); implementation of an intervention to improve medication adherence in adult renal transplant recipients (Russell, 2010); development of clinical pathways for cardiac patients resulting in trends in decreased median time to myocardial infarction intervention, decreased length of stay, and a stronger connection between cardiac and community rehabilitation (Avery & Schnell-Hoehn, 2010); and early extubation in patients after open heart surgery, resulting in decreased length of stay and pulmonary complications (Soltis, 2015). CNSs mentor staff in the use of EBP as well. For example, one academic hospital system used a CNS-led council to mentor nurses in promoting evidence-based nursing care (Becker et al., 2012). CNSs had a leadership role in transforming a policy and procedure committee into a clinical practice council to promote practice that was evidence based.

Participation in Collaborative Research

Although the number of PhD-prepared CNSs with the training to conduct research is increasing, most CNSs are prepared at the master's and DNP level and can be partners in collaborating on research relevant to practice. Collaborative research between a CNS and researcher increases the likelihood of translating research findings to clinical practice. Researchers provide CNSs with new evidence for patient care practices and the assessment of their impact. The PhD-prepared CNS collaborates with peer CNSs by using advanced research skills to appraise journal articles critically and set up research study designs, as well as facilitate contacts with other faculty. They can be the bridge between basic research and patient care. In turn, master's- and DNP-prepared CNSs stimulate researchers to investigate the science that explains their observations of patients and populations. A CNS-led initiative to foster collaboration between hospital staff nurses and university faculty resulted in increased partnerships between faculty and nursing staff and the initiation of research projects focusing on quality improvement (Zinn et al., 2011).

Typically, novice CNSs are not immediately involved in collaborative research because they are focused on mastering their newly acquired competencies. For experienced CNSs, collaborative research is often a realistic goal. Whether novice or experienced CNSs become involved in research depends on the setting, pregraduate and graduate school experience, resources within the setting, and access to research expertise. Many CNSs find satisfaction with involvement in research as a consultant or coinvestigator. A CNS is the clinical expert, understands clinical issues, has access to patients, and can anticipate clinical and system challenges that may occur throughout the research process. A nurse researcher is a research expert, knows research methodology, and has access to the resources that support research. The CNS is optimally positioned to stimulate a researcher's interest because of her or his direct clinical association with patients or participant populations. Before participating in a research project, a CNS must determine whether there is readiness and receptiveness in the practice setting and administrative support, and whether research activities are a realistic performance goal.

Interprofessional collaborative research offers opportunities for innovative solutions to complex issues, improved collaboration, richness of expertise and perspectives, and more comprehensive care improvements (Tracy & Chlan, 2014). CNSs know the organizational and social facilitators and barriers to clinical research, can bridge the academic-clinical gap, and can assist in recruiting and retaining research participants.

In addition to applying research findings to clinical practice, CNSs can use research to influence public policy. Although conducting prospective research to address statutory or regulatory initiatives occurs infrequently, research results can provide substantive and objective facts that are more powerful and meaningful than impassioned pleas. Professional, state, and national databanks contain extensive data, but these data must be translated into language that is understandable and easily communicated. Whatever the model, a CNS is a key player in developing and implementing relevant nursing-sensitive and interprofessional quality indicators for measuring patient and system outcomes through EBP, quality improvement, and research.

Leadership

CNSs serve as leaders of interprofessional quality improvement teams because of their unique preparation at the graduate level (NACNS, 2012b), using advanced communication and leadership skills to evaluate practice and effect change in complex health care delivery systems (AACN, 2006b). It is because of these very leadership skills that CNSs are often pulled away by administrators to lead other initiatives. Leadership is integral to the role because a CNS has responsibility for clinical innovation and change within the patient care system. A CNS has significant formal and informal impact and must be visionary yet realistic. Through a CNS's clinical and systems leadership, change strategies are implemented to improve outcomes and advance nursing practice.

CNSs have an important role in helping a hospital achieve and maintain Magnet status (Hanson, 2015;

Muller et al., 2010; Walker, Urden, & Moody, 2009) because of their education in the three spheres of influence (Lewandowski & Adamle, 2009; Newhouse, 2009). The nurses and nursing practice sphere of influence of the CNS role is already recognized by many hospitals seeking to obtain or maintain Magnet status and should make this role even more valuable in the future. CNSs lead and mentor nurses to lead projects that meet the Magnet standards. Particular strengths lie in the areas of nursing education, EBP, and process improvement, which are key concerns for attaining Magnet status (Muller et al., 2010).

A CNS is the link between many disciplines and resources and asserts clinical and professional leadership in the practice setting or health care system, in health care policy and delivery decisions, and in the administration of direct care programs. Using direct practice, EBP, and consultation, the CNS identifies and plans for changes in practice and care delivery; however, it is through the CNS's leadership skills that change is actually effectively implemented. Clinical and professional leadership competencies are integrated with the other CNS competencies to support an organization's purpose and goals.

Most health care organizations are a bureaucratic maze. A CNS works with and advocates for staff, patients, and families to help them understand the complexities and navigate their way through the system. Because of the CNS's communication skills and knowledge of diplomacy, a CNS can be a facilitator among staff, administration, and patients during organizational change, problem solving, or conflict resolution. As leaders, CNSs also help the members of one discipline understand the priorities of another discipline and often negotiate agreements that bring diverse perspectives into alignment. This mediation benefits patients, promotes communication, and creates an environment that fosters collaboration.

Collaboration

CNSs must be skilled at collaboration because the CNS regularly interacts with a variety of people in order to achieve quality improvements and optimal outcomes (see Chapter 12). A CNS collaborates with nurses, physicians, other health care providers, and patients and their families, providing an interface among them (AACN, 2006b). Depending on the project, the CNS can literally interact with any department in the hospital over time depending on the project—for example, supply chain, finance,

security, operations, and facilities. The Institute of Medicine (IOM) report, *The Future of Nursing: Leading Change, Advancing Health,* has recommended that opportunities be expanded for nurses to "lead and diffuse collaborative improvement efforts" (IOM, 2011, p. 11). Many patients have such complex health care needs that no one health care professional can independently manage them all; this increasing complexity requires more interdependence to adequately manage (Brooten, Youngblut, Hannan, & Guido-Sanz, 2012). CNSs understand the knowledge and skills of other team members and actively participate in and lead interprofessional teams. A CNS can partner with patients and family members to determine their needs, help them ask questions and assess treatment options, and facilitate timely referrals to other disciplines to ensure a positive outcome. Collaboration between a CNS and other health care professionals leads to effective and efficient health care, especially for complex patient populations. CNSs can integrate the insights of many individuals with different perspectives, with each providing theoretical and applied knowledge. Throughout her or his interactions with patients and colleagues, a CNS models the communication and collaboration skills that help teams mature and be effective.

Collaboration is an essential competency—the well-earned result of clinical competence, effective communication, mutual trust, the valuing of complementary knowledge and skills, collegiality, and a favorable organizational structure (see Chapter 12). A model highlighting the need for interprofessional collaboration and coordination is the transitional care model, which is a nurse-led, evidenced-based approach to transitioning chronically ill, high-risk adults from the hospital to home, an ideal role for the CNS (Naylor, Aiken, Kurtzman, Olds, & Hirschman, 2011).

CNSs often identify potential or actual conflicts when collaboration is not working well, and CNS advocacy often prevents or ameliorates adversarial situations and their negative sequelae. A CNS must be skilled in helping team members address and negotiate conflicts to optimize patient care. The outcome of CNS-coordinated collaboration is the empowerment of nurses and recognition of the nurse as a critical member of the health care team. This results in team building, synergy, and integrative solutions. Some practice settings and working relationships are more conducive to partnership than others. The IOM report *The Future of Nursing* has recommended that nurses be educated with medical and other health care professional students and that interprofessional experiences occur throughout their careers (IOM, 2011). Ongoing research has shown that quality care and patient outcomes improve when CNSs collaborate as equals with other health care providers (Naylor et al., 2011), and early joint education may facilitate that partnership.

Blurring of boundaries between health care professionals can occur as the CNS role develops. Boundaries can overlap between the CNS and staff nurse, between the CNS and physician, or between the CNS and another APRN. It is important that clear communication occurs between collaborators in order to ensure that the blurring of boundaries does not result in either gaps in or duplication of care due to unclear accountabilities. CNSs must avoid being territorial; this limits their effectiveness, and they are unlikely to develop positive relationships that can help patients and families navigate the health care system efficiently. Chapters 9 and 12 provide further information on clarity in roles with consultation and collaboration, particularly related to direct care of patients.

Ethical Decision Making

CNSs often identify or consult on ethical issues and facilitate their resolution. In some cases, a CNS is consulted on what staff perceive is a clinical issue but really turns out to be an ethical concern. Being able to recognize, name, and address the moral distress and ethical concerns that are inherent in clinical care is a crucial part of CNS practice. A CNS can significantly influence the acknowledgment and negotiation of moral dilemmas, direction of patient care, access to care, and allocation of resources. CNSs consider numerous factors such as professional and religious codes, cultural values, bioethical principles, and ethical theories when making decisions that may have ethical implications (see Chapter 13).

CNSs have similar responsibilities when applying ethical decision-making skills to patient and organizational issues. They recognize clinicians' experiences of moral distress and articulate moral dilemmas, often serving as advocates for patients, families, and staff. They interpret and mediate patient, family, and team members' views to ensure as complete a discussion of the dilemma as possible. They recognize when there is a need to consult an ethics committee and often initiate that consult. When necessary, CNSs validate nurses' concerns and help nurses present their concerns to other team members, ensuring that the nursing perspective is considered when ethical issues are discussed. When CNSs are excluded from interprofessional ethical decisions, opportunities for effective nursing care are minimized and outcomes, such as timely and appropriate end-of-life care, can be compromised (Hamric & Delgado, 2014). Because CNSs facilitate optimal care for complex patients who are more frail and sick, the ethical challenge is to balance the expectations for quality care with the limitations of appropriate care and assist in articulating the moral dilemmas for patients, nursing personnel, and organizations. When CNSs optimize their knowledge and expertise in the ethical competency domain, they can advance beyond resolution of ethical issues on a case-by-case basis to leading the building of an ethical environment for all patients, families, and health care providers in the setting (Hamric & Delgado, 2014).

Exemplar 14.2, a composite case, illustrates the multidimensional and complex nature of CNS practice, implementing the substantive clinical areas of CNS practice and including the seven competencies across three spheres of influence.

| EXEMPLAR 14.2 | Advanced Practice Competencies and Spheres of Influence: Clinical Nurse Specialist Practice With a Complex Patient[a] |

HH, an 82-year-old woman, was brought by paramedics to the emergency department with acute abdominal pain and severe pulmonary congestion. For the past few weeks, HH had been experiencing dyspnea on exertion and was unable to walk more than a few steps. These symptoms progressively worsened. She was having severe respiratory distress at rest and slept elevated on three pillows.

HH's medical history included insulin-dependent diabetes mellitus, hypertension, atrial fibrillation, coronary artery disease, critical aortic stenosis, severe heart failure, mild chronic obstructive pulmonary disease (COPD), chronic renal insufficiency, chronic urinary tract infections, and obesity. On admission, HH was alert and oriented but somnolent, and she had labored breathing. Pertinent diagnostic results from the chest x-ray examination showed mild cardiac enlargement, pulmonary edema, left pleural effusion, and calcification of the aortic valve. A cardiac catheterization showed severe calcification of the aortic valve not amenable to valvuloplasty.

EXEMPLAR 14.2   **Advanced Practice Competencies and Spheres of Influence: Clinical Nurse Specialist Practice With a Complex Patient[a]—cont'd**

In discussing the results of the examinations with HH, it became clear that she wanted the valve replaced surgically, despite the extensive risks of the surgery at her age and in her condition. The surgeon and staff nurses expressed discomfort with the patient's request; therefore, the CNS was consulted.

PSAS met the patient and her family to assess the situation. HH seemed withdrawn, with poor eye contact and limited interaction. PSAS quickly recognized that English was the patient's second language. HH had a son and two daughters. Her son was very vocal about preferences for his mother's care, but the older daughter had multiple personal crises and tended to defer to her own two sons (HH's grandsons). The younger daughter was hesitant to voice opinions about medical decisions. HH stated that she did not want to continue living as a "cardiac cripple" and continued to demand the surgery.

PSAS believed that several interventions needed to occur to ensure that HH was making an informed decision and that risks had been taken into consideration by everyone involved. PSAS facilitated a health team care conference with all disciplines to review the case and clarify the risks of proceeding with the surgery. Because there was concern about the language barrier, PSAS also facilitated a patient/family care conference with the health care team, HH, her family, and an interpreter. This satisfied the health care team that HH clearly understood her options.

PSAS performed a literature search and spoke with the surgeon to clarify the risks versus benefits of this surgery in an octogenarian. She initiated an ethics committee consult with the staff to discuss concerns related to moral distress about performing surgery in an older patient with such a high risk for a poor outcome. She held multiple in-services to discuss the literature search results and ethical principles involved in proceeding with the surgery. She used the expertise of her psychiatric CNS colleague to help staff identify communication techniques for maintaining optimal relationships with the patient and family.

PSAS also recognized that HH had not completed an advance directive. She initiated a consult with the palliative care team, who discussed with HH how she envisioned her postoperative care. As a result, HH completed an advance directive and made her wishes known not to be indefinitely dependent on external life support.

HH underwent the high-risk surgery to replace her aortic valve with a tissue valve. Postoperatively, she required another surgery to control bleeding, and her postoperative course was complicated by hypotension requiring pharmacologic support, complete heart block requiring a pacemaker, and low urine output. Because of her COPD, HH had difficulty weaning from the ventilator and required a percutaneous tracheostomy placement. Because of her diabetes, her sternal wound failed to heal. An episode of sepsis resulted in renal failure, requiring continuous renal replacement therapy (CRRT). PSAS was active in assisting the novice and experienced nurses to provide direct care to this complex patient and teaching them new procedures, such as assisting with placement of a tracheostomy at the bedside, managing fluid balance in a cardiac patient with CRRT, and managing skin care needs for a sacral pressure wound.

HH's family continued to have difficulty reaching a consensus about the best path for her care and showed frustration with the situation. They had unrealistic expectations related to the likelihood of HH's recovery and believed that staff should "cure her," despite the extensive discussions before surgery regarding the high surgical risks and poor prognosis. PSAS facilitated multiple family care conferences with the health care team and family to keep communication lines open.

Approximately 6 weeks after surgery, it became clear that HH would likely never be weaned from the ventilator and would need to be placed in a long-term care facility. PSAS facilitated one final care conference with the health care team and family to discuss HH's poor likelihood of improvement and review her advance directive. With assistance from the health care team, the family decided that, in accordance with HH's wishes, she should be transitioned to comfort care and have the ventilator removed and dialysis discontinued. PSAS reassured the family that the patient's pain would be well managed, and she spoke with them about the rituals important to them in facilitating end-of-life care. PSAS ensured that HH's wishes were honored, such as having spiritual music played in the room and a bedside prayer service led by her pastor. With her extended family present, HH died several days after the transition to comfort care. ◎

[a]The authors wish to thank Patricia S. A. Sparacino, PhD, RN, FAAN, for this exemplar.

Current Marketplace Forces and Concerns

Patient safety and quality care continue to be major concerns in health care delivery. Medical errors have been identified as the third leading cause of death in the United States, following heart disease and cancer (Makary & Daniel, 2016). Skilled application of the seven competencies in all three spheres of influence (patient, nurse/nursing practice, systems/ organizations) make CNSs well positioned to contribute to address both patient safety and quality care. Role contributions for expert nurses have focused on improving outcomes primarily for populations of patients through implementing EBP and system improvements. CNSs have demonstrated these contributions in decreasing lengths of stay in the hospital, decreasing costs, reducing complications, and increasing patient satisfaction (Newhouse et al., 2011).

Internationally, the CNS and NP have been identified as the most common APRN roles (Delamaire & Lafortune, 2010; Chapter 6). The role of the CNS is expanding internationally for the same primary reasons: the need for quality care of increasingly complex patients (Bryant-Lukosius et al., 2010). This complexity of patients is seen not only in hospital settings but also in patients' homes, expanding opportunities for CNSs to practice outside the usual boundaries of a hospital, to include transitional care (i.e., transferring care from one health care setting to another health care setting) and outpatient care (Bryant-Lukosius et al., 2015; Coleman & Boult, 2003; Marshall et al., 2015; Naylor et al., 2011). In the latest CNS Census (NACNS, 2017c), CNSs report that the number of CNSs practicing outside of an acute care hospital has increased to 20%. In a systematic review of CNS-led hospital-to-home transitional care compared to usual care, the authors found that the CNS was able to reduce patient mortality in patients with cancer; delay time to and reduce death or rehospitalization, improve patient treatment adherence and patient satisfaction, and decrease costs and length of rehospitalization in patients with heart failure; improve caregiver depression and decrease rehospitalization, rehospitalization length of stay, and costs for elderly patients; and improve infant immunization rates and maternal satisfaction with care and reduce maternal and infant length of hospital stay and costs for high-risk pregnant women and very–low-birth-weight infants (Bryant-Lukosius et al., 2015; see Exemplar 14.3). When patients with rheumatoid arthritis were randomly assigned to either the CNS, an inpatient multidisciplinary team, or a day patient multidisciplinary team, quality of life and utility were equal among groups. However, the cost of care was approximately $6084 less when provided by the CNS (van den Hout, Tijhuis, Hazes, Breedveld, & Vliet Vlieland, 2003). Similarly, when comparing outcomes in an outpatient setting, CNSs were able to demonstrate cost-effectiveness as outpatient alternative providers and as complementary care providers (Kilpatrick et al., 2014).

Although CNSs are very clear about their role, one of the concerns facing them is the clarity of the CNS role to others. Resolution of this lack of clarity is essential for successful implementation of the role (DiCenso et al., 2010). Because of the many facets of the CNS role, from expert clinician to direct care provider to systems change agent, it is challenging to articulate the role succinctly. Although the CNS, NP, CNM, and CRNA are all direct patient care providers, the CNS is a unique APRN role that also focuses on nurses/nursing practice and systems/ organizations as foundational to their work (NACNS, 2004). Ensuring the survival of the role is essential to ensure that all three spheres of influence continued to be addressed at an APRN level. Assurance of this requires action at the professional, regulatory, and systems operational levels.

Scope of Practice and Delegated Authority

Scope of practice are those activities a health care individual is permitted to perform within his or her profession (Federation of State Medical Boards, 2005). Scope of practice is specific to each state and is established by state regulations (Federation of State Medical Boards, 2005). Although the CNS has the education, competence, skills, and expertise to practice, if he or she moves from one state to another state, it is the practice act of the new state that will determine what the CNS can do. Differences in state practice acts have led to a "crazy quilt"of varied and inconsistent licensure laws (Safriet, 2010, p. 453). Adding to the "crazy quilt" approach is the fact that the organization/facility where the CNS practices can further restrict the practice of a CNS despite the state's scope of practice. This has led to particular issues for the federal Veterans Health Administration, where an APRN would have privileges according to the state in which she or he was practicing. To standardize CNS practice despite state differences, a recent ruling by the Department of Veterans Affairs (2016) allows CNSs to work to their full practice authority within Veterans Affairs facilities and not within the individual state's scope of practice.

EXEMPLAR 14.3	**Transitional Care CNSs Navigating Patients Across the Care Continuum**[a]

In rural Vermont, three hospital-based acute care clinical nurse specialists (CNSs) began to design an integrated care delivery system for their community. Based on the Mary Naylor Transitional Care Model developed at the University of Pennsylvania, the CNS team partnered with primary care providers (PCPs) to identify high-risk, chronically ill patients who are high users of the health care system. In this model, expert CNSs navigate patients from the hospital to home, which can include short-term rehabilitation stays and primary and specialty office visits. Gaps in communication and care delivery that negatively impact the patient and family experience are identified. Over 2 years, this team collaborated with community agencies and local/regional resources to improve population health and quality outcomes while decreasing costs. The CNSs created a Community Care Team to support people with addiction and mental illness who frequently use the emergency department. This team devised a community-based wraparound care plan to meet the person's clinical, social, and emotional needs. The team also supported implementation of INTERACT (Interactions to Reduce Acute Care Transfers), recognizing the need to decrease turnaround readmissions from the local nursing homes.

Apprehensive to leave the comfort and familiarity of the hospital setting, this journey into the realities of health care reform has offered the CNSs the challenge of a lifetime. All health care providers must strive to understand what happens with patients outside of their time with them. Building a relationship that allows trust to develop also allows patients to feel safe to confide details of what might negatively impact their recovery and wellness.

The following is an example of how CNSs have been architects of integrated care delivery focusing on shared decision making and goal setting to improve the quality of life for many.

Clinical Example

HJ, a 68-year-old man, has been admitted to the hospital three times in the past 6 weeks with exacerbation of chronic obstructive pulmonary disease (COPD), resulting in treatment with antibiotics and steroids and adjustment of inhaler therapy. Each time, the hospitalist consults with the pulmonologist and the discharge plan includes ongoing care by the specialist. Since the last admission, the CNS (BR) has been consulted by the PCP to evaluate why HJ is unable to be successful when discharged from the hospital. The PCP reports that the patient appears to understand his treatment plan and

medications and seems motivated. BR visits the patient in the hospital, introducing herself and explaining that she works with his PCP, who knows he is in the hospital. BR has access to the PCP record and shares pertinent information with the hospitalist and pulmonologist. She also shares patient information at daily interprofessional rounds. As BR assesses the patient, she recognizes that he seems to have difficulty with simple explanations and is not interested in printed material supplied. HJ is home bound and meets criteria for home care referral but adamantly refuses when it is suggested. BR visits the patient daily in the hospital, meets his family, and develops a relationship.

On day 4, when HJ is being discharged, he reluctantly agrees to let BR see him at home: "Just one visit." BR visits HJ the next day and asks to review his discharge information. He hands her a pile of papers that appear untouched. The discharge packet is 20 pages in length, with information about his chronic disease, inhaler use, and all of his medications. BR asks to see where he keeps his medications and he shows her a grocery bag filled with pills collected over several years. She asks him for the new medications just ordered and he blushes with embarrassment. "I went to pick them up and couldn't afford to get them. I will just take what I already have here." Over two more home visits, the real story of HJ comes together. He has minimal financial resources, minimal social support, limited transportation, and few groceries. BR starts to make a plan to better meet his needs. She finds out what is important to him, what he is looking forward to, and what he would like to do that he has not been able to do. She provides hope that it may be possible for him to walk down the driveway to his mailbox again, and he may even get to bingo at the senior center.

While BR is at his home, she does a targeted physical assessment, checking blood pressure, pulse, and oxygenation. **(Direct Care)** He has crackles in the bases less than 24 hours postdischarge because he has not taken his diuretic or used his inhaler since discharge. She asks him to show her how he uses his inhaler and he tries to do it with the cover on, unable to get any of the medication. BR takes the cover off and demonstrates the proper technique. She draws a picture to remind him after she leaves and tapes it to his refrigerator. BR offers a medication box and demonstrates how to fill it correctly. She recognizes that HJ has difficulty reading and plans to consult the Transitional Care pharmacist to design a notebook with pictures of his

Continued

medications with sun and moon stickers to identify when the medications are to be taken. **(Guidance and Coaching)** As she scans HJ's apartment, BR notices multiple safety hazards. She asks to see his bathroom and identifies the lack of grab bars or safety handles. Little by little, HJ lets her in to his world, sharing what he was ashamed to admit, trusting she is there to help and not judge.

BR asks HJ if he would allow the Transitional Care social worker to visit. She explains that the social worker (NS) might be able to help him access funds for food, medications, and living expenses. **(Collaboration)** NS accompanies BR the next day to see HJ. NS explains potential options and informs HJ what Medicaid can offer him. HJ is at first reluctant, but with gentle persistence, NS helps him understand the improvement he may see in his life if he is willing to accept some assistance. BR and NS are able to access a patient fund at the hospital, which allows them to get HS's medications delivered that day.

At the next visit, BR brings the Transitional Care pharmacist to see HJ. He reviews the medication box and continues to help HJ learn to take his medications safely by explaining the notebook containing pictures of his medications. The pharmacist also examines the grocery bag of pills, identifying them to see if they are still current medications and if they are in date. BR explains that she will bring the outdated medications to be discarded at the police station. HJ agrees reluctantly, commenting that they cost a lot of money! BR leaves that day feeling satisfied that she has made a difference by collaborating with her team and building a workable plan of care. She hopes that HJ is on a path to improved health.

One week later, BR returns. Again she completes a targeted assessment and is dismayed to find HJ with shortness of breath, worsening crackles, and a temperature of 101° F. She inquires how long he has been feeling this way and reminds HJ that he could have called her. He says he did not want to bother her and knew she was coming today. BR is disappointed that she did not clearly explain the COPD action plan in a way that HJ understood. She quickly messages his PCP

with an update and gets new orders to help HJ avoid a repeat hospitalization. She also shares with him that it might be helpful for a home care nurse to see him a few times a week until he feels better. **(Collaboration)** She promises she will come with the nurse the first time.

HJ has an appointment with the pulmonologist the following day. BR offers to meet HJ at the office to help ensure he understands the discussion. She has forwarded a synopsis of her findings to the specialist via phone note prior to the appointment, targeting what he might choose to focus on. BR asks if "high-flow O_2 therapy" may be effective to decrease HJ's bouts of pneumonia and shares an article she researched after attending a conference in Chicago. **(Evidence-Based Practice)** The pulmonologist seems interested, and BR promises to set up a meeting with the vendor to explore this use. **(Consultation)** BR updates the Transitional Care team at their weekly meeting and presents this case to the team.

Over the past 2 years, the Transitional Care team has identified gaps in care delivery and, one by one, implemented solutions. This often involves collaboration with other disciplines, multiple community agencies, and Medicaid case workers. Success has come from bringing all partners to the table, brainstorming solutions, and recognizing that "it takes a village" to create integrated care delivery. Presently, competing home care and long-term care agencies sit together at the table strategizing how to work together and finding cost-effective ways to share resources. Medical home case managers and home care nurses who were initially suspicious of the Transitional Care model negatively impacting their roles now welcome the ability to deploy this resource when they have concerns about a patient at home. PCPs acknowledge the benefit of the model because they have one more tool in their toolboxes to be the eyes and ears across the care continuum. Little by little, the Transitional Care personnel are functioning as a cohesive team, recognizing what each member brings to the table and creating a symphony out of the chaos that is health care today. ◎

[a]The authors wish to thank Billie Lynn Allard, MS, RN, for this exemplar.

All health professions have an autonomous domain of practice as well as delegated authority within the medical domain (Lyon, 2004). Historically, the medical profession developed a broad, overarching scope of practice that encompassed almost all health care activities (Safriet, 2010; see Chapter 1). As a consequence, other health professionals (e.g., nurses, physical therapists, pharmacists) have had to carve their scopes of practice out of the medical scope of practice over time. The ANA's restrictive 1955 definition of nursing (ANA, 1955) reinforced the practice of nursing as having independent functions and being dependent on and delegated to by the profession of medicine. It also prohibited nurses from diagnosing and prescribing pharmacologic and/or durable goods for patients.

This history has contributed to a false dichotomy of what constitutes nursing practice and medical practice. As Chapter 1 has demonstrated, the practice of nursing has evolved over time to take on more responsibility and skills once considered to be the sole domain of medicine. As discoveries about health and illness continue to progress, the knowledge and skills of professional nurses and other health professionals will continue to evolve in their own right with their professional practice advancing into traditional boundaries of medicine (Standards for Supervision of Nursing Practice, 1983). As patients have become more complex and understanding of disease more sophisticated, physicians have become more specialized in treating the most complicated or complex patients. Therefore nursing scopes of practice, educational curricula, and competency validation need to stay flexible to evolve over time (Hartigan, 2011).

For CNSs specifically, delegated authority continues to pose an issue as APRNs establish their independent scopes of practice. Consistent with the IOM's *The Future of Nursing* (IOM, 2011) and the Consensus Model for APRN Regulation (APRN Joint Dialogue Group, 2008), CNSs will need to practice to the full extent of their education to meet the needs of more and increasingly complex patients. Inefficiencies in the health care system are present and patients do not obtain timely care when physician supervision of APRN practice is required, due to either regulations or institutional requirements.

Institute of Medicine *The Future of Nursing* Report

The IOM report *The Future of Nursing: Leading Change, Advancing Health* (IOM, 2011) clearly articulated four key messages and eight recommendations as a blueprint for change in nursing and advanced practice nursing in the United States to meet the health needs of Americans in the era of health care reform. The NACNS (2012b) formulated a response to address pertinent recommendations from the perspective of CNSs (Table 14.2). The National Council of State Boards of Nursing (NCSBN) tracks each state's legislative activities in relation to the major components of the Consensus Model, including APRN title, role, license, education, certification, independent practice and independent prescribing, and the IOM recommendations (NCSBN, 2017). This section addresses the IOM's key messages and recommendations as they pertain to CNSs.

Key Message 1

Nurses should practice to the fullest extent of their education and training.

One of the key messages of the Institute of Medicine's *The Future of Nursing* (IOM, 2011) report was that all nurses, including CNSs, should practice to the full extent of their education. One approach to enabling this is the removal of practice barriers imposed by some states' scopes of practice. In spite of an increase in the number of states that have changed nurse practice acts to support APRNs working to the full extent of their education, a 2015 summary of *Assessing Progress on the Institute of Medicine Report The Future of Nursing* concluded that there needed to be continued work to remove scope-of-practice barriers (IOM, 2015).

Since 2010, independent practice for CNSs (i.e., the authority to practice without a supervising physician) has increased from 20 to 28 states (32% increase), and for independent prescribing of pharmacologic agents, there has been an increase from 13 to 19 states (40% increase) (NACNS, 2015a). In addition, CNSs are eligible prescribers in many federal programs, such as Medicare and Medicaid (Centers for Medicare & Medicaid Services (CMS), 2012; Klein, 2012). However, even though a state's practice act may provide for independent practice, practice may be further restricted by the workplace. For example, New Mexico allows for independent practice and prescriptive authority of APRNs (Petersen, Keller, Way, & Borges, 2015). However, in a recent survey of APRNs in New Mexico, 34% of CNSs identified physician oversight of his or her practice as a requirement in their workplace.

TABLE 14.2	NACNS Strategies for Enacting the Institute of Medicine's (IOM's) *The Future of Nursing* Recommendations Related to the Clinical Nurse Specialist (CNS) Role

IOM Key Message	NACNS Recommendations for Enactment
1. Nurses should practice to the fullest extent of their education and training.	<ul><li>Amend nurse practice acts to allow CNSs to diagnose and treat health conditions.</li><li>Eliminate requirements for physician "collaborative practice agreements."</li><li>Remove prescribing restrictions or limitations imposed by required physician oversight, collaboration, or signature.</li><li>Amend requirements for hospital participation in the Medicare program to ensure that CNSs are eligible for clinical privileges, admitting privileges, and membership on medical staffs.</li><li>Advocate for all insurers, including but not limited to Medicare, Medicaid, and third-party insurers, to include coverage of CNS services that are within their scope of practice under state law.</li><li>Amend the Medicare and Medicaid programs to authorize CNSs to perform admission assessments, certify patients for home health care services, and admit patients to hospitals, hospice, and skilled nursing facilities.</li></ul>
2. Nurses should achieve higher levels of education and training through an improved education system that promotes seamless academic progression.	<ul><li>Advocate for academic institutions to offer research and practice doctorates that support CNS specialty-focused advanced practice nursing.</li><li>Advocate for CNS-focused courses in doctoral programs.</li><li>Develop Bachelor of Science in Nursing (BSN)–to–Doctor of Philosophy and BSN-to–Doctor of Nursing Practice (DNP) programs for CNSs to streamline the process for preparing research and clinical scholars.</li><li>Recommend options for seamless progression to DNP preparation for CNSs.</li></ul>
3. Nurses should be full partners, with physicians and other health care professionals, in redesigning health care in the United States.	<ul><li>Promote interprofessional education at the graduate level to optimize collaboration skills.</li><li>Support entrepreneurial opportunities for CNSs in the design, implementation, and evaluation of innovative care models.</li><li>Optimize education related to technology and technology evaluation.</li><li>Revise or amend regulatory language to recognize CNSs as primary care providers for patients with chronic health problems related to medical diagnoses such as diabetes, heart failure, and mental health or chronic conditions such as chronic wounds, chronic pain, or impaired mobility.</li><li>Actively engage CNSs in health care policy decisions.</li><li>Advocate for organizational support to increase CNSs' responsibility in implementing system improvements.</li><li>Encourage accountable care organizations to include CNS services among all the services provided.</li><li>Facilitate the delivery of CNS specialty services in novel health care delivery systems.</li><li>Foster the use of CNS leadership skills in the redesign of health care delivery across settings.</li><li>Encourage CNSs to design, implement, and evaluate new systems of providing care to specialty populations.</li><li>Advocate for CNS opportunities for continued development of leadership skills (lifelong learning).</li><li>Encourage and mentor CNSs to participate in policy and regulatory bodies.</li></ul>
4. Effective workforce planning and policymaking require better data collection and an improved information infrastructure.	<ul><li>Ensure that the criteria for all future survey designs include CNSs. For example, the Workforce Commission and the Health Resources Services Administration may want to develop an APRN survey focusing on the underserved and vulnerable populations. It is critical that CNSs provide the necessary consultation to ensure that CNS-sensitive outcomes are captured within such a survey.</li><li>Include CNSs in the design of all workforce standardized minimum data sets (MDSs), including work by state licensing boards.</li><li>Increase the sample size and fielding of the survey to every other year, facilitating expanding the data collected on APRNs, and release survey results more quickly.</li><li>Include recommendations by CNSs when establishing a monitoring system that uses data from the MDS to measure systematically and project nursing workforce requirements by role, skill mix, region, and demographics.</li><li>Integrate CNSs when coordinating workforce research efforts with the Department of Labor, state and regional educators, employers, and state nursing workforce centers to identify regional health care workforce needs and when establishing regional targets and plans for appropriately increasing the supply of health professionals.</li></ul>

Adapted from National Association of Clinical Nurse Specialists. (2012b). Response to the Institute of Medicine's *The Future of Nursing* report. Retrieved from http://nacns.org/advocacy-policy/position-statements/response-to-the-institute-of-medicines-future-of-nursing-report/

Consistent with the Consensus Model for APRN Regulation (APRN Joint Dialogue Group, 2008), the NCSBN has drafted a compact that would allow for APRNs to practice in participating states by being issued a multistate license (NCSBN, 2015). The APRN Compact is consistent with the recommendations of the IOM report and was approved May 4, 2015, by the NCSBN delegate assembly. However, states would be required to pass the model legislation without any material differences to be able to be participate in the Compact.

The NACNS was a part of an amicus brief (Supreme Court of the United States, 2014) in the case supporting the Federal Trade Commission's ruling in the U.S. Supreme Court case *North Carolina State Board of Dental Examiners v. Federal Trade Commission,* where restriction in provision of non-dentist teeth whitening services was deemed an unfair method of competition. This ruling had clear implications for APRNs in that it provides a foundation for not allowing physicians to restrict access to the market by another adequately prepared health care provider.

Key Message 2
Nurses should achieve higher levels of education and training through an improved education system that promotes seamless academic progression.

Although the IOM recommends that by 2020 the number of nurses with doctorates should be doubled, in a survey of 3118 CNS respondents, 61.8% had Master's of Science in Nursing degrees and 16.2% had Master's of Science degrees (NACNS, 2017c). Although there are currently more CNSs with PhDs (7.47%) than DNPs (5.89%), it is likely that DNPs will become predominant with the focus on moving to the DNP as the entry for APRN practice.

Consistent with other professional APRN organizations, the NACNS has endorsed the DNP as the entry into practice by 2030 (NACNS, 2015b). The decision was based upon the education required to care for the increasing complexity of patients and health care systems and the future direction of nursing practice. In addition, the NACNS has endorsed and supported CNSs obtaining PhD degrees (NACNS, 2016). However, regardless of the graduate degree obtained, it is important that the CNS pursue lifelong learning in order to maintain credibility and continue to innovate and provide quality care (Bousfield, 1997; IOM, 2015).

A recent white paper by the AACN identified variability among APRN educational programs, particularly for CNSs and NPs (AACN, 2015). This variability is also impacted by each state's scope of practice and licensure requirements. For example, if a CNS is going to school in a state that does not allow for prescriptive practice/authority, the CNS would need to go out of state in order to obtain precepted clinical hours prescribing pharmacologic agents. This would add a burden from both a financial and a logistical perspective for the CNS student.

Another challenge is the requirement, with the APRN Consensus Model and the criteria for CNS education programs, of 500 hours of precepted clinical experience both for the role and for the specific population, for a total of 1000 hours (AACN, 2015). The clinical experience must include the continuum of care from wellness to illness. There are a limited number of CNSs working in nonacute settings, thus it is a challenge to find practicing CNSs to precept CNS students in these settings. The "specialty" education of the CNS is essential in addition to the role and population focus required by the APRN Consensus Model. The debate on the number of clinical hours that is sufficient to cover the role, population, and specialty areas has not been resolved at this point.

Key Message 3
Nurses should be full partners, with physicians and other health care professionals, in redesigning health care in the United States.

Recommendations subsumed in this key message include expanding opportunities for nurses to lead and diffuse collaborative improvement efforts and preparing and enabling nurses to lead change to advance health care. CNSs are educated and trained to lead process improvement and collaborative projects. In addition, they are able to mentor and coach staff in a variety of disciplines to lead changes to improve health care systems. CNSs skills in leadership, collaboration, integration of current evidence, and development and evaluation of innovative interventions make them particularly well suited to actively lead these efforts.

CNSs have been identified as having a role in meeting the goals of a reformed health care system because it requires the expertise of those with specialized knowledge (Bousfield, 1997). Health care policy challenges health care providers to be innovative, including delivering cost-effective care in a patient-centered model (McClelland, McCoy & Burson, 2013). The CNS, with competence in direct care, system improvements, and collaboration, is perfectively poised to contribute to this innovation of the health care delivery system (NACNS, National CNS Competency Task Force, 2010).

Key Message 4

Effective workforce planning and policymaking require better data collection and an improved information infrastructure.

Building an infrastructure for the collection and analysis of interprofessional health care workforce data is the only recommendation in this key message. This is an important IOM recommendation for CNSs because they have been consistently excluded from federal governmental data collection. Every 10 years, the Office of Management and Budget in the federal government revises its Standard Occupational Classification (SOC), a uniform classification system designed to help federal agencies organize the data that they collect, analyze, and disseminate to inform public policy (https://www.bls.gov/soc/; Cosca & Emmel, 2010). Data collected for the SOC include items such as the number of persons by occupation and corresponding salaries. The Standard Occupational Classification Revision Policy Committee did not create a separate detailed occupation for CNSs, stating:

> even though education for Clinical Nurse Specialists is different from that of Registered Nurses, the tasks of Clinical Nurse Specialists are not sufficiently unique from those of Registered Nurses who "assess patient health problems and needs, develop and implement nursing care plans, and maintain medical records. (Cosca & Emmel, 2010, p. 36)

The NACNS has continued to advocate for including the CNS as a separate category in the SOC rather than having it subsumed within the general nursing occupational listing (Horner, 2016).

Similarly, the Health Resources and Services Administration (HRSA) publication on *The U.S. Nursing Workforce: Trends in Supply and Education* (HRSA, 2013) did not include CNSs in a separate category but only identified CNSs in an "NP/Clinical Nurse Specialist" category. This poses a challenge because the HRSA publication does not recognize the CNS as a unique APRN role even though it is clearly defined in educational curriculum and is a unique area of APRN practice.

Without understanding the numbers of CNSs in geographic regions, their practice settings, and salaries, it is difficult to know the steps required to increase the number of specialist APRNs to meet the need for safe and high-quality care. A minimum data set for CNSs could be created and required

when licensees seek renewal of their licensure by the boards of nursing as a way to start tracking CNSs in the field (IOM, 2011).

Consensus Model for APRN Regulation and Implications for the Clinical Nurse Specialist

The main purposes of the Consensus Model are to delineate the scope of practice for APRNs and define the regulation of APRNs in the areas of licensure, accreditation of education programs, certification, and education program requirements. This section focuses on the implications of the Consensus Model as it relates to the CNS role. It is important to note that this regulatory understanding of APRNs does not encompass a full conceptual understanding of advanced practice nursing (see Chapter 2). Some of the debates regarding the CNS role in relation to other APRN roles may trace their points of contention to the differences between a regulatory and a conceptual approach to the CNS. Title protection and scopes of practice for CNSs are highly variable from state to state. The Consensus Model clarifies that the CNS is one of the four APRN roles and that all APRNs have a patient-focused practice and should have the legal authority to perform acts of advanced assessment, diagnosing, prescribing, and ordering. Currently there are some states that do not recognize CNSs as APRNs as well as some states where CNSs are not under authorization by the board of nursing. If CNSs move away from direct patient care and focus solely on nursing education and systems improvements, they are at risk for not being recognized as APRNs in state regulations (Cronenwett, 1995; NCSBN, 2008). CNS practices must incorporate direct care of individuals, especially in specialty patients and families who are complex or vulnerable, to reclaim and maintain the public and professional recognition that CNSs are APRNs.

The Consensus Model requires title protection for CNSs, which would be a step forward for states not having this basic regulatory requirement. A grandfather clause (i.e., recognizing and granting authority to APRNs who graduated from accredited programs and were in practice before the implementation date of the Consensus Model) is included in the model regulatory language. This grandfather clause is important for CNSs because certification examinations are not available for all population foci (see "National Certification for Clinical Nurse Specialists" later). Certification of APRNs at the role and population focus levels will be required for all APRNs who seek licensure for practice at the advanced practice level. CNS certification in a specialty will be voluntary and outside the licensure of APRNs once an individual state adopts the Consensus Model.

Reimbursement for Clinical Nurse Specialist Services

Medicare rules prohibit APRNs (CNSs, NPs, CNMs) from admitting patients to skilled nursing facilities and certifying patients for hospice or home care, despite the fact that they may serve as the patients' primary care provider. In 2016, legislation was placed before Congress that would amend the Social Security Title XVIII to allow NPs, CNSs, and CNMs to certify for home and hospice care. Neither the House nor the Senate is likely to take this legislation up in committee without a Congressional Budget Office score. The legislation was first introduced in the 112th Congress, with subsequent introductions in the 113th, 114th, and 115th (2017-2018) Congresses. Most recently, this legislation has been introduced as S. 445, the Home Health Care Planning Improvement Act. If passed, this Act would allow CNSs, NPs, and CNMs to certify eligibility and make changes to home health plans of care (http://www.rnaction.org/site/PageNavigator/nstat_take_action_home_health.html).

Availability and Standardization of Educational Curricula for Clinical Nurse Specialists

The AACN has identified that variability exists in CNS programs, including the curriculum, expectations for student performance, and evaluation processes and tools (AACN, 2015). The Consensus Model for APRN Regulation (APRN Joint Dialogue Group, 2008) requires, at a minimum, the three Ps (advanced physical and health assessment, advanced pharmacology, and advanced physiology and pathophysiology). In addition, the education program, accredited by a nursing or nursing-related accrediting organization, must prepare the APRN in core, role, and population core competencies.

In 2011, the NACNS published *Criteria for the Evaluation of Clinical Nurse Specialist Master's, Practice Doctorate, and Post-Graduate Certificate Educational Programs*, developed by a convened group of professional nursing organizations that either had CNS members or were involved with accrediting of CNS programs (NACNS, Validation Panel, 2011). Congruent with existing standards

TABLE 14.3 Examples of Competency and Practice Standards That Impact Clinical Nurse Specialist (CNS) Education Curriculum and Practice

Title	Year of Publication	Publishing Organization
Statement on Clinical Nurse Specialist Practice and Education	2004	National Association of Clinical Nurse Specialists
Consensus Model for APRN Regulation	2008	APRN Consensus Workgroup
Essentials of Master's Education in Nursing	1996, 2011	American Association of Colleges of Nursing
Essentials of Doctoral Education for Advanced Nursing Practice	2006	American Association of Colleges of Nursing
Clinical Nurse Specialist Core Competencies: Executive Summary 2006-2008	2010	National Association of Clinical Nurse Specialists, National CNS Competency Task Force
Core Practice Doctorate Clinical Nurse Specialist (CNS) Competencies	2009	National Association of Clinical Nurse Specialists

(Table 14.3), the purpose of the document was to standardize nationally endorsed criteria that could be used for development and/or implementation of CNS programs.

In 2015, the AACN wrote a white paper on the *Current State of APRN Clinical Education* (AACN, 2015). The final recommendations included use of simulation to enhance clinical experience, academic-practice partnerships, competency-based education and assessments, and the development of innovative APRN education models. The knowledge, skills, and clinical experience acquired in a graduate program should prepare a CNS to practice at an advanced level, regardless of setting or patient population. Experience in direct patient care is desirable before entering a CNS program because it provides a foundation on which to develop advanced clinical expertise.

Despite these efforts to standardize CNS graduate preparation, programs vary substantially (AACN, 2015). To ensure that the CNS continues to be a recognized advanced practice nursing role, the need is urgent to clarify competencies, standardize CNS curricula, and reach a rational consensus on how to credential CNSs from multiple specialties. Many initiatives are underway that will directly or indirectly affect future CNS preparation, credentialing, and practice. It is necessary to include the recommendations from the Consensus Model to guide new and existing programs as they modify or update their curricula with the purpose of preparing CNSs to provide expert care to patients and improve patient outcomes through education and system changes. The NACNS is in the process of revising the *Statement on Clinical Nurse Specialist Practice and Education* (NACNS, 2004), and the core competencies for CNSs, regardless of specialty, to help standardize education and practice for the new graduate CNS (NACNS, National CNS Competency Task Force, 2010; see Table 14.1).

Recent initiatives are challenging traditional CNS education. The AACN's DNP initiative and the goal of requiring new APRNs to have a practice doctorate (AACN, 2006b) have engendered considerable debate and discussion within the CNS community. Although the DNP initiative is considered by many to have already been decided, there is debate about its consequences, some of which may be unintended (Chase & Pruitt, 2006). Concerns that it may result in fewer students preparing to be CNSs to meet at least geographic pockets of shortages have been discussed in the literature. The length of the DNP curriculum and inability of some universities to offer doctorates pose a challenge for academic institutions (Chase & Pruitt, 2006). The separation of the profession's practice and research missions, differences in master's- and doctorate-prepared CNS competencies, the acronym's suggestion that a DNP is an NP, and regulatory considerations are additional concerns about the DNP (Chase & Pruitt, 2006; Fulton & Lyon, 2005; Meleis & Dracup, 2005). In 2015, the NACNS endorsed the DNP as entry into practice by 2030 (NACNS, 2015b). However, although DNP programs have rapidly expanded, the majority of CNSs are still prepared at the master's level (Auerbach et al., 2015; NACNS, 2017c).

National Certification for Clinical Nurse Specialists

Certification at the population level for CNSs by examination is available through the American Nurses Credentialing Center and the American Association of Critical-Care Nurses Certification Corporation. Specialty CNS certifications are also available from specialty organizations such as the Oncology Nursing Certification Corporation. However, certification examinations are not available

for many CNS specialties, such as cardiovascular, neuroscience, and perinatal nursing, and these specialty certification examinations do not meet the role and population foci as articulated in the NCSBN Consensus Model Regulatory Language. The lack of certification is a major regulatory barrier for many CNS specialties, especially in the era of the Consensus Model. Although the ANCC created and offered a CNS certification examination in the population focus of the family and individual across the life span, it was only offered twice and is now retired (http://nursecredentialing.org/CNSCoreExam). Such a generic certification is ill-matched to the reality of CNS practice, which is by definition specialty specific. If states are going to adopt the Consensus Model, it is imperative that nationally recognized CNS certification examinations be developed for the role to survive. In 2002 the NCSBN decided to remove alternative mechanisms for granting APRN licensure, such as a portfolio or clinical practice evaluation (Hartigan, 2011). Today, the NACNS encourages states to analyze how the lack of a certification examination for all population foci for CNSs will have an impact on practice within each state before fully implementing the Consensus Model (NACNS, 2012a).

Variability in Individual Clinical Nurse Specialist Practices and Prescriptive Authority

The evolution of the CNS role has been dynamic. CNSs who pioneered the role were specialists in psychiatry and mental health. The CNS was initially conceptualized as an expert clinician, consultant, educator, and researcher (Hamric & Spross, 1989). Direct care, although central, was not the only focus. Integrating these role manifestations has been difficult but essential to sustain the role's effectiveness, yet differentiating these elements has not been sufficient to describe what CNSs do.

Variability exists in requirements for prescriptive authority for CNSs (Stokowski, 2016). While states' scopes of practice are changing to support CNS prescription of pharmacologic agents, not all CNSs were prepared in their original education curriculum to prescribe and states have addressed this in various approaches. For example, Oregon recognized CNSs as APRNs, including prescriptive authority, in 2005 (Klein, 2012, 2015). A task force was convened by the Oregon Board of Nursing where the final requirement to allow CNSs to prescribe was equivalent to requirements for NP programs (Berlin, Harper,

Werner, & Stennett, 2002), and the final Oregon regulation for prescribing included a course in advanced pharmacology and a minimum of 150 hours of supervised pharmacologic management (Klein, 2012).

In Minnesota, CNSs must practice for 2080 hours within the context of a collaborative agreement within a hospital or integrated care setting with a Minnesota-licensed CNP, CNS, or physician who has experience providing care to patients with similar medical problems before she or he can prescribe independently (Stokowski, 2016). In contrast, in Wisconsin, APRNs with prescriptive authority are defined as advanced practice nurse prescribers (APNPs) and must pass an examination on Wisconsin statutes and rules pertaining to practice of APNPs (Stokowski, 2016). In addition, there are annual educational requirements for the APNP and requirements that include obliging the APNP to carry personal liability malpractice insurance.

The Consensus Model supports the prescribing of pharmacologic agents by all APRNs (APRN Joint Dialogue Group, 2008). Most current data show that since 2010, CNSs can prescribe independently in 19 states (NACNS, 2015a). Some CNSs want prescriptive authority, others do not, and both sides have been adamant about their positions rather than saying that it is a privilege that an individual CNS can exercise based on his or her preference and practice. This latter approach is how NPs handled this issue— they want prescriptive authority; whether they will use it or not is up to the individual. Physicians are also the same; most use it, some do not, but all have the authority. The key to moving forward is to publicly support prescriptive authority for CNSs and discuss the positive contributions to patient outcomes based on that authority. This consistent messaging will help regulators and other professionals outside the CNS community understand the possibilities for the role.

Understanding the Similarities and Differences Between Clinical Nurse Specialists and Nurse Practitioners

The origins of the CNS and NP roles arose from very different needs in health care when the roles were created. In response to a need for nurses with specialized knowledge and training in psychiatric nursing, Peplau (1952) created the first CNS educational program (see Chapter 1). In the 1960s, clinical nurse specialization, specifically in psychiatry and mental health as well as in critical care units, took its modern

form as a result of three forces in health care: (1) an increase in specialty-related information, (2) new technologic advances, and (3) a response to public need and interest. In coronary care units, nurses expanded their knowledge and skills by learning how to identify cardiac arrhythmias, administer intravenous medications, and defibrillate patients. These nurses were, in fact, diagnosing and treating patients (Cockerham & Keeling, 2014; Keeling, 2004). Therefore the origin of the CNS role was born out of a need for specialty practices.

Concurrently, in the 1960s, the role of the pediatric NP was formed to help relieve the shortage of physicians in poor rural and urban areas. Physicians were increasingly drawn to medical specialties and leaving primary care. Diagnosing, treating, and providing primary care to patients in outpatient settings were beginning to come under the purview of NPs and were some of the defining characteristics, later termed *competencies,* of the role (see Chapter 1). Today, many NPs are entering specialty practice because the need for specialists has grown (Kleinpell & Goolsby, 2012; McCorkle et al., 2012).

In the 1990s, several forces in health care—a downturn in the fiscal health of hospitals; layoffs or repurposing of CNSs into quality managers, case managers, or nurse educator roles; increased emphasis on primary care and rapid growth of NP programs; and the introduction of acute care NPs—led to a sharp decrease in the number of nurses entering CNS programs (see Chapter 1). The image of the CNS as quality manager, case manager, or nurse educator, combined with CNS leaders insisting that CNSs practice in the domain of nursing and not in medicine (Hartigan, 2011), persists today despite the NACNS's efforts to publicize core competencies and activities (NACNS, 2004; NACNS, National CNS Competency Task Force, 2010).

As noted, the Commission on Collegiate Nursing Education accreditation mandates that all APRN students receive the three Ps (AACN, 2006b). Knowledge of the pathophysiology, assessment, and treatment of sepsis, for instance, is no different if a clinician is a CNS, an NP, or a physician.

There are differences, however, between the two roles. Significantly, the amount of time spent performing a particular competency or activity is different for each. CNSs spend time among the three spheres of influence as outlined by the NACNS (American Association of Critical-Care Nurses, 2014; Lewandowski & Adamle, 2009; NACNS, 2004; Norton, Sigsworth, Heywood, & Oke, 2012; Saunders, 2015), whereas NPs spend most of their time in direct care management of patients (American Association of Critical-Care Nurses, 2014; Buerhaus, DesRoches, Dittus, & Donelan, 2015; Carpenter, Gregg, Owens, Buchman, & Coopersmith, 2012; Kilpatrick et al., 2012; McCorkle et al., 2012). With the introduction of the DNP degree, core competencies for APRNs who graduate from these programs will have a balance of direct care management education and didactic instruction in education and systems changes to produce a more well-rounded clinician. CNSs receive more instruction about direct care management and NPs receive more instruction about education and EBP evaluation and implementation than prior to introduction of the DNP. Although the two roles are receiving similar education content and have some overlap in skills, it is unclear whether the shift of education content will substantially change their daily practice patterns due to the fundamentally different underpinnings of the two roles.

In 2007, the American Psychiatric Nurses Association (APNA) and the International Society of Psychiatric Mental Health Nurses (ISPN) published a job analysis between the psychiatric–mental health CNS (PMH-CNS) and the psychiatric–mental health NP (PMH-NP) that found there was 90% commonality in the two roles (Rice, Moller, DePascale, & Skinner, 2007). However, a subsequent analysis of the items in the job analysis revealed that there was a heavy emphasis on direct care activities and fewer items related to health care system changes, organizational consultation, consultation with nursing personnel, and research, which falls heavily in the CNS domain (Jones & Minarik, 2012). For PMH APRNs, competency must be attained in the APRN, medical, and psychotherapy domains. PMH-CNSs have a strong history of in-depth psychotherapy training, whereas PMH-NPs have more training in psychopharmacology. Based on the job analysis findings, the APNA and the ISPN endorsed the recommendation that educational programs prepare PMH APRNs as NPs educated across the life span (APNA, 2011). The National Organization of Nurse Practitioner Faculties (NONPF), which created the standards for NP education, has recognized that there is a transition phase in having only NP education moving forward while still supporting currently practicing PMH-CNSs (NONPF, 2012).

The NONPF criteria are likely to stay in effect until transitions of programs and certification mechanisms from PMH-CNS to PMH-NP have been completed. To this end, the ANCC offered its final Adult PMH-CNS certification examination in October 2017 and its final Adult PMH-NP examination in December 2016. All PMH APRNs will now take the same examination, now titled as the Psychiatric–Mental Health Nurse Practitioner–Board Certified (PMHNP-BC) certification examination (ANCC, 2017). As the APNA and the ISPN continue to consider implications for CNSs and NPs in psychiatric and mental health, it will be important to continue to incorporate core competencies of the two roles, which include medical, psychiatric, and psychotherapy treatment modalities; educating and supporting interprofessional staff; and facilitating change and innovation in health care systems to provide improved access to high-quality mental health care.

Role Implementation

Because of the potential for lack of clarity in the CNS role, it is imperative that CNSs entering a new position understand and prepare for optimal entry into the role. In a Canadian study, Kilpatrick et al. (2016) had CNSs identify both structure and process factors that can facilitate implementation of the role. Organizational structural factors identified by the CNSs included making certain that orientation is planned and structured rather than having an ad hoc approach with each new CNS, ensuring adequate leadership support and stakeholder involvement, and having a structure that facilitates team support. Something as simple as colocation can facilitate development of team cohesion and complementary role functions (Kilpatrick et al., 2016). The CNSs identified that it was also important that the CNS took personal accountability to obtain certification in a specialty area of practice. Process factors that the CNSs identified that were important to successful role implementation included consistent role titles and expectations, which facilitated both intraprofessional and interprofessional relationship development.

CNSs have different reporting structures in different organizations (e.g., reporting to physicians, Directors of Nursing, Directors of Education, Chief Nursing Officers), all of which have advantages and disadvantages. Understanding the reporting structure and corresponding implications is important for any CNS new to a role. CNSs have identified barriers in fully implementing their role (Mayo et al., 2010): multiple job expectations, lack of time, lack of personnel, and lack of secretarial support. These are not unique solely to the CNS role; however, acknowledging the possibility of these when starting a new position informs the CNS and provides an ability to negotiate resources and expectations when negotiating acceptance of the position.

Use of a framework such as the PEPPA framework is especially important when implementing the nonclinical components of the CNS role, although it will support implementation of all role components (Kilpatrick et al., 2016). Use of a framework can also help the organization in the aspects of identifying when a new APRN role is needed, defining new roles, and promoting clarity among team members.

Evaluation of Practice

Because the full extent of a CNS's impact and outcomes may not always be readily visible, it is important that CNSs consider how to evaluate, track, and demonstrate their outcomes from day one in a new role. Although many CNS specialties develop practice setting–specific evaluation tools, a standardized tool should be developed for expected competencies and the assurance of outcome quality. Lunney, Gigliotti, and McMorrow (2007) have designed a tool for graduate students to use for self-evaluation of CNS competency development, which could be adapted for practicing CNSs. Portfolios can be used as a tool to evaluate CNS practice, as exemplified by a model developed in Ohio that merges the APRN standards, relationship-based care, and Magnet forces to recognize professional development (Hespenheide, Cottingham, & Mueller, 2011). Another example that CNSs can use to quantify and describe their contributions to health care organization is the CNS Cost Analysis Toolkit (NACNS, 2017b).

CNSs may document the components of their clinical practice, including numbers of patients seen, types and frequencies of interventions, and outcomes achieved; educational activities for staff, including one-on-one coaching, in-service programs, orientation, and continuing education; and system initiatives, such as quality improvement activities and interprofessional rounds (AACN, 2006b). To evaluate her or his ability and effectiveness in exercising influence, a CNS may ask nursing and other professional colleagues to comment on her or his communication and collaboration skills. CNSs may use this information for self-assessment to determine whether the allocation of activities is consistent with personal, professional, and institutional goals; to prepare quarterly reports; or to assemble a portfolio for their annual evaluations. Tracking these data enables CNSs to identify recurring events that may require an intervention at the staff or system level and midcourse corrections if schedule demands require a shift in goals or a realignment of expectations.

In the early days of CNS practice, few studies documented the impact of CNSs on patient and family outcomes. The evidence is mounting, however, and the positive impact on patient outcome is irrefutable (see Chapter 23). Some hospitals hire CNSs specifically for their positive impact on patient outcomes (Scherff & Siclovan, 2009). Outcome studies can help CNSs document their activities and their effects on patient and family outcomes. Example studies have shown the impact of CNS interventions on causes of medication errors (Flanders & Clark, 2010) and, specifically, in regard to revising a policy on labeling medications and solutions on the sterile field in the operating room (Brown-Brumfield & DeLeon, 2010). As these topics suggest, CNSs can identify relevant structure, process, and outcome variables that can be used to assess the CNSs' contributions to quality patient care, including use of clinical practice guidelines and the effect on clinical outcomes.

Evaluation of CNS practice often includes outcomes management (AACN, 2006b). One component of outcomes management is the analysis of data regarding care efficiency and cost-effectiveness, the results of which guide systematic and continuous process and performance improvement. CNSs at one institution, for example, were instrumental in developing a hospital-wide process that promoted EBP guidelines through research, patient safety workshops, nursing staff orientation, professionalism, quality of work life, and prevention of falls (Ford, Rolfe, & Kirkpatrick, 2011).

Practice evaluation must be integrated into one's daily work. Although researchers have begun to identify the interventions used most often by APRNs, there continues to be a need for demonstrating the outcomes of CNS interventions in all settings where they practice (see Chapter 23).

Future Directions

Three powerful forces have been converging to influence the practice and regulation of APRNs: the IOM report on *The Future of Nursing* (IOM, 2011), the Consensus Model for APRN regulation (APRN Joint Dialogue Group, 2008), and health care reform. There are many exciting opportunities for CNSs to advance their roles and ensure a unique place in the health care system. At the same time, the CNS role is threatened by wide variability in philosophy, education, and operationalization that continues role confusion or ambiguity among those in the CNS community, regulators, educators, employers, and the public. To combat the forces that threaten the survival of the role, CNSs must engage in five action areas:

1. CNSs need to unify around the NCSBN regulatory affirmation of CNSs as being APRNs, with a significant component of practice in the direct care of individuals and an expanded scope of practice that includes advanced assessment, diagnosing, prescribing, and ordering (NCSBN, 2008). A cohesive voice from the CNS community must advocate for all activities to be legally permissible in state scopes of practice and in individual practices, regardless of individual practices or preferences. Use of common language shared by all APRN groups is essential for identifying shared knowledge, skills, and practices. This reduces the perception of infighting and advances the CNS as an APRN role in collaboration with other APRNs. There is strength in numbers and internal unity.

2. CNSs must clearly articulate their contributions to patients, families, and the health care system in the three spheres of influence (NACNS, 2004). By claiming the definition of CNS practice defined at the beginning of the chapter, CNSs can differentiate themselves from other APRNs and still provide direct and indirect care to patients to improve health outcomes in specialty populations (Goudreau et al., 2007).

3. CNSs must ensure that educational curricula and continuing education programs prepare current and future CNSs with the knowledge and skills to have an expanded practice at the advanced level with specialty populations, educating interprofessional staff, and facilitating change and innovation in health care systems. Adherence to the AACN Essentials for DNP and master's APRN education (AACN, 2006b, 2011) is mandatory for the accreditation of APRN programs and serves as the basis for educational standards, according to the Consensus Model for APRN regulation (APRN Joint Dialogue Group, 2008). The core competencies developed by the NACNS should serve as a guide to didactic courses and clinical practica, with an additional focus area on disease management. Preceptors must have CNS students engage in activities in these three spheres of CNS practice to prepare them for a future successful practice (Lewandowski & Adamle, 2009). CNSs have a strong history of continuing educational conferences focused on nursing education and systems or process improvement. Continuing education programs for CNSs should increase the course offerings to include care management of specialty populations, including disease and medication management.

4. CNSs need to be innovative in partnering with others to enact their role with the opportunities that are appearing related to health care reform. CNS models of population care should be developed and researched, including those that extend beyond the traditional inpatient CNS role. CNSs should collaborate with nurse researchers in conducting and publishing comparative effectiveness studies that test the efficacy of CNS interventions in complex and vulnerable specialty populations, patient outcomes, and innovative new care models. Comparative effectiveness research "is designed to inform health-care decisions by providing evidence on the effectiveness, benefits, and harms of different treatment options. The evidence is generated from research studies that compare drugs, medical devices, tests, surgeries, or ways to deliver health care" (AHRQ, 2012). CNSs continue to need to establish that patient outcomes are improved, safe, and high quality as a result of their interventions compared with other practice models. More studies need to be carried out to compare CNS effectiveness in achieving patient outcomes and system-wide improvements, with CNSs managing care as the intervention.

5. CNSs need to seek recognition as APRNs statewide, nationally, and internationally through involvement in policymaking and health care reform efforts. Local recognition can be obtained by seeking institutional credentialing and privileging and ensuring that institutional job descriptions incorporate the three spheres of influence, with particular attention to the direct care of individuals.

CNSs must become involved in passing regulations and legislation using Consensus Model language and including CNSs as APRNs in state regulations or statutes. CNSs must lobby and advocate for national certification mechanisms that accurately reflect CNS practice. In addition, CNSs need to monitor national changes to regulation in agencies such as the CMS to ensure that CNSs continue to be recognized as APRNs for purposes of reimbursement.

Development of CNS and APRN roles will continue to expand internationally. The International Council of Nurses (ICN) has established the ICN Nurse Practitioner/Advanced Practice Nursing Network (see Chapter 6). The goal, aims, and objectives of this group are:

... to become an international resource for nurses practising in nurse practitioner (NP) or advanced nursing practice (ANP) roles, and interested others (e.g., policymakers, educators, regulators, health planners) by:

1. Making relevant and timely information about practice, education, role development, research, policy and regulatory developments, and appropriate events widely available;
2. Providing a forum for sharing and exchange of knowledge expertise and experience;
3. Supporting nurses and countries who are in the process of introducing or developing NP or ANP roles and practice;
4. Accessing international resources that are pertinent to this field. (ICN, 2016)

CNS titling, education, and regulatory issues continue to be a challenge to establishing the role internationally; however, there are many driving forces that support role creation (see Chapter 6). CNSs should maintain awareness of these international efforts and participate in educational exchanges to standardize and collaborate on continuing to define CNS practice when feasible and learn from each other on how to optimize the role and role utilization.

Conclusion

CNSs have a strong and tumultuous history. Over the past 25 years, the departure from direct patient care as being a main focus to working predominantly in the nursing education and systems improvement domains has created confusion within nursing and the public because non-CNSs (e.g., nurse educators, quality improvement managers) function in the same capacity. However, CNSs are uniquely educated to provide advanced practice and specialist expertise when working directly with complex and vulnerable patients, educating and supporting nurses and nursing and interprofessional staff, and facilitating change

and innovation in health care systems that those in other roles in health care cannot.

As health care reform continues to gain momentum to improve health care system quality, there will be many new opportunities for CNSs. As masters of flexibility and creativity, CNSs can be innovative to meet the needs of patients and health care systems. The possibilities are endless if CNSs understand their role, improve understanding of the importance of this role in advanced practice nursing, and maximize the driving forces and minimize the restraining forces related to the role in the health care system.

Key Summary Points

- CNSs demonstrate the seven competencies of APRN practice across three spheres of influence—patient direct care sphere, nurses and nursing practice sphere, and systems and organizations sphere—regardless of setting or specialty.
- CNSs must be persistent in clearly articulating their unique contributions and role to patients, families, other health care professionals, administrators and the public.
- There need to be continued efforts to ensure standardization of CNS educational curricula and opportunities for certification in specialty practice.
- CNSs need to lead and participate in innovative efforts to improve patient outcomes in the current environment of health care reform.

References

To access the references for this chapter, use your smartphone's QR code reader to scan the code below, or go to http://booksite.elsevier.com/9780323447751.

The Primary Care Nurse Practitioner

Lynne M. Dunphy • *Margaret M. Flinter* • *Katherine E. Simmonds*

> *"I've been asked a lot for my view on American health care. Well, 'it would be a good idea,' to quote Gandhi."*
>
> —**Paul Farmer**

CHAPTER CONTENTS

This chapter highlights the critical and essential position primary care nurse practitioners (PCNPs) now occupy in the US health care system. The historical context and evolution of primary care in the changing American health care system is presented, including innovations such as the patient-centered medical home (PCMH), team-based care, health information technology (HIT), and accountable care organizations (ACOs). The history of the nurse practitioner (NP) role is briefly revisited as well as developments in NP education, such as interprofessional and postgraduate education. Also described is the role of the federal government in primary care and trends in the primary care workforce. NP competencies (National Organization of Nurse Practitioner Faculties [NONPF], 2017) are used to operationalize current PCNP practice, with an emphasis on safety-net setting exemplars from practice. Future directions in practice are also discussed, such as telehealth, transitional care, and postgraduate primary care residency and fellowship programs for PCNPs.

Current and Historical Perspectives on Primary Care and the Nurse Practitioner Role

Current Perspectives on Primary Care

Primary care had its origins in Great Britain about 100 years ago and is the foundation of most international health care systems, yet primary care in the United States has lagged behind that of other developed countries (Davis, Stremikis, Squires, & Schoen, 2014; Macinko, Starfield, & Shi, 2003; Starfield, 1992). Although secondary and tertiary care are essential components of health care systems, they should be viewed as complementary to primary care and not foundational.

Fig. 15.1 illustrates the foundation that primary care holds globally (left pyramid) and in the US health care system (right pyramid). Health outcomes have long been documented to improve when primary care is the foundation of a national health care system. Primary care cannot compensate for all the myriad social determinants of health that affect both

health and life expectancy, but consistent access to high-quality primary health care is clearly a factor when considering the growing discrepancy in life expectancy between the United States and other developed countries (Avendano & Kawachi, 2014; Nolte & McKee, 2012) as well as the growing disparity in lifespan between rich and poor nationally (Braveman & Gottlieb, 2014). Primary care providers (PCPs) comprise the frontline of health care, serving patients and communities and addressing most of their health care needs across the lifespan, in sickness and in health. Noted primary care scholar Barbara Starfield (1992) identified the key tasks of primary care as: (1) first contact with care, (2) longitudinal care, (3) comprehensiveness of care, and (4) coordination of services. Longitudinal care refers to a sustained patient-provider relationship over time. In primary care–oriented health systems, there are fewer disparities in health across population subgroups (Starfield, 2008). In 1996, the Institute of Medicine (IOM) issued a report on primary care, defining it as "the provision of integrated, accessible health care services by clinicians who are accountable

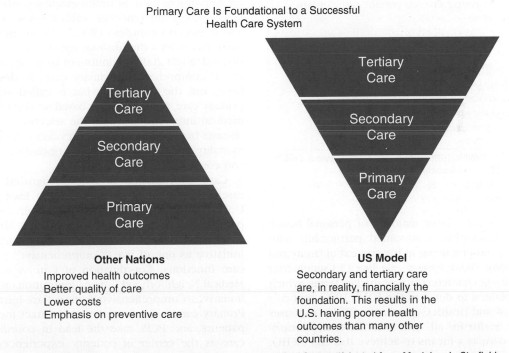

Primary Care Is Foundational to a Successful
Health Care System

Other Nations
Improved health outcomes
Better quality of care
Lower costs
Emphasis on preventive care

US Model
Secondary and tertiary care are, in reality, financially the foundation. This results in the U.S. having poorer health outcomes than many other countries.

FIG 15.1 Models of primary care in other nations and the United States. *(Adapted from Macinko, J., Starfield, B., & Shi, L. [2003]. The contributions of primary care systems to health outcomes within Organization for Economic Cooperation and Development (OECD) countries, 1970-1998.* Health Services Research, 38, *831-865.)*

BOX 15.1 Institute of Medicine Terms Used to Define Primary Care

Integrated
- Comprehensive, coordinated care throughout the life cycle
- Focused on particular needs of patients
- Clinician continuity
- Effective communication of information
- Patient record continuity

Accessibility
- Ease with which care is attained
- Elimination of geographic, cultural, language, reimbursement, and administrative barriers

Clinician
- Uses recognized scientific knowledge base
- Authority to direct the delivery of care

Accountable
- Clinician and system accountability for services provided

Most Personal Health Care Needs
- Competency to manage most health problems
- Use of consultation or referral as needed
- Sustained partnership
- Relationship between patient and clinician over time

Context of Family and Community
- Understanding of the circumstances and facts surrounding the patient (socioeconomic status, family dynamics, work issues)
- Awareness of public health trends
- Need for specific health promotion and disease prevention strategies

From Institute of Medicine. (1996). *Primary care: America's health in a new era.* Washington, DC: National Academies Press.

and environmental factors on health. The WHO identified five key elements in achieving this goal of better health for all: (1) reducing exclusion and social disparities in health (universal coverage reforms); (2) organizing health services around people's needs and expectations (service delivery reforms); (3) integrating health into all sectors (public policy reforms); (4) pursuing collaborative models of policy dialogue (leadership reforms); and (5) increasing stakeholder participation (WHO, 2008). These WHO five elements represent an approach that combines biomedical *and* public health domains. The biomedical approach to illness has dominated the United States over the course of the 20th century, with an individualistic approach to care driven by a fee-for-service payor system. In contrast, public health approaches build on *social determinants of health,* defined by the WHO (2008) as "the conditions in which people are born, grow, live, work and age, including the health system" (WHO, 2008). The WHO further expands this definition to include those circumstances that are "shaped by the distribution of money, power and resources at global, national and local levels, which are themselves influenced by policy choices. The social determinants of health are responsible for most health inequities—the unfair and avoidable differences in health status seen within and between countries" (WHO, 2008). However, there has been a decade-long tension between the original WHO 2008 commitment to what could be called comprehensive primary care, as described here, and the reality of what is called selective primary care, fighting disease based on cost-effective medical interventions, with the selection of target diseases based on four factors: prevalence, morbidity, mortality, and feasibility of control (including efficacy and cost).

Care coordination is now recognized as an essential element of primary care, at least in the United States. It was included as a requirement for participation in the Center for Medicare & Medicaid Services (CMS)-led Comprehensive Primary Care Initiative as one of five "Comprehensive" primary care functions: Coordination of Care Across the Medical Neighborhood (https://innovation.cms.gov/initiatives/Comprehensive-Primary-Care-Initiative). Primary care is the first point of contact for many patients, and PCPs take the lead in coordinating care as the center of patients' experiences with medical care. Individual practices work closely with patients' other health care providers, coordinating and managing care transitions, referrals, and information exchange.

for addressing a large majority of personal health needs, developing a sustained partnership with patients, and practicing in the context of family and community" (IOM, 1996, p. 31). Box 15.1 summarizes the defining characteristics of the key terms, which are explained in detail in the IOM (1996) report.

The World Health Organization (WHO) espouses "better health for all" and uses the term *primary health care* as a means to achieve this end (WHO, 2008). The insertion of the word *health* highlights this broad and aspirational mission and expands the focus from the delivery of primary care services to addressing the broader issue of the impact of societal

Historical Perspectives

Historians remind us that at one time, all health care was primary care. The United States developed a fixation on specialty care in the last century (Howell, 2010). Before World War II, most Americans' health care was provided by a generalist physician. Specialists, who were few and far between, were only rarely seen. Throughout the 1930s and 1940s, generalist care expanded to include pediatricians, internists, and public health nurses (IOM, 1996). However, medical advances in care during World War II and rapid growth of medical technologies, along with the advent of employer-based health insurance, combined to shift the locus of care from the patient's home and family to the hospital (Starr, 1982). The growth of hospital-based care was intertwined with the growth of specialty care and came to dominate our health care system (Stevens, 1989). Indeed, the use of the term *primary care* in the United States began in the late 1960s, as a way of distinguishing it from specialist physician care. Family medicine—essentially primary care—was approved as a specialty in 1969, not long after the first NP programs were established in the United States.

The social tumult of the 1960s and the convergence of multiple powerful social forces such as civil rights, the women's movement, the anti-war movement, and the war on poverty all gave rise to new and transformative systems. Social programs such as Medicare and Medicaid were founded in 1965, and with them came access to health care for millions of people for the first time. These policy innovations were of a magnitude that would not be repeated until the passage of the Patient Protection and Affordable Care Act (ACA) in 2010.

The First Nurse Practitioners

The 1960s saw another innovation that would take root and flourish. The NP role emerged, transforming primary care and nursing by introducing a new role for nurses and a new kind of PCP. This role was based on a person-centric, holistic approach to the care of individuals and families over the lifespan. Dr. Loretta Ford, a public health nurse, and Dr. Henry Silver, a pediatrician, recognized the untapped capability and potential of nurses to expand their practice. They created a demonstration project at the University of Colorado in 1965 to build on and reclaim the role of the public health nurse through the addition of diagnostic, treatment, and management

responsibilities previously limited to physicians. It was distinct from the medical model of that time in that it focused on prevention, health and wellness, patient education, and inclusion of the patient as a partner in making clinical decisions, empowering patients to weigh treatment options (Dunphy, 2013; Silver, Ford, & Day, 1968). More than 50 years later, it seems that primary care medicine has moved much closer to the nursing model, with a concerted focus in medical schools and residency programs on social mission and person-centered, holistic, comprehensive primary care (Englander et al., 2013).

Progress and Change: 1970 to the Present

Issues of health care access and maldistribution of health care resources, along with new federal funding sources, all fueled the continuing development of the NP role. The legislative creation of the National Health Service Corps in 1972 gave early recognition to this new kind of provider, the nurse practitioner, by including NPs in this federal effort to address access to health care and the need for a new kind of community-oriented primary care (Mullan, 1999). Concurrently, on the national scene in the 1970s, there was a rapid influx of capitated group practice models, or health maintenance organizations, which emphasized primary care and prevention and called for expert providers in those domains. Rising costs in health care saw the creation of concepts such as managed care (Bodenheimer & Grumbach, 2016). More recently, the passage of the ACA in 2010 and the expansion of coverage to millions of Americans created further demand for primary care and supported new models of health care delivery.

Primary Care and the Federal Government

An understanding of the US primary care system is essential to an understanding of the role of the PCNP in this system. Thus this section of the chapter discusses important elements of the involvement of the federal government in structuring and financing health care, specifically primary care services for underserved and vulnerable populations. The ACA (2010) established far-reaching goals to expand health care coverage, address access to care, and improve health care quality and safety. It put particular emphasis on primary care, prevention, and health promotion, and laid out an ambitious plan to cover all US citizens through expanding Medicaid coverage for the lowest income earners, subsidizing premiums for individuals with lower incomes to buy health insurance through exchanges, adding requirements for employers of a certain size to offer health insurance, and banning denial of coverage for preexisting conditions by commercial insurance plans (US Department of Health and Human Services [DHHS], 2017). The ACA is considered by many to be the most significant social legislation in a century, and not surprisingly, it has been repeatedly challenged (Hermer, 2016). While the requirement for all states to expand Medicaid coverage was struck down by the Supreme Court in 2014, other requirements such as requiring all Americans to secure coverage or face financial penalties were upheld. The Centers for Disease Control and Prevention (CDC) reported in 2016 that the United States had an uninsured rate below 10%, the lowest since records were first kept (The Advisory Board, 2016). The outcome of the 2016 presidential election and the new administration's focus on repealing and replacing the ACA creates uncertainty as to the future of the ACA, as well as the future of health care coverage and access to health care in the United States.

Health Resources and Services Administration

Through the Health Resources and Services Administration (HRSA), a division of the DHHS, the federal government plays a significant role in supporting systems, organizations, and programs that provide primary care services to vulnerable populations; HRSA works to improve the health care workforce distribution throughout the nation, particularly in underserved, rural, and tribal areas, and supports the transformation of health care delivery by supporting innovative models of care. HRSA also plays an important role in educating and training the health professionals who deliver those services. Comprising 5 bureaus and 11 offices, HRSA provides leadership and financial support to health care providers in every state and US territory (Fig. 15.2). For example, HRSA's Bureau of Health Workforce supports the development and maintenance of an adequate medical, dental, behavioral health, nursing, and public health workforce along with other health care workforce-related programs. In addition to collecting data and providing analysis about the health care workforce, this bureau offers competitive funding for nursing education programs tailored to areas of greatest need, such as rural health and support for innovations in practice.

Health Professional Shortage Areas Designation

The federal government establishes criteria to designate health professional shortage areas (HPSAs) and to use those designations to provide additional resources such as qualifying for National Health Service Corps clinician awards or funding preference. A HPSA is defined as an area in which there are more than 3500 individuals for every primary care physician (PCMD). Of note, the criteria, established decades ago, do not factor in the availability of other PCPs, specifically physician assistants (PAs) and NPs. Similarly, HRSA (2016b) designates Medically Underserved Areas (MUAs) and Medically Underserved Populations (MUPs). The lack of data on the geographic distribution of NPs, their practice settings, and their availability to the populations in HPSAs and MUA/MUPs is a barrier to accurately assessing and planning for workforce needs. Questions have been raised about the validity of using general measures, such as the ratio of provider to population for HPSA scores, or the percentage of elderly persons or poverty in calculating MUAs/MUPs. Butler, Petterson, Phillips, and Bazemore (2013) suggested that measures of social deprivation, such as low education level and exposure to violence, may be more effective as indicators of need and described the wide variation and challenges across the United States in calculating measures of underservice.

The Nation's Primary Care Safety Net

The federal government supports PCNP practice through many different mechanisms, primarily by providing financial assistance to support educational institutions preparing NPs, but also by funding organizations and practices that rely on NPs as PCPs, often in conjunction with care for underserved and vulnerable populations. This support recognizes that the PCNP is ideally prepared to assume responsibility to care for a defined population and a panel of patients in the context of family and community. Significant changes in expectations of patients and providers, in technology and training, and in the way care is organized will usher in future challenges and innovation. We predict that federal support will continue to recognize the critical role of PCNPs in meeting the health care needs of the American people in all settings, but particularly in those organizations often referred to as the health care safety net. The IOM defines the health care safety net as "those providers that organize and deliver a significant level of health

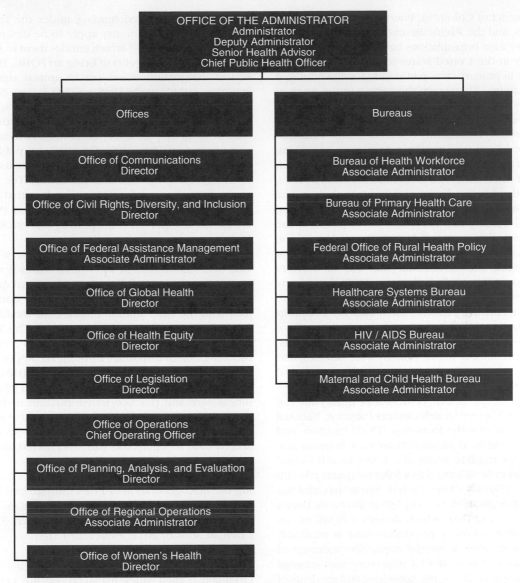

FIG 15.2 Health Resources and Services Administration organization chart. *(From Health Resources and Services Administration. [2016, March]. HRSA organization chart. Retrieved from http://www.hrsa.gov/about/organization/org-chart.html.)*

care and other related services to uninsured, Medicaid, and other vulnerable populations" (IOM, 2000). This term has been in use for more than 30 years, and generally refers to a set of benefits and programs designed for those with no or very low income.

Community Health Centers

For more than 50 years, health centers have delivered affordable, accessible, quality, and cost-effective

primary health care to patients regardless of their ability to pay. During that time, health centers have become an essential PCP for America's most vulnerable populations. Health centers advance a model of coordinated, comprehensive, and patient-centered care, coordinating a wide range of medical, dental, behavioral, and patient services. Today nearly 1400 health centers operate more than 10,400 service delivery sites that provide care in every US state, the District of Columbia, Puerto Rico, the US Virgin Islands, and the Pacific Basin (HRSA, 2016a). These primary care organizations have a dramatic 50-year history in the United States to advance access and quality in primary care, particularly for disadvantaged populations. They trace their roots to the work of Sydney and Emily Kark in South Africa in the 1940s in developing a new model of population-focused, data-driven, community-oriented health care that engaged local community members in organizing and delivering care (Kark & Kark, 1999). Dr. Jack Geiger, then a medical student in the United States, studied with the Karks and brought their model back to the United States. He proposed and secured federal funding that led to the development of the first US health centers in Mound Bayou, Mississippi, and Boston, Massachusetts, as an outgrowth of the civil rights movement and the War on Poverty (Geiger, 2002, 2005; Lefkowitz, 2005). From early on, health centers were defined by a set of core characteristics: private, independent nonprofit organizations with consumer-controlled boards of directors, sliding scale fees for low-income persons, a comprehensive set of primary care services, and a focus on underserved geographic areas and populations.

Community health centers that qualify for the National Migrant Health Centers Program, National Health Care for the Homeless (HCH) Program, and National Public Housing Primary Care Program may apply for funding under the HRSA Health Center Program to be identified as a federally qualified health center (FQHC). The United States has distinct enabling legislation, Section 330 of the Public Health Service Act (2010), which defines a FQHC as "an entity that serves a population that is medically underserved, or a special medically underserved population comprised of migratory and seasonal agricultural workers, the homeless, and residents of public housing" (Legal Information Institute, Cornell Law School, 2012). This is administered through the HRSA Bureau of Primary Care, and enables these safety net organizations to receive enhanced federal support. Nurse-led health centers, as discussed in the next section, may also apply for this federal designation. FQHCs are community-based health centers that receive funds from the HRSA Health Center Program to provide primary care services in underserved areas. They must meet a stringent set of requirements, including providing care on a sliding scale fee based on ability to pay and operating under a governing board that includes patients. Organizations that meet all of the requirements of an FQHC

but have not received funding under the federal health center program may apply to be designated as "FQHC Look-Alikes," which entitles them to some, but not all, of the benefits of being an FQHC. Health center designation is subject to annual rigorous reporting known as the Uniform Data System (UDS). Health centers report on an extensive set of quality of care measures, health outcomes, population and patient demographics, service utilization data, and cost measures (HRSA, 2015). These data are published annually for each individual health center as well as in aggregate by state and nationally. The most recent UDS data are for 2016, reporting that 1376 FHQCs cared for nearly 26 million individuals. PCNPs are a major component of the primary care workforce in this setting.

One of the largest quality improvement projects ever undertaken in the United States was the Health Disparities Collaboratives, a national quality improvement initiative led by HRSA in conjunction with the CDC and the Institute for Healthcare Improvement between 1999 and 2006. This effort engaged hundreds of FQHCs in a rigorous focus on reducing health disparities through the application of quality improvement science (Stevens, 2016). This laid the groundwork for improving both chronic illness care and practice transformation in health centers. Today, more than 95% of FQHCs have implemented electronic health records for all services, and 68% are recognized as patient-centered medical homes.

Health centers have also become leaders in training the next generation of PCPs through residency and fellowship programs for physicians, NPs, dentists, psychologists, and other health care providers (Chen, Chen, & Mullan, 2012; Flinter, 2012).

Nurse-Led Health Centers

Originally called nurse-managed health centers, nurse-led health centers are led and staffed by nurses, and are typically primary care delivery sites located in the communities they serve, many identifying themselves with the name of that community. They are often located in places traditionally lacking access to care, such as homeless shelters, rural areas, or public housing communities (Sutter-Barrett, Sutter-Dalrymple, & Dickman, 2015). Additionally, nurse-led health centers are often associated with academic institutions and provide clinically based educational settings for undergraduates and graduate students across disciplines (Pohl, Tanner, Pilon, & Benkert, 2011). In 2015 there were approximately 258 nurse-led centers nationwide (Hansen-Turton, 2016). In these diverse practices, PCNPs provide team-based care in collaboration with other health care providers such as nurse-midwives, physicians, dentists, registered nurses (RNs), nutritionists, diabetes educators (often nurses), substance abuse counselors, and social workers. In addition, they may partner with community sectors such as legal advocates, housing agencies, peer support, community leaders, and churches.

When explaining why nurse-led centers work, the National Nurse-Led Care Consortium (2017) identifies the community as the place "where national health policy and social reality meet" and notes that as an outgrowth of a neighborhood, these centers are in the unique position of understanding that particular community's needs as well as the diverse needs of its individual residents. Nurse-led centers typically work with community leaders to advance health equity and expand the definition of health care to deal with some of the most serious problems facing American society today, including family, adolescent and neighborhood violence; drug, nicotine, and alcohol addictions; the environmental aspects of diseases such as asthma and birth defects; and problems such as grief, stress, anxiety, and obesity (Austria, 2015). The establishment of trust—with the community as well as individual patients and families—is critical in striving to make the connections between people's lives and health.

A recent integrative review of characteristics of nurse-led centers' quality and outcomes determined that these centers are consistent with the WHO definition of primary health care that includes the social determinants of health (Holt, Zabler, & Baisch, 2014). This study further explained the structure, process, and outcome characteristics of nurse-led health centers to build evidence to inform policy to sustain these centers as safety net providers. Furthermore, Auerbach et al. (2013) posited that nurse-led centers could help mitigate the expected PCMD shortages (see "Primary Care Workforce" later).

School-Based Health Centers

School-based health centers (SBHCs) are an important contributor to the academic and "whole child" success of children and adolescents, particularly in schools with predominantly low-income and ethnic/racial minority population groups. There are 2315 SBHCs in 49 states and the District of Columbia (School-Based Health Alliance, 2015). A systematic review of the literature confirmed that SBHCs improve health and advance health equity, particularly for low-income and racial/ethnic minority groups (Knopf et al., 2016). Lewallen, Hunt, Potts-Datema, Zaza, and Giles (2015) detailed the importance of SBHCs as part of the "whole child/whole school approach to education," and cited improvements across multiple domains from management of chronic illness such as asthma, to decreased emergency room utilization and increased use of contraception among adolescents. Keeton, Soleimanpour, and Brindis's (2012) review of SBHCs noted that SBHCs are not typically a program of the school but rather a partnering organization, such as a community health center (28%), hospital (25%), or local health department (15%), with only 12% operated directly by schools. PCNPs have been the backbone of SBHCs from the start, now joined by PAs in some settings as the main primary care clinical staffing. According to Keeton et al. (2012), more than 75% of SBHCs have behavioral health services, making them a truly integrated model of primary care. They often have advisory boards consisting of community representatives, parents, youth, and family organizations that provide planning and oversight.

Knopf and colleagues' (2016) literature review summarized available evidence of the effectiveness of SBHCs on educational and health-related outcomes and concluded that SBHCs were associated with improved educational outcomes as well as positive health-related outcomes (preventive services, asthma morbidity, and contraception use) and that SBHCs can be effective in advancing health equity (Knopf et al., 2016). Box 15.2 presents a summary of the common characteristics of SBHCs (Keeton et al., 2012).

Care for Homeless and Vulnerable Populations

According to the National Law Center on Homelessness and Poverty (2015), 2.5 to 3.5 million Americans are sleeping in shelters, transitional housing, or public places not intended for sleeping, and another 7.4 million people have lost their homes and "doubled up" with others. Though it may seem obvious, lack of affordable housing is the overwhelming primary cause of homelessness, along with the related factors of unemployment, poverty, low wages, mental illness, and substance abuse. More than 50% of homeless people have a history of mental illness and alcohol and/or substance abuse. For many homeless patients, accessing primary care is complicated by these competing needs, circumstances, and barriers.

BOX 15.2   Characteristics of School-Based Health Centers (SBHCs)

- Being located in schools or on school grounds
- Working within the school to become an integral part of the school
- Providing a comprehensive range of services that meet the specific physical and behavioral health needs of the young people in the community
- Using a multidisciplinary team of providers to care for the students, including nurse practitioners, registered nurses, physician assistants, social workers, physicians, alcohol and drug counselors, and other health professionals
- Providing clinical services through a qualified health provider, such as a hospital, health department, or medical practice
- Requiring parents to sign written consents for their children to receive the full scope of services provided at the SBHC (with the exception of those services in certain states that youth can consent to themselves by law)
- Having an advisory board consisting of community representatives, parents, youth, and family organizations, to provide planning and oversight

From Keeton, V., Soleimanpour, S., & Brindis, C. D. (2012). School-based health centers in an era of health care reform: Building on history. *Current Problems in Pediatric and Adolescent Health Care, 42*(6), 132-156.

While the most important treatment for homelessness is housing, a lack of primary care access makes this vulnerable population even more susceptible to poor health outcomes and leads to an overuse of emergency departments. Research has shown that tailoring medical care to the specific needs of vulnerable populations can increase primary care use and improve chronic disease monitoring and diabetes management (O'Toole et al., 2011). The federal government, through HRSA's HCH Program, itself part of the larger community health center program authorized under Section 330 of the Public Health Service Act, funds grantees across the country. In 2016, federally funded HCH programs provided primary care as well as substance abuse services to 1.2 million people through its multiple healthcare for the homeless program (HRSA, 2016a).

Care for Homeless Veterans

The US Department of Veterans Affairs (VA) system warrants particular attention for its efforts to address homelessness among veterans, who have persistently been disproportionately represented among the homeless. The national outcry over the plight of homeless veterans has led to targeted and innovative programs. Tsai, Link, Rosenheck, and Pietrzak (2016), in looking at barriers to use of primary care by veterans, noted a 9% lifetime rate of homelessness among veterans, with only 17% of them using the VA's health care services. Kushel (2015) found that two low-intensity interventions improved use of primary health care services by homeless veterans: (1) an interview with an RN, followed by motivational interviewing; and (2) an on-site "orientation" to primary care and in particular, the Homeless Patient Aligned Care Teams (PACTs). Whether part of free-standing HCH clinics, FQHC-based programs, in-shelter or mobile clinics, or the VA system, PCNPs are a fundamental component of primary care staffing of services for homeless individuals.

Veterans Affairs System

The VA system is part of the federal government, separate from DHHS. Its mission is to provide care for the nation's veterans. It also has a strong record of innovation. Advanced practice registered nurses (APRNs) are widely used in the VA system in many roles as well as in all branches of the active military. Innovative programs include the VA's Home Based Primary Care program for chronically ill individuals; this program has resulted in cost reductions, reduced hospitalizations and emergency room visits by veterans, and fewer disease exacerbations (Edes et al., 2014). In this program, PCNPs function as the PCP and make home visits. Another example of innovation is a Center for Medicare & Medicaid Innovation (CMS Innovation Center) project, currently testing the Home Based Primary Care approach through the Independence at Home demonstration project. Additionally, the VA system was one of the earliest adopters of electronic health records (EHRs). It also designed the PACT, which includes physicians, PCNPs, PAs, RNs, licensed practical nurses, medical assistants, and administrative clerks on their clinical teams (Edes et al., 2014). This care team was created specifically to address issues of continuity and access to the PCP as part of the VA's national implementation of the PCMH model (Yano, Bair, Carrasquillo, Krein, & Rubenstein, 2014). The PACT became the cornerstone for the way care would be delivered within the VA, and it focused on four key areas: enhanced partnerships between veterans and caregivers, improved access to care, coordinated care among team members, and veteran-centered, team-based care. The VA has also been a leader in the development of postgraduate residency training for new PCNPs (Rugen et al., 2014). The team focus has also served as the basis for the development of interprofessional primary care training such as that undertaken at the West Haven, Connecticut, Center for Excellence in Primary Care, which demonstrated positive outcomes in terms of increased understanding of the role of NPs on the part of internal medicine residents and increased confidence on the part of new NPs relative to their physician counterparts on the team (Meyer, Zapatka, & Brienza, 2015). This interprofessional training project was piloted at five different VA settings across the country. Each site has created new understandings of the challenges of fully implementing team-based care.

Veterans Affairs NPs Granted Full Practice Authority in 2017

In December 2016, following years of advocacy by APRN leaders and others in the VA system, the VA granted full practice authority, starting in 2017, to certified nurse midwives, clinical nurse specialists, and NPs, but excluded certified registered nurse anesthetists (CRNAs). This practice expansion applies to those APRNs regardless of the state in which they practice in the VA system. This important move may accelerate the pace of full practice authority in those states that have not yet made the rule for NPs and strengthens the case for the VA to include CRNAs in the near future.

Practice Redesign in Primary Care

Widespread recognition of the need to improve quality while controlling health care costs has led to serious efforts at reform and transformation both in how care is delivered and how care is paid for. The rapid transformation of health care delivery and payment systems precludes a discussion of all aspects of major changes underway, but some examples such as the PCMH, ACOs, expanded HIT, team based care, shared medical visits, and the rise of convenient care/retail clinics illuminate the rapid changes underway.

Payment Reform

In addition to expanding health insurance coverage to millions of Americans, the ACA also supported

the design, implementation, and evaluation of new service delivery models, largely grounded in primary care (Alliance for Health Policy, 2015). The health care system in the United States has traditionally been dominated by "fee-for-service" reimbursement models that tie revenue to the volume and type of interventions, procedures, and care provided rather than quality and health care outcomes. In 2012 waste in health care was estimated at between $558 and $910 billion per year—from 21% to 34% of total health care expenditures (Berwick & Hackbarth, 2012). The ACA was strategically formulated to turn fee-for-service models around to value-based payment reforms, rewarding prevention of illness and disease, better chronic illness management, and quality care as demonstrated through outcomes. The concept of empanelment, defined as a patient choosing a PCP who is responsible for the quality and acceptability of his or her health care whether delivered directly by that provider or indirectly through referral and coordination. Empanelment is now hard-wired into primary care practice expectations and allows for better tracking of value-based outcomes (Bodenheimer & Grumbach, 2016).

The CMS Innovation Center was established by the ACA with an intent to revitalize and sustain Medicare, Medicaid, and the Children's Health Insurance Program (CHIP) and ultimately improve the health care system for all Americans (Casalino & Bishop, 2015). One of its major initiatives that directly impacts PCNP practice is the Transforming Clinical Practice Initiative, designed to help 140,000 clinicians achieve large-scale health transformation through sharing, adapting, and developing their comprehensive quality improvement strategies. The Transforming Clinical Practice Initiative is consistent with the federal goals to reform both practice and payment structures in ways that support and align with quality measures.

The Medicare Access and CHIP Reauthorization Act of 2015 (MACRA) Quality Payment Program repealed the flawed Sustainable Growth Rate formula used in Medicare billing and initiated the transformation of Medicare payment to a value-based system. MACRA is intended to support clinicians and practices with tools and flexibility to provide high-quality, patient-centered care. Physicians, PAs, NPs, clinical nurse specialists, and CRNAs are all in the MACRA Quality Payment Program (CMS, 2016b).

Other initiatives to reform the primary care component of our health care system since the passage of the ACA in 2010 include the Comprehensive Primary Care initiative, launched by CMS in 2012, a 4-year multipayor initiative designed to strengthen primary care. It involved a collaboration between the CMS and various insurance plans to support the provision of a core set of five "comprehensive" primary care functions: (1) risk-stratified care management, (2) access and continuity, (3) planned care for chronic conditions and preventive care, (4) patient and caregiver engagement, and (5) coordination of care across the medical neighborhood (CMS, 2016a).

While only 20% of health care expenditures flow through new value-based payment models and only 20% of people with employer-sponsored insurance are in high-cost-sharing plans, both segments are expected to grow rapidly. The DHHS plans to shift at least 50% of all its payments to the new payment models by 2018. All of these initiatives are predicted to have a significant impact on PCPs and practices (Sahni, Chigurupati, Kocher, & Cutler, 2015).

Patient-Centered Medical Homes

A significant development in primary care in the United States in recent years has been the degree to which the model of the PCMH has gained traction. Defined standards for certification as a PCMH have taken root as a set of operating principles for the organization and delivery of primary care. First defined in the pediatric medical community decades ago as a strategy to support the coordination of care of children with complex health conditions, in 1978 the WHO created the Alma-Ata Declaration, broadening the definition of health, defining the role of the state, and identifying tenets of the medical home and its key role in primary care. Two decades later in the United States, the IOM published *Primary Care: America's Health in a New Era* specifically identifying the need for a "medical home" for every patient and family (IOM, 1996). After this, the term *medical home* became increasingly evident in the family medicine literature (Robert Graham Center, 2007). The PCMH embraces the patient-provider relationship and the full spectrum of primary care, including standards of accessibility, continuity, comprehensiveness, integrated care, and interprofessional care. Having a personal physician was a requirement in the early days of National Committee for Quality Assurance (NCQA) accreditation as a PCMH, but in 2011 the NCQA expanded its criteria to include nurse-led or other than physician-led PCMHs, shifting the focus to the *patient*. This also led to a shift in primary care delivery models that are patient-centric and include expanded practice hours, weekend availability, more focus on the coordination of care across transitions from home to hospital or vice versa (for example), and the ability to connect with providers electronically, as well as the transparency and availability of medical records to patients.

Currently, many PCMHs include comprehensive integrated care so that mental and physical health needs are met in one setting through the use of interprofessional teams. Box 15.3 lists the concepts for recognition as a PCMH as identified by the NCQA. Blending the well-established principles of primary care—continuity, comprehensiveness, access, and accountability with a patient-centered focus—the PCMH model has been extensively studied, implemented, modified, and highly acclaimed as improving outcomes and management of complex chronic diseases (Nutting et al., 2009). Additionally, despite resource constraints and high-need populations, safety net clinics are transforming care for vulnerable populations through the Safety Net Medical Home Initiative, which has supported the development of replicable approaches to medical home transformation in clinics caring for minority, underserved populations (Sugarman, Phillips, Wagner, Coleman, & Abrams, 2014).

Accountable Care Organizations

The National Academy for State Health Policy defines ACOs as "organizations or structures [that] assume responsibility for a defined population of patients across a continuum of care; they are held accountable through payments linked to value, and reliable performance measurements demonstrate that savings are achieved in conjunction with improvements in care" (Stanek, 2013). ACOs, a key feature of health care reform under the ACA, were originally established as a model for the care of Medicare patients but have since expanded to include state initiatives to create Medicaid ACOs, state employee health plan ACOs, and private ACOs. In 2016 there were 744 ACOs in the United States, covering close to 30 million people (Muhlestein & McClellan, 2016).

ACOs are designed to support coordinated care within their network. Properly coordinated care helps ensure that patients, especially the chronically ill, get the right care at the right time, with the goal of avoiding unnecessary duplication of services and preventing medical errors. When an ACO succeeds in both delivering high-quality care and spending

BOX 15.3 **National Committee for Quality Assurance (NCQA) Patient-Centered Medical Home (PCMH) Recognition Program Requirements**

To earn recognition, your practice must complete criteria in each of these six concept areas:

Team-Based Care and Practice Organization: Helps structure a practice's leadership, care team responsibilities, and how the practice partners with patients, families, and caregivers.

Knowing and Managing Your Patients: Sets standards for data collection, medication reconciliation, evidence-based clinical decision support, and other activities.

Patient-Centered Access and Continuity: Guides practices to provide patients with convenient access to clinical advice and helps ensure continuity of care.

Care Management and Support: Helps clinicians set up care management protocols to identify patients who need more closely managed care.

Care Coordination and Care Transitions: Ensures that primary and specialty care clinicians are effectively sharing information and managing patient referrals to minimize cost, confusion, and inappropriate care.

Performance Measurement and Quality Improvement: Helps practices develop ways to measure performance, set goals, and develop activities that will improve performance.

From National Committee for Quality Assurance. (2017). NCQA PCMH recognition: Concepts. Retrieved from http://www.ncqa.org/programs/recognition/practices/patient-centered-medical-home-pcmh/why-pcmh/overview-of-pcmh/ncqa-pcmh-recognition-concepts.

health care dollars wisely, it shares in the savings it achieves for the Medicare program.

Use of Health Information Technology

HIT is redesigning today's health care system. Data from EHRs, for example, can be used to manage patient populations, track chronic disease management, assure preventive care targets are met, and overall improve patient care outcomes by supporting evidence-based care. Additionally, EHRs have decreased the number of medical errors through oversight of clinical provider order entry and electronic prescribing of medications (Thurston, 2014). In 2016, approximately 78% of ambulatory practices used EHRs (DHHS, Office of the National Coordinator for Health Information Technology, 2016). Cost savings are being achieved by reducing redundant orders and reducing medical errors. Use of EHRs also supports patient privacy. The Health Information Technology for Economic and Clinical Health (HITECH) Act contained significant financial incentives to improve the quality of the health care system through the use of EHRs. To receive these funds, practices need to demonstrate "meaningful use" of their EHRs by meeting thresholds for a number of key objectives, from e-prescribing to communication between providers and across levels of care to the ability to submit clinical quality measures.

Moving Knowledge, Not Patients

Today's PCNPs have access to a novel group of innovations that collectively advance our ability to secure timely consultation from specialists and advance the mastery in caring for patients with highly complex and often high-risk conditions that place considerable strain on primary care practices. Two such innovations, eConsults and Project Echo, warrant particular attention for their contribution to advancing care for special populations, reducing disparities in specialty access for underserved populations, and fostering interprofessional continuous learning and support for NPs as well as all other primary care disciplines.

eConsults were originally developed at San Francisco General Hospital and Trauma Center as an electronic referral and consultation system between PCPs and specialists. Studies confirmed that these electronic consultations could accomplish the goals of reducing wait time for specialty appointments as well as the need for in-person specialty visits and that they allowed PCPs to access the specialty knowledge they needed to care for their patients. The asynchronous nature of eConsults, in which the PCP submits the consult question and relevant data and the receiving specialist reviews and returns recommendations within a mutually agreed upon time period, maximizes flexibility and convenience for both PCPs and specialty care providers (Chen, Murphy, & Yee, 2013; Kim-Hwang et al., 2010). Similar outcomes were reported at the University of California, San Francisco (DiGiorgio et al.,

2015), and in a federally qualified health center (Olayiwola et al., 2016).

Project ECHO provides a different experience of moving knowledge, not patients. Where eConsults are a one-to-one communication between a PCP and a specialist regarding a single patient, Project ECHO brings together multiple PCPs with a team of interprofessional specialists with expertise in a particular clinical area. Project ECHO is a guided practice model that exponentially increases workforce capacity to provide best-practice specialty care and reduces health disparities. The heart of the ECHO model is its hub-and-spoke knowledge-sharing networks, led by expert teams who use multipoint videoconferencing to conduct virtual clinics with community providers. In this way, the primary care workforce learns to provide excellent specialty care to patients in their own communities (Arora et al., 2010). In the Project ECHO model, PCPs "sign up" for weekly brief didactic presentations on a specific clinical problem, followed by discussion, advice, and guidance between the experts and the participating PCPs.

Originally created as a strategy to improve access and outcomes for patients with hepatitis C in rural New Mexico, Project Echo has been embraced by academic medical centers and primary care organizations focusing on vulnerable populations (Arora, Thornton, Jenkusky, Parish, & Scaletti, 2007). The Weitzman Institute of the Community Health Center, Inc., has developed a Project ECHO model that engages clinicians across the country in a number of distinct Project ECHO programs that support practicing PCPs in developing expertise in caring for patients with complex challenges such as chronic pain, human immunodeficiency virus infection, and opioid addiction, to name a few (Bamrick, 2016). Studies have confirmed the effectiveness of the Project ECHO model in improving care and outcomes in certain conditions, particularly hepatitis C (Arora et al., 2010; Khatri, Haddad, & Anderson, 2013).

Team-Based Primary Care

Whether a practice is made up of a single team consisting of one PCP and a medical assistant or a large, multisite organization with both core and extended team members, the evidence base for the advantages of team-based care is well established. Such care improves outcomes, expands access, and contributes to satisfaction (Bodenheimer & Grumbach, 2016; Carter, Rogers, Daly, Zheng, & James, 2009; Coleman, Austin, Brach, & Wagner, 2009;

Willard-Grace et al., 2014). The team-based model has been a particular focus in community health centers and the VA, as discussed earlier, both of which were early adopters of the chronic care model for the management of chronic illness, with adaptation for prevention, health promotion, and routine care (Wagner, 2000). The national PCT-LEAP Project (Primary Care Teams, Learning from Effective Ambulatory Care Practices) studied exemplar practices across the country and published a series of articles highlighting the individual and collective impact of individual team members and the team as a whole (Wagner et al., 2017). Currently, 150 million adults have one or more chronic health conditions, which makes the need for patient self-regulation and family engagement and activation critical in primary care (Bodenheimer & Bauer, 2016).

However, change is difficult. In a discussion paper, the IOM acknowledged openly some of the difficulties, noting "Health care has not always been … a team sport" (Mitchell et al., 2012, p. 17). Drawing on data obtained from participants on successful teams, certain personal values were identified as critical to a high-functioning team: (1) honesty and transparency, (2) discipline, (3) creativity, (4) humility, and (5) curiosity. Acknowledging that each health care team is unique, this paper presented principles of team-based care as well as measurable processes and outcomes and defined a research agenda (Mitchell et al., 2012).

Shared Medical Appointments

Many patients and families struggle to manage chronic diseases. SMAs, originally known as group visits, are defined as care delivery using the chronic care model (Wagner, 2000). SMAs are a type of reimbursable medical appointments format for patients with the same or similar chronic conditions to mutually discuss their health status; the necessary therapeutic regimens and behavioral modifications and how they handle them; and their successes, their failures, and how to cope with each. It is not to be used for acute or initial medical appointments. It extends the time that care providers spend with patients and concurrently provides group/peer support. This format has been used for some time in primary care with evidence of meaningful outcomes (Burke & O'Grady, 2012; Eisenstat, Ulman, Siegel, & Carlson, 2013; Jaber, Braksmajer, & Trilling, 2006; Jones, Kaewluang, & Lekhak, 2014; Watts et al., 2009). Adding APRN-led health coaching within the group visit for chronic care to promote long-term behavioral change and self-management as well as cost-effective care adds a new modality to the traditional group visit model (Jeon & Benavente, 2016). Combining health coaching and SMAs makes conceptual sense because both are effective models to provide and support chronic care management, and adding health coaching within the SMA makes it an innovative delivery system with a supportive environment and peer interactions that are critical to facilitating lifestyle change.

A group visit may be small (6-8 participants) or larger (10-20 participants) and include a lead facilitator (MD, DO, NP, PA, APRN) and/or other members of the care team such as an RN, dietitian, social worker, or psychologist. Ideally one team member would be literate in health coaching. The visit/appointment could last anywhere from 90 to 120 minutes and could be one of an ongoing series of visits or more in the manner of a one-time educational intervention. Culture may be another dimension added to an SMA. Newby and Gray (2016), for example, created a culturally tailored SMA for African-Americans with diabetes. Using a one-time educational group format, they evaluated more than 250 patients with diabetes, half of whom

received the normal standard of care and half of whom participated in a culturally tailored SMA. Newby and Gray demonstrated improved glycemic control in the individuals who participated in the SMAs (Fig. 15.3).

Disruptive Innovation: Convenient Care Clinics

In a classic paper in the *Harvard Business Review* (Christensen, Bohmer, & Kenagy, 2000), disruptive innovations in health care were described as those that are less expensive, that provide more convenient products and services, and that start by meeting the needs of less demanding customers. They specifically cited CVS Minute Clinics, staffed by NPs, as an example of a disruptive innovation in health care, a fundamentally different and new model. Convenient care clinics (CCCs) provide consumers with accessible, affordable, quality health care in retail-based locations, such as pharmacies or grocery chains. As of 2015, there were over 2300 CCCs in the United States, serving more than 35 million patients (Convenient Care Clinic

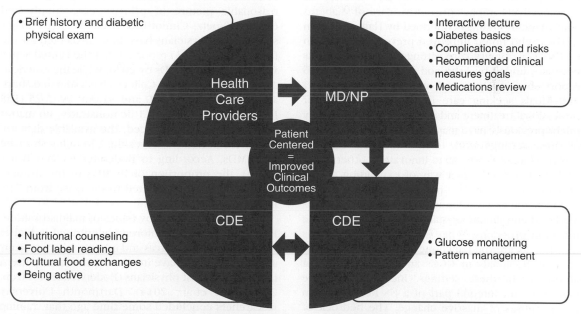

FIG 15.3 Culturally tailored shared medical appointments for diabetic African-Americans that includes an educational component added by a nurse practitioner who is a certified diabetes educator (CDE). *(From Newby, O. J., & Gray, D. C. [2016]. Culturally tailored group medical appointments for diabetic black Americans. JNP: The Journal for Nurse Practitioners, 12[5], 317-323.)*

Association, 2016). These clinics do not require appointments and offer convenient, low-cost basic primary care treatment, screening, and diagnostic services in a variety of settings, with many of these settings also adapting basic chronic care management services and forming partnerships with area health systems, enabled with communicating EHRs. The types of illness treated by CCCs is limited and algorithm driven, and there are questions from the American Academy of Pediatrics (2014) regarding their incentive to overprescribe, lack of longitudinal relationships built with CCC providers, and uneven EHR interoperability with community PCPs. A utilization study found that CCCs may actually increase spending if they drive new health care utilization. The researchers used insurance claims data from Aetna for the period 2010 to 2012 to track utilization and spending for 11 low-acuity conditions. They found that 58% of CCC visits for low-acuity conditions represented new utilization, and visit use was associated with a modest increase in spending of $14 per person per year (Ashwood et al., 2016).

These clinics report high patient satisfaction with short waiting times and appeal to clientele without insurance or those for whom immediate access is needed and not available (Bachrach, Frohlich, Garcimonde, & Nevitt, 2015). They do not negatively impact preventive care or diabetes management, findings confirmed by Hansen-Turton (2016), who noted improved preventive health in CCCs over primary care settings. A more cautious note is sounded by Ashwood and colleagues' 2016 report showing increased utilization and cost by individuals seeking care in CCCs, searching for professional treatment and advice for symptoms they might previously have managed on their own. Some of these settings work to find adequate care for sicker patients as well as to innovate in other ways, such as telehealth, as a way of expanding access to care (Patterson, A., personal communication, 2014). Some CCCs offer additional services such as Medicaid enrollment assistance and access to public nutrition programs. What is unequivocally clear is that PCNPs are the backbone and dominant health care professionals in CCCs and enjoy significant autonomy in these settings. Increasingly, these clinics are an integral part of a US health system in the throes of massive change. The bedrock of CCCs is providing easily accessible, affordable, high-quality health care to consumers who often have to wait days or weeks for basic primary care services.

Primary Care Workforce and the Context of PCNP Practice Today

Primary Care Workforce

Understanding the supply, distribution, and educational pipeline of health care professionals is key to designing programs and policies that will ensure access to culturally congruent and effective health care, yet this information is elusive at best. Although data are available regarding the educational pipeline and the number of graduates of medical and nursing programs, the subsequent geographic distribution of these graduates is challenging to capture and to match with population-based needs. Licensure data at the state level provide a snapshot of the health care workforce, and many states have now transitioned to fully electronic licensure renewal and expanded data collection at the time of license issue and renewal. Additionally, *demand* for health care can be especially difficult to predict due to changing population needs, particularly the aging of the population, insurance coverage, and socioeconomic variables along with the supply and availability of health care resources.

In the absence of an organized national system for collecting and analyzing data on the health workforce in the United States, data from a variety of sources must be assembled to come up with a reasonable picture of primary care supply and demand (Spetz, Cimiotti, & Brunell, 2016). Major shortfalls of physicians have been projected for the future; HRSA (2013) reported that the United States will lack 20,400 PCMDs by 2020, while the American Association of Medical Colleges has estimated shortages of between 12,000 and 31,000 by 2025 (IHS Inc., 2015). As Table 15.1 demonstrates, no matter which source is referenced, the available data are consistent in terms of revealing a looming shortage in PCMDs. According to Bodenheimer and Bauer (2016), the proportion of PCMDs in the primary care workforce is predicted to decrease from 71% in 2010 to 60% by 2025.

This is complicated by issues of maldistribution. Physicians tend to be more concentrated in higher income, more urban areas and in areas where patients are more likely to have insurance; the same pattern holds for specialist physicians (Bodenheimer & Pham, 2010; Meit et al., 2014). Dartmouth University researchers concluded some time ago that training more physicians may increase regional inequities since four of five new physicians will practice in high-supply regions rather than underserved areas (Goodman, Fisher, & Bronner, 2009).

| TABLE 15.1 | Primary Care Workforce Projections for Primary Care Physicians | |

Primary Care Workforce	Estimated Number, 2010	Projected Needed, 2020[a]
General physicians[b]	164,400	187,300
General pediatric physicians (2010)[c]	44,800	49,600
Geriatric physicians (2010)[c]	3,300	4,300
Total	212,500	241,200

[a]Assumes all states expand Medicaid.
[b]Includes general, family, and general internal medicine.
[c]Assumes that the national supply of primary care physicians was adequate in 2010 except for the approximately 7500 full-time equivalents needed to de-designate the primary care Health Professional Shortage Areas.
Adapted from Health Resources and Services Administration. (2013). Projecting the supply and demand for primary care practitioners through 2020. National Center for Health Workforce Analysis. Retrieved from https://bhw.hrsa.gov/sites/default/files/bhw/nchwa/projectingprimarycare.pdf.

Demand

Demand for health care services is rising related to the growth and aging and morbidity of the population as well as a rise in insured persons. Although 2016 marked the first year that we saw a decline in life expectancy for certain segments of the US population, from 1980 to 2015, life expectancy for all Americans increased by 5 years, adding about 38 million Americans in need of care, many with multiple comorbidities. A recent study of PCPs found that patients with a PCNP as a provider were less costly to Medicare than patients with a PCMD as a provider (Perloff, DesRoches, & Buerhaus, 2016). Currently, 150 million adults have one or more chronic health conditions (Bodenheimer & Bauer, 2016). This makes an additional compelling case for the key role that PCNPs can play in alleviating demand for services because, in addition to adding numbers of new PCPs, PCNPs add value given their emphasis on health promotion, disease prevention, teamwork, and skills in care coordination. These findings all confirm the need for more robust efforts to collect accurate information on PCNP practice patterns, distribution, and impact on costs and outcomes.

The Nurse Practitioner Workforce

In contrast to PCMDs, the number of NPs entering the workforce each year has mushroomed from 6600 in 2003 to 23,000 new NPs completing academic programs in 2016, and the number of PCNPs is projected to increase by 84% between 2010 and

2025 (American Association of Colleges of Nursing [AACN], 2017 Bodenheimer & Bauer, 2016). Fig. 15.4 depicts the percentage of NPs in primary care education (85%) versus the 12% of US medical student primary care residency matches and the increase of 1804 NPs per year entering the primary care workforce versus only 19 more US medical school residency matches from 2014-2015 (Pohl, Barksdale, & Werner, 2016). At one time the percentage of PCMDs to PCNPs was approximately 80% to 20%. It is predicted that by 2020 this ratio will fall to 61% PCMDS to 30% PCNPs (Bodenheimer & Bauer, 2016).

Nursing educational institutions provide annual data to the AACN regarding the numbers of NP graduates of their programs. National certification bodies provides data on categories of NPs certified to practice, and state licensure data are provided on the number of NPs licensed to practice in each state. Based on a National Sample Survey of Nurse Practitioners by the HRSA (2012), in 2016 the AANP began assembling a National Nurse Practitioner Database derived from its membership of more than 60,000 NPs. This sample is dependent on its membership's participation and therefore has limitations, but it is an increasingly important data source nonetheless (Box 15.4 and Table 15.2) (AANP, 2017). The AANP documents that as of 2017 more than 234,000 NPs are licensed in the United States, with 89% of these NPs certified in primary care (AANP, 2017). This includes family NPs (always primary care), pediatric PCNPs, adult-gerontology PCNPs, and women's health NPs practicing in primary care. This reflects explosive growth in the number of NPs in the United States. The majority (76%) received certification in a primary care specialty (family, adult-gerontology, pediatric, and women's health). The most widely held primary care certification was Family NP (FNP), reported by almost half of the NP workforce. The lack of diversity was striking, with 87% white and 93% females in the NP workforce. The average age of the NP workforce in 2016 was 49 years (AANP, 2016).

Much needs to be done to diversify the PCNP workforce because the composition of the people doing the care provision is a factor in both access and health outcomes. A body of research has demonstrated that patient outcomes improve in ethnically diverse populations when the patient is cared for by a health care provider who is ethnically and culturally matched, specifically in the areas of use of preventive services, patient satisfaction, and ratings of the physician's participatory decision-making style

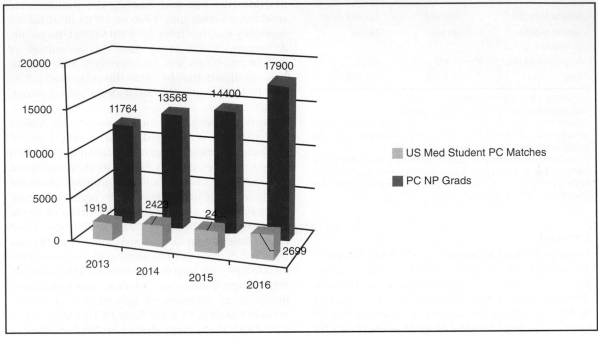

FIG 15.4 Proportions of primary care residents and nurse practitioners, 2013-2016. *(Courtesy of Joanne M. Pohl. Retrieved from http://healthaffairs.org/blog/2016/10/26/primary-care-workforce-the-need-to-remove -barriers-for-nurse-practitioners-and-physicians/.)*

TABLE 15.2   Distribution, Top Practice Setting, and Clinical Focus Area by Area of NP Certification[a]

Area of Certification	Percent	Top Practice Setting	Top Clinical Foci
Acute Care	6.6	Hospital Inpatient Clinic (28.8%)	Surgical (17.1%)
Adult[b]	16.2	Hospital Outpatient Clinic (16.6%)	Primary Care (37.9%)
Adult–Gerontology Acute Care	2.1	Hospital Inpatient Clinic (38.4%)	Surgical (14.8%)
Adult–Gerontology Primary Care[b]	4.5	Hospital Outpatient Clinic (21.4%)	Primary Care (48.0%)
Family[b]	62.4	Private Group Practice (20.9%)	Primary Care (50.0%)
Gerontology[b]	2.3	Long-Term Care Facility (21.3%)	Primary Care (49.5%)
Pediatric–Primary Care[b]	4.8	Hospital Outpatient Clinic (22.4%)	Primary Care (59.3%)
Psychiatric/Mental Health–Adult	1.8	Psych/Mental Health Facility (20.0%)	Psychiatric (97.6%)
Psychiatric/Mental Health–Family	2.4	Psych/Mental Health Facility (31.6%)	Psychiatric (100.0%)
Women's Health[b]	3.5	Private Group Practice (17.4%)	OB/GYN (74.7%)

[a]Data from 2017 AANP National Nurse Practitioner Sample Survey.
[b]Primary care focus.
From American Association of Nurse Practitioners. (2017, June 6). NP fact sheet. Retrieved from https://www.aanp.org/all-about-nps/np-fact-sheet

BOX 15.4 **2017 Facts About Nurse Practitioners**

There are more than 234,000 nurse practitioners (NPs) licensed in the U.S.[a]

- An estimated 23,000 new NPs completed their academic programs in 2015-2016[b]
- 97.7% of NPs have graduate degrees[c]
- 89.2% of NPs are certified in an area of primary care[c]
- Nearly three in four NPs are accepting new Medicare patients and 77.9% are accepting new Medicaid patients[d]
- 49.9% of NPs hold hospital privileges; 11.3% have long term care privileges[d]
- 95.8% of NPs prescribe medications, and those in full-time practice write an average of 23 prescriptions per day[d]
- NPs hold prescriptive privileges, including controlled substances in all 50 states and D.C.
- In 2017, the mean, full-time base salary for an NP was $105,670[c]
- The majority (61.4%) of NPs see 3 or more patients per hour[c]
- Malpractice rates remain low; only 1.9% have been named as primary defendant in a malpractice case[d]
- NPs have been in practice an average of 11 years[c]
- The average age of NPs is 49 years[c]

[a]AANP National Nurse Practitioner Database, 2017.
[b]Fang, D., Li, Y., Kennedy, K. A., & Trautman, D. E. (2017). *2016-2017 Enrollment and graduations in baccalaureate and graduate programs in nursing.* Washington DC: AACN.
[c]2017 AANP National Nurse Practitioner Sample Survey.
[d]2016 AANP National Nurse Practitioner Sample Survey.
From American Association of Nurse Practitioners. (2017, June 6). NP fact sheet. Retrieved from https://www.aanp.org/all-about-nps/np-fact-sheet.

(Marrast, Zallman, Woolhandler, Bor, & McCormick, 2014; Martin, Roter, Beach, Carson, & Cooper, 2013; Saha, Taggart, Komaromy, & Bindman, 2000).

Where Are PCNPs Practicing Today?

According to the AANP (2017; see Table 15.2), the most common practice sites for PCNPs practicing today are hospital outpatient clinics, hospital group practices, and private physician practices. Less frequently, PCNPs practice in settings specifically dedicated to caring for those who have served or are currently serving in our nation's military, as well as in clinics (AANP, 2016). Expanding the presence of PCNPs in primary care is a sound policy strategy for addressing the pressing primary care needs of the United States given the strong evidence that: (1) PCNPs provide care that is safe, effective, and acceptable to patients; (2) they are more likely than PCMDs to work with vulnerable populations, including ethnic or racial minorities, Medicaid or disadvantaged Medicare recipients, and the uninsured; (3) they are more likely to work in small rural and remote rural/frontier areas of the United States; and (4) they provide cost-effective care (Buerhaus, DesRoches, Dittus, & Donelan, 2015; Larson, Andrilla, Coulthard, & Spetz, 2016; Perloff et al., 2016; Stanik-Hutt et al., 2013). Auerbach et al. (2013) suggested that even a modest expansion of nurse-led health centers could mitigate expected PCMD shortages. These authors also discussed the issue of patient-to-provider ratios within a practice (panel size) and its impact on care. Innovations in primary care such as the use of virtual/telehealth visits (Henderson, Carlisle, Smith, & King, 2014) and other technologies, including self-monitoring devices and sensors (Petersen, 2016) and models such as the Hospital at Home project (Klein, Hostetter, & McCarthy, 2016), will all impact the context of primary care practice. SMAs, as previously discussed, and a team-based approach that includes a transformed role for RNs in primary care (Bodenheimer & Mason, 2017) all offer promise of more successful primary care management for complex patients.

Poghosyan, Boyd, and Knutson (2014) found that only one third of the PCNPs in one large primary care organization with both rural and urban practices had their own panel of patients. The lack of PCNP empanelment may be a result of the incorrect understanding of the state regulations governing scope of practice for PCNPs within that state or a result of physician preference in the practice. An earlier study in a different state also confirmed that a number of specific elements of a positive work environment were necessary for productive PCNP practice and that even within the same state, wide variations across settings persist (Poghosyan, Nannini, Stone, & Smaldone, 2013).

The Primary Care Nurse Practitioner

The PCNP is educated to provide the full spectrum of health care services to previously diagnosed and undiagnosed primary care patients and families, including health promotion, disease prevention, health protection, anticipatory guidance, counseling, disease management, and palliative and end-of-life care (National Organization of Nurse Practitioner Faculties [NONPF], 2017). Building on the seven APRN competencies described in Chapter 3, the NONPF (2017) core competencies expand on previous work that identified knowledge and skills essential to Doctor of Nursing Practice (DNP) competencies (AACN, 2006, 2015; NONPF National Panel for NP Practice Doctorate Competencies, 2006) and are consistent with the recommendations of the IOM report on *The Future of Nursing* (2011).

The *Consensus Model for APRN Regulation: Licensure, Accreditation, Certification, & Education* states that the role of the certified NP includes diagnosing, treating, and managing patients with acute and chronic illnesses and disease, with duties including the following: ordering, performing, supervising, and interpreting laboratory, diagnostic, and imaging studies; prescribing medication and durable medical equipment; and making appropriate referrals for patients and families (APRN Joint Dialogue Group, 2008). Further, these role attributes are provided to a specific patient population focus for which the practitioner is specifically educated and licensed (Kleinpell, Buchman, & Boyle, 2012; APRN Joint Dialogue Group, 2008).

The NP community has collaborated to identify competencies for each population focus. Additionally, NPs can be educated and certified as pediatric acute or primary care and adult-gerontology acute or primary care NPs, which incorporates the entire spectrum of adults, including young adults and older adults. Population-focused NP competencies (NONPF and AACN, 2013) with primary care specialization include family/across the lifespan (FNP), pediatric and adult-gerontology primary care, and women's health competencies (NONPF and AACN, 2016). These population-focused competencies are guidelines for educational programs preparing NPs with different populations as licensed practitioners. Foundational to all NP graduates is that they share a generalist nursing foundation, their practice has a base in health promotion, and they have developed advanced assessment and diagnostic reasoning skills. In other words, they have the requisite knowledge, skills, and abilities essential for competent clinical practice, as discussed in Chapter 7 (NONPF and AACN, 2013). These competencies are acquired through mentored patient care experiences while studying a defined curriculum based on role and population focus and occur in clinical settings that support the population focus. Today's curricula

prioritize interprofessional learning and collaborative practice.

A discussion of how these PCNP competencies are enacted within the framework of the seven APRN core competencies follows. Box 15.5 cross-maps the APRN competencies and the NONPF (2017) NP core competencies. In practice, competencies are often executed simultaneously to achieve the best outcome. However, for purposes of didactic discussion, specific competencies are discussed separately. Exemplars from primary care practice illustrate the competencies in action and are used throughout discussion of both the APRN competencies and the NP core and specialty competencies.

Direct Clinical Practice

Direct clinical practice is the central competency of all APRN roles; the delivery of direct care to patients and families is what the PCNP does. In today's hectic care environment, direct clinical practice in primary care includes managing previously diagnosed and undiagnosed increasingly ill and complex patients at a rapid pace, and includes growing numbers of aging patients with a range of chronic diseases and multiple comorbidities. It also requires proficiency in addressing behavioral health problems and the socioeconomic challenges that stress so many families and awareness of ongoing, major health problems in our society. Direct clinical practice in primary care builds on patient-centered approaches applied holistically, formation of therapeutic partnerships, expert clinical thinking, use of reflective practice, and use of evidence as a guide to practice yet having the flexibility to integrate diverse, evidence-informed approaches as needed.

One hallmark of the PCNP's direct clinical practice is the breadth and complexity of health issues encountered in a single day in primary care practice, which necessitates triage and constant decision making. The PCNP compares patient data sets with evidence-informed interventions consistent with current standards of care yet tailored to meet the needs of the individual and family in the context of diversity. As with other APRN roles, PCNPs analyze data and evidence critically to improve practice. PCNPs integrate knowledge from the humanities and sciences within the context of nursing science. In particular, the PCNP has a scientific foundation derived from the natural and social sciences that comprises human biology, advanced physiology, genomics, psychology (including behavioral change), epidemiology (for knowledge of population health),

BOX 15.5 Cross-Mapping of Advanced Practice Registered Nurse (APRN) Competencies and National Organization of Nurse Practitioner Faculties (NONPF) 2017 Nurse Practitioner (NP) Core Competencies

APRN Competencies (See Chapter 3)	NONPF 2017 NP Core Competencies[a]

Direct Clinical Practice (see Chapter 7)
 	
• Use of a holistic perspective
• Formation of therapeutic partnerships with patients
• Expert clinical performance
• Use of reflective practice
• Use of evidence as a guide to practice
• Use of diverse approaches to health and illness management
	Independent Practice Competencies
	• Functions as a licensed independent practitioner.
	• Demonstrates the highest level of accountability for professional practice.
	• Practices independently managing previously diagnosed and undiagnosed patients.
	   • Provides the full spectrum of health care services to include health promotion, disease prevention, health protection, anticipatory guidance, counseling, disease management, palliative, and end-of-life care.
	   • Uses advanced health assessment skills to differentiate between normal, variations of normal and abnormal findings.
	   • Employs screening and diagnostic strategies in the development of diagnoses.
	   • Prescribes medications within scope of practice.
	   • Manages the health/illness status of patients and families over time.
	• Provides patient-centered care recognizing cultural diversity and the patient or designee as a full partner in decision-making.
	   • Works to establish a relationship with the patient characterized by mutual respect, empathy, and collaboration.
	   • Creates a climate of patient-centered care to include confidentiality, privacy, comfort, emotional support, mutual trust, and respect.
	   • Incorporates the patient's cultural and spiritual preferences, values, and beliefs into health care.
	   • Preserves the patient's control over decision making by negotiating a mutually acceptable plan of care.
	   • Develops strategies to prevent one's own personal biases from interfering with delivery of quality care.
	   • Addresses cultural, spiritual, and ethnic influences that potentially create conflict among individuals, families, staff and caregivers.
	• Educates professional and lay caregivers to provide culturally and spiritually sensitive, appropriate care.
	• Collaborates with both professional and other caregivers to achieve optimal care outcomes.
	• Coordinates transitional care services in and across care settings.
	• Participates in the development, use, and evaluation of professional standards and evidence-based care.
	
	Scientific Foundation Competencies
	• Critically analyzes data and evidence for improving advanced nursing practice.
	• Integrates knowledge from the humanities and sciences within the context of nursing science.
	• Translates research and other forms of knowledge to improve practice processes and outcomes.
	• Develops new practice approaches based on the integration of research, theory, and practice.

Guidance and Coaching (see Chapter 8)	Independent Practice Competencies (see above) Technology and Information Literacy Competencies (see below)
Consultation (see Chapter 9)	Independent Practice Competencies (see above) Scientific Foundation Competencies (see above) Ethics Competencies (see below)
Collaboration (see Chapter 12)	Independent Practice Competencies (see above) Scientific Foundation Competencies Ethics Competencies (see below) Leadership Competencies (see below)
Evidence-Based Practice (see Chapter 10)	**Quality Competencies** • Uses best available evidence to continuously improve quality of clinical practice. • Evaluates the relationships among access, cost, quality, and safety and their influence on health care. • Evaluates how organizational structure, care processes, financing, marketing, and policy decisions impact the quality of health care. • Applies skills in peer review to promote a culture of excellence. • Anticipates variations in practice and is proactive in implementing interventions to ensure quality.

Continued

APRN Competencies (See Chapter 3)	NONPF 2017 NP Core Competencies[a]
	Practice Inquiry Competencies • Provides leadership in the translation of new knowledge into practice. • Generates knowledge from clinical practice to improve practice and patient outcomes. • Applies clinical investigative skills to improve health outcomes. • Leads practice inquiry, individually or in partnership with others. • Disseminates evidence from inquiry to diverse audiences using multiple modalities. • Analyzes clinical guidelines for individualized application into practice.
Leadership (see Chapter 11)	**Leadership Competencies** • Assumes complex and advanced leadership roles to initiate and guide change. • Provides leadership to foster collaboration with multiple stakeholders (e.g. patients, community, integrated health care teams, and policy makers) to improve health care. • Demonstrates leadership that uses critical and reflective thinking. • Advocates for improved access, quality and cost effective health care. • Advances practice through the development and implementation of innovations incorporating principles of change. • Communicates practice knowledge effectively, both orally and in writing. • Participates in professional organizations and activities that influence advanced practice nursing and/or health outcomes of a population focus.
	Health Delivery System Competencies • Applies knowledge of organizational practices and complex systems to improve health care delivery. • Effects health care change using broad based skills including negotiating, consensus-building, and partnering. • Minimizes risk to patients and providers at the individual and systems level. • Facilitates the development of health care systems that address the needs of culturally diverse populations, providers, and other stakeholders. • Evaluates the impact of health care delivery on patients, providers, other stakeholders, and the environment. • Analyzes organizational structure, functions, and resources to improve the delivery of care. • Collaborates in planning for transitions across the continuum of care.
	Policy Competencies • Demonstrates an understanding of the interdependence of policy and practice. • Advocates for ethical policies that promote access, equity, quality, and cost. • Analyzes ethical, legal, and social factors influencing policy development. • Contributes in the development of health policy. • Analyzes the implications of health policy across disciplines. • Evaluates the impact of globalization on health care policy development. • Advocates for policies for safe and healthy practice environments.
Ethical Decision Making (see Chapter 13)	**Ethics Competencies** • Integrates ethical principles in decision making. • Evaluates the ethical consequences of decisions. • Applies ethically sound solutions to complex issues related to individuals, populations, and systems of care.

	Technology and Information Literacy Competencies
	 • Integrates appropriate technologies for knowledge management to improve health care.
	 • Translates technical and scientific health information appropriate for various users' needs.
	   • Assesses the patient's and caregiver's educational needs to provide effective, personalized health care.
	   • Coaches the patient and caregiver for positive behavioral change.
	 • Demonstrates information literacy skills in complex decision making.
	 • Contributes to the design of clinical information systems that promote safe, quality, and cost-effective care.
	 • Uses technology systems that capture data on variables for the evaluation of nursing care.

[a]Source: National Organization of Nurse Practitioner Faculties. (2017). Nurse practitioner core competencies content: A delineation of suggested content specific to the NP core competencies. Retrieved from http://c.ymcdn.com/sites/www.nonpf.org/resource/resmgr/competencies/2017_NPCoreComps_with_Curric.pdf.

and advanced pathophysiology and pharmacotherapeutics. Use of "precision medicine" and genetics is essential in today's practice environment. PCNPs integrate elements of care from nursing and medical models in a collaborative approach to clinical practice that enhances the comprehensiveness and quality of the care rendered. The Circle of Caring model for PCNPs (Dunphy, Winland-Brown, Porter, & Thomas, 2015), for example, integrates a biomedical approach to diagnosis and treatment with a nursing-based, person-centered awareness of patient's responses to health and illness across the lifespan (see Chapter 2). This model supports PCNPs' understandings of the social determinants of health that exist within the patient's population and environment and how this relates to the patient's health and illness experience. This comprehensive knowledge base enables PCNPs to authentically meet their patients' needs, to hear their voices or "calls for nursing" and respond holistically. PCNPs synthesize concepts from psychology, sociology, biology, and other forms of the human experience within the context of nursing science (Udlis & Jakubis-Konicki, 2016). This care directly affects the health and lives of individuals, families, and whole communities.

Diagnosing and Managing Disease

The PCNP uses advanced health assessment skills to differentiate between normal findings, variations of normal, and abnormal findings to manage previously diagnosed as well as undifferentiated or undiagnosed patients. Key skills include using deep questioning and listening, history-taking, and use of screening and diagnostic strategies to develop differential diagnoses. This includes obtaining and documenting a relevant health history as well as performing and accurately documenting an appropriate comprehensive or symptom-based physical examination. PCNPs order, perform, and interpret diagnostic tests such as laboratory work and radiographs. Additionally, the PCNP must demonstrate the ability to employ appropriate screening and diagnostic strategies to develop and support diagnoses as well as documenting this through the use of correct diagnostic evaluation and management billing codes. PCNPs are required to independently manage acute and chronic physical and mental illness, including acute exacerbations and injuries, and to minimize the development of complications and promote function and quality of life (NONPF and AACN, 2013). Disease management may include the ability to perform primary care procedures, which

may vary depending on the setting but might include suturing, microscopy, biopsies, Pap smears, joint aspirations and injections, and removal of foreign objects as necessary, to name just a few. PCNPs confirm evidence-informed diagnoses, develop plans of care, prescribe treatments and pharmacotherapeutics, and provide follow up. Often the plan of care requires coordination of care activities or needed services with multiple professionals.

Health Promotion and Disease Prevention

PCNPs also focus on health promotion, disease prevention, health education, and counseling, guiding patients to make better health and lifestyle choices. PCNPs bring an underlying holistic approach to care, grounded in nursing science and philosophy, an approach that integrates the relationship of the social determinants of health to the overall well-being of the population of patients cared for as well as the individual patient for whom care is being provided. The United States continues to lag behind other advanced nations on measures of infant mortality and life expectancy, according to an analysis of more than 300 diseases and injuries in 195 countries and territories (GBD 2015 Mortality and Causes of Death Collaborators, 2016). Drug abuse and diabetes are noted as causing a disproportionate amount of ill health and early death in the United States. PCNPs in primary care today must be able to respond to the unprecedented level of opioid addiction that has resulted in a fivefold increase in deaths over the past 25 years, increasing from 4000 per year in 1990 to more than 21,300 in 2015, and driving an overall reduction in life expectancy for Americans for the first time in many years (GBD 2015 Mortality and Causes of Death Collaborators, 2016). Alcohol and drug addiction, smoking, and access to guns also pose continuing threats. To combat these health risks, the United States will have to go beyond its reliance on a hospital-centric, drug-centric medical system. According to this study, heart disease remains the leading cause of death (532,000) in the United States, with Alzheimer disease in second place (282,530) and lung cancer ranked third (187,390).

These statistics reinforce the need for skills and competencies that support patients to achieve and maintain healthy lifestyles, including addressing the community issues of safety, access to healthy food, and opportunities for physical activity. People need providers with strong communication skills, empathy, and an understanding of the environment in which people live. Nursing as a discipline never abandoned its public health roots; community health nursing and population health are integrated in all nursing curriculum and approaches. PCNPs combine "high-tech" and "low-tech" approaches to deal with these population-based health challenges. Specifically, PCNPs must manage and provide a full spectrum of health care services that includes health promotion, disease prevention, health protection, anticipatory guidance, counseling, disease management, and palliative and end-of-life care (NONPF and AACN, 2013, 2016). Examples of this, building on knowledge about developmental age–related and gender-specific variations, include implementing age-appropriate wellness promotion and disease prevention services, weighing the costs, risks, and benefits to individuals; developing a plan for long-term management of chronic health care problems with the individual, family, and health care team; and evaluating individuals' and/or caregivers' support systems. It is critical that the PCNP promotes safety and risk reduction for vulnerable populations.

Providing Culturally Sensitive, Patient-Centered Care

Care providers who mirror the populations that they care for can be more effective; barring that, cultural humility and a commitment to social justice are critical (The Sullivan Commission, 2004; Valentine, Wynn, & McLean, 2016). PCNPs are educated to provide patients with high-quality, comprehensive, culturally sensitive, and patient-centered care. They use interventions to prevent or reduce risk factors for diverse and vulnerable populations, particularly the young and the frail elderly (NONPF and AACN, 2016). PCNPs counsel and coach as well as educate patients to manage chronic diseases, which are often multiple, and help to guide them through difficult decisions related to lifestyles, prioritization, and choices. PCNPs need to be knowledgeable about and integrate behavioral health, in a team-based approach and/or through sensitivity and cultural humility during their one-to-one encounter with the person/family. They are able to address cultural, spiritual, and ethnic influences that potentially create conflict among individuals, families, staff, and caregivers. They approach persons and families holistically, promote health and hope, and meet persons "where they are." Through the use of reflective practice, PCNPs develop strategies to prevent their own biases from interfering with the delivery of quality care. This may involve educating other professionals and lay caregivers to provide culturally and spiritually sensitive, appropriate care.

Coordinating Transitional Care Services in and Across Care Settings

Strong analytic skills are needed for proper diagnosis, treatment, and care planning and to provide care that is evidence-based and consistent with current standards of care. Part of the role of the PCNP is to discern gaps in care and barriers to care needing resolution during patient encounters. Coordinated, patient-centered care across settings requires advanced knowledge of the health care delivery system as well as an understanding of the payment system. PCNPs apply knowledge of scientific foundations in practice for quality care; they apply skills in technology and information literacy, they use HIT and enhanced EHRs to provide coordinated care and facilitate better communication among health care providers and patients. Even yesterday's nursing care plan has reemerged as a vital tool in the EHR for use by RNs as well as NPs, physicians, social workers, and pharmacists in the coordination of care for our most complex patients—now a billable activity under Medicare. Technology and information literacy competencies also inform NP contributions to the design of clinical information systems that promote safe, quality, and cost-effective care and enable NPs to use technology systems that capture data variables for the purpose of evaluating nursing care.

Primary care practice today is a "team sport." For example, the PCNP must demonstrate sensitivity and good judgment about the interaction of acute and chronic physical and mental health problems and when to "hand off" to other members of the team (Exemplar 15.1). PCNPs use transition of care theory, handing off care of the patient/family to other team members and reporting information necessary for safe team functioning in the care of patients (NONPF and AACN, 2016).

Primary care practices are developing meaningful systems for the coordination of care needed for populations of patients. This involves the integration of technological solutions for care coordination and microlevel as well as macro system-level approaches. PCNPs effect health care change using broad-based skills, including negotiating, consensus building, and partnering. They work to facilitate the development of health care systems that address the needs of culturally diverse populations, providers, and other stakeholders. PCNPs understand that poor communication and lack of patient accountability among multiple providers leads to medical errors, waste, and duplication. PCNPs evaluate the impact of health care delivery on patients, providers, other

EXEMPLAR 15.1 **Family Nurse Practitioner in a Community Health Center**

Jill Winland-Brown, EdD, APRN, FNP-BC
Professor Emeritus, Florida Atlantic University

I volunteer as a family nurse practitioner in a federally funded primary care clinic and see patients from ages 18 to 65. We only accept US citizens living in our county and have an estimated 65,000 uninsured residents who need care in our geographic region.

Several months ago, I had a new patient, JR, a 19-year-old African-American who had just been discharged from the local trauma center. He was sitting on his porch with his girlfriend and was shot four times by a drive-by shooter. He asserts he has had a "clean life" and doesn't know why anyone would want to do that. He does live in an unsafe, drug-infested community. He was shot once in the neck with a "through-and-through" wound, twice in the abdomen, and once in the foot. He should not have been discharged so quickly, but with no insurance, the hospital seems to send patients out "quicker and sicker." JR had difficulty talking and I wasn't sure about his vocal cords. He had a feeding tube in place because his swallowing was suspect, in addition to the two stomach wounds inflicted on his colon and repaired during surgery. His ankle wound was very painful and he had difficulty walking, but he didn't complain. He was mainly very concerned for his safety if the shooter should come back.

With less than a half-hour allotted to care for him, I began to prioritize JR's needs. (Obviously I took longer, but this meant that appointments with other patients were delayed.) He had an order for liquid supplement as a tube feeding and had been shown how to administer it. Because it was very expensive, the hospital only gave him several days' worth. I checked on a website to find affordable drugs, but it was still several hundred dollars for 1 week worth of liquid supplement. I got the navigator involved on that issue while I addressed his other needs. I was going to order speech therapy for him due to his neck injury and physical therapy for his ankle, but he said that when he got home, he was going to stay in because he was extremely fearful of going out. It seemed like a classic case of posttraumatic stress disorder (PTSD). I asked the navigator to explore this issue as well. We do have mental health counselors at our clinic, but there is a long waiting list. The navigator was able to find someone that JR could see, but I could tell that he wouldn't be leaving the house anytime soon. I made sure that he knew how to give himself tube feedings and had enough supplies to change the dressing. The navigator was able to locate a supply house that had some feeding supplement due to expire shortly and they were willing to donate it to JR.

JR's main goal was to get home. My goal was to take care of his throat, his stomach, his ankle, his speech, his supply needs, and his PTSD. It seemed very daunting JR was very thankful and grateful for everything we were able to do. I wanted to see him the next week, but he canceled his appointment. His throat improved dramatically, and he started eating some liquids, then solid foods gradually. In 3 weeks he returned for me to remove his feeding tube, had become plugged. I was grateful for the navigator because she was aware of many more resources than I was, and she saved me so much time. I did see JR one last time (for now) and now that he is "healthy," he is not so afraid anymore. The police never found the shooter. ◎

---

stakeholders, and the environment. Finally, they are competent about analyzing organizational structures, functions, and resources to improve the delivery of care.

Reflective Practice: A Component of Direct Patient Care

Reflective practice enables nurses to manage the impact of caring for other people on a daily basis. It can be defined as the process of making sense of events, situations, and actions in the workplace. Reflective practice has been defined as a process that develops understanding of what it means to be a practitioner and makes the link between theory and practice by means of the practitioner consciously thinking through the experience (Howatson-Jones, 2016). A range of models are available for nurses to use to support reflective practice in clinical practice. Expert clinical thinking and skillful performance are cultivated through repeated evaluation of similar sets of health and illness scenarios and formulating plans of care based on patient expectations, current standards of care, experience, clinical judgment, and current research. Experienced APRNs incorporate this practical wisdom into their decision making, taking actions that they might have been unlikely to take as novice practitioners. Practical wisdom involves knowing what to do and when to do it:

- When is a patient ready to begin home glucose monitoring?
- When is it time to suggest respite or home health care?
- What is the right time to address sexuality issues with a preteen or teenager?
- What is the right time to address an issue directly, and when is it time to back off from confronting difficult issues?

Another important strategy for reflective practice is peer review, if done in a supportive collaborative way; this is included in the NONPF (2017) NP core competencies (see Box 15.5). Open, transparent sharing and review of difficult and complex patient situations can lead to important self-reflection.

A new PCNP especially needs time for reflection, conversation, consultation, and collaboration; but all who practice need time for reflection. Time is needed to keep up with the professional literature and learn how to juggle this into an already busy schedule. Technology takes time and is constantly changing. A supportive environment is critical to success. Increasingly, new graduate NPs of all population foci, be they PCNPs or acute care NPs, report a need for additional education and training to manage today's complex care environments (Hart & Bowen, 2016). In Exemplar 15.2, an NP resident at a FQHC demonstrates reflective practice as she looked back on her experiences in a complex and challenging but supportive care environment.

Guidance and Coaching

The competencies of guidance and coaching have been an identified domain of the NP role since its original iteration and description by NONPF in the early 1990s (see Chapter 2). It is a natural extension of the RN role—a supporter, a facilitator, nonjudgmental in nature, a side-by-side alliance for health or behavioral change, or "getting through" chronic illness, suffering, death, and dying. Many early NPs, all initially in primary care roles, emerged from seasoned RN practice, often as public health or community-based nurses. The relationship between the PCNP and the patient creates a strong foundation for the guidance and coaching competency (see Chapter 8). The PCNP must be skilled at building trust and rapport because the longitudinal nature of primary care relationships can span decades if warmth and trust are established.

Often, an assessment of the chief complaint unearths many issues of which the patient may not be aware. As nurses, NPs are expert clinical thinkers who understand the need to listen carefully to the patient's story. The skilled practitioner helps the patient sift and sort through issues, establish priorities, and understand the interconnectedness of these priorities, often in a limited time frame. Practical wisdom guides the practitioner to use expert clinical thinking, deep listening, and skillful interviewing, but the plan of care must be patient centered and sometimes coordinated with the health care team.

EXEMPLAR 15.2   **Nurse Practitioner Resident at a Federally Qualified Health Center: Reflecting on a Year of Residency**

Delphine Hyppolite, FNP

Prior to my postgraduate residency year, I was certain that I wanted to be a part of an organization that would continue to foster my development as a provider. I also wanted to join an organization that had the mission of meeting the needs of underserved populations; however, one thing that I underestimated was the complexity of those needs. Although I thought I was cognizant of and empathic to the day-to-day distress of such populations, when I encountered their stories I found myself feeling alarmed. Often I found myself wanting an algorithm, a set plan and clarity about what to do and when to do it. As much as this has been a journey for me, I can only imagine what a journey it

has been for many immigrants, former prisoners, substance abusers, and caregivers who have made the first critical step by making *themselves* their first priority. The depression, the trauma, the uninformed and misguided choices, the cyclical family history, and the impoverished environments are all backdrops in these patients' lives. However, the resiliency and milestones all speak to the essence of *true* community health care, my role as a nurse practitioner, and the need for clinics to provide access to care. I meet this next year with a little apprehension due to the continued rigor and complexity of my role, but I also meet the challenge of what lies ahead with confidence that I will rise above it. ◎

This exemplar was abstracted from Dr. Hyppolite's final journal entry at the end of her postgraduate residency year at Community Health Center, Inc., Middletown, CT.

EXEMPLAR 15.3 **A Virtual Medical Home Collaborative Practice**

Sandra Petersen, DNP, FNP
University of Texas, Tyler

Sandra Petersen, DNP, and collaborating physician Kim Dunn, MD, PhD, utilize a virtual medical home to create a patient-centered system of "wired" networks built around the virtual medical home model. Telehealth and patient/provider access to a centralized medical record provide a clinically useful pathway for connecting patients, APRNs, physicians, and third parties (home health, hospice, and physical and occupational therapy services) in the community. The model addresses a major problem in the care delivery system in which care is provided in "silos" and patients do not have direct access to their information. Through automating referral and communication processes to improve patient access, the virtual medical home emphasizes the provision of patient-centered care and provides a sustainable approach to health information exchange. Patients are admitted to the primary care practice (medical home) and provide documentation of all providers (and any third parties) that participate in

their care. Telehealth allows for Health Insurance Portability and Accountability Act–secure virtual visits, "curbside consults" with specialists (such as neurology, cardiology, and psychiatry) or other providers while the patient is at a primary care visit (whether that is in the office or via telehealth); this allows all providers to be "on the same page" with the plan of care for the patient. Patients are provided with a QR code that can be accessed through their smart phone that allows immediate access to a read-only version of their medical record, including laboratory results, recent medical encounters, imaging, diagnostics, and plan of care. Treating providers can access the record through the QR code and have the opportunity to send a message to the primary care medical home, which is the "hub" for communication, to share treatment information. Patient satisfaction is also queried through the system, which automatically sends a survey to patients after a medical home encounter to ensure that the patient understands the plan of treatment and how to take any medications. ◎

PCNPs work to build a plan that is doable and sustainable by the patient and/or her or his family. Patients *must* be at the center of the plan of care for guidance and/or coaching to be effective. As partnerships deepen, the relationship becomes an even more important clinical tool.

Exemplar 15.3 presents a practice in which telecare enhances communication skills of fragile patients and consequently improves the outcomes of care. Today's new PCNPs are entering practice armed with a set of technical competencies unknown to PCNPs just a few years ago. They are trained in complex and sophisticated information management systems via simulation and are increasingly comfortable coaching patients in their use of wearables and home monitoring devices. The PCNP works in teams using actionable clinical dashboards so that data presented may cue the team that more guidance or coaching is needed.

Consultation

To be called on by providers as a consultant requires the PCNP to communicate practice knowledge effectively, both orally and in writing. The consultative activities of the PCNP may take the form of a formal medical consultation but sometimes are

accomplished in more informal exchanges with colleagues. Often the PCNP is the most long-standing member of the team, especially in teaching facilities where students come and go, and the PCNP can provide ongoing care updates. PCNPs have expert background in organizational structure, care processes, financing, marketing, and policy decisions that impact the quality of health care and as such may be called upon to consult in areas related to resources, care delivery, and/or policy, in addition to actual clinical consultation about the management of an individual patient and/or family.

Evidence-Based Practice

Nursing science foundations have contributed to the discipline of nursing, which is characterized by a "unique perspective, a distinct way of viewing all phenomena, which ultimately defines the limits and nature of its inquiry" (Donaldson & Crowley, 1978, p. 113). According to the DNP Essentials (AACN, 2006), specific middle-range theories should be used to guide the practice of NPs. PCNPs use middle-range theories to guide their assessment, decision making, and interventions, particularly when situations call for them (Smith & Liehr, 2014). Evidence-based practice competencies are essential to the PCNP

| EXEMPLAR 15.4 | Olivia Newby's Shared Medical Appointment (SMA) Model |

Olivia Newby, DNP, FN-BC, CDE

Dr. Olivia Newby is a family nurse practitioner and certified diabetes educator (NP-CDE) in a primary care practice located in a low-income, underserved urban community. This community has a high incidence of diabetes, particularly among African-Americans, many of whom are struggling unsuccessfully to manage their type 2 diabetes. Like many primary care providers, Dr. Newby is called upon to improve levels of hemoglobin A_{1c} in her diabetic patients, yet all she has is a 15-minute office visit with each patient.

As a result of her practice experience, Dr. Newby assessed that people with diabetes need a proactive model of care within primary care, so she developed the shared medical appointment (SMA) model. Based on the methodology of a "group visit," planning time begins 1 week before seeing the patient. The patient records are reviewed by an interprofessional team that includes an NP-CDE, a medical assistant, and a social worker. Educational handouts/literature are assessed by the NP-CDE for content and for meeting the diabetes standards of care criteria prior to inclusion in the educational component of this model. The most recent application of the SMA consisted of 14 patients. Patients were directed to the educational area of the practice, where the medical assistant, who "doubles" as a chef, had prepared a sweet potato pie—a commonly eaten food choice in the African-American community—according to American Diabetes Association recommendations. This alternatively prepared food was to serve as an example that people with diabetes have dietary choices that can be tasty, yet meet the American Diabetes Association's recommended nutritional standards.

The design of the educational format consists of patients first being given a short PowerPoint presentation with specific information on diabetes and the impact it can have on their lives. Each patient is then given his or her specific clinical results (hemoglobin A_{1c}, lipid profile, urine microalbumin, and body mass index) as these topics are presented. The participants are counseled by a CDE, who provides interactive demonstrations on using a glucose monitor, reading food labels, and calculating calories and sodium in foods. The educator reviews labels of culturally appropriate healthy food alternatives.

Dr. Newby's SMA model has shown great potential for improving the health of those with diabetes because it allows increased access to care and self-empowerment with education. Group visits occur within a single appointment lasting 90 to 120 minutes and fulfill many gaps in care not addressed in 15-minute office visits. Patients can address multiple questions in one visit as well as take advantage of a peer support group, peer education/motivation, increased time with providers, and the opportunity to discuss myths, concerns, and fears. ◎

---

provider role. Doctorally prepared NPs can integrate middle-range theory and translate research and other forms of information to improve practice processes and outcomes. Ultimately, PCNPs are able to develop new practice approaches based on the integration of research, theory, and practice knowledge. An example of this, discussed earlier, is the clinical practice innovation of an SMA that includes a certified diabetes educator and provides a new and meaningful approach to chronic disease management in primary care (Exemplar 15.4).

Clinical practice guidelines assure that the most current scientific evidence is applied in patient care. Practice patterns, or clinical performance, are evaluated using *process* measures, referring to the types of services delivered by caregivers, as well as *outcome* measures, such as death, symptoms, laboratory studies, health status, and quality of life. The PCNP must participate in measuring outcomes of his or her practice and make adjustments because outcomes are heavily influenced by underlying factors such as severity of illness and patient characteristics (King, 2016).

Leadership

There are many social forces that shape the future health and professional practice environment for PCNPs. PCNPS assume complex and advanced leadership roles to initiate and guide change. That leadership fosters collaboration with multiple stakeholders (e.g., patients, families, community, integrated health care teams, and policymakers) and demonstrates critical and reflective thinking. Given the longitudinal nature of primary care practice, PCNPs are often the long-term member of the team who provides continuity and stability in the care and management of patients over long periods, and thus are ideally suited to lead teams. Nurses continue to be identified as the most trusted professionals

(Norman, 2016). The PCNP's role as a leader in the community—often via membership on boards of health and education, through active participation in community organizations, and as an influential policymaker—provides evidence of her or his suitability and ability to *lead* health care teams, generating transformational practice change. DNPs are prepared to assess systems and organizations and to evaluate and implement system-level change. PCNPs, particularly doctorally prepared NPs, assume advanced leadership roles to initiate and guide change. The IOM (2011) cited leadership as critical to our future as a discipline and profession.

Moreover, PCNPs advocate for improved access, better quality, and cost-effective health care for all populations. They use the development and implementation of innovations that incorporate principles of change to advance practice and promote health at the local, national, and global level. They translate patients' stories. At the local practice level, for example, PCNPs may enact leadership roles when they guide and support staff, triage patients, lead interprofessional teams, coordinate care, and oversee the appropriate use of resources. On a broader level, PCNPs engage in clinical and professional leadership and use effective collaborative skills to assist groups and organizations to envision preferred futures, achieve consensus, and implement change. Where there is need, PCNPs respond.

PCNPs can also demonstrate leadership in advancing practice environments. Bodenheimer and Sinsky (2014) sounded the alarm that the "joy" had gone out of practicing medicine and that a relentless focus on metrics had led to the deterioration of professional practice environments. They called for a redesign of the Triple Aim in health care (Stiefel & Nolan, 2012) to a Quadruple Aim that adds a quadrant for "Improved Clinician Experience." Sometimes called the "Missing Aim" (Fig. 15.5) or the "forgotten aim," it notes that patient outcomes invariably suffer as a result of providers feeling overwhelmed, overworked, and powerless (Chase & Kish, 2015). PCNPs need to lead work to support healthier practice environments that in turn support quality-based outcomes (Exemplar 15.5).

Collaboration

Collaboration and leadership are closely linked in the effort to improve health care delivery systems. The 1996 IOM definition of primary care implies the use of professional collaboration to deliver integrated and accessible care. Effective collaboration

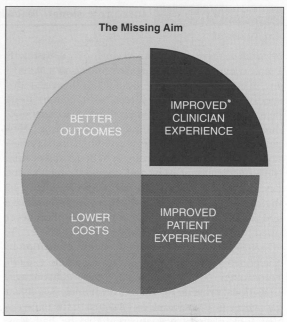

FIG 15.5 The missing aim: improved clinician experience. *(From Sobal, L., & Jaskie, S. [2016]. What's missing from the Triple Aim of health care?* Cardiac Interventions Today, 10*[2], 20-27. Retrieved from http://citoday.com/2016/04/whats-missing-from-the-triple-aim-of-health-care/.)*

within an interprofessional team context results in more comprehensive, patient-focused care promoting a high-quality, cost-effective outcomes both on the local practice level and beyond the walls of the practice, into the community (Bodenheimer & Grumbach, 2016). Effective collaboration improves institutional performance through processes such as continuous quality improvement, which involves the identification of concrete problems and the formation of interprofessional teams to gather data and propose solutions. Computerized information systems assist all of these components, so technological competencies are essential for the PCNP to be an effective collaborator (Exemplar 15.6).

Ethical Decision Making

Illness can create a range of negative emotions in patients, including anxiety, fear, powerlessness, and vulnerability. In the ever-expanding health care system, PCNPs face ethical issues, particularly involving, but not limited to, the allocation of care. How to identify and resolve these ethical issues is an important task for PCNPs. There needs, for example, to be clear separation of financial and clinical

EXEMPLAR 15.5   Interprofessional, Team-Based Education in a Nurse-Led Clinic

Ana Duvnjak

My time at the Florida Atlantic University Christine E. Lynn College of Nursing, Louis and Anne Green Memory and Wellness Center, a nurse-led health center that specializes in the care of patients with memory disorders, fit seamlessly into my interprofessional experience during my third-year medical school rotation. New patients at this center are evaluated by a nurse practitioner (NP) and neuropsychologist to better characterize their medical concerns and memory impairment. Findings are then discussed by an interprofessional team including the NP, social worker, neuropsychologist, and psychotherapist; a therapeutic plan is then developed for the patient and family.

I was able to sit in on a new patient evaluation by Madeline, a primary care advanced practice adult-gerontology NP. A patient, "J," was referred by a transitional program for chronically homeless individuals, where he is a resident. As I listened to the interview that took place, it was apparent that he had some cognitive impairment, which he himself recognized, but it was difficult to determine his reliability as a historian. He had a history of traumatic brain injury

from a vehicle-pedestrian accident as well as substance abuse and an unclear psychiatric history. His perceptions of his relationships and situation gave the impression that he did not realize the severity of his state and did not recognize destructive decisions he had made. He had no contact with his family and could not effectively explain why. As I left, Madeline assured me he would undergo neuropsychological testing to pinpoint his strengths and weaknesses in various cognitive domains. The team would meet to discuss his case and make recommendations.

This rotation allowed me to experience nurse-directed care with heavy involvement from social work and other disciplines. The most striking feature of nurse-led care is an emphasis on continuous communication. Weekly meetings ensure that the team is up-to-date on patient progress and recommendations. The patients seen are medically and socially complex and require a cohesive team approach. I think this is the best example of providing care for the individual as a whole that I have observed so far. It was refreshing and eye-opening. ◎

This exemplar was written while the author was a medical student at the Schmidt College of Medicine, Florida Atlantic University, Boca Raton, FL.

---

decisions. In an era focused on cost containment, the PCNP's accountability to the health care system in which he or she practices may create tension, especially in relation to the use of resources for patient care. PCNPs must always be ethically accountable for their actions, particularly when financial incentives related to resource use are involved (Bodenheimer & Grumbach, 2007). This accountability is aided by increased technology. Despite the familiar pains of adopting new technology and waiting for EHR vendors to "catch up" with practice transformation, technology's impact on primary care has largely been successful.

Additionally, the PCNP will encounter specific patient care concerns that raise ethical issues. Examples include reproductive issues, informed consent, end-of-life-issues, conflict of interest on the part of providers, and conflicting health care goals among family members as well as lack of equity, social disparities of health, and in some cases profound suffering.

PCNP practice must embrace thoughtful reflection on the meaning of moral concepts in terms

of culture and diversity. Operating with a context-sensitive approach can enable PCNPs to understand and name ethical issues in nursing practice more easily and to integrate ethical principles into their decision making (Lützén, 1997). PCNPs evaluate the ethical consequences of decisions and apply ethically sound solutions to complex issues related to diverse individuals, populations, and systems of care. In today's complex care environments, moral distress in care providers as they confront the complexity of people's problems and lives must be confronted.

Going Forward With Shared Competencies for Primary Care

Englander et al. (2016) identified eight domains of general physician competency from the taxonomy used to map what are called core "entrustable professional activities" for entering medical residency. This evolved into a list of 58 competencies within 8 domains (Box 15.6). As can be seen from this list, there is some convergence between these medical domains of competence and the NONPF core NP

| EXEMPLAR 15.6 | Moving Knowledge, Not the Patient: A New Way of Learning, Consulting, and Working With Specialists |

Danielle is a family nurse practitioner (NP) at a rural community health center in Arizona. Like primary care providers across the country, she faces the challenge of caring for patients with chronic pain. She must assess, diagnose, manage, and treat pain in the context of the patient's life and preferences and consider all of the risks and benefits of pharmacologic treatment, especially opioids. But she is not alone in this.

On Thursdays, from noon to 2:00 p.m., Danielle heads to her desk, turns on her computer, and logs into a "zoom" videoconference to join Project ECHO-Pain, where for 2 hours she will take a pause from her intensely busy clinical schedule. She will listen to a didactic lecture on an element of pain management, hearing cases presented by primary care colleagues across the country and the advice given to them by a team of pain management experts. This electronic chat includes 30 participants who share their own clinical experiences and lessons learned. She does this with the support of the rural health center leadership, who recognize how challenging this area of practice can be.

Today, Danielle has asked to present a case and get some guidance. She describes a 60-year-old female patient with chronic and generalized pain who first came to her several months ago. Due to back pain and diffuse joint pain, the patient has been treated with opioid medication for 10 years, along with medication for depression. She is obese (body mass index of 42), post-gastric bypass surgery, and disabled from an injury while working. Danielle's assessment was that the opioid regimen was inappropriate, and she referred the patient to a pain management specialist center. The report from the care provider at that pain center was that the patient "threw a scene" in the office when they attempted to reduce her opioids, and they are returning the patient to Danielle's care.

After Danielle presents the medical, social, and family history, medications and laboratory values, and the results of the patient's physical examination, the Project ECHO team members each comment in turn, ask additional questions, and then pose a second round of queries, making some recommendations. Unlike a consult with "a" specialist, this is a team consult: an orthopedic surgeon and pain specialist, a psychiatrist, a nutritionist, a pharmacist, a physical medicine specialist, an NP pain specialist, and a Chinese medicine specialist. The team concurs that the opioid regimen is inappropriate, and in dialogue with Danielle, they create an action plan of care that Danielle can implement, incorporating behavioral health, physical medicine, pharmacologic, and nutrition-based approaches.

(Project ECHO is a case-based, distance learning strategy first developed by Dr. Sanjeev Arora at the University of New Mexico as a model to support primary care providers in assuming the responsibility for treating patients with hepatitis C in their practices versus referring them to an academic medical center for treatment with a specialist. The model has been replicated around the United States and the world. Danielle is participating in Project ECHO-Pain, sponsored by the Weitzman Institute, a federally qualified health center–based research and innovation center. For Danielle, participation in Project ECHO is a strategy for ongoing learning in a clinically challenging area, expert feedback on specific cases, and support from a community of primary care providers.) ◎

competencies. This promising work from medicine, regardless of specialty, provides clear performance outcomes that are expected of all students receiving an MD degree. Medicine, like advanced practice nursing, is shifting from focusing on *time* and predefined curricula to focusing on *competency-based* medical education. These "guidelines" evolved from a grounding in the literature and were vetted through a process that broadly engaged the medical education community, sparked by a desire to improve the quality and safety of the care that new resident physicians provide to patients. Efforts in the NP community are underway to undertake a journey to better operationalize competency-based learning outcomes.

Future Trends in Primary Care

Telecare: The Patient Will See You Now

No longer does geographic access limit the health care services available. *Telecare*, also known as *telehealth*, is the use of remote health care technology to deliver clinical services; specifically, it is the delivery of health care services and clinical information using telecommunications technology, including a wide

BOX 15.6   The Eight Domains of General Physician Competence[a]

1. Patient care
2. Knowledge for practice (medical knowledge for physicians)
3. Practice-based learning and improvement
4. Professionalism
5. Interpersonal and communication skills
6. Systems-based practice
7. Interprofessional collaboration
8. Personal and professional development

[a]Derived from the taxonomy used to map the core entrustable professional activities for entering residency to their critical competencies.
From Englander, R., Flynn, T., Call, S., Carraccio, C., Cleary, L., Fulton, T. B., et al. (2016). Toward defining the foundation of the MD degree. *Academic Medicine*, *91*(10), 1352-1358.

array of clinical services using Internet, wireless, satellite, and telephone media (American Telemedicine Association, http://www.americantelemed.org/home). Whereas HIT is the generation and transmission of digital health data, often through an EHR, telecare is the delivery of an actual clinical service. HIT can facilitate telecare but it is not a requirement for delivering remote health care. Guided by technical standards and clinical practice guidelines and backed by decades of research and demonstrations, telecare is a safe and cost-effective way to extend the delivery of health care.

Currently, telecare is being delivered in primary care settings, filling a need to improve access to care for anyone, regardless of her or his location. Some examples of specialty care that is delivered in primary care settings include telestroke, teledermatology, and telepsychiatry provided to the underserved, especially more remote and rural populations (Henderson et al., 2014). e-Clinics enable PCNPs to deliver primary care to school-based nursing clinics and employee-based health care in workplaces via telecare. Employers benefit by limiting the loss of productivity and by a reduction in health care costs; healthier children learn better.

Telecare technologies reduce cost through a variety of means of remote patient monitoring. For example, Pekmezaris et al. (2012) demonstrated cost savings in the care of a population of patients with heart failure. Remote patient monitoring devices enabled PCNPs to intervene when there was a change in health status, thus eliminating the need for costly home care visits, lowered exacerbations of chronic illnesses, and fewer adverse events, hospitalizations, and emergency department visits. Patients with diabetes who were living in rural areas were given a computer tablet through the Mississippi Diabetes Telehealth Network; this supported real-time coaching and health education sessions as well as remote monitoring of blood glucose and vital signs and access to specialty care, resulting in better outcomes with cost savings in the primary care context (Henderson et al., 2014).

Use of these virtual modalities, including various remote monitoring devices and sensors—collectively referred to as telecare—is exploding. Increasingly, even unstable patients can be kept at home and managed with the assistance of emerging technologies. Continuous health monitoring for frail elders at home results in timely, quality care and better self-management, keeping patients in their homes longer, more safely, and with better quality of life and decreased costs (Newland et al., 2016). A variant on the hospital-to-home transitional model is equipping assisted living facilities with "smart rooms," complete with smart phones and computer tablets for messaging and sensors to detect injuries, thereby revolutionizing primary care practice (Rantz et al., 2015). PCNPs need to prepare for a more technology-driven practice. Sensor technology has been shown to provide a feeling of connection to the care provider, with the PCNP available by phone or text message or alerted by "pings" that communicate information about the patient's changing status (Petersen, 2016).

Emergence of Postgraduate Residency Models

Over the past 10 years, studies have documented the experience of new NPs and their interest in a postgraduate, intensive period of clinical training following completion of the academic credential that qualifies for certification as an NP, sometimes referred to as an NP residency (Hart & Bowen, 2016). In 2005 a FQHC proposed a model of postgraduate residency designed to support the new PCNPs in their transition to mastery as a PCNP in the safety net setting. Flinter (2005) launched the country's first PCNP residency program in 2007 with a structured, intensive 1-year program focused on training new PCNPs in clinical complexity. A study of the experience of PCNPs showed the effectiveness of the program in the achievement of competence, confidence, and a sense of mastery by the end of the program (Flinter & Hart, 2017). Similar FQHC-based postgraduate programs have been developed in other FQHCs (Norwick, 2016), in the VA system

(Meyer et al., 2015; Rugen et al., 2014), and in private health systems (Bush, 2014; Bush & Lowery, 2016). One study has identified increased levels of NP satisfaction for individuals who have completed an NP residency versus those who have not (Bush, 2014). Further research on outcomes, policy considerations, and academic arrangements of NP residency programs is needed (Harper, McGuiness, & Johnson, 2017).

Conclusion

This is an exciting time to be a PCNP. The future is bright and filled with challenges that demand continued lifelong learning and the opportunity to take more responsibility and accountability for the health and welfare of patients and populations. Technology in the primary care setting is expected to continue as a tool to expand access and lower cost. There is more than enough work for *all* health care professionals in a time of rapid change. The structures of the health care system will continue to change, and PCNPs will be a large part of that evolution.

Key Summary Points

- Historians remind us that all health care was once primary care. The United States developed a fixation on specialty care in the last century, creating an overspecialized tertiary care system with a more fragile primary care system in place.
- Many forces helped create and expand the role of PCNPs:
  - The women's and civil rights movements
  - The legislative creation of the National Health Service Corps in 1970
  - The chronic maldistribution of generalists, leading to the inclusion of NPs in this federal effort to address access to health care
  - The decades-old need for a new kind of community-oriented primary care

- The rapid influx of health maintenance organizations in the 1980s and managed care in the 1990s and the passage of the Patient Protection and Affordable Care Act in 2010
- Full scope of practice for APRNs in the VA system, except for nurse anesthetists
- PCNPs are fundamental to the nation's safety net for health care; in FQHCs, nurse-led health centers, school-based health centers, and the Veterans Administration; and in caring for the homeless, including veterans.
- PCNPs are well positioned to lead highly innovative practice models such as telecare; to promote aging-in-place innovations, wearable technologies, and use of SMAs; and to employ big data to move knowledge, not patients.
- As health care evolves in the United States, it is predicted that PCNPs will continue to be a disruptive innovation, delivering care in nontraditional sites and by nontraditional methods.
- PCNPs are uniquely prepared to provide holistic direct care that is patient centered and outcome directed and is based on evidence in the primary care setting.

References

To access the references for this chapter, use your smartphone's QR code reader to scan the code below, or go to http://booksite.elsevier.com/9780323447751.

The Adult-Gerontology Acute Care Nurse Practitioner

Marilyn Hravnak • Jane Guttendorf • Ruth M. Kleinpell • Brian Widmar • Kathy S. Magdic

> *"How wonderful it is that nobody need wait a single moment before starting to improve the world."*
>
> —*Anne Frank*

CHAPTER CONTENTS

The purpose of the adult-gerontology acute care nurse practitioner (AG-ACNP) is to diagnose and manage disease and promote the health of adult patients with acute, critical, and/or complex chronic health illnesses or injuries who may be physiologically unstable, technologically dependent, and/or highly vulnerable for complications in any geographic setting in which these patients may be found. The AG-ACNP provides comprehensive care in a collaborative model with physicians, staff nurses, and other health care providers as well as with patients and their families. The AG-ACNP not only shares common functions and skills with the other nurse practitioner (NP) subspecialties but also applies unique knowledge and skills in caring for very complex and vulnerable patient populations (American Association of Colleges of Nursing [AACN], 2012;

American Association of Critical-Care Nurses, 2012 and 2017 [in press]). As of 2008, the *Consensus Model for APRN Regulation* (APRN Joint Dialogue Group, 2008) states that the role of the certified NP includes diagnosing, treating, and managing patients with acute and chronic illnesses and diseases, including the following: ordering, performing, supervising, and interpreting laboratory, diagnostic, and imaging studies; prescribing medication and durable medical equipment; and making appropriate referrals for patients and families. Furthermore, these role attributes are used with a specific patient population for which the practitioner is specifically educated and licensed (APRN Joint Dialogue Group, 2008). For NPs caring for patients within the pediatric or adult-gerontology population focus, the scope of practice is further delineated according to a primary or acute care focus within a population focus (National Council of State Boards of Nursing [NCSBN], 2008; AACN, 2012). Thus NPs can be educated and certified as pediatric acute or primary care and as adult-gerontology acute or primary care, which incorporates the entire spectrum of adults, including young adults, middle-aged adults, and older adults. Most AG-ACNPs practice in acute and critical care settings that include subacute care, emergency care, and intensive care settings. These include, but are not limited to, acute and critical care neurology, pulmonology, trauma, transplantation, presurgical and perioperative care, emergency care (excluding pediatrics), pain management services, rapid response teams, and cardiac surgery (Barocas et al., 2014; Collins et al., 2014; Hoyt & Proehl, 2015; Kapu, Wheeler, & Lee, 2014; Kleinpell & Goolsby, 2012; Kleinpell, Ward, et al., 2015). A growing number of AG-ACNPs also practice in specialty-based practice settings such as specialty clinics, medical rehabilitation, home care, long-term care, medical flight program settings, and telehealth (Alexander-Banys, 2014; Kleinpell & Goolsby, 2012; Rutledge, Haney, Bordelon, Renaud, & Fowler, 2014).

New competencies for the AG-ACNP recognize this evolved focus of care, and this chapter provides a framework for this level of AG-ACNP care (AACN, 2012 and 2017). However, there are many adult acute care nurse practitioners (ACNPs) who were certified prior to this titling change who can retain their title as long as they keep their prior certification active. For ease of discussion, we will use the term *adult-gerontology acute care nurse practitioner* and the abbreviation AG-ACNP to include NPs educated with an adult acute care focus since that role's inception. Although all AG-ACNPs share specialty role attributes, there may be intrarole variability based on the nature of the care delivery system, characteristics of a particular employment position or location in which they practice (e.g., private practice versus hospital employee, intensive care unit versus hospital unit or ambulatory care facility) and physiologic specialty (e.g., cardiac, pulmonary, orthopedic, oncology). This chapter presents an overview of the AG-ACNP role, including core and role-specific competencies, scope of practice, issues in practice, and future challenges.

Emergence of the Adult-Gerontology ACNP Role

The role of the AG-ACNP evolved as a result of a number of changes in the delivery of health care, including the need for an advanced practitioner to manage hospitalized patients whose clinical presentations were more complex, changes in the regulations of work hour restrictions for medical residents and fellows, and shortages of intensivist physicians. As early as the 1970s, primary care NPs (family NPs and adult NPs) were recruited to care for adult patients in hospital-based settings, with on-the-job training to provide secondary and tertiary care skills (an example of advanced practice registered nurse [APRN] evolution is described in Chapter 1). By the late 1980s, NPs were increasingly used in tertiary care centers, and it became apparent that a new adult NP specialty was emerging. Education was specifically designed to meet the needs of vulnerable adult patients with acute, critical, and complex chronic illness to ensure consistency in the knowledge, training, and quality of care provided by NP graduates in this new specialty. Master's-level graduate adult ACNP programs began to emerge in the late 1980s, and in 1995, the first national certification examination for ACNPs was administered (AACN, 2012).

Because of these same historical forces, a need for pediatric NPs (PNPs) specifically educated to meet the needs of acutely ill children with complex care needs also emerged. In 2004, the National Association of Pediatric Nurse Associates and Practitioners (NAPNAP) expanded their PNP scope of practice to reflect the acute care role (NAPNAP, 2011). An acute care PNP (PNP-AC) examination from the Pediatric Nursing Certification Board became available in 2005 (AACN, 2012; Bolick et al., 2012; NAPNAP, 2011; Reuter-Rice & Bolick, 2012).

National certification for adult ACNPs began in 1995 in the United States, and as of 2015 there were over 14,000 certified (10,212 adult ACNPs and 4032 AG-ACNPs) in total by the American Nurses Credentialing Center (2016) and the American Association of Critical-Care Nurses (2015). This NP specialty continues to grow as the continued need for the unique services that AG-ACNPs offer becomes recognized. Furthermore, constraints in graduate medical trainee work hour restrictions also provide a growing need for inpatient coverage—a need that can be met by the AG-ACNP (Garland & Gershengorn, 2013; Kleinpell, Ward, Kelso, Mollenkopf, & Houghton, 2015; Pastores et al., 2011; Ward et al., 2013). Finally, increased opportunities for third-party billing for inpatient services provided by the AG-ACNP also facilitates acceptance (Magdic, 2013; Munro, 2013). The AG-ACNP role has spread outside the United States and is being implemented to meet the needs of acutely and critically ill patients in the health care systems of other countries (Aleshire, Wheeler, & Prevost, 2012; Kilpatrick, 2011; Kilpatrick et al., 2010; Kleinpell et al., 2014; Scherr, Wilson, Wagner, & Haughian, 2012; Sung, Huang, Ong, & Chen, 2011).

Competencies of the Adult-Gerontology ACNP Role

Sources That Inform Adult-Gerontology ACNP Competencies

Most recently, in conjunction with the APRN Consensus Model, the focus of care for the adult ACNP has evolved to incorporate adult-gerontology because ACNP practice includes the spectrum of adults, including young adults, middle-aged adults, and older adults (Auerhahn, Mezey, Stanley, & Dodge, 2012). The AG-ACNP provides care to adult patients who are or may be at risk for physiologic instability. These patients may be encountered across the continuum of care settings because the role is not setting specific but is dependent on patient care needs. As a result, the practice of the AG-ACNP can span outpatient to hospital settings, urgent care, subacute care, and rehabilitation. The central and core competencies for the APRN, as explained in Chapter 3, form the foundations of ACNP practice. The central competency for all APRNs is direct clinical practice in concert with the other six core competencies of guidance and coaching consultation, evidence-based practice, leadership, collaboration, and ethical decision making. The ways in which ACNPs enact these core competencies are consistent with other APRN specialties, as discussed in Parts II and III of this text. In addition, AG-ACNPs share common entry-level competencies in accordance with the NP core competencies (National Organization of Nurse Practitioner Faculties [NONPF], 2014). Although the ACNP may need to use specialty skills and knowledge in the care of acutely, critically, and complex chronically ill adults, ACNPs have the following factors in common with the other NP specialties: (1) a generalist nursing foundation, (2) a health promotion basis to their practice, and (3) the development and appreciation of diagnostic reasoning skills. AG-ACNPs prepared at the Doctor of Nursing Practice (DNP) level may have additional knowledge and skills consistent with *The Essentials of Doctoral Education for Advanced Nursing Practice,* including refined communication skills, in-depth scientific foundations, analytic skills for evaluating and providing evidence-based practice, advanced knowledge of health care delivery systems and population-based care, knowledge of the business aspects of practice, and an emphasis on independent

and interprofessional practice (AACN, 2006). The practice-focused doctorate prepares graduates for clinical scholarship, including generation of transferrable evidence through innovation of practice changes, the translation of evidence, and the implementation of quality improvement processes to improve health or health care (AACN, 2015).

Adult-Gerontology ACNP Specialty Competencies

The *Nurse Practitioner Core Competencies* (NONPF, 2011b) outline competencies that are relevant to NP practice regardless of population focus. In addition, each of the NP specialties has unique competencies that differentiate practice. AG-ACNP entry-level competencies are illustrated in the *Adult-Gerontology Acute Care Nurse Practitioner Competencies* for entry into practice (AACN, 2012) and the *Scope and Standards for Acute Care Nurse Practitioner Practice* for expert practice (American Association of Critical-Care Nurses, 2017). A discussion of how AG-ACNP competencies are carried out within the framework of the APRN core competencies described in Chapter 3 follows.

Direct Clinical Practice

Direct clinical practice, the central competency of AG-ACNP practice, is the function that consumes the greatest percentage of AG-ACNP practice time. Prior clinical nursing expertise is essential for the AG-ACNP role because even the novice AG-ACNP cares for acutely and critically ill patients who may precipitously manifest life-threatening conditions that mandate an immediate response. These situations demand a strong clinical practice foundation.

Goals of AG-ACNP care include patient stabilization for acute and life-threatening conditions, minimizing and preventing complications, attending to comorbidities, and promoting physical and psychologic well-being. Additional goals include the restoration of maximum health potential or providing for palliative, supportive, and end-of-life care, as well as an evaluation of risk factors in achieving these outcomes (American Association of Critical-Care Nurses, 2017). AG-ACNPs achieve these goals through performing cognitive skills such as patient assessment, critical thinking, diagnostic reasoning, case management, and prescription of therapeutic interventions. Assessing and intervening in complex, urgent, or emergency situations are key components of AG-ACNP specialty competencies.

The central competencies of direct clinical practice as they apply to AG-ACNP specialty practice can be broadly characterized as those related to diagnosing and managing disease and those related to the promotion and protection of health (AACN, 2012; American Association of Critical-Care Nurses, 2012, 2017).

Diagnosing and Managing Disease

For AG-ACNPs to achieve the specialty competencies to diagnose and manage disease in their specialty patient population, they must demonstrate mastery of advanced pathophysiology, completion of a prioritized health history and comprehensive and focused physical examinations, rapid assessment of unstable and complex health problems, implementation of diagnostic strategies and therapeutic interventions to stabilize health care problems, demonstration of technical competence with procedures, modification of the plan of care based on a patient's changing condition and response to interventions, and collaboration with other care providers to facilitate positive outcomes (AACN, 2012; American Association of Critical-Care Nurses, 2017). The varied practice settings of individual AG-ACNPs across the continuum of health care delivery services result in associated variance in some of the competencies that they perform (Kapu, Thompson-Smith, & Jones, 2012).

Although individual elements of the AG-ACNP role differ, depending on these varied practice settings and on the specialty patient populations served, the basic elements necessary to function as a generalist AG-ACNP remain. The top 22 work activities in an AG-ACNP role delineation study performed by the American Nurses Credentialing Center (ANCC, 2012), arranged by criticality, are listed in Box 16.1.

BOX 16.1   Adult-Gerontology Acute Care Nurse Practitioner List of Top Work Activities Arranged by Criticality

1. Maintains patient privacy and confidentiality (including, but not limited to, Health Information Portability and Accountability Act [HIPAA] compliance)
2. Assesses the patient for urgent and emergent conditions
3. Assesses for rapid changes in physiological and psychological status
4. Differentiates between normal and abnormal findings
5. Prescribes and/or manages nonpharmacologic and pharmacologic treatment (via invasive and noninvasive routes)
6. Formulates differential diagnoses based on synthesized clinical findings
7. Modifies plan of care according to patient's response to treatment
8. Evaluates the safety and efficacy of pharmacological, behavioral, and other therapeutic interventions
9. Manages rapid pathophysiological changes
10. Prescribes and/or manages intravenous (IV)/intraosseous (IO) medications (including, but not limited to, cardiac medications, pain medications, insulin drips, thrombolytics, chemotherapy, intravenous dyes, radiocontrast agents)
11. Delivers care based on current evidence-based guidelines
12. Conducts a comprehensive or problem-focused history and physical examination
13. Conducts a pharmacologic assessment addressing pharmacogenetic risks, complex medical regimens, drug interactions and other adverse events; over-the-counter; complementary or alternative medications
14. Orders interventions to minimize risk and promote safety (including, but not limited to, devices to promote mobility and prevent falls, cognitive and sensory enhancements, restraint-free care, monitoring devices, venous thromboembolism and stress ulcer prophylaxis)
15. Prioritizes differential diagnoses
16. Obtains personal protected health information from collateral sources (including, but not limited to, electronic health records, databases, and other health care providers and family members)
17. Establishes therapeutic relationships in acute, urgent, or emergent care situations
18. Interprets diagnostic tests to formulate diagnoses
19. Advocates for the patient's right to self-determination, sense of safety, autonomy, worth, and dignity
20. Prescribes and/or manages blood-based products
21. Determines need for specialty consultation
22. Manages life-threatening conditions

From the American Nurses Credentialing Center's 2015 Adult-Gerontology Acute Care Nurse Practitioner Role Delineation Study Comprehensive Report. In all, 22 work activities were rated by respondents (N=343) as highly critical.

TABLE 16.1   **Procedures Performed as Reported by 962 Acute Care Nurse Practitioners (ACNPs)**

Procedures Performed in Hospital	Frequency of Performance of Procedures by ACNPs (No. of Procedures)
High Reported Frequency	
Radiologic studies	79.3% (619)
Vasoactive intravenous drips	67.1% (516)
Resuscitative efforts	67% (516)
Defibrillation	63.4% (512)
Wound care	49.9% (480)
Suture	40.7% (392)
Incisions	40.7% (392)
Ventilation	39.8% (295)
Medium Reported Frequency	
Cardioversion	38.2% (283)
Pacemakers	31.3% (230)
Arterial catheters	25.2% (182)
Central venous catheters	25% (182)
Pulmonary artery catheters	21.7% (157)
Intracardiac catheters	20.3% (165)
Cardiac assistive devices	18.8% (135)
Endotracheal	17.7% (128)
Chest tubes	15.9% (113)
Lower Reported Frequency[a]	
Lumbar puncture	14.4% (103)
Surgical first assist	9.5% (91)
Thoracostomy tubes	7.8% (75)
Cutdowns	5.4% (21)
Bladder aspiration	2.8% (16)

[a]In addition, other procedures that were performed with lower frequencies included bone marrow biopsies ($n = 6$), removing intra-aortic balloon pumps ($n = 4$), paracentesis ($n = 4$), joint aspirations ($n = 3$), and splinting fractures ($n = 3$).
Adapted from Kleinpell, R., & Goolsby, M. J. (2012). American Academy of Nurse Practitioners National Nurse Practitioner sample survey: Focus on acute care. *Journal of the American Academy of Nurse Practitioners, 24,* 690-694.

The performance of patient procedures, some of which are invasive, also constitutes a portion of the AG-ACNP's direct clinical practice. Technical procedures commonly performed by AG-ACNPs are listed in Table 16.1. The literature, including AG-ACNP role delineation studies, corroborates AG-ACNP technical skill performance as related to care focus: endotracheal intubation, central line placement, pulmonary artery line placement, needle thoracotomy, chest tube insertion and removal, and cricothyrotomy for the trauma critical care focus; nerve block, joint needle aspiration, diagnostic peritoneal lavage, needle decompression of the chest, lumbar puncture, chest tube insertion, cricothyrotomy and tracheostomy, suturing of lacerations and wounds, and splinting of injuries for the emergency care focus; and endotracheal and nasotracheal intubation (including rapid sequence), chest tube insertion and removal, insertion of central venous and arterial lines, and bronchoscopy for the critical care focus (ANCC, 2012; Dalley et al., 2012; Kleinpell & Goolsby, 2012; Kleinpell, Hravnak, Werner, & Guzman, 2006; NONPF, 2011a). The AG-ACNP procedural role has expanded to include nonvascular radiology procedures such as paracentesis, thoracentesis, and biopsy procedures (Duszak et al., 2015).

A NONPF publication, *Integrating Adult Acute Care Skills and Procedures into Nurse Practitioner Curricula* (NONPF, 2011a), outlines a number of psychomotor skills and procedures most commonly taught in AG-ACNP education programs, including the following: monitoring intracranial pressure, 12-lead electrocardiogram interpretation, defibrillation and cardioversion, pacemaker interrogation, hemodynamic monitoring, central venous line insertion, arterial puncture or cannulation, interpretation of a chest radiograph, performing thoracentesis for pleural effusions, chest tube insertion and removal, airway management for the non–anesthesia provider in procedural sedation, spirometry and peak flow assessment, paracentesis, local anesthesia application, and cutaneous abscess drainage. The increasing acceptance of invasive procedural skills as within the AG-ACNP scope of practice is supported by demonstration of complication rates no greater than those of physician providers (Sirleaf et al., 2014) as well as increasing employment of AG-ACNPs in critical care (Kleinpell & Goolsby, 2012) and improved third-party payment for APRN-performed procedures (Squiers, King, Wagner, Ashby, & Parmley, 2013).

It must be understood that procedural skill performance is not limited to the task itself but also includes knowledge of the indications, contraindications, complications, and skill in managing complications. When performing a procedural skill to derive physiologic data, such as mean arterial pressure, pulmonary artery pressure, or lumbar cerebrospinal fluid pressure, the AG-ACNP must use this information skillfully for patient diagnosis and management. AG-ACNPs are also compelled to collect their individual practice data related to procedure performance, including number and type of complications, and use these data to document ongoing skill competence, to assure positive patient outcomes and patient safety. The practice of an AG-ACNP in a cardiothoracic surgical intensive care unit (ICU), which illustrates the integration of technical skills within the context of diagnosis and management of disease, is provided in Exemplar 16.1.

Promoting and Protecting Health and Preventing Disease

In addition to disease diagnosis and management, AG-ACNPs also provide services to promote and protect health and prevent disease (AACN, 2012; American Association of Critical-Care Nurses, 2012, 2017). Inevitably, some of the methods that AG-ACNPs use to implement health promotion and protection and disease prevention vary from those used by NPs in the primary care specialties, since variations in application are related to the prioritization of needs during acute and critical illness. Moreover, in some practice models the episodic nature of the relationship between the AG-ACNP and patient and family is limited to a single acute

| EXEMPLAR 16.1 | Adult-Gerontology Acute Care Nurse Practitioner (AG-ACNP) Practice in an Intensive Care Unit |

In the cardiothoracic intensive care unit (CTICU), Marie, the adult-gerontology acute care nurse practitioner (AG-ACNP), functions as a leading member of the critical care provider "intensivist" team consisting of the AG-ACNP, attending physician (intensivist), one or two critical care medicine fellows, clinical pharmacist, and other members of the delivery team, including bedside nurses, primary care nurses, registered dietitian, and respiratory therapists. The team works in collaboration with the surgeons, surgical fellows, and residents on the cardiac, thoracic, transplant, vascular, and trauma services. As a CTICU AG-ACNP, Marie manages the patient from admission to the CTICU to discharge from the unit.

The day begins with a report from the team members who provided care during the previous night, highlighting changes in patients' conditions and providing information on new patients. Marie participates in dynamic patient-focused rounds, during which each patient is examined at the bedside and interviewed, when possible. During rounds, a wealth of other data are reviewed, including vital signs, hemodynamic data (e.g., pulmonary artery pressures, central venous pressures, cardiac outputs), ventilator settings and results of previous weaning trials, chest radiographs, diagnostic testing, laboratory and culture data, and a complete list of medications, continuous infusions, and fluid balances. Based on the clinical examination and review of data, and with input from members of the provider and delivery team, a comprehensive plan of care is devised for the patient. Marie assumes varying roles during these patient-focused rounds (e.g., presenting and reviewing data, performing the physical examination, writing orders, calling consultants). During this time, Marie is noting and prioritizing issues to be addressed later, treatment outcomes to be evaluated, planned procedures, culture and diagnostic test results

for review, family conferences, and anticipated admissions and discharges. Once rounds are complete, Marie will begin to address some of the specific issues on her work list.

Marie begins by seeing the four patients who are to be transferred out of the CTICU that morning. She briefly examines each of the patients and reviews their data to ensure that the patients' responses to interventions are appropriate. She verifies that these patients have been weaned from their vasoactive medicines and removes their chest tubes. Marie reviews each patient's history and physical and restarts home medications that are appropriate to the patients' cardiac conditions and comorbidities. She writes transfer orders and collaborates with the bedside nurse to ensure that all patient care issues have been addressed in the orders. One patient has a history of active smoking, and Marie discusses the relationship between smoking and heart disease with the patient as well as smoking cessation strategies. One patient needs to maintain a central intravenous access on the hospital ward. Marie converts the 16-gauge introducer in the patient's right internal jugular vein to a triple-lumen catheter. One patient has developed an arrhythmia with some hemodynamic instability, and Marie initiates appropriate treatment, cancels the patient's transfer to the floor, and informs the intensivist of the change in condition. Marie inserts an arterial line in this patient's left radial artery for closer hemodynamic monitoring. One patient is being transferred to a subacute care facility. Marie collaborates with the unit case manager to finalize transfer plans, speaks with the patient's family before discharge, and speaks with the receiving team in the subacute care facility to ensure continuity of care. During the course of the day, Marie might perform other invasive procedures, such as inserting central venous lines, dialysis

Continued

| EXEMPLAR 16.1 | Adult-Gerontology Acute Care Nurse Practitioner (AG-ACNP) Practice in an Intensive Care Unit—cont'd |

catheters, chest tubes, and nasoduodenal feeding tubes and performing thoracentesis, endotracheal intubation, and removal of intra-aortic balloons. Health promotion and protection assessment and intervention are integral to Marie's role but in different areas than one might expect in the primary care setting. For example, in the CTICU, Marie addresses stress ulcer prophylaxis, preventing complications from immobility, promoting skin integrity, and optimizing nutritional support.

Marie will continuously monitor the patients on the unit throughout the day and provide problem-focused care in response to changing patient needs and condition. She will be contacted by the nurse who is providing bedside care for the patient to address patient problems such as hypotension, hypertension, low cardiac output, low urine output, bleeding, low oxygen saturation, fever, difficulty with ventilation or ventilator changes, agitation and delirium, mental status changes, inadequate pain management, arrhythmias, electrolyte abnormalities, and problems with lines or catheters. She will see patients multiple times throughout the day in response to these concerns, each time assessing possible causes, performing directed physical examinations, formulating a treatment plan, and reassessing clinical findings to evaluate response to therapy. Marie initiates some treatments independently, but other, more complex situations may require her to consult with the intensivist and/or surgeon to review the management options. Marie will communicate with consultants from other teams, such as cardiology, nephrology, and infectious diseases, to coordinate care and treatment plans.

During the day, Marie also participates in the care of patients newly admitted after surgery. As patients arrive from the operating room, Marie receives a brief report from the anesthesia care provider and surgical fellow. She reviews the chart, examines the patient, and reviews initial laboratory results, electrocardiographic

results, and chest radiography results. She reviews the plan of care with the critical care nurse and respiratory therapist, targeting hemodynamic management and ventilator weaning. She documents a progress note, writes orders, and then returns frequently to reassess the patient's status and adjust the plan. One postoperative patient is bleeding severely. Marie alerts the surgeon, orders and reviews a coagulation profile, and ensures that the patient is being rewarmed. She orders blood products to correct the abnormality and monitors the patient to determine whether this therapy is effective or whether the patient will have to return to the operating room for mediastinal exploration.

At the end of the day, the team makes rounds again, seeing the new patients, evaluating the progress of and plans for other patients, and developing a plan for the next 12-hour period. The dynamic environment of the CTICU and the changing CTICU team members require the AG-ACNP to assess and reassess patient conditions frequently, remain flexible and responsive to subtle changes, and carefully organize and manage time.

As a permanent member of the critical care team, Marie provides needed continuity to care. She is instrumental in developing clinical protocols and communicating care expectations to other members of the team. She is available to interact with social services, case managers, physical and occupational therapists, and nutritional consultants. She is able to participate in discharge planning. She is readily available to the nursing staff for questions or problem solving. She participates in the CTICU's continuous quality improvement activities. She participates in research protocols, screens patients for eligibility criteria, and educates others concerning the research initiatives. Marie plays an important role in communication with patients and families and has a unique opportunity for teaching and reinforcing teaching. ◎

illness event. However, hospitalization can also provide a critical window of opportunity for AG-ACNPs to address health promotion and disease prevention with patients.

AG-ACNPs are skilled in a unique form of health promotion and protection and disease prevention—recognizing and modifying health risk factors associated with an inpatient stay. The AG-ACNP is qualified to identify the additional health problems for which the acutely, critically, and complex chronically ill are at risk and implement strategies to minimize or prevent that risk. As direct care providers, AG-ACNPs

have the ability to activate strategies and systems to implement primary, secondary, or tertiary prevention initiatives related to these unique inpatient risk factors. For example, some risk factors imposed by an inpatient stay are physiologic in nature, such as immobility, decreased nutritional intake, fluid and electrolyte imbalance, altered immunocompetence, impaired self-care ability, existing or developing comorbid disease states, and risks associated with invasive diagnostic and therapeutic interventions. Other risks have a psychologic foundation, such as psychologic consequences of alterations in the patient's physical abilities and alteration of his or her environment, sleep deprivation, communication impairment, alteration of self-image, role reversal, financial challenges, knowledge deficits, and the consequences of medication administration, including but not limited to delirium and depression. Families are also influenced by many of these risks and require AG-ACNP services.

In addition, there are risk factors related to hospitalization itself and the multiplicity of caregivers, including discoordination of care, polypharmacy, system inefficiency and redundancy, miscommunication with families, and miscommunication among caregivers (AACN, 2012; American Association of Critical-Care Nurses, 2012, 2017). The AG-ACNP is competent to assess patients for these unique risks and implement interventions to prevent their occurrence or minimize their consequences. As related in the previous section, 2 of the top 11 critical activities performed by AG-ACNPs are associated with minimizing health care–associated risks (i.e., evaluating patients for the safety and efficacy of interventions and ordering interventions to minimize risk) (ANCC, 2012). Although these skills are common to all AG-ACNPs, those prepared at the DNP level are equipped to assume leadership roles in developing, implementing, and evaluating evidence-based interventions to address and improve population health and clinical prevention to aggregate patient populations and across care systems (AACN, 2006, 2015).

Guidance and Coaching

Providing expert guidance and coaching of patients, families, and other health care providers is a core competency that is also an essential part of AG-ACNP practice. In the primary care area, the plan of care may be mutually determined and fully implemented between the NP and patient-family dyad. In contrast, the process of assessment and diagnosis, care planning, implementation, and evaluation in the acute care setting, although still centering on the AG-ACNP and patient-family dyad, will likely involve a number of other individuals, including but not limited to physicians, other nurses, respiratory therapists, dietitians, pharmacists, physical and occupational therapists, social workers, and clergy. In this complex setting, the AG-ACNP's ability to plan, interpret, and explain the plan of care while educating others about disease processes is a valued aspect of the AG-ACNP role. Often, critical illness can require many complex treatments and AG-ACNPs can provide teaching to families, nursing staff, and other members of the health care team to facilitate knowledge of indicated care. The core competency of guidance and coaching is played out at the highest levels when AG-ACNPs prepare patients for discharge after serious illness or when they assist and prepare family members to care for loved ones who have undergone catastrophic or debilitating health problems. ACNPs are particularly adept at communicating with families and patients during times of critical stress, when facilitating ethical decision-making, or when assisting families in communication with neurologically depressed or deteriorating patients. AG-ACNPs may also follow up with patients after hospital discharge to monitor and treat symptoms, facilitate care transition (Sawatsky, Christie, & Singal, 2013), and assess for and mitigate post-ICU syndrome. At times, patients (particularly the poor and uninsured) may not have a consistent primary care provider in the outpatient setting, and the AG-ACNP becomes an important source for health information and health promotion and protection interventions during the inpatient encounter. Some patients may be more receptive to health teaching and coaching that occurs in proximity to an acute health event (e.g., diet and exercise information after an acute myocardial infarction). AG-ACNPs also provide coaching for experienced and inexperienced nurses in complex care settings.

Consultation

The consultative activities of the AG-ACNP may take the form of a formal medical consultation. Sometimes consultative services by the AG-ACNP are delivered in more informal exchanges regarding the patient's condition and plan of care with other health care providers, including other APRNs. This aspect of the AG-ACNP's practice is invaluable in the teaching hospital setting. In this environment, attending physicians and medical trainees rotate on and off the service, and staffing patterns may result in inconsistencies in bedside nursing care. As the consistent member of the health care provider team, the AG-ACNP can use consultative skills to keep the team informed of the patient's condition and changing plan of care throughout the entire length of stay.

Evidence-Based Practice

Evidence-based care competencies are essential to the AG-ACNP provider role and may also vary among AG-ACNP providers. AG-ACNPs work to facilitate individual practice and health care system change through evidence-based practice initiatives (Kapu & Kleinpell, 2013; Kapu, Kleinpell, & Pilon, 2014; Liego, Loomis, Van Leuven, & Dragoo, 2014; McCarthy, O'Rourke, & Madison, 2013). All AG-ACNPs draw from the literature to deliver evidence-based medical and nursing care and actively participate in evidence-based quality improvement initiatives. AG-ACNPs have been instrumental in both adopting and leading initiatives for implementation of practice standards and guidelines (Fox, 2014) and core-measures documentation (Aleshire et al., 2012). Some AG-ACNPs, particularly those prepared at the DNP level, lead interprofessional teams focused on evidence-based practice initiatives (Aleshire et al., 2012). With the launch of the Value-Based Purchasing Program in 2011, hospitals have been required to improve outcomes and maximize reimbursement for Medicare patients, and the AG-ACNP is a valuable provider in applying evidence-based practices to achieve these goals (Kapu & Kleinpell, 2013; Liego et al., 2014). The AG-ACNP may partner with researchers to facilitate conduct of research and in some cases may serve as a clinical member of the research team. AG-ACNPs must be adept in evaluating research findings to assess for their suitability to support clinical practice change (American Association of Critical-Care Nurses, 2012, 2017).

Leadership

All AG-ACNPs provide some form of professional, clinical, and systems leadership in their provider role by serving as mentors and role models for staff nurses, taking on selected administrative responsibilities in the health care agency and acting as care facilitators and change agents within the health care system. An important competency of the AG-ACNP is to function as a leader in overseeing, coordinating, and directing the delivery of comprehensive clinical services within and across the health care system (AACN, 2012). Several studies have demonstrated that this aspect of AG-ACNP practice reduces inpatient length of stay and reduces emergency department return and hospital readmission rates (Collins et al., 2014; David, Britting, & Dalton, 2015; Kartha, Restuccia, Burgess, Benzer, Glasgow, Hockenberry, Mohr & Kaboli, 2014; Kilpatrick, 2013; Landsperger, Semler, Wang, Bryne, & Wheeler, 2015). The AG-ACNP promotes a positive healing environment and espouses assertiveness and conflict negotiation skills. Providing leadership in the planning and implementation of system-wide cost containment or cost-effective initiatives is also an aspect of the AG-ACNP role. AG-ACNPs prepared at the DNP level perform these activities at an even higher level of specificity and autonomy.

In addition to each individual AG-ACNP having leadership competencies, some may have leadership responsibilities for groups of AG-ACNPs or other APRNs (as well as physician assistants [PAs] and others). AG-ACNPs may work within teams of APPs and function as the "lead APP," having responsibility for overseeing the practice, performance, productivity, and scheduling of other APPs on the team, using leadership competencies to perform this role. It is also common in large health systems employing large numbers of NPs to have a centralized NP leader serve as a point of contact, liaison, and expert for all matters specific to NP practice (Bahouth et al., 2013).

Collaboration

Collaboration is one of the most frequently practiced core competencies of AG-ACNPs. Collaborative practice in the clinical setting involves working together, with shared responsibilities for clinical decision making for patient care (see Chapter 12). In the acute care setting, care delivery is always a collaborative effort among interprofessional members of the health care team. Therefore the ability to collaborate successfully is one of the critical components of the AG-ACNP role. In a collaborative practice model, the emphasis is on patient outcomes, with each professional responsible for providing the care for which he or she is best prepared. A collaborative practice model in acute care focuses on the concept that each patient needs the services of different types of providers simultaneously. The advantage to this model is the ongoing continuity and coordination of care. More recently, there is a focus in health care systems to provide patient-centered care or patient and family–centered care, which relies on care being collaborative, holistic, and responsive (Sidani et al., 2014), and AG-ACNPs are prepared to provide this focus.

Although there has been much evidence and support for collaborative practice between nurses and physicians, barriers still exist. Unfortunately, these barriers are created between those for whom collaborative practice should be the focus—other nurses and physicians. However, there is growing recognition that the AG-ACNP role promotes a collaborative model of care (D'Agostino & Halpern, 2010; Kleinpell, Buchman, & Boyle, 2012).

Ethical Decision Making

Ethical decision making in practice comprises another core competency. AG-ACNPs often act as advocates for patients in care dilemmas. Because AG-ACNPs are often involved in planning and implementing end-of-life care, ethical decision-making skills are an essential component of AG-ACNP practice (AACN, 2012; American Association of Critical-Care Nurses, 2012, 2017). In helping facilitate ethical decision making, AG-ACNPs can be instrumental in resolving moral issues and building ethical practice environments (see Chapter 13).

Shaping the Scope of Practice for the Adult-Gerontology ACNP

The scope of AG-ACNP practice is influenced from five levels: national (professional organizations), state (government), local (health care institution), service-related, and individual. In common with other APRNs, the AG-ACNP's scope of practice is broadly set forth in statements by professional nursing organizations. State governments, as regulatory agencies, further delineate the scope of practice in statutes such as nurse practice acts or title protection statutes. Because AG-ACNPs frequently provide their services within hospitals, subacute care facilities, nursing homes, and clinics, their scope may be defined further by policies within these institutions, organizations, and health care entities and even by the needs of a clinically specialized patient population. Finally, individual AG-ACNPs will further define the scope of their practice based on their own talents, strengths, and attributes. How AG-ACNP practice is configured at each of these levels is described in the following sections.

National Level (Professional Organizations)

At the national level, the scope of AG-ACNP practice is influenced by the following: the *AACN Scope and Standards for Acute Care Nurse Practitioner Practice* (American Association of Critical-Care Nurses, 2012 [being revised at time of press]), which describes expert AG-ACNP role performance; the *Adult-Gerontology Acute Care Nurse Practitioner Competencies* for entry into practice (AACN, 2012); and the Nurse Practitioner Core Competencies (NONPF, 2011b, 2014, 2017).

The *AACN Scope and Standards for Acute Care Nurse Practitioner Practice* was initially developed jointly by the American Nurses Association and American Association of Critical-Care Nurses in 1995 and later revised by the American Association of Critical-Care Nurses in 2012 to reflect the focus on AG-ACNP practice, as well as the pediatric ACNP (American Association of Critical-Care Nurses, 2012). It is intended to describe the scope of practice and standards of clinical and professional performance of the *expert* AG-ACNP. The population for which the AG-ACNP provides care includes acutely and critically ill patients experiencing episodic illness, stable and/or progressive chronic illness, acute exacerbation of chronic illness, or terminal illness.

The AG-ACNP's focus is the provision of curative, rehabilitative, palliative, and maintenance care. Short-term goals include stabilizing the patient for acute and life-threatening conditions, minimizing or preventing complications, attending to comorbidities, and promoting physical and psychologic well-being. Long-term goals include restoring the patient's maximum health potential, providing palliative and end-of-life care, and evaluating risk factors in achieving these outcomes. The practice environment for the AG-ACNP is identified as any inpatient or outpatient setting in which the patient requires complex monitoring and therapies and high-intensity nursing interventions or continuous vigilance within the range of high-acuity care (American Association of Critical-Care Nurses, 2012, 2017). Examples include acute and critical care environments, emergency care, and procedural and interventional settings. This continuum of health care services spans the geographic settings of home, ambulatory care, urgent care, long-term acute care, rehabilitative care, and hospice and/or palliative care. The practice environment extends into the mobile environment and virtual locations such as the tele-intensive care unit and areas using telemedicine (American Association of Critical-Care Nurses, 2017 [in press]). The standards of clinical practice and standards of professional performance, along with measurement criteria examples for the *expert* AG-ACNP as specified in this document, are summarized in Box 16.2. These standards, which are closely aligned with the APRN core competencies in Chapter 3, describe a competent level of care and professional performance common to all AG-ACNPs regardless of setting, whereby the quality of *expert* AG-ACNP practice can be judged. Some common themes in the standards of AG-ACNP clinical practice and professional performance that distinguish the practice of AG-ACNPs from other NP specialties are the dynamic nature of the patient's health and illness status, vulnerability of the patient population, need for continuous assessment and adjustment of the management plan in the face of rapidly changing patient conditions, and complexity of the required monitoring and therapeutics. Additional themes include the collaborative nature of the practice and interactive relationship between the AG-ACNP and the health care system.

While the American Association of Critical-Care Nurses document delineates competencies for the *expert* AG-ACNP clinician, two educational organizations—the AACN and the NONPF—have collaborated to define in their document *Adult-Gerontology Acute Care Nurse Practitioner Competencies* (AACN,

BOX 16.2   Standards of Clinical Practice and Professional Performance for the Expert Acute Care Nurse Practitioner

Standards of Clinical Practice

Standard I: Advanced Assessment

The acute care nurse practitioner elicits relevant data and information concerning patients with acute, critical, and/or complex chronic illness or injury.

Standard II: Differential Diagnosis

The acute care nurse practitioner independently analyzes and synthesizes the assessment data in determining differential diagnoses for the patient with acute, critical, and/or complex chronic illness or injury.

Standard III: Outcome Identification

The acute care nurse practitioner identifies individualized goals and outcomes for the patient who has acute, critical, and/or complex chronic illness or injury.

Standard IV: Care Planning and Management

The acute care nurse practitioner develops an outcome-focused plan of care that prescribes interventions for the patient with acute, critical, and/or complex chronic illness.

Standard V: Implementation of Interventions

The acute care nurse practitioner implements the interventions identified in the interprofessional plan of care for the patient with acute, critical, and/or complex chronic illness or injury.

Standard VI: Evaluation

The acute care nurse practitioner evaluates the patient's progress toward the attainment of goals and outcomes.

Standards of Professional Performance

Standard I: Professional Practice

The acute care nurse practitioner evaluates his or her clinical practice in relation to institutional guidelines, professional practice standards, and relevant statutes and regulations.

Standard II: Education

The acute care nurse practitioner maintains current knowledge of best practices.

Standard III: Collaboration

The acute care nurse practitioner collaborates with the patient, family, and members of the interprofessional team across the continuum of care.

Standard IV: Ethics

The acute care nurse practitioner integrates ethical considerations into all areas of practice congruent with patient and family needs and values and the ANA Code of Ethics.

Standard V: Systems Thinking

The acute care nurse practitioner engages in organizational systems and processes to promote optimal patient outcomes.

Standard VI: Resource Utilization

The acute care nurse practitioner incorporates evidence-based diagnostic strategies, therapies, and complementary health alternatives to achieve optimal fiscally responsible outomes.

Standard VII: Leadership

The acute care nurse practitioner leads in the practice setting and the profession.

Standard VIII: Collegiality

The acute care nurse practitioner promotes a respect for colleagues and the interprofessional team through the implementation of standards supporting a healthy work environment.

Standard IX: Quality of Practice

The acute care nurse practitioner evaluates and enhances the quality, safety, and effectiveness of care delivery across the continuum of acute care services.

Standard X: Clinical Inquiry

The acute care nurse practitioner enhances knowledge, attitudes, and skills through participation in research, translation of scientific evidence, and promotion of evidence-based practice.

Adapted from American Association of Critical-Care Nurses. (2012 and 2017). *AACN scope and standards for acute care nurse practitioner practice.* Aliso Viejo, CA: Author.

2012) those minimum competencies necessary for safe *entry into AG-ACNP practice.* As such, they provide guidance to educational programs preparing AG-ACNPs (AACN, 2012). Built on generic role competencies for nurse practitioners (NONPF 2011b, 2014), the entry-level competencies delineate the population-specific AG-ACNP competencies (Box 16.3) for (1) health promotion, health protection, disease prevention, and treatment; (2) NP-patient relationship;

(3) teaching-coaching function; (4) professional role; (5) managing and negotiating health care delivery systems; and (6) monitoring and ensuring the quality of health care practice.

Finally, a resource that does not define scope of practice but does specify the knowledge and skills necessary to perform within the specialty scope is the AG-ACNP national certification examinations. APRN specialty certification serves as a primary

BOX 16.3   Adult-Gerontology Acute Care Nurse Practitioner (AG-ACNP) Competencies at Entry to Practice

I.   Health Promotion, Health Protection, Disease Prevention, and Treatment

A.   Assessment of Health Status

These competencies describe the role of the AG-ACNP in terms of assessing the individual's health status, including assessment of the health promotion, health protection, and disease prevention needs of the acute, critical, and chronically ill or injured patient. Activities include risk stratification; disease-specific screening activities; diagnosis, treatment and follow-up of acute illness; and appropriate referral to specialty care.

B.   Diagnosis of Health Status

The AG-ACNP is engaged in the diagnosis of health status in patients with physiologic instability or the potential to experience rapid physiologic deterioration or life-threatening instability. This diagnostic process includes critical thinking, differential diagnosis, and the identification, prioritization, interpretation, and synthesis of data from a variety of sources. These competencies describe the role of the AG-ACNP related to the diagnosis of health status.

C.   Plan of Care and Implementation of Treatment

The objectives of planning and implementing therapeutic interventions are to return the individual to stability and optimize the individual's health. These competencies describe the AG-ACNP's role in stabilizing the individual, minimizing physical and psychologic complications, maximizing the individual's health potential, and assisting with palliative and end-of-life care management.

II.   Nurse Practitioner-Patient Relationship

Competencies in this area demonstrate the nurse practitioner–patient collaborative approach, which enhances the AG-ACNP's effectiveness of care. The competencies speak to the critical importance of the interpersonal transaction as it relates to therapeutic patient outcomes considering the cognitive, developmental, physical, mental, and behavioral health status of the patient across the adult life span.

III.   Teaching-Coaching Function

These competencies describe the AG-ACNP's ability to impart knowledge and associated psychomotor and coping skills to individuals, family, and other caregivers. The coaching function involves the skills of interpreting and individualizing therapies through the activities of advocacy, modeling, and teaching.

IV.   Professional Role

These competencies describe the varied role of the AG-ACNP, specifically related to advancing the profession and enhancing direct care and management. The AG-ACNP demonstrates a commitment to the implementation and evolution of the AG-ACNP role. Also, the AG-ACNP implements clinical reasoning and builds collaborative intra- and interprofessional relationships to provide optimal care to patients with complex acute, critical, and chronic illness. The AG-ACNP advocates on behalf of the patient population and profession through active participation in the health policy process.

V.   Managing and Negotiating Health Care Delivery Systems

These competencies describe the AG-ACNP role in achieving improved health outcomes for individuals, communities, and systems by overseeing and directing the delivery of clinical services within an integrated system of health care. In addition, the AG-ACNP addresses the development and implementation of system policies affecting services.

VI.   Monitoring and Ensuring the Quality of Health Care Practice

These competencies describe the AG-ACNP role in ensuring quality of care through consultation, collaboration, continuing education, certification, and evaluation. The monitoring function of the role is also addressed relative to examining and improving one's own practice and engaging in interdisciplinary peer and colleague reviews.

Adapted from American Association of Colleges of Nursing. (2012). *Adult-gerontology acute care nurse practitioner competencies.* Washington, DC: Author.

criterion for APRN practice (see Chapter 22). In addition, Medicare regulations stipulate completion of a national certification examination as a requirement for AG-ACNPs to obtain reimbursement. AG-ACNP certification examinations are offered by the American Nurses Credentialing Center (ANCC, 2016) and the American Association of Critical-Care

Nurses (2015). Although it is evident that the content of a certification examination should not drive educational standards or curriculum development, the topics and content for the AG-ACNP certification examinations have been validated by role delineation studies and are consistent with the other documents delineating AG-ACNP practice scope (ANCC, 2012).

As such, they serve to further articulate the scope of AG-ACNP practice.

State Level (Government)

Each state's government provides the second mechanism whereby the AG-ACNP's professional scope of practice is defined. The nurse practice statute for each state governs nursing practice. Practice rules and regulations that are intended to define NP practice vary from state to state (Kleinpell, Hudspeth, Scordo, & Magdic, 2012; NONPF, 2012b).

In all states, APRN regulation for practice is based on basic nursing licensure, but many states have additional rules and regulations that delineate specific requirements and define and limit who can use a specific advanced practice nursing title with protection (see Chapter 22). Although at the state level it is relatively easy to define limitations in scope of practice based on the age of the patient population, it is somewhat more difficult to determine scope based on patient acuity and practice setting, which have an impact on population focus (Kleinpell, Hudspeth, et al., 2012; NONPF, 2012b). Nevertheless, more state boards of nursing are taking a stronger stance to assure that NP scope of practice at state levels is defined in ways consistent with the APRN Consensus Model, particularly in differentiation between primary and acute care (Blackwell & Neff, 2015). This is of particular importance in ensuring that AG-primary care NPs and AG-ACNPs, as well as primary care PNPs and PNP-ACs, are caring for the population for which their education has prepared them. States are bound to do so in order to ensure the public safety of their citizens (Blackwell & Neff, 2015).

Institutional Level

As noted, most AG-ACNPs provide care in health care institutions, which may further delineate the institutional AG-ACNP scope of practice by identifying the subpopulation (specialty population) that the AG-ACNP serves and the process and requirements for collaboration with other health care providers in the institution (Kleinpell, Hudspeth, et al., 2012; Magdic, Hravnak, & McCartney, 2005). Further specification of the AG-ACNP's practice scope may be in job descriptions, in hospital policy, or through the institutional credentialing and privileging process.

Employers and hospitals have the right to define a specific health care provider's scope of practice within the employment situation. Documentation of initial training and ongoing provider competence in the application of specific skills is needed. This scope of employment may not exceed the scope of practice specified by the state's nurse practice act, but it may curtail the AG-ACNP's scope of practice based on the needs and mission of the employer. The institutional scope of employment may take the form of a job description, hospital policy, or both. In general, the job description should include AG-ACNP performance standards and responsibilities as they relate to patient care, collaborative relationships, professional conduct, and professional development; these institutional performance standards can provide a template for AG-ACNP performance evaluation.

When providing care within a health care institution, the AG-ACNP will also undergo the process of provider credentialing and privileging by the institution, whether she or he is an employee of the hospital or of a hospital-affiliated or private practice plan (see Chapter 22). For credentialing, the AG-ACNP is required to provide proof of licensure, certification, educational preparation, (typically) malpractice insurance, and skill performance (training, numbers of procedures performed, proof of competence). Institutional credentialing is necessary for the AG-ACNP to provide care to patients within the institution, although the AG-ACNP may or may not hold a medical staff appointment.

Once an individual is credentialed, a determination is made regarding the clinical privileges that may be granted; this is the process whereby the institution determines which medical procedures may be performed and which conditions may be treated by physician and nonphysician providers (Magdic et al., 2005). Although an appropriately educated provider may be permitted by statute to perform certain acts or skills, the hospital is not required to grant the provider this privilege. The clinical privileges of the AG-ACNP are based partly on the AG-ACNP's professional license, certification, and inherent scope of practice as well as documented training, experience, competence, and health status. For example, the AG-ACNP who has received educational preparation for performing invasive diagnostic procedures (e.g., insertion of central line catheters, endotracheal intubation) may request that these privileges be a part of his or her institutional scope of practice if he or she can provide proof of training and competency along with documentation that the skill is required for the job. An AG-ACNP may periodically request new privileges based on evolving mastery of skills, further training, and changes in services needed by the patient population and institution. AG-ACNPs must understand that although they may be qualified to perform certain procedures, privileges to perform these acts may not necessarily be granted or renewed (usually on a biannual basis) if the patient population that the AG-ACNP currently serves does not require these skills or if ongoing application and competency in the skill during the renewal period cannot be documented. A number of specific institutional examples of AG-ACNP role development, including discussion of formal orientation programs, are available that further outline considerations for competency assessment, credentialing and privileging considerations, and ongoing professional practice evaluation (Bahouth & Esposito-Herr, 2009; D'Agostino & Halpern, 2010; Farley & Lathan, 2011; Foster, 2012; Goldschmidt, Rust, Torowicz, & Kolb, 2011; Kapu et al., 2012; Kilpatrick et al., 2010; Kirton et al., 2007; Pascual et al., 2011; Shimabukuro, 2011).

Service-Related Level

AG-ACNP functions are also adjusted according to the needs of the specialty patient population served or the care delivery team (i.e., service) in the organization. This may be inpatient or outpatient based. This service-related scope of practice outlines the clinical functions and tasks that may be administered by the AG-ACNP specific to the service team with which the AG-ACNP works and the needs of the specialty patient population served. Examples of service-related functions include:

- An AG-ACNP working with a cardiology service may initiate treatment for myocardial ischemia or infarction.
- An AG-ACNP working in a pulmonary hypertension clinic may see patients on a regular basis to assess response to vasodilator therapy.
- An AG-ACNP working with an oncology service may perform bone marrow aspirations or order antibiotics for a suspected opportunistic infection.
- An AG-ACNP on a renal medicine service may write orders for hemodialysis and insert central venous dialysis catheters.
- An AG-ACNP with the cardiovascular surgery service may harvest the vein grafts for coronary artery bypass surgery.
- An AG-ACNP in the medical ICU may intubate and place arterial and central venous catheters.

Therefore service-related scope of practice may vary among AG-ACNPs affiliated with various services or specialties within the same institution and even among those who function under the same generic job description. The service-related scope of practice outlines a more detailed and specific description of the types of activities that the AG-ACNP will perform as a member of the practice.

Though an increasing number of state practice acts no longer require formal or written collaborative agreements, in states in which physician collaboration is a requirement or in cases in which the health care organization has collaborative guidelines, the AG-ACNP's institutional and service-related scope of practice and clinical privileges may be determined collaboratively by the physician and AG-ACNP and set forth in a written agreement. This written agreement for collaborative practice then provides the source document on which the hospital makes privileging decisions (see Chapter 22). Written agreements, often formatted as a checklist, are frequently helpful because the detail included in a written agreement cannot be spelled out in a job description. The agreement might also specify the level of communication or degree of supervision between the AG-ACNP and physician that is required before the performance of a specific function (D'Agostino & Halpern, 2010; Kleinpell, Buchman, et al., 2012). For example, an AG-ACNP with novice skills in central line insertion may require direct supervision for a specified period of time or number of successful attempts but, as the AG-ACNP approaches expert status, the level of supervision may be decreased to minimal or none. Eventually, as the AG-ACNP's expertise continues to advance, she or he may supervise medical trainees or novice AG-ACNPs in these skills. As skills progress, the written agreement, if required, will also need to be modified. In some cases, the written agreement may be used to communicate the AG-ACNP's scope of employment to other members of the health care team such as staff nurses and pharmacists.

When negotiating the written agreement, the AG-ACNP must ensure that no function conflicts with the state's nurse practice act or institutional policies. Nevertheless, the agreement should not be a barrier to practice but be written as broadly as reasonable to allow for practicality, flexibility, and optimization of practice within the context of experience and safety.

Individual Level

The final determinant of scope of practice is role individualization by each AG-ACNP. Experience, specialization, interest, motivation, self-esteem, personal ethics, personality traits, and communication style affect the employment opportunities, clinical specialties, skills, practice arrangements, and degree of autonomy that the AG-ACNP will seek out and/or apply in her or his uniquely personal enactment of the role (Kapu et al., 2012). AG-ACNPs are encouraged to engage in self-reflection and performance appraisal, as well as evaluate their own practice against identified benchmarks, in order to continually assess and improve individual knowledge and skills (AACN, 2012). In addition, AG-ACNPs are encouraged, as they move along the continuum from novice to expert, to be aware of patient care situations that exceed their current skill set and seek advice or assistance to ensure patient safety.

Profiles of the Adult-Gerontology ACNP Role and Practice Models

Although most AG-ACNPs practice in acute and critical care settings, there are a variety of role implementation models in ever-expanding specialty area practice sites. One AG-ACNP role implementation model focuses on episodic management of patients in a single clinical specialty unit; one model follows a caseload of patients throughout their hospitalization or on providing specialty care such as rapid response team care; and one focuses on managing patients across the entire continuum of acute care services, from hospitalization to home.

The AG-ACNP model focusing on episodic care of patients on a specialty clinical inpatient unit provides the earliest model of AG-ACNP practice (Howie-Esquivel & Fontaine, 2006; Kleinpell & Hravnak, 2005). The AG-ACNP, in collaboration with a physician specialist, might manage the care of a patient admitted to a specialty inpatient unit with an acutely unstable medical or surgical condition.

Once the patient is stabilized, the patient is transferred to another clinical unit under the care of another provider. Under this model, AG-ACNPs confine their practice to episodic care at a defined level of acute care, permitting them to develop their skills and knowledge about specific conditions in a delineated setting (see Exemplar 16.1). The limitation of this model is that it does not allow for continuity of care across the continuum.

In a hospital caseload model, the AG-ACNP directly manages a caseload of patients throughout their entire hospitalization, providing individualized ongoing care with continuity to the patient and family. The goal in this model is to facilitate and coordinate a patient's hospital stay to provide high-quality, cost-effective care (Farley & Lathan, 2011; Kapu & Kleinpell, 2013; Kapu et al., 2012; Landsperger et al., 2011). In this model, the AG-ACNP will admit the patient to the hospital, complete the admission history and physical examination, assess the patient's initial clinical status, order and interpret diagnostic and therapeutic tests, perform procedures, evaluate and adjust the plan of care, and prepare the patient for discharge. The AG-ACNP will provide care continuously for patients as they move from high-acuity to lower acuity inpatient care units, facilitate patients' movement through the acute care system, and plan for and implement discharge. Exemplar 16.2 illustrates this model.

In a specialty care model, the AG-ACNP delivers comprehensive specialty care to a group of patients across the entire continuum of care services. For example, an AG-ACNP member of a heart failure care team may oversee patient management during hospitalization, provide postdischarge clinic follow-up, and ultimately manage home-based infusion therapy. The number of AG-ACNPs working in this

---

EXEMPLAR 16.2   **Adult-Gerontology Acute Care Nurse Practitioner (AG-ACNP) Practice in an Inpatient Specialty Service**

On the inpatient thoracic surgery service of a large university teaching hospital, patients are assigned to the AG-ACNP team, which manages the care of each patient throughout her or his hospital stay. The AG-ACNP team is responsible for seeing patients who have undergone elective thoracic surgery, from the immediate postoperative recovery phase until discharge (regardless of the hospital unit in which the patient is housed), as well as completing new patient consultations and following up on existing consults. The team is composed of a total of six full-time AG-ACNP positions and is

responsible for providing care 7 days a week, from 6:00 AM until 6:00 PM, when the service is signed out to night coverage, usually provided by a thoracic surgery fellow.

The day begins when Jennifer, who is the leader of the two-member AG-ACNP team for the day, receives a sign-out of patients from the thoracic surgery fellow covering the previous night. The fellow reports on the status of the patients on the inpatient census and also adds two new patients to the list who were admitted overnight. Jennifer and her AG-ACNP colleague each add one new patient to their existing census. Jennifer then reviews her 10 patients and begins to plan her day, prioritizing her tasks. A computer census is generated and she reviews the daily laboratory results, vital signs, intake and output, surgical drainage totals, weight, and current medication list for each patient.

Jennifer begins to see her patients, starting with the newly admitted patient from the previous night. She reviews this patient's data, reviews the history and physical (H&P) examination findings, and looks at the chest radiograph and admission laboratory results. She interviews and examines the patient, validating the H&P findings. This 74-year-old man, with a history of recent pneumonia, alcohol abuse, and non–insulin-dependent type 2 diabetes, was admitted with fever, cough, and shortness of breath and was found to have a right pleural effusion on chest radiograph. During the night, admission laboratory tests and blood and sputum cultures were obtained, and the patient was treated with antipyretics, broad-spectrum antibiotics, supplemental oxygen, and inhaled bronchodilators. An infectious disease consultation was placed for antibiotic therapy recommendations. Jennifer discusses her concern for empyema with the attending surgeon. She describes her plan for ordering a computed tomography (CT) scan to identify a loculated effusion and to guide chest tube insertion for appropriate drainage. She then returns to the patient to inform him of this plan. She describes the CT scan, explaining the reasons for doing the study as well as the rationale for possible insertion of a chest tube. After answering his questions, she communicates the plan of care to the bedside nurse. Next, she writes orders for the studies and carefully reviews the medications, adjusting as needed. She writes a progress note, then notifies the patient's primary care physician of the patient's admission and discusses the planned course of action. She also contacts the infectious disease team to discuss her initial plan for management with them.

Jennifer next turns her attention to two patients who are to be discharged. After examining the patients and reviewing their data, she writes discharge orders, completes necessary prescriptions, writes final progress notes, and dictates discharge summaries. In coordination with the bedside nurse, she identifies discharge teaching points and arranges postdischarge follow-up appointments with the thoracic surgeon. One patient, now post-esophagectomy, will require home enteral nutrition, so she also arranges for home care and nutrition infusion services.

Over the remainder of the morning, Jennifer sees the other seven patients in similar detail. One postoperative patient has new-onset atrial fibrillation with rapid ventricular response, a common complication after thoracic surgery. The patient requires electrolyte correction and heart rate control but becomes hypotensive and must be transferred to the surgical intensive care unit (SICU). Jennifer will continue to follow the patient in the SICU, but only peripherally, because the patient will be directly managed by the SICU intensivist team. Jennifer provides a verbal report to the accepting intensivist team. Jennifer completes progress notes on her other patients and follows up on the interventions she has ordered throughout the day. She also evaluates patients on the monitored step-down unit for transfer to a nonmonitored unit, but she continues to follow the patients as they move through the system.

During the day, Jennifer has fielded multiple calls regarding patient needs, as well as new admissions to the service, and she has assigned the new admissions to herself or her colleague accordingly. An H&P is completed and dictated on each newly admitted patient, admission orders are written, and a plan of action is coordinated with the attending physician. Jennifer has collaborated with the other AG-ACNP team member who is stationed in the postanesthesia care unit in the afternoon and is coordinating the transfer of new surgical patients to the postprocedure unit or SICU after their elective procedures.

At the end of the day, both AG-ACNPs complete a sign-out to the night coverage fellow and a computer-generated census is completed for their reference. The AG-ACNP team updates an electronic database daily that tracks patient volumes, admissions and discharges, and case mix. The AG-ACNPs are also involved in precepting AG-ACNP students, providing formal lecturing and teaching, and enrolling patients in research protocols. ◎

---

type of model of care is increasing. Exemplar 16.3 illustrates this model with an AG-ACNP in a pulmonary practice who also bills for her services.

Diagnostic reasoning and advanced therapeutic interventions, consultation, and referral to other physicians, nurses, and providers are intrinsic components of this role, as described by the AG-ACNP scope of practice (American Association of Critical-Care Nurses, 2012, 2017). Although AG-ACNPs might require some variation in skills

| EXEMPLAR 16.3 | Adult-Gerontology Acute Care Nurse Practitioner (AG-ACNP) Practice Across the Continuum of Health Care Services |

A community-based pulmonary practice consists of three physicians and Suze, an AG-ACNP. Suze has been with the practice for 4 years. When she was hired, Suze applied for her Medicare national provider identifier (NPI) number, which she then assigned to the practice. This means that when Suze bills for her services, the bill is submitted under her number but payment is made to the practice. Suze's reimbursement rate is at 85% of the physician fee schedule, regardless of whether she bills in the office or in the hospital.

Each member of the practice sees patients in the office and the hospital on a rotating basis. During morning conference, Suze participates with the physicians in reviewing the schedule of that day's office appointments and list of inpatients who need to be followed. Suze sees those patients who have specialized needs relative to learning, treatment adherence, smoking cessation, and caregiver burden or unavailability. Although each one of them has his or her own daily office schedule of patients, the list of inpatients is divided between Suze and the physician assigned to cover inpatients for the week.

Today, Suze will follow up on 15 inpatients who have specialized needs relative to learning, treatment adherence, smoking examination findings, chest radiograph, and additional diagnostic results. For each of these follow-up visits, she first interviews the patient to confirm and gain additional historical information and then conducts a physical examination. As an example, she sees a 55-year-old man admitted for exacerbation of his chronic obstructive pulmonary disease (COPD) and possible pneumonia. He was treated overnight with broad-spectrum antibiotics, intravenous steroids, oxygen, and a nebulizer and is currently less dyspneic. Suze discusses with the pulmonologist her plan to order a chest computed tomography (CT) scan because this is the patient's third COPD exacerbation in the past 8 weeks. She is concerned that an underlying condition may be causing the exacerbations. In addition, knowing that he is a current cigarette smoker, she adjusts the antibiotic therapy regimen to cover organisms more likely to occur in smokers. She discusses smoking cessation with the patient and they agree to collaborate on

developing a smoking cessation strategy at his first office appointment after hospital discharge. Suze and the pulmonologist review the case and treatment plan. He agrees and states that he will also look at the chest radiograph from the office computer but has no need to see the patient that day. Suze writes her progress note and additional orders. At the end of the day, Suze submits her bill for this inpatient under her NPI number to the office manager. Payment will be made to the practice at 85% of the physician fee schedule.

The following day, Suze sees this patient again. She interviews him, performs a physical examination, and reviews the laboratory results and the CT scan. She calls the pulmonologist to tell him that the CT scan is normal. The pulmonologist reviews the CT scan with Suze and visits the patient, asks a few questions related to symptoms, and listens to the patient's lung sounds. He agrees that the chest CT scan is negative; writes a note, which refers to Suze's note and opinion; and documents his history and physical examination findings and interpretation of the CT scan. Because Suze and the pulmonologist have each seen the patient and performed some part of the service, the total work is combined and Suze submits this day's bill as a shared visit under the physician's number. In this case, the practice will be paid at 100% of the physician fee schedule. Had the pulmonologist not seen the patient and performed and documented a part of the service, the bill would have been submitted only under Suze's NPI number.

The patient is discharged to home on his routine metered-dose inhalers, a steroid taper, and oral antibiotic. He returns in 2 weeks for a follow-up office appointment scheduled with Suze. Suze interviews the patient, who states that he is feeling much better; she performs a physical examination. She finds his lung sounds are much improved. They discuss smoking cessation and the patient agrees to set a stop smoking date. Suze writes a prescription for a drug to help reduce nicotine cravings and also writes refill prescriptions for his inhalers. She documents the events of the visit and later discusses the plan with the pulmonologist. Suze submits the bill under her own NPI number and the practice is reimbursed at 85% of the physician fee schedule. ◎

depending on the care model, strong commonalities exist. As with other APRN roles, all AG-ACNPs are proficient in advanced physical assessment, clinical decision making (diagnostic reasoning), ordering and interpreting laboratory studies and procedures, and

collaborating in the development and implementation of a treatment plan that includes prescribing medication. Using diagnostic reasoning, the AG-ACNP diagnoses the origin of a complex medical problem that develops in an acutely or critically ill patient (see Chapter 7). The skills inherent in effective diagnostic reasoning include the fundamental skills of the AG-ACNP role: history taking, physical examination skills, pattern recognition, ability to analyze and synthesize data, and ability to generate a working diagnosis. A number of factors affect the quality of diagnostic reasoning when applied to the acutely and critically ill, such as multisystem deterioration, hemodynamic instability, depressed level of consciousness, and unavailability of significant others to supply, corroborate, or supplement patient information. All these factors challenge the AG-ACNP's ability to diagnose an acutely or critically ill patient's ever-changing physical condition accurately and expeditiously.

Another inherent portion of the AG-ACNP practice profile is the performance of technical skills, as indicated earlier. Patient needs within a specialty practice ultimately influence the type and level of therapeutic and diagnostic psychomotor skills that an individual AG-ACNP performs (Kapu et al., 2012; Kleinpell & Goolsby, 2012). The AG-ACNP role is one of evidence-based practice, which should be evident in clinical decision making and intervention selection.

As AG-ACNP education increasingly transitions to DNP preparation, emphasis on promoting evidence-based practice for patients with acute, critical, and complex chronic illness and the use of information systems and technology for improving health care, as well as leadership opportunities focused on systems change, quality improvement, and translating research into clinical practice changes, will bring new challenges for the role of AG-ACNPs and the models in which they function.

Comparison With Other Advanced Practice Nurse and Physician Assistant Roles

The AG-ACNP role differs from other APRN roles with regard to the type of patient care problems encountered, acuity of the patient's condition, need for rapid and continuous assessment, planning and intervention, and setting in which the care is delivered. For example, the clinical nurse specialist (CNS) enacts the APRN role through three spheres of influence (e.g., at the patient level in direct care, at the nurse level as with staff development, and at the organizational level, leading system changes to improve patient care). In comparison, the AG-ACNP uses clinical assessment skills to assess complex and acutely ill patients through health history taking, physical and mental status examination, performing

procedures, and risk appraisal for complications. Both the AG-ACNP and CNS roles target a patient-centered approach to care for patient populations, but the continuous on-unit presence of the AG-ACNP at the bedside often differentiates the role of the AG-ACNP from the CNS role, while staff education and development and system change responsibilities represent a larger percentage of the CNS's role. Conversely, CNSs do not generally carry out many of the procedures and interventions that characterize the AG-ACNP role. Although institutional variations in role implementation for CNSs and AG-ACNPs sometimes lack clear-cut differentiation in role responsibilities, it is acknowledged that the CNS and NP roles are different, with distinct practice foci (Becker, Kaplow, Muenzen, & Hartigan, 2006).

Table 16.2 can assist readers in conceptualizing where the main focus of AG-ACNP practice falls within the health care continuum and where there might be differences or overlap with the primary care NP role. The table presents examples of management strategies for common patient health care problems encountered in the traditional geographic primary, secondary, and tertiary health care settings. With diabetes care, for example, AG-ACNP practice predominantly involves strategies directed toward management of the patient during an acute exacerbation of the diabetes. Because of the severity of symptoms, the patient must be admitted to the hospital, where she or he can be continuously monitored and where management strategies may change from hour to hour (tertiary care). During this same hospitalization, the patient may need to have an infected foot ulcer treated with intravenous antibiotics (secondary care). Once the crisis is over, but while the patient is still hospitalized, the AG-ACNP may provide discharge teaching on routine foot care (primary care) as well as diabetic diet and glucose monitoring. At this point, the patient may be referred back to his or her primary care provider for further follow-up and management.

In comparison, the primary care NP's practice is predominantly directed toward management of the patient's diabetes when it is stable (primary care). This would include ongoing surveillance, guidance and coaching of the patient's self-management of the diabetes, education on diabetes risk factors, and assessment of signs of disease progression and complications. The primary care NP may also assess when the patient's diabetes is not well controlled and requires adjustment of insulin or oral hypoglycemic agents (secondary care). At the point when the patient is not responding or becomes acutely

TABLE 16.2   Patient Care Problems and Nurse Practitioner Management Interventions Traditionally Associated with Various Health Care Delivery Settings

Delivery Setting	Health Problem and Interventions		
	Diabetes	Hypertension	Pneumonia
Tertiary care management (ICU setting)	Diabetic ketoacidosis management Fluid replacement Electrolyte titration IV insulin	Continuous vasoactive drugs Arterial pressure monitoring Evaluation and management of possible CVA	Mechanical ventilation and artificial airway Pulmonary toilet Culture assessment Sepsis management Continuous monitoring
Secondary care management (inpatient unit)	Diabetic exacerbation management Sliding-scale insulin administration and monitoring Hydration Workup of cause(s)	Hypertensive crisis management Additional antihypertensives Adjunct therapy as needed	IV antibiotics Oxygen therapy Advanced assessment CXR, arterial blood gases, SpO₂
Primary care management (outpatient setting)	Initial Dx or stable management Oral antihyperglycemics or subcutaneous insulin Diet Prevention and assessment of associated complications Foot care Risk factor management	Diet Oral agents Lifestyle changes Prevention and assessment of associated complications Risk factor management	Oral or intramuscular antibiotics

CVA, Cerebrovascular accident; *CXR,* chest x-ray; *Dx,* diagnosis; *ICU,* intensive care unit; *IV,* intravenous; *Sp0₂,* peripheral arterial oxygen saturation.

ill, the primary care NP will recognize the need for the patient to be referred to a setting in which continuous monitoring and management is provided (tertiary care).

Using these examples helps educators and clinicians understand that there is a natural overlap in some areas of knowledge and practice between acute care and primary care NPs. However, each NP specialty also has its own distinct focus. The knowledge base and practice of the AG-ACNP cannot be limited only to unstable conditions requiring complex technologic diagnostic and management strategies for which the acutely or critically ill patient may be admitted to the hospital; the AG-ACNP also needs to be prepared to manage the range of health care problems that accompany the patient. This includes not only the acute illness or exacerbation of chronic illness that requires acute care services but also the patient's comorbidities, which also must be cared for while in the acute care setting. For example, the hospitalized diabetic patient discussed earlier may also have stable hypertension, stable asthma, osteoarthritis, and an acute episode of mild vaginitis. While the patient is hospitalized, the AG-ACNP must simultaneously attend to these stable comorbid health conditions to maintain their quiescence.

APRNs, including AG-ACNPs, are different from PAs. The PA role is under the jurisdiction of the physician's license. Some overlap exists between the AG-ACNP and PA in terms of the management of disease; however, the AG-ACNP's direct clinical practice competencies also provide for nursing's holistic perspective as well as the promotion and protection of health. Whereas PAs are trained in the medical model to focus on providing illness-based care to patients, AG-ACNPs, with their nursing background and practice, bring expertise in patient and family education, communication, collaboration, and health promotion and disease prevention for individuals and populations. A further differentiation is that AG-ACNP practice also incorporates additional APRN core competencies related to leadership and coaching. A growing number of facilities are integrating PA and AG-ACNP practitioners on hospital-based teams to manage care for hospitalized patients (Moote, Krsek, Kleinpell, & Todd, 2011).

Adult-Gerontology ACNPs and Physician Hospitalists

The hospitalist is an internal medicine physician responsible for managing the care of hospitalized patients. The physician hospitalist role is now being incorporated in many academic teaching centers and community settings, and the AG-ACNP has been added as a member of this team (Rosenthal & Guerrasio, 2009). Some AG-ACNPs function as members of the hospitalist team and manage patients independently or in collaboration collaboration with the physician hospitalist (Winne et al., 2012).

A primary care physician refers the patient to the hospitalist team for management during the acute care admission. The hospitalist team provides care for the patient during hospitalization and refers the patient back to the primary care provider at the time of discharge. The goal of this service is to provide seamless, cost-effective care. This can be an advantage for a primary care physician with busy office hours who may have limited time to make hospital visits and may not be sufficiently familiar with acute care management. The specific role of the AG-ACNP, as a member of the hospitalist team, is similar to the roles previously described, including obtaining an admission history and physical examination, performing daily physical examinations, making rounds with the physician, developing a treatment plan, reviewing laboratory studies and radiographs, and performing procedures. Furthermore, coordinating patient care management when many consultants are involved in decision making is a significant part of the role, as is consultation with the case managers to facilitate discharge planning effectively (Cowan et al., 2006). Exemplar 16.4 illustrates the model of an AG-ACNP serving on a hospitalist service.

Adult-Gerontology ACNP Practice Models

As described previously, the AG-ACNP role can be enacted in service-based, unit-based, or specialty-based practice. Each of these roles comprises different practice models for the AG-ACNP. The exemplars in this chapter further provide descriptions of these practice models. Other practice models involve physician/APP team-based care, often provided in 24 hours, 7 days a week (24/7) coverage models of care. As more ICU settings adopt a 24/7 model of care, in part to meet workforce demands due to a decrease in resident coverage, the AG-ACNP is now an acknowledged component of such models in the ICU (Garland & Gershengorn, 2013; Ward et al., 2013). The impact of AG-ACNP team-based practice models can be further delineated. Several studies have demonstrated the impact of AG-ACNP team-based models of care provided on a 24/7 basis,

validating that AG-ACNP team-based care is similar to care provided by medical teams (Collins et al., 2014; Costa, Wallace, Barnato, & Kahn, 2014; Gershengorn, Johnson, & Factor, 2012; Landsperger et al., 2015; McCarthy et al., 2013). Differences exist, however, in the specific roles and functions of AG-ACNP practice in different models of care, including differences in provider-to-patient ratios (Kleinpell, Ward, et al., 2015).

Outcome Studies Related to ACNP Practice

Measuring practice outcomes (see Chapter 23) is a component of establishing the value of any APRN role (Newhouse et al., 2011). Positive outcomes of AG-ACNP care have been demonstrated in a number of settings, including emergency care (Li, Westbrook, Callen, Gregiou, & Braithwaite, 2013), inpatient medical services, geriatric inpatient care, cardiovascular care (David et al., 2015; Kleinpell, Avitall, et al., 2015), trauma care (Collins et al., 2014; Morris et al., 2012), intensive care (Costa et al., 2014; Gershengorn et al., 2012; Kapu et al., 2012; D'Agostino & Halpern, 2010; Farley & Lathan, 2011; Fleming & Carberry, 2011; Landsperger et al., 2015; Moote et al., 2011; Shimabukuro, 2011; Sonday & Grecsek, 2010; Yarema & Judy, 2011), and oncology and palliative care (Hutchinson, East, Stasa, & Jackson, 2014; Kilpatrick et al., 2014), and as rapid response team leaders (Barocas et al., 2014; Kapu, Wheeler, et al., 2014; Sonday & Grecsek, 2010). These demonstrated positive outcomes of AG-ACNP care include decreased costs, shorter hospital lengths of stay, decreased rates of hospital readmission, decreased emergency room admissions, decreased use of laboratory tests, lower rates of urinary tract infections and skin breakdown, time savings for house physicians, similar care outcomes compared with physician practices, patient and family satisfaction, and an increased role in discussing patient outcomes with nurses and families.

Although these studies exploring AG-ACNP effectiveness have been conducted in several types of care settings, continued research on the impact of AG-ACNP practice is needed. Most studies on the use and outcomes of AG-ACNPs have focused on comparing AG-ACNP care with physician care, reducing costs, or the impact of AG-ACNP care on a focused area of care (Kleinpell, Hanson, & Buchner, 2008). However, more research would be helpful. Because ACNPs are practicing in a number of different roles that span the trajectory of acute and critical illness—across the inpatient ICU to the

Adult-Gerontology Acute Care Nurse Practitioner (AG-ACNP) Practice on a Hospitalist Team

John is one of three nurse practitioners (NPs) working on a hospitalist team at a community hospital. He is prepared as an AG-ACNP and his colleagues are prepared as adult NPs. They work with a 10-member hospitalist team to provide care to hospitalized patients. The hospitalist service is the primary admitting service for the hospital and provides medical inpatient consultations. John's role consists of managing a group of patients, following up on newly admitted patients, performing a history and physical examination for new admits, discharging patients, and responding to consultation requests. Consultations vary from medical comanagement of surgical patients to the evaluation of acute condition changes and follow-up of diagnostic tests. Condition changes can vary from alterations in vital signs to onset or worsening of symptoms such as nausea, vomiting, shortness of breath, or chest pain, and laboratory results may require further follow-up for possible changes to the treatment plan (e.g., supplemental potassium).

Because he is prepared as an AG-ACNP, John is also called for consultations in the intensive care unit (ICU) or to evaluate patients who might need transfer to the ICU, and he works in collaboration with intensivists to manage acute changes in ICU patients. In addition to serving on the code team, he is a member of the hospital's rapid response team and may be called to further evaluate a patient who has had an acute change in condition anywhere in the hospital.

John will see patients independently but has a hospitalist physician in house with whom he can further consult for patient care management issues, including generating differential diagnoses, evaluating different treatment options, and discussing care progression in outliers. Often, patients are discussed among the entire team, using the expertise of each member on the hospitalist team.

Other roles of the hospitalist NP include providing patient status updates to family members, explaining the plan of care to clinical nurses, reporting the status of a hospitalized patient to the patient's primary care physician (improving transitions of care communication), planning goals of care for patients being discharged, transferring patients for rehabilitation, ensuring documentation and reporting of core measures (e.g., pneumonia, venous thromboembolism prophylaxis), implementing patient satisfaction activities, planning advance directive care, incorporating integrative and complementary therapies (e.g., acupuncture, healing touch, stress reduction interventions), and coordinating care across the spectrum of consultants who are treating the patient.

Working as a hospitalist AG-ACNP requires John to keep current with requirements for documentation and billing, focused professional practice evaluation (FPPE), and ongoing professional practice evaluation (OPPE). He finds that attending the annual national NP conference and the national hospital medicine conference provides him with essential updates for his practice as well as valuable continuing education. He has negotiated with the hospitalist group to cover travel, registration, hotel costs, and paid time off for these annual conferences. Most recently, John submitted an abstract to present at the national NP conference to speak about the role of the NP on the hospitalist team.

John currently serves on the advanced practice committee for the institution, which reviews the applications for medical staff appointment of advanced practice providers. He also serves on the acute and critical care quality committee, which meets monthly to review quality data such as infection rates and development of acute care protocols.

Although several physician assistants also serve on the hospitalist team, John's role is different in that in addition to managing patient care, he is also involved in several performance improvement initiatives. As an APRN, John brings a strong performance and quality improvement perspective to the team, often identifying opportunities to improve care and care delivery, examining possible solutions, and generating consensus among the interprofessional team. One recent initiative targeted the reduction of unplanned readmissions for heart failure patients at risk for rehospitalization within 30 days by initiating a discharge clinic that will be run by the hospitalist NPs. Building on their educational preparation, AG-ACNPs also promote, mentor, and facilitate evidence-based practice by identifying clinical issues, critically examining the literature, and disseminating findings to improve EBP, minimize variances among providers, and evaluate clinical and administrative outcomes related to practice changes.

As an AG-ACNP on a hospitalist team, John enjoys the flexibility of the role because he is involved in direct patient care management. He also serves in advanced practice consultation roles for committee work for implementing FPPE and OPPE practice standards and for developing NP-run initiatives such as the discharge clinic for heart failure patients. John's role represents a growing opportunity for AG-ACNPs as hospitals develop and expand hospitalist services to assist in the management of hospitalized patients. ◎

hospitalist team, to the post–acute care area, and on to rehabilitation, and with specialty services such as cardiac arrest, rapid response, and critical care transport teams, among others—research is needed to delineate the impact of ACNP practice in these broader and less geographically circumscribed areas. More research delineating AG-ACNP practice impact across the full spectrum of acute care services, or in more than a single center, might be helpful to improve generalizability of results. Also, research examining the impact of doctoral preparation would be helpful to support any added benefit to the profession, to patients, and to employers of AG-ACNPs. If AG-ACNPs are to delineate the impact of their care and justify their existence, it is imperative that their worth be supported by careful research (see Chapter 23).

Specialization Opportunities Within the Adult-Gerontology ACNP Role

As mentioned previously, the AG-ACNP might participate as a member of a specific clinical specialty or consult service practicing in an acute care setting. Some examples of specialty service expansion are highlighted below.

Bone Marrow Transplantation Services

The AG-ACNP working as a member of the bone marrow transplantation service has an autonomous role while functioning as a part of a collaborative practice model; the team may be composed of a resident, fellow, attending physician, and AG-ACNP. The AG-ACNP provides continuity of care for the service by being the only consistent member of the academic health care team, in which physicians rotate between clinical and research activities. The AG-ACNP carries a caseload of patients and follows them through their hospital stay until discharge. Role responsibilities include carrying out preliminary daily rounds on each patient, performing physical examinations, interpreting laboratory tests (e.g., electrolytes, radiology studies), performing marrow aspirations, and consulting specialists (e.g., gastroenterology, infectious disease, pulmonary medicine) to assist in patient management. On the basis of the information gathered, the AG-ACNP collaborates with the other provider team members during daily rounds to develop the daily and long-term treatment plan. In addition, the AG-ACNP teaches the house and nursing staff and incorporates health teaching and health promotion and protection activities into her

or his practice, especially related to risks associated with immunosuppression.

Diagnostic and Interventional Services

In preadmission surgical services, the clinical functions of an AG-ACNP include history taking and physical examinations; performing preprocedure evaluations; providing patient and family education; obtaining and interpreting laboratory, electrocardiographic, and radiologic data; identifying at-risk individuals in need of preadmission discharge planning; initiating contacts with social services; discharge planning; and management recommendations for patients in the surgical holding area. The AG-ACNP consults with the anesthesiologist and surgeon regarding patient health problems that may affect or preclude anesthesia delivery or surgery. AG-ACNPs may provide similar services to patients in the cardiac catheterization suite or the gastrointestinal procedure laboratory. AG-ACNPs may not only support diagnostic and interventional services but may also perform some invasive diagnostic procedures (Duszak et al., 2015).

Heart Failure Services

On the heart failure service in a university medical center, a team of three AG-ACNPs may collaborate with each other and with physician team members to optimize continuity of care for their patients. Each AG-ACNP has a caseload of patients for whom he or she assumes responsibility in the outpatient area. They see each patient in clinic on a regular basis, examine patients, and adjust the treatment plan. They perform follow-up by phone contact on a weekly basis, helping patients assess their symptoms, follow daily weights, discuss dietary changes, and adjust oral medications as needed. Based on information gleaned in follow-up contacts, the AG-ACNP may have the patient come to the outpatient clinic for further clinical assessment and treatment (e.g., a dose of intravenous diuretic, adjustment of continuous inotropic medication infusions). Each AG-ACNP team member provides in-hospital coverage on a weekly rotating basis. When a patient requires admission to the hospital for an acute exacerbation of heart failure, one AG-ACNP, along with the physician, manages the hospitalized patient. They know the patient's problems and treatment plan, can provide continuity, have established a trusting relationship with the patient and care team, and readily facilitate discharge planning and follow-up care.

Orthopedic Services

The AG-ACNP working with patients with orthopedic problems covers a full spectrum of practice settings, including the emergency room, orthopedic clinic, and inpatient orthopedic service. The orthopedic AG-ACNP works closely with the attending physicians, staff nurses, and residents to coordinate care from preadmission testing to discharge. Each AG-ACNP carries a caseload of hospitalized patients and outpatients undergoing short procedures. The role may include perioperative management as first assistant in the operating room.

Critical Care Teams

An emerging AG-ACNP role is working as an active member and leader within interprofessional critical care teams. As a critical care expert, the "intensivist" AG-ACNP works closely with attending physician intensivists, critical care staff nurses, residents and fellows, pharmacists, respiratory and physical therapists, and dietitians to provide care to high-acuity patient populations (Kleinpell, Ward, et al., 2015; Squiers et al., 2013). Each AG-ACNP on the intensivist team will manage a caseload of patients, including a variety of patient acuities, new admissions, postoperative recoveries, and transfers. The AG-ACNP will perform selected invasive procedures such as central venous line insertion or chest tube insertion. The AG-ACNP may also lead the rapid response team or evaluate and manage unstable patients on stepdown units.

Rapid Response Teams

A more recent role for the AG-ACNP may be as team leader or team member of a hospital medical emergency or rapid response team. When hospitalized patients develop sudden physiologic instability outside of critical care areas, a mismatch between patient needs and available supportive resources occurs. Rapid response teams deploy personnel and other resources to meet patient needs in a crisis in any area of the hospital (Aleshire et al., 2012; Barocas et al., 2014; Kapu, Wheeler, et al., 2014; Scherr et al., 2012). These teams consist of multidisciplinary members such as AG-ACNPs, physicians, critical care nurses, respiratory therapists, and nursing supervisors. The team might be activated to respond to conditions such as hypotension, acute mental status changes, bleeding, respiratory distress, chest pain, or oliguria. The AG-ACNP may be

the team leader, coordinating the assessment, triage, and treatment plan, or he or she may participate as a team member enacting problem-focused response protocols, placing peripheral or central venous lines, assisting with airway management, and coordinating transfer to another level of care, if necessary (Barocas et al., 2014; Kapu, Wheeler, et al., 2014).

Supportive and Palliative Care

The AG-ACNP may serve on inpatient palliative care teams. Working with palliative care attending physicians and consulting services, the AG-ACNP may provide expert consultations, assessing and planning for patient palliative care needs (Fox, 2014). The AG-ACNP helps facilitate discussions of goals of care between the consulting service and the patient and family, in high-risk preoperative situations, or in situations involving the unstable critically ill patient. The inpatient palliative care AG-ACNP can also serve as a clinical resource for acute and critical care teams in planning and evaluating palliative care interventions or the de-escalation of care, in recommending comfort measures, and by facilitating transition from one level of care to another such as to an inpatient palliative care unit or hospice setting.

Preparation of Adult-Gerontology ACNPs

Education of NPs should be in one of the six population foci outlined in the APRN Consensus Model (APRN Joint Dialogue Group, 2008) and should prepare the student to sit for the certification examination consistent with the appropriate practice population. AG-ACNPs are registered nurses who are prepared at the master's or DNP level of graduate nursing education. All AG-ACNP programs should provide for program requirements as outlined in the Criteria for Evaluation of Nurse Practitioner Programs (NONPF, 2012a).

All AG-ACNP programs should build on either *The Essentials of Master's Education in Nursing* (AACN, 2011), or *The Essentials of Doctoral Education for Advanced Nursing Practice* (DNP Essentials) (AACN, 2006). The AG-ACNP curriculum incorporates the graduate core, advanced practice core, NP population curricula, and AG-ACNP specialty curricula. Programs that prepare AG-ACNPs at the DNP level do not negate the master's core but, rather, build on it (AACN, 2006). DNP curricula combine foundational or core competencies for all DNP program graduates as well as AG-ACNP specialty competencies for the practice doctorate, aligned with the Practice Doctorate Nurse Practitioner Entry-Level Competencies (National Panel for NP Practice Doctorate Competencies, 2006).

The AG-ACNP specialty content should focus on the knowledge and skills essential to diagnose and manage the episodic and chronic problems commonly experienced by adult patients with acute, critical, and complex chronic illness while performing health promotion and protection and disease prevention activities within the context of the continuum of the health care delivery system (AACN, 2012). As illustrated in the conceptual model of care services previously presented in Table 16.2, AG-ACNPs diagnose and manage not only the acute health problems associated with the patient's chief complaint but also quiescent, stable, and comorbid health conditions. Because AG-ACNPs must be prepared to manage health problems across the full continuum of acute health care services, their didactic information and clinical experiences should provide for this broad focus. Similarly, the program should provide didactic and clinical preparation in the NP competencies as delineated in the Adult-Gerontology Acute Care Nurse Practitioner Competencies (AACN, 2012), the *AACN Scope and Standards for Acute Care Nurse Practitioner Practice* (American Association of Critical-Care Nurses, 2012, 2017), and the *Nurse Practitioner Core Competencies* (NONPF, 2011b).

Teaching skills in screening and prevention specific to acute care practice are also essential. Because AG-ACNP graduates must be competent in critical incident management, clinical simulation and use of standardized patients are helpful strategies to facilitate translating knowledge to practice in AG-ACNP education (Hravnak, Beach, & Tuite, 2007; Pascual et al., 2011). More recently, interprofessional education models facilitate role definitions and assist AG-ACNP students to integrate into care teams (Corbridge, Tiffen, Carlucci, & Zar, 2013). Technical skills training is also commonly incorporated into AG-ACNP programs, as indicated in Table 16.1. The NONPF has published a skills manual to standardize the teaching of clinical skills in ACNP programs (Melander & Settles, 2011).

AG-ACNP education has been actively transitioning to the DNP preparation as entry into practice or as a post-master's program. DNP programs prepare graduates with the additional didactics and experiences to achieve the level of competence indicated in *The Essentials of Doctoral Education for Advanced Nursing Practice* (AACN, 2006). This expansion in direct practice abilities includes advanced communication (interpersonal and technologic), use of an expanded scientific foundation to provide an evidence basis for practice across settings, advanced participation, collaboration and leadership within the health care delivery system and the business of health care, and a focus on independent practice (NONPF, 2012b). The 2011 Institute of Medicine (IOM) *The Future of Nursing* report called for an increase in the number of doctorally prepared nurses, and the number of enrollees in DNP programs increased from 7034 in 2010 to 18,352 in 2015 (IOM, 2016). An example of the practice skills of an AG-ACNP who has received practice doctorate education is presented in Exemplar 16.5.

NPs who have been educated in another NP specialty but who are now caring for patients in the population focus specific for adult-gerontology acute care, and for which additional competencies and skills are required for the quality and safety of practice, must ensure that their educational preparation is consistent with this population focus (Kleinpell, Hudspeth, et al., 2012). Since neither certification nor licensure grants universal practice rights, it is important that NP practice be substantiated by the appropriate education. Individuals with master's preparation in another APRN specialty may enroll in an AG-ACNP post-master's or DNP completion program to ensure that they undergo didactic and supervised clinical practica to prepare adequately for caring for this unique and vulnerable patient population (Kleinpell, Hudspeth, et al., 2012). Employers are increasingly aligning with requiring AG-ACNP educational preparation as a mandate for practice with adults with complex acute, critical, and complex chronic health conditions, including the delivery of acute care services regardless of the geographic practice setting (Kleinpell, Hudspeth, et al., 2012), and as consistent with the state boards of nursing (NCSBN, 2008) and the IOM *The Future of Nursing* recommendations (IOM, 2011, 2016).

In spite of the recent efforts to standardize entry-levels standards for competence at the completion of AG-ACNP programs, there is still some variation in the quality of programs and the practice-readiness of graduates. Because of the complexity and vulnerability of the patient population, some health care systems have established onboarding programs and postgraduate residencies or fellowships to extend the practice supervision period and transition to practice (Bahouth et al., 2013; Schofield & McComiskey,

Adult-Gerontology Acute Care Nurse Practitioner (AG-ACNP) Role Implementation Following Doctor of Nursing Practice (DNP) Preparation

Joyce is a DNP-prepared AG-ACNP currently working in a nephrology practice. The practice consists of one AG-ACNP and five physicians. The practice is organized so that each provider has his or her own caseload of patients and follows these patients in the office and in the hospital. In addition, Joyce is responsible for one of the outpatient dialysis clinics, where she sees patients 3 times per week. This particular dialysis clinic is located in a neighborhood consisting mainly of Hispanics and African-Americans. Every month, members of the practice meet for breakfast to discuss issues related to patient care and the logistics of the practice. Her usual schedule consists of daily morning rounds on her hospitalized patients followed by afternoon office hours on Tuesdays and Thursdays and outpatient dialysis clinic patients on Mondays, Wednesdays, and Fridays.

To track her patients, Joyce uses an application on her Smartphone. As she makes her rounds, she enters the patient data and, at the end of the day, uploads the information into her office computer. Having patient data on a Smartphone or tablet allows Joyce to access patient information quickly when, for example, she admits a patient who was seen in the office a week ago but she herself was not in the office.

Recently, Joyce launched a new set of standard admission orders for patients admitted to the hospital with a diagnosis of chronic renal failure. Development of these standard orders resulted from a series of complications that occurred when new medical residents did not order the appropriate laboratory tests or all the routine medications used to treat renal failure. These complications resulted in increased hospital stays and costs. Joyce searched the literature to provide evidence to support orders that she believed were necessary and then collaborated with the medical staff, nurses, dietitian, pharmacist, and manager of the laboratory to develop this order set. Consensus was reached in 6 months and the orders were approved. Joyce then collaborated with the nursing staff to develop a quality improvement project that looked at whether these orders influenced patient outcomes positively.

In addition to seeing clinical patients, every third month Joyce sits on the credentialing and privileging committee at the hospital. She participates in the review of applicants to ensure that they are qualified to provide competent, safe patient care. Joyce's unique role is to provide peer review on the applications of NPs.

At the dialysis clinic, Joyce is the administrator and patient care provider. Physicians from the practice also provide patient care on a rotating basis and are available for consultation. The staff is composed of registered nurses, nursing assistants, and secretarial support. To maintain optimal patient care, Joyce has implemented policies and evidence-based procedures. A quality improvement committee, led by Joyce, periodically reviews charts for compliance with selected quality indicators. In addition, Joyce coordinates a bimonthly journal club for the clinic's staff as one mechanism to ensure that the staff members are current in their practice. Because of the clinic's location, Joyce sits on the local neighborhood board. Her goal is for the clinic to be a good neighbor. Joyce collaborates with the board members to provide culturally appropriate educational opportunities on topics such as hypertension and diabetes in an effort to reduce the incidence of renal failure in that community.

Joyce serves as adjunct faculty at the local university. She lectures to the AG-ACNP students on renal disease and also serves as a clinical preceptor for AG-ACNP students. In addition, she is a member of the AG-ACNP program's local advisory board, which meets annually. The purpose of this board is to provide consultation to the AG-ACNP faculty on ways to recruit and graduate outstanding students who can meet the needs of the community. At the last meeting, Joyce pointed out that students had poor recall of current guidelines related to the management of diabetes, a leading cause of renal disease. Joyce suggested ways to integrate this information into the curriculum. She pointed out that current guidelines on diabetes management can be found on diabetes professional organization websites and can be accessed through a Smartphone application for easy reference in the clinical area. ◎

2015). This serves to assure care delivery that is at local standards and mitigate institutional liability. Even once they are established in practice, the competence of the care delivered by AG-ACNPs working in entities credentialed by The Joint Commission will need to undergo both focused and ongoing professional practice evaluations, as is required for all licensed and credentialed providers (Hravnak, 2009; Makary, Wick, & Freischlag, 2011).

Reimbursement for Adult-Gerontology ACNPs

AG-ACNPs must be knowledgeable about billing and payment mechanisms for professional services and about policy issues that affect AG-ACNP reimbursement. Obtaining reimbursement for services provided by NPs continues to be a universal challenge for every NP specialty, particularly AG-ACNPs. Some of these challenges include securing admission to provider panels, determining whether a service is covered, billing for critical care time, and deciding which billing option to use: direct, "incident to," or shared (see Chapter 21). The complexities of how federal and state laws apply to specific practice situations can deter groups from fully utilizing AG-ACNPs (Buppert, 2015). In addition, how an AG-ACNP demonstrates financial productivity affects an employer's decision to hire and/or retain AG-ACNP providers.

Although there are many considerations as to which billing option to use, there are compelling reasons why AG-ACNPs should bill directly under their own provider number, including recognition of the AG-ACNP's financial worth as a result of produced income and tangible recognition of the AG-ACNP's professional standing, which in turn leads to professional satisfaction and peer recognition (Magdic, 2013). Direct reimbursement also brings visibility to the quantity and type of care for which an AG-ACNP is compensated. Visibility is accomplished through documentation and monitoring of billed services in the National Claims History file established by the Centers for Medicare & Medicaid Services (CMS, 2006; Magdic, 2013). Through evaluation of services billed by AG-ACNPs at the national level, an aggregate profile of AG-ACNP practice with respect to billable direct patient care activities can be developed (Magdic, 2013).

Almost every encounter between an AG-ACNP and a patient can be associated with a payor. The five major categories of payors, each with its own policies and legal structures, are Medicare, Medicaid, indemnity-type insurance, managed care organizations, and businesses that contract for certain services (Buppert, 2015; Sample, Britton, Brown, & Munro, 2014). Reimbursement for AG-ACNP services within the Medicare framework is a focus in this chapter. Although Medicare serves as the most common form of reimbursement of AG-ACNP services, other payors have their own unique variations. However, the AG-ACNP who understands Medicare regulations is better equipped to navigate the policies of other payors. New health policy changes in the Patient Protection and Affordable Care Act (2010) will bring new reimbursement configurations for AG-ACNPs. Detailed descriptions of third-party payors and related issues are described in Chapter 21.

When Medicare legislation was enacted in the 1960s, the regulations specified that NPs could receive direct reimbursement only when they provided care in certain geographic locations such as skilled nursing facilities and federally designated rural medically underserved areas. The 1997 Balanced Budget Act removed the geographic restrictions on the direct reimbursement option for NPs. However, there are still complex issues in regard to reimbursement and it is important that AG-ACNPs understand the rules surrounding the direct, "incident to," and shared billing options. Any or all of these options may be used by the AG-ACNP in certain situations.

Medicare Reimbursement for Adult-Gerontology ACNPs

Office and Nonhospital Clinic Setting

Although AG-ACNPs typically provide services to patients in hospital and hospital-affiliated offices and clinics, a portion of their practice may occur in a non–hospital affiliated setting, as described earlier in the discussion of AG-ACNP role implementation models. In the office setting, an AG-ACNP must decide whether to bill directly or "incident to" the physician. Direct billing means the AG-ACNP provides the evaluation and management (E/M) services and submits the bill under her or his own provider number. In this option, Medicare reimburses at 85% of the physician fee schedule. "Incident to" is the part of Medicare law providing for coverage of services and supplies furnished incident to the professional services of a physician. Deciding which option to use is often a business decision. More information regarding "incident to" billing can be found in Chapter 12 of the *Medicare Claims Processing Manual* (CMS, 2016) (see also Chapter 21).

A third option addresses cases in which the AG-ACNP and the physician share the E/M service in the outpatient setting in which the AG-ACNP performs a portion of an E/M encounter and the physician completes the E/M service. In this situation, the "incident to" requirements are met and the shared outpatient service should be billed under the physician's number. If the "incident to" requirements are not met, the shared outpatient service must be reported using the AG-ACNP's number. Of note, there is no "incident to" billing option for AG-ACNPs who provide services to patients in the hospital, emergency department, or hospital-affiliated clinics (CMS, 2016).

Hospital Inpatient, Hospital Outpatient, and Emergency Department Settings

Hospitals and emergency departments are common practice sites for AG-ACNPs, but billing for their services in these settings can be challenging (Magdic, 2013). Whether an AG-ACNP can bill for services delivered in the hospital is first dependent on whether the AG-ACNP's salary is listed on the hospital's Medicare cost report. If it is, then the AG-ACNP's services are already paid for under Medicare Part A. Transmittal 1168, issued by the CMS on January 26, 2007, updated the *Medicare Claims Processing Manual* regarding "Direct Billing and Payment for Non-Physician Practitioner Services Furnished to Hospital Inpatient and Outpatients" (CMS, 2007). According to this transmittal, payments for professional services of NPs (as well as CNSs and PAs) can be unbundled from the payment to the hospital for hospital services billed under the hospital's cost report. However, the hospital still bills the fiscal intermediary for the facility fee associated with NP, CNS, or PA services (Buppert, 2015). Direct payment for the AG-ACNP's professional services furnished to hospital inpatients and outpatients are made to the AG-ACNP at 85% of the physician fee schedule unless the AG-ACNP reassigns payment to the hospital (Buppert, 2015).

Shared billing is another option for AG-ACNPs in the hospital inpatient, outpatient, and emergency department settings (Magdic, 2013). High patient acuity in these areas fosters a close collaborative relationship with physicians, and it is not uncommon for both the AG-ACNP and physician to provide services to hospitalized patients on the same day. On October 25, 2002, CMS issued change request 2321, which updated the *Medicare Carriers Manual* §15501 guidelines for E/M services (CMS, 2002b). These guidelines were further clarified by Transmittal 178 in May 2004 (CMS, 2004) and provide direction for billing and reimbursement of E/M services provided by both the physician and AG-ACNP when they are in the same group practice and provide services on the same day, either at the same or different times. A shared visit in these circumstances means the physician has a face-to-face encounter with the patient, provides some portion of the E/M service, and provides supporting documentation which he or she links to the AG-ACNP's documentation. For shared billing between the AG-ACNP and

physician to occur, the AG-ACNP should be employed by the physician practice and have a contractual relationship with the physician or both should be employed by the same entity (CMS, 2004).

Key issues regarding shared E/M services are as follows (CMS, 2004):

- If the AG-ACNP provides a medically necessary service and there is no face-to-face encounter between the patient and physician, the service must be billed under the AG-ACNP's provider number. A physician simply reviewing the chart and creating or adding to a note does not constitute a face-to-face encounter.
- If both the AG-ACNP and physician provide portions of the E/M service on the same calendar day at the same or different times and there is a face-to-face encounter between the patient and physician, then the physician and AG-ACNP may combine their services and bill for a shared visit under the physician's or AG-ACNP's provider number at the level supported by their combined documentation.

The preceding discussion also applies to billing for AG-ACNP services provided within the hospital outpatient or emergency department. For more information regarding "incident to" and shared billing, refer to the CMS *Medicare Carriers Manual*—Part 3, Claims Process, Transmittal 1764 (CMS, 2002a) and Chapter 12, Section 30.6.4, of the *Medicare Claims Processing Manual* (CMS, 2016). An example of billing activities of an AGACNP in the inpatient setting is provided in Exemplar 16.3, which illustrates the billing practices of an AG-ACNP in a pulmonary specialty practice who sees patients in the hospital and office.

Critical Care Reimbursement for Adult-Gerontology ACNPs

Critical care involves high-complexity decision making to assess, manipulate, and support vital system functions, and requires extensive interpretation of a number of data sources and application of advanced technologies (CMS, 2016). Reimbursement for critical care services can occur in any location in which such services are performed, including ICUs, emergency departments, and general medical-surgical floors (CMS, 2016). Critical care services are billed using time-based Current Procedural Terminology (CPT) codes (Sample et al., 2014). The first 30 to 74 minutes of critical care services on a given calendar date are billed under one specific CPT code (99291). For each additional 30 minutes, a second CPT code is used (99292). A physician may not link to an AG-ACNP's note for either code. The AG-ACNP or the physician—but only one—may provide the initial 30 minutes of critical care time. For each additional 30 minutes, the service is billed by whomever provided the service (CMS, 2016). If the total time spent providing critical care services is less than 30 minutes, other E/M codes must be used (American Medical Association, 2016).

It is important to note that rapid changes in health care affecting Medicare, Medicaid, and private payers are occurring at the federal and state levels, especially with the introduction of the Patient Protection and Affordable Care Act in 2010. Readers are referred to current Medicare and Medicaid rules and regulations for guidance.

Challenges Specific to the Adult-Gerontology ACNP Role

The role of the AG-ACNP is continuing to evolve and gain recognition. The increased need for AG-ACNPs to manage patient care directly in an expanding health care arena will continue to provide unique practice opportunities. The practice doctorate will provide additional opportunities to expand and increase the emphasis on promoting evidence-based practice and organizational and systems leadership (AACN, 2006; NONPF, 2015). The IOM report (2011) highlighted the importance of practicing to the full scope of NP practice, and this has direct implications for the AG-ACNP role. Practicing AG-ACNPs continue to report that physicians and hospital administrators are unfamiliar with the full practice role and the differences between the AG-ACNP and primary care NP specialties. Also, some physicians may feel threatened by the role. Misunderstandings about AG-ACNP practice and labeling of the role as a so-called physician extender or midlevel provider have stemmed from the misperception that AG-ACNPs are replacements for house staff and function as resident replacements or hold a practice role "more than a nurse" but "less than a physician." Many of these misperceptions and perceived threats can be addressed through education. AG-ACNPs can use formal and informal opportunities to educate the professional public about the purpose and practice of AG-ACNPs, providing clear and concrete examples of their use and efficacy. To articulate their role, it is extremely important for AG-ACNPs to frame their practice within the nursing paradigm, one that uses the admitting history and physical examination to develop a plan of care that includes the following:

recognizing the patient's holistic problems and the medical diagnosis; addressing these nursing and medical problems throughout the hospital stay; using interventions that not only diagnose and manage disease but also promote and protect health; framing the discharge summary so that patients have a continuum of nursing and medical care as they return to the community; and applying all the AG-ACNP role competencies, not only those related to direct clinical care, to their practice.

Exposure to the comprehensive care that AG-ACNPs provide and the education of the health care team about the role will lead to continued role recognition and acceptance. Educating administrators and other health care professionals can facilitate acceptance of the role, which will in turn provide an opportunity for independent contracting for AG-ACNP professional services. Awareness of worth in terms of billable revenue and the care that AG-ACNPs can provide is imperative for successful contract negotiations and marketing purposes.

Changing employment trends have also affected AG-ACNP practice. Originally, AG-ACNPs were hired predominantly in tertiary medical center settings. AG-ACNPs now report increased employment with physician practice groups, managed care organizations, accountable care organizations, independent subacute care facilities, and even individual contractual relationships. However, these opportunities also bring the challenges of negotiating legal contracts, multiorganizational credentialing and privileging, group practice, managed care and accountable care organization policies, and reimbursement issues (Kleinpell, Buchman, et al., 2012; see Chapters 21 and 22).

AG-ACNPs need to continue to develop strong collaborative relationships with physicians and others to provide optimal patient care. The DNP AG-ACNP is especially prepared to advocate for advanced interprofessional collaboration for improved health outcomes (AACN, 2006). Working to negotiate a collaborative practice partnership can be a challenge. In working to establish collegial interactions and by sharing successful practice models, AG-ACNPs can promote enhanced collaborative relationships (see Chapter 12).

Future Directions

New forecasts for the need for AG-ACNPs identify that continued role expansion will be needed (Auerbach, 2012) and that the future of AG-ACNP practice will provide a world of opportunity (Aleshire et al., 2012). The AG-ACNP role is also advancing globally (Kleinpell et al., 2014). In alignment with the APRN Consensus Model, there is more awareness of the importance of ensuring consistency between NP education, certification, and clinical scope of practice (Kleinpell, Hudspeth, et al., 2012). The IOM initiative to ensure that this occurs through fostering adoption of the APRN Consensus Model by all boards of nursing is gaining traction, thereby further promoting the AG-ACNP as the appropriate preparation for those caring for acutely and critically ill adults (IOM, 2016). New models of care continue to expand for AG-ACNP practice such as hospitalist team roles as well as 24/7 ICU team-based models of care (Kapu, Kleinpell, et al., 2014). NPs working in hospital inpatient settings are also among the most highly compensated, and this may serve to attract individuals to this role (American Association of Nurse Practitioners, 2015).

In the future, AG-ACNPs may practice in multiple settings with individually negotiated contracts. Managing episodes of acute illness or exacerbation of chronic illness in home health care, subacute care, and outpatient settings might be directed by the AG-ACNP, as is already the case in some areas. These areas are natural extensions of acute care services and encompass the scope of AG-ACNP practice and the stabilization of acute and complex chronic disease. There are myriad opportunities relative to acute and chronic therapeutic management—for example, the management of renal dialysis or ventilator-dependent patients.

Cost reduction in acute care services will continue. Currently, collaborative teams composed of a physician, resident, and AG-ACNP are popular in many practice settings (Costa et al., 2014; Gershengorn et al., 2012; Landsperger et al., 2015). Some patient populations may be managed by teams composed of several AG-ACNPs with one physician, as in the heart failure service example described previously.

Monitoring outcomes of AG-ACNP practice remains essential. Although a growing number of utilization and outcome-based studies of AG-ACNP practice have been conducted and published, there is still the need to demonstrate the impact of AG-ACNP care in a growing number of specialty practice arenas. The emphasis on continuous quality improvement will continue to mandate the need for AG-ACNPs to become proactive and involved in measuring the impact of their care.

With more AG-ACNPs being educated at the DNP level, there is an increased potential to apply scientific knowledge to clinical practice and establish and uphold evidence-based practice as well as apply research to clinical practice. Information on the impact of the AG-ACNP role at the DNP level is also needed. AG-ACNPs are expected to assume leadership roles in evaluating the scientific literature and applying their findings to change and improved care (see Chapters 10 and 11).

AG-ACNPs must accept the challenge to improve and advance themselves and their profession continually. Strategies for success in the AG-ACNP role include maintaining competency, networking, demonstrating outcomes of practice, and communicating about the role. To provide safe, high-quality, and efficient care, the AG-ACNP must persistently pursue ongoing education and professional development to be knowledgeable about recent advances in health care and be judicious in the application of research findings. AG-ACNPs should not only read the literature but also publish on clinical and role topics. Sharing their clinical expertise and experiences can benefit their peers as those peers seek to develop and enhance their roles. It is important that AG-ACNPs be involved in their NP professional and clinical specialty organizations so that the issues unique to AG-ACNP practice gain recognition by the leaders of national organizations and also to ensure that AG-ACNPs have a voice in the legislative and political decision-making process. Collaboration with public policymakers to influence legislation issues related to the AG-ACNP role or, on a larger scale, health policy issues, is also an imperative for all AG-ACNPs (AACN, 2012; American Association of Critical-Care Nurses, 2012, 2017); see Chapters 11, 12, and 19).

Conclusion

The AG-ACNP role provides an opportunity for NPs to have a significant impact on patient outcomes at a dynamic time in the health trajectory of patient populations as well as in the history of health care delivery. As the role continues to evolve, and as health care systems respond to market forces and economic change, opportunities to further develop the AG-ACNP role will arise. Future development of the AG-ACNP role should be based on the evaluation of the need for the role, an understanding of the scope of the role, and role outcomes assessment. Ensuring that AG-ACNPs practice to the full scope of their education and training is in alignment with the recommendations of the IOM (2011). The role of the AG-ACNP is now well established, but because the role continues to evolve, participation in national organizations to refine consensus regarding role components, program curriculum, marketing, and role evaluation is ongoing. AG-ACNP educators and clinicians must work together to ensure that the preparation and practice of AG-ACNPs is safe, effective, and fully represented as the movement of doctoral APRN education evolves. AG-ACNPs also need to thoroughly understand as well as be proponents of the APRN Consensus Model (APRN Joint Dialogue Group, 2008) to ensure that licensure and education match the practice setting in order to assure public safety as well as educate employers in those practice settings where the population focus demands the AG-ACNP as the most appropriate APRN provider. AG-ACNPs must be strong activists in efforts to gain broader recognition of their role within their full scope of practice across acute care settings. In this evolving health care arena, AG-ACNP practice is rapidly expanding and holds unlimited potential. Ongoing challenges include ensuring expansion of the AG-ACNP with a focus on advanced practice nursing, rather than as a physician replacement model of care.

Key Summary Points

- The purpose of the AG-ACNP is to diagnose and manage disease and promote the health of patients with acute, critical, and complex chronic health conditions across the continuum of health care services.
- Although all AG-ACNPs share specialty role attributes, there may be intrarole variability based on the nature of the care delivery system, characteristics of a particular employment position, location in which they practice, and physiologic specialty.
- For AG-ACNPs to achieve the specialty competencies to diagnose and manage disease in their specialty patient population, they must demonstrate mastery of advanced pathophysiology, completion of a prioritized health history and comprehensive and focused physical examinations, rapid assessment of unstable and complex health problems, implementation of diagnostic strategies and therapeutic interventions to stabilize health care problems, technical competence with procedures, modification of the plan of care based on a client's changing condition and response to interventions, and collaboration with other care providers to facilitate positive outcomes.
- Although the AG-ACNP role is the newest NP specialty, there is evidence demonstrating that AG-ACNPs deliver care that is safe and cost-effective.

References

To access the references for this chapter, use your smartphone's QR code reader to scan the code below, or go to http://booksite.elsevier.com/ 9780323447751.

The Certified Nurse-Midwife

Melissa D. Avery • *Melissa A. Saftner*

> *"Everyone has been made for some particular work, and the desire for that work has been put in every heart."*
>
> *—Rumi*

CHAPTER CONTENTS

The purpose of this chapter is to describe nurse-midwifery practice in the United States, including a historical perspective as well as current education, accreditation, and certification of nurse-midwives, along with trends in professional practice. A brief discussion of other models of midwifery in the United States as well as midwifery's place internationally are provided. Although other classifications of midwives in the US are identified, the focus of the chapter is on certified nurse-midwives (CNMs). CNM competencies, standards and quality metrics, and evidence of outcomes of CNM practice are discussed and numerous interprofessional efforts are emphasized.

We wish to acknowledge the previous chapter authors Maureen Kelly, PhD, CNM, and Jane Mashburn, PhD, CNM, for their excellent work in previous editions.

These partnerships continue to advance excellent clinical care for women.

Nurse-midwifery is approaching 100 years since its initial formal development as a profession in the United States when Mary Breckinridge brought the British model of midwifery, nurse plus midwife, to rural areas of Kentucky in 1925 (Burst, 2015). Nurse-midwifery in the United States has made many contributions that have paved the way for advanced practice registered nurses (APRNs). The American College of Nurse-Midwifery was incorporated in New Mexico in 1955. In 1969, the American College of Nurse-Midwives (ACNM) was formed by the merger of the American College of Nurse-Midwifery and the American Association of Nurse-Midwives. By 1970, the ACNM had developed functions, qualifications, and midwifery standards of practice; within the next several years the ACNM also established criteria for the accreditation of nurse-midwifery education programs and a national certifying examination. Nurse-midwifery activities have been instrumental in securing prescriptive authority and direct reimbursement by insurers for CNMs. These activities have had a favorable direct or indirect impact on all APRNs. Pioneering efforts of CNMs have helped cultivate a clinical and political climate of acceptance, not only for themselves but also for clinical nurse specialists, certified registered nurse anesthetists, and nurse practitioners as highly valued and visible providers of care across all settings.

Midwife Definitions

Because midwifery and nurse-midwifery in the United States and globally represent different definitions and preparation, it is appropriate to begin by defining the terms internationally and within the US context. The common denominator for all midwives is providing care to women during pregnancy and birth. The word *midwife* comes from the Old English and means "with woman." Although midwifery includes certified midwives (CM), certified professional midwives (CPM), and licensed midwives (LM), this chapter focuses on the profession of nurse-midwifery. Midwives and midwifery practice are distinct from the medical practice of obstetrics and gynecology based on an emphasis on woman-centered care and a strong belief in pregnancy and birth, as well as other normal life transitions, as physiologic events to be supported as such, utilizing medical interventions only as indicated by the woman's health status.

International Definition

The International Confederation of Midwives (ICM) defines a midwife as

> ...a person who has successfully completed a midwifery education program that is duly recognized in the country where it is located and that is based on ICM Essential Competencies and Global Standards for Education; who has acquired the requisite qualifications to be registered and/or legally licensed to practice midwifery and to use the title "midwife," and who demonstrates competency in the practice of midwifery. (ICM, 2011)

Midwifery is a unique profession distinct from nursing and medicine and is combined with nursing in some countries. Midwifery education is recommended to be a minimum 3 years if direct entry (not combined with nursing) and at least 18 months if the midwifery program is completed following basic nursing education (ICM, 2013).

US Midwife Definitions

In the United States, three groups of professionals aim to meet the ICM definition of a midwife. CNMs are educated in the two disciplines of nursing and midwifery and must earn a graduate degree, complete a midwifery education program accredited by the Accreditation Commission for Midwifery Education (ACME), and pass the national certification examination administered by the American Midwifery Certification Board (AMCB) to receive the professional designation CNM (ACNM, 2012b). Certified midwives (CMs) are individuals educated in the discipline of midwifery who earn graduate degrees, meet health and science education requirements, and complete an ACME-accredited midwifery education program. They pass the same national certification examination as CNMs to receive the professional designation CM (ACNM, 2012b). The CM direct entry (not combined with nursing) route was developed by ACNM in the mid-1990s in an effort to develop an equivalent midwifery credential (Burst, 2015). With the same accreditation requirements and same certification credential as CNMs, the ACNM standards for practice and other ACNM documents such as the Code of Ethics also apply to CMs. The regulatory processes are developing; CMs can be credentialed in six states and have prescriptive authority in two (ACNM, 2016d). An ACNM priority is to make CM practice opportunities and prescriptive authority the same as CNMs in all states.

A certified professional midwife (CPM) is "an individual who is a knowledgeable, skilled, and professional independent midwifery practitioner and who has met the standards of certification set by the North American Registry of Midwives (NARM)" and passes the examination administered by NARM. Graduation from an accredited midwifery education program is not required for the NARM examination (NARM, 2016). In addition to CNMs, CMs, and CPMs, there are also individuals who use the title "direct entry midwife (DEM)," lay midwives (also known as "granny midwives"), traditional midwives, traditional birth attendants, empirical midwives, independent midwives), and licensed midwives (Midwives Alliance of North

America, 2016). Some of these practitioners are legally recognized in some states, some have had formal training, and some have had apprenticeship training.

Historical Perspective

Midwifery predates nursing and medicine. Throughout time, and in all cultures, the midwife has played an important and highly respected role in the community. In Biblical times, the midwife assisted a woman in labor, helped birth the baby, and provided for aftercare of the mother and infant. Novice midwives acquired knowledge and skill by apprenticing with experienced midwives and through their own observations and experiences.

In colonial times, midwives were an integral part of community life and were highly respected members of society. In the early 1900s, a number of developments in the United States considerably diminished that respect and led to a decline in the practice of midwifery. The immigrant population was served by European immigrant midwives and African-American women from the South were cared for by traditional African-American midwives. These midwives lacked a national organization, methods of communication, access to the health care system, and legal recognition (Burst, 2015). During this same time frame, physicians took over the role of birth attendant, obstetrics became a medical specialty, and birth moved into the hospital setting. The medicalization of birth did much to eliminate midwifery and continues to influence and regulate the practice of nurse-midwifery today.

Although midwifery remained part of mainstream health care in many European, Asian, and African countries, US nurse-midwifery was reborn in the 1920s, with more growth of nurse-midwifery practice and education in the United States occurring in the 1940s and 1950s. Initial midwifery graduates worked in nursing education and public health because there was a lack of clinical practice opportunities. Like other forms of advanced practice nursing that emerged later, the resurgence of midwifery and the evolution of nurse-midwifery occurred in response to the need for care of the underserved. By the late 1960s and 1970s, the opportunities for nurse-midwives in clinical practice increased. Demand for nurse-midwifery services for all women grew and the profession responded by opening more education programs and more midwifery practices (Burst, 2015; see Chapter 1).

The Nurse-Midwifery Profession in the United States Today

Recognition of Nurse-Midwifery

In the United States, the Institute of Medicine (IOM) released its report on *The Future of Nursing* (IOM, 2011), the impetus of which was the passage of the Patient Protection and Affordable Care Act (ACA, 2010; see Chapter 19). The report identified CNMs as one of four types of APRNs and called on nurses and midwives to be full partners in redesigning health care in the United States. A 2015 updated report highlighted progress in obtaining full practice authority for APRNs in the 5 years between the reports and noted that there was still more work to be done (IOM, 2015). Shortly after the passing of the ACA, Childbirth Connection, a national nonprofit organization dedicated to improving maternity care through consumer engagement and health system transformation, sponsored the Transforming Maternity Care Partnership with participation by CNMs and the ACNM as well as other interdisciplinary professionals. The resulting report, *Blueprint for Action: Steps Toward a High-Quality, High-Value Maternity Care System* (Angood et al., 2010), called for expanding access to midwives and reducing barriers to midwifery practice, among other system-critical focus areas for improvement. The ACNM and Childbirth Connection are also partners with the Centers for Medicare and Medicaid Services (CMS) in *Strong Start,* an initiative designed to improve maternity care outcomes through evaluating new models of prenatal care, including group prenatal care, birth center care, and woman- and family-centered maternity care homes (Urban Institute, 2016). All of this activity in the United States related to maternity care and midwifery signals increasing opportunities for CNMs as health care reform continues in the United States with a goal of achieving the Triple Aim of improved patient experience, improved population outcomes, and reduced costs (Berwick, Nolan, & Whittington, 2008). These global and domestic initiatives aim to mobilize and intensify worldwide action toward transforming the care that is available to all women and children.

In 2015, the most current year for which data are available, CNMs/CMs attended 338, 663, births (the data do not separate CNM from CM), which constituted 12.5% of vaginal births and 8.5% of all births in the United States (Martin, Hamilton, Osterman, Driscoll, & Matthews, 2017). Of these midwife-attended births, 94.2 % occurred in hospitals, 3% in freestanding birth centers, and 2.7% in women's homes (Martin, Hamilton, Osterman, Driscoll & Matthews, 2017).

Nurse-midwifery practice is legal in all 50 states, and CNMs have prescriptive authority in 50 states and the District of Columbia (ACNM, 2016d). As with all APRNs, prescriptive authority is regulated by individual states. CNMs are also defined as primary care providers under federal law (ACNM, 2012d).

Education and Accreditation

The ACNM established a national mechanism for the accreditation of nurse-midwifery education programs in 1962 in order to foster a consistent approach to quality education. Because the organization wanted to have its process subject to peer review and recognition, it applied to the US Department of Education for recognition as an accrediting agency. The ACME is the official accrediting body of the ACNM and has been recognized since 1982 by the Department of Education as a programmatic accrediting agency. ACME-accredited programs must receive preaccreditation status before enrolling students and apply for accreditation following graduation of the first class of students. Once the initial accreditation has been granted, the program must be reviewed at least every 10 years (ACNM, 2013).

Although the American Association of Colleges of Nursing (AACN) recommended in 2004 that the Doctor of Nursing Practice (DNP) be the entry level for clinical practice, neither the ACNM nor the ACME has endorsed that position. The ACNM supports a graduate degree as basic preparation for midwifery practice consistent with certification requirements, and it does not support the DNP as the entry-level requirement for midwifery education (ACNM, 2015d). Midwifery education has always been more broadly based than nursing. Even at the master's level, degrees may be awarded from schools of nursing, midwifery, public health, or allied health. The ACNM's Division of Education has developed competencies for the practice doctorate in midwifery, recognizing the practice doctorate as one possible option for doctoral preparation for midwives (ACNM, 2011c). There currently is no ACNM or AMCB statement about mandatory doctoral preparation, although the ACNM supports and values the attainment of doctoral degrees for CNMs. The lack of a recommendation for a specific degree beyond requiring graduate educational preparation is the result of a long history of evidence documenting that CNMs provide competent care, a lack of evidence of the impact of doctoral education for midwives, increased cost of doctoral education, and support of midwifery educators for multiple routes of achievement of the Core Competencies (Avery & Howe, 2007).

As of 2017, there are 40 nurse-midwifery graduate programs in the United States accredited or preaccredited (2) by the ACNM's Accreditation Commission for Midwifery Education (ACNM, 2017a). Of these, 36 are located in schools of nursing, 3 in other graduate programs, and 1 in a freestanding institution of higher education. Evolving along with other APRN programs, as of 2017, 9 ACME-accredited programs offer master's and DNP options, 22 culminate in a master's degree, and an additional eight offer the DNP only (ACNM, 2017a).

Certification and Certification Maintenance

A national certification examination for entry into nurse-midwifery practice was instituted in 1971 and serves to protect the public by assuring a common standard for entry into practice. The AMCB credential is required by most states for licensure and by many institutions for credentialing (AMCB, 2013). Certification is time limited for all CNMs; recertification requires completing three modules provided by the AMCB plus two approved continuing education units or taking the AMCB Certification Examination (AMCB, n.d.) every 5 years. As of August 2016, 11,475 nurse-midwives were nationally certified as CNMs by the AMCB, and 103 midwives were certified as CMs; of these, 56 CNMs and 2 CMs were male (AMCB, 2016). Of AMCB-certified midwives, 128 had earned a Doctor of Philosophy (PhD) (AMCB, 2016).

Reentry to Practice

CNMs may occasionally leave the workforce for a period of time and thus be out of practice. Certification may be maintained during this time by following the AMCB processes described previously. The ACNM has provided guidance to help midwives demonstrate safe competent practice following a period of time away, which may include didactic learning and precepted clinical practice; a written plan describing the individual identified process is recommended (ACNM, 2016a).

Regulation, Reimbursement, and Credentialing

CNMs are regulated on a state-by-state basis and there are numerous regulatory and reimbursement barriers at the local, state, and federal levels regarding the full deployment of all APRNs. These barriers are discussed in Chapter 19. Therefore, this section highlights the regulatory, reimbursement, and credentialing considerations that may be distinct to nurse-midwifery. CNMs are regulated by boards of nursing in a majority of states and are regulated by boards of medicine, health/public health, and midwifery in others (ACNM, n.d.-g).

The ACNM endorsed the Consensus Model for APRN Regulation (APRN Joint Dialogue Group, 2008) and made additional recommendations specific to midwifery practice (ACNM, 2011a). The first recommendation strongly supports the foundational Consensus Model principle that APRNs be licensed as independent practitioners with no regulatory requirements for collaboration, direction, or supervision. The ACNM has released an official statement about independent nurse-midwifery practice (ACNM, 2012e; Box 17.1). In addition, the 2011 ACNM–American College of Obstetricians and Gynecologists (ACOG) report, *Joint Statement of Practice Relations Between Obstetricians and Gynecologists and Certified Nurse-Midwives/Certified Midwives,* is a model document that recognizes each group as licensed independent providers who may collaborate based on the needs of their patients (ACNM, 2011c; Box 17.2). The ACNM advocates that nursing boards support separate boards of midwifery or boards of nurse-midwifery. The ACNM also recommends that the consensus document clarify that a graduate *nursing* degree is not required to take the AMCB Certification Examination, which is an effort to support nurse-midwifery programs accredited and located in other programs or separate institutions of higher learning (e.g., public health or allied health programs) (ACNM, 2011a).

CNMs achieved equitable reimbursement for their services under Medicare effective January 2011. In other words, under Medicare, CNMs are paid at the same fee schedule rate as physicians for doing the same work. This long-awaited provision was part of the ACA (see Chapter 19). Because of this provision, the CNM reimbursement rate increased from 65% of the physician's fee to 100% of the Medicare Part B physician fee schedule (ACNM, 2012c). CNMs have not yet been included in the wellness examination provision of the ACA, but the ACNM continues to work to change this (ACNM, 2012c). Medicaid mandates reimbursement for nurse-midwives in all 50 states; the level of reimbursement ranges from 65% to 100% of the Medicare reimbursement rate (ACNM, 2016g). Most states also mandate private insurance reimbursement for midwifery services

---

BOX 17.1   Independent Midwifery Practice

The following represents the position of the American College of Nurse-Midwives (ACNM):

- Midwifery practice is the independent management of women's health care, focusing particularly on common primary care issues, family planning and gynecologic needs of women, pregnancy, childbirth, the postpartum period, and care of the newborn.
- The practice occurs within a health care system that provides for consultation, collaborative management, and referral, as indicated by the health status of the woman or newborn.
- Independent midwifery enables CNMs and CMs to use their knowledge, skills, judgment, and authority in the provision of primary health service for women while maintaining accountability for the management of health care in accordance with the ACNM *Standards for the Practice of Midwifery.*

Background

Independent practice is not defined by the place of employment, the employee-employer relationship, requirements for a physician's co-signature, or the method of reimbursement for services. Further, independent practice should not be interpreted to be alone, because there are clinical situations in which any prudent practitioner would seek the assistance of another qualified practitioner.

Collaboration is the process whereby health care professionals jointly manage care. The goal of collaboration is to share authority while providing quality care within each individual's professional scope of practice. Successful collaboration is a way of thinking—a relationship that requires knowledge, open communication, mutual respect, a commitment to providing quality care, trust, and the ability to share responsibility.

From the American College of Nurse-Midwives. (2012). *Position statement: Independent midwifery practice.* Silver Spring, MD: Author.

(ACNM, 2016d); similar variability in the level of reimbursement occurs for private insurance reimbursement for CNM services. The ACNM remains vigilant during ongoing health care policymaking and advocates for "common-sense policy solutions that ensure women and newborns have guaranteed

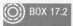 **BOX 17.2   Joint Statement of Practice Relations Between Obstetrician-Gynecologists, Certified Nurse-Midwives, and Certified Midwives**

The American College of Obstetricians and Gynecologists (the College) and the American College of Nurse-Midwives (ACNM) affirm our shared goal of safe women's health care in the United States through the promotion of evidence-based models provided by obstetrician-gynecologists (OB-GYNs), certified nurse-midwives (CNMs), and certified midwives (CMs). The College and the ACNM believe that health care is most effective when it occurs in a system that facilitates communication across care settings and among providers. OB-GYNs, CNMs, and CMs are experts in their respective fields of practice and are educated, trained, and licensed independent providers who may collaborate with each other based on the needs of their patients. Quality of care is enhanced by collegial relationships characterized by mutual respect and trust, as well as professional responsibility and accountability.

Recognizing the high level of responsibility that OB-GYNs, CNMs, and CMs assume when providing care to women, the College and the ACNM affirm their commitment to promote the highest standards for education, national professional certification, and recertification of their respective members and to support evidence-based practice. Accredited education and professional certification preceding licensure are essential to ensure skilled providers at all levels of care across the United States.

The College and the ACNM recognize the importance of the options and preferences of women in their health care. OB-GYNs, CNMs, and CMs work in a variety of settings, including private practice, community health care facilities, clinics, hospitals, and accredited birth centers. The College and the ACNM hold different positions on home birth. Establishing and sustaining viable practices that can provide broad services to women requires that OB-GYNs, CNMs, and CMs have access to affordable professional liability insurance coverage, hospital privileges, equivalent reimbursement from private payers and under government programs, and support services, including but not limited to laboratory testing, obstetric imaging, and anesthesia. To provide highest quality and seamless care, OB-GYNs, CNMs, and CMs should have access to a system of care that fosters collaboration among licensed, independent providers.

Adapted from the American College of Nurse-Midwives. (2011). *Position statement: Joint statement of practice relations between obstetrician-gynecologists and certified nurse-midwives/certified midwives.* Washington, DC: Author.

health coverage and access to a full range of preventative, reproductive and sexual health services under state Medicaid programs and coverage and access to essential health benefits (EHBs), including maternity and newborn care." (ACNM, 2017b, p. 2).

Multiple authors have called for greater flexibility in state licensing laws (Dower, Moore, & Langelier, 2013; Safriet, 2011; Yang & Kozhimannil, 2015). CNMs and other advanced practice nurses face barriers in state laws and care reimbursement policies that vary widely across the United States. Known barriers to midwifery practice across the US states comprise various levels of physician supervision, including written practice agreements and restrictions to prescriptive authority preventing midwives and others from practicing their full scope of professional practice. Researchers recently demonstrated that in states where CNMs practiced independently (no requirement for physician supervision or practice agreement for overall practice), more CNM-attended births occurred and there were more midwives per 1000 births. Twenty-six states and the District of Columbia met the definition of independent CNM practice in 2017; 13 require a written practice agreement, 5 require a written practice agreement for prescribing only, and 6 require supervision (A. Kohl, personal communication, August 2017).

In addition to state regulation, hospitals and health plans have established credentialing requirements for health care professionals. These credentialing standards determine who may have hospital admitting privileges, be employed by health care systems, and be listed on managed care provider panels. Ideally, health systems would have a mechanism consistent with the profession's standards, recognizing nurse-midwifery as distinct from other health care professions, and have processes that guide CNMs in building on entry-level competencies within their scope of practice. Credentialing is a particularly thorny issue for CNMs, as revealed in a 2011 online survey conducted by the ACNM. A total of 1893 responses were received; 80% of the CNM respondents stated that they did not have full voting privileges within the medical staffs of their local facilities, almost 50% reported that employment by a physician practice or the hospital was a requirement of privileging, and 65% stated that they had privileges to practice but limitations or supervisory restrictions on scope of practice (; Bushman, 2014). Medical staff membership is denied in 17 states and allowed in the remaining states (ACNM, 2016g). Although CNMs have made significant strides in full participation in the health care system, continued work is needed to be able to practice their full scope in all jurisdictions and health systems

The federal government, through the CMS, exerts a strong influence over hospitals through its conditions of participation. These are rules with which hospitals are required to comply to maintain eligibility to participate in Medicare and Medicaid programs. In 2012, the CMS issued medical staff participation rules clarifying that hospitals may grant privileges to physicians and nonphysicians and that regardless of whether they were granted medical privileges, practitioners in the institution are required to adhere to the bylaws and regulations of the institution (Cooney & Johnson, 2012). The conditions of participation document urges hospitals to use "nonphysician providers" to help them care for the health of the public and requires that an application for credentialing be reviewed by the medical staff and governing body of the hospital. In all, these regulations send a strong signal about the use of CNMs and other APRNs in hospital settings but fall short of requiring that CNMs be credentialed as members of the medical staff (Cooney & Johnson, 2012). Of course CNMs, like all health professionals, advocate for being referred to by their title rather than as a "non" other professional.

American College of Nurse-Midwives

The National Organization of Public Health Nurses established a section for nurse-midwives in the 1940s. During the reorganization of national nursing organizations, the National Organization of Public Health Nurses was absorbed into the American Nurses Association (ANA) and the National League for Nursing; however, these two organizations did not include a recognizable entity for nurse-midwives. Midwives at the 1954 ANA convention formed the Committee on Organization. This committee approved the definition of a nurse-midwife but the National League for Nursing and the ANA could not find a place for the nurse-midwives (for various reasons). Subsequently, at their May 1955 meeting, the Committee on Organization voted to form a separate nurse-midwifery organization—the ACNM (Burst, 2015).

The growth and development of American nurse-midwifery has been fostered by the ACNM, founded in 1955 as the professional organization for CNMs. The ACNM vision is a midwife for every woman and the mission is advancing the practice of midwifery in order to achieve optimal health for women throughout their life spans (ACNM, 2012d). The organization supports members by establishing evidence-based clinical standards, creating liaisons with state and federal agencies and members of Congress, providing continuing education, supporting midwifery-relevant research and practice, promoting midwifery globally, and supporting the accreditation of midwifery education programs. In 2016 the ACNM represented 7781 active and student members (S. Chairez, personal communication, April 2016), approximately 54% of US CNMs.

The ACNM Philosophy (ACNM, 2004; Box 17.3), Code of Ethics (ACNM, 2015b; Box 17.4), Standards for the Practice of Midwifery (2011e; Table 17.1) and Core Competencies for Basic Midwifery Practice (ACNM, 2012a; Box 17.5) are important documents that guide the profession and practitioner. The ACNM is currently actively promoting a focus on physiologic birth through its national *Healthy Birth Initiative,* including a specific effort to reduce cesarean births (ACNM, 2016e). Midwives are increasingly recognized in the United States for their high-quality care, patient satisfaction, and high-value care—indeed, the parameters of the Triple Aim. This recognition has led to partnerships and recognition from the Alliance for Innovation on Maternal Health, the ACOG, and the Association of Women's Health, Obstetric and Neonatal Nurses (AWHONN) (ACNM, n.d.-a; AWHONN, 2016). Current national legislative objectives include identification of maternity care shortage areas (in partnership with the ACOG); interprofessional quality improvement initiatives; and reimbursement for CNMs who teach learners, including midwifery students, medical students, and residents (ACNM, n.d.-c, n.d.-d, n.d.-f).

Midwifery Internationally

In 2000 the United Nations set the Millennium Development Goals, increasing the world's attention on women's and children's health. Improvements have been made, and the maternal mortality ratio has declined 44% from 1990 levels to 216 maternal deaths per 100,000 live births in 2015 (World Health Organization, 2015). The new target in the United

> ### BOX 17.3 Philosophy of the American College of Nurse-Midwives
>
> We, the midwives of the American College of Nurse-Midwives, affirm the power and strength of women and the importance of their health in the well-being of families, communities, and nations. We believe in the basic human rights of all persons, recognizing that women often incur an undue burden of risk when these rights are violated.
>
> We believe that every person has a right to the following:
>
> - Equitable, ethical, accessible quality health care that promotes healing and health
> - Health care that respects human dignity, individuality, and diversity among groups
> - Complete and accurate information to make informed health care decisions
> - Self-determination and active participation in health care decisions
> - Involvement of a woman's designated family members, to the extent desired, in all health care experiences
>
> We believe that the best model of health care for a woman and her family does the following:
>
> - Promotes a continuous and compassionate partnership
> - Acknowledges a person's life experiences and knowledge
> - Includes individualized methods of care and healing guided by the best evidence available
> - Involves the therapeutic use of human presence and skillful communication
>
> We honor the normalcy of women's life cycle events. We believe in the following:
>
> - Watchful waiting and nonintervention in normal processes
> - Appropriate use of interventions and technology for current or potential health problems
> - Consultation, collaboration, and referral with other members of the health care team as needed to provide optimal health care
>
> We affirm that midwifery care incorporates these qualities and that women's health care needs are well-served through midwifery care.
>
> Finally, we value formal education, lifelong individual learning, and the development and application of research to guide ethical and competent midwifery practice. These beliefs and values provide the foundation for commitment to individual and collective leadership at the community, state, national, and international levels to improve the health of women and their families worldwide.

Adapted from the American College of Nurse-Midwives. (2004). *Philosophy of the American College of Nurse-Midwives.* Silver Spring, MD: Author.

Nations Sustainable Development Goals, approved in 2015, is to reduce the maternal mortality ratio even further to below 70 per 100,000 live births by 2030. Midwifery has emerged as a key human resource to help achieve this goal. Internationally, publications such as *The Lancet's* Series on Midwifery (Renfrew et al., 2014) and the State of the World's Midwifery 2014 (United Nations Population Fund, 2014) highlight midwifery as key to continue to reduce maternal and neonatal mortality. Authors call on the United Nations and world governments to invest in educating and retaining midwives. In addition to these important reports, the ICM has developed a set of core documents to "strengthen midwifery worldwide in order to provide high-quality, evidence-based health services for women, newborn, and childbearing families" (ICM, 2014a). The ICM documents represent essential competencies for basic midwifery practice, education, regulation, and association strengthening. As a result, midwives from around the world have a common standard against which they can evaluate their profession. Taken together, these reports and ICM documents reflect the urgent need for more and better prepared midwives in developed and developing countries and are a call to action and a blueprint for taking the agenda forward (see Chapter 6).

Implementing Advanced Practice Nursing Competencies

Overview of APRN and Certified Nurse-Midwife Competencies

Nurse-midwifery is constantly evolving and has a broader scope of practice now than it did 90 years ago. Nurse-midwifery has six core competencies (see Box 17.5) that are similar to the six identified APRN competencies in addition to direct care (see Chapter 3). As with the APRN model in Chapter 3, the direct care role is integral to CNM practice and is well substantiated in both exemplars presented later in this chapter. Consistent with advanced practice nursing, nurse-midwives assume responsibility and

BOX 17.4   American College of Nurse-Midwives: Code of Ethics

CNMs and CMs have three ethical mandates in achieving the mission of midwifery to promote the health and well-being of women and newborns within their families and communities. The first mandate is directed toward the individual women and their families for whom the midwives provide care, the second mandate is to a broader audience for the public good for the benefit of all women and their families, and the third mandate is to the profession of midwifery to ensure its integrity, and in turn its ability, to fulfill the mission of midwifery.

Midwives in all aspects of professional relationships will:

- Respect basic human rights and the dignity of all persons.
- Respect their own self-worth, dignity, and professional integrity.

Midwives in all aspects of their professional practice will:

- Develop a partnership with the woman in which each shares relevant information that leads to informed decision making, consent to an evolving plan of care, and acceptance of responsibility for the outcome of their choices.
- Act without discrimination based on factors such as age, gender, race, ethnicity, religion, lifestyle, sexual orientation, socioeconomic status, disability, or nature of the health problem.
- Provide an environment where privacy is protected and in which all pertinent information is shared without bias, coercion, or deception.
- Maintain confidentiality, except where disclosure is mandated by law.
- Maintain the necessary knowledge, skills, and behaviors needed for competence.
- Protect women, their families, and colleagues from harmful, unethical, and incompetent practices by taking appropriate action that may include reporting as mandated by law.

Midwives as members of a profession will:

- Promote, advocate for, and strive to protect the rights, health, and well-being of women, families, and communities.
- Promote just distribution of resources and equity in access to quality health services.
- Promote and support the education of midwifery students and peers, standards of practice, research, and policies that enhance the health of women, families, and communities.

Adapted from the American College of Nurse-Midwives. (2015). *Code of ethics with explanatory statements.* Silver Spring, MD: Author.

accountability for their practice as primary health care providers (ACNM, 2012f). Patient-centered assessment and management are hallmarks of all aspects of CNM care. CNMs have, in common with all APRNs, the characteristics of using a holistic, evidence-based perspective. CNMs use research methodologies and ethical decision making to support a caring, low-technology, woman-centered approach to childbirth. The ACNM has a well-defined position statement on consultation and collaboration in midwifery practice (ACNM, 2014b) that has helped inform APRN practice (see Chapters 9 and 12). CNMs have demonstrated leadership in the development of freestanding birth centers, facilities for normal, healthy women who desire a wellness model of pregnancy and birth. It is informative to take a closer look at the competencies related to advocacy and patient education to understand nurse-midwifery practice further. The ACNM-defined competencies in advocacy and patient education parallel the advanced practice core competencies of ethical decision making, guidance, and coaching CNMs enact the seven competencies of advanced practice nursing, as described in the following sections.

Direct Clinical Practice

CNMs demonstrate a high level of expertise in the assessment, diagnosis, and treatment of women's life cycle events. They approach these events, such as puberty, pregnancy, birth, and menopause, as physiologic transitions that are best supported by education and midwifery expertise. Nurse-midwives form partnerships with the women that they care for, empowering them to be active participants in their own health care. Nurse-midwives incorporate scientific evidence into clinical practice, are familiar with complementary and alternative therapies, exercise expert clinical thinking and skillful performance, and demonstrate a holistic approach in the care they provide.

TABLE 17.1	**Standards for the Practice of Midwifery**

Midwifery practices, as conducted by certified nurse-midwives (CNMs) and certified midwives (CMs), are the independent management of women's health care, focusing particularly on pregnancy, childbirth, the postpartum period, care of the newborn, and the family planning and gynecologic needs of women. The CMN and CM practice within a health care system that provides for consultation, collaborative management, or referral, as indicated by the health status of the patient. CNMs and CMs practice in accord with the *Standards of the Practice of Midwifery,* as defined by the American College of Nurse-Midwives (ACNM).

Standard I Midwifery care is provided by qualified practitioners.	The midwife: • Is certified by the ACNM-designated certifying agent. • Shows evidence of continuing competency as required by the ACNM-designated certifying agent. • Is in compliance with the legal requirements of the jurisdiction in which the midwifery practice occurs.
Standard II Midwifery care occurs in a safe environment within the context of the family, community, and a system of health care.	The midwife: • Demonstrates knowledge of and uses federal and state regulations that apply to the practice environment and infection control. • Demonstrates a safe mechanism for obtaining medical consultation, collaboration, and referral. • Uses community services as needed. • Demonstrates knowledge of the medical, psychosocial, economic, cultural, and family factors that affect care. • Demonstrates appropriate techniques for emergency management, including arrangements for emergency transportation. • Promotes involvement of support persons in the practice setting.
Standard III Midwifery care supports individual rights and self-determination within boundaries of safety.	The midwife: • Practices in accord with the Philosophy and Code of Ethics of the ACNM. • Provides patients with a description of the scope of midwifery services and information regarding the patient's rights and responsibilities. • Provides patients with information regarding, and/or referral to, other providers and services when requested or when care required is not within the midwife's scope of practice. • Provides patients with information regarding health care decisions and the state of the science regarding these choices to allow for informed decision making.
Standard IV Midwifery care is composed of knowledge, skills, and judgments that foster the delivery of safe, satisfying, and culturally competent care.	The midwife: • Collects data, assesses patients, develops and implements an individualized plan of management, and evaluates outcome of care. • Demonstrates the clinical skills and judgments described.
Standard V Midwifery care is based on knowledge, skills, and judgments reflected in written practice guidelines that are used to guide the scope of midwifery care and services provided to patients.	The midwife: • Maintains written documentation of the parameters of service for independent and collaborative midwifery management and transfer of care when needed. • Has accessible resources to provide evidence-based clinical practice for each specialty area, which may include, but are not limited to, primary health care of women, care of the childbearing family, and newborn care.
Standard VI Midwifery care is documented in a format that is accessible and complete.	The midwife: • Uses records that facilitate communication of information to patients, consultants, and institutions. • Provides prompt and complete documentation of evaluation, course of management, and outcome of care. • Promotes a documentation system that provides for confidentiality and transmissibility of health records. • Maintains confidentiality in verbal and written communications.

Continued

TABLE 17.1 | **Standards for the Practice of Midwifery—cont'd**

Standard VII	The midwife:
Midwifery care is evaluated according to an established program for quality management that includes a plan to identify and resolve problems.	• Participates in a program of quality management for the evaluation of practice within the setting in which it occurs. • Provides for a systematic collection of practice data as part of a program of quality management. • Seeks consultation to review problems, including peer review of care. • Acts to resolve identified problems.
Standard VIII	The midwife:

Midwifery practice may be expanded beyond the ACNM core competencies to incorporate new procedures that improve care for women and their families.	• Identifies the need for a new procedure, taking into consideration consumer demand, standards for safe practice, and availability of other qualified personnel.
	• Ensures that there are no institutional, state, or federal statues, regulations, or bylaws that would constrain the midwife from incorporation of the procedure into practice.
	• Demonstrates knowledge and competency, including the following:
	  a. Knowledge of risks, benefits, and patient selection criteria
	  b. Process for acquisition of required skill
	  c. Identification and management of complications
	  d. Process to evaluate outcomes and maintain competency
	• Identifies a mechanism for obtaining medical consultation, collaboration, and referral related to this procedure.
	• Maintains documentation of the process used to achieve the necessary knowledge, skills, and ongoing competency of the expanded or new procedures.

Adapted from the American College of Nurse-Midwives. (2011). *Standards for the practice of midwifery.* Silver Spring, MD: Author.

BOX 17.5 | **Core Competencies for Basic Midwifery Practice**

The *Core Competencies for Basic Midwifery Practice* include the fundamental knowledge, skills, and behaviors expected of a new practitioner. Accordingly, they serve as guidelines for educators, students, health care professionals, consumers, employers, and policymakers.

Major headings and examples/summaries of each include:

Hallmarks of Midwifery
Highlights include recognizing developmental and physiologic processes as normal, women as partners in care, cultural humility, health promotion, and evidence-based care.

Components of Midwifery Care: Professional Responsibilities of CNMs and CMs
Includes knowledge of legal basis for practice, engagement in policy related to women's health, international issues in women's health, bioethics, collaboration in research, practice according to standards, professional engagement, business knowledge, and supporting the profession through midwifery education.

Components of Midwifery Care: Midwifery Management Process
Defined process of gathering information, planning care in partnership with women, evaluating care, consultation as needed, and adapting care as indicated.

Components of Midwifery Care: Fundamentals
Basics underlying care, including anatomy, physiology/pathophysiology, epidemiology, genetics/genomics, phamacotherapeutics, nutrition, and growth and development.

Components of Midwifery Care of Women
Includes specific competencies in each of the areas of primary, preconception, gynecologic, antepartum, intrapartum, and postpregnancy care.

Components of Midwifery Care of the Newborn
Competencies for basic care during the first 28 days of life, including facilitating transition to extrauterine life, assessment of newborn, basic care (including feeding and parent education), interventions and referral for abnormal conditions, and support of the family.

Adapted from American College of Nurse-Midwives. (2012). *Core competencies for basic midwifery practice.* Full document available at http://www.midwife.org/ACNM/files/ACNMLibraryData/UPLOADFILENAME/000000000050/Core%20Comptencies%20Dec%202012.pdf

The ACNM updated its position statement on CNMs as primary care providers and leaders of maternity care homes in 2012 (ACNM, 2012f). Primary care is included as a core competency for midwifery practice (ACNM, 2012a); it includes the provision of primary health care for women from the perimenarchal through postmenopausal phases as well as primary care for newborns. This care is provided on a continuous and comprehensive basis by establishing a plan of management with the woman. The maternity care home is a concept to address women-centered care before, during, and after pregnancy. It is patterned after the patient-centered medical home (see Chapter 15) and aims to improve neonatal and maternal health outcomes. Twenty-seven awards were granted through the Strong Start Initiative in 2013, and 12 were focused on maternity care homes. Since the grant funding began in 2013, rates of preterm birth and cesarean birth have decreased and breastfeeding rates have increased (Urban Institute, 2016). Maternity care homes are influencing health outcomes, and the ACNM regards midwives as well positioned to lead patient-centered maternity care teams (ACNM, 2012f). Midwives approach health care holistically and assess the woman's environment, relationships, and health status in order to develop a plan of care specific to each woman. Nurse-midwives juxtapose nursing knowledge and skills with advanced education in midwifery to enhance outcomes for women across the life span. DNP-prepared nurse-midwives in particular have additional training and preparation to organize and lead maternity care homes to improve quality and facilitate change in practice delivery in accordance with DNP Essential II (AACN, 2006).

Guidance and Coaching of Patients, Families, and Other Care Providers

Guidance and coaching are APRN functions that assist patients through life transitions such as illness, childbearing, and bereavement (see Chapter 8). Nurse-midwives offer skillful communication, guidance, and counseling throughout the nurse-midwifery management process (ACNM, 2012a). Client education is a cornerstone of nurse-midwifery practice. Evidence that nurse-midwives invest time in patient education is supported by Paine (2000), who has reported that nurse-midwives spend more time during office visits providing patient education and counseling than is spent by physicians. For example, when a nurse-midwife counsels a pregnant woman regarding antenatal genetic screening, she or he not only educates the patient about how the test is done but also advises the woman as to what the results might indicate, what further testing would then be offered, and what decisions the woman and her partner may need to make, and offers to provide additional coaching as the process unfolds. In the instance of the first-trimester screen, a combined screen that includes a blood test and ultrasound measurement of the fetal nuchal translucency, the woman would learn that it is a screening test for certain chromosomal conditions, such as Down syndrome, in the fetus. She is informed that it is not diagnostic and that a positive screen means that there is increased risk for the problem, not that the fetus has the problem. A positive result would lead to further decision making on whether to have further testing such as an amniocentesis or high-level ultrasound. The procedures, risks, and benefits of these tests would then be explained. If the woman opts for further testing and the results indicate a complication, she would then need to decide whether to continue or terminate the pregnancy. This level of guidance requires time, expertise, skill, and commitment.

As noted in Chapter 8, guidance is an interaction between an expert coach (the nurse-midwife) and the learner (the patient) that enables the learner to develop knowledge and skills within an area of the coach's expertise. An example of this application of knowledge includes health promotion for weight management. Nurse-midwives are trained to understand nutritional needs of women across the life span. Caloric requirements, appropriate food choices, and healthy weight range recommendations are within the scope of care that midwives provide. Nurse-midwives are expected to apply their knowledge to guide women through the natural life transitions. In addition to obesity prevention, nurse-midwives apply their knowledge and skills to support women during pregnancy transitions, childbirth, breastfeeding, grief and loss, parenthood, changes in family constellation, family planning, primary care, and women's health-related issues.

Consultation

Nurse-midwives use consultation in their practice, both as the consultant and as the consultee. Patients consult with CNMs regarding health care and health promotion. For example, a woman may see a nurse-midwife regarding back pain during pregnancy. She wants to know what she can do at home to alleviate the discomfort and support a healthy pregnancy. The nurse-midwife may consult with a physical therapist, massage therapist, or other expert in alleviating back pain to get recommendations about activities or exercises the woman can safely perform at home to decrease her pain. Nurse-midwives often provide consultation in the hospital setting to residents, physicians, and nurses. During a labor and birth, nurses and nurse-midwives may consult each other regarding the interpretation of a fetal monitor tracing. Nurse-midwives serve on hospital quality improvement committees, where they can advocate for evidence-based policies and patient-centered care. Physicians often consult nurse-midwives regarding complementary therapies, breastfeeding, and/or alternative birthing options such as water birth.

Nurse-midwives also consult other professionals. There are many cases in which a nurse-midwife would make use of another's expertise to provide the best care for his or her patients. For example, a CNM caring for a pregnant woman with a low platelet count might consult with the midwife's collaborating physician or a hematologist to decide on the appropriate care and provider for this woman and her fetus. Nurse-midwives frequently consult with lactation consultants to assist women who are having breastfeeding difficulties or with physical therapists to advise on mobility and discomfort problems. Nutritionists, psychologists, chiropractors, acupuncturists, endocrinologists, and cardiologists are other health care providers who may be part of the health care team of an individual pregnant woman.

Evidence-Based Practice

Since the early days of the United States, midwives have contributed to knowledge regarding women and infants. Martha Ballard's diary from 1785 to 1812 detailed the care that she gave to women and their families in her rural community; it demonstrated skills, knowledge, outcomes, and political forces that influenced the practice of nurse-midwifery (Ulrich, 1990). The CNM evidence base has grown significantly since Martha Ballard's time. With more nurse-midwives advancing their education in DNP and PhD programs, nurse-midwifery–driven research, theory development, and evidenced-based practice projects are enhancing clinical care and patient outcomes.

As an example, Julia Seng has conducted extensive research on posttraumatic stress disorder (PTSD), childhood abuse, and childbirth outcomes (Seng, Low, Sperlich, Ronis, & Liberzon, 2011; Seng et al., 2013). She has extended her research to include a physiologic and biologic focus related to PTSD and trauma that informs care for nurse-midwives and other maternity care providers (Choi & Seng, 2016; Seng, D'Andrea, & Ford, 2014; Lopez & Seng, 2014). Seng and colleagues argued that pregnancy is a critical time to interrupt the cycle of intergenerational trauma and violence and advocated for intervention when trauma is identified. Additionally, they noted that women with a past history of violence and trauma may be retraumatized during the birth experience. Holly Powell Kennedy is another example of a CNM researcher who has focused her work on topics important to CNM practice, such as normalizing birth (Kennedy, 2010; Kennedy, Grant, Walton, Shaw-Battista, & Sandall, 2010), cesarean birth and vaginal birth after cesarean (Dahlen, Downe, Wright, Kennedy, & Taylor, 2016; Kennedy, Grant, Walton, & Sandall, 2013; Shorten, Shorten, & Kennedy, 2014; Shorten et al., 2015), and extending midwifery care to all women (Renfrew et al., 2014). In addition to distinguished individual midwifery researchers, research is incorporated as a core competency of the ACNM foundation documents. Nurse-midwives are charged with infusing scientific evidence into clinical practice to evaluate, apply, interpret, and collaborate in research (ACNM, 2012a).

The ACNM recognizes the importance of building and translating evidence into CNM practice. One mission of the ACNM Division of Research has been to contribute to knowledge about the health of women, infants, and families and advance the practice of midwifery. The Division of Research promotes the development, conduct, dissemination, and translation of midwifery research into practice (ACNM, 2016c). The ACNM is developing a research agenda that includes a strategic focus on six distinct areas: policy, evidence-based practice, education, collaboration, visibility and message, and organizational and leadership development (ACNM, 2016c). Nurse-midwifery has its own journal, the *Journal of Midwifery & Women's Health,* a peer-reviewed, clinically focused publication that publishes research pertinent to pregnancy, well-woman gynecology, family planning, primary care of women, and health care policies. The ACNM also keeps members up to date via continuing education series and weekly e-newsletters on emerging health crises, such as the Zika and Ebola viruses, and cooperates with federal agencies and other professional organizations to improve health nationally and internationally.

Leadership

Leadership skills are professional responsibilities that are core competencies for nurse-midwives. DNP-prepared nurse-midwives receive additional education and training related to leadership within organizations and systems. Not only are nurse-midwives knowledgeable regarding national and international issues and trends in women's health and maternal-infant care but also they are expected to be leaders in bringing those issues to the forefront. Nurse-midwives are expected to exercise leadership for the benefit of women, infants, and families; the profession of midwifery; and the ACNM. To this end, the ACNM has state- and federal-level resource centers aimed at advocacy for issues related to women's and children's health as well as for tracking professional and interprofessional issues. Federal advocacy includes participating in the Coalition for Quality Maternity Care, which endorses legislative initiatives and strengthens outreach to the grassroots level. It also includes leadership at the federal level to support women's reproductive rights by urging legislators to reject funding cuts that limit access to and information about reproductive choice. For example, in 2013, the ACNM filed an amicus brief in the *Burwell v. Hobby Lobby* case in collaboration with other women's health organizations to emphasize a woman's right to contraceptive access. Additionally, the ACNM enhances the ability of CNMs to function as independent practitioners through state-level advocacy and supporting full practice authority consistent with the *Consensus Model for APRN Regulation* and the IOM's *The Future of Nursing* report (ACNM, n.d.-b, 2014a; IOM, 2011). The ACNM has deepened its leadership and advocacy by representation in external organizations. In the 2014 Annual Report, 79 CNMs were noted as ACNM representatives in external organizations, including key partnerships with the ANA, the ACOG, the ICM, the Midwives Alliance of North America, and Childbirth Connection (ACNM, 2014a).

Collaboration

Interprofessional collaboration is critical to improving patient and population health outcomes in the complex health care environment. Nurse-midwives, particularly those prepared at the doctoral level, have the training and expertise to build interprofessional collaborative teams and facilitate team work and often lead these teams to set goals and improve outcomes (AACN, 2006). The ACNM has a series of position statements on collaboration. The 2014 statement focuses on midwifery management as independent, primarily intended for healthy women; however, in the event of complications, collaborative management or referral to a physician may be an appropriate pathway to ensure a patient's well-being (ACNM, 2014b). The *Joint Statement of Practice Relations Between Obstetrician-Gynecologists and Certified Nurse-Midwives/Certified Midwives* (ACNM, 2011c; see Box 17.2) includes shared agreement on high standards of education, certification, and accreditation as well as mutual support for ensuring that both professions have access to affordable professional liability insurance coverage, hospital privileges, and equivalent reimbursement from private payers, and support services for their work. There is also agreement that these provider groups have access to a system of care that fosters collaboration among licensed independent providers. The 2011 statement also recognized the need for nurse-midwives and physicians to collaborate but stressed the working relationship, respect for each other's abilities and knowledge, and professional responsibility and accountability. In its position statement *Collaborative Agreement Between Physicians and Certified Nurse-Midwives and Certified Midwives,* the ACNM (2011b) clarified its position regarding collaborative agreements in a continuing attempt to delineate the nature of collaboration between physicians and CNMs. This document notes the limitations of collaborative agreements—they do not guarantee effective communication, may wrongly imply that CNMs need supervision, and also may restrict midwives from exercising their full scope of practice (ACNM, 2011b; Box 17.6).

When a complication occurs, the nurse-midwife can continue to be instrumental in the woman's care while benefiting from collaboration with an obstetrician-gynecologist. This involves the nurse-midwife and physician jointly managing the care of a woman whose case has become medically, gynecologically, or obstetrically complicated. The collaborating physician and nurse-midwife mutually agree on the scope of care that each will provide. If the physician needs to assume the main role in the woman's care, the nurse-midwife will still participate to some degree in the physical care and emotional support and, to a large degree, in counseling, guidance, and teaching. For example, a nurse-midwife caring for a pregnant woman identifies that inadequate fetal growth may be an issue. The nurse-midwife then consults with the collaborating physician and, together, they decide on what further

BOX 17.6   Position Statement: Collaborative Agreement Between Physicians and Certified Nurse-Midwives and Certified Midwives

It is the position of the American College of Nurse Midwives (ACNM) that safe, quality health care can best be provided to women and their infants when policymakers develop laws and regulations that permit certified nurse-midwives (CNMs) and certified midwives (CMs) to provide independent midwifery care within their scope of practice while fostering consultation, collaborative management, or seamless referral and transfer of care, when indicated. ACNM affirms the following:

- Requirements for a signed collaborative agreement do not guarantee the effective communication between midwives and physicians that is so critical to successful collaboration:
  - They do not ensure physician availability when needed.
  - There is no evidence that they increase the safety or quality of patient care.
  - In certain circumstances, such as in the aftermath of a natural or declared disaster, such requirements have hampered the ability of CNMs and CMs to provide critically necessary emergency relief services.
- Collaborative agreements signed by individual physicians wrongly imply that CNMs and CMs need the supervision of those individuals in all situations. Based on this misconception:

- Professional liability companies have used signed agreements, with their implied requirements for supervision, as the rationale for raising physician premiums, citing increased risk related to such unneeded supervision.
- CNMs and CMs may be restricted from exercising their full scope of practice or from receiving hospital credentials, clinical privileges, or third-party reimbursement for services that fall within the scope of their training and licensure.
- Requirements for signed collaborative agreements can create an unfair economic disadvantage for CNMs and CMs:
  - They have been used to limit the number of midwives who can practice collaboratively with any one physician, effectively barring CNMs and CMs from practice in some cases or restricting the ratio of CNMs and CMs to physicians
  - They allow potential economic competitors to dictate whether or not midwives can practice in a community
  - They restrict access to care and choice of provider for women. This is of particular concern in underserved areas.

Adapted from American College of Nurse-Midwives. (2004). *Philosophy of the American College of Nurse-Midwives.* Silver Spring, MD: Author; and American College of Nurse-Midwives. (2011). *Position statement: Collaborative agreement between physicians and certified nurse-midwives and certified midwives.* Silver Spring, MD: Author.

testing and care are required under these circumstances. In this case, the testing does show inadequate growth; therefore, the woman will alternate her prenatal visits between the physician and nurse-midwife so that together they can provide frequent fetal surveillance and the best possible outcome for mother and baby. Effective communication is essential in ongoing collaborative management to maintain a healthy working relationship and provide comprehensive care to the individuals under the collaborators' care.

In addition to obstetrician-gynecologists, nurse-midwives collaborate with other providers. During labor, nurse-midwives may collaborate with a doula to provide the laboring woman with the best birth experience possible and to meet the goals of her individual birth plan. Doulas are labor support persons who work with the woman and her family

to ensure that she is well supported during the labor process. Doulas do not offer medical advice or care. Nurse-midwives collaborate with nurses and maternity unit managers to develop unit policies for the optimal care for the pregnant woman and her fetus during the intrapartum and postpartum periods. Nurse-midwives collaborate with other nurse-midwives, labor and delivery nurses, and physician colleagues to develop practice standards and guidelines. These are just a few examples of the myriad ways in which nurse-midwives collaborate in delivering evidence-based care.

Ethical Decision Making

The goal of ethical midwifery practice is to do the right thing for the right reason. Codes of ethics guide moral behavior and are considered to be part of the criteria that make a practice a profession (Thompson, 2002). The ACNM Code of Ethics, reviewed and approved by the ACNM Board in 2015, has three mandates (ACNM, 2015b; see Box 17.4). The first is directed toward the individual woman and her family, the second is for the benefit of all women and their families, and the third is to the profession of midwifery. These mandates are reflected in the Core Competencies for Basic Midwifery Practice (see Box 17.5), the Philosophy of the ACNM (see Box 17.3), and Standards for the Practice of Midwifery (see Table 17.1). The ACNM Code of Ethics aligns with the ICM Code of Ethics, which overviews the ethics of midwifery relationships, the practice of midwifery, professional responsibilities of midwives, and the advancement of midwifery knowledge and practice (ICM, 2014b).

Nurse-midwives are faced with ethical decisions in their daily practice, especially in regard to use of interventions; providing competent, evidence-based, client-centered care; informed consent and protecting privacy; and equitable access to health care (ACNM, 2015b; Brauer, 2016). Whether and when to use electronic fetal monitoring is an example of a care dilemma. It has become a standard of care to monitor the fetal heart rate during labor by electronic fetal monitoring. Most places of birth (mainly hospitals) have guidelines regarding this practice. Many nurse-midwives care for women in hospital settings with implied and explicit expectations to use routine fetal heart rate monitoring, even though the monitor may be intrusive to the woman and not part of her birth plan. However, current evidence does not support routine continuous electronic fetal heart rate monitoring; instead, intermittent auscultation is supported for healthy women without risk factors (ACNM, 2015c; Cox & King, 2015). Informed consent may not be part of the conversation about various options for monitoring the status of the fetus during labor.

Traditional biomedical ethics developed after the atrocities of World War II. Biomedical ethics is a discipline focused on moral philosophy, normative theory, abstract universal principles, and objective problem solving in dilemmas (Thompson, 2002). The over-medicalization of natural life span transitions in health care has directed the education and practice of nursing and midwifery, and bioethics has guided their codes of ethics. The essence of ethical midwifery practice occurs through human engagement, relationships, and the equilibrium of power within those relationships. Midwives create partnerships with women where the woman has autonomy to make informed choices about her health care. This relationship is a collaborative, supportive relationship rather than the patriarchal, provider-dominated interaction that has characterized medical care. In addition, it has been proposed that the ethics of engagement foster ethical midwifery practice by encouraging practitioners to focus on being with women through human engagement (Thompson, 2003).

Client advocacy is part of the ACNM code of ethics that is central to nurse-midwifery practice. Client education and support of clients' rights and self-determination inform every aspect of nurse-midwifery care. These values have been challenged by the burgeoning growth of medical technology over the past two decades and the incursion of managed care in the 1990s. The availability of highly technical interventions for many aspects of childbearing—such as infertility and monitoring pregnancies and birth—conflicts with the traditionally low-technology, low-interventionist approach of nurse-midwives. However, by becoming part of key national movements, such as the Alliance for Innovation on Maternal Health and the US Midwifery Education, Regulation, and Association (US MERA, a group tasked with expanding access to high-quality midwifery care and development of a more cohesive US midwifery presence informed by ICM global standards and competencies), CNMs leverage their ability to ensure that the care being provided to women is woman centered and evidence based. As structures for care delivery continue to evolve from the creation of the ACA, such as health exchanges and accountable care organizations, it will be crucial for CNMs to be involved in the governance of these entities.

Current Practice of Nurse-Midwifery

Scope of Practice

Nurse-midwifery practice encompasses a full range of health care services for women, from adolescence to beyond menopause. These services include the independent provision of primary care, gynecologic and family planning services, preconception care, pregnancy care, care during childbirth and the postpartum period, care of the normal newborn during the first 28 days of life, and treatment of male partners for sexually transmitted infections. CNMs provide initial and ongoing comprehensive assessment, diagnosis, and treatment. They conduct physical examinations; prescribe medications, including controlled substances and contraceptive methods; admit, manage, and discharge patients from birth centers or hospitals; order and interpret laboratory and diagnostic tests; and order the use of medical devices. CNMs' care also includes health promotion, disease prevention, and individualized wellness education and counseling. CNMs must demonstrate that they meet the ACNM Core Competencies for Basic Midwifery Practice (ACNM, 2012a) and must practice in accordance with the ACNM Standards for the Practice of Midwifery (ACNM, 2011e). With constant changes in health care, CNMs may need to expand their knowledge and skills beyond those of basic CNM practice. Advanced CNM skills, such as level 1 ultrasound or acting as first assistant in surgery, may be incorporated into a CNM's practice as long as the CNM follows the recommendations for acquiring these skills by obtaining formal didactic and clinical training to ensure that the advanced skill is acquired and monitored to ensure patient safety. These steps are outlined in Standard VIII of the ACNM standards for practice (ACNM, 2011e; see Table 17.1).

Practice Settings

There are many different settings in which a CNM may practice. A CNM may engage in full-scope practice: care of women from adolescence though the postmenopausal period, including attending women during labor and birth. She or he may also choose one segment of practice—for example, ambulatory care or hospital care—or work exclusively with a population of interest, such as human immunodeficiency virus–positive women or young adolescents. Nurse-midwives practice in urban, suburban, and rural areas. Practice settings can include private practice (nurse-midwife–owned or physician-owned), hospitals, freestanding birth centers, clinics, or homes. Nurse-midwifery practice can be part of a group practice, with any combination of physicians, nurse practitioners, physician assistants, or other health care providers, or a solo practice. The nurse-midwife's actual practice depends on the needs of the population and community being served, interest in specific practice models, preferences of the women being cared for, and availability of physicians and nurse-midwife colleagues for consultation and collaboration as well as personal philosophy of the individual midwife.

A nurse-midwife–assisted birth can take place in homes, freestanding birth centers, birth centers in hospitals, or traditional hospital settings (community, regional, or tertiary). For nurse-midwives and the women for whom they provide care, the choice of setting may be a matter of philosophy, comfort, convenience, or degree of medical risk, or a combination of these factors. Each setting has unique advantages and disadvantages.

Home births are very family and woman centered. Risks of iatrogenic and nosocomial infections are minimized. Nonpharmacologic techniques are used to support women during labor because analgesia and regional anesthesia are not available in the home setting. After the birth, the woman can rest or sleep in her own bed, nurse her infant at will, and enjoy the attention and support of her family and friends. A study by Cheyney, Bovbjerg, et al. (2014) documented the outcomes associated with planned home births among low-risk women attended by midwives in the United States. Eighty-six percent of women who gave birth at home were exclusively breastfeeding 6 weeks postpartum. Additionally, women in the planned home birth group had a cesarean rate of 5.2%, well below the national average of 32% (Martin, Hamilton, Osterman, Driscoll, & Mathews, 2017 2015). Finally, the rates of intrapartum, early neonatal, and late neonatal mortality were quite low at 1.3, 0.41, and 0.35 per 1000, respectively. Access to emergency transfer is critical to safe care and good outcomes, as is an integrated maternity care system with excellent, respectful communication among providers (Cheyney, Everson, & Burcher, 2014; Home Birth Summit, 2016).

The freestanding birth center has a homelike environment, with some select emergency equipment. Birth centers can be accredited by the Commission for the Accreditation of Birth Centers, which ensures that birth centers are meeting standards for safety and care. Most birth centers do not use analgesics or narcotics. Local anesthesia may be used for perineal repair. Disadvantages are similar to those of a home birth in that emergency transport to a hospital may be necessary if the mother or baby develops complications during labor or birth. Most families are discharged within 6 to 12 hours of birth.

Current US hospital units for labor and birth tend to be dual-purpose rooms; women labor and give birth in the same room, and almost all rooms are private. The room may have a rocking chair, pull-out couch, and private bath, with a tub or shower. Although individual and nicely appointed, these rooms are part of the larger medical environment, with fetal monitoring, operating rooms, anesthesia services, and immediate access to neonatal intensive care. The other support people available (nurses, physicians) may not hold the same philosophy of birth as a midwife. Even for a woman without risk factors, there can be more of a tendency to intervene than to support a normal physiologic birth. Pressure to keep things moving and a reliance on the use of technology can be palpable on a busy obstetric unit. The traditional hospital labor, delivery, and maternity units are designed to care for many women at a time, making the units easier for staff to function but not necessarily conducive to the normal labor process. These units are well suited for high-risk women who need access to higher levels of care and infants who may need special care nurseries. However, midwife-attended births in the United States primarily occur in hospital environments where most US women give birth. Therefore, it is incumbent on the midwife to help create an atmosphere of normalcy and trust in the midst of a culture of technology. The nurse-midwifery philosophy of the normalcy of pregnancy and birth in most siutations is beginning to be embraced more widely by the broader health system.

Certified Nurse-Midwife Practice Summary

Nurse-midwives in the United States have a unique approach to care continuity. Nurse-midwives provide prenatal care for a designated caseload of women, attend those women during labor and birth (often shared in a group care model), see them in the postnatal period, and can then provide primary, interconceptional, or gynecologic care for these same women over their life spans. Not all US or international practice models function using this form of continuity; however, women and CNMs have embraced such a model in the United States, similar to the obstetric model of care. Nurse-midwives have many opportunities to influence women's health care through direct care, their broad scope of practice, and through administrative and other leadership positions and by engaging in legislative and policy work. As the number of doctorally prepared midwives continues to increase, whether by virtue of the DNP, PhD, or other related degrees, the scope of influence of midwives on the care system as well as on individual care will continue to increase. Nurse-midwifery care is uniquely woman focused, independent, and collaborative. It offers women the opportunity to obtain accessible, understandable, high-quality care that is safe, satisfying, and individualized to their and their families' needs throughout their lives and during the reproductive years.

Exemplar 17.1 describes Margaret Dorroh's experience in a freestanding birth center. CNM care in the Indian Health Service is highlighted by Ann Debeaumont Doll in Exemplar 17.2.

Professional Issues

Image

The image of the nurse-midwife in the United States varies across communities and health care settings. As noted, many practitioners call themselves midwives, although there is no single standard for education, regulation, and practice, which leads to confusion. Some US citizens continue to believe that midwives lack an educational credential and that they help women give birth at home, that a midwife is a practitioner rooted in the past. Although our students reported this response when announcing to some friends and family about becoming a nurse-midwife, there is considerable evidence of change. CNM-attended births continue to increase. *U.S. News & World Report* (2016) ranked nurse-midwifery at #80 of the 100 best jobs, and job growth of 31% is anticipated from 2014 to 2022 according to the United States Department of Labor (2016). In addition, previous medical resistance at the organizational level has dissipated, exemplified by the 2011 joint statement of practice relationships between the ACNM and the ACOG (ACNM, 2011b) and other ongoing partnerships. The ACNM is moving boldly forward in the 2015-2020 Strategic Plan in support of members and advancing midwifery and women's health by expanding access to midwifery care to all women (ACNM, 2015a). Consumer outreach, including the Healthy Birth Initiative (ACNM, 2016b) and recent ACNM-produced promotional videos of midwives providing care in multiple settings—Healthy Birth with a Midwife (https://www.youtube.com/watch?v=spxWiXbbB0w&list=PLEvd72S0tC-qiAfeXjGdgjRvB7HeybHM9&index=4, 2015), Midwives & the Care They Provide (https://www.youtube.com/watch?v=MLVwdmlZU_8, 2014), and Midwives in Hospitals: A Great Choice for Childbirth (https://www.youtube.com/watch?v=15YAObX_lrM, 2015)—are evidence of increasing visibility and influence.

Work Life

CNMs provide a full range of primary health care services for women, from adolescence through menopause. There is variety in the way these services can be offered and CNMs are fortunate to have options from which to choose. Full-scope women's health care services encompass ambulatory and

The patient education process begins before a patient is accepted into the practice. Orientation sessions are held to provide prospective patients with information to assist them in determining whether they want to have their baby in a birth center. These sessions, conducted by the certified nurse-midwife (CNM), are designed to provide information and a tour of the facility. Prospective patients can see firsthand the comfort measures (e.g., the whirlpool tub) and equipment to handle normal deliveries and emergencies. Finances are discussed, because the cost of care in the birth center is approximately half of that for obstetric care in a hospital setting with a physician. Many insurers, Medicaid, and Medicare cover birthing center care.

In an autonomous setting such as this, clinical documentation must be meticulous, and an individualized health record ensures that accurate, consistent, and complete information is obtained. Thorough health and family histories are taken, including information about the woman's physical health and her psychological well-being:

- Any recent health concerns, including exposure to infectious agents?
- What type of support system does she have in place?
- What resources might she have that are not currently being called on?
- Was the pregnancy planned or a surprise?
- What are her family circumstances?
- Is there a stable relationship, including past or current history of abuse?
- Are there other children?

It is important to document positive and negative influences that can have an impact on the patient's health and the health of her baby. Once the assessment is complete, risk factors that would prevent us from being able to accept a patient are reviewed; if we cannot accept a patient, we make a referral. If no risk factors are identified, we schedule the patient's first visit.

When patients are accepted into the practice, they are told that they are equal partners in their care. It is the goal of patient education to make this a reality. To be active participants in their care, patients are taught to weigh themselves and do their own urine dipstick tests. They participate in charting the information, thus noting the progress of their pregnancy firsthand. The program of care for pregnant patients at our birth center includes 10 to 15 prenatal visits, childbirth classes, labor and delivery in the birth center, a home visit within 72 hours of birth, and two office follow-up visits

for mother and baby, one at 1 week and the other at 6 weeks after birth.

Clinical hours are held daily. The CNMs in the practice share in-office visits, teaching classes, and on-call time. Other responsibilities include administration and facility maintenance. We see pregnant patients, postpartum patients with their babies, and gynecologic patients. The amount of time scheduled for a visit is based on need. A first visit for a pregnant patient is 1 hour long. An established gynecologic patient who is coming for her contraceptive medication requires only a few minutes, long enough to establish that she is having no problems.

When a patient is in active labor or her membranes have ruptured, she calls the CNM on duty. We attribute this largely to the educational process that has taken place. She is met at the birth center and examined. On the rare occasion of false labor or very early labor, we are able to individualize care. If a patient lives far away, we may elect to observe progress for a number of hours. If the woman is sleep deprived, she and her labor may benefit from some sedation. We remain with our patients in the birth center during labor. A registered nurse (RN) is on call for every delivery. If the CNM attending the patient is tiring from having been up for a long labor, or several labors, the RN can be called to come in early to care for the patient while the CNM rests. Sometimes, the RN is not needed until close to time for the birth.

The mother-to-be helps us accommodate her wishes by preparing a birth plan. As her due date nears, one of her tasks (along with packing a bag to bring to the birth center and readying her home for a baby) is to write a birth plan, which will become part of her record. This allows her to tell us who she wants with her during labor, what she imagines labor will be like, what she hopes labor will be like, and what comfort measures would assist her during labor. We use this tool in several ways. We evaluate the effectiveness of our teaching by reading what the woman thinks labor will be like and helping her manage expectations. Mention of fears not previously revealed gives us an opportunity to resolve any emotional factors that could hinder a successful labor. Knowing the person(s) that the patient wants with her during labor informs us about her support system. The people present during labor are an important factor in enhancing the woman's experience of labor.

The list of comfort measures is mainly a reminder to us, although it is a key contribution from the patient.

Continued

In the midst of labor, a woman may forget that she was looking forward to the whirlpool tub for relaxation and pain relief. A glance at the birth plan helps us try the things that the patient has already identified as being potentially helpful to her. The birth plan helps emphasize to the patient that this is her labor, with its inherent responsibilities and rights. Her dignity and worth as a human being are of highest priority, as are the well-being of mother and baby. We try to nourish the woman's self-esteem and strengths that help in labor, life, and motherhood. The stronger the woman is in every way, the better will be the outcome.

Patients are given ample written material to help with their recall of information covered in classes. (If a patient is unable to read, extra time is spent providing information verbally and making sure that the patient understands it.) To help the patient assume responsibility for herself and her labor, she is expected to bring food and beverages with her to the birth center that she would like to have available during labor and certain supplies, such as perineal pads, bed pads, and diapers. Patients take their babies home dressed in their own clothes and wrapped in their own blankets. They take with them an instructional booklet that they were given in the postpartum class. The booklet describes mother and baby care for the first few days in detail. Because mothers and babies are discharged early, often in 4 to 6 hours, it is imperative that the mother be prepared to check the baby's temperature and respirations, check her own uterus, and be able to recognize signs of complications that require attention. These are all enumerated in the instructions, and there is room for notes and questions. Having a reference helps new moms feel more secure. If something needs attention, they can always call the nurse-midwife, but they usually find what they need to know in the booklet. It often confirms what they sensed—that everything was okay or that they need to get in touch with the nurse-midwife. Thus new mothers start out having faith in their own perceptions regarding their infants being reinforced.

Empowering our patients, enhancing their decision-making abilities, reinforcing the mind-body connection, and enhancing family life by helping women find their personal power are goals of CNM care at the birth center. When I think of the enormous effects of empowerment, two new moms come to mind.

ML's case is positive proof of the benefits of teaching new mothers to trust their feelings and make decisions based on them. On the third or fourth day after delivery, ML's baby ceased nursing well. He had been nursing vigorously and now was not. Nursing poorly is one of the signs listed in our booklet that requires professional help. ML insisted to her husband that they had to go to the emergency room immediately. They lived a long distance from the birth center and it had been decided earlier that if there should be a problem that seemed serious, she should go to a nearby emergency room rather than try to get to the CNM. Initially, doctors could find nothing wrong, but ML insisted they keep looking. As it turned out, the baby had a congenital heart defect that does not show up on a clinical examination until 3 or 4 days after birth. ML said she was glad she had been given the information at the birth center; it gave her the confidence to trust her feelings that something was seriously wrong. The baby had heart surgery and is doing well.

A woman with confidence and trust in herself can do almost anything, as shown by the case of SJ. She was 26 years old and came to the birth center soon after it opened, to have her fourth child. SJ had a high school education and was home with her children, all of whom were younger than 5 years. Her self-esteem was negligible. Her husband came to a few of the prenatal classes but was sullen and unsupportive. SJ seemed to droop, but she was an excellent mother and was an attentive and fast learner regarding everything to do with childbirth, child rearing, and health in general. Her interest and enthusiasm grew as we reinforced her abilities and strengths. By the time she gave birth to her son, she seemed a different person from the withdrawn, self-effacing young woman we had met 7 months earlier. Two years after this baby's birth, SJ visited the birth center. "I just wanted to thank you," she said. "Before I came here, I never felt I was any good at anything. You told me I was a good mother, you noticed how well cared for my children were, and you encouraged me to learn all about birth and even let me borrow books and tapes. Well, I learned I was good—at a lot of things! You all showed me that. And I wanted you to know I'm in nursing school now because I want to be able to do what you do—not just take care of people physically, but help people grow." ◎

[a]We wish to acknowledge Margaret W. Dorroh, CNM, for this exemplar.

EXEMPLAR 17.2   **Nurse-Midwifery Practice in an Urban Indian Health Service Hospital[a]**

In 1973, one of the largest Indian Health Service (IHS) hospitals employed the first nurse-midwife. This service unit, located in the southwestern United States, serves 14 surrounding Native American tribes. It is the largest urban referral center for IHS clinics and hospitals located on tribal reservations, many of which are remote with limited resources. The practice has since grown to a midwifery service that employs nine certified nurse-midwives (CNMs) and two family nurse practitioners (FNPs). The CNMs provide in-hospital maternity care around the clock, including labor and delivery and obstetric triage, with full hospital admitting privileges. The midwifery service has recently expanded with the addition of an FNP and a dual-certified FNP/CNM to better serve our population in the full-scope clinical practice located on site. The service unit employs eight obstetrician-gynecologists (OB-GYNs) who care for high-risk patients with more complex medical problems and provide consultation to the midwifery service. In 2013 the Women and Infant Service Line was formed incorporating pediatrics, women's health, obstetric medical services, nursing, and all the supportive ancillary services under the direction of a doctorally prepared CNM.

The IHS has a long-standing and rich history of midwifery care. The midwifery model of care that values women supporting women through the normal process of pregnancy and childbirth is aligned with indigenous women's practice of receiving birth assistance from women within their communities and from tribal midwives. The IHS, established in 1955, recognized the value of midwifery care to Native American women early on and began incorporating midwifery care in IHS facilities in the late 1960s. Midwives are afforded a high level of respect and are valued within the IHS for their ability to provide culturally attentive care for Native American women. CNMs at this site are medical staff members with full voting privileges. CNMs are integrated in leadership positions, serve on committees, participate in quality assurance, take part in clinical decision making that impacts the obstetrics and women's health medical services, and are involved in program development and implementation. The majority of CNMs precept student nurse-midwives and greatly appreciate giving back to the profession in this way. The midwifery service has participated in the American College of Nurse-Midwives (ACNM) Benchmarking Project with a twofold purpose as stated by the ACNM: (1) to provide members with a platform for monitoring, maintaining, and improving the quality of midwifery care; and (2) to provide a national snapshot of midwifery quality metrics, related to perinatal outcomes in all settings where CNMs/CMs are involved in full-scope maternity care. The midwifery service has consistently met benchmarking goals and received commendations as a best practice throughout the years of participation. CNMs are encouraged to expand their scope of practice. For instance, opportunity exists for colposcopy training if desired. CNMs first-assist for cesarean births and are trained to provide limited ultrasound, also expansions of basic scope of practice. Innovation and creativity are encouraged and supported. A recent example of such innovation was the implementation of nitrous oxide for pain management in labor and delivery. This effort was midwifery driven and has been well received by staff and appreciated by our patients.

Collaborative practice between CNMs and OB-GYNs within the IHS has been the long-standing standard of care since the mid-1970s (Indian Health Service Manual, Chapter 13: Maternal and Child Health). The midwifery practice enjoys a collaborative practice of mutual respect with physician colleagues. Delineation of services between the OB-GYN services and the CNM services are defined in the policies. Low-risk women are admitted to the CNM service and high-risk women, as defined in the policies, are admitted to the OB-GYN services. If complications develop during the course of care that cannot be resolved with physician consultation, care is transferred to the OB-GYN services.

In 2015, 98% of the spontaneous vaginal births at this service unit were attended by CNMs. The primary cesarean rate of women admitted to the midwifery service was 13.2% and the overall cesarean rate for the midwifery service was 15.7%. The overall cesarean rate of the combined OB-GYN and CNM services was 28.3%. This combined services cesarean rate is consistently below the national average of 32.2% for 2014, as reported by the Centers for Disease Control and Prevention (http://www.cdc.gov/nchs/fastats/delivery.htm). The vaginal birth after cesarean success rate was 85%. Considering that 25% of the patients who gave birth at this service unit in 2015 had gestational diabetes, and thus were at increased risk of complications, the improved outcomes are even more indicative of the benefits of the midwifery care. The presence of the CNMs to support normal physiologic labor and birth has driven a midwifery model of care that includes nursing and physician support. Laboring women typically have

Continued

| EXEMPLAR 17.2 | Nurse-Midwifery Practice in an Urban Indian Health Service Hospital[a]—cont'd |

a robust family support system that is present for the labor and birth. Women are in an atmosphere that is sensitive to their culture and traditions and often voice a sentiment of "coming home" to the Indian hospital. The total epidural rate is 33%, which is relatively low, enabling women to be active with intermittent monitoring and utilize laboring in water, the birthing ball, frequent position changes, and choices regarding how they position themselves to birth. Nitrous oxide and narcotic analgesia are available if desired.

The Baby Friendly Initiative was mandated IHS-wide, and accreditation was achieved at this service unit in 2013. In 2015, 89% of women were breastfeeding at time of discharge from the maternity services. Significant evidence supports decreased incidence of diabetes and obesity—two major health disparities among the Native American population—in infants who are breastfed. Antibodies and nutrition obtained through breast milk are known to improve infant well-being and overall health with potential for decreased risk for diabetes and obesity in adulthood. The educational component related to the Baby Friendly Initiative, both prenatally and during the course of postpartum care, is readily provided by CNMs. The transition to meet the requirements for Baby Friendly accreditation on the obstetrics/postpartum ward were fairly seamless because they mirrored long-held midwifery practice at our site, such as delayed cord clamping, immediate skin-to-skin contact with the newborn placed on the maternal chest, early

initiation of breastfeeding, infant rooming-in with the mother, and feeding on demand. The more difficult transition was initiating skin-to-skin contact in the operating room following a cesarean birth. However, it was quickly incorporated into routine practice when the benefits to parents became evident. If we are unable to place the newborn on the mother's chest skin-to-skin, the newborn is received by the father of the baby or the support person present in the operating room suite.

The midwifery service conducted 10,930 outpatient visits in 2014. The outpatient clinic is structured to provide CNMs with adequate time to facilitate coordination of care and provide education; however, our patients often have complex needs requiring coordination of care that is time consuming and often met with obstacles. The CNMs are integrally involved in the current IHS mandate to implement a medical home model of care, which has provided us with the opportunity to have services readily available in the clinic, such as obstetrics, social services, and a nutritionist. These additional services have removed some of the barriers to facilitating care. The midwifery model of care lends itself well to this practice that is scarcely resourced and continues to demonstrate cost-effective care and positive outcomes. We continue with our commitment to rally to provide all available resources to ensure a positive outcome for Native American mothers and their newborns. ◎

[a]We wish to acknowledge Ann Debeaumont Doll, MS, CNM, for this exemplar.

in-hospital care for a group of women, and midwives in full-scope practice usually work the highest number of hours per week compared with midwives in other practice models. Salaries range from $50,310 to $132,270 (median, $92,510), according to the United States Department of Labor (2016).

A 2010 survey of California nurse practitioners and CNMs provides a sample of CNM work hours; respondents reported an average work week of 33.5 hours for CNMs, including an average of 11 on-call hours per week (California Board of Registered Nursing, 2011). Almost 35% of CNMs reported working 33 to 40 hours per week, and 22% reported working 25 to 32 hours per week. Approximately 52% of CNMs reported working 5 to 8 hours per day on average, thus a portion of CNM respondents were working part time. Over 73% of midwives said

that they always or almost always work to the full extent of their scope of practice, and over 85% reported being satisfied with their APRN career. Average CNM salaries reported in this survey were similar to those reported by the United States Department of Labor (2016).

If a practice has several nurse-midwives and the call is shared (e.g., one or two nights of call a week for each midwife), along with 2 to 3 days in the ambulatory clinic setting, the workload can be manageable. To give their best to their patients and stay healthy, nurse-midwives with a heavier on-call schedule need to develop self-care strategies that enable them to balance work with personal responsibilities and relationships. Perhaps more importantly, there is increasing evidence about the relationship between fatigue and medical errors, affecting the call schedule of medical residents and prompting numerous organizations to issue alerts and position papers. Professional midwifery organizations and employers need to be proactive in making recommendations about this aspect of quality and safety. The ACNM published a document with recommendations for sleep and safety for midwives and midwifery students (ACNM, 2017).

Some nurse-midwives may choose an alternative practice model to enhance their personal interests or maximize work-life balance. They may choose to be a laborist, working specific shifts and providing maternity services in the hospital, including triage and the management of labor and birth of women whose provider may be unavailable or who have not enrolled with a provider before labor. An ambulatory women's health position is also an option and gives the advantage of regular hours, although the labor and birth component would be missing in this position. Some midwives engage in teaching in midwifery programs and may also follow an academic research trajectory. Others have positions in medical program education, teaching medical students and obstetric and family medicine residents about preventive health care and normal pregnancy and birth. For those who love it, the satisfaction of providing care to a pregnant woman, following her through her pregnancy, assisting her through the physical and mental demands of labor and birth, anticipating the unpredictability of birth, and seeing the joy of a family greeting their newborn make nurse-midwifery fascinating, exciting, and personally worth the physical and emotional investment of oneself that may be required. It is a privilege to be with families experiencing pregnancy and birth. The opposite kind of experiences, when a woman experiences a stillbirth or a newborn with a major genetic or anatomic abnormality, can be difficult for the midwife and families. Yet even in these difficult situations, there is satisfaction in supporting a woman and her family as they cope with complex life situations.

Professional Liability

Midwives need to clarify critical details of professional liability insurance, including the type of policy, whether the policy from an employer is institutional or individual (and individual vs. group limits of coverage), if the employer is self-insured or works with a specific insurance company, whether the employer will pay tail coverage for a claims-made policy, and if the employer provides legal counsel if a claim is made, are critical details for midwives

to clarify. Nurse-midwifery liability insurance rates are generally higher than those for other APRNs because of the malpractice climate of maternity care (ACNM, 2014a). Professional organizations and individual nurse-midwives work to stay abreast of legislative and practice changes that may help reframe the current litigious environment in which health care occurs, especially for practitioners of midwifery and obstetrics. According to the most recent survey of ACNM members in 2009, 32% of respondents had been named in at least one lawsuit (Guidera, McCool, Hanlon, Schuiling, & Smith, 2012).

The ACNM, through its state and federal legislative offices, supports tort reform that would cap non-economic damages, limit the number of years in which a plaintiff can file a health care liability action, place reasonable limits on punitive damages, and expand alternative dispute resolution methods. In addition to supporting tort reform, the ACNM has developed a professional liability resource packet that seeks to keep CNMs updated on these issues. The organization also emphasizes quality and safety in practice and risk management strategies that help prevent adverse events from occurring. Finally, it seeks to ensure that midwives have a medical liability insurance option available with a strong underwriter and national coverage endorsed by the professional organization; such an option currently exists (ACNM, n.d.-e).

Quality and Safety

Quality and safety are important topics to nurse-midwives; the ACNM has increased its activity through a position statement, *Creating a Culture of Safety in Midwifery Care* (ACNM, 2016f). This document outlines the principles of evidence-based practice, interprofessional team communication, patient-centered care, and participation in quality management programs. The ACNM is a core member of the Alliance for Innovation on Maternal Health program, a national partnership of organizations dedicated to reducing maternal mortality, improving postpartum care, and providing resources for consistency in providing well-woman care in the United States (ACNM, n.d.-a). The ACNM is also a member of the Council on Patient Safety in Women's Health Care (http://safehealthcareforeverywoman.org), providing information to members of collaborating organizations to provide safe care to every woman. Partnership with multiple national women's health professional groups on the development of a safety bundle for postpartum hemorrhage, a common cause of maternal morbidity and mortality, exemplifies this work. The resulting paper was published in several professional journals simultaneously, including the *Journal of Midwifery & Women's Health* (Main et al., 2015). Similarly, the ACNM again partnered with multiple professional organizations in publishing *Transforming Communication and Safety Culture in Intrapartum Care: A Multiorganizational Blueprint* (Lyndon et al., 2015).

Nurse-midwifery has a sustained history of reducing health disparities among disadvantaged groups, starting in rural Eastern Kentucky where, over a 30-year period, low-birth-weight and maternal mortality rates dropped from levels that were among the highest in the country to those among the lowest. From 1925 to 1958, the maternal mortality rate was 9.1 per 10,000 for the Frontier Nursing Service and 34 per 10,000 for the United States as a whole (Metropolitan Life Insurance Company, 1960). A recent Cochrane review continues to document that midwife-led care models result in fewer medical interventions, greater maternal satisfaction, and a trend toward lower costs with outcomes at least equivalent to other care models (Sandall, Soltani, Gates, Shennan, & Devane, 2016).

Conclusion

Positive advances in nurse-midwifery and between nurse-midwifery and the broader health care system are evident. The ACNM has been extending its reach and has been invited to collaborate broadly with professional nursing, other midwifery groups, medicine (including obstetrics and gynecology), policy, and public health colleagues nationally and internationally. The need for more midwives has been recognized internationally to continue to reduce maternal and neonatal mortality. In the United States the IOM report *The Future of Nursing,* passage of the ACA, increased consumer demand, an improved public image, a growing CNM research evidence base, and strong national quality and educational standards have placed CNMs and other APRNs in a visible leadership role in redesigning the health care system for the future. From a midwifery perspective, it is anticipated that a future health care system will honor all women and offer support in realizing the satisfaction that comes with a truly woman-centered health care system.

Key Summary Points

■ CNMs are primary care providers who are educated in and practice the two distinct disciplines of nursing and midwifery

■ CNMs are educated in graduate programs accredited by the Accreditation Commission for Midwifery Education and are certified by the American Midwifery Certification Board.

■ The midwifery model of care practiced by CNMs includes a strong focus on woman-centered care and supporting the normalcy of pregnancy and birth as well as other life transitions.

■ Midwifery has been recognized internationally as a key resource for improving maternal and newborn health in developed and developing countries.

■ CNMs practice and have prescribing authority in all 50 states, practice in all types of health care settings (including the US military), and attend births in hospitals, homes, and freestanding birth centers.

■ As the number of CNMs and CNM-attended births continues to grow, nurse-midwives continue building the required evidence base for practice and are fully engaged in collaborative policy efforts to reform the US health care system.

References

To access the references for this chapter, use your smartphone's QR code reader to scan the code below, or go to http://booksite.elsevier.com/ 9780323447751.

The Certified Registered Nurse Anesthetist

Margaret Faut Callahan • Michael J. Kremer

"As a nurse, we have the opportunity to heal the heart, mind, soul, and body of our patients, their families, and ourselves. They may forget your name, but they will never forget how you made them feel."

—*Maya Angelou*

CHAPTER CONTENTS

Nurse anesthesia is the oldest organized advanced practice registered nurse (APRN) specialty. Standardized postgraduate education, credentialing, and continuing education are all areas pioneered by these APRNs. In 1989, certified registered nurse anesthetists (CRNAs) were the first nurse specialists to receive direct reimbursement for their services. This chapter discusses the professional definitions of nurse anesthesia practice and issues important to this APRN specialty. A profile of current CRNA practice is described and challenges and future trends are proposed. The American Association of Nurse Anesthetists (AANA) is described and a model of professional competence for CRNAs is presented. The transition of nurse anesthesia education to the practice doctorate and the associated competencies

for CRNAs prepared at the doctoral level are also reviewed.

Brief History of CRNA Education and Practice

Education

Nurses have provided anesthesia since the American Civil War (1861-1865). The first organized program in nurse anesthesia education was offered in 1909. Alumnae from nurse anesthesia programs formed the National Association of Nurse Anesthetists (NANA) in 1931; the organization was renamed the American Association of Nurse Anesthetists (AANA) in 1939. In 1952, the AANA established a mechanism for accreditation of nurse anesthesia education programs that has been recognized by the U.S. Department of Education since 1955 (Bankert, 1989).

At this writing there are 118 accredited nurse anesthesia programs, with over 2121 clinical sites in the United States and Puerto Rico. In addition, there are six new nurse anesthesia programs in the accreditation capability review process. These APRN education programs are affiliated with or operated by schools or colleges of nursing, allied health, or other academic entities (Gerbasi, 2015).

Certification

Nurse anesthetists were among the first APRNs to require continuing education. The AANA implemented a certification program in 1945 and instituted mandatory recertification in 1978. The CRNA credential came into existence in 1956 (Bankert, 1989). Until 2016, CRNAs required recertification every 2 years, which included meeting practice requirements and obtaining a minimum of 40 continuing education credits (National Board of Certification and Recertification of Nurse Anesthetists [NBCRNA], 2016b). In 2016, a major shift in CRNA credentialing occurred.

In 2012, the NBCRNA announced a Continued Professional Certification (CPC) program that became operational in 2016. The CPC program reflects the principles of competency-based medical education utilized by the American Board of Medical Specialties certification and maintenance of certification programs as well as the Maintenance of Certification in Anesthesiology program used by the American Society of Anesthesiologists (Carraccio et al., 2017; Culley et al., 2013). It took 4 years to develop a reliable and valid mechanism to assess continued professional competence. The CPC program is an 8-year program comprising two 4-year CPC cycles and consists of four major components (NBCRNA, 2016b):

- Class A credits (assessed continuing education): 60 credits every 4 years
- Class B credits (professional development): 40 credits every 4 years
- Core modules: four every 4 years, one in each of four core areas
- CPC examination: once every 8 years

Because the CPC program requires not only continuing education credits but also mandatory retesting, many concerns had to be addressed over the previous 4 years. Both the NBCRNA and the AANA focused on patient safety as well as what was in the best interest of the CRNA community. The resultant program provides opportunities for CRNAs to become accustomed to the new approach while moving to the most robust CPC program in advanced practice nursing today (NBCRNA, 2016a). Thus the CRNA is the only APRN role that requires evidence of continued competency through an examination every 8 years.

Practice

CRNAs provide anesthesia for approximately 32 million surgical and diagnostic procedures in the United States each year (AANA, 2016d). The impact of the aging population, coupled with implementation of the Patient Protection and Affordable Care Act (ACA, 2010; US Department of Health and Human Services, 2016), if operationalization continues as planned, will result in more surgical and diagnostic procedures being performed because more citizens will have insurance coverage.

The Institute of Medicine (IOM) report on *The Future of Nursing* (2010) noted that

> … transforming the health care system to meet the demand for safe, quality and affordable care will require a fundamental rethinking of the roles of many health care professionals, including nurses. The ACA represents the broadest health care overhaul since the 1965 creation of the Medicare and Medicaid programs, but nurses are unable to fully participate in the resulting evolution of the U.S. health care system. (p. 5)

The IOM report expressed concern that physicians challenge expanding scopes of practice for nurses and that "given the great need for more affordable health care, nurses should be playing a larger role in the health care system, both in delivering care and decision making about care" (p. 7). The IOM report concluded that

> [N]ow is the time to eliminate outdated regulations and organizational and cultural barriers that limit the ability of nurses to practice to the full extent of their education, training and competence. … Scope of practice regulations in all states should reflect the full extent of … each profession's education and training. (IOM, 2010, p. 96)

Reflecting on progress addressing the issues identified in the 2010 IOM report, Hassmiller (2015) noted:

> We are proud of the solid progress made in increasing the number of nurses with advanced degrees,

expanding the number of states with broader scopes of practice, bringing more nurses into leadership positions and increasing workforce diversity. We have built the infrastructure needed to make continued progress in all of these areas through an active, engaged network of nurses and other key stakeholders participating in Campaign for Action coalitions in all 50 states. Yet we have a great deal of work left to do. We must increase the number of nurses serving in leadership positions and further expand the number of states in which nurses can practice to the full extent of their education and training.

Nurse anesthetists have been the main providers of anesthesia care to US military men and women on the front lines of combat since World War I. Documentation of nurses providing anesthesia to wounded soldiers dates back to the American Civil War (Bankert, 1989). Currently, 4% of US nurse anesthetists serve in the military or at US Department of Veterans Affairs (VA) facilities (Wilson, 2015).

Regarding malpractice coverage, the average 2016 malpractice premium for self-employed CRNAs was 33% lower than in 1988, or 65% lower when adjusted for inflation. This decline in malpractice premium rate reflects the safe care provided by nurse anesthetists and is impressive given inflation and our litigious society (AANA, 2016c).

Men have historically been more represented in nurse anesthesia practice compared with nursing as a whole. Gender distribution among nurse anesthetists and student nurse anesthetists is 45% male, compared with fewer than 10% of males in the US nursing profession. Currently, more than 90% of the 49,000 US nurse anesthetists are members of the AANA (AANA, 2016c).

Role Differentiation Between CRNAs and Anesthesiologists

CRNAs provide anesthesia services in collaboration with surgeons, anesthesiologists, dentists, podiatrists, and other qualified health care professionals. When anesthesia is administered by a nurse anesthetist, it is recognized as the practice of nursing; when administered by an anesthesiologist, it is recognized as the practice of medicine. Regardless of their educational backgrounds, all anesthesia providers adhere to the same standards of care (AANA, 2016b).

Profile of the CRNA

A CRNA is a registered nurse who is educationally prepared at the graduate level and certified as competent to engage in practice as a nurse anesthetist, rendering patients unable to sense pain with anesthetic agents and related drugs and procedures. Anesthesia services are delivered by anesthesia providers on request, assignment, or referral by the operating physician or other health care provider authorized by law, usually to facilitate diagnostic, therapeutic, or surgical procedures. In addition to general or regional anesthesia techniques, as well as monitored anesthesia care, a referral or request for consultation or assistance may be initiated for the provision of obstetric anesthesia services, ventilator management, or treatment of acute or chronic pain through the performance of selected diagnostic or therapeutic blocks or other forms of pain management. Education, practice, and research within the specialty of nurse anesthesia promote competent anesthesia care across the life span at all acuity levels. CRNAs practice according to their expertise, state statutes and regulations, and institutional policy (AANA, 2016b). CRNAs work collaboratively with all members of the perioperative team, including nurses, technicians, surgeons, and anesthesiologists.

CRNAs are responsible and accountable for their individual professional practices and are capable of exercising independent judgment within the scope of their education (credentials), demonstrated competence (privileges), and licensure. CRNAs are recognized in all 50 states by state regulatory bodies, primarily boards of registered nursing. Nurse anesthesia is a recognized nursing specialty role and is not a medically delegated act (AANA, 2016g).

Compensation, along with role-related autonomy and responsibility, continues to attract qualified applicants to this advanced practice nursing specialty. Recent annual CRNA salary data for all full-time CRNAs showed a median annual salary of $170,000. CRNAs employed by hospitals had higher median annual compensation rates ($180,000) than did those CRNAs employed by anesthesia practice groups ($160,000). The median annual compensation for military or VA-employed CRNAs was $170,000 (Wilson, 2015).

The CRNA practice profile is influenced by the work of the AANA Practice Committee and AANA Professional Practice Department. The Professional Practice Department participates in safety and quality issues, including reduction of needlestick injuries and safe injection practices. The AANA is represented at the National Patient Safety Foundation and is involved with the Ambulatory Surgery and Office Surgery Initiative. The AANA is a major stakeholder and participant in the National Quality Forum (NQF), addressing patient safety issues (AANA, 2016f). For example, the NQF's Serious Reportable Events in surgical or invasive procedures include surgery or another invasive procedure performed on the wrong site or patient as well as intraoperative or immediately postoperative/postprocedure death in an American Society of Anesthesiologists Class 1 (healthy) patient (NQF, 2016).

The AANA works with accrediting bodies to review standards revisions. There is CRNA representation on The Joint Commission (TJC) Technical Advisory Committees. TJC has created credentialing requirements for all categories of clinicians, a process into which the AANA had input. CRNAs are surveyors for the Accreditation Association for Ambulatory Health Care.

Scope and Standards of Practice

The *Scope of Nurse Anesthesia Practice,* as set forth by the AANA, is comprehensive and includes all aspects of anesthesia care (AANA, 2016e). Regardless of the setting in which CRNAs practice, their role includes meeting the individual anesthesia care needs of patients in the perioperative period, including the following (AANA, 2013b):

- Performing and documenting a preanesthetic assessment and evaluation of the patient, including requesting consultations and diagnostic studies; selecting, obtaining, ordering and administering preanesthetic medications and fluids; and obtaining informed consent for anesthesia
- Developing and implementing an anesthetic plan
- Initiating the anesthetic technique, which may include general, regional, and local anesthesia and sedation
- Selecting, applying, and inserting appropriate noninvasive and invasive monitoring modalities for continuous evaluation of the patient's physical status
- Selecting, obtaining, and administering the anesthetic, adjuvant and accessory drugs, and fluids necessary to manage the anesthetic
- Managing a patient's airway and pulmonary status using current practice modalities
- Facilitating emergence and recovery from anesthesia by selecting, obtaining, ordering,

and administering medications, fluids, and ventilator support
- Discharging the patient from a postanesthesia care area and providing anesthesia follow-up evaluation and care
- Implementing evidence-based acute and chronic pain management modalities
- Responding to emergency situations by providing airway management, administering emergency fluids and drugs, and using basic or advanced cardiac life support techniques

Additional nurse anesthesia responsibilities delineated in the *Scope and Standards of Nurse Anesthesia Practice* (AANA, 2013b), which are within the expertise of the individual CRNA, include the following:

- Administration and management—scheduling, material and supply management, development of policies and procedures, fiscal management, performance evaluations, preventive maintenance, billing, data management, and supervision of staff, students, or ancillary personnel
- Quality assessment—data collection, reporting mechanisms, trending, compliance, committee meetings, departmental review, problem-focused studies, problem solving, intervention, and document and process oversight
- Education—clinical and didactic teaching, basic cardiac life support and advanced cardiac life support instruction, in-service commitment, emergency medical technician training, supervision of residents, and continuing education
- Research—conducting and participating in departmental, hospital-wide, and university-sponsored research projects
- Committee appointments—assignment to committees, committee responsibilities, and coordination of committee activities
- Interdepartmental liaison—interface with other departments such as nursing, surgery, obstetrics, postanesthesia care units (PACUs), outpatient surgery, admissions, administration, laboratory, and pharmacy
- Clinical and administrative oversight of other departments—for example, respiratory therapy, PACU, operating room, surgical intensive care unit, and pain clinics

The *Standards for Nurse Anesthesia Practice* (AANA, 2013c) serve these functions:

1. Assist the profession in evaluating the quality of care provided by practitioners.
2. Provide a common base for practitioners to use in their development of a quality practice.

3. Assist the public in understanding what to expect from the practitioner.
4. Support and preserve the basic rights of the patient.

There are 11 standards of practice for CRNAs that "apply to all anesthetizing locations and may be exceeded at any time at the discretion of the CRNA. Although the standards are intended to promote high-quality patient care, they cannot assure specific outcomes" (AANA, 2013c). The standards are found in Box 18.1.

Anesthesia care is provided by CRNAs in four general categories: (1) preanesthetic evaluation and preparation; (2) anesthesia induction, maintenance, and emergence; (3) postanesthesia care; and (4) perianesthetic and clinical support functions. Parallels between nursing and nurse anesthesia are apparent. CRNAs perform preanesthetic assessment, plan appropriate anesthetic interventions, implement planned anesthetic care, and evaluate patients postoperatively to determine the efficacy of their interventions. CRNAs working independently routinely perform all these aspects of clinical practice. When CRNAs and anesthesiologists work together, a variety of factors, such as billing arrangements and local anesthesia practice patterns, determine the extent each practitioner is involved in specific anesthesia care areas (AANA, 2016b).

Preoperative evaluation has become more complex with the increasing acuity of surgical patients. Thorough preanesthetic assessments, combined with specialty consultation as needed, are essential activities at which nurse anesthetists must be proficient (AANA, 2016b).

Developing and implementing an anesthetic care plan is another important aspect of CRNA practice. This care plan is formulated with input from the patient, surgeon, and anesthesiologist in those settings in which CRNAs and anesthesiologists work collaboratively. Input from the patient, surgeon, and anesthetist is relevant when making the important decision about which type of anesthetic to administer in a given situation. Compromise and flexibility may be necessary to achieve the goals of surgery and anesthesia to maximize safety and minimize risks during the procedure and postprocedure period.

The scope of practice for CRNAs varies depending on institutional credentialing. Although most CRNAs provide general anesthesia and monitored anesthesia care (local anesthesia, intravenous sedation, and monitoring by an anesthesia provider), regional anesthesia may be administered less frequently than general anesthesia due to institutional credentialing and local practice patterns. Placement of invasive monitoring lines and pain management techniques may also be less commonly performed by nurse anesthetists, also due to institutional credentialing and local practice patterns. Practice restrictions may not always be imposed via the credentialing process; some providers choose not to perform certain types of procedures. The AANA's *Guidelines for Core Clinical Privileges for Nurse Anesthetists* (AANA, 2013a) include CRNA qualifications and recommended core clinical privileges, which are found in Box 18.2.

Education, Credentialing, and Certification

To become a CRNA, the following requirements must be met (AANA, 2016c):

- Complete a Bachelor's of Science in Nursing degree or other appropriate baccalaureate degree.
- Hold current licensure as a registered nurse (RN).
- Complete at least 1 year as an RN in a critical care setting.
- Graduate with a minimum of a master's degree from an accredited nurse anesthesia educational program. Nurse anesthesia programs range from 24 to 36 months, depending on university requirements. All nurse anesthesia programs include clinical training in academic medical centers or large community hospitals.
- Successfully complete the National Certification Examination (NCE) offered by the NBCRNA for CRNAs.

In order to be recertified, CRNAs must meet the ongoing CPC program requirements (described previously), document substantial anesthesia practice, maintain current state licensure, and certify that they have not developed any conditions that could adversely affect their ability to practice anesthesia (AANA, 2016c).

Since 1998, all nurse anesthesia programs have been at the graduate level. As of January 1, 2022, all students entering accredited nurse anesthesia educational programs must be enrolled in a doctoral program (Gerbasi, 2015). Practice doctorates offered in nurse anesthesia programs include the Doctor of Nursing Practice and the Doctor of Nurse Anesthesia Practice. The Doctor of Nursing Practice is typically offered for programs housed in schools of nursing, and the Doctor of Nurse Anesthesia Practice may be the exit degree for nurse anesthesia programs located in schools of health sciences or other

BOX 18.1 Standards for Nurse Anesthesia Practice

Standard I: Perform and document a thorough preanesthesia assessment and evaluation.

Standard II: Obtain and document informed consent for the planned anesthetic intervention from the patient or legal guardian, or verify that informed consent has been obtained and documented by a qualified professional.

Standard III: Formulate a patient-specific plan for anesthesia care.

Standard IV: Implement and adjust the anesthesia care plan based on the patient's physiologic status. Continuously assess the patient's response to the anesthetic, surgical intervention, or procedure. Intervene as required to maintain the patient in optimal physiologic condition.

Standard V: Monitor, evaluate, and document the patient's physiologic condition as appropriate for the type of anesthesia and specific patient needs. When any physiologic monitoring device is used, variable pitch and threshold alarms shall be turned on and audible. The certified registered nurse anesthetist (CRNA) should attend to the patient continuously until the responsibility of care has been accepted by another anesthesia professional.

  a. **Oxygenation:** Continuously monitor oxygenation by clinical observation and pulse oximetry. If indicated, continually monitor oxygenation by arterial blood gas analysis.

  b. **Ventilation:** Continuously monitor ventilation. Verify intubation of the trachea or placement of other artificial airway devices by auscultation, chest excursion, and confirmation of expired carbon dioxide. Use ventilator pressure monitors as indicated. Continuously monitor end-tidal carbon dioxide during controlled or assisted ventilation and any anesthesia or sedation technique requiring artificial airway support. During moderate or deep sedation, continuously monitor for the presence of expired carbon dioxide.

  c. **Cardiovascular:** Continuously monitor cardiovascular status via electrocardiogram. Perform auscultation of heart sounds as needed. Evaluate and document blood pressure and heart rate at least every 5 minutes.

  d. **Thermoregulation:** When clinically significant changes in body temperature are intended, anticipated, or suspected, monitor body temperature in order to facilitate the maintenance of normothermia.

  e. **Neuromuscular:** When neuromuscular blocking agents are administered, monitor neuromuscular response to assess depth of blockade and degree of recovery.

  f. **Positioning:** Monitor and assess patient positioning and protective measures, except for those aspects that are performed exclusively by one or more other providers.

Standard VI: Document pertinent anesthesia-related information on the patient's medical record in an accurate, complete, legible, and timely manner.

Standard VII: Evaluate the patient's status and determine when it is safe to transfer the responsibility of care. Accurately report the patient's condition, including all essential information, and transfer the responsibility of care to another qualified health care provider in a manner that assures continuity of care and patient safety.

Standard VIII: Adhere to appropriate safety precautions as established within the practice setting to minimize the risks of fire, explosion, electrical shock, and equipment malfunction. Based on the patient, surgical intervention, or procedure, ensure that the equipment reasonably expected to be necessary for the administration of anesthesia has been checked for proper functionality and document compliance.

Standard IX: Verify that infection control policies and procedures for personnel and equipment exist within the practice setting. Adhere to infection control policies and procedures as established within the practice setting to minimize the risk of infection to the patient, the CRNA, and other health care providers.

Standard X: Participate in the ongoing review and evaluation of anesthesia care to assess quality and appropriateness.

Standard XI: Respect and maintain the basic rights of patients.

Adapted from American Association of Nurse Anesthetists. (2013). Standards for nurse anesthesia practice. Retrieved from http://www.aana.com/resources2/professionalpractice/Pages/Standards-for-Nurse-Anesthesia-Practice.aspx.

BOX 18.2 Suggested Core Clinical Privileges for Certified Registered Nurse Anesthetists (CRNAs)

- Preanesthetic preparation and evaluation of the patient, including a focused history and physical examination; recommending or requesting appropriate diagnostic studies and evaluating the results; and selecting, obtaining, ordering, and administering preanesthetic medications. CRNAs document their preanesthetic evaluation and obtain a comprehensive informed consent for anesthesia and related services.
- Intraoperative care: CRNAs obtain, prepare, and use all equipment, monitors, supplies, and drugs used for anesthesia; select, obtain, or administer the anesthetics, adjuvant drugs, fluids, and blood products; perform the necessary skills with airway management, with general, regional, monitored anesthesia care, and with invasive line placement; and maintain physiologic homeostasis throughout the perioperative course.
- Postanesthesia care: CRNAs provide postanesthesia follow-up and evaluation of patient responses to anesthesia and surgery,

taking corrective actions and requesting consultation as needed; initiate and administer respiratory support as necessary; provide pharmacologic or fluid support to maintain hemodynamic stability; initiate postanesthesia pain management strategies; and discharge patients from the postanesthesia care unit according to institutional policy.
- Clinical support functions: CRNAs manage emergency situations, including initiating or participating in cardiopulmonary resuscitation; provide airway management; insert invasive monitoring lines; and are consulted for sedation and analgesia management in postoperative and critically ill patients.
- Special requests may include interventional pain management for CRNAs credentialed to perform those procedures.
- Nonclinical responsibilities include administrative functions, quality assessment, education, and research.

Adapted from American Association of Nurse Anesthetists. (2013). Guidelines for core clinical privileges for nurse anesthetists. Retrieved from http://www.aana.com/resources2/professionalpractice/Pages/Guidelines-for-Core-Clinical-Privileges.aspx.

academic units. Regardless of the degree offered, nurse anesthesia practice doctorates must comport with the Council on Accreditation of Nurse Anesthesia Educational Programs (COA) Standards for Accreditation of Nurse Anesthesia Programs—Practice Doctorate (COA, 2015b). These criteria include a minimum program length of 36 months, demonstration of adequate numbers of faculty prepared at the doctoral level, and completion of a final scholarly work (COA, 2015b).

Nurse anesthesia education occurs in diverse settings, including schools or colleges of nursing, allied health, science, and medicine. However, the relative value of this diversity has never been quantified in terms of an academic power base or educational credibility. This diversity exists because the nurse anesthesia educational community values various undergraduate degrees for entrance into nurse anesthesia programs and because of the initial difficulty nurse anesthesia educators met when trying to move certificate nurse anesthesia programs into schools of nursing.

The requirement for advanced degrees does not dictate the movement of programs into one academic discipline. A reason for this may stem from those

programs that in the 1970s established relationships with whichever academic unit was open to affiliating with a nurse anesthesia program. Programs that pioneered nurse anesthesia education at the graduate level established relationships with those departments in colleges and universities that were willing to take risks with the small numbers of students in nurse anesthesia programs. This diversified model of nurse anesthesia education has proliferated in the last 30 years, and many of these long-established programs would find it strategically and operationally difficult to change their academic affiliations (i.e., from allied health to nursing).

In the mid-1970s, over 170 nurse anesthesia educational programs existed. A rapid decline in the numbers of nurse anesthesia programs occurred in the 1980s, a change that was of great concern to the role. The closures were attributed variously to physician pressure, declining support, the inability of hospitals to continue support of small programs, and lack of geographically accessible universities with which a nurse anesthesia program could affiliate (Faut-Callahan, 1991). Those who argued that nurse anesthesia programs closed solely because of the graduate degree mandate offered little evidence to support that claim. One can surmise that if the requirement for graduate education was the only reason for program closures, those programs would have remained open until 1998, when the master's degree was required. Despite the decline in the overall numbers of nurse anesthesia programs, many of which were certificate programs with enrollments of fewer than five students, the level of educational programs changed dramatically. After an initial decline in graduates, the newer graduate programs increased their admissions. To accomplish this, programs had to increase the numbers of clinical training sites. This resulted in a strengthened educational system, deeply entrenched in an academic model.

Colleges of nursing now house 64% of nurse anesthesia education programs in the United States (COA, 2015b), reflecting increasing collaboration between all APRN groups on education, legislative, and policy matters. Because AANA founder Agatha Hodgins unsuccessfully sought a place for CRNAs within the American Nurses Association (ANA), a separate professional organization (the AANA) was formed (Bankert, 1989; Thatcher, 1953). However, rapprochement between nursing and nurse anesthesia has resulted in effective collaboration (Munguia-Biddle, Maree, Klein, Callahan, & Gilles, 1990). Coalitions of APRNs have effectively worked together at the state and federal levels on health reform and other issues for many years.

Programs of Study

Nurse anesthesia educational curricula include time requirements for didactic and clinical activities that reflect minimum standards for entry into practice. Academic content areas are crucial to the preparation of practitioners for beginning-level competence in a highly demanding, rapidly changing specialty. Various colleges and schools that administratively house nurse anesthesia programs may have additional academic requirements. Nurse anesthesia programs in colleges of nursing include core graduate-level courses taken by all graduate-level nursing students. These courses include graduate-level nursing theory, nursing research, advanced physical assessment, pathophysiology, and pharmacology. The COA Standards for Accreditation (2015b, p. 21) state that "the curriculum is designed to focus on the full scope of nurse anesthesia practice including:

- Advanced physiology/pathophysiology, advanced pharmacology, basic and advanced principles in nurse anesthesia, and advanced health assessment."

The curricular content required by COA in the Practice Doctorate Standards includes:

- Physiology/pathophysiology—120 contact hours
- Advanced pharmacology—90 contact hours
- Basic and advanced principles in nurse anesthesia—120 contact hours
- Research—75 contact hours
- Advanced health assessment—45 contact hours
- Human anatomy, chemistry, biochemistry, physics, genetics, acute and chronic pain management, radiology, ultrasound, anesthesia equipment, professional role development, chemical dependency and wellness, informatics, ethical and multicultural healthcare, leadership and management, business of anesthesia/practice management, health policy, health care finance, integration/clinical correlation (COA, 2015b, p. 21)

The COA practice doctorate accreditation standards require that students administer a minimum of 600 anesthetics. The NBCRNA requires that graduates of accredited nurse anesthesia programs who seek to take the NCE have completed the clinical experiences specified in the COA accreditation standards, as described previously. All nurse anesthesia graduates must have cared for patients across the lifespan at all acuity levels undergoing procedures of varying complexity. There are required numbers of specific clinical experiences, such as endotracheal intubations or thoracic surgical cases, that must be met for nurse anesthesia graduates to be eligible to take the NCE. Most programs exceed these minimum requirements. In 2015, the average nurse anesthesia graduate in the United States provided 865 anesthetics and completed 2619 clinical hours while enrolled in accredited nurse anesthesia programs (NBCRNA, 2016c).

The COA accredits nurse anesthesia education programs in the United States and its territories (COA, 2015a). COA members include nurse anesthesia educators and practitioners, nurse anesthesia students, health care administrators, and university and public representatives. The COA conducts mandatory on-site program reviews, with a maximum accreditation period of 10 years. Nurse anesthesia educators and the COA have found that retaining a prescriptive curriculum in terms of hours and types of clinical experiences has helped the survival of educational programs, through ensuring that quality improvement processes and accreditation standards are consistently utilized by accredited nurse anesthesia programs.

Nurse Anesthesia Educational Funding

Despite growth in the national debt, Title VIII funding has continued. The Nurse Anesthetist Traineeship (NAT) program provides support for student RN anesthetists who are enrolled full-time in a master's or doctoral nurse anesthesia program. Traineeship funds may be used to offset costs for tuition, books, fees, and reasonable living expenses for students during the period for which the traineeship is provided. In 2012, the NAT program changed to include first-year nurse anesthesia students, who previously were eligible for traineeship funding under the Advanced Education Nurse Training program. The total NAT funding available for 100 estimated applicants in 2016 was $2,250,000 (US Department of Health and Human Services, 2016).

External funding, such as federal Title VIII nursing workforce development traineeships, has helped offset expenses for nurse anesthesia students and helped meet CRNA workforce needs. The AANA closely monitors each proposed federal budget for potential changes in Title VIII funding and has advocated for additional funding in this area. Nurse anesthesia educational programs collectively receive about $3 million each year through the Title VIII Nurse Workforce Development Program.

The AANA Division of Federal Government Affairs promotes nurse anesthesia workforce development through legislative advocacy in Congress and through representation before the Health Resources and Services Administration and its Division of Nursing, which administer the Title VIII NAT program. Title VIII funding can lessen the debt load experienced by nurse anesthesia students. Students are not typically encouraged to work as RNs while enrolled in nurse anesthesia programs because the rigor of these programs usually entails 60 or more hours per week of committed time.

Practice Doctorate

Historically, nurse anesthesia curricular requirements have overloaded the typical master's curriculum. The current required minimum length of nurse anesthesia programs is now 24 months, but that will change by 2025 because all nurse anesthesia programs will be a minimum of 36 months in length, which is required by the COA accreditation standards (COA, 2015b). The vision of legendary nursing leader Luther Christman, PhD, RN, FAAN, for nurses to be

prepared with advanced degrees, both in their discipline and in a basic science, is reflected in the move to doctoral entry degrees in anesthesia and other advanced practice specialties. At this writing, nurse anesthesia is the only APRN specialty to have a timeline requiring the transition of all programs to the practice doctorate level despite earlier advocacy in academic nursing for advanced practice nursing education to move to the practice doctorate by 2015.

Although nurse anesthesia faculty previously described limitations such as time and finances that would interfere with their pursuit of a doctoral degree (Jordan & Shott, 1998), the number of CRNAs prepared at the doctoral level has more than tripled in the recent past, from 1.2% to 4% (Wilson, 2015). Many CRNAs are currently pursuing practice or research doctorates, which bodes well for the future of the specialty and its transition to doctoral education.

Certification

Nurse anesthesia was the first nursing specialty to have mandatory certification. This process began in 1945, when the first certification examination in nurse anesthesia was given (Bankert, 1989). The NBCRNA (2016a) noted that

> [C]ertification is a process by which a professional agency or association certified that an individual licensed to practice a profession has met certain standards specified by that profession for specialty practice. The purpose of certification is to assure the public that an individual has mastered a body of knowledge and acquired skills in a particular specialty.

The NBCRNA uses psychometricians, an academy of test item writers, and computer adaptive testing to assess beginning-level competence in nurse anesthesia practice. A professional practice analysis is performed at regular intervals by the NBCRNA to determine which entry-level competencies are necessary for a new nurse anesthesia graduate.

The AANA Continuing Education Department is responsible for the review and approval of continuing education programs sponsored by the AANA and other organizations, maintenance of attendance records of continuing education activities, and preparation of continuing education transcripts and certificates of attendance for AANA-sponsored programs (AANA, 2016a).

Institutional Credentialing

CRNAs practice according to their expertise, state statutes or regulations, and local institutional policy. Institutional credentialing procedures may require additional evidence of clinical and didactic education in areas such as cardiothoracic or regional anesthesia. State nurse practice acts and practice patterns in the anesthesia community contribute to variability in the scope of nurse anesthesia practice in different settings.

Competence can be partially ensured through institutional credentialing processes, including ongoing professional practice evaluation. A hospital or other facility may delineate procedures that the CRNA is authorized to perform by the authority of its governing board. Suggested core clinical privileges are in the AANA Guidelines for Core Clinical Privileges for Nurse Anesthetists (AANA, 2013a; see Box 18.2).

The COA has required the master's degree as the exit degree for nurse anesthesia programs since 1998 and will not approve any new master's degree programs for accreditation beyond 2015. Students accepted into an accredited program on January 1, 2022, and thereafter will need to complete the program with a doctoral degree. The COA standards require that program administrators and assistant administrators will be required to have a doctoral degree by 2018 (COA, 2015b).

Current CRNA Practice

Workforce Issues

Some 50,000 CRNAs currently practice in the United States (AANA, 2016c). Data that comprise CRNA practice profiles are derived from annual practice surveys completed by CRNAs when they pay their AANA dues. The response rate to these surveys has been as high as 72%, providing a reasonable degree of generalizability. AANA membership has almost doubled in the last 20 years, from 25,000 CRNAs in 1996 to 49,000 CRNAs in 2016. This growth rate bodes well for the future of nurse anesthesia, along with the continued availability of high-quality, cost-effective anesthesia services, especially to citizens in rural and medically underserved areas. This growth reflects the work of the National Commission on Nurse Anesthesia Education (Maree, 1991), which provided the profession with workforce data projections and related strategies to ensure that the market demand for nurse anesthetists will be met. The growth in nurse anesthesia programs and graduates over the last 20 years can be attributed to the advocacy of the AANA, through the National Commission on Nurse Anesthesia Education, for the development of new educational programs to meet increasing needs for anesthesia services (Mastropietro, Horton, Ouellette & Faut-Callahan, 2001). Successful efforts to increase the number of nurse anesthesia programs and graduates resulted in programs expanding from 89 in 1994 to 115 in 2016. In 1995, there were 1054 nurse anesthesia graduates, while 2469 students completed nurse anesthesia education programs in 2015 (Gerbasi, 2015).

The current and future needs of nurse anesthesia programs mandate a faculty cadre to teach the rigorous didactic and clinical portions of nurse anesthesia programs and to manage the transition to the practice doctorate. Most nurse anesthetists are practicing clinicians; fewer than 10% of CRNAs serve in clinical leadership or educator roles. The salary differential between academic and clinical settings can be a significant barrier to the recruitment of academic faculty. For example, the average salary for a master's-prepared assistant professor in a school of nursing is $77,022 (AACN, 2016), while the average clinical CRNA salary is $173,875 (Salary.com, 2017). Given the aging CRNA workforce, projected CRNA retirements between 2016 and 2021, and the requirement for movement of nurse anesthesia education programs to the practice doctorate by 2025, more CRNA educators are needed (AANA, 2016c).

The average age of CRNAs reported in the AANA 2015 membership survey was 48 years, similar to the average age for RNs in the United States. Regarding the duration of time spent in the specialty, 32% of CRNAs who responded to this survey had been in practice longer than 20 years. AANA member survey data show that 10% of AANA members plan to retire between 2016 and 2018, while another 15% anticipate retiring between 2019 and 2021 (Wilson, 2015). The market demand for CRNAs will also be affected by shifting payer mixes and research findings that support the safe and cost-effective anesthesia services provided by CRNAs (Dulisse & Cromwell, 2010; Hogan, Seifert, Moore, & Simonson, 2010; Lewis, Nicholson, Smith, & Alderson, 2014; Needleman & Minnick, 2009; Negrusa, Hogan, Warner, Schroeder, & Pang, 2016).

Projected nurse anesthetist retirements, the aging population, and the impact of the ACA, with over 30 million additional people covered, demand a health care workforce sufficient to deliver patient access to high-quality health care. It is essential that nurse anesthesia education programs continue to produce adequate numbers of graduates to meet workforce needs. The ACA included a 4-year pilot project for Graduate Nursing Education intended to support the clinical practice education of APRNs for the growing Medicare patient population. The Graduate Nursing Education project seeks to ensure that the education of APRNs has funding opportunities similar to those provided for physicians under Graduate Medical Education (Centers for Medicare & Medicaid Services [CMS], 2012).

The high demand for nurse anesthetists in clinical and academic settings is not expected to change. The safety, cost-effectiveness, and high quality of nurse anesthesia care, coupled with the advocacy provided by members through the AANA, keep nurse anesthesia at the forefront of the health care workforce. Recognition of the impending increase in demand for CRNAs by professional leaders resulted in increased numbers of accredited programs and graduates to address workforce needs (Mastropietro et al., 2001).

Practice Settings

At one time, CRNAs were primarily hospital employed. However, employment arrangements for CRNAs have changed over time. CRNAs provide services in conjunction with other health care professionals such as surgeons, dentists, podiatrists, and anesthesiologists in diverse clinical settings. These APRNs practice in a variety of clinical environments. Nurse anesthetists provide anesthesia services on a solo basis, in groups, and collaboratively. Some CRNAs have independent contracting arrangements with physicians or hospitals. In 2015, 38% of AANA member survey respondents were hospital employed, 36% worked for anesthesia group practices, 11% were independent contractors, and 4% were employed in the military or VA facilities (Wilson, 2015). Nurse anesthetists have provided most anesthesia services in rural areas since the inception of the specialty. Currently, 14% of AANA member survey respondents provide anesthesia services in hospitals that perform fewer than 800 surgeries per year (Wilson, 2015).

Today, most surgery is performed on a same-day admission or outpatient basis. Anesthesia practices have adapted to this change from a predominantly inpatient model for surgery. A number of mechanisms, ranging from preoperative telephone interviews to preanesthesia clinics, are used to conduct preanesthesia assessment and allow anesthesia providers an opportunity to discuss care options, procedures, and risks with patients. However, detailed physical assessment and establishing a rapport between the anesthesia provider and patient often still occur on the day of surgery.

Access to Health Care

Access to health care remains an ongoing concern across the country, with geographic maldistribution of anesthesia providers being a major factor; nurse anesthetists provide the bulk of anesthesia care in rural America. US manpower trends in anesthesia have been studied, with the demand for CRNAs expected to grow by 16% between 2013 and 2025 (HRSA, 2016).

An anesthesia workforce study conducted by Rand Health (Daugherty, Benito, Kumar, & Michaud, 2010b) had two major questions:

1. Is there a shortage or surplus of anesthesia providers?
2. What are the demographic patterns, employment arrangements, usages of time across different types of procedures, and working patterns present in the anesthesia provider workforce?

This study, commissioned by the American Society of Anesthesiologists, demonstrated a current shortage of anesthesia providers but estimated a surplus of CRNAs by 2020. The latter finding is inconsistent with AANA member survey data, estimating a significant number of projected retirements between 2016 and 2021 (Wilson, 2015). The Rand study described a 9.6% anesthesiologist vacancy rate and estimated the vacancy rate for CRNAs as 3.8%. Geographic maldistribution of providers was noted, with 95% of anesthesiologists reported to be working in urban locations but only 44% of CRNAs practicing in urban settings. This reinforces the contributions of CRNAs in the care of rural and medically underserved citizens. The Rand study reported the average annual salary for an anesthesiologist to be $337,551, versus $151,380 for a CRNA, reinforcing the cost-effectiveness of nurse anesthetists (Daugherty, Benito, Kumar, & Michaud, 2010a).

Epstein and Dexter (2012) noted that anesthesia groups may wish to decrease the supervision ratio for nontrainee providers (e.g., CRNAs). Because hospitals offer many first-case starts and focus on starting these cases on time, the number of anesthesiologists needed is sensitive to this ratio. The number of operating rooms that an anesthesiologist can supervise concurrently is determined by the probability of multiple, simultaneous, critical portions of cases requiring the presence and availability of cross-coverage. The authors conducted a simulation study that demonstrated peak occurrence of critical portions during first cases and frequent supervision lapses. These predictions were tested using actual data from an anesthesia information management system. The practical implication of this research is that it is logistically difficult for anesthesiologists supervising concurrent cases with the same start times to be physically present for the start of those cases. Depending on the billing arrangement, presence of an anesthesiologist for certain portions of a case may not be a requirement.

CRNAs provide 32 million anesthetics annually in the United States (AANA, 2016c). Using CRNAs to the full extent of their education allows for greater efficiencies in the delivery of safe and cost-effective anesthesia care. A growing body of outcomes research has demonstrated that full implementation of APRNs, including CRNAs, is safe and cost-effective (Dulisse & Cromwell, 2010; Hogan et al., 2010; Lewis et al., 2014; Negrusa et al., 2016).

CRNAs have traditionally provided anesthesia to rural and medically underserved populations. The presence of CRNAs allows these hospitals and other health care facilities to provide services to patients who might otherwise need to travel long distances for essential care. In some rural settings in some states, 100% of anesthesia, trauma stabilization, and obstetric anesthesia services are provided by nurse anesthetists (AANA, 2016d). Without the services of CRNAs in rural communities, many small hospitals would close, leaving few alternatives for health care. Some rural CRNAs have completed additional training in the management of acute and chronic pain and offer services such as pain clinics so that patients do not have to travel to distant centers for pain treatment.

Academic medical centers and government-operated facilities also rely heavily on nurse anesthetists. Many CRNAs practice in the VA hospital system, dealing with high-acuity patients undergoing complex surgical procedures. The military relies heavily on and actively recruits nurse anesthetists. A CRNA may be the only anesthesia provider on a naval vessel. This essential access to anesthesia care for military men and women is part of nurse anesthesia history, dating back to the Civil War. In combat zones, knowledge of regional anesthesia and the ability to practice autonomously enable the CRNA to respond capably to mass casualty situations, in which many trauma victims require anesthesia simultaneously (AANA, 2016d).

American Association of Nurse Anesthetists

Organization and Structure

The AANA was among the first nursing specialty organizations. At a 1931 regional nurse anesthesia meeting, AANA founder Agatha Hodgins described her vision of the essential elements for a national nurse anesthesia organization (Thatcher, 1953, p. 183):

> Improvement of the present situation is in the hands of the nurse anesthetists themselves. If the work is to be properly safeguarded and hoped-for progress attained, it is necessary that remedies be applied to certain conditions now acknowledged to exist. It would seem that the first step should be the awakening of deeper interest and the development of constructive leadership. Following in logical order would be: self-organization as a special division of hospital service ... educational standards, postgraduate schools of anesthesia ... required to conform to an accepted criterion of education; state registration, putting right the nurse anesthetist to practice her vocation beyond criticism; constant effort toward improving the quality of work by means of study and research, thus affording still greater protection to the patient; [and] dissemination of information gained through proper channels.

Early efforts of nurse anesthetists to affiliate with the ANA were not successful because each organization had different ideas of what such an affiliation would entail (Gunn, 1991; Thatcher, 1953). With time, the breach between nursing and nurse anesthesia has narrowed considerably. Since its inception as the National Association of Nurse Anesthetists (NANA) in 1931, the AANA has placed its responsibilities to the public above or at the same level as its responsibilities to its membership. The association has produced education and practice standards, implemented a certification examination for nurse anesthetists in 1945, and developed an accreditation process that was implemented in 1952. The AANA has been a leader in the formation of multidisciplinary councils with public representation to fulfill the autonomous credentialing functions of the profession, including accreditation, certification, and recertification.

When AANA founder Hodgins became ill, Gertrude Fife, who provided anesthesia for pioneering heart surgeon Claude Beck, assumed the role of developing

NANA in its early days (Thatcher, 1953). The name of the association was changed to the American Association of Nurse Anesthetists in 1939. Helen Lamb, who served two terms as AANA president (1940-1942), provided anesthesia exclusively for the patients of Dr. Evarts Graham, one of the first modern thoracic surgeons (Bankert, 1989). The first anesthetic administered for the correction of tetralogy of Fallot was provided by a nurse anesthetist, Olive Berger, at Johns Hopkins Hospital. Early nurse anesthesia leaders were involved in complex practice settings with surgeons who were also influential in their fields. In addition to the development of a professional identity for nurse anesthesia, early nurse anesthetist leaders developed curricular standards for nurse anesthesia educational programs. These standards initially included a minimum program length of 6 months, with subsequent institution of mandatory certification and recertification policies.

The AANA Board of Directors oversees and governs the association in its efforts to be the preeminent association of anesthesia providers by putting patients first and taking a leadership role in policy making, nurse anesthesia education, and research to ensure high-quality, safe anesthesia. A number of committees and task forces support the work of the AANA. Several committees have student representatives.

John F. Garde was a distinguished health care leader who served as AANA Executive Director from 1983 to 2001, and again on an interim basis from February 2009 until his untimely death in July 2009. A statement of his holds true today (Garde, 1998, p. 15):

> The profession has an optimistic future. I point out with pride the commitment that AANA members have toward the future of their profession—a commitment that encompasses being outstanding anesthesia practitioners who belong to their Association. I am reminded, too, what Dick Davidson, President of the American Hospital Association, said when asked about what will remain in health care 100 years from now: "There will always be personal contact and caring. We will always have hands touching patients. Everything we do is about human need. That's the constant over time." And, that is the legacy of the nurse anesthesia profession.

Mission and Vision

The AANA vision statement describes being "a preeminent professional association for healthcare and patient safety." The accompanying mission

statement states that "AANA advances patient safety, practice excellence and its members' profession." The core values of the profession are quality, professionalism, compassion, collaboration, wellness, and diversity (AANA, 2017). The association seeks to support its members and protect patients.

Current areas of federal advocacy activity for the AANA include ensuring that US military veterans have access to high-quality health care. The Veterans Health Administration proposal for full practice authority is being advanced through legislation seeking to recognize the full practice authority of all APRNs, including CRNAs, working in the VA health care system. This policy change would enable all CRNAs to practice to the full extent of their education and training, standardizing policy across the VA (AANA, Office of Federal Government Affairs, 2017a).

The AANA advocates for APRN and CRNA workforce development through the Title VIII Nurse Workforce Development Program. The AANA requested that the 2017 fiscal year Title VIII budget be increased to $244 million, to provide additional funding for NAT grants. Title VIII funding also facilitates APRN workforce development (AANA, Office of Federal Government Affairs, 2017b).

Nongovernmental regulation of nurse anesthesia practice is closely monitored by the AANA. It is related to the activities of TJC, the Accreditation Association for Ambulatory Health Care, and other agencies whose policies may affect nurse anesthesia practice.

Reimbursement issues related to Medicare, Medicaid, and other payers are closely monitored by AANA because changes in reimbursement can have a major impact on CRNA earnings. The AANA also provides members with resources on how to start a business, contracts, reimbursement, practice models, management and staffing, pain management, and disability. Practice trends monitored by the AANA include pain management and scope of practice issues. Provision of sedation and analgesia, including propofol, by nonanesthesia providers, is closely monitored by the AANA. Other areas in which the AANA provides support to its members include strategies to address workplace harassment, expert witness identification, development of skills and resources for the possibility of mass casualty events, and bioterrorism situations.

An AANA subsidiary, AANA Insurance Services, provides malpractice coverage for many nurse anesthetists. Trends monitored by this agency include the decreasing number of insurers covering CRNAs and all health care providers. The remaining insurers are being more selective about whom they cover. Consequently, malpractice liability insurance premiums have increased. The principal insurer for CRNAs who need to obtain coverage, as opposed to those who work for self-insured entities, is now CNA Insurance. Applicants must meet underwriting guidelines and criteria.

The AANA also closely monitors trends in patient safety and malpractice litigation. There are numerous continuing education meetings across the country that provide content on practice innovations and patient safety topics, which is integral to the mission of the association. Reinforcing the 11 standards of care described in the *Scope and Standards for Nurse Anesthesia Practice* (AANA, 2013b), such as performing preanesthesia assessments, routine use of pulse oximetry, and end-tidal carbon dioxide monitoring, is central to these presentations.

Relationships Within Nursing

The AANA is represented at meetings of many nursing organizations, including the ANA, the American Association of Colleges of Nursing, the National League for Nursing, the Federation of Specialty Nursing Organizations, the International Council of Nurses (ICN), and the International Federation of Nurse Anesthetists (IFNA). CRNAs have played leadership roles in the development of the APRN Consensus Model, which includes state-level determination of the following (National Council of State Boards of Nursing, 2008):

- APRN legal scope of practice
- Recognized roles and titles of APRNs
- Criteria for entry into advanced practice
- Certification examinations for entry-level competence assessment

Representatives of the AANA, the ANA, the Association of Perioperative Registered Nurses, and the ICN frequently attend meetings of these nursing organizations, fostering cross-disciplinary collaboration. The AANA is a long-time member of the Federation of Specialty Nursing Organizations ("On the Federation," 1980). CRNAs were involved in the development of the second edition of the ANA's *Scope and Standards for Nurse Anesthesia Practice.*

International Practice Opportunities

The IFNA was founded in 1989 by 11 countries in which nurse anesthetists were educated and practicing. The IFNA now has 40 member countries. The IFNA mission "is dedicated to the precept that its members are committed to the advancement of educational standards and practices which will advance the art and science of anesthesiology and thereby support and enhance quality anesthesia care worldwide" (IFNA, 2017). The IFNA establishes and maintains effective cooperation with institutions that have a professional interest in nurse anesthesia. The IFNA (2017) seeks

- To promote continual high quality of patient care
- To serve as the authoritative voice for nurse anesthetists and nurse anesthesia internationally
- To provide a means of communication among nurse anesthetists throughout the world
- To promote the independence of the nurse anesthetist as a professional specialist in nursing
- To advance the art and science of anesthesiology

The IFNA describes these organizational objectives (IFNA, 2017):

- To promote cooperation between nurse anesthetists internationally
- To develop and promote educational standards in the field of nurse anesthesia
- To develop and promote standards of practice in the field of nurse anesthesia
- To provide opportunities for continuing education in anesthesia
- To assist nurse anesthetists' associations to improve the standards of nurse anesthesia and the competence of nurse anesthetists
- To promote the recognition of nurse anesthesia
- To establish and maintain effective cooperation between nurse anesthetists, anesthesiologists and other members of the medical profession, the nursing profession, hospitals, and agencies representing a community of interest in nurse anesthesia

IFNA member countries include European, Scandinavian, African, and Asian nations. Since its inception in 1989, the IFNA has developed Standards of Education, Standards of Practice, Standards of Monitoring, and a Code of Ethics for Nurse Anesthetists. Model nurse anesthesia curricula have been developed, along with an approval process for educational programs. The IFNA was initially recognized as a professional resource group by the ICN, and the IFNA is currently an affiliate member of the ICN. Research findings have shown that nurse anesthetists participate in 80% of the anesthetics administered worldwide and are sole providers of 60% of the anesthetics (Ouellette & Horton, 2011).

Role Development and Measures of Clinical Competence

Horton (1998) conducted a comprehensive study of the views of CRNAs to determine implicit and explicit ideas about the culture of nurse anesthetists. Dominant rules of behavior were identified. CRNAs identified two major domains of professional activity: (1) remaining active and vigilant in defending and maintaining practice rights; and (2) dedication to patient care. Demonstrating their dedication to patient care, CRNAs note the following as key elements of proactive patient care: individualized care, technology, touch, surveillance, vigilance, and honesty. Horton (1998) found that CRNA dominant values include autonomy, education, continuing education, achievement, group cohesiveness, identity as a CRNA, membership in the AANA, political activism, and technology.

The role of the nurse anesthetist encompasses many facets (Exemplar 18.1). Callahan (1994) described a competency-based model for nurse anesthesia practice that demonstrated areas in which nurse anesthetists must strive to achieve competence. The unifying themes of caring, collaboration, communication, and technology were identified. Many of the characteristics of advanced practice nursing described in Chapter 3 are found in this model. Munguia-Biddle and colleagues (1990) defined components of the model and suggested that the process of care provided by nurse anesthetists uses a problem-solving model that employs assessment, analysis, planning, implementation, and evaluation in the complex decision making and actions that exemplify CRNA practice in the health care environment. They further defined lifelong learning as part of the nurse anesthesia process of care. This essential component reflects the changing nature of nurse anesthesia practice.

The advanced practice of nursing in the specialty of nurse anesthesia has special attributes that speak to the strength and uniqueness of the CRNA role in the provision of anesthesia care in the health environment (Fig. 18.1). Caring for the patient as a holistic

---

EXEMPLAR 18.1   A Day in the Life of a Certified Registered Nurse Anesthetist

K.M. has been a certified registered nurse anesthetist (CRNA) for 10 years. Prior to that, he worked as a registered nurse in the emergency department of a busy city hospital in the Midwest, followed by 2 years of medical intensive care unit experience in a tertiary medical center. Since completing his nurse anesthesia program, K.M. has worked at a level I trauma center in a large Midwestern city. His case mix includes patients across the life span at all acuity levels. K.M. frequently works with students from a nearby nurse anesthesia program who rotate through his department. His work day is 10 hours a day but, with setup time and other activities, such as postoperative visits, the day can be closer to 12 hours. The CRNAs in this facility are unionized county employees.

K.M. and his colleagues receive their clinical assignments for the next day by 2:00 PM the preceding day. Some patients seek care at this public facility because they have no health insurance but are otherwise healthy. Other patients are of markedly high acuity, with complex comorbid conditions such as intravenous drug abuse, reactive airways disease, morbid obesity, and hypertension.

There are 20 operating rooms in this facility. On a given day, K.M. may do five cases if he is working in an area such as general surgery. If he is the trauma CRNA, he will be assigned to patients from the trauma unit who have experienced blunt and/or penetrating trauma. Skills in airway management, vascular access, and volume resuscitation are essential for anesthesia providers who deal with trauma patients. When assigned to urology cases, K.M. may do up to 20 cases, mostly under spinal anesthesia, for that surgical service. K.M. enjoys the ability to provide care to high-acuity patients who undergo complex surgical procedures. He is able to use other regional anesthesia skills, including placement of thoracic epidural blocks and peripheral nerve block catheters. Many of the patients at this facility have challenging airway anatomy, so K.M. has become skilled at placing endotracheal tubes in sedated patients using fiberoptic bronchoscopy, a safe technique.

K.M. values collegial relationships with the physicians and other CRNAs with whom he works. Areas in which he would like to see changes are CRNA compensation, which is lower than in the private sector, and the turnover time between cases, which is longer than in the private sector. However, the benefits associated with government employment exceed many of those available in the private sector. K.M. is also an instructor in a nearby nurse anesthesia program. His day off is spent teaching and mentoring students in this program. ◎

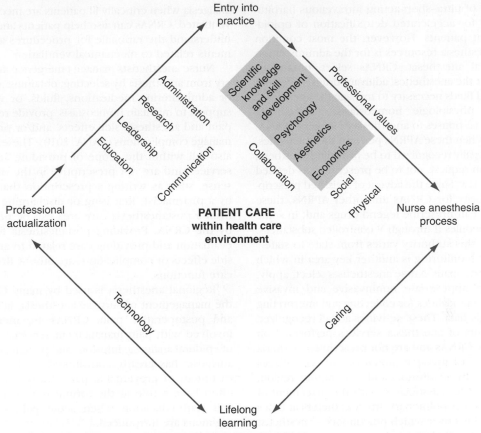

FIG 18.1 Nurse anesthesia practice model. *(From Munguia-Biddle, F., Maree, S., Klein, E., Callahan, L., & Gilles, B. [1990]. Nurse anesthesiology competence evaluation: Mechanism for accountability [unpublished document]. Park Ridge, IL: American Association of Nurse Anesthetists.)*

being is an important tenet of CRNA professional behavior. CRNAs strive to be altruistic human beings, believing that caring is essential to one's personal development (Munguia-Biddle et al., 1990).

Collaboration between the nurse anesthetist and other members of the health care team takes place in separate and joined activities and responsibilities directed at attaining mutual goals of excellence in patient care. Communication is sharing information to achieve mutual understanding. Communication skills are a cornerstone of patient interviews, imparting information to other health professionals, documentation of practice, and participation as a contributory member in meeting society's health needs. Technology denotes an area rich in advances and scientific content that requires strengthening and updating throughout the CRNA's professional life. Practitioners have the ability to apply the nursing

process to complex problems at a high level of competence (Munguia-Biddle et al., 1990).

The process of care for nurse anesthetists parallels the nursing process and emphasizes the importance of this approach to comprehensive anesthesia care following the model and its components. CRNA practice is based on the APRN competencies found in Chapter 3. Some of these competencies are discussed here and in the three exemplars of CRNA practice.

Direct Clinical Practice

Anesthesia services can facilitate diagnosis, as in the case of the so-called curare test for myasthenia gravis. Anesthesia as a therapeutic modality is seen in the treatment of acute and chronic pain; it is also used in psychiatry for conducting interviews under the influence of ultra–short-acting intravenous barbiturates and for accelerated detoxification of opioid-dependent patients. However, the most common use of anesthesia resources is for the administration of surgical anesthesia. CRNAs select, obtain, or administer the anesthetics, adjuvant drugs, accessory drugs, and fluids necessary to manage the anesthesia; maintain physiologic homeostasis; and correct abnormal responses to anesthesia or surgery (AANA, 2016d). When these APRNs perform these activities, they are legally recognized to be providing anesthesia services on request, not to be prescribing as defined by federal law. Since the advent of legislated prescriptive authority for CRNAs and other APRNs, these providers can prescribe legend drugs and, in some cases, Schedules II through V controlled substances. However, this authority varies from state to state.

Patient monitoring is another key area in which CRNAs participate. Nurse anesthetists select, apply, and insert appropriate noninvasive and invasive monitoring modalities for collecting and interpreting physiologic data. These activities are all recognized components of anesthesia services performed on request by CRNAs and are not prescriptive. Criteria for the use of invasive monitors and who places them vary by institution and geographic region. Professional fees associated with the placement of devices such as pulmonary artery catheters at times lead to conflict over which practitioner—anesthetist or surgeon—will place invasive monitors and receive the associated reimbursement.

Nurse anesthesia practice also includes airway management, with modalities ranging from mask ventilation to placement of laryngeal mask airways or endotracheal intubation. CRNAs are knowledgeable about mechanical ventilation options and the pharmacologic support needed to maintain mechanical ventilation within and outside of the operating room. In some settings, these APRNs are the sole providers of ventilator management oversight. A combination of technical skills required for airway management using a variety of instruments (e.g., rigid laryngoscope, fiberoptic bronchoscope, video laryngoscope) and knowledge of respiratory anatomy and physiology and pharmacology are all important.

Clinicians continue to develop an array of approaches to sedation and analgesia for ventilator-dependent patients. Opportunities exist for collaborative research in this area (Weinert & Calvin, 2007). The expertise that CRNAs can provide in the management of ventilator-dependent patients includes reinforcing the need for appropriate sedation and analgesia when critically ill patients are mechanically ventilated. CRNAs can also help patients and families understand the rationale for procedures and treatments related to mechanical ventilation.

Nurse anesthetists manage emergence and recovery from anesthesia by selecting, obtaining, ordering, or administering medications, fluids, or ventilator support to maintain homeostasis, provide relief from pain and anesthesia side effects, and/or prevent or manage complications (AANA, 2010). These activities also fall within the scope of providing anesthesia services and are not prescriptive in the traditional sense, such as writing a prescription that is filled by a pharmacist. Releasing or discharging patients from a postanesthesia care area can be performed by the CRNA. Providing postanesthesia follow-up evaluation and providing care related to anesthetic side effects or complications are other CRNA direct care functions.

Regional anesthesia is used by many CRNAs in the management of surgical anesthesia, labor pain, and postoperative pain. CRNAs are increasingly involved with pain management services. The use of epidural analgesic infusions and patient-controlled analgesia has greatly contributed to the effective treatment of preventable pain. Nurse anesthetists often have a role in the formulation of protocols and staff education when acute pain treatment regimens are introduced.

Anesthesia services are frequently used in obstetrics for providing analgesia and anesthesia to women in labor. Regional anesthesia and applied pharmacology have greatly advanced obstetric anesthesia, which in the past relied on systemic drugs that could cause neonatal depression. Epidural analgesia has become increasingly common for vaginal and cesarean section delivery, often obviating the need for general anesthesia and its attendant risks. In addition to using regional anesthesia in obstetric and postpartum settings, CRNAs have long worked collaboratively with other clinicians in these areas to manage intrapartum and postpartum pain with various pharmacologic and nonpharmacologic modalities (Faut-Callahan & Paice, 1990).

Nurse anesthetists respond to emergency situations by providing airway management skills and implementing basic and advanced life support techniques. These APRNs can provide leadership in these settings, away from the operating room, reinforcing the need to apply nationally promulgated standards of anesthesia care. An example of one of these standards of care is the measurement of end-tidal carbon dioxide to rule out esophageal intubation (AANA, 2016d). Nurse anesthetists are bound by the standards of practice adopted by their specialty.

Palliative Care

CRNAs possess expert skills in pain and symptom management. Building on experience in acute and critical care nursing, nurse anesthetists have extensive experience with end-of-life care. CRNAs value the close relationship that develops with patients and their families in the critical care environment and may develop close relationships with patients for whom they care during complex surgeries related to serious illness. The knowledge, skills, and experiences of CRNAs have made them uniquely qualified to assist with palliative and end-of-life care (Callahan, Breakwell, & Suhayda, 2011). Although palliative care is not typically a part of CRNA practice, there has been recent interest in exploring this area of care.

There are tremendous gaps in palliative and end-of-life care resources that have been identified by the IOM (IOM, National Cancer Policy Board, 2001), most notably in rural areas. Over the past decade, there have been many efforts to identify gaps and develop strategies to fill them (American Association of Colleges of Nursing, 2012; Emanuel, 2012; Locate a Hospice, 2017; National Hospice and Palliative Care Organization, 2012; Palliative Care Program, Medical College of Wisconsin, 2017). Those in need of palliative and end-of-life care often do not receive adequate care by qualified providers (Locate a Hospice, 2017; National Hospice and Palliative Care Organization, 2012).

CRNAs have many skills needed to participate in palliative care but do not typically work in these settings. CRNAs' extensive knowledge in pain and symptom management could enhance existing or new palliative care practices. CRNAs, especially those who have recently entered anesthesia practice and have current critical care knowledge and experience with palliative care, may embrace this additional form of patient care because it provides them an opportunity to develop long-term relationships with patients.

Student RN anesthetists have reported an interest in this type of patient care and noted that they are often asked by families about plans of treatment and resources available to them (Callahan et al., 2011). After taking an interprofessional palliative care course, student nurse anesthetists demonstrate significant knowledge in all domains of palliative care.

In many rural settings, 100% of anesthesia is delivered by CRNAs. These are the same communities that often do not have palliative and end-of-life services. Recognition of the experience of CRNAs and the knowledge and skills they develop in pain and symptom management may lead to an increase in providers who can assist with the significant gap in palliative care services in the United States.

Guidance and Coaching

Because surgery and diagnostic procedures are performed primarily on an outpatient or same-day admission basis, CRNAs are challenged to develop a rapport with their patients rapidly and develop a mutually agreed on plan for anesthesia care. Part of the development of the anesthesia plan involves the CRNA coaching the patient and family. The anesthetic options for the involved surgery or procedure need to be thoroughly discussed, along with the associated risks and benefits. This process can involve teaching the patient and family about postoperative analgesic options and coaching patients to avail themselves of the full benefits of the analgesic regimen, whether the treatment for pain entails patient-controlled epidural or intravenous analgesia.

Patients who undergo outpatient surgery receive coaching from CRNAs about activity, dietary limitations, and use of postoperative analgesics. Patients and their families in these situations also need coaching about when it may be appropriate for them to contact the office of the surgical or anesthesia provider.

Families of infants and children who undergo surgery and anesthesia need to be coached by the CRNA regarding the assessment and management of pain, postoperative nausea, and vomiting. Parameters for advancing activity and diet need to be clearly conveyed to the family or caregiver as part of this coaching process.

Consultation

Clinical consultations provided by CRNAs include interactions with other clinicians regarding pain management in postoperative patients. In some settings, CRNAs provide consultation in the area of sedation and analgesia for ventilator-dependent patients and management of respiratory care, including ventilator settings, and selection of vasoactive medications for critically ill patients.

In Exemplar 18.2, CRNA J.R. has a practice focused on the assessment and treatment of acute

EXEMPLAR 18.2   Certified Registered Nurse Anesthetist's Role in Pain Management

J.R. has been a practicing certified registered nurse anesthetist (CRNA) for 17 years. The strongest influences in her professional development are "believing in our profession, my knowledge, skills and competencies, while seizing any and all opportunities for professional advancement that crossed my path."

Her interest in nurse anesthesia was stimulated by early exposure to the CRNA role. Her father was an otolaryngologist who practiced in a Midwestern city with a population of 60,000. At the hospital in which he practiced, there were three anesthesiologists and a CRNA on staff. At that time, the surgeons were allowed to post their cases to the surgery schedule and choose the anesthesia provider. Most of the time, J.R.'s father chose the CRNA to provide anesthesia care for his patients. He stated that the CRNA had excellent skills and was wonderful with pediatric patients.

J.R. has practiced as a staff CRNA in a large physician-owned anesthesia group with 11 physicians and 26 CRNAs in the Midwest. She has also been a hospital-employed chief CRNA for an obstetric anesthesia practice involving three network hospitals in another Midwestern city. Most recently, her practice has moved into the realm of interventional pain management for a neurosurgical group. Her time currently is divided among direct patient care (80%), teaching (10%), administration (5%), and professional activities (5%). J.R. acknowledges that working as an employee of a large neurosurgical group in an office-based interventional pain practice is very unique. A 2011 American Association of Nurse Anesthetists (AANA) survey of members showed that 2% of respondents worked in pain management (AANA, 2016c). CRNA involvement in this specialty has been contested in multiple states by other providers.

J.R.'s current practice developed following an initial contact by another advanced practice registered nurse (APRN) who was employed by the neurosurgical group, demonstrating the value of professional networking. J.R. was asked to meet with the group to discuss a practice opportunity. The group was interested in hiring a CRNA to reopen an interventional pain clinic that had been closed for over a year. J.R. was contacted because of her experience with regional anesthesia and her leadership activities in her state nurse anesthesia association. After she met with the physician who championed this effort, she was interested in accepting the challenge. The position "gave me an incredible opportunity for clinical growth and I strongly felt this was a perfect example of how CRNAs are beneficial in an area outside the traditional operating room setting."

A typical day in J.R.'s practice begins with a quick review of her schedule and a safety check of equipment and medications. Her day usually consists of a mixture of diagnostic and therapeutic interventional procedures, such as epidural steroid injections, nerve root blocks, joint blocks, trigger point injections, and lumbar discography.

"In our pain clinical, a patient checks in at the front desk and an escort assesses his or her vital signs and brings the patient to an exam room. A nurse will interview the patient, answer questions, and ensure informed consent." During that time, J.R. "reviews the chart, imaging studies, assessment forms, and the order for treatment." She also interviews the patient prior to the procedure to answer questions or obtain additional information pertinent to the treatment plan before deciding on the type and targeted site of injection.

The patient is taken to the fluoroscopic suite and is prepped and draped under sterile technique. J.R. then performs a diagnostic or therapeutic injection under fluoroscopic guidance. The patient is assessed immediately after the injection and returned to the examination room for 30 minutes for observation. Prior to discharge, the patient is reassessed and information is recorded concerning the type and amount of pain relief provided by the injection. The patient is educated concerning the onset and duration of action of the injected medications and possible complications of the medication and injection and is given discharge and follow-up information.

J.R. describes the greatest challenges in her practice as "initially … obtaining the necessary knowledge, skills, and competencies to perform the procedures requested by the group that oversees me because there was no other employment situation identical to this practice. Overall, it is dealing with the political environment because there are physicians who feel a CRNA should not be providing pain management care."

J.R.'s story demonstrates the value of professional collaboration, mentoring, networking, and organizational involvement. Her willingness to take risks and improve care elevates the profession. ◎

and chronic pain. In her consultative role, she provides interventional pain management services to a wide array of patients.

CRNAs who serve as clinical managers or administrators of educational programs frequently consult with colleagues in similar positions. Members of the CRNA educator community often are generous in sharing curricular or policy information with colleagues.

Some CRNAs serve as expert witnesses in medical malpractice actions. This consultation activity helps legal counsel determine whether the actions of a defendant CRNA comport with the applicable standards of anesthesia care. CRNAs also serve as editors and editorial reviewers for peer-reviewed journals. In these roles, CRNAs advise colleagues on information ranging from the suitability for publication of an unsolicited manuscript and recommend additions, deletions, or corrections of submitted papers. Also, CRNAs serve as peer reviewers for traineeship grants submitted to the Health Resources and Services Administration. Some CRNAs with active programs of research sit on grant review panels of the National Institutes of Health.

As on-site reviewers for the COA or other programmatic or institutional accreditation agencies, CRNAs have opportunities to serve as consultant evaluators. Those who have been involved as on-site reviewers frequently express satisfaction with participation in this peer review process.

Evidence-Based Practice

Reports in peer-reviewed journals have continued to document the safety and cost-effectiveness of care provided by CRNAs, dating to 1899 (Dulisse & Cromwell, 2010; Hogan et al., 2010; Lewis et al., 2014; Needleman & Minnick, 2009; Negrusa et al., 2016; Pine, Holt, & Lou, 2003; Simonson, Ahern, & Hendryx, 2007; Magaw, 1899; Magaw, 1906). Nurse anesthetist Alice Magaw collected and analyzed data related to her clinical practice. She noted that while other anesthetic techniques had been utilized, the most satisfactory approach at the time was the "open method" of ether administration. By 1906, the clinical practice outcomes of Miss Magaw included over 14,000 anesthetics administered without anesthesia-related mortality, which was otherwise unheard of in that era (Bankert, 1989).

Findings reported in more recent papers demonstrate that there is no difference in the quality of care provided by CRNAs and their physician counterparts. A cost-effectiveness analysis of anesthesia

providers found that CRNAs are less costly to train than anesthesiologists and can perform the same set of anesthesia services, including those for relatively rare and difficult procedures such as open heart surgery, organ transplantation, and pediatric procedures. In concert with the IOM report, the investigators noted that "as the demand for health care continues to grow, increasing the number of CRNAs and permitting them to practice in the most efficient delivery models, will be a key to containing costs while maintaining quality of care" (Hogan et al., 2010, p. 159).

Research is a core APRN competency that is valued by CRNAs. Nurse anesthetists have long advocated the use of evidence in their daily practice. Outcomes research has confirmed the high quality and reasonable cost of anesthesia services provided by CRNAs (Dulisse & Cromwell, 2010; Hogan et al., 2010; Lewis et al., 2014; Negrusa et al., 2016; The Lewin Group, 2016). The AANA Professional Practice Division has resources for anesthesia practice as well as evidence-based practice documents and position statements that address practice issues, including the following:

- Scope of Nurse Anesthesia Practice
- Office-Based Anesthesia Practice
- Postanesthesia Care Standards for the Certified Registered Nurse Anesthetist
- Core Clinical Privileges for Certified Registered Nurse Anesthetists
- Management of the Obstetrical Patient for the Certified Registered Nurse Anesthetist
- Expert Witness for Nurse Anesthesia Practice
- Documenting Anesthesia Care
- Informed Consent for Anesthesia Care
- Infection Prevention and Control Guidelines for Anesthesia Care
- Latex Allergy Management
- Management of Waste Anesthetic Gases

These documents can be found in the AANA Practice Documents resources on the AANA website (http://www.aana.com/resources2/professionalpractice/Pages/Professional-Practice-Manual.aspx#Guidelines).

Nurse anesthetists have been adopting the principles of evidence-based practice and teaching advocated by the IOM (Grenier & Knebel, 2003). Nurse anesthesia education and practice reflect patient-centered care, delivered by an interprofessional team. Nurse anesthetists are increasingly using the best available evidence when planning and implementing anesthesia care. CRNAs are also committed to quality improvement and the use of data to improve practice and education. Anesthesia practice involves competencies in technology and informatics; CRNAs use these information systems to support and improve patient care. Nurse anesthesia educational programs and continuing education opportunities emphasize the critical evaluation of clinical and research databases that can be used as clinical decision support resources (Kremer, 2011).

CRNAs have written seminal evidence-based texts that provide the foundation for practice. *Nurse Anesthesia,* now in its fifth edition, is a comprehensive compendium of topics ranging from scientific foundations to practice-related technology and intraoperative management (Nagelhout & Plaus, 2014). *Pharmacology for Nurse Anesthesiology,* a text written by CRNAs, is used in many nurse anesthesia programs (Ouellette & Joyce, 2011). *Case Studies in Nurse Anesthesia* (Elisha, 2011) is a valuable resource for students and clinicians. The text of record for professional issues in nurse anesthesia is *A Professional Study and Resource Guide for the CRNA* (Foster & Faut-Callahan, 2011). Major content areas in this text include the essence of professionalism, understanding the responsibilities of clinical practice, the health care environment, the politics of health care, and challenges in professional practice.

The *AANA Journal* routinely publishes evidence-based continuing education courses on key topics of importance to the overall mission of promoting patient safety. CRNAs are increasingly making contributions to peer-reviewed literature through case studies, review articles, reports of research findings, and continuing education courses. The common theme is emphasis on continued competency, patient safety, and the development of scholarship, consistent with the values described by Horton (1998). As scholarly publications authored by CRNAs proliferate, useful data-based information is shared that benefits the diverse practice settings where CRNAs serve as solo practitioners or work collaboratively with other providers.

Leadership

Nurse anesthesia has grown and prospered as an advanced practice nursing specialty because of the clinical competence and leadership demonstrated by generations of CRNAs. Despite challenges from organized medicine and initial lack of acceptance by the ANA, CRNAs were undeterred in their forward movement. The leadership provided by nurse anesthetists in the clinical area (see "American Association of Nurse Anesthetists" earlier), along with dedication to a rigorous credentialing process and health care policy activism, accounts for achievements such as the attainment of billing rights under Medicare Part B in 1989.

The clinical expertise demonstrated by Alice Magaw at the Mayo Clinic and Agatha Hodgins on the battlefields of France during World War I resulted in leadership roles for these women, whose anesthetic techniques were taught to physicians and nurses from around the world. Military CRNAs also provided leadership in the development of rigorous, didactically front-loaded curricula that prepared military nurses to provide anesthesia as new graduates in austere environments (Gunn, 1991; Horton, 2007).

CRNA leadership often involves participation in elected and appointed positions at the local, regional, and national levels. At the local level, CRNAs may serve on or chair committees in the clinical and/or academic areas in which they practice. The level of responsibility shouldered by CRNAs in the clinical area provides skills in rapid information processing and decision making, which may be helpful in governance activities, such as committees. In Exemplar 18.3, CRNA FM demonstrates leadership in his practice group and across the clinical settings for which his anesthesia group provides clinical services.

Collaboration

As with other advanced practice nursing roles, nurse anesthesia practice is based on a collaborative model. Collaboration, one of the seven APRN competencies described in Chapter 3, is defined as a dynamic process in which individuals interact with genuine intent to inform each other and solve problems to achieve outcomes. Every day, CRNAs collaborate with other nurses, APRNs, physicians, physician assistants, and technicians. Partnerships are formed that provide the best care to patients. Collaborative practice has been described as the practice of forming partnerships to accomplish care for patients. Baggs and colleagues (1997) identified six critical elements in physician-nurse collaborative practice: cooperation, assertiveness, shared decision making, communication, planning together, and coordination. As noted earlier, the IOM report on *The Future of Nursing* (2010) called for nurses to be full partners with physicians and other health professionals in redesigning health care in the United States. This is a logical extension of collaboration from the bedside to the health care policy level.

Certified Registered Nurse Anesthetist Role: Leadership and Autonomy

F.M. has been a certified registered nurse anesthetist (CRNA) for 17 years. His interest in the profession was initiated by a family friend who was a CRNA and who encouraged F.M. to pursue a career as a nurse anesthetist. The factors that have most influenced F.M. in his professional development are his interests in a number of areas, including complex pathophysiology, matching anesthesia techniques to complex patient presentations, pharmacology, and the desire for autonomous practice. F.M. notes, "I get paid to do anesthesia!" This enthusiasm for his specialty is typical of many practicing CRNAs.

F.M. was an active-duty military CRNA and practiced at several military medical centers. As a civilian CRNA, he moved into a group practice based at a rural critical access hospital and other facilities in the Midwest. He spends 90% of his time in direct patient care. Some of that time he oversees a student rotating through his facility because he remains with the student and patient at all times. The balance of F.M.'s time is spent "in the business of anesthesia," related to being part owner of his practice.

A typical day in F.M.'s practice includes meeting in the group's office with colleagues for coffee at 6:00 AM. Following that, he prepares for anesthetics that he will administer that day. He then meets, interviews, plans, and administers the anesthetic for the first and subsequent cases of the day until the cases are done. If he is on call, he spends the afternoon in the preoperative clinic performing preoperative assessments and interventions for complex patients who will be coming to the operating room in the future.

Some of the unique aspects of F.M.'s practice include autonomy and the use of regional anesthesia techniques. He and his practice partners were early adopters of ultrasound-guided regional block techniques, including interscalene and femoral nerve blocks. He enjoys the challenges of caring for high-acuity patients undergoing complex surgical procedures in a small community hospital.

F.M. describes the greatest challenges in his practice as "autonomy—having to make decisions while caring for very sick and complicated patients with no input from other anesthesia providers [and] the complexity of the patients and the procedures we are performing on them." He also notes that managing a very busy private practice anesthesia group is challenging, "ensuring that we cover all the surgeons and hospitals but at the same time protecting our staff from overwork."

The practice in which F.M. is a partner evolved from a small hospital-employed group of one anesthesiologist and two CRNAs. As the workload grew and more surgeons were added, the group grew larger. "We eventually ended up with three anesthesiologists and six CRNAs. Unfortunately, several members decided to move closer to family. At this point we decided to take advantage of the turmoil and go independent. We formed our own private practice group, a service corporation. We have been functioning like this for the last 9 years."

F.M.'s military background provided knowledge about infrastructure and resources for personal and professional development that carried over into his later career. His CRNA practice partners are all former military CRNAs and their principal clinical site is a clinical affiliation site for military and civilian nurse anesthesia programs. F.M. has had extensive involvement with his state and national professional organizations and presents to these groups on clinical and nonclinical topics. ◎

Nurse anesthetists first formed collaborative relationships with surgeons in the late 19th century. At the request of surgeons, nurses were called on to administer anesthesia because of the then-high surgical and anesthetic mortality rates. Today, approximately 80% of nurse anesthetists collaborate with physicians–consultant anesthesiologists in daily practice. There are no statutory requirements for the supervision of nurse anesthetists by anesthesiologists. Therefore, CRNAs also legally collaborate with surgeons, podiatrists, and dentists. There is no increased legal liability for surgeons who collaborate with CRNAs because CRNAs are responsible for their own actions.

CRNAs collaborate with other physicians by sharing their patient assessments and plans for anesthesia care. At the same time, collaboration occurs with the patient, so a mutually agreeable anesthetic plan can be developed; procedures, risks, and benefits associated with the anesthetic are discussed. Nurse anesthesia services are always provided in collaboration with the operating physician, dentist, podiatrist, or consultant anesthesiologist, which has proved to be a beneficial collaborative practice model.

CRNAs work collaboratively with surgeons, physician anesthesiologists, and other health care professionals. CRNAs practice in all settings where anesthesia is delivered: hospital operating rooms, nonsurgical interventional procedure rooms and delivery rooms; critical access hospitals; ambulatory surgical centers; the offices of dentists, podiatrists, ophthalmologists, plastic surgeons, and pain management specialists; and the US military, US Public Health Service facilities, and VA health care facilities (AANA, 2016d).

Accountability and Ethics

CRNAs are legally liable for the quality of the services that they render (Blumenreich, 2007). They make independent judgments and decisions about the appropriateness of their professional services and the probable effects of those services on the patient. A CRNA who believes that the anesthesia care plan for a particular patient is inappropriate should seek consultation for more appropriate direction. CRNAs should be patient advocates and always seek resolution to situations involving ethical conflicts in patient management and other ethical issues. If reasonable doubt continues, it is the responsibility of the CRNA to consider withdrawal from rendering the service, provided that the well-being of the patient is not jeopardized. The expected behaviors associated with CRNAs are found in the AANA's "Code of Ethics for the Certified Registered Nurse Anesthetist" (AANA, 2005).

Bosek (2011) noted that "ethical situations require CRNAs to consider professional and personal values, think about what is the right thing to do, identify options, and act upon the selected 'right' option." This nurse ethicist believes that nonmaleficence, or to "do no harm," is a fundamental goal that should guide the actions of CRNAs. In concert with the values identified by Horton (1998), Bosek (2011) indicated that advocating for the welfare of patients is a responsibility that CRNAs must uphold.

Reimbursement

Reimbursement is one of the most complex aspects of anesthesia practice. From the inception of this specialty through the 1950s, CRNAs were often paid as employees of the surgeon or hospital that employed them. In rural areas, CRNAs often contracted with hospitals to provide services based on fee-for-service structures—that is, a set amount of compensation per case as opposed to a straight salary for hours worked. The advent of private payers such as Blue Cross Blue Shield has led to the compensation of only physicians and hospitals through these plans. Other health care providers, such as APRNs, psychologists, and physical therapists, would submit charges to the hospital or treating physician. The hospital or physician would then obtain reimbursement for these services as incident to their own and pass this on to the nonreimbursed provider (e.g., APRN).

In the 1980s, escalating health care costs caused Medicare to institute a prospective payment system. This legislation initially affected only Medicare Part A (hospital costs), and subsequently also affected Medicare Part B (physician and nonphysician costs). Prospective payment system legislation mandated a fixed payment rate for all hospital care, covering Part A services paid to hospitals based on the diagnosis-related classification group of the patient. This fixed rate was to cover all costs associated with hospital admission, including services provided by nonphysician health care providers. CRNAs were in great jeopardy under this system. In their cost-cutting efforts, hospitals had no incentive to hire CRNAs because the related employment costs would come directly from the hospital diagnosis-related group payment. Congress inadvertently created reimbursement disincentives for the use of CRNAs while bolstering incentives to use anesthesiologists. AANA lobbying efforts resulted in the Health Care Financing Administration (now the CMS), rewriting portions of this legislation, enabling all CRNAs to obtain Medicare reimbursement or to sign over their billing rights to their employer (Broadston, 2001).

Historically, anesthesia charges have been based on direct time involvement as a charge for simple time or as a charge based on a combination of time and the complexity of the anesthetic procedure. The resource-based relative value scale, developed in the 1960s, is used to determine anesthesia charges based on the complexity of a surgical procedure. The result is charges for base units, or surgical procedures described by anatomic or functional units. Additional modifier units can be added to base units for factors such as emergency procedures, extremes of age, or anesthetic risk. After adding base and modifier units, time units are calculated at one unit per 15 minutes. The value of time units is determined by the payer, such as Medicare or Blue Cross Blue Shield, and the market. The total of base, modifier, and time units determines the professional fee for administration of anesthesia. One unit of anesthesia time may be billed at from $15 to more than $70.

A conversion factor is a dollar amount per unit used to convert the relative value scale intensity measurement into an actual charge for services. Medicare publishes conversion factors annually.

Private practices may charge three to four times the Medicare conversion factor. For calendar year 2016, the National Anesthesia Conversion factor determined by the CMS was $22.44 (CMS, 2016). The gross charge for services provided is determined by multiplying the total procedure base and time units by the conversion factor (Walker & Broadston, 2011). Many third-party payers, such as Medicare and some Blue Cross insurers, completely ignore the charges of the practitioner and determine payments from their own fee schedules. These payments are often determined by what providers charge on average for their services (Broadston, 2001; Walker & Broadston, 2011).

Medicare Part A provides pass-through funding to eligible rural and critical access hospitals for CRNA services. CRNAs cannot receive direct reimbursement from Medicare Part A. Medicare Part B provides direct reimbursement to CRNAs for anesthesia services. Key differences exist between reimbursement models using medical direction, medical supervision, and nonmedical direction. Many third-party payers, including state Medicaid and private insurers, use reimbursement mechanisms similar to those used by Medicare (Walker & Broadston, 2011).

Teaching CRNAs and teaching anesthesiologists have specific reimbursement considerations that influence the education of future anesthesia providers. There is no parity in the reimbursement for teaching cases involving physician residents versus student RN anesthetists (Walker & Broadston, 2011). CRNAs receive national provider identifier numbers that are used in the billing process. Billing services are frequently responsible for the generation of anesthesia charges, but anesthesia groups are responsible for ensuring accurate diagnosis and procedural coding on all submitted claims.

CRNAs can value their clinical and financial outcomes through data collected, often by billing services, over specified time periods (e.g., monthly, quarterly, or annually). The total number of anesthetics administered during the specified time frame needs to be determined. Then the total number of relative value units generated is calculated by multiplication of the total number of anesthetics administered by the average number of relative value units per case, which might be 10.5 units. The surgical case mix, payer mix, and breakdown need to be determined—for example, 15% commercial, 35% Medicare, and 10% Medicaid. Finally, the specific reimbursement rates per relative value unit per section of the case mix–payer mix are calculated. Payor mix will vary with practice settings; this information is helpful as part of the assessment of a potential new practice setting (Broadston, 2001).

Attempts to control spiraling health care costs and improve access to care have resulted in the development of accountable care organizations (ACOs) and patient-centered medical homes and resurgent interest in health maintenance organizations with capitated payment schemes. Fee-for-service reimbursement structures may become less common because of the imposition of additional cost containment measures by payors and the national economy. Unfortunately, cost containment in health care does not ensure patient access to APRNs based on cost-effectiveness. Transition mechanisms in vertical integration strategies, such as combining payors, providers, and a wide spectrum of network services, still focus on physicians and hospitals as the principal health care resources.

An average reduction of 21.2% in Medicare reimbursement rates was implemented in 2015 (Matthews, 2015). Issues such as hospital readmissions deemed to be unnecessary decrease Medicare reimbursement to providers. Medicare pays health care providers, including CRNAs, about 80% of the private health insurance rate. In contrast, Medicaid pays about 56% of what is paid by private health insurance (Matthews, 2015). These trends in reimbursement are tracked closely by professional organizations, such as the AANA, to determine the impact on provider compensation.

Health care providers receive an additional 1.5% incentive payment in exchange for reporting quality measures to Medicare. These quality measures include the maintenance of perioperative normothermia, appropriate timing of prophylactic preoperative antibiotics, and pain management planning.

Currently, anesthesiologists can bill for 100% of physician reimbursement on each case when supervising two concurrent cases. In settings in which nonmedically directed CRNAs supervise two nurse anesthesia students concurrently, the nonmedically directed CRNA can also bill for 100% on each case. However, in a scenario that may be more common, if an anesthesiologist is supervising two CRNAs who are in turn each supervising two student RN anesthetists, the anesthesiologist can only bill for 50% on each of the four concurrent cases and the CRNAs would receive only 50% of the anesthesia fee provided (Walker & Broadston, 2011). This creates a disincentive for organizations to support nurse anesthesia education. From a policy perspective, it is desirable that the Medicare anesthesia payment rules treat CRNAs and anesthesiologists similarly.

Legislation passed by Congress in 1986 provided direct billing for CRNAs under Medicare Part B. In 2001, the CMS allowed states to opt out of the Medicare Part A reimbursement requirement that a surgeon or anesthesiologist oversee anesthesia services provided by CRNAs. To date, a total of 17 states have opted out of Medicare Part A CRNA supervision requirements (AANA, 2016d). Efforts by some state medical societies to overturn these opt-outs have been unsuccessful. An analysis of Medicare data for 1999 to 2005 found no evidence that opting out of the oversight requirement resulted in increased inpatient morbidity or mortality (Dulisse & Cromwell, 2010). Negrusa et al. (2016) found that there was no measurable impact of expanded CRNA scope of practice on anesthesia-related complications.

Future of Reimbursement

There is speculation that changes in anesthesia reimbursement, driven by legislation and market economics, may result in payment being limited to the services of one provider. This has generated concern that graduates of all nurse anesthesia programs will need to have the knowledge, skills, and abilities of a full-service provider, such as one who can work without a collaborating physician, when they complete their educational program. Although current accreditation and certification standards do not mandate that graduates of nurse anesthesia programs have the ability to function at this level when they graduate from an accredited program, proposed changes in reimbursement for health care services, such as the implementation of ACOs, need to be monitored so that the education and practice of CRNAs and other APRNs adapt to a dynamic market.

ACOs are proposed as a new payment model under Medicare and foster pilot programs to extend the model to private payors and Medicaid. Proponents believe that ACOs will allow providers to work more effectively together to improve quality while decreasing spending. The success of ACOs will depend on whether the CMS, private payors, and clinicians can collaborate on the development of a tightly linked performance measurement and evaluation framework that ensures accountability to patients and payors and supports timely learning for key participants. A robust, comprehensive, and transparent performance measurement system that accurately accounts for the contributions of all clinicians will be necessary

to assure the success of ACOs. Studies to date on the cost-effectiveness and safety of services provided by CRNAs should help ensure that CRNAs are represented in ACOs (Fisher & Shortell, 2010).

The incentive for health care providers to implement ACOs successfully is that failure to control health care costs will likely result in Medicare payment reductions by the federal government (see earlier). Under such a scenario, providers may try to negotiate higher payment rates from private payors to compensate for lower Medicare rates. Although this scenario does not guarantee successful implementation of ACOs, looming, significant price reductions may result in focused efforts to contain costs through increased collaboration in the delivery of health care (Emanuel, 2012).

Continued Challenges

Nurse anesthesia has dealt with challenges since the inception of the specialty. However, the number of CRNAs in the United States is now at an all-time high, which is a tribute to the safe, cost-effective care provided by these clinicians. Nurse anesthesia education has rapidly moved from certificate-level training to degree-granting institutions that initially offered baccalaureate and later master's- and now doctoral-level programs.

Reimbursement will continue to be a significant challenge for CRNAs as the health care system continues to evolve. An increasing proportion of Medicare and Medicaid in payer mixes begs the question of whether a fee-for-service system is sustainable in US health care. Medicare reimbursement is a significant portion of the payor mix in many clinical settings. Population demographics ensure that this trend will continue. In addition to affecting Medicare patients directly, these potential reimbursement reductions also affect all insurance plans whose rates are tied to Medicare, including the Tricare plan for military personnel and their dependents.

The potential effects of Medicare Part B payment reductions are significant. Although Medicare reimburses most physician services at 80% of market rates, Part B provides reimbursement for anesthesia services at about 45% of market rates. According to AANA member surveys, each CRNA on average provides anesthesia for about 900 cases per year. The potential exists for reductions in compensation for all anesthesia providers if decreases in Medicare reimbursement are implemented.

Conclusion

Nurse anesthetists provide surgical and nonsurgical anesthesia services in a variety of settings in the United States and other parts of the world. CRNAs work collaboratively with physicians, as do other APRNs, and are capable of providing the full spectrum of anesthesia services. Nurse anesthesia, the earliest nursing specialty, was also the first nursing specialty to have standardized educational programs, a certification process, mandatory continuing education, and recertification and the first to convert to a doctoral timeline. At this writing, 46 nurse anesthesia educational programs have been approved by the COA to offer entry-level doctoral degrees and 24 programs provide post-master's doctoral degree completion programs for CRNAs. A remaining 69 nurse anesthesia programs have yet to be approved for offering doctoral degrees for entry to practice by 2022. In the same way that this profession has dealt with education issues ranging from initial standardization of education in the 1930s to subsequent requirements for academic degrees, the move to doctoral entry education will be completed by dedicated CRNA educators.

Nurse anesthetists have been involved in the development of anesthetic techniques along with physicians and engineers. CRNAs have been nursing leaders in obtaining third-party reimbursement for professional services and in coping with challenges such as the prospective payment system, managed care, and physician supervision. Economics and control of practice continue to be areas of challenge that CRNAs meet proactively, state by state. Hostile bills in state legislatures introduced by other provider groups (i.e., curtailing CRNA pain management activities, proposing licensure of anesthesiologist assistants) are addressed by advocacy efforts from state nurse anesthesia associations.

Key Summary Points

- Activism at the state and federal legislative and regulatory levels is a recognized and necessary activity.

- Increasing coalition building among nurse anesthetists, other APRNs, and nurse educators is congruent with a shared nursing vision.
- Market demand for CRNAs is high, and additional evidence of the safety, quality, and cost-effectiveness of anesthesia care provided by CRNAs supports the needs of third-party payors, ACOs, legislators, and the public for outcome data.
- Efforts to allow CRNAs to function at the full scope of their education and training, at the state and federal levels, are often opposed by other provider groups. A growing body of knowledge regarding the safety and quality of anesthesia care provided by CRNAs refutes contentions by others that existing anesthesia care delivery models are optimal.
- Nurse anesthesia was the first APRN specialty to adopt a timeline for conversion of educational programs from master's- to doctoral-level entry.
- CRNAs will continue to provide high-quality anesthesia care as practice, education, and reimbursement models evolve to reflect new economic models for the delivery of health care.

References

To access the references for this chapter, use your smartphone's QR code reader to scan the code below, or go to http://booksite.elsevier.com/ 9780323447751.

CHAPTER

Maximizing APRN Power and Influencing Policy

19

Eileen T. O'Grady • *Gene E. Harkless*

> *"People always say that I didn't give up my seat because I was tired, but that isn't true. I was not tired physically... No, the only tired I was, was tired of giving in."*
>
> —*Rosa Parks*

CHAPTER CONTENTS

The purpose of this chapter is to build advanced practice registered nurse (APRN) policy competency. Readers will be reminded of nursing's core historical function in policymaking and given three different frameworks to explore the policymaking process. Current and emerging APRN policy issues will be emphasized, and the chapter ends with a discussion on APRN policy leadership skills and defines the specific attitudes and behaviors necessary to be influential in the policy realm. These skills are highlighted in the exemplars. It is the authors' great hope that students reading this chapter will be moved to expand their roles beyond the clinical and broaden their circle of influence on how health care gets paid for, measured, and delivered.

Policy: Historic Core Function in Nursing

Florence Nightingale spent much of her career walking the halls of Parliament promoting policy change to improve quality, dignity, and equity, first for the Crimean war soldiers and later for the poor of London. Her 3 years of clinical practice gave her clinical expertise and credibility to assume the role of policymaker. She embraced that role because of her high degree of moral distress and concern about the needless suffering and premature death of her patients (Jameton, 1993; Whitehead, Herbertson, Hamric, Epstein, & Fisher, 2015). She believed she knew the right thing to do for the soldiers, and the constraints she faced were significant. Empowered by her clinical practice during the Crimean war, she used data that she had collected systematically to persuade Parliament to make needed military and civic law reforms that promoted health. In 1858, Nightingale became the first woman elected as a member of the Royal Statistical Society, and she later became an honorary member of the American Statistical Association (Gill & Gill, 2005). Her work and prestige were Victorian era validations of the importance of using evidence to inform policy. Nightingale's activism presaged the APRN as patient advocate and policy shaper. She leveraged statistics and clinical expertise to become an effective advocate for influencing policy. She expected nurses to have a high degree of social interest in the human condition and to be involved in the policymaking process. As Nightingale's work demonstrated, health policy challenges and opportunities can be found in both "big P" policies such as formal laws, rules, and regulations at the local, state, national, and/or international level and in the "small p" policy arena such as nongovernmental organizational guidelines, decisions, and social norms guiding behavior (Brownson, Chriqui, & Stamatakis, 2009).

This historic covenant with the public must be strengthened. APRNs must deepen their commitment to and become masterful at critiquing, formulating, and influencing policies that interfere with human wholeness and health. Most APRNs in practice today have experienced the effects of polices that lead directly to poor health care. We must substantively weave policy into the core APRN roles so that those experiences move APRNs into leadership roles and they become advocates for change.

Policy: APRNs and Modern Roles

Powerful APRN clinical experiences, when effectively communicated, serve to deepen policymakers' understanding of health-related issues. APRN practice experiences are poignant stories that enlighten policy issues by providing a human context while bringing nursing's value to the health policy arena. Most APRNs in practice today have experienced the effects of ill-conceived policies that lead to needless suffering, poor resource use, and poorly coordinated, highly specialized, fragmented health care. This practice experience, coupled with the ability to analyze the policy process, provides a strong foundation to propel APRNs into politically competent action and advocacy.

Engaging in policymaking is a core element of leadership to be cultivated by all APRNs (see Chapter 11). The Institute of Medicine (IOM) report *The Future of Nursing* (2010) has determined that "nurses have a key role to play as team members and leaders for a reformed and better integrated patient-centered health care system" (p. xii). Major health reform legislation in 2010—the Patient Protection and Affordable Care Act (ACA)—mandated health insurance coverage, which has swept nearly 20 million additional people into the US health care delivery system and lowered the US uninsured rate to less than 10%, the lowest in 50 years (Obama Care Facts, 2016). The system had to accommodate the surge in demand, but the ACA also required a change in the way care was delivered, focusing on value-based care that improves the health of the population and de-emphasizing fee for service, while lowering costs. The election of Donald Trump to the Presidency in 2016 was in part based on a platform that promised repeal and replacement of the ACA; this has created uncertainty in the future direction of health care reform. However, the movement toward value-based care preceded the ACA and has bipartisan support (Muhlestein, Burton, & Winfield, 2017). The approach under the Trump administration may be different, but the goals of achieving better care, a healthier population, and lower costs will likely remain the same. Meeting these goals poses significant challenges to APRNs. Addressing this challenge, Altman, Butler, and Shern (2016) identified three specific recommendations that are highly pertinent to APRNs engaging in policymaking:

- **Recommendation 1:** *Build Common Ground Around Scope of Practice and Other Issues in Policy and Practice* (Altman et al., 2016, pp. 51-52). Removal of scope-of-practice barriers will require a broader and more diverse stakeholder base. Interprofessional practice requires all members of the team to function at the top of their license and is becoming the new standard of care, so more common ground must be sought. In order for APRNs to function at the highest level of their education and training, garnering common ground will require persistence and a strong degree of political competency because more than 50% of the states have outdated nurse practice acts that do not reflect national APRN education standards and current APRN practice that focus on full practice authority. It will take a significant degree of political organizational networking, coalition building, campaigning, and educating the public to remove the barriers to practice that are embedded in many states' nurse practice acts. There has been a growing chorus of agencies working to lift these and other barriers to APRN practice. At the federal level, the Centers for Medicare & Medicaid Services (2012) issued a final rule broadening the concept of medical staff, permitting hospitals to allow other practitioners (e.g., APRNs, physician assistants, and pharmacists) to perform all functions within their scope of practice. Despite this rule, medical staff membership and hospital privileges remain subject to existing state laws and business preferences. One major concern is that APRN regulatory practice constraints are restraint of trade. Importantly, the Federal Trade Commission (2014) has engaged in advocacy for APRNs' scope of practice expansion in order to promote healthy competition in many states, providing letters, comments, and/or testimony to this end.

- **Recommendation 7:** *Expand Efforts and Opportunities for Interprofessional Collaboration and Leadership Development for Nurses* (Altman et al., 2016, p. 155). APRNs should enact, support, and promote interprofessional collaboration and programs that focus on leadership. Health care professionals from all disciplines should work together in building improved health care systems, particularly in an interprofessional and collaborative environment. Preparing and enabling nurses to lead change to advance health will require APRNs to develop leadership skills, which include having a high degree of respect for other professions and shaping and influencing policymaking at all levels. This recommendation will require APRNs to become insightful and politically savvy, know how to find common ground, and translate research/best practices into practice. This recommendation emphasizes

that nurses must hold key leadership positions across decision-making bodies in the government and private sector.

- **Recommendation 8:** *Promote the Involvement of Nurses in the Redesign of Care Delivery and Payment Systems* (Altman et al., 2016, p. 156). APRNs must work with payors, health care organizations, providers, employers, and regulators in the redesign of care delivery and payment systems. To this end, APRNs are encouraged to serve in executive and leadership positions in government, for-profit, and nonprofit organizations; health care delivery systems (e.g., as hospital chief executive officers or chief operations officers); and advisory committees.

Among the recommendations in *The Future of Nursing* (IOM, 2010) is Recommendation 8: Build an infrastructure for the collection and analysis of interprofessional health care workforce data. This requires APRNs to be involved in improving the research enterprise around quality and safety metrics, payment models, and the health care workforce to better inform policymaking. To that end, Altman et al. offered three themes for nursing that will drive the IOM's recommendation further (2016, p. 4):

1. The need to build a broader coalition to increase awareness of nurses' ability to play a full role in health professions practice, education, collaboration, and leadership;
2. The need to continue to make promoting diversity in the nursing workforce a priority; and
3. The need for better data with which to assess and drive progress.

Politics Versus Policy

Health Policy

All policy involves decisions that influence the daily life of citizens. Longest (2016) has defined health policy as the authoritative decisions pertaining to health or health care, made in the legislative, executive, or judicial branches of government, that are intended to direct or influence the actions, behaviors, or decisions of citizens.

Although there are many definitions of policy and politics, policy generally refers to decisions resulting in a law or regulation. Politics refers to power relationships. It is the responsibility of a multitude of policymakers, whether mayors, county supervisors, government employees, legislators,

BOX 19.1   How to Find a Legislative Bill and Determine Bipartisan Support

To find a federal bill, go to the Library of Congress website (https://www.congress.gov/) and find the current legislative session. Search keywords or enter the bill number. Once you get to the bill summary, do an analysis to determine whether the bill has any chance of passing by going to the list of cosponsors. The Library of Congress does not list political affiliation next to the cosponsor's name, which requires looking up each member to find out to which party he or she belongs. Be sure that members of Congress from each party are cosponsoring the bill in equivalent numbers. If it is only one party sponsoring the bill, you may conclude that the bill is largely partisan, with small chance of passage. A politically competent APRN will always look for bipartisan cosponsorship of bills, which have the highest chance of actually becoming law. The same method will work for a bill in any state legislature (found on each state's government website).

governors, or presidents, to make health policy. Overall responsibility generally places authority with the legislative branch to craft laws (Box 19.1); the executive branch crafts rules to implement the laws, and the judicial branch interprets conflicts among the spheres of government, citizens, and a public or private entity.

Politics

Politics is the process used to influence those who are making health policy. Politics introduces nonrational, divisive, and self-interested approaches to policymaking, often along ideologic lines. In the United States, the core disagreement between the two political parties comes down to what the role of the government should be (if any) in resolving the conflicting viewpoints. Any political maneuvering to enhance one's power or status within a group may be described as politics. Politics in a democracy is the nonviolent way of reaching agreement between differing points of view and requires compromise in which neither party gets precisely what it wants. Compromise and deal-making are the only alternatives to coercion or authoritarianism (Crick, 1962). Politics is largely associated with a struggle for ascendancy among groups having different priorities and power relationships. Preferences and interests of stakeholders and political bargaining (favor swapping) are

important and extremely influential political factors that overlie the policymaking process. The self-interest paradigm suggests that human motives are not any different in political arenas than they are in the private marketplace. This behavioral assumption implies that it is rational for people and organizations to use the power of government to achieve what they cannot accomplish on their own. Ideally, elected officials seek office to serve the public interest, not their own. However, to be successful in the electoral process, they need electoral support through financial contributions, rendering them beholden to fundraising and funders (Feldstein, 2006). Highly politicized decisions often create outcomes that have little to do with efficient use of scarce resources and what is best for the general public. These forces, which may or may not be based on evidence, contribute to the lack of coordination among health policies in the United States, making policy formulation highly complex and exceedingly interesting.

APRNs must engage in the political process to influence public policy and resource allocation decisions within political, economic, and social systems and institutions. APRN political advocacy facilitates civic engagement and collective action, which may be motivated by patient-centered moral or ethical principles or simply to protect what has already been allocated. Advocacy can include many activities undertaken by a person or organization, such as media campaigns, public speaking, commissioning and publishing policy-relevant research or polls, and filing an *amicus curiae* (friend of the court) brief. Lobbying as a political advocacy tool is only effective if a relationship between the lobbyist and legislator influences or shapes a policy issue. Social media for political advocacy is playing an increasingly significant role in modern politics (Rim & Song, 2016).

United States Differs From the International Community

The US health system and political process for creating health care policy is unique in that the system is decentralized, fragmented, and complicated. In the United States, there is no single entity responsible for health care delivery, payment, or policymaking. There are many spheres of policymaking with overlapping authority involving a wide diversity of people, cultures, traditions, and illness patterns. Although the federal government may create broad guidelines, the 50 states, for the most part, have the autonomy to create policies that best serve their citizenry—hence the large patchwork of public, private, local, state, and federal entities. These can be operating as governmental, nonprofit, or for-profit entities, all of which are creating policies and/or delivering care. Moreover, unlike other developed nations, US health care policy is highly political and can shift dramatically from one administration to another, creating further instability.

The US federal government is a provider of health services via the prison system and the Department of Veterans Affairs. In the United States, the creation of the ACA was a contentious effort to solve deep, underlying problems in the nation's health care system. Many of the ACA provisions encouraged innovating and testing new models and payment mechanisms for care delivery, creating new challenges for APRN influence. As was heard by a policymaker, "if you've seen one accountable care organization, you've seen one accountable care organization." However, for the most part, health care delivery is still largely under private sector control, making US health policy development incremental, fragmented, highly politicized, and far more decentralized than in the rest of the world.

For most of the rest of the world, and in countries such as China, Canada, Great Britain, Switzerland, and the Netherlands, there is a highly centralized health authority for policymaking and a more integrated care delivery system. These nations, with centralized systems of care, are able to track the impact of their policy decisions more closely and build more tightly controlled surveillance systems to follow epidemics, immunization rates, spending, workforce, and other important markers of a strong health care system. Moreover, centralized health care systems limit the number of policymakers that need to be influenced, which can be a great advantage. Although there are a smaller number of people to influence, if those policymakers are strongly opposed to issues such as expanded APRN practice, centralization becomes disadvantageous. The unique US public-private, federal-state, nonprofit, and for-profit arrangements in which the majority of people get their insurance through their employer make it difficult to enact programs that are highly effective in other nations in the United States. Exemplar 19.1 depicts the experience of nurse practitioners (NPs) who practice across the boundaries of the health care systems of two countries, Canada and the United States.

Sadly, but consistently, the US health care outcomes are not what would be expected given that

| EXEMPLAR 19.1 | A Tale of Two Countries, Two Nurse Practitioners, and Two Health Care Systems |

Nancy Brew and Mark Schultz

A husband-and-wife nurse practitioner (NP) team, Nancy (Brew) and Mark (Schultz), had been living and practicing in Alaska for over 20 years when they emigrated to British Columbia (BC), Canada, in 2006. Nancy had worked as a family nurse practitioner (FNP) in Alaska for many years and experienced increasing moral distress[a] (see Chapter 13) from trying to provide equitable and quality care to uninsured and underinsured patients in the expensive, private-payor US health care system. Mark was working in an Anchorage intensive care unit and wanted to pursue his graduate degree to become an FNP. They were both drawn to the concept of health care for all, so the idea of working in a country in which everyone had access to health care and no one had to fear bankruptcy or losing their home if medical disaster struck was compelling. Together, they decided

to stretch their professional wings and embark on an international practice adventure.

Universal health care access to physician and hospital services was established in Canada in the 1960s. The Canadian health care system is chiefly administered via provincial and territorial governments. NP-authorizing legislation is now present in all 13 Canadian provinces and territories, and in 2016, 4500 NPs were licensed and practicing in Canada. Similar to NPs in the United States, Canadian NPs are regulated on a province-by-province basis, so there are some variations in scope across the country. The majority of jurisdictions do not require NPs to establish collaborative agreements with a physician or a group of physicians. Many provinces have also given NPs the authority to admit, treat, and discharge patients in a hospital. As of 2016, NPs in all but one province could prescribe controlled substances.

[a]Moral distress—when one knows the right thing to do, but institutional constraints make it almost impossible to pursue the right course of action (Hamric, 2009; Jameton, 1984).

Continued

A Tale of Two Countries, Two Nurse Practitioners, and Two Health Care Systems—cont'd

Funding in a socialized health care system presents unique challenges to moving advanced nursing practice forward. Each regional government determines how to fund advanced practice nurse (APN) practice. In British Columbia (BC), almost all primary care is still provided by small physician group practices in a fee-for-service model in which each patient visit is individually billed to BC's Medical Services Plan. To date, BC NPs have not gained authorization to bill; thus, APNs in BC are fiscally unable to open their own practices or freely join existing physician practices, even in the most underserved rural areas. A limited number of salaried positions have been created for BC NPs, but many of these are in specialty areas because the primary care physicians resist APN practice. Hence Mark has worked predominantly in cardiology and orthopedic surgery since becoming an NP, although he was trained in family practice. This is ironic because the NP role in BC was initially legislated to improve access to primary care. There is a great need for primary care providers in BC, with a significant number of patients unable to find one. NPs could be doing more to address the Canadian primary care shortage, but Canadian health care, as a single-payor, government-run system, lacks a market-based approach to workforce shortages.

Nancy and Mark found it interesting to have worked in health care on both sides of the border during the 2010 American health care reform debate. The Canadian health care system was held up as a cautionary tale, that the Canadian system was an egregious example of poor care, long waits, and unaccountable all-empowering bureaucracy that ran health care into the Canadian ground. Although it is true there can be months' long wait times to see specialists for nonurgent conditions, Nancy and Mark have found that appropriate specialty referrals are given rather freely. Nonurgent computed tomography scans can occur in a week, nonurgent magnetic resonance imaging may take a few months, and the wait times for hip and knee replacements can approach 6 months. The couple found that in Canada, visits are shorter and charting is more concise, but Canadian health care is similarly evidence based and equal in quality. In contrast to in the United States, all Canadian residents and citizens have full access to inpatient and outpatient health care but are likely to pay a monthly premium depending on personal income level. For example, in BC in 2016, the monthly premium for a single individual was $0 to $75.00 and that for a family of three or more was $0 to $150.00. Canadians are responsible for the cost of outpatient prescriptions, which are subsidized to varying degrees by provincial governments.

As they reflect on 10 years of Canadian practice, while still "locuming" during the summers in the Alaska bush, they have seen firsthand the strengths in each system and how the different health care policies play out. In the United States, they see poor care as a result of an individual's inability to pay and cite the example of an uninsured man from a rural fishing village with advanced heart failure. He cannot afford the ferry ride to the clinic and cuts his pills in half or often runs out of them altogether. When he succumbs to cardiac decompensation, he is flown to a regional hospital where he spends several days in the intensive care unit ($40,000) only to return to his village without medication, to repeat the cycle. These costs are ultimately absorbed by the government and health care system. Were he in the Canadian system, he would be followed more closely, possibly by a cardiac outreach team, provided with filled prescriptions, and offered a transportation subsidy. However, Canadian NPs have witnessed the moral hazard[b]

of unlimited access to health care, in the form of occasionally frivolous visits, such as seeking a bandage for a minor cut or scrape rather than going to the store, or long waits to see a dermatologist for acne that could have been treated in primary care. Both private pay cost barriers and system overuse issues are policy driven and have enormous impact on the larger economy and lives of individuals.

Although they recognize the grass is not greener in Canada for APN practice, these two NPs are grateful to live and work in Canada for its all-inclusive health care system, provided at a per capita cost that is considerably less than in the United States. There are times when they wish they could take the best parts of both systems and combine them to decrease the moral distress in the United States and the moral hazard in Canada. ◎

[b]Moral hazard—when a party insulated from risk behaves differently than he or she would behave if he or she were fully exposed to the risk (Jameton, 1984).

the United States spends at least 50% more per capita on health care. Compared with other developed nations, life expectancy in almost all age groups—up to age 75 years—is shorter than their counterparts in 16 other wealthy, developed nations. The scope of the US health disadvantage is pervasive and involves more than life expectancy: the United States ranks at or near the bottom in both prevalence and mortality for multiple diseases, risk factors, and injuries. The US health disadvantage spans many illness and injuries. When compared to peer countries, Americans fare worse in at least nine areas:

1. Infant mortality and low birth weight
2. Injuries and homicides
3. Adolescent pregnancies and sexually transmitted infections
4. HIV/AIDS
5. Drug-related deaths
6. Obesity
7. Heart disease
8. Lung disease
9. Disability

These findings suggest no support for the oft-repeated claim that US health care is the best in the world. The reason for the US disadvantage has been attributed to four factors: a fragmented health system, poor health behaviors, poor social and economic conditions, and automobile domination of the built environment, minimizing walking as an important physical activity. These challenging problems require a robust public health system (Woolf & Aron, 2013). The APRN is well qualified to lead change in this area.

Key Policy Concepts

Federalism

It is essential to understand the different responsibilities and authorities of the state and federal governments because these are highly relevant to most health care programs, such as Medicare, Medicaid, and the State Children's Health Insurance Program, as well as to the creation of an interoperable health information system. Federalism refers to the allocation of governing responsibility between the states and federal government. The states and the federal government have a complex relationship governing health policy, which explains a large part of our chaotic and fragmented approach to health care in place today. Passage of the ACA in 2010 required states to expand access, enhance quality, and lower costs, albeit with a great degree of flexibility. The ACA has greatly amplified the tensions between

federal mandates and states' rights, to the degree that the US Supreme Court had to clarify the constitutionality of the federal government's powers in requiring individuals to purchase health insurance. With the decision handed down in the Supreme Court case *National Federation of Independent Business v. Sebelius* (2012), the Court upheld most provisions of the ACA, declaring the individual mandate and the expansion of Medicaid constitutional; however, it was ruled that Congress may not link all Medicaid funds based on participation in the expansion. In May of 2017, the US House of Representatives voted in the American Health Care Act (AHCA), the first step toward dismantling the ACA federalist approach. This included, but was not limited to, eliminating taxes imposed by the ACA, removing individual and employer mandates, allowing states to waive the ACA's essential health benefit requirement, and allowing insurers to deny coverage to those with preexisting health conditions if they do not maintain continuous coverage (Jost, 2017a).

The US Constitution unambiguously gives the federal government absolute power to preempt state laws when it chooses to do so. However, the 50 states are also granted unfettered authority, such as regulation of health care professionals and health insurance plans (Bodenheimer & Grumbach, 2012). Ambiguity between state and federal authority allows states to experiment with policy solutions. The "states as learning laboratory" concept has grown out of local health policy problems and enables states to experiment with innovative policy solutions that could not be done on a national level. Moreover, states have local health care problems, requiring local, flexible, and humane solutions. Many federal health policy decisions are devolving decision making to the states. Because health care is experienced at the local level, APRNs must be aware of the overlapping state and federal spheres of government and the tension between their authorities.

Incrementalism

Although the policymaking process is a continuous interrelated cycle, most efforts to change policy stem from the negative effects of an existing policy. In the United States, we rarely reform, but we frequently modify. This concept of continuous, often modest modification of existing polices is termed *incrementalism*. Major reforms of health policy are seen rarely, usually once in a generation, such as Medicare and Medicaid in 1965 and the ACA in 2010. Minor changes of existing policies play out slowly over time and are therefore more predictable. Incrementalism promotes stability and stakeholder compromise. A good example of incrementalism is the gradual increase in federal spending for biomedical research from $300 in 1887 to more than $33 billion in 2017, going to the 27 institutes and centers within the National Institutes of Health. Within that structure, the National Center for Nursing Research was created in 1985 by a congressional override of a presidential veto as a result of the influence of strong nurse leaders. In 1993, the Center was elevated to the National Institute for Nursing Research and funded with $50 million; funding levels in 2017 will exceed $146 million.

Presidential Politics

US presidential politics is playing a larger role in health care in the United States. The presidential candidates frame health issues that greatly influence the public perception regarding the severity of the problem and responsibility for the problem. These candidates are trying to win support for their health care priorities and are often unaware of the evidence regarding what is driving cost or disease burden. Even though the United States faces serious health concerns, largely driven by poor health behaviors and a chronic disease epidemic, there is very little political will to address the root cause of these drivers. For example, many of the US agriculture policies subsidize corn, which is used in many processed foods (high-fructose corn syrup). Those processed foods are a large part of the poor American diet, leading to obesity and the long list of health issues that cascade from obesity (Stanhope et al., 2015). The very first presidential primary is held in Iowa, a large agriculture state that produces more corn (2.5 billion bushels) than any other state (IowaCorn.org, 2016). This essentially shuts down any conversation on aligning US farming policy with health policy. Of the 12 presidential candidates caucusing in Iowa in 2016, not a single candidate addressed America's eating and food problems and their link to chronic disease.

Moreover, the Republican-controlled House of Representatives had voted on defunding, crippling, or repealing the ACA 55 times between 2010 and 2015 (Haberkorn, 2015). In May 2017, with the Republicans controlling the Congress and the presidency, the House was finally able to pass the AHCA (an ACA "repeal and replace" bill) by a 217 to 213 vote (Jost, 2017a). However, further efforts to repeal and replace the ACA came to a halt in July 2017

with a 49 to 51 Senate vote (Jost, 2017b). At that time, the Republicans left the door open for another attempt to "repeal and replace" but, as demonstrated by this failed effort to bring about this major Republican legislative initiative, American congressional and presidential politics have become a continuous cycle, making it difficult for candidates to address complex problems that are too big or too unpopular. This exemplifies the difficult and complex nature of health policy, which requires considerable political capital to address.

APRNs, Civic Engagement, and Money

Without question, and regardless of one's political affiliation, there is widespread agreement that money has enormous influence on elections, the wealthy have more influence on elections, and candidates who win office promote policies that help their donors. Some of the more effective interest groups do not align with one political party but give equally to both parties so that they can gain access to important decision makers. It is estimated that members of Congress spend anywhere from 25% to 50% (and sometimes more) of their time fundraising, especially as an election approaches (Sherb, 2012). APRNs have come a long way in supporting candidates. In 2016, there were 5 nurses and 17 physicians elected to Congress. The easiest form of civic engagement is to vote for or donate to a candidate or political action committee (PAC); next is to work on a campaign, followed by running for office. Table 19.1 outlines health professions lobbying spending, donations to PACs, and how they distributed those funds across political parties.

Policy Models and Frameworks

Longest Model

Longest (2016) has conceptualized policymaking as an interdependent process. The Longest model defines a policy formulation phase, an implementation phase, and a modification phase (Fig. 19.1). Importantly, this model illustrates the incremental and cyclical nature of policymaking, two of the most important features of the US health care policymaking process with which APRNs must be familiar. Essentially, all health care policy decisions are subject to modification because policymaking in the United States involves making decisions that are revisited when circumstances shift. The US system is not

TABLE 19.1 Selected APRN and Other Health Professions Organizations Political Action Committee (PAC) and Lobbying Donations, 2016[a]

Health Professions Organization	PACs (Partial Cycle as of February 28, 2016)	Lobbying
American Association of Nurse Anesthetists	$1,241,000 [55% Republican]	$830,000
American College of Nurse-Midwives	$468,000 [21% Republican]	$90,000
American Association of Nurse Practitioners	$108,000 [50% Republican]	$401,000
National Association of Clinical Nurse Specialists	No PAC Reported	0
American Medical Association	$2,000,000 [64% Republican]	$15,290,000
American Nurses Association	$262,649 [15% Republican]	$855,000

[a]Total lobbying spending for health professionals, 2016: $65,000,00; total number of health professional clients reported, 2016: 208; total number of health professions lobbyists reported, 2016: 726.
Adapted from Center for Responsive Politics. (2016, December 2). Retrieved from http://www.opensecrets.org/.

designed for big bold reform. Rather, it considers intended or unintended consequences of existing policy and tweaks changes (Longest, 2016).

Policy Modification

The US system is based on continuous policy modification. Almost every policy results in some form of unintended consequence, which is only learned through implementation of a prior policy. Policies that are appropriate and relevant at one point in time become highly inappropriate as time passes and economic, social, demographic, and commercial circumstances shift. Policy consequences are the reason that stakeholders and policymakers seek to modify policy continually. These policy changes can be driven by stakeholders when a policy negatively affects a group or by members of Congress or rulemakers when policy does not meet their objective. Understanding the process of policy modification and amendment of earlier polices is a key to mastering political competency (Box 19.2).

The Kingdon or Garbage Can Model

Agenda setting is a major component of the Longest policy formulation phase. With so many health policy problems in the United States, why do some problems get attention and others languish at the bottom of the policy agenda for decades? Kingdon (1995) conceptualized an open policy window, with three conditions streaming through the open window at once. First, the problem must come to the attention of the policymaker; second, it must have a menu of possible policy solutions that have tae very real potential to solve the problem; and third, it must have the right political circumstances. If all three of these conditions occur simultaneously, the policy window opens and progress can be made on the issue (Fig. 19.2). Conversely, once shut, this policy window (opportunity) may never open again.

Policy Activators

Policy problems come to the attention of policymakers in a number of ways, including through constituents, litigation, research findings, market forces, fiscal environment, crisis, special interest groups, and the media, singly or collectively. Wakefield (2008) has identified policy dynamics particular to agenda setting (Table 19.2). Additional dynamics have been added, and each dynamic has one or more so-called accelerator, which drives the agenda setting or triggers policymakers to take action on an issue. The political circumstances that push problems onto the agenda must have a high degree of public importance and low degree of stakeholder conflict surrounding the policy solution. If there is a great deal of stakeholder disagreement, competing proposals may be put forth, weakening the likelihood that the problem will be addressed. Strong health services research can provide the evidence base to help policymakers specify and therefore accelerate agenda setting (Longest, 2016).

Knowledge Transfer Framework

APRN research must be robust enough and highly relevant to be useful for policymakers. Not all research can or should have an impact. The nature of the political process compels researchers to link their work to policy formation. APRNs could more forcefully link their research to policymaking by framing it in a policy context. Gold (2009) has created

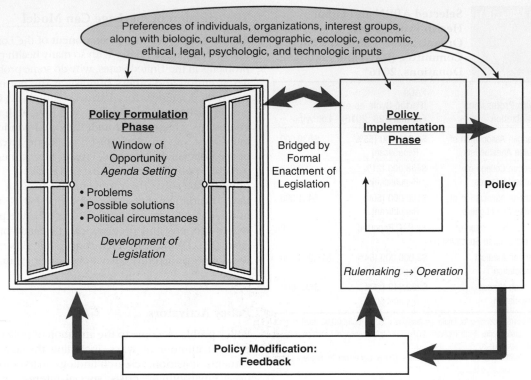

FIG 19.1 The Longest model. *(From Longest, B. B., Jr. [2010]. Health policymaking in the United States [5th ed.]. Chicago, IL: Health Administration Press.)*

BOX 19.2   Role of Public Comment

Public laws do not contain specific language about how the policy or program is to be carried out. For health-related issues, the executive branch agency, usually the Department of Health and Human Services, must publish its proposed rules in the daily *Federal Register*, seeking public comment. The public comment opportunity is usually limited to 60 days; however, stakeholder groups can exert an enormous degree of influence in the rulemaking process during this limited period. This public comment stems from two important American principles: (1) that democracy can only work if its citizenry is informed and participates, and (2) the federal government does not hold all the expertise but must solicit comment from experts involved in the issue to alert the agency to unforeseen options or consequences (Regulations. gov, 2016). Advanced practice registered nurse (APRN)

organizations can powerfully influence rulemaking by submitting evidence-based public comment and by activating the APRN grass roots to launch a public comment campaign. The *Federal Register* will tally the number of responses received and report how many were in favor of or opposed to the proposed rule. Thoughtful, well-crafted public comments submitted by an APRN organization have been directly incorporated into final rules, rendering submission of public comments and the rulemaking process crucially important activities for APRNs. For example, when the *Federal Register* published rules removing Medicare payment restrictions for APRNs, excerpts of a letter submitted by the American College of Nurse Practitioners were quoted and used as an evidence source to support the payment expansions.

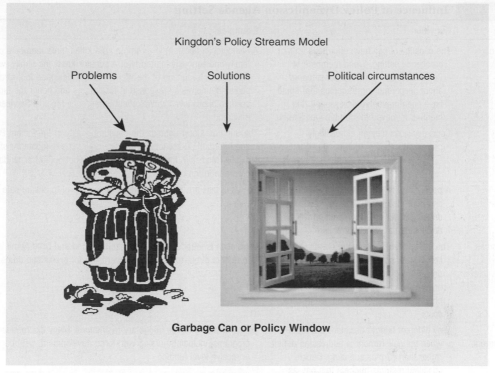

Kingdon's Policy Streams Model

Problems Solutions Political circumstances

Garbage Can or Policy Window

FIG 19.2 Kingdon's policy streams model. *(From Kingdon, J. [1995]. Agendas, alternatives, and public policies [2nd ed.]. New York, NY: Harper Collins College.)*

a framework for researchers to increase the likelihood that their findings will reach some "take-up" of new ideas to be useful and implementable in the policy sphere. It opens up a pathway through the unexplored "black box" between health research and its use by policymakers. Such pathways can help stakeholders bridge between the research and the end user by asking five questions. An example of high-quality, nurse practitioner–led research is the well-designed study by Chao, Grilo, White, and Sinha (2015) in which they found that chronic stress had a significant direct effect on food cravings and food cravings had a significant direct effect on body mass index. The highly relevant policy link is that interventions aimed at lowering obesity rates must address the underlying emotional and stress landscapes that cause food cravings and not merely focus on food habits. This may well explain why the obesity epidemic is exploding, because current interventions are primarily dietary. Addressing the questions in Fig. 19.3 makes it more likely the research will be transferred into policy.

Current Advanced Practice Nursing Policy Issues

Framing Current Issues: Cost, Quality, and Access

The cost-quality-access triad (Fig. 19.4) focuses on the drivers of health policy, across all levels of health care, whether it is at the international, national, state, local, community, institutional, or corporate level. Cost, quality, and access, as health policy drivers, are inherently interdependent; a shift in one inevitably affects the others. Cost, quality, and access issues are not tangential problems to the US health care challenges—they are the challenge.

Cost

The ACA enactment in 2010 stands alongside the passage of Medicaid and Medicare in 1965 as a grand and challenging change in US health care policy. This massive bill aimed to improve access, improve quality, and, most importantly, control the rate of

TABLE 19.2   Influence of Policy Dynamics on Agenda Setting

Dynamic	Activator	Examples
Constituents	The constituent can have enormous impact on agenda setting. When members of Congress learn from their constituents about deeply moving tragedies that could have been prevented or lessened, the member is moved to introduce legislation.	An automobile accident in a remote area killed three members of a family and seriously injured two. A senator knew the family, which prompted introduction of the Wakefield Act, designed to improve pediatric emergency response in rural areas and honor the family. It became public law, the Wakefield Emergency Medical Services for Children.
Litigation	Court decisions play an increasingly prominent role in setting health policy.	The Supreme Court upholds the constitutionality of the Patient Protection and Affordable Care Act (ACA) but removes the mandate for states to expand Medicaid, thus allowing states to "opt out" of expanding coverage to the poor.
Research findings	A pediatrician in Flint, Michigan, investigated and published her findings on the toxic drinking water and its impact on the developmental growth of children.	Scores of bills are introduced at the federal level to ensure safe drinking water.
Market forces	The pharmaceutical industry greatly expands commercial advertising/marketing of prescribed drugs to consumers. This direct advertising creates higher demands on pharmaceuticals, driving up health care costs.	Legislation is introduced to authorize the Food and Drug Administration to restrict direct-to-consumer advertising for prescribed drugs.
Fiscal environment	Very different budget decisions are made when the government is addressing deficit rather than surplus spending. Deficit spending restricts budgets to a pay-as-you-go policy.	Deficit financing forces budgetary restrictions. Many discretionary health programs, including nursing workforce development, get budget cuts or receive level funding.
Special interest groups	Well-organized special interest groups with a clear message can have an enormous impact on government action or inaction.	The autism advocacy community frames the increase in autism spectrum disorders as a public health emergency, motivating Congress to pass legislation spanning a wide range of provisions for those with autism, including research, treatment, and services (https://www.autismvotes.org/advocacy).
Crises	Crises can promote rapid response policy changes, usually centered on quality and access.	Startling opioid and heroin addiction rates across the United States led to scores of bills on tightening opioid prescribing, making naloxone available to first responders, and funding treatment centers.
Political ideology	The majority party (Democrats versus Republicans) has a large impact on agenda setting. The divide centers on what role the government should play in US society.	The newly installed 112th Republican-controlled US House of Representatives introduced the second bill of the session in January 2011, the Repealing the Job-Killing Health Care Law Act, a failed attempt to repeal the ACA.
Media	The lay press, reporting on policy issues or crises, often compel policymakers to take action.	Major news outlet report that millions of unencrypted personal health care records were stolen or mistakenly made public. Tensions rise between added reporting requirements and privacy. Legislation is introduced on strategies to enforce the Health Insurance Portability and Accountability Act (HIPAA) and mandate encryption.
U.S. president with a high degree of commitment	When the occupant of the White House sets health reform as a major domestic policy agenda by linking unsustainable health care costs to the health of the macroeconomy, the power of that office becomes evident.	In March 2010, President Obama signs the historic ACA, despite a 2-year debate, town hall meetings across the nation, and multiple national speeches explaining to the public why reform is necessary. It becomes the major initiative of his presidency.

Adapted from Wakefield, M. K. (2008). Government response: Legislation. In Milstead, J. (Ed.), *Health policy and politics: A nurse's guide* (3rd ed., pp. 65-88). Sudbury, MA: Jones & Bartlett.

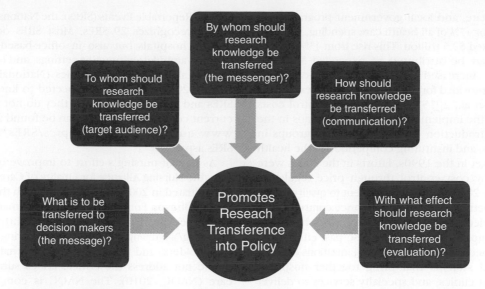

FIG 19.3 Pathway to move and accelerate effective research into policy.

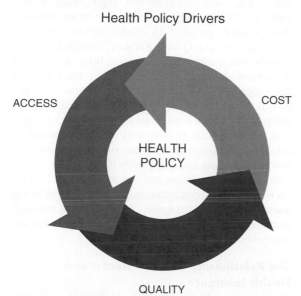

FIG 19.4 Cost-quality-access schema.

cost increase in health care. At the time the ACA was signed in 2010, the total amount spent on health care in the United States was $2.6 trillion, up from $2 trillion in 2005 (Centers for Medicare & Medicaid Services [CMS], 2011). By 2013, the amount had increased by another $300 billion to $2.9 trillion or $9255 per capita (Hartman, Martin, Lassman, & Catlin, 2015). For 2015, the national health expenditures

were estimated at $3.2 trillion, another $300 billion increase in 3 years (Keehan et al., 2015). To put this in perspective, if you take the $600 billion anticipated increase in health care cost from 2010 to 2015, you could provide a family income of about $52,000 for about 11.5 million families (McCormally, 2011).

Although the expanded coverage anticipated by the ACA has been put in jeopardy by the goals of the Trump administration, improved economic growth and the increasing need for health care services by the baby boomer population will likely cause health care spending to outpace the annual growth of the US gross domestic product (GDP) in the next decade and beyond. Even with focused efforts to bend the cost curve of health care, increases in health spending are expected to be 5.8% per year until 2024, with the GDP growing only 4.7% per year during the same period (Keehan et al., 2015). By 2024, the health share of the GDP may reach 19.6%. The proportion of the country's GDP expended on health care is of importance to the future of the United States because every dollar spent on health care is a dollar less spent on education, transportation, housing, food, and other essentials. In comparison with the current percent of GDP, the cost of health care in 1960 was about 6% of the GDP and in 1980 it was about 9% of GDP (Kaiser Family Foundation, 2011).

Policymakers have a large stake in continuing policies to control the cost of health care. By 2024, federal, state, and local government programs will account for 47% of all health care spending, reaching an estimated $2.5 trillion. This rise from 43% in 2013 can in part be attributed to expanded Medicaid eligibility, increased enrollment in Medicare, and subsidies provided for the health insurance exchanges (Keehan et al., 2015). Past efforts to control costs included the implementation of health plans in the 1970s, introduction of diagnosis-related groups in the 1980s, and instituting competition in the health care market in the 1990s. Efforts in the 2000s were marked by cost control through price regulation and in the 2010s by linking payment to quality (using clinical metrics) and continuing price controls. Even these varied attempts to control costs have had limited impact. Building on these past efforts, the ACA created accountable care organizations (ACOs), integrated systems that bring together hospitals, outpatient clinics, and specialty services to deliver better care coordination and quality of service. ACOs are a vehicle to implement the intent of the ACA by creating more integrated systems that can coordinate care better, thus improving quality and managing costs more effectively.

It remains to be seen how the ACA will be modified and which mechanisms will be deployed to control costs under the Trump administration, but as stated earlier, the movement toward value-based care preceded the ACA and has bipartisan support (Muhlestein et al., 2017). Many health care delivery organizations have made great strides in improving the value of care and will likely continue to improve care delivery and coordination based on ACA principles.

Quality

Attention to quality became a national issue following the IOM's series of reports, *To Err is Human* (Kohn, Corrigan, & Donaldson, 2000) and *Crossing the Quality Chasm* (IOM, 2001), focusing on the problems in the health care system leading to poor care. Linking quality to payment is how government and private companies try to ensure that quality of care is not compromised because of cost-saving measures. Linking quality to cost control is referred to as value-based purchasing. As part of value-based purchasing, the CMS (2006) identified 27 so-called never events and established a policy that hospitals would not get paid for taking care of patients experiencing an event that *should never happen,* such as wrong-site surgery and any stage 3 or 4 or pressure ulcers acquired after admission or presentation to a health care setting. "Never events" are now referred to as

Serious Reportable Events (SREs); the National Quality Forum recognizes 29 SREs. Most SREs occur not only in hospitals but also in office-based surgery centers, ambulatory practice settings, and long-term care or skilled nursing facilities (National Quality Forum, 2011). APRNs are expected to know these SREs and work to ensure that they do not occur. A current compilation of SREs can be found at http://www.qualityforum.org/Topics/SREs/List_of_SREs.aspx

As part of nursing's effort to improve quality of care, the Nursing Alliance for Quality of Care (NAQC) was initiated in 2009 and funded through the Robert Wood Johnson Foundation and is now managed by the American Nurses Association (http://www.naqc.org/). Nursing had no alliance to bring together stakeholders, and there was concern that nursing would not address the critical issues surrounding care (NAQC, 2010). The NAQC is composed of nursing organizations and consumer groups. Policy-makers recognize the contributions of nurses in advancing consumer-centered, high-quality health care. The NAQC was modeled after other alliances that primarily focused on improving the quality of care. The Hospital Quality Alliance, founded in 2002, was the first quality alliance formed, bringing together numerous stakeholders supported by the CMS and the American Hospital Association, primarily to get hospitals on board to report quality measures. In the past decade, several more alliances have emerged that focus on the review and/or development of quality measures. APRNs can obtain information about advancing nursing quality through the American Nurses Association and the work of the NAQC, their professional organizations, and, in general, being aware of the work in quality improvement through organizations such as the Institute for Healthcare Improvement.

The Relationship Between Access and Health Insurance

Access to health care has been linked to health insurance, and the ACA has made important strides to make insurance accessible to individuals and families. Although average annual premium increases for family coverage are well below the rate of increases from 1999 to 2005, the 2016 increases in premiums and deductibles have risen much faster than inflation and worker's earnings (Fig. 19.5). However, for those purchasing insurance on the ACA's Health Insurance Marketplaces, the benchmark plans' premiums stayed relatively flat in 2014-2015 (Kaiser Family Foundation, 2016b).

RECENT TRENDS IN EMPLOYER-SPONSORED HEALTH INSURANCE PREMIUMS

Average Annual Premium Increases for Family Coverage, 1999–2015

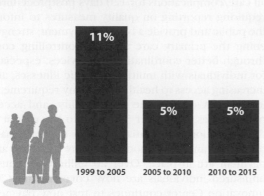

11%	5%	5%
1999 to 2005	2005 to 2010	2010 to 2015

Average Premiums Increased by 4% Between 2014 and 2015

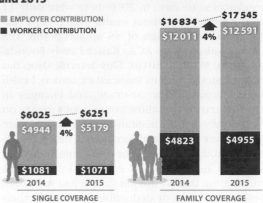

- ■ EMPLOYER CONTRIBUTION
- ■ WORKER CONTRIBUTION

SINGLE COVERAGE: 2014 $6025 ($4944 / $1081), 2015 $6251 ($5179 / $1071), 4%

FAMILY COVERAGE: 2014 $16 834 ($12 011 / $4823), 2015 $17 545 ($12 591 / $4955), 4%

Increases in Premiums Between 1999 and 2015 Have Outpaced Inflation and Workers' Earnings

CUMULATIVE INCREASE

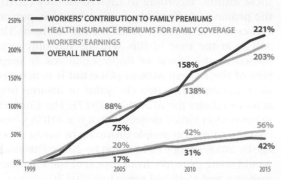

- — WORKERS' CONTRIBUTION TO FAMILY PREMIUMS
- — HEALTH INSURANCE PREMIUMS FOR FAMILY COVERAGE
- — WORKERS' EARNINGS
- — OVERALL INFLATION

221% / 203% / 56% / 42% (2015)
158% / 138% / 42% / 31% (2010)
88% / 75% / 20% / 17% (2005)

Over the Past 5 Years, Deductibles Have Risen Much Faster Than Premiums and Wages

CUMULATIVE INCREASE

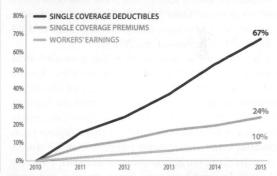

- — SINGLE COVERAGE DEDUCTIBLES
- — SINGLE COVERAGE PREMIUMS
- — WORKERS' EARNINGS

67% / 24% / 10% (2015)

Distribution of Annual Premiums for Workers With Family Coverage, 2015

PERCENTAGE OF COVERED WORKERS

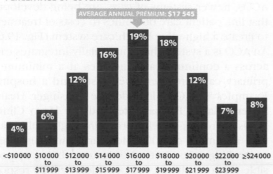

AVERAGE ANNUAL PREMIUM: $17 545

<$10 000	$10 000 to $11 999	$12 000 to $13 999	$14 000 to $15 999	$16 000 to $17 999	$18 000 to $19 999	$20 000 to $21 999	$22 000 to $23 999	≥$24 000
4%	6%	12%	16%	19%	18%	12%	7%	8%

Many Employers Took Action in 2015 to Address Anticipated Excise Tax on High-Cost Plans

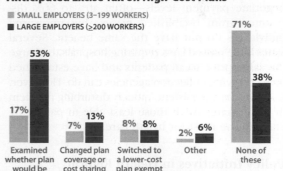

- ■ SMALL EMPLOYERS (3–199 WORKERS)
- ■ LARGE EMPLOYERS (≥200 WORKERS)

	Small	Large
Examined whether plan would be subject to tax	17%	53%
Changed plan coverage or cost sharing to avoid tax	7%	13%
Switched to a lower-cost plan exempt from tax	8%	8%
Other	2%	6%
None of these	71%	38%

Authors: Michelle Long, MPH; Matthew Rae, MPH, MPA; Gary Claxton; Anne Jankiewicz; and David Rousseau, MPH; for the Kaiser Family Foundation

Source: Kaiser Family Foundation analysis. Original data and detailed source information are available at http://kff.org/JAMA_01-05-2016. Please cite as JAMA. 2016;315(1):18. doi:10.1001/jama.2015.17349.

THE HENRY J. KAISER FAMILY FOUNDATION

The JAMA Network

FIG 19.5 Trends in employer-sponsored health insurance. *(From Long, M., Rae, M., Claxton, G., Jankiewicz, A., & Rousseau, D.; Kaiser Family Foundation. [2016]. Eligibility and coverage trends in employer-sponsored insurance. JAMA, 315, 1824.)*

As a direct result of the ACA provisions that expand access to care, in 2016 there were only 11 million Americans without health insurance, a dramatic drop from a high of 45 million before the implementation of the ACA (Kaiser Family Foundation, 2016b; Marken, 2016). This dramatic drop has been attributed largely to Medicaid expansion, health insurance marketplace coverage, and changes in private insurance that allow young adults to stay on their parent's health insurance plans and require plans to cover people with preexisting health conditions. Although the number of uninsured has dropped, a new issue has emerged from a 2014 survey finding that 31 million people had such high out-of-pocket costs or deductibles relative to their incomes that they were underinsured (Collins, Rasmussen, Beutel, & Doty, 2015). Over 10% of adults enrolled in a private health insurance plan had a deductible of $3000 and 41% of those had debt loads of $4000 or more. Over 50% of underinsured individuals reported problems paying medical bills or had medical debt (Collins et al., 2015).

A hazard for the uninsured is that they are often charged the full price for health services (Kaiser Family Foundation, 2016a). In a study of Medicare cost reports, the top 50 US hospitals with the highest ratios of charges over Medicare-allowable costs (markups) had markups about 10 times higher than allowable costs. Uninsured patients may be asked to pay the full charges, and out-of-network patients and casualty and workers' compensation insurers are often expected to pay a large portion of the full charges (Bai & Anderson, 2015). Insurance companies negotiate payment levels—often 40% to 60% discounted from established prices—but uninsured individuals do not have the same benefit. Several states have passed laws requiring hospitals to charge the same price to all patients and have established limits on what collection agencies can do. However, this remains a persistent, morally disturbing problem in many states, with those least able to pay being charged the most for health care.

Policy Initiatives in Health Reform

The ACA and the Health Care and Education Reconciliation Act of 2010, which amended some provisions in the ACA, represent the most far-reaching legislation enacted since the passage of Medicare and Medicaid in 1965. Major elements of the ACA included the creation of a high-value health care system through payment reform mechanisms such as bundled payment (e.g., Medicare pays $30,000

for coronary artery bypass graft surgery, including all care/complications for 120 days postprocedure); requiring reporting on quality measures to inform the public and provide a basis for payment; strengthening the primary care system; controlling costs through better coordination of services, especially for individuals with multiple chronic illnesses; and increasing access to health care. Many requirements in the ACA overlap the cost, quality, and access policy issues. Now over 5 years into the rollout of the legislation, substantial gains in coverage have been met and new models of care delivery and payment are in place. Over 20 million previously uninsured individuals are now covered, the CMS Innovation Center continues to test new payment models focused on improving value, and more people are cared for in systems that emphasize value over volume (Bauchner & Fontanarosa, 2016). Even with these efforts, according to Lavizzo-Mourey (2016), the promise of affordable, comprehensive, person-centered care is still a point on the horizon. The AHCA, at the time of this writing, has only been passed by the House of Representatives; it keeps 90% of the original ACA in place but it is believed to substantially threaten the gains in insured lives achieved under the ACA (Jost, 2017). The Congressional Budget Office projected that the AHCA would result in 14 million people dropping or losing coverage by 2018, rising to 24 million by 2026. The losses would come primarily from repeal of the individual mandate and Medicaid cuts (Jost, 2017).

Cost and Quality

ACOs, newer systems of care, are being developed that link patient care outcomes to costs of treatment to create a high-value health care system (Fig. 19.6). An ACO is a system that horizontally integrates care across a continuum and includes at a minimum a primary care provider, specialists, and a hospital. Examples of ACOs include the Geisinger Health System, Kaiser Permanente, and the Mayo Clinic. ACOs are responsible for providing high-quality care to a minimum of 5000 Medicare enrollees while controlling costs. Instead of insurers being responsible for controlling cost, providers will be responsible. Based on reduced costs of care, savings are then shared with the providers. Although there have been previous attempts to create coordinated care systems, a new requirement—that ACOs must report quality measures—is transformational.

According to the American Association of Nurse Practitioners (AANP, 2012), ACOs create incentives

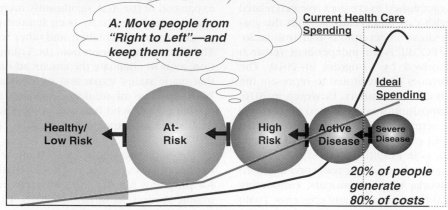

FIG 19.6 Value-based health care delivery system. *(Adapted from Nursing Alliance for Quality Care. [2010]. Strategic policy and advocacy roadmap. Retrieved from http://www.naqc.org/Docs/NewsletterDocs/2010-SPAR. pdf.)*

for health care providers to work together to treat an individual patient across care settings. ACOs agree to lower the cost of health care while meeting identified performance standards by sharing resources and coordinating care. NPs are authorized to be ACO professionals. However, a last-minute change in the Shared Savings section of the ACA for Medicare patients limits the assignment of patients for this program to those who are being cared for by primary care physicians. Therefore, patients who choose an NP for their primary care provider cannot be counted as beneficiaries and any shared savings are not assigned. Thus although this does not prevent NPs from joining an ACO, it does prevent their patients from being assigned to a Medicare ACO and then gaining any subsequent benefits that result from participation. Essentially, APRNs are locked out of the governance structures, leadership, and cost savings (profit) from these structures that are set up to greatly benefit from APRN service. Each ACO is governed differently, and it will be important for APRNs to be involved in leading, governing, and sharing the ACO savings and not become employees of these emerging structures. At this time, the AANP and other nursing advocacy groups continue to push

for a statutory fix to reinstate assignment of patients of all ACO professionals, including NPs, by adding provider-neutral language.

Medicare bundled payments, in which payment for care is based on a lump sum payment for an episode of care rather than on an individual visit, procedure, or service, began in April 2016 for hip and knee replacements, to include all surgery costs through full recovery for hospitals in 67 geographic areas. In 2014, more than 400,000 Medicare recipients had hip or knee replacements costing more than $7 billion for just the hospitalization (Delbanco & de Brantes, 2015). Through this new payment model, hospitals will benefit financially from high-quality, lower cost service but may have to repay Medicare if quality and cost targets are not achieved. In addition to efforts to provide better coordination through bundled payments, the ACA also specifies a program to reduce readmission. Hospitals are required to report on all readmissions over a specific time period, and the readmission rates are made public and posted on the Hospital Compare website (https://www.medicare.gov/hospitalcompare/search.html?). Both the bundled payment model and the requirement to reduce admissions are areas in which APRN practice can contribute significant savings and improved outcomes (Newhouse et al., 2011).

The Patient-Centered Outcomes Research Institute (PCORI) was established to conduct research related to testing health care interventions, with the goal of identifying those interventions that truly make a difference. PCORI is an independent research institute authorized by Congress in 2010. The Board of Governors is constituted to represent the broader health care community. However, in 2016, the board composition was dominated by 12 physicians and the remaining 9 members represented a variety of health care constituencies, including one APRN. The focus in PCORI is to fund comparative effectiveness research to answer real-world questions about what works best for patients, considering their individual circumstances and concerns. To do this, PCORI requires the engagement of patients and other stakeholders throughout the research process, and they require a partnership with the target community. PCORI funds studies on diverse topics such as comparing self-management and peer support communication programs among patients with chronic obstructive pulmonary disease and their family caregivers, testing telehealth for those with Down syndrome, and translating and incorporating older adult opinions into meaningful research. By 2019, PCORI will have spent $6 billion on comparative effectiveness research (Reichard, 2013).

Access

Access to health care is emphasized in the ACA through many policy mechanisms. A controversial section of the ACA is the requirement for individuals to purchase health insurance, known as the *individual mandate.* Anyone not covered by an employer or government program must purchase health insurance or pay a penalty. Twenty-six states challenged this requirement in court and on June 28, 2012, the Supreme Court issued a historic decision that upheld the individual mandate by considering it a tax that was within the power of the federal government to levy. The ruling was masterful in bridging different philosophic views among the justices and many different political agendas. To make the required insurance affordable to those who are not covered through employment or a government program, health insurance exchanges have been established by states. These provide marketplace information about costs and benefits so that individuals can transparently choose the best

plan. In addition, the ACA required an expansion of the Medicaid program to all individuals younger than 65 years with incomes up to 133% of the poverty level ($32,319 for a family of four). The Medicaid expansion of the ACA significantly increased coverage that had previously been limited primarily to pregnant women, children, and other select groups. The AHCA, with support from the Trump administration, aims to eliminate the enhanced funding levels that made states' expansion of Medicaid possible. With this loss of funding, coverage for over 11 million people who have gained eligibility through ACA Medicaid expansion is at stake (Rosenbaum, 2017).

The Supreme Court decision allowed states to opt out of the expansion and not lose federal funding for programs already in existence, thus finding a middle ground. As of January 2016, 19 states were not expanding their programs. According to Garfield and Damico (2016), Medicaid eligibility for adults in states not expanding is severely limited. In 2016, the median income limit for parents is about 44% of poverty, or an annual income of $8840 a year for a family of three, and in nearly all states not expanding, childless adults are ineligible. These individuals and families are caught in a coverage gap because they have incomes above Medicaid eligibility limits but below the lower limit for marketplace premium tax credits. The ACA expected that low-income people would receive coverage through Medicaid, so there is no financial assistance to people in poverty for other coverage options. A promising and expanding opportunity for APRNs to increase access to care is working for or developing nurse-managed clinics (NMCs). The ACA provides funds to help support expansion of NMCs. There are currently over 250 NMCs, with most clinics being part of an academic nursing program. Most NMCs are recognized as patient-centered medical homes approved through the National Committee for Quality Assurance (Kennedy, Caselli, & Berry, 2011). To be recognized, a clinic must comply with all the quality reporting requirements and have electronic health records (see Chapter 24).

Emerging Advanced Practice Nursing Policy Issues

APRN Payment Issues

There are continued challenges for APRNs related to payment rates. Medicare continues with their long-standing policy of paying APRNs 85% of the Physician Fee Schedule (PFS). However, when services are billed as "incident-to" physician care, billing can be at the 100% rate (see Chapter 21). As of 2011, certified nurse-midwives (CNMs) are the only APRN group to receive 100% of the PFS. This increase from 65% was initiated in 2011; however, CNMs are not yet eligible to participate in some Medicare services such as conducting/billing a Medicare initial or annual wellness visit. Certified registered nurse anesthetists (CRNAs) have a specific fee schedule established by Medicare that defines payment that is modified by the level of independence of practice, ranging from supervision by a physician to no supervision by a physician.

Over the years, there has been considerable discussion about the 85% rate, with many APRNs advocating for same pay for the same service (comparable worth). Others have argued that having reduced payment makes APRNs a cost-effective solution to high health care costs. A study of Medicare Part A (inpatient) and Part B (office visit) compared claims for 2009-2010 submitted by NPs with national provider identifier (NPI) numbers and primary care physicians. After adjusting for demographic characteristics, claims for beneficiaries assigned to an NP were $207, or 29%, less than for the primary care physicians. This held for inpatient and total office visit paid amounts as well, with 11% and 18% less for NP patients, respectively. This suggests that increasing access to NP primary care had not increased costs for the Medicare program and may be cost saving (Perloff, DesRoches, & Buerhaus, 2016). The findings from an older study of CRNA cost-effectiveness found that when simulated under high-use, ideal conditions with 12 stations and 4 cases per station, an anesthesiologist would generate yearly revenue minus costs of $1,285,945, whereas the independent CRNA generated $3,277,945. When lower demand was simulated with 12 stations and 2 cases per station, only the independent CRNA had a positive net revenue of $702,690, whereas the anesthesiologist model lost $1,289,310 (Hogan, Seifert, Moore, & Simonson, 2010). Clearly, independent CRNAs provide the best economic benefit.

Overall, Medicare is a huge program and only growing bigger because of the large US aging demographic shift. From a policy perspective, the cost increases from ACA-mandated changes to the Medicare program, coupled with pressures to control the health care cost curve, have created a difficult policy situation. Legislators view the Medicare program as untouchable, believing that limiting

benefits significantly would likely end political careers. For many years, Medicare had in place a sustainable growth rate formula that required "mandatory" fee cuts that were always averted by last minute congressional action. No savings were attained but no other solution was offered to replace the imaginary cuts until 2015, when the formula was finally repealed and replaced by the Medicare Access and CHIP Reauthorization Act of 2015 (MACRA).

MACRA established a new schedule of Medicare fee updates for APRNs, physicians, and other eligible health care providers. Payment rates are increased by 0.5% a year now, but there will be no rate changes between 2020 and 2025. In 2019, APRNs, physicians, and other eligible providers will need to choose to be paid under the new Merit-based Incentive Payment System or to join the Alternative Payment Model (APM) program. APRNs and other providers who receive a substantial portion of their payments from an ACO, medical home, or another APM will receive 5% annual increases in Medicare payments through 2024. Payments to medical professionals who instead participate in the Merit-based Incentive Payment System will be adjusted upward or downward according to measures of their performance quality using a variety of indicators. Clinicians rated as exceptional on these indicators are eligible for additional payments through 2024. Then from 2026 on, Medicare will have two separate fee-update systems: APRNs and others participating in the APM program will receive annual increases of 0.75%, while nonparticipants will receive increases of 0.25% (Oberlander & Laugesen, 2015).

Payment to APRNs by private insurers continues to be challenging in many states. Because insurers are regulated at the state level, approval of APRNs as part of a network has to be done state by state. There are many examples of private insurers cutting payment rates to APRNs. In 2009, a large insurer in Oregon cut payment rates to APRNs for mental health care and other insurers followed. Soon after this, notices were sent to APRNs that primary care rates would also be cut. To address this arbitrary policy, Oregon became the first state to require insurance companies follow "equal pay for equal work" rules on insurance reimbursements for NP, physician assistant, and physician services in primary care and mental health care (Oregon Nurses Association, n.d.).

The economic benefits of APRNs are clear. The Perryman Group issued a report in 2012 that found substantial economic benefits for Texas when APRNs provide health care. Assuming a modest net savings of about 6.2% when health care is provided by

APRNs, the money not spent on health care would create 97,205 permanent jobs and each year generate $8.0 billion in gross product. Tax receipts to the state from those newly created jobs would increase by almost $700 million (The Perryman Group, 2012).

More recent work by Perloff et al. (2016) found that Medicare evaluation and management payments for those patients receiving NP services were 29% less than for services provided by primary care physicians. According to these authors, this is the first national-level data set to examine the cost of primary care services provided by NPs and primary care physicians over a 12-month time frame (2009-2010). However, challenges remain in using the Medicare data for analyzing APRN practice. To capture the practice of APRNs accurately, all APRNs need to be billing under their own NPI number. Use of "incident-to" billing, although it generates 100% of the PFS, hides the work of APRNs and attributes the service to another's NPI number. In some situations, supervision requirements set by organizations, employment arrangements, or scope of practice requirements may limit APRNs' ability to bill under their own NPI number. The importance of APRNs using their NPI for all services cannot be overstated.

APRN Full Practice Authority

The National Council of State Boards of Nursing (NCSBN, 2014) has proposed a model nurse practice act that would achieve full practice authority for all APRN roles. This model practice act explicitly describes APRNs as licensed independent practitioners within standards established or recognized by the NCSBN. The challenge is that achieving this or similar legislation requires that many state licensing laws be re-legislated. State licensing laws define the permissible scope of practice for the health care professions. The purpose of state health professions laws are to protect the public and to assure consumers that health care workers conduct their practices in areas for which they are properly trained. However, according to LeBuhn and Swankin (2010), scope of practice laws too often are unnecessarily restrictive and serve to protect the economic interests of another group. These authors reiterated the 1995 Pew Health Professions Commission's Task Force on Health Care Workforce Regulation report, which recognized the blurred boundaries between professional scopes of practice as technology has advanced and workforce innovations have been embraced and called for increased regulatory flexibility. The Pew Commission noted that varying objectives and levels of specificity are found in different professions' scopes of practice without rationale and that the system "treats practice acts as rewards for the professions" rather than as rational mechanisms for safe and effective care by competent practitioners. Importantly, the Pew report stressed that practice acts should be based on demonstrated initial and continuing competence and that it should be expected that different professions share overlapping scopes of practice.

With the publication of *The Future of Nursing: Leading Change, Advancing Health* (IOM, 2011), the support for full practice authority has accelerated with support from the National Governors Association, the National Conference of State Legislatures, the American Association of Retired Persons, and the Federal Trade Commission, among others. In contrast to this support, the American Medical Association and other state and national medical organizations continue to be formidable opponents. In *The Future of Nursing* report (2011), Safriet addressed the historical and political context for much of organized medicine's opposition. Physicians were the first to gain legislative recognition of their practice and essentially claimed the entire health-illness continuum as their exclusive purview, and it was interpreted as solely under their control. It is within this context that other health professions have had to carve out their practice acts, as illustrated by the efforts by APRNs to expand their scope of practice in Florida (see Exemplar 19.2).

To change this paradigm, in 2006 Safriet worked with six professional licensing boards, including the Federation of State Medical Boards and the NCSBN, to achieve consensus on a position paper addressing scope of practice legislation. Notably, the six organizations agreed that the criteria related to who is qualified to perform functions safely without risk of harm to the public are the only justifiable conditions for defining scopes of practice (NCSBN, 2009). In spite of these efforts, full practice authority remains a goal for many states. The NCSBN compiles a state-by-state report tracking status of practice and prescribing across all APRN roles (NCSBN, 2016a). Provider-neutral language in all rules and regulations would go far in removing artificial barriers to practice that lack an evidence base.

In 2013, the Veterans Health Administration (VHA) drafted a new nursing handbook that would grant its 3600 APRNs with full practice authority, even in states that require physician oversight. The proposal was designed to "reduce variability in practice across the entire VA health care system," among other

EXEMPLAR 19.2   An APRN Cliffhanger in Florida: Political Competence in Action

Janet DuBois

Advanced practice registered nurses (APRNs) in Florida have been waging a political battle for over 20 years to gain the authority to prescribe controlled substances, and Florida is the only state in the United States to prohibit APRNs from prescribing them. This not only contributes to decreased access to care but also adds to the financial burden of both the patient and the health care system. According to the US Census Bureau (2010), 86% of the state falls within the definition of a rural area, affecting over 1.6 million residents, many of whom have limited access to primary care services. This is due to the common barriers that rural-dwelling Americans experience, including lack of access/primary care provider services, transportation, lack of insurance, and language and culture barriers (US Census Bureau, 2010). Limiting APRNs' ability to prescribe controlled substances adds to these barriers and makes it difficult to provide comprehensive care for all citizens. Many APRNs report having to schedule another visit for their patients to coincide with a physician presence or having to refer their patients to a primary care physician just to prescribe a much needed medication that is a controlled substance. This includes those used to treat common conditions such as coughs, diarrhea, anxiety, sleep disorders, weight loss, and psychiatric illnesses.

Coalition Building

Many of the APRN organizations in Florida have come together to form the Florida Coalition of Advanced Practice Nurses, to address advanced practice nursing scope of practice issues within the state. Members include the Florida Nurse Practitioner Network, the Florida Association of Nurse Anesthetists, the Certified Nurse Midwives, the Florida Association of Nurse Practitioners, and the Florida Nurses Association, to name a few. The Coalition meets quarterly as a group and many members participate in weekly meetings during the active legislative session, called the "huddle," to discuss ongoing legislation and issues and to strategize to achieve the mutually agreed upon goals, the primary one being full scope of practice. A critical early step was to get all APRN groups to have a unified voice so they could strengthen and better serve more than 14,000 advanced practice nurses in Florida.

During the 2016 Florida legislative session, coalition members agreed to promote the Florida House bill to eliminate practice barriers around prescribing controlled substances. Throughout the session, each organization's key leaders worked closely with their lobbyist and both the Florida Senate and House bill sponsors to promote this legislative goal, craft appropriate language, and offer their clinical knowledge and expertise to ensure the best outcomes. Much of the dialogue surrounded negotiating with the opposition and what compromises we were willing to make in order to pass favorable legislation. In the past, the Florida Medical Association had agreed to support similar legislation if we were willing to have joint board oversight (Board of Nursing and Board of Medicine), or the anesthesiologist group pressured our bill sponsor into adding limitations on what certified registered nurse anesthetists could do, taking away privileges they already had. We were not willing to compromise on either of these points, which resulted in the bill not passing in previous years. On the other hand, we did compromise by agreeing to limitations on the amount of Schedule II opioids and psychotropics we would be authorized to prescribe.

Effective use of APRN Power
Persistence and Activating the Grass Roots
The initial version of the House bill (HB 423) was filed in October of 2015 (presession) and passed through multiple committees prior to coming before the full House for a final vote. The bill went through the various required House committees with little opposition and was presented for a full House vote on March 2, 2016, passing with 117 Yeas and 2 Nays. We considered this a victory but knew we still had to get the Senate companion bill (SB 1250) passed before our long-awaited controlled substances prescribing authority could become a reality. We anticipated that this would be an uphill battle with the Senate because there was more fierce opposition there to the bill. The Senate delayed scheduling, and the Senate president was opposed to scheduling the bill for a final Senate vote should it pass through all committees. Two weeks before the end of the session (February 26th), the Senate Appropriations Committee received the bill but delayed voting on it. Naturally we were getting extremely nervous and decided it was time to put some pressure on the committee members. We sent out email blasts through the Coalition instructing them to call or email all 19 members of the Appropriations Committee to support our bill and schedule it for a vote. Finally, on March 1st, the Appropriations Committee passed the bill with a very positive 17/0 vote. While the session was winding down, SB 1250 was still in committee and the Senate President was stalling and refused to allow the bill to be put on the calendar for a final

Continued

reading and vote. That's when the bill really stalled. Three days before the end of the 2016 legislative session, we began to really panic; we were so close to this landmark legislation and yet it looked like we may not get the bill passed! We started calling in favors we had among legislators and sending urgent emails to all the APRNs in Florida, our colleagues in practice (including our physician supporters), academia, and friends and family to call and email the Senate President to implore him to place the bill for a final Senate vote. The Senate President received hundreds of emails and calls from APRNs, physicians, patients, and friends and family urging him to place the bill on the calendar. Still, he didn't budge.

Engaging a Champion

In a last ditch effort, a few of the larger organization's lobbyists called on another, more seasoned lobbyist who in the past had always supported or represented APRNs. He made a call to a powerful former governor of Florida, who intervened on our behalf, instructing the Senate to place the bill for a vote. At last, 2 days before the end of the session, the bill was voted on in the Senate and passed unanimously. However, it still needed to be reconciled with the House version before becoming law. In the last 2 days of the session, the

bill went back and forth between the House and the Senate four times before the final vote in the House at approximately 5:33 p.m. on the very last day of the session. Needless to say, the victory was sweet but the process was long and tedious. The bill was signed into law by the Governor of Florida on April 14, 2016.

While the final bill authorized APRNs with national certification and a master's degree in their specialty field to prescribe controlled substances, there are some caveats. The bill only allows for a 7-day supply of any Schedule II drugs and only allows psychiatric nurse practitioners to prescribe Schedule II psychotropic drugs for children under 18 years of age, aimed at limiting the prescribing of attention-deficit/hyperactivity disorder medications to children. In addition, the law stipulated that a formulary committee, consisting of three APRNs, three physicians, and one pharmacist, was to meet and establish any further limitations on the prescribing of controlled substances. The law became effective January 1, 2017, and all APRNs who meet the standards are able to register with the DEA and are prescribing controlled substances II-V. We still consider this a landmark victory, and we will continue to work with policymakers, stakeholders, and legislators to reach our goal of full practice authority in Florida. ◎

---

issues, according to the VHA. Organized medicine responded with 104,256 comments against the proposed rule, including 43 state medical organizations and others strongly denouncing the proposed change and urging that "VHA policies support physician-led health care teams and state-based licensure and regulation remain unchanged" (Basu, 2014). However, the VHA received a total of 223,296 comments on the proposed rule, mostly in favor of expanding APRN practice. It is clear to see that an engaged citizenry had an impact on this ruling. It is a disappointment that the final ruling did not include CRNAs, and the exclusion of this APRN category is counter to the evidence on CRNA safety and effectiveness. The APRN Full Practice Authority was granted in 2016 for NPs, CNMs, and CNSs, and more work will need to be done to get CRNAs included in a future ruling.

APRN Workforce Development

Data about the US nursing workforce has been critical to formulating rational policies related to APRNs.

Lack of data has been a major issue in defining the benefits of APRNs. The primary source of valid and reliable data has been the Health Resources and Services Administration, which in 2012 began a national survey of NPs, the *National Sample Survey of Nurse Practitioners.* However, this survey does not sample other APRNs beyond NPs. Another data source about the NP practice environment is the *National Nurse Practitioner Practice Site Census,* which has been conducted by the AANP every 2 to 3 years to characterize and review trends in the NP workforce (AANP, 2015). CRNA and CNM data are of higher quality because each of these advanced nursing practice specialties has a single organization and national certifying body tracking its workforce over time, essentially a census. They are able to analyze their data to answer policy-relevant questions quickly, with a few keystrokes. CNS data have been more difficult to accurately obtain and track. In states where CNSs do not have title protection, they may self-identify as CNSs but do not meet the criteria of an APRN as defined by the Consensus statement or the American Association of Colleges of Nursing.

The National Association of Clinical Nurse Specialists did its first CNS census survey in 2014, and CNS surveys are done jointly every 2 years by the NCSBN and the National Forum of State Nursing Workforce Centers (NCSBN, 2016b).

The Bureau of Labor Statistics also reports occupational employment statistics for NPs, CRNAs, and CNMs; however, CNSs are not separated from the registered nurse category (Bureau of Labor Statistics, Department of Labor, 2012). Some data may be available through nursing organizations, current NCSBN national data, and some state nursing workforce centers. The quality of data from these sources is variable.

A policy issue to which APRNs need to continually attend is ensuring that APRN data are identifiable for quality evaluation and outcome assessment. When APRN services are billed "incident-to" the physician services, the value of the APRN work is attributed to the physician. A model for data collection for APRNs is NMCs, which have effective data collecting

and reporting systems and are recognized by the National Committee for Quality Assurance as patient-centered medical homes. Having strong, current, reliable APRN workforce data is essential for overcoming invisibility and building political power.

APRN Political Competence in the Policy Arena

The move to doctoral education for APRNs elevates the need for APRN involvement in policy development because effective leadership demands it. Policy competence is clearly emphasized in the Doctor of Nursing Practice (DNP) competencies as Essential V: Health care policy for advocacy in health care and is embedded in all of the other DNP Essentials (American Association of Colleges of Nursing, 2006). Policy competency requires APRNs to incorporate policy strategies continuously among the practice, research, and policy nexus in all practice settings (Table 19.3). As DNP programs explode in both

TABLE 19.3	Doctor of Nursing Practice (DNP) Competencies[a] for Health Policy and Politics	
DNP Essential[b]	**Policy Skill**
I. Scientific underpinnings for practice	• Analyze policy and the practice of politics, political systems, and political behavior with nursing science to effect policy-level change.
II. Organizational and systems leadership for quality improvement and systems thinking	• Create and sustain coalitions (policy communities) on health care quality and access via policy development at institutional, community, corporate, regional, national, or international levels.
III. Clinical scholarship and analytic methods for evidence-based practice	• Participate in design, translation, or dissemination of APRN practice inquiry within the context of health services research. • Use evidence/best practices to inform policymakers about APRN practice and quality.
IV. Information systems/technology and patient care technology for the improvement and transformation of health care	• Influence sensible metric development. • Ensure that nursing's values are captured. • Overcome APRN invisibility by ensuring the inclusion of nursing and APRNs in all administrative and clinical databases. • Provide policy leadership to link meaningful data on nursing activity electronically to cost, quality, and health outcomes.
V. Health care policy for advocacy in health care	• Engage in political activism and policy development, mentor activism, and participate on boards that affect health policies.
VI. Interprofessional collaboration for improving patient and population health outcomes	• Promote interprofessional practice. • Build interprofessional coalitions as a powerful advocacy tool to promote positive change in the health care delivery system. • Communicate across disciplines to build common ground.
VII. Clinical prevention and population health for improving the nation's health	• Promote the financing and delivery of evidence-based clinical preventive and population health services in all health policy arenas.
VIII. Advanced nursing practice	• Function as a content expert and a policy change leader and serve as steward for advanced practice nursing.

[a]Relevant to all advanced practice registered nurses (APRNs).
[b]Adapted from American Association of Colleges of Nursing. (2006). The essentials of doctoral education for advanced nursing practice. Retrieved from http://www.aacn.nche.edu/publications/position/ DNPEssentials.pdf.

numbers of programs and graduates, policy analysis and political competence must be integrated into every course, content area, and project so that the DNP graduate has the ability to assume a broad leadership role on behalf of the public and nursing profession. The solutions to today's social injustices, politicized delivery systems, perverse financing, and uneven quality in the health care system are difficult. APRNs are well positioned with clinical credibility to inform, design, and influence policy solutions, but this will happen *only if* they expand their arena of influence beyond the clinical setting (see Exemplar 19.3 on the nation's largest nursing PAC).

Political Competence

Politically competent APRNs serve as content experts with policymakers and their staff. Often, policymakers in the legislative branch are generalists who have a working knowledge on a broad range of topics such as immigration, transportation, energy, agriculture, and tax policy. However, in the regulatory branch, the policymaker will be far more knowledgeable on a narrower range of topics. At the institutional level, the corporate, or "C suite," executive is also broad based, focusing on the institution's profit margin, reputation in the community, and public reporting profile. These wide-ranging knowledge bases make it imperative for the APRN to use core nursing skills to determine the policymaker's baseline level of knowledge before launching into information sharing or making suggestions. Serving as a resource to policymakers with evidence-based information and helpful suggestions that are in the public interest is crucial and requires a thoughtful, skillful approach. When serving in this capacity, it is important to avoid a self-serving posture. To influence or participate meaningfully and effectively in policy development, APRNs must be aware of the policymaking process from idea conception to implementation as well as the open windows of political opportunity. Being effective in policy influence requires having deep knowledge about the problem the policy is intending to solve. Furthermore, intentionally developing and maintaining strong relationships with policymakers and other health care interest groups are important APRN activities. This requires asking many questions, building rapport, and seeking to understand where the policymaker is coming from before pushing an APRN or a patient-centered agenda forward. Heeding the US policy process, policymakers seek advisement on highly specific policy modifications rather than

major reform recommendations. Elected officials turn over at a far higher rate than civil servants or health care executives, who make careers out of formulating and implementing health policy. Because of the longevity of their careers, the strong trustworthy relationships APRNs make with the policymaker's staff as well as regulatory professionals can yield great results over time.

Individual Skills

Deep Knowledge

Self-Awareness

The value of APRNs is an important idea but, to be heard effectively, a great degree of maturity, discipline, humility, restraint, and respect for self and others must be practiced. Most political careers are created with small steps; when the person is effective, she or he is elevated into larger and larger spheres of influence. The politically competent APRN will have a long history of developing strong relationships with individuals inside and outside of nursing. The prerequisites for this level of maturity are knowing the self, staying focused on the long-range goals, and avoiding being shrill or bringing emotionally charged energy into policy formulation.

For the most part, the APRN must be held in high regard and be extremely knowledgeable, highly competent, and authentic, with solid integrity and a great degree of personal warmth. The APRN must have the trust of others to serve from a universal posture of problem solving and not make decisions solely to elevate the nursing discipline (effective use of power). The locus of responsibility for a politically competent APRN must be far broader than just nursing interests (see Exemplar 19.4 and Box 19.3). There must be a commitment to practical problem solving to increase access to care, lower costs, and improve quality of care. This requires the APRN to be careful about burning bridges so that there are no individuals or communities of people who want to see the APRN fail.

Content Expertise

Journalists Buresh and Gordon (2006) describe three communication challenges that are common across nursing:

1. That not enough nurses are willing to talk about their work.
2. Nurses, media, and health organizations often unwillingly project an inaccurate portrait of nursing as a "virtue" rather than a scientifically based, unique body of knowledge.

EXEMPLAR 19.3	The Anatomy of a Successful Political Action Committee, From One of the Nation's Strongest[a]

The American Association of Nurse Anesthetists (AANA) has the largest federal nursing political action committee (PAC) in the nation by far. With donations of over $1.3 million per 2-year election cycle, it is also one of the top federal health care PACs in the country. They are very proud of their thoughtful process for governing their PAC and making distributions. The certified registered nurse anesthetist (CRNA)-PAC Mission is *to Advance the Profession of Nurse Anesthesia through Federal Political Advocacy,* and they place a strong emphasis on being highly strategic, inclusive, and thoughtful. All operations related to the PAC, including fundraising, research, marketing, communication, and disbursements, stem from strategy and input from the mission, member leadership, and advocacy agenda of the AANA. The PAC is governed by eight CRNAs and one CRNA student. They are assisted by one full-time AANA staff member who regularly works with the PAC committee to serve as liaison and share compliance and political knowledge to make the most informed decisions. There are five key reasons why their PAC is so highly successful.

Grassroots Driven

First, they deploy a highly inclusive process asking grassroots CRNAs for local information about congressional campaigns. Making highly strategic disbursement decisions, they begin with the CRNA community and involve them in identifying key campaigns. Their sole criteria are directed at making disbursements to candidates who will move the CRNA agenda forward. Because the CRNA community is politically diverse, they do not formally endorse candidates. The PAC bases its financial support on the candidate's familiarity with and support of the CRNA profession and ability to influence the overall health care agenda in Congress. The PAC remains in close contact with individual CRNAs through the process.

Educating Policymakers

What the PAC disbursements gain for the AANA is access to federal elected officials and other leading policymakers. Policymakers are dealing with a wide breadth of issues and may not know how a policy is being played out in their community. Making PAC donations provides access to policymakers and opportunities for CRNAs to educate them about the benefits of CRNA care and how restricting CRNA practice impacts patients and increases health care costs. With the demanding schedule placed on lawmakers, the PAC affords one-on-one opportunities to discuss issues important to CRNAs that are otherwise unattainable.

Inspire and Acculturate CRNA Students *Early* Into Policy Engagement

A strong value and part of the culture of the AANA is to involve its student members, which reflects the fact that the AANA has over 90% of all CRNAs as paid members. Nurse anesthesia students learn that their jobs providing anesthesia can be legislated away in an instant, making CRNA students aware of and engaged in policy from the start. The AANA presents policy engagement as having a visible and practical relationship to the students' practice and livelihood and encourages early donating to the PAC so that it becomes a pattern as they mature in their careers.

Common Single Threat

Another key aspect of the success of the AANA's CRNA-PAC is that the American Society of Anesthesiologists (ASA) is a very real and outspoken opponent to CRNA practice and has unfortunately tried to block CRNA practice and reimbursement at every turn. While there are decades of peer-reviewed research documenting the safety and efficacy of CRNA practice, the ASA clings to its ideologic agenda that CRNA practice is "unsafe." Moreover, as a physician organization, the ASA has a $3.8 million PAC, nearly double the size of the AANA's CRNA-PAC. A large number of AANA members agree that the ASA opposition is a very real threat to their livelihood. AANA members see PAC contributions as a way to gain access to lawmakers so that they may educate them to more sound, patient-centered, and evidence-based policymaking.

Bipartisan Giving

Policymakers are carefully vetted, and disbursements target legislators who will carry the CRNA agenda forward. The CRNA-PAC typically gives equally to the Republicans and Democrats with a slight skew toward the party that is in power in the US House of Representatives and the US Senate. This way the CRNA-PAC is not viewed as being aligned with a single political party, giving members and AANA leadership access to and an information channel with bipartisan legislators and candidates. ◎

[a]Dr. Eileen O'Grady would like to thank Kate Fry of the AANA Staff and PAC Liaison, who was generous with her time in being interviewed for this exemplar.

From Diploma Registered Nurse to North Carolina State House: What Pulled Gale Adcock Into Public Office

Gale Adcock

It has been said, "If you are not at the table, then you are on the menu."

Gale Adcock graduated from nursing school with her nursing diploma. How did this small town Virginia girl, a first-generation college graduate raised in an apolitical family, evolve into a state and nationally recognized advanced practice registered nurse (APRN) thought leader, director of a primary care practice for a global corporation, and an elected official? In 1980, the North Carolina Nursing Practice Act was preparing to sunset (expire at a predetermined date). A statewide call to action was made for nurses to partner with a member of the General Assembly, acting as their conduit of information and influence as the bill made its way (successfully) through the General Assembly. Gale jumped with both feet into this effort and was immediately very interested in the process. She sought out a position on the North Carolina Nurses Association (NCNA) Board of Directors and soon became its president. She accepted opportunities to chair the North Carolina Center for Nursing, the NCNA Council of Nurse Practitioners, the American College of Nurse Practitioners Public Policy Committee, and a 7-year term on the North Carolina Board of Nursing. She was part of the successful lobbying effort for direct third-party reimbursement to North Carolina APRNs.

In the mid-1990s, Gale was the sole nurse appointed by the governor to the North Carolina Health Planning Commission and, as a spin-off the following year, she cochaired the Preventive Services Task Force. In 2009 she was again the sole nurse appointee (the governor's only appointment, representing business, no less) to the Blue Ribbon Task Force on the State Health Plan for Teachers and State Employees. She was elbow to elbow with the state's business leaders, insurers, and legislators who made up most of the task force members.

Over the next decade, Gale was urged by many in her community to run for political office. In 2007, when her local town council seat was vacated by a two-term incumbent, she was recruited to run by a group of determined supporters. Gale won her first race against two opponents, with 55% of the vote. In 2011 she ran for reelection to the Cary Town Council against a single opponent and won handily, with 66% of the vote. Immediately after being sworn in for her

second 4-year term, she was unanimously elected as the town's Mayor Pro-Tem (she stands in for the mayor when the mayor is unavailable).

Next up for Gale was running for and winning a seat in the North Carolina State House. As the House Representative for the 41st district of North Carolina, her platform issues are based on inclusion, preserving public education, quality and accessible health care, protecting the environment, and growing the economy, including expanding women's rights, the LGBT community, and others.

Gale firmly believes that every level of elected office offers opportunities to make decisions that affect health care and that raise the profile of APRNs as informed and decisive policymakers with a broad range of interests. No longer can or should APRNs be content to see themselves as players on only one field.

From Gale's Playbook: Fail-Safe Behaviors

After more than 30 years working up and down the health policy pipeline, from diploma nurse to elected official, Gale has learned to serve with the following skill sets:

A Content Expert: Get to know the APRN statutes and rules in your state. Be unshakable in your understanding of APRN authority to practice. Question every incidence of misinterpretation of APRN authority to practice, regardless of intention. It is astonishing how often others are misinformed about APRN practice. On at least this issue, strive always to be the expert in the room.

A Student of Process: Know how things actually get done in your setting—the committee structure, unwritten norms, and other operational nuances. Learn the faces and names of those with influential power. Become familiar with parliamentary procedure and read the local political pundits.

A Trusted Partner: There is no place for partisanship at any table you join. Do not make assumptions about motivation. Give everyone the benefit of the doubt and form partnerships with everyone possible. Party affiliation does not tell you what an individual actually believes or how she or he will operate.

EXEMPLAR 19.4 **From Diploma Registered Nurse to North Carolina State House: What Pulled Gale Adcock Into Public Office—cont'd**

A Well-Rounded Advocate: Seek out and use new venues to share the APRN message of wellness, primary prevention, and unencumbered access to health care. Consider running for a local elected office, such as school board (making decisions about cafeteria meals, how much gym time is included in the school day, health curriculum, presence of vending machines); county commission (funding for the local health department, substance abuse programs, mental health services, schools); and town or city council (greenways, bike lanes, parks, walkable communities, air and water quality). ◎

BOX 19.3 Four Ways to Build and Stay Current With Health Policy Knowledge

1. News Feeds

The best way to stay informed about current and emerging news is to subscribe to a few news feeds that get pushed to you from reputable, bipartisan policy sources. Glance at the headlines and read only what is of interest. Advanced practice registered nurses (APRNs) must be aware of the larger context of health care delivery and develop telescoping skills, in which one hooks smaller institutional policy issues onto what is happening in the larger world. Having knowledge of the larger policy world positions the APRN's capacity to participate more powerfully in institutional policy. Subscribe to three of the following (free) news feeds from the list below:

- Agency for Healthcare Research and Quality (AHRQ)— https://www.ahrq.gov/news/newsletters/e-newsletter/index.html
- Institute of Medicine news—http://www.nationalacademies.org/hmd/Global/Media%20Room/News.aspx
- Commonwealth Fund—http://www.commonwealthfund.org/
- Robert Wood Johnson Foundation news digests—http://www.rwjf.org/en.html
- Kaiser Family Foundation—http://www.kff.org/
- Rand Corporation—https://www.rand.org/
- Medicare Payment Advisory Commission—http://www.medpac.gov/

2. Watch the *PBS News Hour*

See local listings for your TV station (http://www.pbs.org/newshour/). This hour-long program is usually on twice an evening (repeated). It differs from network news in that there are long conversations with policy experts and the viewpoint is balanced and of the highest quality. It avoids news by sound bites, and there is frequent emphasis on health policy issues. Moreover, listening to the conversations with experts in the field, with a high degree of civility, on topics related to the economy or politics will assist the APRN to become a more informed citizen and raise the level of political competency. This is an easy way to stay informed and experience depth behind the issues.

3. Read and Glance at Newspapers

Newspaper articles may seem old-fashioned, whether in print or online, but almost every daily regional print outlet has at least one current health policy article. Often, these are found in the business or opinion sections. Read the Sunday opinion pages and the health section of your regional news source.

4. Read Abstracts From *Health Affairs*

Health Affairs is the leading journal of health policy thought and research (http://www.healthaffairs.org/). The peer-reviewed journal explores current health policy issues. Its mission is to serve as a high-level, nonpartisan forum to promote analysis and discussion on improving health and health care and to address such issues as cost, quality, and access. The journal reaches a broad audience that includes government and health industry leaders; health care advocates; scholars of health, health care, and health policy; and others concerned with health and health care issues in the United States and worldwide. Everybody involved in health policy reads it, so scanning the titles and abstracts is a great way to stay current.

3. When nurses do speak up about nursing, they often bypass, downplay, or devalue the work of human caring.

These communication challenges capture the central dilemma of modern nursing: that nurses are caring for the sickest or most vulnerable members of society without the resources or authority to carry it out. They are unable to fully promote health in the over-medicalized, overspecialized health delivery systems that do not focus on, value, or otherwise profit from early intervention measures that align with nursing core values. Nurses' political competency must be enhanced, and APRNs must fully inhabit the policy realm and move from silence to powerful voice. APRNs must be seated at tables of power where government, academic, and corporate decision making occurs. As the ACA has further decentralized health care in the United States, there are now many more tables at which APRNs may be seated. The most pressing health care problems in society, especially the chronic disease epidemic, require an intelligence that advanced practice nurses fully own.

Bringing APRN wisdom through a polarity thinking lens can enhance one's expertise. Many of the most persistent health care problems are not really problems to be solved but tensions that need to be leveraged. For example, the problems of cost cutting and improving quality create tensions when one focuses only on one without attention to the other. Polarity thinking helps bring APRN pragmatic wisdom to complex problems. The APRN can identify these polarities and find solutions by connecting interdependent pairs, pointing out that we cannot have one tension without its opposite. Other such examples include inhaling versus exhaling, patient care versus self-care, and technology versus human caring. These issues do not go away over time; rather, they are tensions that need to be managed (Wesorick, 2016). APRNs can motivate groups who may be stuck by approaching challenging dilemmas by getting them to move from "either-or" solutions to "both-and" solutions, which may be a more thoughtful way for APRNs to bring their expertise to policy tables.

Seek Out Experts

A great degree of humility is required on the part of the politically active APRN; one effective way to embody humility is to seek out respected individuals with expertise (content experts), including those whose political agenda may be different from one's own. Consulting experts along the way to gain insight and knowledge builds trust because the seeker of expertise does not presume to be an expert in all matters related to health care. The APRN must integrate all sides of an issue (stakeholder analysis) and then make a determination about how and whether to use that expertise. That means seeking out and engaging experts who may oppose one's policy agenda.

Political Antenna
Policy Process

Content expertise is not the only skill set required to be effective in influencing policy in an interprofessional arena. The APRN must be always extremely mindful of the policy process and carefully measure how one participates in discussions to maximize being heard (political antennae). Developing political antennae can be strengthened by engaging stakeholders who may oppose or support an action that the APRN may want to take. This stakeholder analysis, done privately before issues become public (or before a meeting), is an effective way to learn about all the issues, especially the opposition viewpoint, so that a creative strategy can be developed to inoculate the opposing ideas with an evidence base or a creative idea. Knowing how others are motivated and what their agenda is places the APRN at an advantage in negotiating a mutually agreeable outcome. By learning others' opinions about contentious issues, the APRN can carefully garner support.

Conduct at Meetings

In terms of public meetings and how APRNs conduct themselves, impromptu remarks should be avoided because they could be used against the person, the nursing profession, or other interests in the future. It is important to continuously gauge the other stakeholders at the meeting; if, for example, a physician has made a point about nursing that the APRN wanted to make, let that external validation stand as a comment that is supportive of nursing, rather than repeating the point. It is important to show restraint in meetings, waiting until an insightful thought comes that forwards the discussion, or to bring more accurate factual data to the conversation, or to help clarify the polarizing issues and areas of agreement in a policy discussion. To be successful, the APRN must keep cool, responding factually, and avoiding rhetorical inflammatory comments, which might diminish other disciplines (no bashing other provider groups). By participating in meetings with this respectful approach, deep content expertise, and a focus on process, the APRN is well positioned to encourage others to support nursing issues.

Use Power

Contribute to Public Discourse

Another essential responsibility for APRNs is to inform and contribute to the public discourse on important health policy issues because APRN interests and public interests are not at odds. Gaining public support and influencing public opinion can help get the attention of policymakers or propel issues onto the policy agenda. Submitting an op-ed (meaning "opposite the editorial page" in the publication) to major news outlets is a powerful way to do this (Box 19.4). This requires writing that links the health issues to society, uses poignant stories to bring the problem to life, and incorporates evidence to build a strong case about why a policy change is needed. APRNs must use their professional credentials and expertise with a sense of responsibility toward educating the public and not be hesitant to act as advocates based on their knowledge and experience. This could include seeking out media invitations to news programs or starting a podcast to inform the public about the APRN's expertise on major issues of the day.

Serve on Boards

There are numerous opportunities for APRNs to serve on federal, corporate, and health-related advisory boards, which are crucial to integrating APRNs into policymaking. A coalition of nursing stakeholders has created an organization, Nurses on Boards Coalition (http://www.nursesonboardscoalition.org) with the sole purpose of getting 10,000 nurses on boards by 2020. This is an effort to correct the fact that nurses are underrepresented on a number of policymaking boards, including those of hospitals and health centers. Serving on boards allows APRNs to expand their influence from the front lines to the boardroom

and to use that frontline clinical knowledge to inform the boardroom. Often, APRNs are appointed because they have strong working relationships with people who happen to be on boards and are familiar with the APRN as a compelling knowledge source who is effective in groups. A definite set of behaviors is required to serve on national advisory or corporate boards and a high degree of mastery is necessary to be reappointed or invited back (Fig. 19.7).

Use Power Instead of Force

Power accomplishes with ease what force, even with extreme effort, cannot accomplish. On the interpersonal front, it is important for APRNs to avoid using force in advancing their positions in the policy arena. Doing so can diminish one's power. This is commonly done by nurses who participate in interprofessional policy or problem-solving meetings. The twin approaches of being judgmental and parochial can quickly compromise effectiveness. *Judgmentalism*—criticizing other people or disciplines—distracts from effective problem solving and, in the process, can reflect poorly on the person who judges, greatly diminishing the power to influence. Diminishing others or the work they do can provoke defensiveness and consequently limit the capacity to influence others meaningfully. *Nursing parochialism* occurs when nurses present a narrow, restricted scope or outlook in which only nursing and nursing's interests are offered as solutions. These postures in the policy arena (or any other setting) do not build wide-based support or strong relationships.

Everyone has seen nurses and other leaders who become shrill and consistently present positions that reflect pure self-interest in public arenas, whereby each person in the room knows what the individual will say before she or he speaks. This is a posture

---

BOX 19.4 **Op-Ed Suggestions**

Op-eds are not formulaic, but some general guidelines may enhance the potential for publication. Op-eds and letters to the editor are both unsolicited, but letters to the editor are usually shorter and in direct response to a story or article that has previously been published. Op-eds are longer opinion pieces (generally opposite the editorial page) that are usually related to some current event or news story. A strong 750-word op-ed piece starts with the credentials and experience of the author. The policy problem is hooked to a leading current problem or news story.

Add a specific poignant story to describe how the problem affects people. Offer policy solution(s) backed up by three points of evidence. Add a "to-be-sure" segment, which anticipates and counters opponents' views and inoculates against those stakeholders who oppose your ideas. Finally, provide a conclusion with possible action items for members of the public (e.g., call or write legislator, support a bill). Ask at least five people with strong writing skills to critique the piece prior to submission.

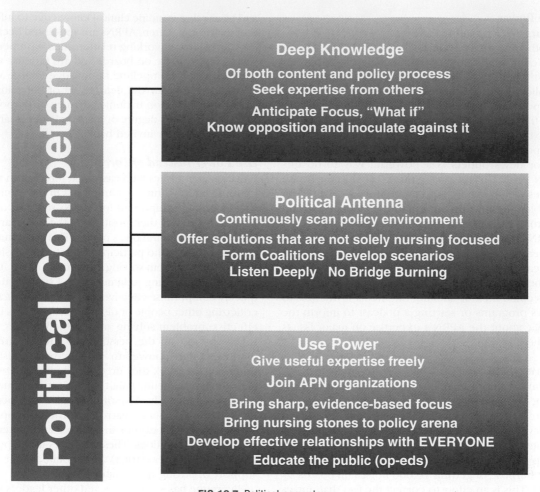

FIG 19.7 Political competence.

of parochialism that APRNs must work hard to avoid. To be effective in interprofessional and influential arenas and to pursue larger roles, APRNs must build strong relationships founded on trust and respect. In policy-related meetings, APRNs must demonstrate that nurses can solve problems in the health care system, not just for nurses' sake. APRNs will inhabit a more powerful stance and become most effective when they bring a broader perspective to all of health care, not just nursing. This may require sharing one's own expertise freely, with a generous spirit, and avoiding the hoarding of information.

The value of APRNs and their potential impact on cost, quality, and access, if fully unleashed, is an enormously powerful solution to some of today's most significant health care problems. Power is characterized by humility and truth, which needs

no defense or rhetoric; it is self-evident. Force is divisive and exploits people for individual or personal gain (Hawkins, 2002).

Take Action to Create Public Trust

In a study of nursing and power among Canadian nurse practitioners, Quinlan and Robertson (2013) described a form of nonauthoritative power called "communicative power" as the mutual understanding achieved between pairs of individuals by the efforts of a third. It differs from most kinds of informal power in that communicative power is oriented to the collective good, whereas informal power focuses on individual gain. Their study showed that NPs have the greatest amount of communicative power because they were able to mobilize their holistic practice and bridge the medical and nursing frames

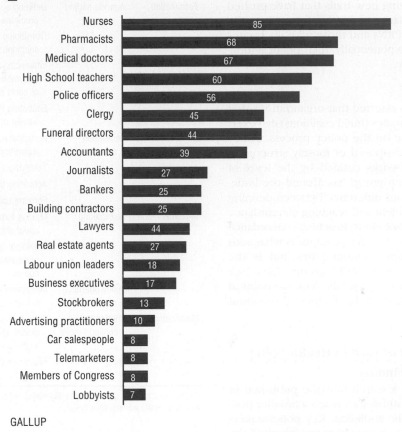

Please tell me how you would rate the honesty and ethical standards of people in these different fields -- very high, high, average, low or very low?

Dec. 2-6, 2015

■ % Very high/High

Nurses	85
Pharmacists	68
Medical doctors	67
High School teachers	60
Police officers	56
Clergy	45
Funeral directors	44
Accountants	39
Journalists	27
Bankers	25
Building contractors	25
Lawyers	44
Real estate agents	27
Labour union leaders	18
Business executives	17
Stockbrokers	13
Advertising practitioners	10
Car salespeople	8
Telemarketers	8
Members of Congress	8
Lobbyists	7

GALLUP

FIG 19.8 Gallup Poll on honesty/ethics in professions.

of knowledge and so are better able to contribute to the knowledge exchange within the teams. It was concluded that NPs have the potential to fully realize their role as knowledge-boundary spanners. The move to doctoral education raises this potential for APRNs even more. Communicative power in the policy arenas could be more fully deployed in light of the public trust. For 15 years in a row, when the public has been asked which professions they trust the most, nurses have ranked at the very top (Fig. 19.8). This trust creates a social covenant with the public and, by extension, trust in APRNs in the policymaking context. The public trusts nurses to be advocates on their behalf.

Build APRN Unity

There are numerous ways for APRN organizations to exert influence continuously on the policymaking process. Forming coalitions with other APRNs and other nursing, health care, and consumer groups strengthens political effectiveness. Although there is a rich diversity of nursing organizations (more than 120 nationally and scores of state and regional organizations), none has a membership base that is more than a fraction of the more than 3 million nurses. Forming coalitions and strategic plans around policy is necessary to maximize impact. APRN organizational leaders can play a role in defining health policy problems and designing possible solutions. The APRN movement has advanced tremendously, but a greater degree of policy solidarity would significantly strengthen the political effectiveness and power of APRNs. APRNs are characteristically pioneers, blazing new trails that have pushed the role and boundaries of nursing forward. As the total numbers of APRNs and those with doctorates continue to grow exponentially, their political influence will also grow.

Build Coalitions

Longest (2016) has asserted that organizations that form policy communities (build coalitions) can exert enormous influence on the policy process. Policy communities are composed of loosely structured, heterogeneous networks defined by the level of investment that each group has around the issue. There is an enormous difference between defining a health policy problem and reaching concordance on policy positions/solutions. Reaching concordance in the development of policy positions is what adds great power to policy communities and is the organizational challenge for APRN groups. Table 19.4 depicts the policy process and the requisite political competency skills that can be deployed throughout the process.

Moving APRNs Forward in Health Policy

Communicating Findings

Findings on APRN research must be published in journals outside of nursing to reach a broader policymaking and public audience. Key policymakers and the public must be made more aware of the contributions that APRNs make in reducing health care costs and improving access and quality of care. Achieving broader recognition, reducing APRN invisibility, and removing barriers to APRN practice will be contingent on APRNs communicating methodologically sound APRN research, which produces results that are generalizable to the larger delivery system. Moreover, APRNs must expand publications to journals outside of nursing, which have a much broader readership. Fig. 19.9 shows an abstract of APRNs publishing in the highly regarded journal, *Health Affairs.* This journal reaches a wide and highly influential audience. It is read by and used as a reliable knowledge source by health policymakers.

Resources and Challenges in Evidence-Informed Policy Development

As evidence-based clinicians, APRNs may assume that policy is formed by conducting good research,

TABLE 19.4	Influencing Health Policy Throughout the Process	
Policy Area	**Skill**	**Examples**
Formulation	Agenda setting	Defining and documenting problems
		Developing and evaluating solutions
		Influencing political circumstances by lobbying or court decisions
		Educating the public (e.g., writing op-eds)
	Legislation development	Participating in drafting legislation
		Testifying at hearings
		Activating the grassroots
		Forming coalitions
Implementation	Rulemaking	Making formal comments about draft rules
		Providing input to rulemaking advisory bodies
	Policy operation	Interacting with policy implementers
Modification	Unintended consequences	Creating a case for modification through evaluation and evidence
		Educating the public about need for change

Adapted from Longest, B. (2016). *Health policymaking in the United States* (6th ed.). Chicago, IL: Health Administration Press.

disseminating the findings, and building best practices in a rational, linear process. Another assumption is that once a policy is specified, people on the ground will simply implement it. As noted earlier in this chapter, in practice, policy is messier than this. Clearly, evidence needs to influence policy up front. This requires a much better relationship between policymakers, researchers, and practitioners and a deeper understanding of each other's priorities and ways of working. The following insights from Glasby (2011) address the challenges of the evidence, policy, and practice interaction:

1. Evidence is only one voice competing for attention, so researchers need to be committed and passionate.
2. Evidence needs to influence policy early on—not after the policy is formulated or rolled out.

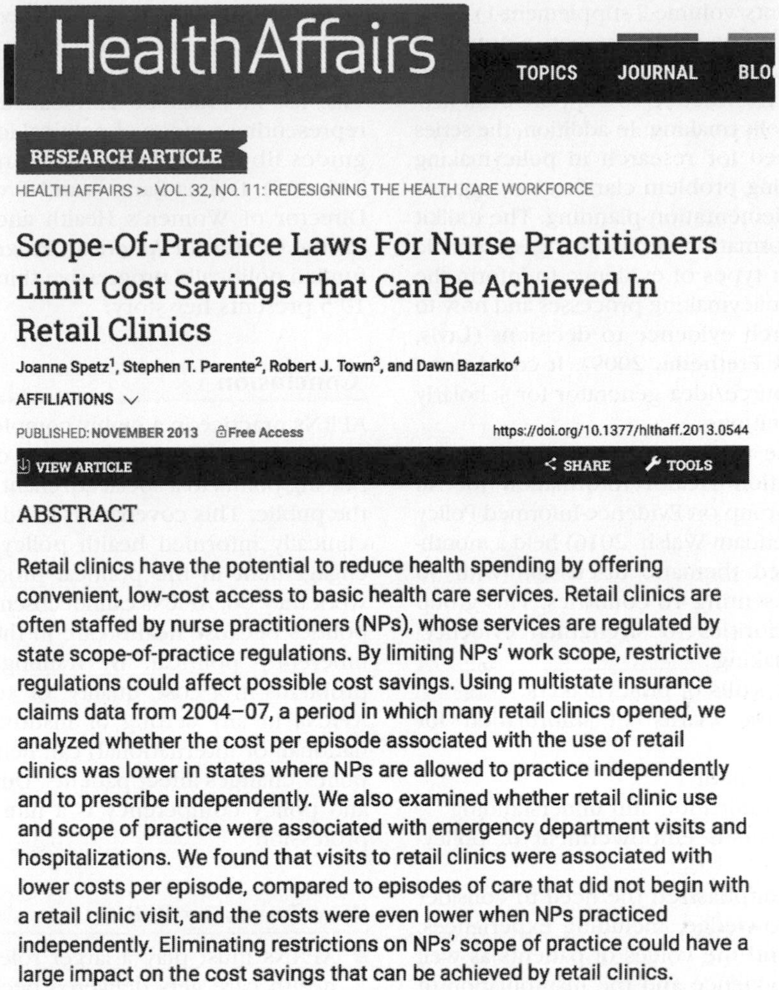

HealthAffairs

TOPICS JOURNAL BLO

RESEARCH ARTICLE

HEALTH AFFAIRS > VOL. 32, NO. 11: REDESIGNING THE HEALTH CARE WORKFORCE

Scope-Of-Practice Laws For Nurse Practitioners Limit Cost Savings That Can Be Achieved In Retail Clinics

Joanne Spetz[1], Stephen T. Parente[2], Robert J. Town[3], and Dawn Bazarko[4]

AFFILIATIONS

PUBLISHED: NOVEMBER 2013 Free Access https://doi.org/10.1377/hlthaff.2013.0544

VIEW ARTICLE SHARE TOOLS

ABSTRACT

Retail clinics have the potential to reduce health spending by offering convenient, low-cost access to basic health care services. Retail clinics are often staffed by nurse practitioners (NPs), whose services are regulated by state scope-of-practice regulations. By limiting NPs' work scope, restrictive regulations could affect possible cost savings. Using multistate insurance claims data from 2004–07, a period in which many retail clinics opened, we analyzed whether the cost per episode associated with the use of retail clinics was lower in states where NPs are allowed to practice independently and to prescribe independently. We also examined whether retail clinic use and scope of practice were associated with emergency department visits and hospitalizations. We found that visits to retail clinics were associated with lower costs per episode, compared to episodes of care that did not begin with a retail clinic visit, and the costs were even lower when NPs practiced independently. Eliminating restrictions on NPs' scope of practice could have a large impact on the cost savings that can be achieved by retail clinics.

FIG 19.9 A peer-reviewed abstract in a widely read policy journal on policy issues related to nursing scope of practice. *(From Spetz, J., Parente, S. T., Town, R. J., & Bazarko, D. [2013]. Scope-of-practice laws for nurse practitioners limit cost savings that can be achieved in retail clinics.* Health Affairs, 32, *1977-1984. Retrieved from http://content.healthaffairs.org/content/32/11/1977.long)*

3. Policymakers and researchers need to understand each other's worlds and priorities.
4. Sometimes it may be necessary to gather the best evidence in the time available rather than all the evidence.
5. Simply "disseminating" more research will not necessarily help to embed evidence in practice. Instead it may be more fruitful to support local leaders to make sense of emerging policy and help to create receptive local contexts.
6. Asking the right question is crucial—asking "Does this work?" requires a different approach from asking "If I do this, what might be the implications?"

Evidence-informed health policy is a growing field and one that APRNs can tap for knowledge and skill development in policy development and implementation. The World Health Organization (2017) sponsors the Evidence-informed Policy Network (EVIPNet). In 2009 the SUPporting Policy Relevant Reviews and Trials (SUPPORT) project published a series of articles in *Health Research Policy and Systems* that serve as a toolkit for evidence-informed health policymaking (https://health-policy-systems.biomedcentral.com/

articles/supplements/volume-7-supplement-1). Each of the 18 articles in the series presents a proposed tool that can be used by those involved in finding and using research evidence to support evidence-informed health policymaking. In addition, the series highlights the need for research in policymaking processes, including problem clarification, options framing, and implementation planning. The toolkit also provides information on assessing systematic reviews and other types of evidence to inform the aforementioned policymaking processes and how to move from research evidence to decisions (Lavis, Oxman, Lewin, & Fretheim, 2009). It could serve an important resource/idea generator for scholarly projects or dissertations.

Building on the work by Lavis et al., the international organization Health Information for All (HIFA) Working Group on Evidence-Informed Policy and Practice (Pakenham-Walsh, 2016) held a month-long Internet-based thematic discussion with 36 participants representing 16 countries. This group identified five priorities to strengthen evidence-informed policymaking:

1. Building the skills of policymakers
2. Improving the clarity of information for policymakers
3. Public engagement
4. Better communication and understanding
5. Persuasion versus empowerment of policymakers

The participants emphasized the need to consider tacit forms of knowledge, including experiences, lessons learned, and the voices of patients as well as the biases of evidence and the manipulation of facts for political purposes. Furthermore, the need to engage stakeholders up front so as to formulate the key questions necessary for making decisions is a first step in any research. Finally, the report focused on the importance of empowerment through evidence in contrast to persuasion using emotional appeal. These priorities can be directly translated to APRN health policy work locally and globally.

The development and evaluation of health policy often takes place in organizations referred to as think tanks. They can be small, local organizations or large, international, multi-million dollar organizations such as the Kaiser Family Foundation, the Heritage Foundation, and the Center for American Progress. These organizations seek to shape governmental policy by offering expertise in various areas, including health care. Recognizing the value bias that is often held by a think tank is essential when drawing on its

work to inform policy. The University of Pennsylvania maintains a list of public policy think tanks according to areas of research, including health. This list includes US and Canadian organizations representing a range of political ideologies (https://guides.library.upenn.edu/c.php?g=476482&p=3254052). Donna Barry is an NP who served as the Director of Women's Health and Rights Program for the Center for American Progress, a large, well-funded politically progressive think tank. Exemplar 19.5 presents her story.

Conclusion

APRNs practice in a highly complex, ever-changing environment. The high degree of public trust in nursing points to a social covenant APRNs have with the public. This covenant is to advocate for sound, clinically informed health policy, which requires engagement in the political process. By the very work they do, APRNs cannot absent themselves from politics because health care in the United States is inherently political. By framing all health care problems in a cost, quality, or access framework, APRNs in any setting or institution (local, state, national, or international) can help others see how policy changes affect patients. Developing political and policy competency is a must to advance the profession.

Key Summary Points

▪ APRNs must play a larger role in shaping how health care gets delivered because they have a social covenant with the public to serve as patient advocates in the broadest sense. To be able to do this, APRNs must resist the pull of the familiar and overcome invisibility and passivity.

▪ Policymakers are looking for solutions to escalating costs and continued patient safety problems. Political competency needs to be part of every APRN's professional role.

▪ Membership in professional organizations that advance issues critical to APRN practice and the health of the United States is vital to the continued viability of APRNs. The first step to being involved in policy formulation is to be knowledgeable about the policy process and the current and emerging issues relevant to APRNs. To be involved, APRNs need to understand the details related to funding issues, measures of quality, how they reflect APRN practice, and specific programs designed to improve access (Table 19.5).

| EXEMPLAR 19.5 | Think Tanks to Influence Policy: The Journey of Donna Barry |

Donna Barry

In 2002, I was directing a Partners In Health project to treat multiple-drug-resistant tuberculosis in Russia when Representative Sherrod Brown from Ohio visited our treatment program in Siberia. That visit and work on that project were my first steps into the world of policy and opened my eyes to the crucial role that advanced practice registered nurses (APRNs) need to take on in policy development.

One of the main points of our project in Russia was to update treatment and show better treatment outcomes using multiple drugs for longer treatment periods and less surgical intervention. The Russia project was part of a bigger policy focus on global treatment policy at the World Health Organization. Senator Brown's visit to the Siberian clinic was to give him on-the-ground stories and experience to shore up his annual defense of increased money for tuberculosis treatment in the State and Foreign Operations budgets in the US House of Representatives and the US Senate.

Eventually I became the first Director of Policy and Advocacy at Partners In Health. During 6 years in that role, I worked alongside several team members and a large coalition, spending our efforts on the following topics, among many others:

- Working on policy related to improving treatment for undernutrition/malnutrition in low-income countries
- Increasing the number of health care providers in low-income countries as well as improving their training and retention rates
- Updating outdated US foreign assistance laws and rules that made foreign aid less effective and often more expensive to deliver

- Increasing foreign aid budgets for HIV/AIDS and tuberculosis
- Encouraging the United Nations to consider preventing and treating noncommunicable diseases such as cancer and heart disease as important as preventing and treating infectious diseases

I have since been named the director of the Women's Health and Rights Program at the Center for American Progress (CAP) in Washington, DC. One of the first issues that came up after starting that position was the Supreme Court case on contraceptives and the religious liberty of private corporations *(Hobby Lobby v. Burwell)*. There were multiple court cases related to contraception, abortion, the Affordable Care Act, and other key health issues that arose during my time at CAP. Understanding the US court/judicial system was never covered in nursing school or my public health training, but learning how that system works and affects policy is key to comprehending much of US health policy. It is also very important that APRNs understand how laws, regulations, and rules governing health care in our country are made—we APRNs can favorably impact them if we are engaged when they are drafted, reviewed, debated, and implemented.

Change in the domestic and global policy arena is usually incremental and very slow. However, it is critical that nurses, especially APRNs, stay engaged in policy change that affects the fields in which we work, whether that policy is local, state, federal, or global. Our voices and experience are deeply valued by policymakers but also unique and vital for sound policy. ◎

| ◎ TABLE 19.5 | Selected Health Policy Experiences for Advanced Practice Nurses |

Policy Experience, Internship, Fellowship Opportunity	Contact
Academy Health	http://www.academyhealth.org
Nurse in Washington Internship	http://www.nursing-alliance.org/Events/NIWI-Nurse-in-Washington-Internship
National Academy of Social Insurance	https://www.nasi.org/studentopps
Robert Wood Johnson Health Policy Fellowship	http://www.healthpolicyfellows.org/
White House Fellows Program	https://www.whitehouse.gov/participate/fellows
American Association of Nurse Practitioners Health Policy Fellowship	https://www.aanp.org/legislation-regulation/federal-legislation/health-policy-fellowship
Health and Aging Policy Fellowships	http://www.healthandagingpolicy.org/about-the-fellowship/partnerships/

■ An important truth for APRNs and policy is that a single person, with deep understanding of an issue along with highly developed political skills, can make a difference. An individual backed by organizational strength, particularly by coalitions of organizations, can make an even more significant difference.

References

To access the references for this chapter, use your smartphone's QR code reader to scan the code below, or go to http://booksite.elsevier.com/ 9780323447751.

Marketing and Negotiation

Susanne J. Phillips

> *"So never lose an opportunity of urging a practical beginning, however small, for it is wonderful how often in such matters the mustard-seed germinates and roots itself."*
>
> —*Florence Nightingale*

CHAPTER CONTENTS

The current changes in the health care environment for advanced practice registered nurses (APRNs)—brought about by the Institute of Medicine's (IOM's) report on *The Future of Nursing* report (IOM, 2011, 2015), the Patient Protection and Affordable Care Act (ACA, 2010), and the changes in regulation based on the *Consensus Model for APRN Regulation* (APRN Joint Dialogue Group, 2008)—all impact the way that APRNs market themselves and negotiate practice contracts. Marketing one's self is an important skill for APRNs to develop in order to become viable members of and achieve stature as principal players in the health care arena during these unsettled times.

In marketing themselves successfully, APRNs must integrate clinical expertise, leadership, collaboration, and other APRN competencies and business skills. In addition to understanding reimbursement payment mechanisms, and regulatory and credentialing requirements (discussed in Chapter 22), all APRNs—new graduates, seasoned professionals, and those striving to develop and maintain independent practices—must understand marketing and negotiation.

This chapter focuses on marketing the role of the APRN both as a new graduate and as an experienced clinician. It includes a discussion on entrepreneurship/intrapreneurship, and the need for innovation, marketing, and negotiation skills for all APRNs.

Self-Awareness: Finding a Good Fit

Success in and satisfaction with one's APRN role revolve around the right match between APRNs and the work they do and the ability to be flexible and innovative within the scope of that role. Adaptability to the changing health care marketplace is one of the role's greatest strengths. APRNs participate in both direct and indirect care processes in any practice setting. Examples of indirect processes are the steps taken to market the practice, register a patient and collect demographics; the process of third-party billing; meeting regulatory, safety, and quality imperatives; and the interaction with medical, pharmaceutical, and office supply vendors. Box 20.1 provides examples of clinical and administrative processes

BOX 20.1   Examples of Direct and Indirect Advanced Practice Registered Nurse Processes and Skills

Clinical/Direct Processes and Skills	Administrative/Indirect Processes and Skills
• Disease management	• Community outreach
• Health promotion/disease prevention	• Risk management and assessment
• Patient education	• Reporting mechanisms
• Staff education	• Quality and safety initiatives
• Wound management	• Support staff supervision
• Childbirth education	• Presentation/teaching/precepting
• Lactation consultation	• Grant writing
• Chronic disease consultation	• Computer literacy
• Prenatal, delivery, and postpartum care	• Budget development and implementation
• Adhering to opioid prescribing rules	• Billing for services
• Anesthesia	• Word processing/desktop publishing
• Patient engagement—group visits	• Compliance monitoring, Health Insurance
• Minor procedures	Portability and Accountability Act
• Rapid response policy to emerging public	• Quality/safety monitoring and reporting
health threats (e.g., Ebola, Zika)	

and skills in the APRN role. Both direct and indirect processes are essential to the successful management of any health care system, whether it be a small, self-contained APRN or physician practice or a large multihospital network.

Over an APRN's career, the balance between direct and indirect process involvement and the size of the system in which these processes occur may vary. At any given time, such shifts in balance and size of the system may require that APRNs adopt an entrepreneurial approach, an intrapreneurial approach, or a mixture of both (Dayhoff & Moore, 2005). An *entrepreneur* plans, organizes, finances, operates, and participates in a new health care delivery organization. Entrepreneurs have control over and responsibility for an increased proportion of indirect processes of care in their roles compared to intrapreneurs. An *intrapreneur* is generally an employee in an existing health care system, in which many of the indirect processes of the care delivery system may be controlled and managed by other employees or departments. The intrapreneur improves, redesigns, or augments an employer's current direct care processes, with a lesser role in day-to-day business administrative functions. Entrepreneurs function within the context of the larger, societal health care system. Intrapreneurs function within an institutional health care system—a microcosm of the larger arena. Both entrepreneurs and intrapreneurs are risk takers; however, entrepreneurs are likely to take bigger risks and have a higher tolerance for the accompanying uncertainty. Both

entrepreneurs and intrapreneurs are individuals who continually search for and who are receptive to opportunities and innovation. Innovation comes through the creation of a new process (whether direct, indirect, or both) or through radical changes to an existing process so that it seems "like new."

When embarking on program or practice oversight, the APRN needs to understand the balance between direct and indirect processes as well as how much time the APRN wants to devote to each of these. A large portion of time is dedicated to clinical visits and must be financially productive, so there must be a realistic balance between time spent in direct and indirect care. The decision about the proportion of one's role to devote to direct care versus indirect processes is based on the professional and personal values and goals of the APRN and the needs and demands of the practice.

A self-assessment may assist the APRN in clarifying professional and personal values. Types of questions to consider include the following, which are intended to be illustrative only and are not assumed to be exhaustive:

• ***Philosophical basis for practice.*** What type of nursing practice or approach to care delivery best describes how I perceive my own nursing practice? What do I value most and how does that value get expressed in my practice? Do the options before me favor this model or some other approach? If they favor another approach, how compatible is it with my own beliefs and values? (See Chapter 2.)

- **_Preference for intrapreneurial or entrepreneurial approach._** Do I thrive on risk taking, like some risk, or prefer situations with a conservative level of risk involved? How is a "loss" or being "unsuccessful" defined? If I like taking risks, how much of a loss can I afford to take—both professionally and personally—if my venture proves to be unsuccessful? (The more risk one is willing to take, the more entrepreneurial one is likely to be.) Do I prefer being a part of a team or being on my own? If I like being on a team, what other team members would I like to be included on this team? How big a team am I most comfortable with? If I prefer working on my own, how will I interact with my colleagues? (See Chapters 7, 9, and 11.)

Choosing Between Entrepreneurship/ Intrapreneurship

Many nurses seek APRN education with the clear intention of pursuing entrepreneurial or intrapreneurial work. The very first decision an APRN must make is whether to be an employee-intrapreneur, a freelancer, or an entrepreneur. As an employee, the changing health care landscape requires APRNs to approach their work with an intrapreneurial spirit. The APRN intrapreneur has the requisite APRN approach that questions the status quo and hunts for innovative solutions that promote health, wellness, and wholeness. Intrapreneurship refers to the APRN who assumes the role to develop new ideas in established organizations, facilitating translation of research, evidence, and evidence-based product evaluation into clinical practice with an acute eye on cost reduction, patient outcomes, and revenue generation (Dayhoff & Moore, 2002; Hewison & Badger, 2006). Intrapreneurship provides the APRN with flexibility to be entrepreneurial within the stability of an employee relationship, while providing transformational leadership in the context of the organization (Hewison & Badger, 2006; Manion, 2001).

The APRN entrepreneur/freelancer is a free agent who often gets paid by the hour or project. The APRN freelancer is able to choose the work and the population that is most meaningful to him or her, who can set her or his own hours, terms, and conditions. It is possible to have steady work with no overhead, little risk, and a great degree of practice autonomy. Freelancing is a way for APRNs to do the highest quality work with the populations best suited to their skill set. Being successful requires building a strong reputation and cultivating mastery as a clinician. It often requires a contract with the practice or facility and can create an uneven flow of work, and often there are no benefits such as health insurance, malpractice insurance. and paid time off. Nurse entrepreneurs are encouraged to seek professional liability insurance for their business.

The APRN entrepreneur has been described as "an individual who identifies a patient's need and envisions how nursing can respond to that need in an effective way, then formulates and executes a plan to meet that need" (Ieong, 2004, p. 1). In addition to assuming risks of a business, the self-employed entrepreneur is directly accountable to the client or patient (Wilson, Averis, & Walsh, 2003). Entrepreneurs build a business larger than themselves, and earn money when they are not providing services or products themselves. It requires a sharp focus on growth and developing systems that are scalable.

Characteristics for Entrepreneurship/ Intrapreneurship

New APRNs, with prior nursing experience and expertise, may develop interest in entre- or intrapreneurship opportunities following graduation. Prepared with doctoral competencies in business and health care delivery, organizational and systems leadership, collaboration, health care policy, and a unique and acute awareness of patients' unmet needs, Doctor of Nursing Practice (DNP)–prepared APRNs are uniquely positioned to identify innovative opportunities and gaps in service within the current health care system (American Association of Colleges of Nursing, 2006; Wilson, Whitaker, & Whitford, 2012). Likewise, experienced APRNs, motivated by life events, boredom, lack of autonomy, burnout, role constraints, or a general feeling of being stuck in the medical model, may find themselves pursuing these opportunities following years of APRN service (Shirey, 2007). Whether an APRN is a new graduate or a seasoned clinician, advanced practice nurses seek innovative practice settings out of love of nursing and a desire to make a difference (Shirey, 2007). Additionally, strong self-efficacy and influence of mentors and family motivate nurses to pursue an innovative work environment (Shirey, 2007).

APRNs seeking innovative and transformative practice settings envision their individual potential for making a difference in patients' lives and have a desire to stay close to patient care delivery; however, being entrepreneurial or highly innovative within an organization requires tolerating a higher degree of risk taking. These APRNs desire to solve a problem through a unique business or practice venture, providing an alternate and perhaps more flexible professional lifestyle. The bedrock of any entrepreneurial endeavor is for the APRN to have strong clinical competence. This must precede and override all APRN business arrangements regardless of specialty or setting. Characteristics of clinically competent nurse entrepreneurs/intrapreneurs include strong leadership and assertiveness, along with self-confidence and willingness to take risks (Hewison & Badger, 2006; Wilson et al., 2012). Self-discipline, creativity, a need to achieve, and integrity drive their creative vision, providing the necessary motivation to network and market oneself (Hewison & Badger, 2006), and above all, entrepreneurs are mission driven, placing values above profits (Shirey, 2007).

National Call for Innovators

The IOM, in its original *The Future of Nursing* report (IOM, 2011) and in the 2015 update (IOM, 2015), initiated a national call for nurses to engage in entrepreneurial practice to improve health care delivery. This imperative provides a firm basis and renewed recommendation for new and experienced APRNs to implement innovative ideas with a focus on accessibility and affordability. In fact, these opportunities exist across all settings where health care is delivered. Graduate-prepared APRN roles, with formal education in health systems, health economics, and business concepts, are better prepared to engage in self-employment or opportunities within an organizational framework to pursue innovative and transformative solutions to improve health outcomes. Rewards of entrepreneurship/ intrapreneurship include personal and professional freedom, desired lifestyle, professional legacy, a larger circle of influence, and expert status, which, according to research, outweigh the disadvantages of running one's own business in the entrepreneurial setting or managing organizational conflict within the intrapreneurial setting (Hewison & Badger, 2006; Shirey, 2007; Wilson et al., 2012).

Entrepreneurial/Intrapreneurial Success

Success is defined individually by attainment of professional goals. Successful APRNs cite a number of reasons for their entrepreneurial achievement:

the importance of acquired expertise and skill acquisition through education and consultation, identification of a professional mentor, and assistance from outside experts to provide necessary legal, financial, and business guidance as they embark on their innovative journey (Doerksen, 2010; Shirey, 2007). Exemplar 20.1 provides an example of APRN entrepreneurial success.

Intrapreneurship success is largely dependent on organizational environment and support (Dayhoff & Moore, 2003b). Removal of bureaucratic barriers, multidisciplinary support, access to resources, and organizational flexibility drive success of intrapreneurial initiatives (Dayhoff & Moore, 2003b). The American Association of Colleges of Nursing (AACN), in its publication *The Essentials of Doctoral Education for Advanced Nursing Practice* (AACN, 2006), emphasizes successful entrepreneurship/ intrapreneurship through organizational and systems leadership competencies as well as health care policy and interprofessional competencies. Attainment of entrepreneurial/intrapreneurial competencies provides nursing expertise in organizational assessment and facilitation of organization-wide changes in practice delivery (AACN, 2006). Utilizing political skills, systems thinking, and business analysis, DNP-prepared APRNs are prepared to excel in innovative practice settings. Examples of entrepreneurship/ intrapreneurship opportunities across the APRN competencies are provided in Table 20.1.

Challenges of Innovative Practice

Innovative practice arrangements are not without challenges. Factors contributing to difficulty with entrepreneurial and intrapreneurial practice include the APRN's perceived lack of business skills, especially in the areas of health care finance, legal and regulatory policies, and business operations (Johnson & Garvin, 2017; Shirey, 2007). Lack of formal educational preparation in traditional APRN master's programs has contributed to this lack of knowledge; however, with the recent move to DNP preparation across APRN roles, business and systems competencies have been addressed in the curriculum.

External forces creating larger systems challenges include organizational strategies that suppress intrapreneurial thinking and lack of APRN identification as a key stakeholder in the development of organizational, local, state, and national health policy. This has created a system of unequal partnership and contribution (Wilson et al., 2012). This particular challenge has led to lack of or limited APRN

EXEMPLAR 20.1   Clinical Nurse Specialist Consultant and Education Business: Making the Leap

Kathleen Vollman, MSN, RN, CCNS, FCCM, FAAN

Two journeys helped prepare me to launch a successful consultation and education business. The first involved my experience through my master's thesis work of designing, developing, and researching a device that helped position critically ill patients into the prone position (Vollman, 1999; Vollman & Bander, 1996). The clinical and business skills I developed in order to take an idea and bring it to market were completely transferable to intrapreneurial activities while serving as a CNS at a large urban medical center and then later when I launched the business full time (Vollman, 2004). While working as a CNS within the hospital, I was able to gather a wealth of knowledge and experience related to leadership, frontline and organizational change in large systems, lean technology, teamwork, and process management as well as a passion for creating safe work cultures that empower nurses to own their practice. During that time, I also reached out beyond the walls of the organization to share the success of our clinical project work on reducing infections and pressure injury and improving nurse retention. I wrote abstracts to present at local, regional, and national conferences alone and in partnership with staff nurses. I published articles within my areas of expertise. Through this work, I began to develop an international reputation for speaking and consulting on various pulmonary/critical care, reducing health care–acquired injury, and professional nursing topics. This help set the foundation for the development of an independent consultation and education business (Vollman, 2014). Prior to making the official leap to a completely independent business, I straddled the two worlds for 5 years. In 2003 I left my position at the hospital and launched Advancing Nursing, LLC, a company that creates empowered work environments for nurses through the acquisition of greater skills and knowledge to advance the profession of nursing.

In reality, my business parallels the CNS role within a hospital system. If the expectations are unrealistic, the ability of the person to achieve the expected outcomes is limited. Through my CNS journey, I had developed four areas of expertise that serve to guide the scope of the education and consultation product/service:

- Clinical critical care in care of pulmonary and septic patients
- "Back-to-basics" using evidence-based nursing care to prevent patient harm
- Care of the nurse and work environment
- CNS role development and entrepreneurship

In each of these a common thread exists. The goal and the vision for the business are to provide frontline nurses with the necessary knowledge, skills, and resources to enable them to advocate for their patients, the patients' families, and themselves and be fulfilled in their professional work. The next step was to set up the structure (Dayhoff & Moore, 2003a). The structure that best suited Advancing Nursing was a limited liability corporation, a hybrid legal structure that provides the limited liability features of a corporation and the tax efficiencies and operational flexibility of a partnership (Small Business Association, 2016). Once I received the submission document from the state that the business name was official, I set up a separate business checking account at the bank. Minimal capital was required for business start-up, and overhead was very low.

Development of a graphic representation of the business and communication strategies and creating a website were the next steps. Having developed the mission statement made designing the graphic image easier. The image is an inert triangle going from dark to lighter, representing growth as the nurse gains knowledge and skill to increase her or his personal power to take care of patients and advance the profession of nursing. For a business website, the web address is frequently the business name, but with an already established professional name it was easy to choose the domain: www.vollman.com.

One of the lessons learned in starting a business is the importance of networking and being comfortable in admitting your limitations. Through networking, I found someone like me but in the tech world who was just starting out and who helped me build the business website. Marketing was done by word of mouth, scientific publications, networking, and ensuring that someone could always connect with me to ask questions, to request a talk or visit, or to comment. As CNSs, we are taught to measure outcomes, and that is true in business as well. I measured both process components and outcomes in a variety of ways, including business growth (new clients), number of referrals, revenue versus expenses, invitations to speak, hits to the website, number of downloads, email follow-through, conference evaluations and posters, and individual clinician and organizational feedback.

One of the largest hurdles I had was determining fee structures for various activities. Determining your

Continued

Clinical Nurse Specialist Consultant and Education Business: Making the Leap—cont'd

worth and asking to be compensated for it is difficult for most nurses, myself included. My colleagues across the country were instrumental in this area because the information is not published anywhere. Through discussion with clinicians who were doing similar work nationally and internationally I was able to come up with a fee I was comfortable with and that was accepted well by customers. As the business grows, remember to increase your rates based on demand, success of your product/service, and what the market can bear.

There were some decisions I made early on. I chose not to be the continuing education provider. I prepare all the materials necessary but allow the inviting organization to take over all continuing education tasks.

I made a conscious decision to work with selected industry partners. Companies that I formed relationships with had products and services that supported the nurse's ability to perform evidence-based care in an effective and efficient manner. To help maintain life balance, 5 years into the business, I added a 2-day-a-week assistant to help manage invoices, accounting, article retrieval, and some additional activities.

I feel I am one of the most fortunate people in the world because I am living my dream and sharing my passion of evidence-based practice with other nurses and health care practitioners to make an impact in patients' lives. Take the risk of becoming an entrepreneur; you will never regret the journey. ◎

TABLE 20.1   Examples of Entrepreneurship/Intrapreneurship Activities Across the Advanced Practice Registered Nurse (APRN) Competencies

Entrepreneurship Activities		Intrapreneurship Activities	
Direct Clinical Practice	Nurse-owned primary care clinics, specialty ambulatory practice, birth centers Nurse-owned health screening company Nurse-owned telehealth company Interdisciplinary health care business ventures APRN-owned health care practices	Direct Clinical Practice	Development of nurse-triage and telemedicine services Development and implementation of group visits Nurse-managed chronic disease management clinics Transition care Development of interdisciplinary care teams Facilitation of research results into practice CRNA-managed anesthesia provider services CNM-managed antepartum services
Guidance and Coaching	Nurse-owned health promotion/disease prevention company Nurse-owned chronic disease management company Nurse-owned health coaching company Nurse-owned continuing education services	Guidance and Coaching	Development and implementation of health coaching programs, quality assurance programs Nurse-triage programs
Leadership	Nurse-owned businesses Development of new models of reimbursement for nursing care delivery APRN executive organizational leadership	Leadership	Use of informatics to develop and implement new models of care delivery Nurse-managed transitional care programs Development of nursing care policies Nurse-managed palliative care teams Development of organizational tele-ICU centers
Consultation	Wound care Health navigation Chronic disease management Gerontology Telehealth Advance care planning Legal nurse consultant APRN staffing businesses Nurse-midwifery consultants	Consultation	Nurse-led initiatives on quality and safety Clinical expert in area of specialization—examples: pain management, childbirth, lactation, regulatory issues

CNM, Certified nurse-midwife; *CRNA,* certified registered nurse anesthetist; *ICU,* intensive care unit.

recognition and reimbursement as an independent profession, a challenge that is particularly difficult when seeking funding for innovative health care delivery ideas.

Despite numerous challenges, new and experienced APRNs have risen to the challenge, providing necessary organizational and political leadership. As APRNs enter the world of innovative practice, they will find these opportunities more rewarding with careful attention to collegial working relationships, mentorship, and connectivity from seasoned APRN entrepreneurs and intrapreneurs and active participation in health care policy reform.

Marketing for the New APRN

Preparing the New APRN to Market Core Competencies

Graduates of accredited APRN programs are well prepared to market their detailed and often colorful recounting of clinical practicum and procedural portfolios attained during school as well as newly acquired national certification and state licensure. New graduates may find the less-recognized role competencies, such as guidance and coaching, consultation, leadership, collaboration, and ethical decision making, more difficult to market because many people outside of advanced practice nursing are not familiar with these broad APRN competencies (Spoelstra & Robbins, 2010). As described in Chapter 4, acquisition in each of the core competencies is crucial, with attention to documenting these experiences via a professional portfolio. A guided student self-reflection exercise designed to connect didactic and clinical practicum experiences to APRN role development provides documentation of competency acquisition (Latham & Fahey, 2006). Table 20.2 provides examples of educational activities new APRN graduates may highlight during the interview process with prospective employers or business investors. Marketing the unique skill set of the APRN will enable the applicant to stand out in an interview from other clinicians from different health care disciplines. Demonstrating the unique value of APRN care to a practice or organization is essential to a successful job search.

Professional Networking

Professional networking through membership in local, state, and national APRN organizations is of great benefit to APRNs seeking employment or to build a business. Many APRN education programs strongly recommend attendance at a local APRN role-specific meeting for social introduction into the profession, which begins well before graduation. A successful job search incorporates several active strategies and a strong personal organizational approach. Early reflection and identification of clinical strengths, work values and interests, and professional goals as well as personal areas for growth is crucial when considering various employment opportunities. As a preliminary step in a job search, it is crucial for each APRN to understand the market for his or her APRN role within the desired geographic employment area; researching potential employers' opportunities and hiring practices from their websites provides this vital initial information (Vilorio, 2011). In addition to online research of potential employers, a vital search strategy includes personal networking, from which professional relationships are built and which takes time. Networking with faculty, fellow students, and alumni at local, state, and national APRN events, in addition to networking with preceptors and clinicians during clinical rotations, residencies, fellowships, and volunteer opportunities, may lead the novice APRN to her or his first job as a new graduate or build a client base for the new entrepreneur. Vilorio reported that "Organizations tend to hire people they know or who are referred to them by someone they trust" (2011, p. 5) and often fill new positions before positions are publicized.

Career centers within APRN academic institutions offer additional assistance with the preparation of cover letters, résumés, and curricula vitae (CVs), as well as interview coaching. Local and regional employment opportunities for APRNs are commonly provided by local and state APRN organizations through webpages, electronic newsletters, and group email. Many of the national APRN organizations offer substantial career assistance to new, recently graduated, and seasoned APRNs. In addition to networking opportunities, these organizations offer national certification preparation resources, mentorship opportunities, scholarship information, online learning, salary surveys, and career resources, including job centers. Some of this information is publicly available and some requires student membership. Table 20.3 lists national APRN organizational websites pertaining to student and new graduate career resources.

Web-Based Resources

Web-based professional networking sites are available and routinely utilized by APRN recruiters, employers,

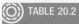 **TABLE 20.2   Advanced Practice Registered Nurse (APRN) Competencies With Associated Essentials to Highlight During an Interview**

APRN Core Competency	Essentials*	Educational Activities to Highlight During the Interview Process
Direct Clinical Practice	I, III, VI, VII, VIII	Population of patients seen during clinical rotations Number of patient encounters by level of complexity Diagnoses managed demonstrating application of evidence-based care Pharmacotherapeutics prescribed Referrals provided Procedures performed Variability of patient care settings appropriate to APRN role preparation Health promotion and disease prevention activities performed specific to APRN role APRN role-specific competencies related to direct clinical practice Entrepreneurship opportunities
Guidance and Coaching	IV, V, VI, VII, VIII	Anticipatory guidance activities Entrepreneurship/intrapreneurship opportunities Population-specific APRN-led patient education and monitoring programs (obesity management, pain management, diabetes management, family planning, etc.) Development and implementation of tailored patient education materials and programs Team-based care activities Group visit participation Motivational interviewing training and experience Transition care coordination and intervention activities Self-reflection through journal writing
Consultation	II, IV, V, VI, VII, VIII	Consultant role as clinical expert with other health care professionals (peers, nurses [entrepreneurs/intrapreneurs], physicians, allied health personnel) in setting where clinical experiences occur Consultation with expert clinicians with comanagement or referral to ensure positive patient outcome Team-based reflective practice training Telehealth consultation training and clinical experiences Development of legal/regulatory documents pertaining to consultation
Evidence-Based Practice	I, III, IV, V, VI, VII, VIII	Doctor of Nursing Practice or Capstone projects Clinical research activities, completed abstracts or proposals, completed literature reviews, projects/posters Evidence-based practice (EBP) presentations given pertinent to APRN role Examples of incorporating EBP in the clinical setting during educational program Practice guideline projects and presentations Projects demonstrating evaluation of clinical guidelines Clinical questions formulated to investigate when in practice
Leadership	II, IV, V, VI, VII, VIII	Entrepreneurship/intrapreneurship clinical practice experiences Group visit facilitation experience Project planning and management experiences Mentorship of other health professions students Formal and informal networking opportunities Active student membership on curricular or evaluation committees Membership on campus-wide student committees Policy development and implementation Podium and poster presentations Local, state, or national policy fellowships Student leadership roles in professional organizations Development of electronic educational materials/applications Patient advocacy activities

TABLE 20.2 Advanced Practice Registered Nurse (APRN) Competencies With Essentials—cont'd

APRN Core Competency	Essentials*	Educational Activities to Highlight During the Interview Process
Collaboration	II, IV, V, VI, VII, VIII	Development of legal/regulatory collaboration agreement documents if appropriate for state regulation
		Interprofessional case-based learning activities
		Interprofessional patient care clinical experiences
		Conflict negotiation and resolution workshops and activities
		Team-leading, team-building, and teamwork experiences
		Group visit experiences
Ethical Decision Making	I, II, IV, V, VI, VII, VIII	Demonstration of creating an ethical environment during the practicum experience
		Case-based ethics simulation activities reflective of the APRN role
		Reflective evaluation of clinical cases encountered in practicum
		Obtaining informed consent experiences
		Reporting of patient concerns to administration
		Student participation on institutional or academic ethics committees
		Integration of APRN role-specific Code of Ethics into APRN role
		Interprofessional educational experiences focusing on ethical decision making
		Participation in quality improvement activities during clinical practicum experiences
		Development of institutional review board protocols for research activities
		Local, state, and national patient advocacy activities pertaining to safety and patient rights

*Essentials as specified in American Association of Colleges of Nursing. (2006). The essentials of doctoral education for advanced nursing practice. Retrieved from http://www.aacn.nche.edu/publications/position/DNPEssentials.pdf.

TABLE 20.3 National Advanced Practice Registered Nurse (APRN) Organizations: Student Information

National Association/Organization	Main Webpage Address	Student Webpage Address
American Association of Nurse Anesthetists	http://www.aana.com/Pages/default.aspx	http://www.aana.com/ceandeducation/students/Pages/default.aspx
American Association of Nurse Practitioners	https://www.aanp.org/	https://www.aanp.org/education/student-resource-center
American College of Nurse-Midwives	http://www.midwife.org/	http://www.midwife.org/Midwifery-Students
National Association of Clinical Nurse Specialists	http://nacns.org/	All resources may be found on the main webpage
Gerontological Advanced Practice Nurses Association	https://www.gapna.org/	https://www.gapna.org/just-students
National Association of Pediatric Nurse Practitioners	https://www.napnap.org/	https://www.napnap.org/students
Nurse Practitioners in Women's Health	https://www.npwh.org/	All resources may be found on their main webpage
American Nurses Association	http://nursingworld.org/	http://www.nursingworld.org/EspeciallyForYou/AdvancedPracticeNurses/APRN-Education

and potential investors. Approximately 85% of employers report that online profiles influence hiring decisions (University of California, Irvine, 2016b), and thus APRN students are well advised to review their personal social media to ensure content such as profiles, images, and communication reflect professional values. All profile pictures should be presentable and photographs that may not reflect

these values should be "untagged" (University of California, Irvine, 2016b). Preparation of an electronic professional profile, such as a LinkedIn profile, is a great resource for APRN students as well as experienced APRNs. Although business networking sites have numerous similar functions, the advanced job search feature on LinkedIn allows the professional to search by function, geographic area, organizational

TABLE 20.4	Web-Based Networking Resources for Advanced Practice Registered Nurses

Web-Based Resources	Link
LinkedIn A networking tool to find connections to recommended job candidates, industry experts, and business partners	https://www.linkedin.com/
MedMasters A comprehensive professional networking and career management site for the medical community	http://medmasters.com/
Monster Source for career opportunities nationwide	http://www.monster.com/
For Entrepreneurs **National Nurses in Business Association**	https://nnbanow.com
NP Business Development NP business blog and podcast	http://barbaracphillips.com/home/
Nurse Entrepreneur Network Business solutions for nurse entrepreneurs	http://www.nurse-entrepreneur-network.com/

level, and industry, leveraging employment and entrepreneurial opportunities with online and mobile application capability (Fertig, 2012). With faculty guidance and peer review, students and new entrepreneurs can promote the ideal job they are seeking or business they are marketing while providing a professional profile highlighting unique skills, expertise, experience, and education. This LinkedIn profile allows recruiters, potential employers, and investors looking for specific skills to easily find a suitable candidate (Fertig, 2012). This activity allows an APRN to build a professional network and provides marketing opportunities in one place that have lasting value. Table 20.4 provides a list of social networking sites for professionals, entrepreneurs, and business owners.

Professional Recruiters

Utilizing a professional recruiter who is well versed in APRN practice is another avenue to ensure a successful job search. APRNs may enlist the services of a recruiter for assistance in finding a position or may be contacted by a recruiter who is searching for qualified candidates. In either case, the recruiter fees are typically paid by the employing agency.

Networking through LinkedIn or other professional networking websites will provide an opportunity for recruiters looking for specific APRN qualifications to quickly pull together a pool of prospective employees. An APRN may be directly contacted by an internal recruiter, an external recruiting agency or temporary staffing agency, or an executive "headhunter." Regardless of the type, these recruiters are paid by the employer typically when and if they refer the candidate who gets hired. Although professional recruiters have an interest in the interviewee's success, they may have a greater interest in the practice for which they are recruiting. After all, the recruiter or recruiting agency is paid based on a percentage of the annual salary of the recruited individual and the number of candidates placed within a practice.

Some of the advantages of enlisting a recruiter for a job search include the fact that these professionals are generally well connected and may have job opportunities that are not published. They typically understand the organizational culture, patient volumes, population, and expectations of the practice or organization and can provide valuable information in preparation to the interviewee. Regardless of whether the APRN seeks the services of a recruiter or a recruiter approaches an APRN for a position, recruiters and recruiting agencies decide which candidates to put forward for interviews, which may result in missing out on opportunities for those who do not use recruiters. The recruiter may be expected to spend time vetting interviewee qualifications through behavior-based interview questions and clinical-based queries, as well as verification of current certificates, licenses, and privileges, before presenting candidates to a potential employer.

Communication

Expert written and communication skills are vitally important whether conducting a job search or pitching a business proposition or organizational innovation. Business and recruitment experts recommend utilizing a cover letter regardless of the route of communication, including electronic mail; failure to do so may be viewed as unprofessional (Gallo, 2014). The tone of all communication must remain professional at all times (Arndt & Coleman, 2014). Before corresponding with a potential employer, a thorough analysis of the mission and purpose of the organization, including its leadership, must be undertaken (Gallo, 2014). Methods of communicating one's expertise, introduced in a cover letter, may

BOX 20.2   Template Cover Letter

May 19, 2016

Name & Address of Company

I am a (university) educated certified registered nurse anesthetist (or recent graduate of a CRNA program at [university]). I am writing in response to the CRNA position recently posted through the California Association of Nurse Anesthetists website. The skills and experience I gained through my clinical education as a CRNA, as well as my experience as a CRNA in a Level 1 Trauma Center in Southern California and as a critical care registered nurse, will enable me to provide both comprehensive and quality anesthesia care to patients at your outpatient surgical center.

I am also an ACLS instructor and have taught this content to a range of intraprofessional specialists. My experience as first an ICU nurse and then a CRNA provided the opportunity to work on or lead interdisciplinary teams. I have become a very effective team member of all health care teams that I work on. I believe that interprofessional practice offers the highest quality health care.

Thank you for your time and consideration in review of my qualifications. I look forward to hearing from you.

Signature

Contact information

Adapted from University of California, San Francisco, Office of Career & Professional Development. (2013). Advanced practice nurse job search. Retrieved from http://career.ucsf.edu/sites/career.ucsf.edu/files/PDF/NuringAPNJobSearchHandout.pdf.

include a professional portfolio comprising multiple documents, such as a résumé or CV.

Cover Letters

Cover letters typically contain detailed information describing why the applicant is qualified for the position, providing an explanation of interest in the specific organization and identification of relevant skills or experiences the applicant possesses. Business experts agree it is important to briefly emphasize personal value to the organization and limit the letter to one page (Gallo, 2014). This is not the format to restate items described in the résumé or CV but rather to highlight relevant experiences. Cover letters are typically sent via electronic mail or uploaded as a document within an electronic application. The literature describes cover letters as referral letters or query letters. *Referral letters* include the individual who referred the applicant to the practice or organization. Referral bonuses may be overlooked if the potential employer is not aware that a referral has been made. *Inquiry (query) letters* typically accompany a résumé and can be sent to organizations or practices that may be hiring but have not advertised a formal job opening. Inquiry letters contain information on why the company is of interest and why the APRN's skills and experience would be assets to the organization. Inquiry letters allow the APRN to expand on his or her CV by focusing on a few qualifications, using specific examples, and forming a connection between past experience and the position. APRN applicants have to convey why they are motivated to apply for this position and how

they will fit in with, and what value they will uniquely bring to, the organization. Box 20.2 provides an example of a cover letter; however, a simple electronic search will yield many excellent examples.

Professional Portfolio

A professional portfolio is an electronic presentation of an APRN's qualifications and accomplishments. An electronic professional portfolio is often compiled during the APRN program and maintained after graduation, building content as professional opportunities and skills are attained. The portfolio serves to educate prospective employers on the APRN role, scope of practice, and impact on patient outcomes and cost savings, while providing evidence of the individual's professional knowledge, skills, expertise, experience, accomplishments, and scholarly work (Beauvais, 2016). When professionally presented, the portfolio highlights the APRN's potential contribution to the organization, providing a strong base for negotiation (Hespenheide, Cottingham, & Mueller, 2011). A portfolio differs from a CV in that a portfolio houses multiple documents, including a résumé or CV, necessary to communicate the APRN's qualifications. Box 20.3 provides a basic list of the documents to be included in a portfolio. An electronic link to the portfolio can be sent to a potential employer prior to the interview.

Résumés and Curricula Vitae

A curriculum vitae (which means "course of life" in Latin) or a résumé, which is often submitted with a cover letter, is usually the first introduction and

---

BOX 20.3 Components of a Professional Portfolio

- Curriculum vitae and/or résumé
- Biographical sketch or professional introduction
- Professional development and educational activities
- Clinical practice/practicum experience
- Competencies and evaluations
- Pertinent statutes and regulations
- Role-specific professional scope of practice and standards of care

- Collaborative practice agreements (if required)
- Reimbursement guidelines
- Color copies of professional license(s), certifications, diplomas, certificates, awards, Drug Enforcement Agency (DEA) registration, national provider identifier (NPI) registration
- Scholarly work: publications, papers, abstracts, presentations, posters, etc.
- References

BOX 20.4 Components of a Résumé (1 Page, Double-Sided Maximum)

- **Contact information:** name, degree, license, certifications, email address, phone number with area code (top of page)
- **Summary of Qualifications:** specific, meaningful description of the type of position desired (optional)
- **Education:** Postsecondary only; name of school, major, degree received, graduation date (or projected), honors. Be sure to put graduation date and month because credentialing committees need it to verify degrees
- **Experience:** Describe using action verbs. Job title for all paid, volunteer, or internship positions; emphasize duties/responsibilities, skills, abilities, significant/relevant achievements; quantify accomplishments; include job title, employing organization, dates

of employment (month & year). Avoid listing nonmedical work experience; avoid complete sentences, abbreviations, or acronyms, and do not begin phrases with "I"; avoid medical abbreviations; do not list unrelated, detailed duties or controversial activities or associations
- **Licensure and National Certification:** with expiration dates for states in which a license was held (current, inactive, or expired); avoid listing numbers
- **Professional Memberships or Affiliations:** Optional
- **Other Skills:** Bilingual/multilingual (list all languages); proficiency in electronic medical record (EMR) platforms if pertinent; advanced skills: suturing, casting, first assist, etc.
- **References:** "Available upon request"

---

provides the first impression to a prospective employer.

Described as a marketing document in which the hiring agency is the buyer and the APRN is the product, a *résumé* is a concise introduction of education, experiences, and career-related skills, tailored to a specific job opportunity (Lees, 2013). A résumé typically begins with a short summary of the candidate and why the candidate is the right person for the job. Experts recommend emphasizing accomplishments over responsibilities as a technique in creating a résumé that stands out. Although various types of résumés exist, a document that concisely combines both the chronology of the APRN's work history and the applicant's unique skills and strengths targeted to the employer is recommended (CAREER-wise Education, 2016). Box 20.4 provides a detailed description of the components of a résumé.

A *curriculum vitae* is a document in longer format typically used by those searching for academic, research, or executive leadership positions that require a more comprehensive review of qualifications. Without a page limitation, the CV provides a detailed review of a person's professional accomplishments over a lifetime, listed in reverse chronologic order and added to throughout her or his career. With components similar to a résumé, the CV adds experiences such as research, teaching, mentoring, professional activities, professional memberships, publications, presentations, honors, and awards. Preparing a comprehensive CV from which a concise résumé can be adapted for individual employment opportunities is advisable. Potential employers or interested clients will indicate whether they require a CV or résumé to be provided with the initial application. Box 20.5 describes the components of a CV.

⊙ BOX 20.5 Components of a Curriculum Vitae (No Page Limitation)

- **Personal Data:** Contact information: name, degree (highest degree in each discipline), license, certifications, email address, phone number with area code
- **Education:** name of schools, major/minor, degree received, graduation date (or projected), honors; may also include title of dissertation or DNP project here, including university and date
- **Professional Experience:** date, position, institution/city/state
- **Academic Experience:** date, position, course number, course description, institution/city/state; Additional education/training including title/institution/city/state
- **Professional Certification:** APRN national certification, certifying organization, expiration date
- **Professional Licensure:** RN and/or APRN license, state (list all), expiration date; Controlled substances (state and DEA), state, expiration date
- **Awards and Honors:** Date, award, organization
- **Professional Activities:** Organization name, role, date
- **Consultations:** Date, organization, city/state, description
- **Expert Panel Validation Member:** Name, date, title, city/state, organization

- **Peer Reviewed Journal Articles:** American Psychological Association (APA) or other publication format; the name of the person who is the subject of the CV should be emphasized in bold print
- **Book Chapters/Editor:** APA or other publication format
- **Newsletter Editor/Author:** Organization newsletters with date, volume number, issue number and title
- **Peer Reviewer**
- **Published Commentaries**
- **Published Abstracts**
- **Grants:** date, name of program, funding source, amount, primary investigator name credentials, name funded %
- **Research:** title, role, date, awarded name organization
- **Presentations:** date, title, name conference/event, location, city/state
- **Committee Work:** institution, dates, role, name of committee
- **Program Coordination:** date, university, title of program, role
- **Community Volunteer Work:** dates, name of organization, project, title/role

Adapted from National Association of Pediatric Nurse Practitioners. (n.d.). Sample PNP CV. Retrieved from http://www.napnapcareerguide.com/sample-pnp-cv/.

Interview Process

There are many types of job interviews and, depending upon the practice, group, or organization APRNs choose to work for, they may experience one or more types of interviews during their job search. The interview is an opportunity both for the employer or business to get to know the prospective employee and for the candidate to ask important questions about information unavailable through general job postings and exploration. It is vital that a new APRN is empowered to interview the prospective employer and demonstrates active participation in the process (Kador, 2010). Failure to ask questions during the interview may give the impression that a candidate lacks interest, may not ask questions once hired, or worse, may accept a position that is a bad fit for the APRN (Warner, 2011). Box 20.6 and Box 20.7 provide examples of questions to be prepared for as well

as questions to ask potential employers. Questions related to contracts, salary negotiation, malpractice insurance, on-call responsibility, reimbursement, and billing are discussed later in this chapter.

One-on-one interviews are the most common, in which the candidate is interviewed by one person who represents the employer and who will ask questions of the candidate and, more importantly, provide an opportunity for the APRN to ask questions about the culture and the company. *Telephone interviews* may occur initially and are held with a recruiter or manager of a practice. Some of the advantages to this type of interview include the ability to refer to notes and talking points; the disadvantages include the inability to see and interpret body language and facial expressions. If English is a second language for the candidate or interviewer, it may be difficult for them to understand each other over the phone. *Video interviews* are a recent trend

BOX 20.6   Types of Interview Questions and Strategies

Open-Ended Questions: Assess motivation, training, skills, and experiences
- *Example:* "Why should we hire you?"
- *Strategy:* Summarize relevant training, experience, and skills in 2 minutes.

Behavior-Based Questions: Based on premise that past behavior is a predictor of future performance; ask for an example of a particular situation you handled or skill you used
- *Example:* "Tell me about a time when you disagreed with a professional colleague on a course of treatment and how it got resolved."
- *Example:* "Tell me about a time when you did or said something that had a negative impact on a customer, peer, or direct report. How did you know the impact was negative?"
- *Strategy:* Give a SHARE Model® response (see Box 20.9).

General Questions: Frequently asked in an interview

- *Example:* "How do you handle conflict?"
- *Example:* "Tell me about a situation when you discovered that you were on the wrong course. How did you know? What did you do? What, if anything, did you learn from the experience?"
- *Strategy:* Give an example demonstrating your approach to handling a situation.

Hypothetical Questions: A vignette common in the practice/organization presented to assess how well you solve problems
- *Strategy:* Give a SHARE Model® response.

Clinical Questions: General or open-ended questions about a particular clinical experience or a vignette aimed at assessing your problem-solving skills
- *Strategy:* Discuss your thought process, the questions you would ask, investigation/ exploration of the situation you would conduct, and how you might present the case to a more experienced clinician.

Adapted from Bielaszka-DuVernay, C. (2008). Hiring for emotional intelligence. *Harvard Business Review*. Retrieved from https://hbr.org/2008/11/hiring-for-emotional-intellige; and University of California, San Francisco, Office of Career & Professional Development. (2013). Advanced practice nurse job search. Retrieved from http://career.ucsf.edu/sites/career.ucsf.edu/files/PDF/NuringAPNJobSearchHandout.pdf.

utilizing web-based technology to screen and interview a candidate from a distance. Although similar to an in-person interview, unique points to consider include technologic availability and location, including clarifying the time zone for the scheduled interview time. Candidates will be notified if this type of interview will be conducted and typically provided instructions on the software installation in advance. Web-based platforms such as Skype or Adobe Connect are easy to install and operate. Candidates should ensure that the software and web camera are installed and tested ahead of time. Candidates should also consider the reliability of their Internet connection and ensure a clean, quiet interview location free of distraction and interruption. Box 20.8 provides important reminders for interviewees.

Committee or panel interviews are common in APRN practice and allow an opportunity for the employer to observe how candidates respond in a team scenario. A group of providers, administrators, and staff will typically take turns asking questions. Eye contact by the APRN with all panel members is important during this process. In academic settings,

the APRN might be asked to interview with a group during a meal; although less formal, it is still an interview.

Second interviews are common in the health care profession. This interview may take place in the unit or office where the candidate would be assigned and can take up a significant portion of the day. A series of interviews with various executives, administrators, and health care providers should be anticipated. Second interviews are a further indication that the company is interested in hiring the candidate.

Preparation for the Interview

Interview preparation is essential. An APRN's self-reflection on his or her strengths, weaknesses, interests, deal breakers, and career goals will prepare him or her for initial, basic interview questions. An APRN should prepare three to five copies of her or his résumé or CV, a copy of her or his transcript and diploma, a reference list, and a professional portfolio with an electronic link (or thumb drive). A notebook with a list of questions is helpful in guiding the question-and-answer period of the

BOX 20.7   Questions to Ask in an Interview

General Questions

- Is this an employee or an independent contractor position?
- Has the organization hired an APRN in this position in the past?
- What would a typical day/week be like for the candidate? Is overtime expected?
- How will the selected candidate's performance be evaluated? Is there a formal process? What constitutes success in this position?
- What is the orientation process at your organization? Are there scaled productivity requirements or transition-to-practice expectations?
- How would you describe the level of autonomy you expect from APRNs in this practice/at this institution?
- What are some changes and challenges you have seen here in the past year, and what are some changes and challenges you forecast in the next year?
- How would you describe the culture and management style of the organization?
- Are there prospects for growth and advancement?
- Is continuing education compensated or reimbursed?
- What are the next steps in the process?

Practice- or Position-Specific Questions:

- How is productivity measured in this practice setting?
- What electronic medical record program is utilized at this facility? Is there on-site technical assistance following orientation to the program?

- Will the candidate for this position see overflow patients or be expected to develop his/her own panel of patients?
- Is relief provided during extended surgical procedures (CRNA-specific)?
- Does this position have call or after-hours responsibilities?
- What training, support, or mentorship can I expect during the first year with this organization?
- Who will I be assigned to as a supervising or collaborating physician or APRN (if required by state regulation)?
- Will the candidate be employed or paid during the credentialing and privileging process? If so, what responsibilities will the candidate have during that time?
- How long does the credentialing and privileging process take? When would you expect the candidate to begin patient care responsibilities?
- What is the process to implement initiative ideas for improvement?
- What is the reporting structure?
- Will there be staff that report to an APRN?
- How will my services be marketed within the organization?
- What are some of the leadership opportunities for this position?
- Is there ability to infuse evidence into practice? What is the process?
- Ethical dilemmas: how are they named and handled?

NOTE: Questions related to benefits and salaries are typically discussed during the negotiation phase of the job search process.

Adapted from Buppert, C. (2014). 20 questions to ask a prospective employer. *The Journal for Nurse Practitioners, 10*(1), 62-63; Konop, J. (2014). The 10 questions you should be asking a potential employer. *Huff/Post 50*. Retrieved from http://www.huffingtonpost.com/2014/06/21/interview-questions-to-ask-employer_n_5492147.html; University of California, San Francisco, Office of Career & Professional Development. (2011). APN employment interviewing. Retrieved from https://career.ucsf.edu/sites/career.ucsf.edu/files/PDF/NursingAPNinterviewing.pdf; and Warner, S. (2011). Interview the employer. *Advance Healthcare Network*. Retrieved from http://nurse-practitioners-and-physician-assistants.advanceweb.com/Features/Articles/Interview-the-Employer.aspx.

interview (University of California, Irvine Career Center, 2016a).

The résumé or CV will provide evidence of APRN role-specific direct practice competencies by documenting licensure and certification. In addition to these competencies, health care executives and administrators are also interested in one's ability to self-regulate, work well in teams, and be an effective communicator. Emotional intelligence—the ability

to be aware of one's own feelings and to read accurately the emotions of others—emerges during the interview process and can be confirmed during reference checking. Research suggests that the top 10 skills perceived to be most important to business executives include integrity, communication, courtesy, responsibility, social skills, positive attitude, professionalism, flexibility, teamwork, and work ethic (Robles, 2012). APRNs can exemplify these

BOX 20.8   Tips for a Successful Interview

- Treat all staff members with respect before, during, and after the interview.
- Speak confidently.
- Be prepared with questions for which you are not able to obtain answers from researching other sources.
- Summarize your relevant skills and restate your interest at the end of the interview.
- Ask about next steps and contact information.
- Alert your references that they may be contacted.

- In-Person Interviews:
  - Arrive early with your cell phone silenced.
  - Dress in business attire regardless of the setting or culture.
  - Be prepared with copies of your résumé/curriculum vitae.
- Phone/Video Interviews:
  - Ensure a reliable, hands-free connection.
  - Conduct the interview alone in a quiet place.

Adapted from University of California, Irvine Career Center. (2016). Types of interviews. Retrieved from http://www.career.uci.edu/docs/students/Types-of-Interviews.pdf.

skills by preparing for interview questions in advance. Interview questions designed to elicit information on the applicant's emotional intelligence include questions about one's self-awareness and self-regulation, the ability to recognize the impact of one's behavior on others, and the ability to learn from mistakes (Bielaszka-DuVernay, 2008). Box 20.6 provides sample questions designed to identify those with high emotional intelligence.

The APRN can be asked behavioral and technical or clinical skills questions during the interview. Technical skills will center on the APRN role and response to common clinical scenarios. Behavior-based questions in an APRN interview will focus on interpersonal and communications skills. Preparing for the interview should include reflection on situations in which the APRN has experience with conflict resolution (patients and coworkers), working with team members, intrapreneurial experience (i.e., developing and implementing innovative solutions and practices), leadership abilities, stressful or difficult decision making, nursing philosophy or approach, project management skills, learning curve, and personal motivation (University of California, San Francisco, Office of Career & Professional Development, 2011; University of California, Irvine Career Center, 2016a). The SHARE Model® described in Box 20.9 provides a strategy for answering behavior-based and hypothetical questions. With practice, the APRN candidate can demonstrate and highlight competencies unique to the APRN profession during the interview.

Demonstrating the Value of APRN Care

The core of the nursing profession, the human caring relationship with attention to human experiences and environments (American Nurses Association,

BOX 20.9   SHARE Model®

1. Describe a *specific* **S**ituation.
2. Identify **H**indrances or challenges.
3. Explain the **A**ction taken.
4. Discuss the **R**esults or outcome.
5. **E**valuate or summarize what was learned.

Adapted from Mayo Clinic. (n.d.). Preparing for an interview. Retrieved from http://www.mayoclinic.org/jobs/how-to-apply/preparing-for-interview.

2010), distinguishes APRN care from that of other health care providers. Articulating the value of APRN care within the context of a distinct model of care, as described in Chapter 2, is essential when interviewing for a new APRN position. Describing how the APRN will contribute to access, patient satisfaction, improved quality, and enhanced safety within the practice setting will set the APRN apart from other health care professions. In addition to the humanistic contribution to patient care, productivity and outcomes are important metrics in demonstrating value to practice. A new graduate's productivity will grow rapidly over the first year, and understanding how a potential employer defines productivity is essential. Value to a health care practice or organization is multifaceted and is not strictly a measure of volume but also involves complex payor reimbursement calculations tailored to the health care setting (Rhoads, Ferguson, & Langford, 2006). The candidate should ask the interviewer how productivity and value are measured in the organization for the specific APRN role.

The APRN should review, identify, and select a few recent role-specific resources to be included in her or his portfolio, demonstrating APRN-specific outcomes and emphasizing whole-person, nursing-focused care.

An important systematic review of APRN outcomes to read and discuss with potential employers is a sentinel article by Newhouse and colleagues (2011). In addition, the *APRN Reading List*, containing research and published reports on quality, safety, and cost-effectiveness outcomes of APRN care, is compiled and updated by the National Council of State Boards of Nursing (2016). The candidate should be prepared to discuss how the APRN role provides complementary and value-added resources to the care provided by the health care team. Finally, the candidate should avoid delivering a message that the APRN role is "better than" another health care provider role. As Newhouse et al. (2011) suggested, APRNs in certain roles have better outcomes in certain areas than providers trained in a separate health discipline, but conveying that an APRN is better than another type of provider may be distasteful and might result in a lost job opportunity. Referring to other members of the health care team with a great deal of respect is imperative.

Negotiation and Renegotiation

The process of negotiation begins in the initial interview, although it is rare to ask for specific items,

including salary, at this time. A candidate should consider the interview process as a time to gather information about the organization. By the end of the interview process, the APRN should ensure a clear understanding of the employment or independent contractor arrangement; the scope of the job; the organization, management, and the direct work team; an idea of the salary and benefits; opportunities for professional growth; and how this job meets short- and long-term goals (University of California, San Francisco, Office of Career & Professional Development, 2013). Negotiations may occur informally, initially, with discussion of each party's needs and desires through in-person meetings and/or telephone or email correspondence.

Once a formal written offer is received, the APRN should take an agreed-upon time to consider all aspects of the offer, paying close attention to concerning clauses. Box 20.10 describes concerning elements to consider when negotiating a new agreement or contract. The Office of Career & Professional Development at the University of California, San Francisco (2013) recommends selecting two aspects of the offer to negotiate, starting with the most important aspect first. When negotiating points for the contract, the APRN candidate should provide

---

BOX 20.10   Contract and Negotiation Red Flags

- Negative discussion about the organization or employees during the interview process
- Hesitation or refusal by the employer or organization to provide an employment contract or written agreement
- Lack of reasonable amount of time to review contract or pressure to accept a job offer on the spot
- Financial penalties for leaving the organization or practice
- Lack of mentorship for new APRN
- Lack of APRN recognition on/in marketing materials
- Collaboration/supervision fees
- "Incident-to" billing of services for APRN care
- Lack of understanding of the APRN role
- "Noncompetition (no-compete)" clause: legal and enforceable in some but not all states; a promise not to compete or practice in the APRN role, during or after employment; may include restrictions from practicing within specialty, within a geographic area, within a

certain time frame (during and after the employee leaves the business); must be "reasonable," or acceptable by a judge if the clause were questioned in litigation (Buppert, 2008a, 2015).
  - If required and the employment opportunity is necessary or desired, may negotiate something of value in return
- "Termination without cause" clause: allows the employer to terminate the employee any time with 30-day notice (Buppert, 2008a, 2015); defeats the purpose of a contract; no job security
  - Employers are less likely to delete this clause
  - Ensure termination of contract circumstances are clearly stated
- Nonsolicitation provisions: prohibit former employees from soliciting patients or remaining employees when the provider leaves the practice/business
- Supervision requirements in a full practice authority state

a brief rationale for the request, explaining the candidate's understanding of the current offer and then asking for what the candidate wants, avoiding an apologetic tone. A period of "residency" or "transition" is one potential important area for negotiation. As a new clinician or an experienced clinician moving into a new clinical area, it is likely that productivity as defined by the employer may be lower with time built in to orient to the organization and systems. Negotiating ongoing expert clinical mentorship and possibly a reduced workload for a defined period is a reasonable and important request,

with evidence suggesting optimal transition to the new role (Davis, Little, & Thornton, 1997; Hill & Sawatzky, 2011). Exemplar 20.2 provides case study examples of the importance of mentorship during a new APRN role transition.

In an employment contract, the salary and compensation package typically includes benefits that add value of up to 30% to 40% of the salary (University of California, San Francisco, Office of Career & Professional Development, 2013). The methodology for determining pay structure may be an hourly rate, a straight salary, a percentage of net receipts, or a

---

EXEMPLAR 20.2   New Graduate Nurse Anesthesia Mentorship

Karyn Karp, MS, CRNA

Newly graduated registered nurse anesthetists (RNAs) are required to meet, and typically exceed, minimum numbers of practice experiences in general and specialty anesthetics for patients of every age group and acuity presenting with multiple combinations of coexisting diseases. However, certified registered nurse anesthetist (CRNA) staffing varies widely among health care facilities, ranging from a solo anesthesia practitioner, to operating practitioner (surgeon) supervision, to full medical direction by anesthesiologists.

California has been fortunate to have a long tradition of autonomous practice by nurse anesthetists, who led the nation in 1936 by proving that anesthesia is the practice of nursing as well as the practice of medicine in the Supreme Court of California. Should a new graduate RNA, or only experienced CRNAs, practice in an "independent" setting? A host of factors should be considered carefully before making this decision. Anesthesia services are provided in a range of settings that vary widely, even in health care facilities in the same locale. Important questions to ask involve the ability, clinical experience, and confidence of the RNA provider; the type and size of the facility and its staffing, equipment, and resources; and resources available in the immediate area and the community at large. It is critical to consider how many providers make up the anesthesiology department and who will be present and/or available for backup when procedures are scheduled as well as during on-call hours. Patient demographics and surgical service type and caseload are also important as well as whether the RNA possesses enough experience to administer specialty services competently.

Consider the following real-life case examples that occurred over a 3-month period in a designated Critical

Access Hospital (CAH) and Level IV trauma center offering multiple services, including obstetric and pediatric care. The facility experienced difficulty in attracting qualified, experienced CRNA providers due to its remote location and limited resources. A new graduate RNA was contracted to provide anesthesia services. In the following cases, the senior CRNA was outside the facility on backup call, serving as a mentor to the RNA.

Case 1, Obstetric anesthesia consult: A 39-year-old, gravida 7, para 4, parturient was referred by a family practice physician for an anesthesia consult at 35 weeks' gestation, calculated from estimated delivery date at 40 weeks. The patient was 59.5 inches tall and weighed 432 pounds (196 kg); body mass index (BMI) was 62.9 and met the criteria for super morbid obesity (BMI > 60). Prepregnancy weight was 409 pounds. Examination revealed a Mallampati class II airway (partial view of uvula and soft palate) and inability to palpate lumbar landmarks or iliac crests bilaterally due to a thick fat layer. The patient was prescribed glyburide for type A2 gestational diabetes mellitus, with poor compliance. She received a continuous labor epidural for a prior spontaneous vaginal delivery with documented difficult placement and had a prior cesarean section for arrested fetal descent due to macrosomia with a 12-pound infant. When questioned about anesthetic complications, the patient stated, "The epidural just made me itch." She had complained of terrible, unabated pain during labor and her cesarean section. Should the patient be permitted to have her baby at the CAH hospital?

| EXEMPLAR 20.2 | New Graduate Nurse Anesthesia Mentorship—cont'd |

Case 2, General surgery anesthesia consult: A male patient, age 82, with a history of hypertension, coronary artery disease with anterior myocardial infarction, chronic microcytic anemia, and chronic obstructive pulmonary disease was scheduled for a complex colectomy for colon cancer. The RNA had excellent experiences delivering neuraxial postoperative pain techniques for multiple patients managed in the intensive care units of community hospitals and had placed over 100 arterial lines and 30 central lines. Should the patient receive his surgery at the CAH?

Case 3, Pediatric patient, status post fall: A male patient, age 6, with no prior medical or surgical history was brought to the emergency department (ED) after a 20-foot fall from a treehouse. Pupils were round, equal, and reactive to light. The patient appeared to respond appropriately to questions but was crying, restless, and inconsolable, complaining of pain where his head was hit. He also had a deep, 6-inch leg wound and would not permit any examination; the ED physician believed it should be sutured. Should the CRNA provide sedation or anesthesia so the ED physician can examine and suture the patient's leg wound?

The new graduate RNA considered providing anesthesia for the general surgery and pediatric patients, while the parturient was referred to an alternative facility to deliver her baby. However, after consulting with the senior CRNA, both the general surgery and pediatric patients were referred to a higher level facility for care.

The CAH floor nursing staff was not familiar with the epidural management of postoperative pain. If the colectomy patient were to require postoperative ventilation in the two-bed intensive care unit for any reason, it is unknown whether experienced nursing staff would be available to care for the ventilator, an indwelling epidural, or invasive monitoring. The pediatric patient was transferred via Life Flight to a university medical center 60 miles away for a referral to the neurosurgery department.

The parturient surprised everyone by coming into the CAH in active labor dilated to 8 cm. Under the Emergency Medical Treatment and Active Labor Act (EMTALA), the definition of an emergency medical condition includes a pregnant woman having contractions, and transfer of an unstable emergency medical condition from another hospital is a violation of the law. The patient requested a labor epidural. After several unsuccessful attempts, the RNA called the backup CRNA; the patient required a 6-inch epidural needle to place the block. A shoulder dystocia and thick meconium were present at delivery. The CRNA and RNA successfully intubated and resuscitated the neonate. The mother experienced a postpartum hemorrhage requiring 14 units of blood products, which exhausted the local blood bank supply.

These cases illustrate the unique challenge of providing independent anesthesia services and the clear advantage appropriate mentorship provides to new graduate RNAs, their patients, and the facilities in which they practice. Strengths and attributes of the RNA provider, the health care facility, and its resources, location, and setting all have important consequences for the new graduate and should be considered carefully when selecting an initial practice location. ◎

---

base salary plus percentage (Buppert, 2015). Some employers or organizations may base the salary on a pay range developed by the organization commensurate with experience, or provide an open offer. APRNs are familiar with hourly and straight salary methods of payment, but they may find their contract written with either payment based on percentage of net receipts or a base salary plus a percentage of net receipts (Buppert, 2015). When salary is based on a percentage of net receipts, the salary calculation is based on the amount billed for the APRN service, minus the amount received from the payor and the practice expenses for the APRN (Buppert, 2015). Each APRN should understand the local salary range

for his or her APRN role prior to asking for flexibility in salary. Highlighting APRN core competencies that may exceed expectations of the role and will immediately add value to the setting is essential when negotiating salary, benefits, and work environment. Some contracts will offer bonuses, and the criteria for calculating bonuses vary greatly. Buppert (2015) described four types of bonus formulas: productivity based, quality based, profit based, and patient satisfaction based. If a bonus is offered in the employment contract, the APRN must be sure there is a clear understanding of how the bonus will be calculated, realized, and paid. Evidence-based salary negotiation tips offered by Deepak Malhotra, a Harvard Business

School professor, recommend the following (Gallo, 2015):

- Be prepared to answer a potential employer's question regarding salary expectations and to justify your rationale if there is a significant difference.
- Research what other providers are making in similar institutions and be prepared to ask questions that would be helpful in determining a fair salary.
- Once an offer is made, inquire about what went into calculating the figure.
- Avoid making threats; come prepared with collaborative and creative ideas and a rationale for your perceived worth.
- Consider the overall package, including responsibilities, location, flexibility in work hours, opportunities for growth and promotion, support for continued education and mentorship, bonus opportunities, and tuition reimbursement.

When renegotiating a compensation package, the experienced APRN must clearly articulate, with supporting data, her or his organizational and financial contributions in the past year. The professional portfolio provides a place to document and store data demonstrating excellence in practice, clinical leadership, and personal and professional development (Hespenheide et al., 2011). Data such as patient encounters/visits, individual billing and reimbursement data specific to payor mix, quality metrics, administrative responsibilities, projects, leadership opportunities, patient satisfaction surveys, continuing education, and competency verification can be included for showcase during renegotiation. A wise APRN negotiator will be able to articulate both his or her financial contribution and his or her expenses (salary, benefits, continuing education, overhead, etc.) to the practice. APRNs should begin collecting these data as soon as they begin their new job so they are prepared for renegotiation during the periodic review.

In a recent randomized, controlled field experiment conducted in Australia, Leibbrandt and List (2015) found that when potential employees are explicitly told that salary or pay is negotiable, both women and men negotiate equally for a higher wage. In contrast, when salary determination is ambiguous, men are more likely to negotiate for a higher wage and women are more likely to express willingness to work for lower pay. To avoid gender discrepancy in salary negotiations, the APRN should ask if the salary is negotiable early in the negotiation phase

of the interview process. The entrepreneurial environment is unique with respect to negotiation of fees for work as a consultant. Development of the consultant's contract and fee proposal, including terms and conditions for payment, must be tailored to the scope of work and expected outcomes of the work or project (Stichler, 2002). Experienced entrepreneurial mentors can assist new APRN entrepreneurs in identifying and placing a dollar value on the APRN's unique knowledge, experience, expertise, and skill.

Business and Contractual Arrangements

Depending on the APRN role, new graduates will likely accept their first position as an employee, but in some cases it will be as an independent contractor. The nature of these two business relationships is significantly different with respect to taxation and professional liability. As a new graduate, it is essential to have a basic understanding of the business arrangement and the state-specific laws surrounding that arrangement.

Employment Contracts

Employment arrangements may be offered with or without a contract. Employment contracts are recommended and provide a professional platform for negotiation and discussion of issues, offering some protection for the APRN as well as the employer (Buppert, 2015; Hanson & Phillips, 2014). The complexity of an employment contract warrants careful review by an attorney hired by the APRN before it is accepted and signed. Negotiation of the terms of the contract is common and considered a professional imperative. Buppert (2015) described the issues commonly addressed in an employment contract, as shown in Box 20.11.

Independent Contractor

Commonly utilized by certified registered nurse anesthetists, certified nurse-midwives, and in some cases certified nurse practitioners, APRNs use this arrangement to contract their services with a business entity and are generally considered to be self-employed (Buppert, 2015; Hanson & Phillips, 2014; Internal Revenue Service, 2015). The US Internal Revenue Service (IRS) has strict regulations pertaining to qualification as an independent contractor, and development and review of the contract by an attorney is advised (Buppert, 2010). To be considered an independent contractor, several business matters are examined, including behavioral and financial

---

BOX 20.11   Elements of APRN Employment Contract

- Scope of services: productivity requirements; on-call requirements; hospital/nursing home/satellite responsibilities; administrative responsibilities
- Duration of employment arrangement or contract
- Performance evaluation terms
- Compensation: salary or hourly; bonus or incentive plans (productivity- or quality-based formulas)
- Benefits: health insurance, life/disability insurance, workers compensation, retirement, continuing education expenses, liability

- insurance, professional dues, license/registration fees, credentialing fees, vacation, holidays, sick time/bereavement, cell phone, mileage, pager
- Malpractice coverage
- Collaboration/supervision requirements (if required by state law)
- Mentorship, consultation, and staff support
- Restriction on outside professional activities
- Termination clause
- Revision and renegotiation provisions
- May specify conflict resolution processes
- Noncompete clause

Adapted from Buppert, C. (2015). *Nurse practitioner's business practice and legal guide* (5th ed.). Sudbury, MA: Jones & Bartlett.

---

control of the services provided and the type of business relationship. The APRN must control how and what services she or he performs and may be paid a flat fee or, in some professions, may be paid hourly (IRS, 2016). Independent contractors are not considered employees; are responsible for paying their own state and federal taxes; provide their own benefits, uniforms, and equipment (and possibly supplies); and receive an IRS 1099 form compiled by the employing organization at the end of the year (Hanson & Phillips, 2014; IRS, 2015). The rights of the contractor and organization are specified in the contract.

There are advantages and disadvantages to each type of contractual relationship, but professional consensus recommends having a contract agreement in professional business relationships. Careful review of the employee or independent contractor contract by an attorney knowledgeable in APRN practice is essential to ensure that the APRN's interests are taken into account (Buppert, 2008a). Exemplar 20.3 provides real-life examples of contractual language that could have been avoided if the APRN had sought counsel and review of the contract.

Professional Issues

Marketing and negotiation also involves discussion of professional issues such as state practice authority and malpractice insurance requirements. Both issues have legal implications and warrant a unique place in the discussions during negotiation of a potential position. Chapter 22 provides additional details.

Practice Arrangements

APRN laws and regulations vary widely from state to state. New APRNs must be able to articulate statutory and regulatory practice and prescriptive authority, licensure and certification requirements, and controlled substance registration requirements specific for their APRN role. The APRN should not assume that the employer understands nursing scope of practice laws in the state. This knowledge can be highlighted during the interview process, demonstrating leadership in APRN policy—a unique contribution to a future practice or organization. An APRN should provide future employers with sample documents pertaining to the appropriate laws, which can be easily stored in the professional portfolio.

Future employers often have questions surrounding practice laws during the interview process. When appropriate, the APRN should articulate the difference between full practice authority, independent practice (particularly in states where the roles are defined separately), collaborative practice, and supervisory practice. The APRN should be ready to answer questions regarding collaborative and supervisory practice agreement specifications and should ask the interviewer about the physicians or APRNs who will serve in those roles. Regardless of the state's practice authority, an employer may restrict APRN practice or require collaboration or supervision as an organizational policy. This is allowable, and it is a personal decision of the APRN whether or not to work in a more restrictive environment than the state requires. Many states have adopted "transition-to-practice" laws in which

EXEMPLAR 20.3   **Detrimental Clauses in APRN Contracts That Should Not Have Been Signed**

Melanie Balestra, JD, MN, PNP

(http://balestrahealthlaw.com/)
Ms. Balestra's law practice focuses on legal and business issues that affect physicians, physician assistants, nurse practitioners, nurses, and other health care providers as well as representing them before their respective regulatory boards. With a specialization in the legal aspects of starting entrepreneurial practice, Ms. Balestra has assisted over 200 health professionals throughout the United States and has presented numerous workshops on this subject. Ms. Balestra is the only practicing nurse practitioner licensed to practice law before the U.S. Supreme Court and serves as counsel of record for the California Association of Nurse Practitioners. She has supplied the following examples of detrimental clauses in employment contracts that should not have been signed.

Computer License Fee

"The Employer will guarantee the fee for the computer software license for use of the Employer's electronic medical record. This fee will be forgiven after three years of employment. However, Employee agrees that if termination of this Agreement is at Employee's request, a prorated fee for use of the computer license will be incurred and due upon effective termination date. This fee will be calculated based on total cost of license at time of employment divided by 36 months. If the fee is not paid upon termination of contract, it will be withheld from the final paycheck. The fee repayment in no manner authorizes Employee use of software license after employment ceases with Employer." This clause requires the employee to pay a prorated fee for use of the computer license if the employee leaves the practice early. Use of this license during the provision of professional services is required for creating documentation in the medical record and should be covered by the employer.

Meaningful Use/Other Incentives

"Employee expressly understands that the Employer is responsible for providing and maintaining edges that all income fees and incentives obtained by use of software and hardware shall belong to the Employer. This includes government incentives for meaningful use. If Employee elects to terminate employment, incentives will remain with the Employer. Employee expressly agrees to reimburse Employer for incentives paid directly to Employee for incentives earned while employed with Employer." This clause requires the APRN to give all Meaningful Use incentive fees received to the employer. In many group practices, incentive fees are often part of a negotiated bonus rate.

Covenant Not to Compete

"Employee covenants to and with Employer that for a period of 12 months after termination of the Contract, whether by expiration of its term or otherwise, the Employee will not, directly or indirectly, engage in providing healthcare to children (including government or private entities, clinics that provide care to children such as pediatric or family practice clinics) within a radius of 25 miles of either campus of _____." Non-compete clauses are not uncommon. The APRN should seek legal advice on how to negotiate this clause if the employer refuses to remove it.

Salary

"Salary is $50 per hour based on productivity of seeing 40 patients per 8-hour day. Productivity will be reviewed on a monthly basis and adjusted according." There are a number of issues with this clause, including (but not limited to) a requirement to see 5 patients per hour or 1 patient every 12 minutes; lack of specificity when patients do not show up for their appointment or cancel; and quality, safety, and potential malpractice issues.

Independent Contractor

"Contractor cannot work for any other medical practice within a twenty-five mile radius unless approved by Contractee." As an independent contractor, limitations on the APRNs ability to work outside of this contract are constraining and must be considered. ◎

a period of oversight is required prior to the APRN enjoying full autonomous practice authority (Phillips, 2016). In states that require "transition-to-practice" collaboration or supervision, APRNs should discuss this regulatory requirement with potential employers and clarify who will provide the oversight and attestation of this experience once completed. The APRN must interview the person who will be overseeing his or her practice before a position is accepted.

Malpractice Insurance

Employer-based malpractice insurance coverage is typically provided to APRN employees; however, these policies serve to protect the practice or organization as a whole and, when utilized, the APRN has little or no say in how the claim is resolved (Fetcho, 2013). It is important for the candidate to inquire about the terms of coverage during the interview and negotiation process. Two types of policies exist for malpractice coverage: *claims-made* and *occurrence*. *Occurrence* policies cover the insured for a malpractice claim that occurs during the policy period regardless of when it is reported as long as the policy was in force when the alleged malpractice occurred. *Claims-made* policies cover the insured for a malpractice claim made during an active policy period only if the claim is also made during the active policy period. *Tail coverage* can be purchased and added to a claims-made policy if the insured decides to end the policy. Tail coverage extends the time a claim can be reported as long as the claim occurred while the policy was active. Chapter 21 provides additional detail.

Independent contractors, like employees, are encouraged to purchase individual professional liability insurance. Depending upon the business structure of the practice, additional employees or contractors, corporate status, and other variables, the APRN entrepreneur must also consider additional coverage such as premises, workers compensation, unemployment, disability, and health insurance (Buppert, 2008b). It is essential that APRN entrepreneurs seek legal counsel when setting up a business to determine specific needs.

Medical malpractice policies covering a health care organization or practice may restrict APRN practice, such as by requiring cosignature of patient records or physician presence during care delivered by the APRN, and rarely cover expenses related to license discipline or administrative review (Fetcho, 2013). An individual APRN malpractice insurance policy, paid for separately by the APRN, in addition to employer-based coverage, is recommended by Carolyn Buppert (2015), an attorney and APRN. Citing "fracture [in] collegial alliances" (p. 283), Buppert noted that malpractice lawsuits damage the relationship between the APRN employee and the organization. When named in a lawsuit, the organization may blame the APRN, necessitating individual defense (Buppert, 2015). A recent regulatory trend to require APRN liability coverage has passed in some states and is being considered in a majority of the full practice authority legislation (Phillips, 2016). The APRN should ensure that she or he is versed in the legislation as well as statutory requirements for malpractice coverage in the state where she or he intends to provide care.

Overcoming Invisibility

Novice APRNs or seasoned entrepreneurs must be able to demonstrate their unique value to an organization whether interviewing for their first position or marketing their entrepreneurial/intrapreneurial practice improvement idea. This is important because often the APRN role is invisible to external funding agencies such as insurers, foundations, and governmental bodies. As a result, APRNs' services may also be invisible to potential employers and organizations.

There are a number of situations in which APRNs are invisible. One example is Medicare policy, by which physicians can bill nurse practitioner (NP) services "incident-to" in order to receive 100% reimbursement from Medicare. During the interview or negotiation process, the NP should emphasize the restrictions placed on the physician when doing this, including mandated physician presence during NP-provided patient care and physician-only access for new patients or existing patients with new complaints. Other examples of invisibility include the National Ambulatory Medical Care Survey, the Center for Studying Health System Change, and the Area-Resource File. None of these survey studies or databases includes APRN distinctions in their data. This is significant because they are used to determine such things as service need, federal funding, and provider shortage areas. Beyond obtaining employment, doctorally prepared APRNs should strive to be involved in local, state, and national policymaking so that future studies and databases will include such APRN-specific data. This will enable APRNs to demonstrate value, enhance health care delivery, and assist in obtaining federal and private funding and reimbursement.

Marketing the APRN's services once established within the organization or practice is an essential step in overcoming invisibility. In addition to including the APRN on organizational signage, the APRN should be prepared to provide a succinct APRN role description, educational background, and skill set for incorporation into print and electronic marketing materials. Skilled in organizational and systems leadership competencies, DNP-prepared APRNs are uniquely qualified to assist in the development of an organizational APRN marketing strategy.

Conclusion

Developing skills to market the unique practice and contribution of the APRN role is important to enable APRNs to become viable members of and achieve stature as principle players in the health care arena. Evolution of these skills is established in APRN education, and it is important for academic institutions to include such activities for successful acclimation into the professional world. As a new graduate searching for one's first position or a seasoned clinician seeking to redefine one's professional role, reflection and self-assessment of one's philosophical basis for practice and preference for an intrapreneurial or entrepreneurial approach is an important exercise to determine the right professional fit.

Increasingly, educational institutions are preparing APRNs to leverage the innovative call described in the IOM's *The Future of Nursing* report (2011, 2015). Doctoral and APRN role-specific competencies addressing concepts of entrepreneurial and intrapreneurial practice have been implemented into APRN education, preparing APRNs to execute innovative ideas with a focus on accessibility and affordability. Although challenging, innovative practice setting opportunities are increasingly sought by new APRN graduates as well as experienced APRNs.

This chapter provides the new APRN with practical information and resources needed for a successful job search. Demonstrating the unique value of APRN care to an organization in an era of invisibility is an essential marketing skill that is practiced and refined during the job search and interview process.

Key Summary Points

■ Attention to and reflection on personal professional goals is essential to finding a good career fit as an APRN entrepreneur.

■ Despite challenges, APRNs are increasingly prepared for and seeking employee-intrapreneur, entrepreneur, and freelancing career opportunities that provide innovation and flexibility.

■ Highlighting and marketing APRN core competencies during the job search process enables the APRN applicant to stand out in an interview.

■ Professional networking through professional association membership and utilization of web-based business networking sites increases the success of a job search and supports growth and success of a business.

■ Electronic professional portfolios highlight the APRN's potential contribution to an organization, providing a strong base for negotiation.

■ Articulating the value of APRN care within the context of a distinct model of care with careful attention to the humanistic contribution to patient care, productivity, and outcomes is essential when interviewing for a new APRN position or when negotiating with investors.

■ Negotiation is a two-way street; the APRN applicant should take an agreed-upon time to carefully consider all aspects of the employment offer, including salary compensation, benefits, and time alternatives. Review of contract agreements by an attorney is recommended.

References

To access the references for this chapter, use your smartphone's QR code reader to scan the code below, or go to http://booksite.elsevier.com/ 9780323447751.

Reimbursement and Payment for APRN Services

Nancy Munro • Kathy S. Magdic

> *"You may have to fight a battle more than once to win it."*
> — *Margaret Thatcher*

CHAPTER CONTENTS

By their expanded knowledge and skill set built on a nursing framework, advanced practice registered nurses (APRNs) within the roles of certified nurse practitioner, clinical nurse specialist (CNS), certified registered nurse anesthetist (CRNA), and certified nurse-midwife (CNM) are uniquely poised to fill a niche beyond a traditional physician provider. Four national initiatives have accelerated the interest in and necessity for APRN reimbursement: (1) the Institute of Medicine *The Future of Nursing* reports (IOM, 2011, 2015); (2) the Patient Protection and Affordable Care Act (ACA, 2010); (3) the *Consensus Model for APRN Regulation* (APRN Joint Dialogue Group, 2008); and (4) the evolution of APRN doctoral education (American Association of Colleges of Nursing [AACN], 2006). Reimbursement for health care services is a very complex issue, and it is imperative that the APRN understands the process. The goal of this chapter is to provide an overview of the complicated reimbursement process in the United States, with an emphasis on the role of the Centers for Medicare & Medicaid Services (CMS). It is important to note that at the time of the publication of this textbook, there are anticipated major changes in the reimbursement process in the United States due to the 2016 presidential election results. Medicare and Medicaid will remain in place, but it is not clear currently what changes will occur in these reimbursement structures as well as other models.

Historical Perspective

In order for the APRN to understand the US reimbursement system, a brief review of its history will be helpful. The vision of a national health care system was a goal of both Presidents Roosevelt and Truman. Neither President was able to successfully pass legislation, but in 1965, President Lyndon Johnson signed the Social Security Amendment, which included the creation of Medicare and Medicaid. Medicare was created to assist those individuals greater than 65 years of age as well as individuals with other specific diseases or conditions (AACN, 2006). Initially, physician services were the target for reimbursement using a fee-for-service model. Nurse practitioners (NPs) were paid primarily as employees. A legislative attempt was made to provide for reimbursement of NPs who worked in rural underserved areas through the Rural Health Care Protection Act of 1997, which was not passed into law. Finally, through passage of the Balanced Budget Act of 1997, the CMS authorized NPs and CNSs, collectively referred to as nonphysician providers (NPPs), to bill for their professional services for both hospital inpatients and outpatients regardless of geographic setting. *NPP* is a term that is used by others to define all of those that are not physicians in the clinical sphere. The term "non physician provider" is considered a pejorative by the APRN community. Despite continuous unified APRN efforts to use different language that is provider neutral, the term is still used. Payment would be at 85% of the physician fee schedule (American Association of Nurse Practitioners, 2013). Although this was a major legislative accomplishment, it continues to be a point of contention regarding reimbursement for APRN services. When APRN services are reimbursed at 85% of what a physician would receive caring for the same patient, it implies that the APRN is "doing less" than a physician in the same situation. The loss of the remaining 15% is considered a loss in income for the practice but does not take into account the positive patient outcomes of the APRN. Reimbursement of CNM and CRNA services was initiated in the 1980s, and they are able to bill at 100% depending on the clinical situation (CMS, 2017e).

Decades of research consistently support the excellent outcomes and high quality of care provided by APRNs. A landmark study was conducted by the Office of Technical Assessment in 1986 that confirmed that APRNs provide "services that both substitute for and complement physicians' services, depending on the particular service or type of practice" (US Congress, Office of Technology Assessment, 1986, p. 49). The systematic review by Newhouse and colleagues (2011) evaluated NP outcomes such as functional status, hospitalizations, emergency department visits, and biomarkers and concluded that NP patient outcomes are comparable to those of physicians. The relationship between the NP practice environment and state-level health outcome measures of Medicare and Medicaid patients was evaluated in another important study (Oliver, Pennington, Revelle, & Rantz, 2014), which found that states with full practice authority (where NPs were the primary care providers for patients without the need for physician oversight) had decreased hospitalizations and better overall health outcomes. This research significantly strengthens the position of the APRN as the United States continues to evolve and focus on patient outcomes and health care costs. Yet, in today's health care economic marketplace, APRNs continue to face major obstacles in reimbursement, including barriers related to scope of practice (see Chapter 22). From a systems thinking approach, APRNs must continue efforts to rectify these inequities through an understanding of state rules and regulations for APRNs and engage in active participation and knowledge-based improvements to the current processes of reimbursement.

Reimbursement in the United States

Reimbursement Process

The reimbursement process has multiple steps. APRNs practice state to state directly based on rules and regulations within the state's nurse practice act. The entire process begins by knowing the APRN state scope of practice rules and regulations, followed by obtaining the required documents needed to practice within a given state. The patient's clinical encounter with an APRN provider follows along with posting of the patient's payment through out-of-pocket payment or third-party reimbursement. Once the clinical encounter is completed, the APRN documents the clinical encounter in the patient's record and completes the appropriate forms required for reimbursement. Proper coding for a clinical encounter is discussed later in the chapter. The documentation in the medical record needs to provide sufficient data to support the level of service that is billed.

Scope of Practice

The reimbursement process for APRNs begins with understanding one's scope of practice. Regulatory bodies expect that patient care provided by any health care professional is commensurate with the education and licensure of that professional. One of the major criteria for reimbursement listed by the CMS is that the APRN must be practicing within his/her scope of practice. The term *scope of practice* describes the procedures, actions, and processes that a health care practitioner is permitted to undertake in keeping within the terms of the professional license issued by each state. It is founded in state law with the intent to protect the public (American Association of Critical-Care Nurses, 2012). Some states define scope of practice in statutes enacted by the state legislature, while in other states boards of nursing are given the authority to define scope of practice by the state's legislature (Buppert, 2014). There are many ways that states regulate APRN scope of practice. For example, in some states CNMs are regulated by the Board of Medicine or a Board of Midwifery. A second example of variable state regulation is the CNS role. It is not defined in some states, which means the CNS is held to the same scope of practice as a registered nurse in that state (American Nurses Association [ANA], 2017). It is important for the APRN to be aware of his or her state's law regarding scope of practice related to reimbursement (see Chapter 22). Medicare will pay for services that are "medically necessary," and the service must be within the scope of practice for a "non-physician provider in the state in which he/she practices" (CMS, 2017f).

Obtaining a Provider Number

In order to be considered a provider by an insurer, all health care professionals must obtain a national provider identifier (NPI) number, which is a unique number provided by the CMS for all covered professionals, including APRNs (CMS, 2016c, 2017f). Additional information on NPI numbers can be found in Chapter 22. Each insurance company has its own process for becoming a "recognized provider," which results in payment for care delivered to its beneficiaries. The basic process for a provider to be reimbursed is illustrated in Fig. 21.1. The APRN must become familiar with this process to ensure the successful completion of all documentation needed to practice and bill properly for services performed. Compliance departments in health care practices are valuable resources to help guide the APRN through the complicated documentation that is required by insurance companies to receive reimbursement for care.

Documentation of Services: ICD-10 and CPT Codes

Documentation is the operative word for billing one's services. In other words, if it is not documented, it was not done. When documenting in the patient's medical record, there are two issues to consider: (1) the diagnosis for which services are provided (the ICD code) and (2) the actual service being provided (the CPT code). The International Classification of Diseases (ICD), maintained by the World Health Organization, forms the basis for why a service is provided; it lists up to 69,000 ways the human body hosts diseases, signs and symptoms, abnormal findings, complaints, social circumstances, and external causes of injury or diseases. The ICD concept has an ancient origin, dating back to the 1700s, and has evolved to an international database to study causes of mortality. The World Health Organization holds intellectual property rights and conducts ongoing revisions of these classifications of diseases; the most current version is the International Classification of Diseases, 10th Revision, Clinical Modification (ICD-10-CM) (Centers for Disease Control and Prevention, 2015). The ICD-10-CM tabular list consists of categories, subcategories, and codes. All categories are 3 characters while subcategories are either 4 or 5 characters. Codes may be 3, 4, 5, 6, or 7 characters. Codes may start with a letter to signify a disease, followed by 6 numeric digits that specify etiology, anatomic site, and severity. There may be an additional character that helps identify injuries, obstetrics, or external causes of injury (Centers for Disease Control and Prevention, 2015). An example of an ICD-10 code would be as follows: S32.010A – wedge compression fracture of first lumbar vertebra, initial encounter for closed fracture. The longer the code, the more specific the information about the diagnosis. Currently, there are approximately 69,000 ICD-10 codes. Fig. 21.2 indicates how the ICD codes are incorporated into the process of documentation for billing.

The Current Procedural Terminology (CPT) forms the basis for specific services performed in relation to the diagnosis. The CPT code is a numeric code used to report medical procedures and services under public and private health insurance programs. It is a 5-digit number that is used to indicate a level of service. These codes are developed by the American Medical Association (AMA) and reviewed by a CPT editorial panel that meets three times per year to review codes, develop new codes, and publish the codes (AMA, 2016). There are approximately 78,000

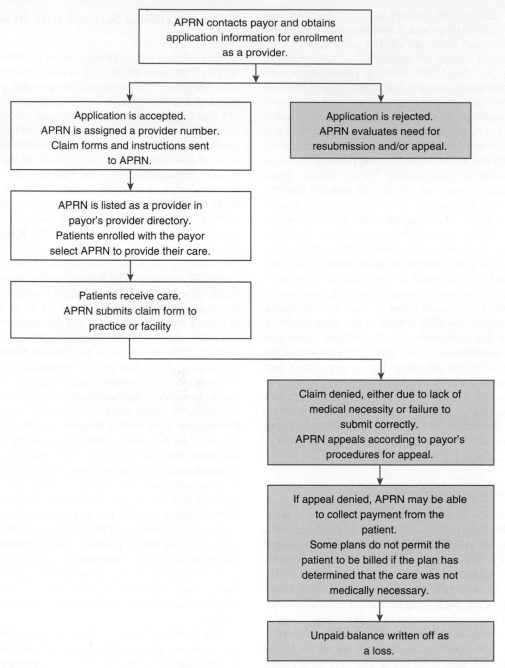

FIG 21.1 Basic third-party payor reimbursement process.

CPT codes that define inpatient and outpatient services. There are six sections to the CPT code manual: Evaluation and Management (E/M); Anesthesia; Surgery; Radiology; Pathology and Laboratory; and Medicine. The codes used most frequently by APRNs for each patient encounter are the E/M codes.

Billing for an E/M code requires the selection of a CPT code that best reflects the patient type, the setting of the service, and the level of E/M service performed. The care can be very simple and straightforward or very complex. It is important to remember that the CPT code must link to the ICD code in

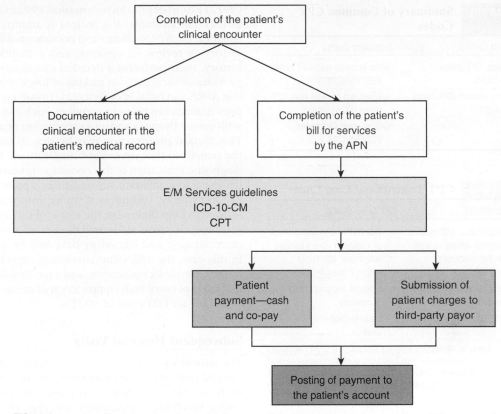

FIG 21.2 Overview of reimbursement showing how any clinical encounter is processed through the payment system.

order to establish medical necessity. Without this link to establish medical necessity, it is likely that the claim will be denied.

Commonly Used CPT Codes

Evaluation and Management (E/M) Codes

CPT codes that describe provider-patient encounters are often referred to as "E/M codes" and can be thought of as the building blocks of documentation for all patient encounters. There are different E/M codes for different types of encounters, such as office visits or hospital visits, and multiple E/M codes can be used when billing for services. There are seven factors to consider when deciding on which E/M code to choose. However, of those seven, the three key factors that help determine which code to use are the history, the physical examination, and medical decision making. In addition, the CMS provides a typical time period to be spent with the patient. Except for CPT codes used for critical care time and

counseling and coordination of care, use of other CPT codes does not require that the duration of time spent with the patient be documented.

Within each type of encounter, there are different levels of care. For example, the 99214 CPT code may be used to charge for an office visit with an established patient. There are five levels of care for this type of encounter. The 99214 code is often called a "level 4" office visit because the code ends in a "4" and because it is the fourth "level of care" for that type of visit (with the 99215 being the fifth and highest level of care). Each patient care encounter is unique and requires specific documentation.

Outpatient Codes: New and Established Patients

There are a series of outpatient E/M codes that include new patients to the practice (99201-99205) and established patients (99211-99215). A new patient is a patient "who has not received any professional services, i.e., E/M service or other face-to-face

TABLE 21.1	Summary of Common CPT Codes
Outpatient Codes	**Inpatient Codes**
New patient: CPT codes 99201-99205	Initial hospital visit: CPT codes 99221-99223
Established patient: CPT codes 99211-99215	Subsequent hospital visit: CPT codes 99231-99233
	Critical care: CPT codes 99291-99292

TABLE 21.2	CPT Transitional Care Codes
CPT Code 99495	**CPT Code 99496**
• Communication with patient or caregiver (direct contact, telephone, electronic) within 2 business days	• Communication with patient or caregiver (direct contact, telephone, electronic) within 2 business days
• Medical decision of at least moderate complexity	• Medical decision of high complexity
• Face-to-face visit within 14 days	• Face-to-face visit within 7 days

Adapted from Centers for Medicare & Medicaid Services. (2016). Transitional care management services. Retrieved from https://www.cms.gov/Outreach-and-Education/Medicare-Learning-Network-MLN/MLNProducts/downloads/Transitional-Care-Management-Services-Fact-Sheet-ICN908628.pdf.

service (e.g., surgical procedure) from the physician or physician group practice (same physician specialty) within the previous 3 years" (CMS, 2017f, p. 50). The CPT codes for the new patient are dependent on documentation of the level of history, physical examination, and medical decision making, with the more complex services covered in the codes 99204 and 99205. An established patient is one who has been followed to some degree by the practice within a 3-year time period. Again, the CPT code used (99211-99215) should reflect documentation of the level of service provided, with the higher number codes reflecting more intense data collection of the history, physical examination, and medical decision making processes. Specific rules are described in the Evaluation and Management Services documentation guidelines (CMS, 2017b). Table 21.1 and Table 21.2 summarize the most commonly used CPT codes.

Initial Hospital Visit

The CPT codes applied to a patient admitted to the hospital include the codes for an "initial hospital visit" and range from less complex documentation

(99221) to in-depth documentation (99223) (CMS, 2017f). For example, if a patient is admitted with dyspnea, the APRN obtains and documents a detailed history, a review of systems, and a family/social history, then performs a detailed examination and provides medical decision making of low complexity; that APRN can bill E/M code 99221. However, patient presentations can be more complex, such as a patient with severe dyspnea and an exacerbation of asthma. This clinical presentation may be due to failure of the patient to take prescribed medications. Further diagnostic evaluation of this condition reveals a new left lower lobe infiltrate. As the patient's presentation becomes more complicated, more information is needed to help determine the cause of the infiltrate. An in-depth physical examination is required and more imaging and laboratory data may be needed. In this case, the APRN documents a comprehensive history, physical examination, and a medical decision making process of high complexity that meets criteria to bill for an E/M code of 99223.

Subsequent Hospital Visits

The patient's progress and need for further diagnostics and treatment must be assessed and documented each day after the admission date. The E/M CPT codes involving "subsequent hospital visits" are 99231-99233 (CMS, 2017f). Documentation of these services does not require repetition of content in the notes on admission but should reflect the patient's status and evolution of medical decision making as more data are evaluated. For example, when referring to the patient with an asthma exacerbation, the plan of care for this patient, who was not taking the prescribed medications, may include education on the importance of taking the prescribed medications as well as a change of medications to those that require once-daily dosing to improve compliance. However, if a left lower lobe infiltrate is discovered on a chest radiograph, pneumonia may be an additional diagnosis, which will increase the complexity of the medical decision-making process, necessitating the use of a higher CPT code. Daily examination of the patient should be more detailed because of the complication/additional diagnosis. As the patient's symptoms worsen, further diagnostic testing may be needed. A chest computed tomography scan may reveal even more complicated issues (bronchiectasis) that may require a pulmonary consult. Time spent with this type of patient will be longer and will require the highest code of subsequent hospital care (CPT code 99233). It is important for the APRN to remember that documentation details must support the service provided. Additional imaging may be required, and interpretation of that test should be included in the daily note. If the imaging requires expertise above the level of the APRN's proficiency (i.e., a complicated chest computed tomography scan), the APRN's note should include the discussion of the test interpretation with an expert (e.g., a radiologist).

Critical Care Codes

Two CPT codes are used to bill for critical care services: 99291 and 99292. CPT code 99291 refers to the services provided in the first 30 to 74 minutes when caring for a critically ill patient; CPT code 99292 is used for every additional 30 minutes of critical care time and is referred to as an "add-on" code. The time period of 30 to 74 minutes is a frequent time reference used by the CMS when time spent by the provider is required in their documentation (CMS, 2017f). These codes were developed in the early 1990s when it was recognized that different codes were needed for critically ill patients. The criteria for documentation of these services is very different from that which is required for subsequent hospital visits. Time spent in the evaluation and management of critically ill patients is a major requirement in the documentation (e.g., "I spent 45 minutes caring for this patient"). There are no specific components needed in the note, but two concepts must be present: (1) description of the instability of the patient and (2) description of the complex medical decision making involved. The wording used in describing these concepts becomes very important in the CPT codes. The CMS provides examples for conveying instability such as: "high probability of imminent or life threatening deterioration in the patient's condition." (CMS, 2017f, p. 63). An example of complex medical decision making would be: "in order to preserve and optimize cardiac function, a milrinone drip will be added and cardiac function will be monitored using the bedside echocardiogram." Critical care services require direct personal management by the physician or APRN. Training personnel (resident or fellow as well as APRN student) can participate in the care, but the physician or APRN must document correctly and cosignature of a trainee's note is not acceptable. Any procedures performed must be documented separately and cannot be included in the time of care calculation (CMS, 2017f). Using the prior example of a patient with an asthma exacerbation

and new left lower lobe infiltrate, appropriate use of the critical care codes come into play when the patient becomes hypoxic and develops respiratory distress, which requires transfer to the intensive care unit.

While it is known that the first 30 to 74 minutes (CPT code 99291) of critical care time can only be delivered by one provider (physician or NPP), there was controversy about which provider can use CPT code 99292. The CMS clarified this issue in Transmittal 1548: If a physician or a qualified NPP provides "staff coverage" or "follow-up" for each other after the first hour of critical care services was provided on the same calendar day by the previous physician or qualified NPP, the subsequent visits provided by covering physician or qualified NPP in the group shall be billed using CPT critical care add-on code 99292 (CMS, 2008). The interpretation of this statement has been inconsistent among payors and is currently under review by the CMS (personal communication, June 2015).

Medicare Reimbursement

Medicare Structure

The CMS is the regulatory body of the Department of Health and Human Services that administers Medicare and develops regulations that govern reimbursement practices for all health care providers specifically regarding Medicare. These regulations are guidelines that also provide direction for reimbursement practices by other insurance companies or third-party payors; however, other payors may also establish their own guidelines. There are four parts to Medicare (CMS, 2014; see Table 21.3). It is important that APRNs understand the difference between Part A, which covers hospital expenses, and Part B, which covers medical expenses such as physician services. Direct reimbursement for APRNs can only occur when submitting the claim through Medicare Part B. Part A does not reimburse the APRN directly because those services are already paid for as part of the hospital expense and to bill under Part A would be considered "double dipping."

APRNs must be aware of how claims are processed and how to seek information, get clarification, or resolve a billing issue. Chapter 12 of the CMS Medicare Claims Processing Manual is an excellent reference dedicated to rules governing reimbursing APRNs (CMS, 2017f). However, the first point of contact for any questions about a Medicare claim is the Medicare Administrative Contractor (MAC).

⊙ TABLE 21.3	Medicare Coverage	
Definition of Coverage	**Description of Coverage**	**Funding for Coverage**
Part A includes inpatient care received in a hospital or skilled nursing facility.	Part A covers critical access hospitals, short-term care in skilled nursing facilities, postinstitutional home health care, and hospice care. Those individuals eligible for Social Security are automatically enrolled in Part A.	Funded primarily through payroll taxes, although beneficiary cost sharing in the form of deductibles and coinsurance also fund the program.
Part B includes coverage of physician services and outpatient care.	Part B covers physician and nonphysician provider services; outpatient hospital services; home health care not covered by Part A, such as physical and occupational therapy; and other medical services, such as diagnostic testing, durable medical equipment, and ambulance costs. Enrollment in Part B is voluntary to beneficiaries receiving Part A.	Payment into the system through monthly premiums that are established yearly based on system expenses and through deductibles and coinsurance programs for various services.
Part C offers an alternative program similar to a health maintenance organization (HMO) or a preferred provider organization (PPO).	Medicare Part C, also referred to as Medicare Advantage Plan, is not a separate benefit. Part C is a part of the Medicare policy that allows private health insurance companies, such as HMOs and PPOs, to provide Medicare benefits. Medicare Advantage Plans must offer the same benefits as Medicare, but may have different rules, costs, and coverage restrictions.	May require a monthly premium in addition to Part B.
Part D is prescription drug coverage.	Beneficiaries must join a drug plan to receive coverage under Part D. Commercial insurance companies run the drug plans, which must meet or exceed standard drug plan benefits as defined by the government. This coverage is provided in an attempt to lower prescription drug costs.	Payment is a monthly fee that varies by plan and is in addition to the Part B premium. May be embedded in Part C premium.

Adapted from Centers for Medicare & Medicaid Services. (2014). Introduction to Medicare. Retrieved from: https://www.cms.gov/Medicare/Coordination-of-Benefits-and-Recovery/Coordination-of-Benefits-and-Recovery-Overview/Medicare-Secondary-Payer/Downloads/Introduction-to-Medicare.pdf.

MACs are private health insurers that have been assigned a geographic jurisdiction to process Medicare Part A and Part B medical claims and durable medical equipment claims for Medicare fee-for-service beneficiaries. Multiple states are included in each jurisdiction, and each MAC may interpret CMS regulations slightly differently (CMS, 2016e). Currently, there are 12 Medicare Parts A and B MAC jurisdictions in the United States. Fig. 21.3 illustrates the current CMS reimbursement structure in the United States. When considering this structure, it is understandable how regulations can have variable interpretations.

Resource-Based Relative Value Scale

Medicare reimbursement for services provided by health care professionals has historically been based on the work that each provider documents. Medicare used to pay for provider services using "usual, customary, and reasonable" rate setting, which led to payment variability. The quantification of *all* facets of the work involved in providing a health care service was addressed when the resource-based relative value scale was developed in 1989 as a payment model for physician reimbursement. This system considers three aspects of the work involved: (1) the physician's time or work, (2) the costs of running a practice, and (3) the physician's professional liability insurance premiums (Laugesen, 2014). A mathematical calculation, known as the sustainable growth rate (SGR), was formulated and addressed each service that may be provided. Because the cost of running a practice and liability insurance can vary due to geographic location, the formula includes a conversion factor. This number is referred to as a relative value unit (RVU) (Laugesen, 2014). The RVU is recognized as a measure of productivity that can be incorporated into salary negotiations, especially when an APRN is employed by a physician group. Although the RVU is a common component of salary negotiation with physicians, the RVU portion of a salary is highly variable and can be difficult to appreciate because often this information is not readily available. The ACA promoted many service delivery mergers, so many physician practices are being purchased by corporations, resulting in changes in the way that salaries are being negotiated. If physicians are required to meet a certain level of RVUs to attain a certain level of salary, the APRN's billing practices

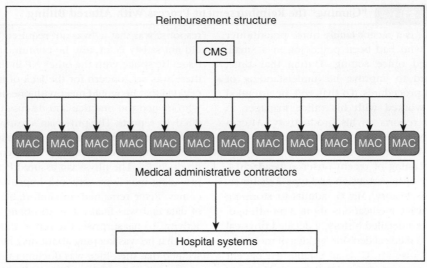

FIG 21.3 CMS reimbursement process, detailing the complexity of interpretation and application of CMS rules with 12 medical administrative contractors (MACs) interpreting the rules individually.

may be altered so that physicians can gain those RVUs, thus increasing their own salaries. This is very difficult to document, but reports of this process are increasing as more APRNs are billing directly for their services. The remedy for this kind of "gaming" is to meticulously document APRN-delivered care and patient outcomes. While the reimbursement process is in transition from quantity (RVUs) to quality (outcomes) as the basis for reimbursement, the transition from RVUs to outcomes is still in the formative stage so the RVU mechanism will be in place for the near future. Exemplar 21.1 addresses possible "gaming" issues.

Medicaid

Medicaid provides health insurance benefits and other assistance for eligible low-income individuals and families. Medicaid is jointly funded by the states and the federal government and administered by the states within broad federal guidelines. This means that both the states and the federal government have key roles as responsible stewards of the program, but the states decide eligibility for patients and review and process Medicaid claims. Historically, payment was usually lower than that which is available through other insurance groups. However, implementation of the ACA has led to many changes in Medicaid and will continue to institute change over time. For example, in calendar years 2013 and 2014, Medicaid

payments for primary care services were increased to be equivalent to Medicare rates. This allowed family medicine physicians, general internal medicine physicians, and pediatricians to qualify for this increased payment. In 1989, Congress mandated that state Medicaid agencies provide direct reimbursement to family NPs, pediatric NPs, and CNMs. Some states cover the services of other APRNs as well. The resulting inconsistencies have caused significant confusion.

Most states are expanding coverage for low-income adults; all states are modernizing their Medicaid/Children's Health Insurance Program (CHIP) eligibility, enrollment, and renewal processes. The Medicaid website offers links to individual states and their Medicaid rules and regulations (Medicaid. gov, 2014).

The Children's Health Insurance Program

CHIP is a partnership between the federal and state governments that provides health coverage to uninsured children whose families earn too much to qualify for Medicaid but too little to afford private coverage. All states provide immunizations and well-baby/well-child care at no cost to enrollees. The federal government establishes general guidelines for the administration of CHIP benefits. However, specific eligibility requirements to receive CHIP benefits, as well as the type and scope of services

EXEMPLAR 21.1   "Gaming" the Reimbursement Process With Altered Billing

Peter, APRN-BC, is a recent family nurse practitioner (NP) graduate who had been practicing in a small, community-based office setting. During that time, he worked hard to improve his understanding of reimbursement procedures. To that end, he attended seminars and worked with his office manager to understand the reports on his productivity. After a year, Peter moved and joined a practice in a busy metropolis. He is scheduled to see Mr. G., a 70-year-old male complaining of recent onset of headaches. He has a history of hypertension and type 2 diabetes. While taking his history, Mr. G. admits to stopping his antihypertensive medications about a month ago. Peter documents a detailed history, a detailed physical examination, and medical decision making of moderate complexity. Because Mr. G. is an established patient and according to Centers for Medicare & Medicaid Services (CMS) 1995 documentation guidelines, Peter bills E/M code 99214. Because the physician was not in the office at the time of Mr. G.'s visit, Peter billed the visit under his own national provider identifier number.

Peter has continued to follow the suggestion of his former office manager, who recommended that he keep track of all his services, including the associated International Classification of Diseases, 10th Edition, and Current Procedural Terminology codes. Initially Peter did not receive any productivity reports from his new officer manager in the metropolitan practice. When he inquired why he was not receiving reports, the response was that it "was not required." This response did not satisfy Peter, and he continued to pursue this issue. He spoke with the other NP in the practice, but there was no concern for the lack of information. He decided that he would meet with one of the physicians who owned the practice and discuss the lack of productivity reports. The physician's response was similar to that of the office manager, and he tried to explain to Peter that he did not need to be concerned about productivity. The physician assured Peter that he was providing excellent care and improving patient outcomes. Peter remained uncomfortable with this lack of data and was finally able to obtain a report of his activity. To his surprise, the report did not match the data that he was keeping about his billing practices. It seemed that the office was documenting higher levels of care, which was disturbing to Peter.

The best option for Peter would be to meet with the physician owners of the practice and discuss his concerns. The discrepancies in data could have been an unintentional error, which could be easily clarified. However, intentional upgrading of services is a fraudulent practice. If there was an investigation of billing procedures for this practice, even though Peter did not upgrade the codes himself, he would be held responsible. This is a very difficult position for an APRN to be in, but if there is no clarification or resolution of questionable billing practices, Peter should resign his position and should report intentional up-billing practices to the CMS. ◎

---

provided, are determined by each individual state (Medicaid.gov, 2016).

The Medicare Access and CHIP Reauthorization Act of 2015

The CMS is continuing to make changes in the Medicare payment programs that focus on quality and not purely the quantity of care. The Medicare Access and CHIP Reauthorization Act of 2015 (MACRA) reforms the existing payment system (CMS, 2017d). The highly complicated SGR formula (mentioned earlier) for determining Medicare payments for health care providers' services will be phased out and replaced with a reimbursement system based on measurable patient outcomes. This legislation will create a new framework for rewarding health care providers for giving *better* care, not *more* care. The existing quality reporting programs are cumbersome and difficult to use, so all quality reporting systems will be combined into one new system. These changes will be referred to as the Quality Payment Program (QPP) and will link quality with payment. Eligible professionals include NPs, CRNAs, CNSs, physician assistants, and physicians, who will be paid based on quality, resource use, clinical practice improvement, and meaningful use of certified electronic health record technology. These new changes will require significant transformation in approach to reimbursement and care delivery. Therefore the APRN must document her or his care and patient outcomes and be highly flexible and adaptable to demonstrate the effectiveness of the APRN in this new system.

Other Reimbursement Models

Private Health Insurance Fee-for-Service Plans

Private health insurance plans include carriers such as Blue Cross Blue Shield, Aetna, Prudential, and Metropolitan. These traditional fee-for-service plans reimburse providers for patient charges according to the usual and customary charges for that local area. (An insurance policy does not explicitly need to include the coverage of nursing services for APRNs to be reimbursed for their services.) APRNs' direct reimbursement by private insurance carriers varies from state to state and from carrier to carrier. When considering application for third-party reimbursement, the APRN needs to be familiar with the state's nurse practice act, state insurance laws and codes (including reimbursement amendments), judicial decisions, and opinions by the attorney general. The state APRN organizations would be the best source for this type of information (ANA, 2014).

State health insurance laws do not necessarily prohibit third-party reimbursement to APRNs. The individual APRN applies to the third-party insurer and requests "provider status." If reimbursement is rejected, familiarity with the state's nurse practice act and the state's health insurance laws can assist the APRN in appealing the decision. Some third-party payors reimburse under the APRN's collaborating physician's name. APRNs should contact each insurance company directly for credentialing and reimbursement protocols. When choosing to become a participating provider with a third-party insurance company, reimbursement is from a negotiated fee schedule. The APRN or practice manager has the ability to negotiate for the best fee possible.

Managed Care Contracts

Managed care contracts encompass various prepaid group practice arrangements. These programs usually offer health care services to members enrolled in the plan for a predetermined, prepaid, or discounted fee. Prepaid means that the group practice receives a fixed payment or premium to care for members of a certain population and that the organization bears the financial risk for the care that members receive. That is, they are paid a fixed amount and if the cost of care exceeds the fixed amount, the delivery system is responsible or "at risk." Participating providers are required to provide services for contracted reimbursement amounts.

Bundled Payment

Bundled payment, also known as *global bundled payment,* is defined as the reimbursement of health care providers (such as hospitals and APRNs) on the basis of expected costs for clinically defined episodes of care (see Exemplar 21.2). It has been described as "a middle ground" between fee-for-service reimbursement (in which providers are paid for each service rendered to a patient) and capitation (in which providers are paid a "lump sum" per patient regardless of how many services the patient

---

EXEMPLAR 21.2   **Midwifery Billing**[a]

Elise Rodriguez, CNM, DNP, is a certified nurse-midwife in a private practice that contracts directly with insurance companies. She has seen L.J. for all her prenatal visits and attended her delivery at Community Hospital. The pregnancy and delivery were uncomplicated, and Dr. Rodriguez provided independent midwifery management throughout. After the delivery, Dr. Rodriguez billed the insurance company for a global fee using code 59400 with diagnosis codes of O80, Z37.0, and Z3A. XX. The global fee covered all of the routine prenatal visits, Dr. Rodriguez's management of the delivery, and routine postpartum care. Community Hospital submitted a separate bill to the insurance company for the facility fee for the labor and delivery.

At 5 weeks postpartum, L.J. came to the office for a visit complaining of fever and breast pain. Dr. Rodriguez examined her, diagnosed her with mastitis, and prescribed appropriate medication and other therapeutic measures. Because this visit was for a specific problem and not part of routine postpartum care, Dr. Rodriguez submitted a separate bill for it, coding the visit as a 99213-24 (office visit–established, modifier shows outside regular postpartum care) with a diagnosis code of O91.23. The next week, L.J. returned for her routine 6-week postpartum visit. Because this visit was included in the global fee billed for after the birth, no separate bill was submitted. ◎

[a]The authors would like to thank Nancy A. Niemczyk, CNM, PhD, and Kimberly J. Abersold for their contribution of this exemplar.

receives). Bundled payments are being used as a strategy for reducing health care costs and improving the quality of care and the patients' journey of care. In this model, a payor will, for example, provide the delivery system $30,000 for a coronary artery bypass graft surgery, and that fee includes all the necessary preoperative, surgery, and inpatient care and all the services, including any complications up to 6 months' postoperative. In this model, the health care delivery system takes on the financial risk of the patient, assuming any costs related to complications. It forces the delivery system to enhance quality and coordination of care. The bundled payment model offers many opportunities for APRNs to play a major role in improving quality and cost efficiency. It incentivizes systems to deliver the care that truly meets the Triple Aim (Berwick, Nolan & Whittington, 2008).

Value-Based Purchasing

The CMS is now focused on linking quality of care to payment for services that are of value to patients, a shift from reimbursement for volume to reimbursement for value. A major criticism of the US health care system has been the lack of coordination of care, which can lead to fragmentation, an unacceptable rate of medical errors, overuse, and incomplete care of patients. The Hospital Value-Based Purchasing program is a CMS initiative that rewards acute care hospitals with incentive payments for the quality of care they provide to Medicare beneficiaries (CMS, 2017c). CMS is linking the Medicare payment system to a value-based system and dropping payments based purely on costs (CMS, 2015). The program uses the hospital quality data reporting infrastructure developed for the Hospital Inpatient Quality Reporting program (CMS, 2013). With the advent of the Doctor of Nursing Practice, the APRN could demonstrate advanced levels of clinical judgment, systems thinking, and accountability in designing, delivering, and evaluating evidence-based care to improve patient outcomes (AACN, 2006). *Value-based purchasing* is the current term that many APRNs have known as pay-for-performance, and this program is likely to continue to expand and become the new reimbursement model. Many APRNs within the acute care setting are reimbursed under a value-based purchasing plan. Individual states and private insurers have followed the CMS lead and have established guidelines linking quality of care and improved outcomes with payment.

Accountable Care Organizations

Accountable care organizations (ACOs) are groups of physicians, hospitals, and other health care providers who form an organization to give coordinated, high-quality care to the Medicare patients they serve. Coordinated care helps ensure that patients, especially the chronically ill, get the right care at the right time, with the goal of avoiding unnecessary services, hospital readmissions, and medical errors (CMS, 2017a). An ACO provides patient-centered, integrated health care across all settings (e.g., home, office, hospital) from prevention through rehabilitation by a variety of health care providers. This model presents an excellent opportunity for the APRN to demonstrate the ability to diagnose, manage, and coordinate care for every type of patient population. Chronically ill patients with conditions such as diabetes, hypertension, and hyperlipidemia are excellent examples of health care situations where the APRN has established expertise in improving outcomes and promoting patients' accountability for their own care (Newhouse et al., 2011). Accountable care models are structured to ensure optimal outcomes of care. A well-configured ACO must have a panel of at least 5000 patients and ensure that all the providers caring for a patient know the patient's condition and preferences and work together to optimize tests, procedures, referrals, and education in order to provide coordinated and efficient care (CMS, 2017a). There are reportable measures that ACOs must demonstrate, and electronic health records must be in place. CMS is continuing to develop different ACO programs to address various patient populations, including end-stage renal disease and congestive heart failure. ACOs that demonstrate advanced coordination of care for higher risk patient populations will be eligible for a higher level of financial reward (CMS, 2017g). APRNs must establish a position in these systems to ensure recognition of their contributions to optimal coordinated patient care that allows for financial recognition for their positive outcomes. This requires involvement in governance and leadership structures so that APRNs are formulating ACO policy and sharing in financial incentives, not merely serving as employees (National Academies of Practice, 2009).

Medical Homes

Another health care model to support complex patients with multiple chronic conditions is the patient-centered medical home (PCMH). The original concept of the medical home was developed by the American Academy of Pediatrics in the 1960s. The primary care physician was the proposed leader of patient-centered primary care who would focus on the person and provide coordinated and integrated care. This model has been revisited in order to provide access to health care and manage chronic care more effectively in today's health care system. The Medicare Improvements and Extension Act of 2006 provided for the initiation of the Medicare Medical Home. Demonstration projects were developed to reward primary care physicians who were originally targeted to lead care. In 2008, Medicare began including NP-led, PCMH practices for reimbursement (Schram, 2010). The ACA has provisions designed to promote improved access, increased quality of care, and decreased costs, including PCMHs. Medical homes focus on primary care and shared common elements, including a primary care clinician (physician, NP, or physician assistant) to coordinate care. APRNs are gaining recognition as being leaders in the medical home model of care. The National Committee for Quality Assurance, in conjunction with physician groups, has developed a process—the Physician Practice Connections—Patient Centered Medical Home, now known as Q-PASS (Quality Performance Assessment Support System)— that recognizes practices that are able to deliver services consistent with the PCMH model of care (National Committee for Quality Assurance, 2016). In 2010 this organization implemented recognition of "nurse-led" primary care practices as PCMHs; several NP-run practices have earned this recognition (ANA, 2010). In addition, nurse-managed health centers, which are community-based primary care under the leadership of an APRN, have been established. These not-for-profit centers usually have sliding scales for payment. A few nurse-managed health centers are designated as Federally Qualified Health Centers.

There are also several variations of the medical home in the private sector that may or may not include APRN providers. It is critical that APRNs become familiar with and support practice designs that allow ARPNs the ability to lead and coordinate care efforts (National Academies of Practice, 2009).

Current and Emerging Reimbursement Issues for APRNs

Overcoming Invisibility

The overarching goal of APRN reimbursement is to have the APRN bill the insurer directly for services provided. The first barrier to this goal is that the APRN is reimbursed at 85% of the physician fee, even though the practice costs and the care provided are the same. Some physicians who employ APRNs consider this reduction in reimbursement a disadvantage and want to find ways to capture the additional 15%. Two reimbursement "models" are used to eliminate this gap. These models are referred to as "shared visits" and "incident-to" services. These are not codes but a method of billing that results in reimbursement of APRN services at 100% of the physician fee as long as certain criteria are met. However, in order to obtain the 100% reimbursement, the APRN services must be submitted under the physician's billing number and the APRN becomes an "invisible provider." Being an invisible provider means that the data documenting the work of the APRN become lost, thereby losing the demonstrated effectiveness of the APRN role.

"Shared Visits"

"Shared visits" are patient E/M services that are jointly performed between a physician and an APRN in the same group practice (CMS, 2017f). The APRN must be practicing within his or her scope of practice when providing the service, which may occur jointly with the physician or independently on the same calendar day. The APRN's and physician's documentation must reflect the level of service. The key components for 100% reimbursement are that the physician is required have a *face-to-face encounter* with the patient (no particular length of time required); the encounter needs to be documented by the physician, who should link his or her note with the APRN's note; and the physician's note needs to include *one of the three components* of evaluation and management (history, physical examination, or medical decision making). The physician's note does not have to be long or complicated. An acceptable example might be: "I have examined the patient and discussed the plan for the day. Crackles present bilaterally posteriorly and agree with diuresis and monitoring electrolytes." There is no required format for the physician's note, and it can be linked electronically as long as there has been face-to-face contact with the patient. Discussion with the family is not an allowable substitution to a face-to-face visit with the patient. As long as the criteria for billing a shared visit are met, the bill may be submitted under the physician's billing number for 100% of the physician fee. The shared visit model applies to hospital inpatient, hospital

BOX 21.1   APRN Shared Visit Concept Summary

Criteria for 100% reimbursement:
- Same day encounter
- Physician-APRN same service
- APRN within scope of practice
- *Face-to-face physician encounter*
- *Proper physician note that is linked to APRN note*

    If any of the above criteria are not met, the visit is billed at 85% under the APRN's National Provider Identifier number.

Adapted from U.S. Centers for Medicare & Medicaid Services. (2017). Medicare claims processing manual. Chapter 12—Physicians/nonphysician practitioners. Retrieved from https://www.cms.gov/Regulations-and-Guidance/ Guidance/Manuals/downloads/clm104c12.pdf.

BOX 21.2   "Incident-to" Concept Summary

Criteria for 100% reimbursement:
- Physician to see patient on initial visit
- Physician presence in office suite if APRN sees patient in subsequent visits
- Some frequency of physician participation in plan of care

    If any of the above criteria are not met, the visit is billed at 85% under the APRN's National Provider Identifier number.

Adapted from Centers for Medicare & Medicaid Services. (2017). Medicare claims processing manual. Chapter 12—Physicians/nonphysician practitioners. Retrieved from https://www.cms.gov/Regulations-and-Guidance/ Guidance/Manuals/downloads/clm104c12.pdf.

outpatient, or emergency department situations. Box 21.1 presents a summary of concept components of shared visits.

"Incident-To" Billing

The term *incident-to* is a shortened version of the phrase "incident to the services of a physician." It is considered an integral, although incidental, part of a physician's professional service (CMS, 2017f). This billing method applies to clinic or office visits in the outpatient setting. In order for an APRN to bill 100% for this type of visit, the physician must see any patient new to the practice or any established patient with a new problem in order to formulate the plan of care. In addition, the physician must be physically present within the suite of service, which means the physician cannot be available by phone or outside the suite of service for any reason. Once the plan of care is established, the APRN can then continue to see the patient on subsequent visits and alter the plan of care depending on the condition of the patient. In this situation, the encounter may be billed under the physician's provider number at 100% of the physician fee schedule. The physician must perform subsequent services at a frequency that reflects active participation in management of treatment (CMS, 2017f). If the APRN sees the patient in a succeeding visit and a physician is not present in the suite of service, the APRN can only bill for 85% of the physician fee under the APRN's provider number. Box 21.2 provides a summary of this concept, and Exemplar 21.3 contains a detailed example of an "incident-to" visit.

Advanced Care Planning and APRNs

The APRN provides a unique skill set that is different from that of other health care providers and can enhance patient care. The health care environment is becoming more complex and coordination of care is imperative. The APRN is prepared to envision and operationalize patient care from a holistic perspective. The IOM issued a report entitled "Dying in America: Improving Quality and Honoring Individual Preferences Near the End of Life" (IOM, 2014) that emphasized the need for improved shared decision making and advance care planning that reduces the utilization of unnecessary medical services and those not consistent with a patient's goals for care. In 2016 two new CPT codes (99497 and 99498) were developed that acknowledge the need for better understanding and discussion of end-of-life care. The hope is that these codes will develop advanced care planning as an *optional* component of the annual wellness visit and will provide financial incentives for medical and social support services that decrease the need for emergency department and acute care services. Code 99497 is used for the first 30 minutes of face-to-face advanced care planning with the patient, including explanation and discussion of advanced care directives. The add-on code 99498 is used for any additional 30 minutes needed to achieve improved care planning. Currently, there are no limits on the number of times these codes can be used, but if they are used multiple times there must be the appropriate documentation about the change in the patient's condition and/or the patient's wishes regarding end- of- life care (CMS, 2016b). This service can greatly expand and accelerate the process of identifying patients' wishes in the event they can no longer make decisions about their health care. APRNs are well suited to lead these discussions

Ms. Beatty is a nurse practitioner who sees patients in the office of an internal medicine practice. DH, a 66-year old male covered under Medicare, presents to the office as a new patient for evaluation of increasing shortness of breath. In addition, he has a history significant for hypertension and diabetes. Initially, the office staff scheduled DH to be seen by Ms. Beatty, but because DH is new to the practice and the billing is to be done under the "incident-to" rules, he can only be seen by the physician, Dr. Waters. Dr. Waters does the initial history and physical examination followed by writing orders for laboratory and diagnostic testing. He codes the visit as a 99204 (office visit–new patient), submits the bill, and receives 100% reimbursement of the physician fee schedule. He has DH schedule a return visit in 2 weeks. Because the plan of care has been established, DH is scheduled to be seen by Ms. Beatty. She sees DH, does a focused history and physical examination, and reviews the results of the tests. Dr. Waters is in the office but he does not see the patient. Ms. Beatty codes the visit as a 99213 (office visit–established). The requirements for "incident-to" billing have been met, and the bill is submitted under the physician's number and is reimbursed at 100%. Ms. Beatty schedules the patient to return again in 1 month. During this encounter, Dr. Waters has to leave the office for a meeting. Ms. Beatty again does a focused history and physical examination and codes the visit as a 99213 (office visit–established). Because Dr. Waters is not in the office, the rules for "incident-to" have not been met, and the visit must be submitted under Ms. Beatty's number and will be reimbursed at 85% of the physician fee schedule.

A second patient, AG, is a 73-year-old female who is covered under Medicare and has a history of coronary artery disease. AG presents to the same internal medicine practice as a new patient because her original primary care provider retired. Dr. Waters is busy seeing other patients, so the staff asks if Ms. Beatty can see the patient. She agrees, performs a detailed history and physical examination, and bills the visit as a 99204 (office visit–new patient). Even though Dr. Waters is in the office, Ms. Beatty submits the bill under her own number because the rules for "incident-to" billing have not been met (i.e., a physician must see all new patients to establish the plan of care). Reimbursement, in this case, will be at 85%.

The concepts of "shared visit" and "incident-to" billing provide an option that allows advanced practice registered nurses (APRNs) to bill 100% for the service provided. However, the financial drive to bill 100% under the physician's number has led to some highly questionable practices. Frequently, the face-to-face encounter required for shared visits is not fulfilled or the physician's documentation is not correct. With "incident-to" services, the absence of the physician in the suite of service and/or failure of the physician to see a new patient or an established patient with a new problem has also been problematic. The Centers for Medicare & Medicaid Services (CMS) monitors the use and frequency of these billing practices, and if suspicious patterns are noted, investigation for fraudulent practices may be pursued. The APRN must always be aware that he or she is responsible for his or her own practice.

Allowing an APRN to bill under her or his own number, in addition to making the APRN's services visible, eliminates any intentional or unintentional billing inaccuracies. Moreover, shared visit or "incident-to" practices are not creating value for APRNs as a profession because they render APRN practice invisible. If APRNs cannot measure their value, they will be marginalized in the new health care climate in which value is emphasized over volume. ◎

---

and increase the number of people who receive patient-centered and highly individualized care.

Transitional Care and APRNs

There is a growing body of evidence that suggests that patients coping with multiple chronic conditions and complex therapies are vulnerable to deficits in care (Newhouse et al., 2011). Inadequate patient and caregiver education, poor continuity of care, and lack of communication among providers lead to negative quality and increased costs when providing care (Newhouse et al., 2011). Effective care management

of these populations is needed to prevent hospital readmissions, improve health care outcomes, and enhance patients' experience with care as well as reduce total health care costs (CMS, 2016d). Medicare now pays for transitional care management services (CMS, 2016a). These services may be provided by a physician or qualified APRN and include a combination of remote as well as face-to-face care for patients following discharge back to the community (patient's home, assisted living, nursing home, etc.) from a hospital, skilled nursing facility, or community mental health center or from outpatient observation or partial hospitalization (CMS, 2016d). There are three components of transitional care management: (1) an interactive contact, (2) certain remote or off-site services, and (3) a face-to-face visit. The interactive component consists of communication with the patient or caregiver within 2 business days following hospital discharge and may be done by telephone, by email, or face to face. The remote services include reviewing discharge information or need for follow-up, interaction with other health care professionals who will assume care of the patient, providing education to family or caregiver, or establishing referrals and arranging needed community resources (CMS, 2016d). The face-to-face component of care is required in these codes to reflect a level of medical decision making and a face-to-face encounter between 7 and 14 days after hospital discharge. These codes will allow for the required face-to-face encounter to be furnished through telehealth, building the foundation for electronically delivered care (CMS, 2016d) (see Table 21.2).

Conclusion

The health care reimbursement system in the United States is very complex. It has developed over many years as the system has expanded. The APRN is responsible for understanding the rules and regulations that all health care providers must follow. Billing for health care services can be a strategic practice for the APRN and can assist with the visibility of the position. Because the APRN provides an expanded holistic perspective to patient care, the APRN needs to remain a viable component of total patient care, and reimbursement will contribute to the financial viability of the position.

The health care reimbursement system, overall, is in transition. The change of focus from quantity of care to quality of care is very logical but unsettling to a system that functioned on the premise that more care is better care. As MACRA is being implemented, the structure for the QPPs is going to require documentation of patient outcomes as a basis for reimbursement. In time, all health care provider outcomes will be given equal consideration and the 85% versus 100% reimbursement principle will no longer exist—a significant advantage for the APRN, validating outcomes of APRN practice such as decreased length of stay and fewer readmissions (Newhouse et al., 2011). It is imperative that APRNs in any practice continue to become visible through documentation of their practice outcomes, assuring that these data are presented to the QPP reporting system. APRNs clearly demonstrate the contributions of their role at all levels of the evolving system, from the institution where they work to the state and national level. Becoming part of the governing process of heath

care institutions and practices allows the APRN to understand and participate in decision-making processes. The competition for reimbursement will continue to be intense and will test the endurance of APRNs, but the successful history of patient-centered care will position the APRN to be highly successful.

Key Summary Points

■ APRNs must have a basic understanding of the reimbursement system in the United States. However, change in the existing system is anticipated, and the APRN needs to be alert for changes and how those changes will affect her or his practice. National and state APRN organizations will be excellent resources for this information, especially regarding the final rules of MACRA.

■ Tracking outcomes will be the major mechanism for APRNs to document their contribution to health care to increase their visibility. All APRNs need to develop a method in their practice to document outcomes. Ongoing research on outcomes is needed to support APRN reimbursement (see Chapter 23).

■ The APRN is responsible for his or her reimbursement practices. The entire reimbursement process is a team effort, but ultimately the APRN will be held responsible for any care or procedures for which he or she bills.

■ It is important to know the rules and regulations of reimbursement. The reimbursement system will remain complex, so it is imperative that the APRN become familiar with the process used at her or his place of employment. A relationship with the compliance department or practice manager will assist in a better understanding of all aspects of reimbursement pertinent to her or his practice.

References

To access the references for this chapter, use your smartphone's QR code reader to scan the code below, or go to http://booksite.elsevier.com/9780323447751.

Understanding Regulatory, Legal, and Credentialing Requirements

Charlene M. Hanson • Maureen Cahill

"The surest test of discipline is its absence."

—*Clara Barton*

CHAPTER CONTENTS

This chapter describes advanced practice registered nurse (APRN) credentialing and regulation and provides updates on the status of the *Consensus Model for APRN Regulation: Licensure, Accreditation, Certification and Education* (APRN Joint Dialogue Group, 2008). The Nursing Model Act and Nursing Model Rules (National Council State Boards of Nursing, [NCSBN], 2014a, 2014b), their implications and implementation, and emerging issues that are anticipated in the changing health care environment. The purpose of this chapter is to help the reader understand the multiple steps and the legal and regulatory framework for licensure as an APRN.

The current health care environment requires that any discussion of regulatory issues be fluid, dynamic, and subject to rapid change. National events have coalesced to bring about important effects on the regulation of APRNs. In the previous edition of this text, work concerning the Consensus Model was in its early stages. Today, this important regulatory change has been implemented in part or in whole across states and the District of Columbia. APRN coalitions and stakeholders continue efforts to align state statutes and rules with the APRN Consensus Model.

The Consensus Model for APRN Regulation: Licensure, Accreditation, Certification, and Education

Credentialing, which is used to ensure that APRNs meet competency and safety standards to protect the public, evolved haphazardly. State nursing societies and nursing boards became aware some time ago that the evolution of nursing practice included advanced and expanded roles. Idaho became the first state to attempt regulation at this level in 1971 (Nurse Practitioners of Idaho, 2016). As other states also attempted regulation of advanced nursing practice, legislation applied regulatory processes to these evolving roles. Unfortunately, regulatory changes that pertained to advanced practice nursing occurred at different time points in different states, and with varied elements of what was to be regulated (Rounds, Zych, & Mallary, 2013). Dialogue began that embraced all credentialing stakeholders and was a major step toward a uniform plan to educate and regulate APRNs. The eventual result of that work was an agreement among educators, certifiers, and regulators as to the most significant elements in the preparation and regulation of advanced nursing practice as well as regarding exactly which roles would fall under regulation and what populations they would address. State boards of nursing, working through the NCSBN, agreed to the elements of the APRN Consensus Model as their uniform licensure requirements for the regulation of the four APRN roles. To assist with implementation of these requirements, NCSBN created model language for bills that would align states with APRN regulations to facilitate state Boards of Nursing in carrying out the new regulations. All states would work toward adoption of this preparatory and regulatory standard (NCSBN, 2014a, 2014b).

Through discussion, brainstorming, and reaching consensus on a plan, the APRN Consensus Model was born (APRN Joint Dialogue Group, 2008). Forty-eight nursing organizations endorsed the work. The vision in the creation of the APRN Consensus Model was to implement one national regulatory scheme that allowed APRNs to be innovative and meet patient needs. A detailed history of this work can be found in the Institute of Medicine's (IOM's) report *The Future of Nursing: Leading Change, Advancing Health* (IOM, 2011).

Implementation of Consensus Model Regulation

Now, some 9 years after the publication of the APRN Consensus Model, the NCSBN's *APRN Campaign for Consensus,* which tracks states' alignment with the Model, reports that all states and jurisdictions have achieved 75% of the elements needed to align with the APRN Consensus Model (APRN Joint Dialogue Group, 2008). Based on this seminal work, the Consensus Model is being implemented across the United States. It is important that readers access the Consensus Model documentation and familiarize themselves with the elements of the Model and the progress toward implementing them. The reader must understand that although the target date for implementation was 2015, transition to the new regulation will take years to implement fully in all states (Madler, Kalanek, & Rising, 2012).

The organizations that make up the LACE communication network (licensure, accreditation, certification, and education) have continued to meet regularly to move forward of implementation of the Consensus Model, keep lines of communication open, maintain transparency, advance APRN regulation, and identify and strategize about important and ongoing issues. The LACE network is a virtual social networking configuration. A platform is in place whereby LACE member organizations pay a membership fee to belong to the working group that sustains the core components of the Consensus Model (LACE, 2010).

All four LACE organizational categories (licensure, accreditation, certification, and education) are aimed at meeting any new requirements and assisting with state implementation. Information about APRN regulation can be found on the respective state board of nursing websites (NCSBN, 2017a). There are five accreditation programs that can have oversight of APRN education, and there are two accrediting bodies that have oversight of APRN certification programs or examinations (Table 22.1).

For questions about up-to-the-minute, current APRN rules and regulations, especially those that pertain to specific state statutes regarding licensing of APRNs, prescriptive authority, and reimbursement, the reader should refer to individual state regulatory bodies for practice requirements and to the continuously updated NCSBN Maps project (NCSBN, 2016b).

TABLE 22.1 APRN Accrediting Bodies	
Accrediting Bodies That Oversee APRN Education Programs	Accrediting Bodies That Have Oversight of APRN Certifying Examinations
Commission on Collegiate Nursing Education (CCNE)	American Board of Nursing Specialties (ABNS)
Accreditation Commission for Education in Nursing (ACEN)	National Commission for Certifying Agencies (NCCA), a division of the Institute for Credentialing Excellence (ICE)
Commission for Nursing Education Accreditation (CNEA)	
Council on Accreditation of Nurse Anesthesia Educational Programs (COA)	
Accreditation Commission for Midwifery Education (ACME)	

The Need for Education and Credentialing of APRNs in the US Health Care System

During the years since 2008, national focus has turned sharply toward health care outcomes and costs following astounding annual data, most recently from 2017, comparing US health outcomes and costs with those of other high-income countries (The Commonwealth Fund, 2017a). Americans had among the worst health outcomes, though the United States spent considerably more on health care than any of the comparison countries. On review, it seemed insurability, access to care—and in particular primary care—socioeconomic disparities, and health policy lay at the root of the issue (Squires & Anderson, 2015). Interestingly, there is an association with state health outcomes as measured in the 2017 Commonwealth Fund state scorecard when compared with APRN state full practice and prescribing (The Commonwealth Fund, 2017b). Using the APRN Maps methodology, the highest rated one-third of US states has the greatest percentage of full practice and prescribing authority for APRNs, and the lowest scoring one-third of states has the lowest percentage of full practice and prescribing for APRNs (NCSBN Maps, 2016b).

By 2010, US policymakers were well aware that the ranks of the uninsured had climbed steadily since 2000. Availability of employer-sponsored insurance had declined and more than one in six people less than 65 years of age were without coverage (The Henry J. Kaiser Family Foundation, 2012). This data prompted passage of the broadest health reform legislation since the enactment of Medicare in 1965, entitled the Patient Protection and Affordable Care Act (ACA, 2010). The ACA would extend coverage to millions of uninsured, improving access to care, while intending to control costs. APRNs were included as primary care providers, members of accountable care organizations (ACOs), leaders of medical home configurations, and providers in nurse-managed clinics. These changes drive the need to ensure the highest levels of education and effective regulation for the advanced nursing roles. Finally, the IOM's *The Future of Nursing* report (IOM, 2011) and the subsequent *Assessing Progress on the Institute of Medicine Report: The Future of Nursing* made a recommendation that APRNs "should practice to the full extent of their education and training" (National Academies of Sciences, Engineering, and Medicine [NASEM], 2015a, pp. 4-6). State-by-state regulation of APRNs is affected by education provided to legislators and the public about the ways in which APRN autonomy could contribute to cost-effective and outcomes-enhancing solutions in health care that were provided through these and other publications.

Advanced Practice Registered Nurse Master's and Doctoral Education

The first criterion that any new APRN must meet is successful graduation from an approved, accredited APRN program. Education programs for APRNs must be at the graduate nursing level, resulting in a Master's Degree in Nursing or a Doctor of Nursing Practice (DNP); many programs are transitioning from master's to DNP education. In fact, the American Association of Nurse Anesthetists (AANA) and the National Association of Clinical Nurse Specialists (NACNS) have declared their endorsement of the doctorate for entry into certified registered nurse anesthetist (CRNA) practice by 2025 and for entry into the clinical nurse specialist (CNS) role by 2030 (AANA, 2007; NACNS, 2015). The Consensus Model and the NCSBN Nursing Model Act and Model Rules, describing state uniformity in adopting the Model, do not establish a timeline for the move to doctoral education for APRNs, and currently no state requires a DNP as eligibility for APRN recognition. Eligibility to sit for national certification and obtain APRN licensure or recognition by the state requires a transcript showing successful completion of a graduate degree from an accredited university that specifies the role and population focus of the graduate;

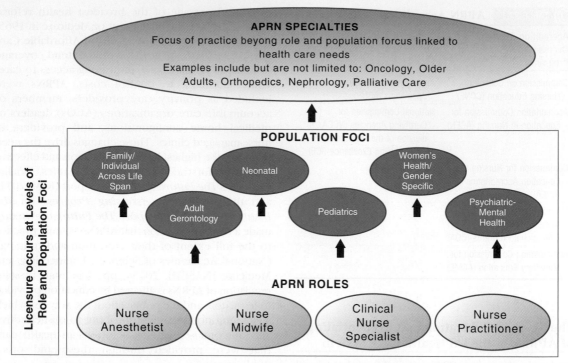

FIG 22.1 Advanced practice registered nurse (APRN) regulatory model. *(Adapted from National Council of State Boards of Nursing. [2008]. Consensus model for APRN regulation: Licensure, accreditation, certification and education [APRN Consensus Work Group and NCSBN APRN Advisory Committee]. Retrieved from https://www.ncsbn.org/Consensus_Model_for_APRN_Regulation_July_2008.pdf.)*

includes the core advanced pathophysiology, advanced health and physical assessment, and advanced pharmacology courses (the "three Ps") and sufficient clinical hours; and further specifies that the program must have national nursing accreditation (NCSBN, 2014a, 2014b). This is the standard for APRN licensure or recognition in all states.

Benchmarks of Advanced Practice Nursing and Education

Three components of APRN education and practice are related to scope of practice and provide additional important benchmarks—advanced practice nursing core competencies, the APRN role and population competencies, and Master's or Doctor of Nursing (DNP) Essentials. (AACN, 2006, 2011) These three benchmarks form the foundation on which boards of nursing develop APRN statutes. The Consensus Model delineates six population designations for practice for NPs and CNSs. They are adult/gerontology, neonatal, pediatric, family (primary care and acute),

psychiatric/mental health, and women's health and/gender-related (Fig. 22.1). Specific population foci for CNMs and CRNAs are not delineated in the Consensus Model. Specialty areas such as palliative care, oncology, and orthopedics are additional certifications above the roles and population foci at which APRNs are licensed. Specialty certification can indicate expertise in a subject area for an APRN, and is encouraged as further role development, when appropriate (NCSBN, 2008). Specialty certification is voluntary and is additive to the education and certification requirements for licensure. The APRN Consensus Model intended that licensure be congruent with the educational preparation and focus of the role and population (APRN Joint Dialogue Group, 2008).

Advanced Practice Registered Nurse Competencies

Nursing program accreditation requires that the program be structured based on either *The Essentials* of *Master's Education in Nursing* or *The Essentials of Doctoral Education for Advanced Nursing Practice,* created by the American Association of Colleges of Nursing (AACN, 2006, 2011). These documents support scope of practice for APRNs by providing the requirements for graduate core content, the APRN core, and "three Ps." At the DNP level, a stronger foundation in population-based care, organizational leadership, interprofessional collaboration, public policy, information systems, and translating research into practice enhances APRN roles (AACN, 2006). Taken together, the graduate essentials, the common core "three Ps" courses, and the role- and population-specific preparation are an educational blueprint, as laid out in the APRN Consensus Model. Importantly, students must graduate from a program with specific nursing accreditation that aligns with the Model in order to meet eligibility criteria to sit for certification and to attain licensure or recognition as an APRN (AACN, 2013; Commission on Collegiate Nursing Education, 2013). In order to add APRN populations or to change role or role focus, the APRN can complete a post-graduate certification program that has nursing accreditation, as described in the APRN Consensus Model (APRN Joint Dialogue Group, 2008).

Professional APRN Competencies

Professional organizations such as the NONPF, the NACNS National CNS Competency Task Force, the American College of Nurse-Midwives, and the AANA support each role and population focus with their own set of competencies. These more specific competencies provide benchmarks particular to the role and population focus (see Chapters 14 to 18 for examples of and sources for these competencies). APRN program structure builds its foundation on the Master's or DNP Essentials and the core courses (pathophysiology, physical assessment, and pharmacology), then incorporates the professional organization competencies in the portion of the program that is specific to the APRN role and population (Fig. 22.2).

APRN Program Oversight and Accreditation

For a graduate nursing program (master's or DNP) preparing APRNs, credentialing has a somewhat different meaning. Program credentialing includes accreditation for the educational program by one of the four APRN education accrediting organizations.

Education programs must also meet state education approval and requirements through each state's department of education or though multistate agreements. In many states the boards of nursing also approve graduate nursing education leading to the APRN roles (NCSBN, 2017c).

The Accreditation Commission for Education in Nursing and the Commission on Collegiate Nursing Education, as well as Council on Accreditation of Nurse Anesthesia Educational Programs (COA) and the Accreditation Commission for Midwifery Education (see Table 22.1), have aligned their standards with the requirements for APRN education outlined in the Consensus Model. The accreditation process provides an overall evaluation of the graduate nursing and APRN curricula and clinical programming.

Pre-accreditation review, based on the work of the NCSBN and consensus groups that was suggested by Hanson and Hamric (2002), has been adopted by the accreditors. Pre-accreditation procedures before the start of new programs are now the norm. Pre-accreditation will ensure that all new programs are well developed with appropriate curricula in place before students are admitted and that the program prepares graduates who can be licensed as APRNs.

The review and monitoring of NP and CNS education at the population focus level is more complex than for CRNAs and CNMs because of the multiplicity of program foci, including the population subcategory of acute or primary for the adult/gero and pediatric nurse practitioners. The NONPF, Pediatric Nursing Certification Board (PNCB), NACNS, and other similar bodies provide curriculum guidelines, program standards, and competencies to assist APRN programs with curriculum planning.

APRN Role and Population Certification

Agencies that offer APRN certification exams such as the American Nurses Credentialing Center and the American Academy of Nurse Practitioners Certification Program review programs to determine eligibility for APRN graduates to sit for national APRN certification examinations.

National certification for APRNs is a primary vehicle used by state boards of nursing to ensure a basic measure of competence. Advanced practice nursing certification is national in scope, and it is a mandatory requirement for APRNs to obtain and maintain credentialing in most states (NCSBN, 2014a, 2014b). Certification examinations for APRNs must be psychometrically sound and legally defensible to

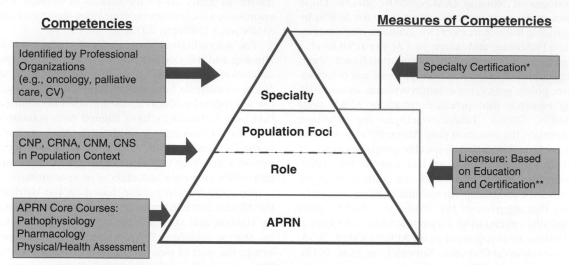

Relationship Between Educational Competencies, Licensure and Certification

FIG 22.2 Relationship between educational competencies, licensure, and certification. *APRN,* Advanced practice registered nurse; *CNM,* certified nurse-midwife; *CNP,* certified nurse practitioner; *CNS,* clinical nurse specialist; *CRNA,* certified registered nurse anesthetist; *CV,* cardiovascular. *Certification for specialty may include examination, portfolio, peer review, etc. **Certification for licensure will be psychometrically sound and legally defensible examination by an accredited certifying program. *(Adapted from National Council of State Boards of Nursing. [2008]. Consensus model for APRN regulation: Licensure, accreditation, certification and education [APRN Consensus Work Group and NCSBN APRN Advisory Committee]. Retrieved from https:// www.ncsbn.org/Consensus_Model_for_APRN_Regulation_July_2008.pdf.)*

be utilized as an element of advanced nursing licensure (AACN, 2017). Additionally, APRN certification programs must be accredited by the National Commission for Certifying Agencies (Institute for Credentialing Excellence, 2016) or by the American Board of Nursing Specialties. Certification organizations base content for their exams on role delineation studies that assist in defining the knowledge, skills, abilities, and framework required by the APRN in their role or population focus. CRNAs were credited with the first national certification in 1945, with other APRN specialties following suit, although few standards for certification were in place prior to 1975 (see Chapters 1 and 14 through 18). Certifications exist today for each of the described APRN roles and populations, with the exception of the Women's Health CNS, for which competencies are written (NACNS, 2014) but no examination exists. Certification programs rely on a certain number of potential test takers to offset the expense of creating and maintaining an examination. APRN national

certification websites identify the criteria for eligibility, test outlines, and recertification and practice requirements.

Certification organizations share information on those who hold and maintain certification required for state licensure/recognition with Boards of Nursing. The APRN Nursys database, maintained by NCSBN, houses licensure and certification information for ease of access among state Boards of Nursing and is increasingly in use across states. (NCSBN, APRN Nursys, 2017).

Postgraduate Education

Targeting postgraduate APRN programs to students who have already attained a graduate degree in nursing but who wish to add an additional population focus is common practice. However, many individuals who choose to return to school now pursue DNP education. The Consensus Model requires that post-master's education programs obtain formal graduate nursing accreditation. It is important that master's-prepared nurses who aspire to do postgraduate work and to acquire a new or additional APRN credential identify programs that offer curricula that meet the standards of eligibility for national certification and state licensure.

Continued Competency Measured Through Recertification

Overall, APRNs must fulfill continuing education (CE) and practice requirements to maintain their national certification(s) successfully, although requirements differ according to the role. Each advanced practice nursing certification entity clearly lays out the requirements and time frame for recertification. Generally, national certification lasts from 2 to 5 years and requires that the candidate be retested unless the established didactic and clinical parameters are met. All APRNs must maintain certification that is used for licensure eligibility. In some cases in which early exams have been retired, there may not be a testing option left for some who let their credential lapse (American Nurses Credentialing Center [ANCC], 2017).

Mandatory Continuing Education and Clinical Practice Requirements

CE requirements differ as to the type and amount of CE needed to maintain current national certification in a particular population focus. CE may also be a requirement of licensure renewal, which in some cases may be in addition to those requirements needed for certification renewal. Each role and focus requires a certain number of clinical hours for successful recertification. These are established by the certification program. CE should be consistent with the role and population, although it may be interprofessional. For example, CRNAs may choose to attend a conference with collaborating anesthesiologists, or family NPs may attend a conference with family practice physicians. It is encouraging to note that more conferences are offering interprofessional speakers and panels at specialty-specific conferences. APRN expert clinicians are serving as conference faculty for medical CE and vice versa. Ongoing CE hours can be met by attending CE courses and workshops, working toward degree requirements, completing journal CE offerings, writing for publication, and completing online offerings, simulations, webinars, and CD-ROM materials. The move to interprofessional offerings has broadened the scope of information available.

Most APRN roles and specialty areas have specific requirements built in for an adequate number of clinical practice hours between the years of recertification to ensure that APRNs remain clinically current and competent through regular practice. Each certification process clearly spells out the clinical hour practice requirement for the specialty. If individuals are not maintaining an APRN practice, they should not represent themselves as APRNs (see Chapter 3). APRNs who do not meet stipulated CE and practice requirements must retake the national certifying examination to continue to practice, if that is an option.

With the transition to the new consensus regulatory model, some certification examinations will no longer be available, so the need to keep certification current is critical. Certification is one way to ensure that APRNs are competent to provide needed health care to patients and families. Therefore, standardization of APRN certification and recertification processes is paramount to ensuring the credibility of advanced practice nursing.

Elements of APRN Regulation and Credentialing

As APRNs become more mobile across state and international boundaries, and as communications allow for increased interaction, it is important that credentialing and regulatory parameters be well understood. Box 22.1 lists the elements of regulation for APRNs. *Credentialing* is an umbrella term that refers to the regulatory mechanisms that can be applied to individuals, programs, or organizations (Styles, 1998). Credentialing represents the process of collecting and verifying an individual's professional qualifications and can occur at a national level by

 BOX 22.1 Elements of Regulation (LACE) for Advanced Practice Registered Nurses

Licensure
- Prescriptive authority (see Box 22.4)

Accreditation of APRN Programs

Certification (National)
- Recertification

Education
- Master's
- Post-master's
- Doctoral

meeting eligibility to sit for and pass a certification examination. It also occurs at the level of state-based regulation with the conferring of recognition or licensure when eligibility, including graduate or postgraduate education, and national certification in an APRN role and population are achieved. Credentialing can occur at the level of employment through an institutional process that grants access to the medical staff and describes the standards and duties one is expected to carry out within APRN employment (Summers, 2012), and it is increasingly occurring through regulators and malpractice carriers who seek assurance that APRN practice is congruent with education and certification.

Documents specified in Box 22.1 create the standard whereby advanced practice nursing is monitored and regulated and deemed safe or unsafe and whereby APRNs are disciplined from state to state. Two credentialing changes have occurred or will occur as states move toward consensus-aligned regulations. First, titling will require that APRNs legally represent themselves as an APRN first and then by their role (CRNA, CNM, NP, or CNS). Many states already use these role and population titles, but some do not (Fotsch, 2016; NCSBN, 2016a). Second, APRNs will need to have a second license. Second licensure means that an APRN must meet criteria established by a state board of nursing and is held to the highest level of regulation. The issues of titling and second licensure are important to all APRNs and to the public, so that it is clear that each APRN role holds regulatory recognition as both an RN and an APRN and shares a core preparation as well as uniform regulatory standards intended to offer the highest levels of public protection.

Use of the umbrella term *advanced practice registered nurse (APRN)* is intended to clarify that advanced practice in nursing is structured on top of the registered nurse platform and requires an additional, approved, scope of practice that is additive to and expands on that of the registered nurse. Data used to assess the nursing workforce and to sort provider characteristics in researching outcomes can distinguish those who are advanced practice nurses and can further distinguish them by role (Kleinpell, Scanlon, Hibbert, Ganz, East, & Fraser, 2014). Statutes define the title that is legally protected (APRN) and define the minimal requirements of recognition of the four included roles.

The scope of an APRN, while structured as additional to the registered nurse platform, is unique and is reflected in the requirement of a second license. Licensure remains the highest level of state-based, professional regulation and reflects the accountability for this evolved and greater nursing scope (NCSBN, 2011).

Language Associated With the Credentialing of APRNs

It is important for APRNs to understand the language and terms used to describe the credentialing process. Credentialing, including education, national certification, and licensure, involves several steps before one has full authority to practice as an APRN. To complicate matters, as noted, the credentialing procedures and requirements vary somewhat among states and practice settings. Definitions for the major components of APRN credentialing are presented in Box 22.2.

Titling of APRNs

The issues surrounding the titling and credentialing of APRNs have been difficult since the inception of APRN roles. The preference is to use the title "advanced practice registered nurse" to indicate the uniform preparation and regulation of the four APRN roles (CRNA, CNS, CNM, and NP). The Consensus Model makes this preference a permanent change. Advanced practice nursing has evolved in differing ways over time, with multiple titles, which confuses policymakers, patients, and the profession. Currently, not all states recognize all advanced practice roles for title protection. The NCSBN Maps project indicates that as many as 14 states use titles such as APN or ARNP instead of the widely recognized and accepted APRN (Fotsch, 2016; NCSBN, 2016a). APRN role and certification programs have aligned title with their credentials, just as they have aligned the Consensus Model educational requirements.

State Licensure and Recognition

Individual state nurse practice acts define the practice of nursing for registered nurses (RNs) throughout the 50 states and territories (NCSBN, 2017). State laws overseeing APRNs are divided into two forms: (1) statutes as defined by the nurse practice act, which are enacted by the state legislature; and (2) rules and regulations, which are made by state agencies under the jurisdiction of the executive branch of state government. Historically, under Amendment X of the US Constitution, states have the broad authority to regulate activities that affect the health, safety, and welfare of their citizens,

BOX 22.2 Advanced Practice Registered Nurse (APRN) Credentialing Definitions

Accreditation: The voluntary process whereby schools of nursing are reviewed by external nursing educational agencies for the purpose of determining the quality of a nursing and/or APRN program.

Certification: A formal process (usually an examination, but may be a portfolio) used by a certifying agency to validate, based on predetermined standards, an individual's knowledge, skills, and abilities. Certification provides validation of the APRN's knowledge in a particular role and population or specialty. It is used by most states as one component of second licensure for APRN practice.

Credentialing (institutional level): The process that an individual institution, or health system, uses to permit an APRN to practice in an APRN position within the institution. Generally, APRNs submit particular documentation to an institutional credentialing committee, which reviews and authorizes the APRN's practice.

Credentialing (state level): The requirements that a state uses to assess minimum standards of competency for APRNs to be authorized to practice in an APRN role. The purpose of credentialing is to protect the health and safety of the public. These requirements include an unencumbered registered nurse (RN) license, graduate education transcripts, and national certification in one of six population foci.

Legal authority: The authority assigned to a state or agency with administrative powers to enforce laws, rules, and policies.

Licensure: The process whereby an agency of state government grants authorization to an individual to engage in a given profession. For nursing, licensure is usually based on two criteria—the applicant attaining the essential education and degree of competency necessary to perform a unique scope of practice and passing a national examination. APRNs are licensed first as RNs and second as APRNs.

Regulations: The rules and policies that operationalize the laws and policies that recognize APRNs and credential them for practice in an APRN role and population focus.

including the practice of the healing arts within their borders. Licensure stems from this history, grounded in public protection, whereby each state creates standards to ensure basic levels of public safety. In the vast majority of states, APRN roles are overseen solely by the Boards of Nursing. The CNS roles are regulated by Boards of Nursing in all states that recognize the role. North Carolina, Virgina, and Alabama have joint subcommittees of Boards of Nursing and Boards of Medicine that regulate CNMs and NPs. CNMs are also subject to regulation by Boards of Medicine in New Jersey and Pennsylvania and Boards of Midwifery in New York, Rhode Island, and North Carolina. Florida requires practice per Board of Medicine approved protocols for APRN roles (NCSBN, 2017c).

Some states require a temporary permit for a new graduate to practice as an APRN while awaiting national certification results or other requirements, such as a required "gradual" transition to practice or added pharmacology education for prescriptive authority. New graduates should contact their state board of nursing and submit the required application for a temporary advanced practice nursing permit if the state allows this practice. With the advent of electronic testing, the time lapse between testing and obtaining results for licensure is minimal and markedly reduces the need for a temporary permit. In some states, temporary permits for APRNs no longer exist.

Institutional Credentialing

The need for hospital privileges for APRNs varies according to the nurse's practice. For example, CNMs and many rural NPs cannot care for patients properly without the ability to admit patients to the hospital should the need arise. Conversely, many CNSs are employed by hospitals and have no need for admitting privileges. It has not been necessary for CRNAs and some NPs to admit patients to the hospital independently to give comprehensive care, but they may need to see patients in the emergency room. Further, with the advent of hospitalist medicine, the need for physicians and APRNs with office-based practices to carry hospital privileges is less necessary.

The rules for practice as part of the hospital staff are even more specific and variable than those for state regulation and are separate from hospital administration; they are bound to the local hospital or medical facility and medical staff of the granting institution. The criteria and guidelines are written exclusively for medical practitioners, and APRNs are admitted or denied privileges based on their competency and experience (Buppert, 2015). Increasingly, medical staff credentialing committees are adding APRN members and facilities are creating APRN advisory committees (CAP2, 2017).

The first step for APRNs seeking hospital privileges is to ask the top-level nurse administrator how the credentials committee is organized, who makes up the membership, and what support there is for APRN applicants. Is there a process for nurses or others to petition for privileges? Nursing administrators are often members of credentials committees, and the APRN should meet with nurse colleagues for advice and support before the application process. A second step is to obtain the application package and begin to collect the necessary documents, which include, for example, licenses and certifications, transcripts, letters of support, and provider numbers. Support from collaborating physicians is key; in some committee structures, a collaborating physician may serve as the petitioner for a nurse colleague. Dialogue among the hospital administration, physician staff, and other stakeholders (e.g., APRN colleagues and other team members) is necessary if admitting privileges are required for the desired practice role. Alliances with consumers often add support to the application. Some hospitals have specific guidelines and protocols for all providers who are not physicians; others do not.

Determination of the specific privileges desired is critical to the process. For example, is it necessary to be able to admit or discharge patients, write orders, perform procedures, visit in-hospital patients, or take emergency room call? The Joint Commission requires that APRNs who provide "a medical level of care" be credentialed through the medical staff process. If they do not function at that level of care, they can be credentialed through an "equivalent process" (The Joint Commission, 2016). In today's market, professional "turf issues" are losing ground and opportunities for hospital privileges are opening the door for new APRN practice alternatives.

The APRN Consensus Model stresses that practice should be congruent with APRN education and national certification. Prior to implementation of the Model, the hiring distinctions of acute and primary care designations and role versus specialty certification were not stressed. Today, alignment with education and certification is vital and, increasingly, facility

BOX 22.3   Timeline for APRN Education, Certification, Licensure, and Practice

1. Final semester in graduate school—Graduate—Get transcript
2. Application for certification from approved certifying organization
3. Application for licensure from state board of nursing
4. Apply, interview, and obtain practice position as APRN
5. Develop practice agreement with precepting physician (if needed)
6. Apply for prescriptive authority from board of nursing (if needed)
7. Apply for Drug Enforcement Administration (DEA) number
8. Apply for national provider identifier (NPI) number
9. Obtain malpractice insurance
10. Apply for institutional/hospital privileges (if needed).

credentialing and risk management entities are checking for such alignment.

Box 22.3 identifies the timeline for establishing APRN credentials for practice.

Prescriptive Authority

Credentialing and licensure for prescriptive authority also occurs at the state level. Pharmacology requirements vary among states, although currently, most states and all certification programs require a core advanced pharmacotherapeutics course (a requirement of the Consensus Model) during the graduate APRN education program and some states require yearly CE credits thereafter to maintain prescriptive privilege. Prescriptive authority may be regulated solely by the board of nursing, as it is in several states; jointly by the board of nursing and board of pharmacy, as it is in several others; or by a triad of boards of nursing, medicine, and pharmacy (NCSBN, 2017c). Prescriptive authority may be included in a state's licensure or recognition of APRNs or it may be conferred as a separate license or authority. As prescriptive authority has evolved over the past several years, certain basic requirements have become fairly standard for APRN prescribers (Box 22.4). These requirements vary among states but provide a core regulatory process for prescriptive

BOX 22.4 **Requirements for Advanced Practice Registered Nurse (APRN) Prescribers**

- Graduation from an approved master's- or doctoral-level APRN program
- Licensure and recognition as an APRN in good standing
- National certification in an APRN population focus area
- Recent pharmacotherapeutics course of at least 3 credit hours (45 contact hours)
- Evidence of a collaborative practice arrangement (in some states)
- Ongoing continuing education hours in pharmacotherapeutics to maintain prescribing status (in some states)
- State prescribing number (in some states) and national Drug Enforcement Administration number

authority. Concerns for prescriptive drug abuse have prompted new and varying restrictions on controlled substance prescribing practices (National Alliance for Model State Drug Laws, 2016; The National Law Review, 2014). It is incumbent upon the APRN to understand clearly the mechanism of legal prescriptive authority in his or her state and to understand whether ongoing continuing education is required (Stokowski, 2013).

As noted, state boards of nursing should clearly document the numbers of hours of pharmacology required for an APRN to receive and maintain prescriptive privilege in terms of the APRN education program and annual CE requirements. APRN programs that previously integrated pharmacologic content in clinical management courses are required to have a stand-alone advanced pharmacotherapeutics course to comply with state requirements and accreditation standards (LACE, 2010). Pharmacology content should be taught by faculty pharmacists or a nurse-pharmacist faculty team who have an in-depth knowledge of therapeutic prescribing. Some states are requiring that APRN nursing programs verify specific course and content hours that can be used in a board of nursing application for prescriptive authority. Furthermore, several states require documentation of the number of hours of CE for pharmacology per year or per cycle. The direction is clearly to require APRNs to attend ongoing CE in pharmacology to maintain prescriptive privileges,

although APRNs should update their knowledge in this area whether or not their state requires it. Timely CE offerings and distance learning modalities (e.g., podcasts, Internet-based offerings) are available to meet the needs of busy clinicians. States will likely continue to move in the direction of interprofessional pharmacology education for nurses and physicians. Mobile applications that work with all types of devices are available to prescribers, and all APRNs must perform due diligence to assure that the applications they use are up to date, accurate, and evidence based (Ventola, 2014).

Identifier Numbers

Drug Enforcement Administration Number

In addition to obtaining prescriptive authority, APRNs who plan to prescribe or dispense controlled substances will need to apply for a Drug Enforcement Administration (DEA) number, as required by federal and state policy (DEA, Diversion Control Division, 2017b). DEA numbers are site specific; therefore, APRNs practicing at more than one site will need to obtain an additional DEA number for each site. The DEA's authority is federal; states have specific regulations pertaining to controlled substance authority. For APRNs who practice in states that enact the APRN Compact, it is important to know that independent prescribing authority under the APRN Compact multistate privilege pertains to legend drugs only and all controlled substance prescribing remains subject to DEA and state controlled substance regulations (NCSBN, 2015a; DEA, Diversion Control Division, 2017a).

National Provider Identifier Number

In addition to prescriber and DEA registration, APRNs will need to apply for a national provider identifier (NPI) number. The administrative simplification provisions of the Health Insurance Portability and Accountability Act (HIPAA) of 1996 mandated the adoption of a standard unique identifier for health care providers.

The National Plan & Provider Enumeration System (NPPES) collects identifying information on health care providers and assigns each provider a unique NPI. Every APRN should go to the NPPES website (https://nppes.cms.hhs.gov/#/) for further information or to apply for an NPI enumerator. NPI numbers are important for APRN prescribers because many drugs are on insurance company formularies and prescriptions are billed via the NPPES system. The attribution of care to a specific provider helps to track outcomes, compile provider workforce data, improve the transparency of care, and prevent fraud.

Scope of Practice for APRNs

By definition, the term *scope of practice* describes practice limits and sets the parameters within which nurses in the various advanced practice nursing specialties may legally practice. Scope statements define what APRNs may do for and with patients, what they can delegate, and when collaboration with others is required. Scope of practice statements tell APRNs what is actually beyond the legal limits of their nursing practice, even if they have the education and skills. The scope of practice for each of the four APRN roles differs (see Chapters 14 through 18). Scope of practice statements are key to the debate about how the US health care system uses APRNs as health care providers (US Department of Veterans Affairs, Office of Public and Intergovernmental Affairs, 2016). Controversies arise when health professionals' overlapping scopes of practice create interprofessional conflict (Federal Trade Commission, 2014). For example, CRNAs who administer general anesthesia have a scope of practice markedly different from that of the primary care NP, although both have their roots in basic nursing and have shared a core curriculum in APRN education. In addition, it is important to understand that scope of practice differs among states and is based on state laws, which impact the state's health care delivery (Xue, 2016).

Recent federal policy initiatives, including the update to the IOM's *The Future of Nursing* report (NASEM, 2015a) and the Federal Trade Commission (Gavil & Koslov, 2016), issued strong recommendations to remove restrictions on APRNs' scopes of practice. Reports from the National Governors Association (2012), the National Health Policy Forum (2010), and the Citizens Action Coalition stated firmly that current scope of practice adjudication is far too technical, subject to political pressure, and therefore not appropriate in the legislative sphere. There must be a more powerful forum so that the public can enter into the dialogue (see Chapter 19).

Accountability becomes a crucial factor as APRNs obtain more authority over their own practices. A scope of practice statement should identify the legal parameters of each APRN role, stating the additional accountabilities beyond that of the RN. These statements are then used by education and certification programs to assure that the student is trained to those additional accountabilities and tested on them

for entry into practice (Buppert, 2015). American society is highly mobile, and APRNs must recognize that their scope of practice will vary among states. In a worst case scenario, one can be an APRN in one state but not meet the criteria in another state (Barton Associates, 2016). States that adopt the APRN Compact will align their multistate practice privilege with the statutory language of the APRN Compact. This will allow for uniform practice among Compact states (NCSBN, 2015a).

APRNs owe Barbara Safriet, former Associate Dean at Yale Law School, a debt of gratitude for her vision and clarity in helping APRNs understand and think strategically about scope of practice and regulatory issues. In her landmark 1992 monograph, Safriet noted that APRNs are unique in that there is a multiprofessional approach to their regulation based on ignorance and on the fallacy that medicine is all-knowing, particularly about advanced practice nursing (Safriet, 1992). As Safriet has implied, restraints on advanced practice nursing result from ignorance about APRNs' abilities, rigid notions about professional roles, and turf protection. She cited reforms in scope of practice laws in Colorado that encouraged solutions to long-time tensions over control of practice between organized medicine and nursing. Colorado's provision defines the term *practice authority* in terms of ability and thus redirects the regulatory focus from providers' status to the APRN's training and skills (Safriet, 2002, 2011). This example and the imminent move to Consensus Model regulation offer hope that, in the future, policies can be formulated to close the gap between what APRNs can do and what they are allowed to do by scope of practice statutes. Scope of practice is hampered in many states where APRN practice is carved out of the medical practice act as a medically delegated act that precludes reasonable autonomy for the APRN. The ability to diagnose disease and treat patients, inherent in the role of the APRN, is fluid and evolving and is often tied to the collaborative relationships that APRNs have with physician colleagues (American Nurses Association, 2016). Barbara Safriet was inducted as an honorary fellow into the American Academy of Nursing in 2013 and became the first honorary fellow of the American Association of Nurse Practitioners that same year.

It is important to note that although APRNs desire autonomous licensure through the state boards of nursing, the need to work interprofessionally as colleagues and team members is essential to attaining high-level patient outcomes (IPEC, 2016).

Standards of Practice and Standards of Care for APRNs

Standards of practice for nurses are defined by the profession nationally and help to further delineate scope of practice. Standards are overarching authoritative statements that the nursing profession uses to describe the responsibilities for which its members are accountable (American Nurses Association, 2016; NACNS, 2016). As such, they complement and enable the APRN core, population focus, and specialty competencies. APRNs are held to the standards of practice of both the nursing profession and the various APRN specialties. At both levels, standards of practice describe the basic competency levels for safe and competent practice (see Chapters 14-18 for the standards of practice for CNSs, NPs, CNMs, and CRNAs). Professional standards of practice match closely with the core competencies for APRNs, outlined in Chapter 3, which undergird advanced practice nursing.

Standards of care differ from the standards of practice set forth by the nursing profession. These standards are often termed *practice guidelines.* Practice guidelines provide a foundation for health care providers to administer care to patients. Ideally, these guidelines crosscut the health professions' disciplines and provide the framework whereby basic safety and competent care are measured. For APRNs, this means that the standard used to evaluate advanced nursing practice is often the same as the standard used to review medical practice. Clinical guidelines are used as the standard of care in legal decisions; therefore, it is essential for APRNs to be part of the team developing new evidence-based guidelines.

Standards of care are derived from evidence-based practice and are continuously evolving. At the federal policy level, the Agency for Healthcare Research and Quality has responsibility for conducting the research needed to evaluate clinical practice guidelines that define a standard of appropriate care in specific areas (National Guideline Clearinghouse, 2016). The Centers for Disease Control and Prevention as well as professional medical and nursing specialty organizations also create guidelines for practice. Organizations such as the National Quality Forum and the Centers for Medicare and Medicaid Services (CMS) measure practice against standards of care, as do many private insurers (Evans, 2016). It is important for APRNs to be part of interprofessional teams that develop and test practice guidelines for care and to participate in the selection of measures (National Quality Forum, 2017).

Issues Affecting APRN Credentialing and Regulation

The definition of an APRN requires that the four established APRN roles be clinically focused and that the APRN provide direct clinical care to patients (Hamric, 2005, 2014). The definition developed in this text goes beyond this requirement and is discussed further in Chapter 3. From a legal and regulatory perspective, inclusion in the designation of what constitutes an APRN is driven primarily by three factors: (1) the diagnosis and management of patients at an advanced level of nursing expertise, (2) the ability of APRNs to be directly reimbursed, and (3) the degree to which nurses wish to hold prescriptive and hospital admitting privileges. As practice migrates from acute care facilities into alternative settings, there must be a well-defined and efficacious way for state boards, insurers, prescribing entities, and similar groups to monitor the scope of practice, prescribing, and reimbursement patterns of APRNs, not only in acute care settings but in all relevant settings (Kleinpell, Hudspeth, Scordo, & Magdic, 2012). These groups need clear criteria that can be validated to ensure patient safety and monitor certification and credentialing.

Collaborative Practice Arrangements

States that have delegated medical authority for APRNs often require what are termed *collaborative agreements* for APRNs who diagnose diseases, manage treatment, and prescribe medications for patients. As implied, collaborative agreements provide a written description of the professional relationship between an APRN and a collaborating physician that defines the parameters whereby the APRN can perform delegated medical acts and are, at their core, supervisory.

A collaborative agreement or arrangement may take many forms, from a one-page written agreement defining consultation and referral patterns to a more exact, prescribed protocol for specific functions, based on state statutes for advanced practice nursing. When collaborations are required for licensure or credentialing, they are supervisory (NCSBN, 2016b). Collaborative agreements need to be written as broadly as possible to allow for practice variations and new innovations. Examples of collaborative practice agreements can be found on the Internet.

The term *protocol* in relation to advanced practice nursing was common several years ago as a physician-directed, specified guideline for the medical aspects of practice that defined each patient problem and the treatment approach. Some states used this so-called cookbook approach to NP practice as a way to oversee prescriptive and other treatment modalities. For the most part, specific protocols for care are no longer used in most settings because it is difficult to update and tailor them to the individual needs of patients and practices. More important, advanced practice nursing has evolved. Numerous studies support the ability of APRNs to provide competent care with positive outcomes and protocols have been replaced by evidence-based practice guidelines within a collaborative arrangement. It is important to note that the specificity of the collaborative arrangement, where required, is usually based on trust and respect between the collaborating APRN and physician colleague. Increasingly, required collaborations have been removed but a trend has been to require a specified transition-to-practice period for newly licensed APRNs. Today such requirements exist in as many as 11 states for practice and/or prescribing, ranging from 30 to 1500 hours for prescribing and from 1000 hours to 4 years for practice (Cahill, 2017, raw unpublished data). Such requirements are arbitrary, are outdated, add to confusion, and entirely lack an evidence base.

Reimbursement

On a par with the need to be able to prescribe medications for patients is the need to be appropriately paid for services delivered and reimbursed for care. Clearly, APRNs should be paid for services rendered for health care whether they work independently, share a joint practice with a physician colleague, or are employed in an institution or provider network (see Chapter 21). Although the insurance industry is regulated by the individual states, many of the private pay insurance standards used to set payment mechanisms are modeled after federal Medicare and Medicaid policy (Clemmons & Gottlieb, 2013). Federal mandates that encourage direct payment of nonphysician health care providers are often blocked at the state level by discriminatory rules and regulations for APRNs. State legislative change is occurring that expands direct payment to these groups (Hain & Fleck, 2014), though changes occurring in CMS pay-for-performance strategies are arguably the most impactful (CMS, 2015).

From a credentialing standpoint, attention to CMS rules, Medicare and Medicaid provider numbers, Clinical Laboratory Improvement Amendments (CMS, 2016) regulations, and provider requirements are extremely important to ensure that APRNs are reimbursed. It is important for APRNs to know how to contract for their services at the individual level as they negotiate employment packages, but even more importantly, they need to be present at the negotiating table as members of executive management teams who are setting the policies for provider services where the rules for payment are made. Exemplar 22.1 describes the many credentialing requirements needed to begin practice as an APRN.

Historically, APRNs have been reimbursed indirectly "incident-to" physicians, and at a considerably lower rate. Incident-to billing came into being after the Balanced Budget Act of 1997 through an amendment that allowed NPs to bill Medicare at 85% of the physician fee. The CMS has attempted clarification in documents such as their 2015 booklet, *Medicare Information for Advanced Practice Registered Nurses, Anesthesiologist Assistants, and Physician Assistants* (CMS, Medicare Learning Network, 2016).

It is important to identify the third-party payors of most patients for whom the APRN will be caring and to learn their requirements for reimbursement of APRNs. Only then are APRNs in an appropriate position to seek status as reimbursable providers with Medicare, Medicaid, and the many private payors (see Chapter 21). There are several areas in which reimbursement schemes directly affect the regulation of advanced practice nursing. Although private payment by the patient is gaining strength, Medicare and Medicaid, commercial insurers, ACOs, and health maintenance organizations cover most health care costs in today's market. These entities build networks of providers by hiring, purchasing services from, or contracting with physicians and APRNs, hospitals, and others to provide health care services to patients. When APRNs join a provider network, they must meet all the requirements, regulations, and standards of care established by the plan. For example, a primary care NP applying for a position would need to meet all the criteria listed in Box 22.4 and obtain appropriate Medicare and Medicaid provider status as well as malpractice history and coverage. It is incumbent on the APRN to have all credentials and regulatory documentation in good and accessible order when preparing to practice because third-party payors are often located in and governed by reimbursement administrators in a distant state.

EXEMPLAR 22.1   **Meeting the Requirements for Credentialing and Regulation**

Laurie is in the final semester of her Doctor of Nursing Practice family nurse practitioner (FNP) program at a state university. She is in the process of negotiating a contract with a provider network of physicians and advanced practice registered nurses (APRNs) in a rural practice. Laurie knows that she must begin the process of acquiring the necessary credentials to be able to practice in her state after she has successfully passed national APRN certification in her population focus area. When she applied to her FNP program, she made sure that the university and graduate program were accredited and in good standing. Now that she is ready to graduate, she must prepare for a new and challenging professional life.

In her seminar class, Laurie received the application to sit for national certification the month after she graduates and has sent the application forward to register the date for her examination. Her next step is to download the advanced practice nursing rules and regulations for her state so that she fully knows the scope of practice she must adhere to. She also obtains the APRN application materials from the state board of nursing. Laurie reviews these documents carefully in order to understand the application process, materials, and fee that she will need to submit to the state licensing board.

Laurie carefully notes that APRNs in her state must show proof that they have completed a 45–contact hour, state-approved graduate nursing course in pharmacotherapeutics. Also, she must complete 6 hours of continuing education in pharmacotherapeutics each

year to maintain her status as a prescriber. She makes a note to request the transcript and syllabus for her pharmacotherapeutics course to attach to the application for her APRN license.

Unless she resides in a state with full practice authority, on signing her contract, Laurie will first need to negotiate a written collaborative arrangement with the precepting physician colleague, who will see the patients who are beyond her scope of practice. Second, she needs a Medicaid provider number to see children in the Medicaid program. She will need to apply for her national provider identifier and Drug Enforcement Administration numbers. In addition, this health care system requires that Laurie apply to the local hospital and nursing home privileging committees so that she can see patients on rounds, do admitting and discharge planning, and follow nursing home patients on a regular basis.

As part of her package, Laurie has negotiated for the employer to pay the premium on her malpractice insurance as an APRN. She also negotiates $3000 per year for continuing education. She needs to call her insurance carrier to discuss the transfer of her student policy to a full malpractice policy to cover her as a certified APRN with the appropriate scope of practice that she will need in her new position. She knows that she wants to purchase an occurrence type of policy. Laurie uses the support of her colleagues and mentors as she works through this important process of preparing her credentials to practice as an APRN (see Box 22.2). ◎

Risk Management, Malpractice, and Negligence

Although malpractice suits involving APRNs are rare, malpractice issues are ever-present for all providers of health care, regardless of credential or setting. In an unstable health care environment, patients look to the tort system to ease the apprehension and anxiety about the care that they receive. Patients are more likely to seek redress if they mistrust their provider or believe that they have been harmed by the system. First and foremost, APRNs need to understand clearly what constitutes negligent practice and grounds for malpractice and to put safeguards in place so they do not have to confront the legal system.

By definition, negligence is the failure to act in a professionally, reasonable way as a health care clinician. Negligence may lead to malpractice and legal action. The following four factors (the "four Ds") must be present for a malpractice suit to be valid (Buppert, 2015):

- A **duty** of care must be owed to the injured party, through direct office or hospital care or through phone or e-mail advice; a patient-nurse relationship must be established.
- The accepted standard of care was breached **(breach of duty)**.
- The patient must have **damage** or have sustained an injury.
- There must be **direct causation (cause)** demonstrated—that is, the patient has suffered

an injury that was caused by the APRN clinician. (Often, there are multiple causative factors based on care by several caregivers over time.)

Within the judicial system, care is evaluated by preset criteria in the form of medical and advanced practice nursing standards. National professional organizations set the standards for appropriate care. APRNs are held to the standard of care explicated by advanced practice nursing standards. However, there is much blurring between medical and nursing standards, creating a dire need for interprofessional standards of care that will hold health care providers to the same standards as their peers. There are several ways that legal standards of care are established in a particular case. The most common is through expert testimony offered by a person who is qualified by education, experience, knowledge, and skill level to judge the actions of the providers in the case. Other mechanisms include review of professional literature, manufacturers' package inserts, and documented professional standards of care. Letz (2002) has suggested four ways to prevent malpractice events: establish a good rapport with patients over time, follow an established standard of care to ensure competence, document accurately and completely, and take a course in risk management.

APRNs can use several risk management techniques to mitigate against malpractice occurrences. First and foremost, APRNs should assure that their practice is congruent with their education and certification, or, if educated pre–Consensus Model (before 2008) and practice is not congruent, they should consider advanced certification in their present practice area, if it is available. For those educated before 2008, it is also wise to maintain a continuing education log and a competency performance record, including a patient profile list and performance review history. It is important to document well and to audit charts frequently for mistakes and omissions. APRNs must be vigilant if asked to give advice by phone or to see patients outside the practice setting. In such instances the APRN should treat these events as an office visit with full documentation in the patient record.

APRNs need awareness of two national issues related to diagnosis. The widespread use of unnecessary diagnostic tests (laboratory and imaging) has contributed to skyrocketing health costs, while the timeliness and accuracy of diagnosis remain a challenge. To address the first concern, a national effort is underway to "choose wisely" in the selection of appropriate diagnostic tests. The ABIM (American Board of Internal Medicine) Foundation hosts the national "Choosing Wisely®" campaign, which advocates for care that is supported by evidence, not duplicative, free from harm, and truly necessary (ABIM Foundation, 2016). To address the timeliness and accuracy of diagnosis, the IOM released a report from the Committee on Diagnostic Error in 2015, adding this area to its Quality Chasm series and elevating concerns regarding patient safety risks in missed or delayed diagnoses (NASEM, 2015b). Diagnostic studies overall show that 5% of adults seeking outpatient care in the United States will suffer a diagnostic error, and such errors will contribute to about 10% of patient deaths (Stempniak, 2015). Claims against APRNs are many fewer than those against physicians, and some studies have suggested no difference in diagnostic reasoning nor in ordering diagnostic tests (Louden, 2015, Pirret, Neville, & La Grow, 2015). However, diagnostic-related issues are the top reason for closed claims cases against NPs in at least one claims analyses (Nurses Service Organization [NSO], 2012). Several studies have suggested that APRNs—in particular, NPs—have diagnostic accuracy comparable to their physician counterparts (van der Linden, Reijnen, & de Vos, 2010). The study of clinical reasoning and diagnostic error is producing valuable information for all diagnosticians to consider. The Society to Improve Diagnosis in Medicine is inclusive of APRNs and has created a "diagnostic toolkit" with checklists and tips to aid in diagnostic improvement (NASEM, 2015b; Society to Improve Diagnosis in Medicine, 2016).

Professional liability claims companies often create advisories for professionals based on analyses of past claims and can be a source of risk avoidance strategies (NSO, 2012). Malpractice carriers offer discounts to APRNs who take risk management courses. Professional websites are a source of comprehensive risk management tools and current discussions of legal questions confronting APRNs.

Malpractice Insurance

APRNs need a thorough understanding of liability insurance coverage, types of policies, and extent of coverage required. It is important to understand the difference between the two most common types of professional liability insurance plans, *claims-made* and *occurrence.* A claims-made insurance policy covers claims made against the APRN only while the policy is in effect. Coverage must be continued indefinitely to ensure coverage for claims filed in the future for actions that occurred in the past. A claims-made policy can be extended through the purchase of additional coverage, referred to as a "tail," that covers the APRN during the switch from one carrier to another (American College of Physicians, 2016). Conversely, with an occurrence policy, the APRN is covered for alleged acts of negligence that occurred during the time that the policy was in effect. The benefit of occurrence coverage is that even if the policy is cancelled at some future date, coverage for events that occurred while the policy was in effect will be honored. More information about advanced practice nursing liability insurance can be found on websites for the major malpractice insurance carriers. Each APRN must understand the extent of coverage per incident and how personal legal costs are covered in the policy. The amount of insurance needed is governed by the type of practice in which the APRN is engaged; CRNAs and CNMs, who are under more risk, need more coverage (Kinzelman & Bushman, 2015).

It is important that APRNs carry their own individual liability coverage, even if they are covered by an employer group practice. Employer-based insurance contracts are geared to protect the institution or practice as a whole and are not targeted to protect the individual APRN. The comfort of having one's own counsel during litigation far outweighs the cost of individual liability insurance. Conferences, workshops, and Internet offerings are available to assist APRNs in choosing the appropriate insurance carrier and plan. Increasingly, state statutes may require liability coverage by APRNs. As APRNs move in and out of what is considered the domain of medicine, serious thought must be given to the standard whereby APRNs will be judged if they are deemed to have made an error. Although not many documented cases have cited APRNs who have injured patients by wrongful action, the question about whether APRNs should be tried by the courts according to medical or advanced nursing practice standards is important and needs to be clarified. Facility malpractice carriers may require that an APRN's practice is congruent with his or her education and certification, including congruence in population focus and the subfoci of acute care and primary care, if they apply. Increasingly, these carriers are concerned about the potential for cases that relate to APRNs practicing outside of their scope of education and certification (NSO, 2012). It is incumbent on APRNs to set clear standards for practice that are based on clinical competency.

Privacy Issues: Health Insurance Portability and Accountability Act

The federal Health Insurance Portability and Accountability Act (HIPAA) became law in 1996. The US Department of Health and Human Services (DHHS) website maintains a section on Health Information Privacy, where the ruling and its latest amendments and documentation can be accessed (https://www.hhs.gov/hipaa/index.html). HIPAA mandates implementation of statewide, uniform, minimum patient privacy standards. The main goal of HIPAA is to protect the privacy of a patient's identifiable health information that is maintained or transmitted by health care providers and insurers (US DHHS, 2013). This includes any information that would identify the patient, the patient's problem, the plan of care, and how care is paid for. The regulations for privacy established by HIPAA have placed a new level of legal responsibility on health providers, including APRNs. If APRNs accept third-party reimbursement or transmit any health information in any form, they are required to comply with HIPAA regulations.

Organizations must conduct security risk assessments to safeguard private health information. Facilities and providers can design their own policies and procedures to meet the needs and scope of their practice, but these policies must adhere to all the standards included in the operating standards of HIPAA (Buppert, 2015). Penalties are severe and include civil monetary fines and, in some cases, felony criminal penalties. The Office of Civil Rights of the DHHS is charged with enforcing the HIPPA requirements (Law360, 2015).

Telehealth and Telepractice and Licensure Portability (The APRN Compact)

No changes in health care delivery in many years are likely to be as impactful as telehealth and licensure mobility. The United States and, indeed, the world is on the precipice of a massive shift in health care. Health care will have moved from the early days of horse and buggy home visits to the digital age of virtual visits, telecare, group- or peer-led visits, and remote monitoring (Weiner, Yeh, & Blumenthal, 2013). Telehealth is predicted to be a $20 billion to $30 billion industry in the next 5 years (Qamar, 2015); thus, never before has licensure portability been more important. The success of telemedicine is dependent upon the ability of health care providers to follow their patients regardless of location.

　Interstate Practice Through Licensure Portability Using the Interstate Compact

Ron Garcia is an advanced practice registered nurse (APRN) clinical nurse specialist who specializes in heart failure. He is a member of a large cardiology team in a multistate health system. Ron leads the heart failure team that includes a pharmacist, a social worker, a physical therapist, home care nurses, and home care aides. Ron's patients are referred to him from cardiologists across this multistate system. His team provides ambulatory and home visits as well as remote monitoring for patients. They have developed a management protocol that has produced remarkable results in improving compliance with home monitoring and reducing readmissions in patients with heart failure. Presently he practices and holds licensure in four states.

Ron is an advocate for interstate licensure. He recognizes that care that is received by his patients can produce benefit or harm. The patients have recourse through their state boards of nursing if they have a complaint with any licensed professional on his teams.

This requires that he and his team members hold licenses in each state where their patients receive care. The health system would like to expand care, under his leadership, to the other states. When his state joins the APRN Compact and the Nurse Licensure Compact, both he and the nurses, if they meet qualifications, will be able to practice in any other state that joins those compacts. Ron knows that innovations and breakthroughs in health care are occurring at an amazing rate. Teams like his are discovering socially sensitive care strategies that produce results. His company chooses to expand Ron's team in Compact states preferentially, while they wait for additional states to join the Compacts.

As geography becomes less relevant in care provision, state geographic boundaries will become irrational in a high-value care delivery system. Ron understands that a system of mutual regulatory recognition (licensure portability) through an interstate APRN Compact for APRNs is vitally important. He considers volunteering with the coalition to help with this issue. ◎

The APRN Compact (NCSBN, 2015a), a model described as mutual recognition, allows an APRN holding a multistate license in her or his home state to practice in any participating Compact state. Another compact, the Nurse Licensure Compact, applies to RNs and licensed vocational nurses. This compact has been in effect for 15 years but, like the APRN Compact, is newly revised and now has been adopted in 26 states. The Enhanced Nurse Licensure Compact will be in place as of January 19, 2018 (https://www.ncsbn.org/enhanced-nlc-implementation .htm). States participating in the APRN Compact need not also participate in the Nurse Licensure Compact, but many states will adopt both compacts. APRNs can actively support passage of Compacts in their state and learn more about them at https:// www.ncsbn.org/aprn-compact.htm and https://www .ncsbn.org/enhanced-nlc-implementation.htm (see Exemplar 22.2).

Physicians have also adopted a state-based licensure portability mechanism through the Federation of State Medical Boards. The Medical Compact license does not eliminate the need to pay multiple state licensure fees, as it does in the nursing compacts, but it does expedite the licensure process (Interstate Medical Licensure Compact, 2017).

Not all telehealth endeavors have evidence of outcomes improvements and/or cost reductions, but some do. Virtual intensive care units have shown remote monitoring to improve outcomes and reduce stays (Hwang, 2014). Other areas showing some benefits have been in chronic care management, mental health care, and physical rehabilitation (McLean et al., 2013). State-based legislation that applies to defining telehealth providers, refining reimbursement requirements, and determining the level of involvement of the various professions in the regulation and delivery of telehealth is mounting year by year (American Telemedicine Association, 2015). Although most legislation passed thus far does not exclude APRNs as providers, it is important that professional nursing groups and APRNs remain informed of and continue working toward improved telemedicine and telehealth bills and implementation of licensure mobility through Nursing Compacts in their states.

Safety and Cost Containment Initiatives

Acts of Congress since the events of 9/11, economic downturns, and federal and state budget crises have cut programs for the poor. These factors, plus the increase in the number of older adults with chronic illness, will augment the need for APRNs, even while funds to pay for this care are reduced, causing increased stress on underserved populations with health problems. Such issues are not just economic but also geographic, as seen in the present loss of rural access hospitals (McCarter, 2015; O'Donnell & Ungar, 2014). The ACA also calls for increased numbers of APRN primary care providers, nurse-managed clinics, and ACO configurations, such as medical or health care homes (Lathrop & Hodnicki, 2014). Bodenheimer and Grumbach (2012) have suggested several alternatives to painful cost controls that APRNs can implement. Initiating simple policies, such as the judicious use of supplies and prudent choice of diagnostic tests and procedures, is a first step. Physician groups have moved quickly to fill the quality gap because they recognize the potential relationship of quality to payment issues, which is now a fact of practice through value-based purchasing. APRNs need to engage and participate in value-based purchasing projects fully as a way to ensure the visibility, quality, and cost-effectiveness of their practice (Johnson, Harper, Hanson, & Dawson, 2007; Revisions to the Physician Fee Schedule, 2016; see Chapter 22).

IOM reports, such as the Quality Chasm series (U.T. Health Science Center at San Antonio, School of Nursing, 2015), have focused on human factors that influence patient safety. In addition to a healing environment for patients, initiatives that enhance patient safety, such as enlarging the safety knowledge base of caregivers and providing technologic assistance in the form of smart phones and tablets, are useful tools. The initiation and resources of nurse-driven initiatives such as the QSEN Institute (http://qsen.org/) and the Nursing Alliance for Quality Care (http://www.naqc.org) are excellent examples of progress toward quality and safer care for patients. Funding opportunities and demonstration projects for APRNs to improve safety outcomes and decrease errors are clearly evident in the national agenda (Agency for Healthcare Research and Quality, 2016). APRNs are active participants in the National Quality Forum, the National Patient Safety Foundation, the Institute for Healthcare Improvement, the Society to Improve Diagnosis in Medicine, and other quality- and safety-related organizations.

Although ongoing data collection is needed to substantiate the positive outcomes by APRN providers, research has shown that APRNs are safe and cost-effective alternatives to physician-based health care (see Chapter 23). Increased APRN visibility makes it imperative that APRNs monitor the value of their own practices and clearly understand the costs of providing care to patients. If APRNs want to be providers of record, they must show positive and safe outcomes of their work to justify Medicare reimbursement and inclusion on all insurance panels as well as to maintain the public's trust.

Influencing the Regulatory Process

As major stakeholders in the regulatory process, it is imperative that APRNs directly influence the process in several ways, including using political strategies. At all levels, regulators are eager to find practicing APRNs and advanced practice nursing educators who will take an active role in assisting them to develop and implement sound regulatory policies and procedures. The information explosion has brought the ability to communicate and connect with others at a moment's notice, which makes it easier for APRNs to influence the system directly. Chapters 11 and 19 provide in-depth discussions of skills needed for leadership and political advocacy. Additional ways for novice and expert APRNs to engage actively in any regulatory process that affects their practice include the following.

Novice or Any APRNs

- Participate in professional organizations and become involved in regulatory activities, such as educating lawmakers, providing public comment on APRN issues, writing letters, and being part of an APRN campaign or coalition activities.
- Monitor current APRN legislation and legislation that affects patients.
- Offer to participate in test-writing committees for national certification examinations as item writers and/or reviewers.
- Respond to offers to review, edit, and provide feedback about circulated draft regulatory policies that directly affect APRN advanced practice nursing education and practice.

Experienced and Expert APRNs

- Seek out a gubernatorial appointment to the board of nursing or advanced practice committee that advises the board of nursing in your state.
- Seek membership as the APRN or consumer member of the advisory council for the state medical board or state board of pharmacy.

- Seek appointment to CMS panels on which Medicare and Medicaid provider issues are decided.
- Seek appointment to hospital privileging committees and ensure that privileging materials are appropriate for APRNs.
- Seek appointment on advisory committees and task forces that are advising the NCSBN and other regulatory and credentialing bodies.
- Provide public comment on draft legislation regarding health care and health care providers.
- Offer testimony at state and national hearings at which proposed regulatory changes in APRN advanced practice nursing regulation, prescriptive authority, and reimbursement schemes will be discussed.

To accomplish these activities, APRNs need to use research data, a powerful tool for shaping health policy (Hamric, 1998). By actively participating in the regulatory process, APRNs ensure themselves of a strong voice in regulatory and credentialing processes. At the very least, it is incumbent on the practicing APRN to monitor the process carefully through APRN networks and social media to stay informed.

Current Practice Climate for APRNs

The Time is Right for True Collaboration Among Health Care Providers

Collaboration is the belief that quality patient care is attained by the contribution of all care providers (Arcangelo, Fitzgerald, Carrol, & Plumb, 1996). Parallel play, or working side by side, is not enough; a true blending of all of the health professionals' unique contributions offers a comprehensive health care approach. Effective teams have been in place in health care for many years. Examples exist in military care and disaster medicine, and also in specialty care teams such as in oncology, as well as in medical home models (Eggenberger, Sherman, & Keller, 2014; IOM, 2011). APRNs do not now, nor have they ever, practiced in isolation. APRNs are RNs who have targeted and focused education in a specific role and with one or more defined populations (NCSBN, 2017b). They are additionally educated as APRNs with a level of nursing practice that extends beyond that of the RN, utilizing all available team members, to the extent that they can contribute to patient outcomes. In their educational preparation and in their nursing roles, APRNs are well aware of their practice boundaries. APRNs are taught how to

effectively consult with others and to make referrals as needed and, more importantly, to fully collaborate with all members of the health care team.

As coordinators of care, nurses at all levels embrace the concept of collaboration, but, unfortunately, along the way, something changed. As APRNs advocated for practice to the full scope of their education and training, states began to adopt legislation that utilized the term *collaboration* to describe a required and supervisory relationship with a physician. This regulatory language "hijacked" the term *collaboration* for APRNs. Such requirements of oversight by another professional group suggest that the scope of APRN practice is somehow subsumed within the scope of medicine. This is not true for APRN practice any more than it would be for any other professional group. The current environment is the right time to move beyond outdated "regulatory collaboration" language and into true collaboration with all members of the health care team.

Visioning for Advanced Practice Nursing

When APRNs seek to change statutes and regulations, it is not because they see themselves as needing to practice in a vacuum of independence apart from the rest of the health care team, but because they desire to be a valued part of the team. It is a hard fact that APRNs must have authority over their own practices and the decisions they make about patient care. They must be able to defend their actions within the legal system based on nursing-driven standards and regulation. Only in this way can an APRN move out of the darkness of being a "shadow provider" (Wilcox, 1995). Issues related to being a shadow provider are best exemplified by "incident-to" billing by NPs using the physician's Medicare number. Advanced practice nursing care is invisible to regulators and insurers with this type of billing procedure. Securing attribution for their unique services in health care reimbursement and outcomes will be vital to enabling APRNs to move out of the shadows and into the light. As care increasingly moves to a team-based model, APRNs are poised to lead teams, when appropriate, and to be valuable team members. Attribution of care to specific team members is an important variable to learn what parts of team-based care contribute to the expected outcomes. This is one example of the challenges APRNs face as they work to clarify state policies. It may be that APRNs will feel comfortable only when their position in the health care community is fully secure in all states;

this will require focused and coordinated political and legislative work related to credentialing and regulatory issues.

APRNs have already achieved impressive strides over time in the areas of credentialing and regulation of APRNs. The health care provided by APRNs has had far-reaching effects on all members of society; thus the evolution of advanced practice nursing in the United States is a source of pride to nurses. The positive excitement of the IOM's 2011 recommendations, revisited in the 2015 update *Assessing Progress on the Institute of Medicine Report: The Future of Nursing* (NASEM, 2015a), the Josiah Macy Foundation's recommendations, and ACA language is countered with the responsibility for higher accountability and the need for more standardized ways to credential, certify, regulate, and sanction competent practice for a growing number of APRNs. This occurs through state-by-state adoption of the elements of the APRN Consensus Model and uniform licensure requirements. In 2017, the Veteran's Health Administration (VHA) began to implement full practice authority in specific VHA facilities across the United States for the CNS, NP, and CNM roles (US Department of Veterans Affairs, Office of Public and Intergovernmental Affairs, 2016). In this same year, the passage of the Comprehensive Addiction and Recovery Act (CARA) added nurse practitioners to those prescribers who could offer medication-assisted treatment for addiction (CARA, 2016). The future for APRNs now includes an APRN Compact that will enable practice mobility aligned with the APRN Consensus elements across state borders (NCSBN, 2015a).

Forces within health care, as well as needs within the regulatory and educational climate of advanced practice nursing, have set the stage for an era of progressive change. The pressing health care needs in the United States have serious implications for education, practice, and regulation of APRNs. Advancing technologies, enhanced mobility of APRNs across state lines, and diversity among state regulatory mechanisms have brought together APRN leaders and stakeholders to craft a new vision for the future of advanced practice nursing.

Future Regulatory Challenges Facing APRNs

Health professions reports published over the past decade have continued to recommend the need for generic benchmarks and standards for health care

education and practice for all health care professions (Grapczynski, Schuurman, Booth, Bambini, & Beel-Bates, 2015). The future requires that APRNs create clear, broad-based, competency-based standards for education and practice to allow for growth and movement across state lines. Regulation for the health professions will require a new approach that dispels notions of exclusivity, exclusion, or independence from other disciplines. This move toward overarching regulation for the health professions, when and if it comes to pass, will require much higher levels of collaboration among the disciplines and specialties than now exist (IPEC, 2016; see Chapter 12) and, most importantly, broad-based standards and regulations for advanced practice nursing. New models of regulation will require strong leadership and increased involvement by practicing APRNs, as exemplified in the current Master's and DNP Essentials, and dynamic, cutting-edge competencies put forth by APRN organizations.

Conclusion

At no time has it been more vital for APRNs to understand and value the important relationships among groups that control the complex processes and systems that regulate practice. New models of health care and varying configurations of how APRNs practice in interprofessional teams have escalated the importance of regulatory considerations. The growth of virtual health care delivery makes the picture even more complex (Eggenberger, Sherman, & Keller, 2014). APRNs will need to provide leadership and clear direction to policymakers to ensure the development of broad-based practice standards that will satisfy state statutes and make sense in all areas of advanced practice nursing. The consensus-derived key elements for the preparation and education of the four described APRN roles are powerful drivers of the inclusion of APRNs at all levels of US health care. The need for APRNs to move into key roles as health care providers in the next decade requires careful vigilance with regard to the LACE components of credentialing and regulation. The ever-changing landscape of America's health system demands vision and a steady hand into the future.

Key Summary Points

■ APRNs are increasingly educated, certified, and regulated in alignment with the APRN Consensus Model (APRN Joint Dialogue Group, 2008) and uniform licensure requirements, such as those included in the APRN Compact (NCSBN, 2015a).

- Credentialing procedures and requirements vary from state to state and determine scope of practice. APRNs must strive to achieve a scope of practice in their state that is commensurate with their education and clinical skills.
- True collaboration among LACE members will be required to provide needed education and regulation models that foster quality health care by APRN providers.

References

To access the references for this chapter, use your smartphone's QR code reader to scan the code below, or go to http://booksite.elsevier.com/ 9780323447751.

CHAPTER

Integrative Review of APRN Outcomes and Performance Improvement Research

23

Ruth M. Kleinpell • Anne W. Alexandrov

> "The obvious is that which is never seen until someone expresses it simply."
>
> —*Kahlil Gibran*

CHAPTER CONTENTS

Measuring the impact of advanced practice registered nurse (APRN) practice is an important component in supporting the value of the role with evidence from quality research studies. This becomes especially pertinent with current initiatives such as the Patient Protection and Affordable Care Act (2010) program of hospital inpatient value-based purchasing and other quality care initiatives that are focused on performance monitoring and the development of operational and clinical performance metrics.

A number of factors have led to the current focus on outcomes of care in health care, including increased emphasis on providing quality care and promoting patient safety, regulatory requirements for health care entities to demonstrate care effectiveness, increased health system accountability, and changes

in the organization, delivery, and financing of health care. APRNs are affecting patient and system outcomes in a number of ways, but too often these outcomes are not quantified or attributed to advanced practice nursing. Employers, consumers, insurers, and others are calling for APRNs to justify their contribution to health care and to demonstrate the value that they add to the system. The Institute of Medicine report *The Future of Nursing* has highlighted the importance of promoting the ability of APRNs to practice to the full extent of their education and training and to identify further nurses' contributions to delivering high-quality care (Institute of Medicine, 2011). Verifying APRN contributions requires an assessment of the structures, processes, and outcomes associated with APRN performance and the care delivery systems in which they practice.

Evaluation of individual APRN impact occurs at multiple levels, with supporting evidence collected during annual performance reviews, outcomes measurement activities, process improvement analyses, program evaluations, and small- and large-scale

We acknowledge the work of the late Gail Ingersoll, EdD, RN, FAAN, FNAP, in advancing the focus on advanced practice nursing outcomes. In addition to writing on APRN outcomes in the previous editions of this book and elsewhere, Dr. Ingersoll was involved in research related to APRN care; her contributions to the state of the science of advanced practice nursing outcomes have been significant.

585

clinical, health systems, and outcomes research. At the least, individual performance review and outcomes measurement are required of all APRNs, regardless of practice setting, population served, or APRN role and position responsibilities.

Outcomes evaluation and ongoing performance assessment are essential to the survival and success of advanced practice nursing. The importance of this dimension of advanced practice is highlighted repeatedly in *The Essentials of Doctoral Education for Advanced Nursing Practice* (American Association of Colleges of Nursing [AACN], 2006). Incorporated within each essential competency is a discussion of the need to evaluate the effect of APRN action and decision making on care delivery outcomes (AACN, 2015). A key rationale supporting the development of the Doctor of Nursing Practice degree has included industry demand for APRNs capable of gauging baseline clinical outcomes, determining gaps in the use of evidence-based practice (EBP), masterfully leading change that is scientifically sound, and measuring the impact of their interventions.

The newly revised Criteria for Evaluation of Nurse Practitioner Programs also highlights the importance of outcome evaluation and ongoing performance assessment for nurse practitioner (NP) programs, including evaluation of students' attainment of competencies throughout the program (National Organization of Nurse Practitioner Faculties, 2016). An evaluation plan to measure outcomes of graduates is a required component, with outcome measures to include, at a minimum, certification pass rates, practice/position in area of specialty, employer/practice satisfaction, and graduate satisfaction with APRN preparation (National Organization of Nurse Practitioner Faculties, 2016).

This chapter focuses on measuring and monitoring the quality of care delivered and the outcomes achieved by APRNs. Performance indicators are discussed at two levels—the aggregate level, at which evidence addresses APRN role impact in one of the four APRN roles, and the individual level, with activities directed at the outcomes of a single APRN's practice. This chapter outlines key terms and describes frameworks for quality and outcomes assessment. Methods supporting comparative effectiveness research led by APRNs are reviewed and strategies for identifying and assessing APRN-sensitive outcome indicators are highlighted. Emphasis is placed on how to use outcomes of APRN practice to showcase impact as well as to promote EBP adoption.

Review of Terms

Numerous interrelated terms are used to define and describe the components of performance appraisal and outcomes assessment. The principal terms used in this chapter are listed alphabetically in Table 23.1.

Why Measure Outcomes?

Measuring outcomes has become a required component of health care, based in part on federal and state regulatory agencies, practice guidelines, employers, and consumer groups. Health care organizations are now actively monitoring outcomes of care as a means of evaluation as well as for requirements for accreditation and certification. Entities including the Centers for Medicare and Medicaid Services (CMS), The Joint Commission, the National Quality Forum (NQF), and the Agency for Healthcare Research and Quality (AHRQ), along with individual state-mandated reporting, are key drivers of the increased focus on improving outcomes. APRN models of care provide the opportunity to demonstrate impact of care and to improve quality of care outcomes for patients.

What Outcome Measures Are Important?

A number of outcomes are important to patients, including perception of the quality of health care, complication rates, return to work after illness/injury, mortality and morbidity rates, patient/family as well as state and federal costs of care. The National Patient Safety Goals of The Joint Commission (2017) outline a number of specific goals that promote quality and safety outcomes for patients, including compliance with hand hygiene, prevention of central line–associated bloodstream infections, prevention of surgical site infections, prevention of indwelling catheter–associated urinary tract infections, and improvement in patient and provider communication, among others. The NQF has endorsed numerous quality measures for the CMS, including provision of venous thromboembolism (VTE) prophylaxis, anticoagulation for atrial fibrillation, patient education for numerous disease states, mortality, early antibiotic administration in sepsis, and smoking cessation counseling; however, the vast majority of these indicators are process based, with very few outcome indicators required at this time. Similarly, the AHRQ has developed numerous inpatient quality indicators and patient safety indicators for NQF endorsement and CMS adoption, including prevention of postoperative sepsis, central line–associated bloodstream

TABLE 23.1 **Definitions of the Components of Performance Appraisal and Outcomes Assessment**

Term	Definition
Benchmark	A point of reference for comparison. Benchmarking is the process used to compare an individual's (or organization's) outcomes with those of high performers. It requires an assessment of the processes used by high-performing practitioners or organizations to achieve their outcomes as well as the strategies and systems used to attain and then sustain performance excellence.
Performance benchmark	An ideal practice standard target that has been achieved by some group or organization known for its quality of services. This process-focused benchmark serves as the gold standard against which others are compared. Some evaluators also use this term to denote achievement of an intermediate outcome (e.g., attainment of desired best practice performance).
Comparative effectiveness research	Research evidence generated from studies that compare drugs, medical devices, tests, or ways to deliver health care. It is designed to inform health care decisions by providing evidence on the effectiveness, benefits, and harms of different treatment options. Comparative effectiveness studies are the gold standard for outcomes research, enabling patients, providers, and payors to determine best practice choices (Agency for Healthcare Research and Quality, Effective Health Care Program, 2012).
Dashboard	A visual representation of data to enable the review, analysis, and tracking of data trends. The dashboard is like a scorecard because it allows for the visualization of performance and outcome information (MEASURE Evaluation, 2010; U.S. Department of Education, 2011).
Disease management	An organized process focusing on the patient's disease as the target of interest, with improvements in outcome seen as a result of attention to the attributes or characteristics of the disease. Quality indicators endorsed and adopted by federal and private health plans commonly target adherence to evidence-based processes that are expected to affect disease management.
Effectiveness	Extent to which evidence-based interventions or programs produce desired or intended outcomes in real life. The principle of effectiveness supports the adoption of standardized health care processes forming the basis for pay-for-performance core measures because it assumes that widespread use of evidence-based methods should demonstrate reductions in disease and complication incidences and, ultimately, health care costs.
Intervention effectiveness	The measurement of results in line with implementation of a specific evidence-based practice. Intervention effectiveness studies are considered *Phase 4 studies* that explore the generalizability of efficacious interventions; specifically, intervention effectiveness studies examine whether results are similar to those produced in *Phase 3* randomized controlled trials that demonstrated initial efficacy of an intervention.
Program effectiveness	Measurement of the results attained through the systematic adoption of evidence-based structures (e.g., systems such as equipment, manpower) and standardized processes.
Efficiency	The effects achieved by some intervention in relation to the effort expended in terms of money, resources, and time.
Evidence-based practice	Integration of research findings (evidence) into clinical decision making and care delivery processes. Evidence-based data are also useful in the development of *practice guidelines,* which are used to assist practitioners' and patients' decisions about appropriate health care for specific clinical care situations (Joanna Briggs Institute, 2012). Practice guidelines are systematically developed recommendations, strategies, or other information to assist health care decision making in specific clinical circumstances (Agency for Healthcare Research and Quality, 2012). The shift to pay-for-performance, based on the systematic implementation of evidence-based practice, provides an example of the power of scientifically sound processes and is driving practitioner viability in the health care market.
Impact measurement	An analysis of the difference in a targeted outcome measure and growth of practice systems resulting from use of the outcomes management process (Alexandrov & Brewer, 2010). Impact measurement enables advanced practice registered nurses (APRNs) to showcase the effectiveness of programs implemented to improve patient outcomes. Analyzing the impact of an outcomes management process can help identify key aspects of the process that led to changes in an outcome (U.S. Department of Health and Human Services, Administration for Children and Families, 2010).

Continued

TABLE 23.1	**Definitions of the Components of Performance Appraisal and Outcomes Assessment—cont'd**
Term	**Definition**
Metric	Also described as a measure or indicator; defines parameters for structure, process, or outcome, depending on its level. For example, a metric for rate-based measures would define population numerators and denominators to ensure that each party using the metric measures the same population (validity) in the same way each time (reliability). The National Quality Forum (NQF) has defined criteria that should support all metrics to be submitted for endorsement by that agency, thereby making them eligible for pay-for-performance adoption by the Centers for Medicare & Medicaid Services and other third-party payors. These criteria include the following: (1) the importance of studying the measures and publicly reporting findings; (2) the scientific acceptability of measure properties—that they measure validity and reliability; (3) usability, the extent to which payors, providers, and consumers can understand results and use them for health care decision making; and (4) feasibility, the extent to which the required data are available or could be captured without undue burden (NQF, 2012).
Outcome	Results produced by inherent characteristics, processes, and/or structures; newly developed processes and/or structures may constitute interventions. Measurement of outcomes will vary according to the intended target. For example, targets may be patients, families, students, other care providers, communities, and in some cases, organizations (if the organization as a whole is the recipient of the intervention). Outcomes may be intended or unintended and reflect positive or untoward results such as complications. Because of this, measurement plans must be cautiously developed to capture all outcomes (positive or negative) that theoretically align with the planned intervention, including the likelihood of no change in pre-intervention status (Alexandrov, 2008; Doran, 2011). Most definitions of outcome have evolved from the original writings of Donabedian (1966, 1980), who defined an outcome as a change in a patient's physiologic health state (i.e., morbidity and mortality) (see Chapter 2). This patient-centered understanding of outcomes is particularly relevant to APRNs, whose actions directly or indirectly affect patients and families.
Outcome(s) assessment	An evaluation of the observed results of some action or intervention for recipients of services. Outcome assessments provide the data needed to support or refute the perceived beneficial effect of some clinical decision, care delivery process, or targeted action.
Outcome indicators	Metrics or measures capable of demonstrating actual results produced by the interaction of inherent characteristics, processes, and/or structures. Outcome indicators are derived from systematic determination of all potential results that could occur; these measures should be clearly defined in terms of their measurement properties to ensure validity and reliability, with consideration of their temporal association to the intervention. Today, a variety of well-defined, tested, and endorsed outcome measures are available for use in outcome and disease management programs; however, there are considerably fewer outcome measures available for use compared to process measures. Because the development of sound process and outcome measures requires extensive expertise and testing, APRNs are encouraged to select NQF-endorsed measures to support many of their projects because these are thoroughly vetted and promote meaningful comparisons (NQF, 2017b). This approach ensures consistency in the methods used to study and improve phenomena of interest.
Outcome(s) management	The active implementation of processes and/or structures that aim to improve targeted results. According to the classic work of Ellwood (1988), a comprehensive outcomes management program does the following: (1) emphasizes the use of standards to select appropriate interventions; (2) measures a broad array of outcomes, including disease-specific, behavioral, functional, and perception-of-care outcomes; (3) pools outcomes data for groups of like patients in relation to processes of care and patient characteristics; and (4) analyzes and disseminates findings to stakeholders (patients, payors, providers) to inform decision making. The goal is to improve care to aggregate populations.
Outcome(s) measurement	The collection, analysis, and reporting of reliable and valid outcome indicators.
Outcome(s) research or *patient-centered outcomes research*	The use of the scientific method to measure the result of interventions on targeted patient health outcomes (Alexandrov & Brewer, 2010; Clancy & Collins, 2010). Outcomes research methods target examination of aggregate results in relation to inherent characteristics and changes in structures and processes. Comparative effectiveness research is the most rigorous form of patient-centered outcomes research, using rigorous randomized clinical trial designs to determine differences in treatment options; these studies provide the basis for fully informed patient decision making.

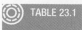 **TABLE 23.1** **Definitions of the Components of Performance Appraisal and Outcomes Assessment—cont'd**

Term	Definition
Performance (process and system) improvement	Activities designed to increase the quality of services provided. The focus of attention shifts to the actions taken by the provider and/or new systems that have been developed rather than the outcomes achieved. Although outcomes may be monitored to determine whether the change in process and/or systems produces a desired effect, primary attention is on the interventions (care delivery processes) delivered. Subsumed within performance improvement activities are those associated with quality improvement initiatives, also described by some as *continuous quality improvement* or *total quality management*. Although subtle distinctions are assigned to each of these terms, the focus and the intent are the same—to ensure the delivery of care that is appropriate, safe, competent, and timely and to maximize the potential for favorable patient outcomes. In most cases, the measurement of performance is guided by the use of established indicators of best practice such as national guidelines for care.
Performance evaluation (assessment)	Assessment of individual achievement and the attainment of personal, professional, and organizational goals. Performance assessment activities for APRNs include those associated with evaluating and improving day-to-day interactions with individual patients and health care colleagues and those involving the measurement of APRN impact on populations, organizations, and communities.
Process indicator (measure)	A measure of visible behavior or action that a care provider undertakes to deliver care. Process indicators measure the fidelity of targeted interventions and are essential to demonstrating a causal link between new care processes and outcome metrics of interest. When outcome measures are evaluated without process fidelity measurement, it is "assumed" that the targeted process that was changed produced the outcome. But, because this may not be the case, process fidelity has become an important aspect of comparative effectiveness research so that clarity of the intervention's contribution to patient outcomes can be established.
Program evaluation	Assessment of overall programmatic performance, including process fidelity, structural adherence and competency, and the reliable performance of all individual and team contributors to the delivery of health care, in relation to key outcomes of interest. Because APRNs play an integral role in supporting and leading programs, APRN contributions are often evaluated in the context of an overall program.
Proxy indicators	An indirect measure used when a direct measure cannot be obtained or when an accurate indicator has not been identified. An example of a proxy indicator is the collection of self-report data from parents or spouses when patients are unable to respond to questions about perceptions of care or previous health. In the acute care hospital setting, case mix index, patient age, and comorbidity often are used as proxy indicators of risk adjustment for given clinical populations, simply because more direct indicators are not readily accessible. Length of stay has been a commonly measured proxy outcome but there are limitations to its use because many factors can affect length of stay.
Quality of care	A term used to convey overall process utilization and structures of care. Quality of care should be considered a "summary" term because measurement of care quality requires the systematic measurement of processes, structures, and outcomes.
Risk and severity adjustment	A process used to standardize groups according to characteristics that might unduly influence an outcome. An example of severity adjustment would involve leveling a heart failure cohort by controlling for their New York Heart Association Functional Classification at baseline so that patients with severe heart failure can be compared equally against patients with less severe failure; without such an adjustment, baseline severity may affect resource use at discharge, cost of care and length of stay, rehospitalization, functional status, and even mortality. The aim of risk and severity adjustment is to level the field among all patients in a sample so that outcomes associated with interventions may be measured more accurately.
Standards	A profession's authoritative statements that describe the responsibilities of its practitioners (American Nurses Association, 2010). Standards focus on the processes of care delivery and scope of practice, serving as criteria for the establishment of practice-related rules, conditions, and performance requirements.
Structural indicators	Measures of human, technical, and other resources used in care delivery. These structures focus on the characteristics of the setting, system, or care providers and include such elements as numbers and types of providers, provider qualifications, agency policies and procedures, characteristics of patients served, and payment sources.

infection, and postoperative respiratory failure (AHRQ, 2017).

The Patient Protection and Affordable Care Act's Value-Based Purchasing Program initiative focuses on a hospital's performance on 25 quality measures related to clinical process-of-care measures and patient experience of care. Under this program, incentive payments are made to hospitals based on quality measure performance as well as improvement in performance over time. Currently, 45 measures are specified under the Hospital Inpatient Quality Reporting program that are possible candidate measures (CMS, 2017). Box 23.1 outlines examples of outcome measures as well as candidate measures for the Hospital Value-Based Purchasing program. Focusing on improving these areas of care has significant implications not only for patient care but also for hospital reimbursement rates. Therefore targeting these identified measures and assessing the impact of APRNs in these areas of care has considerable relevance.

However, measuring the outcomes of APRNs is not a consistent part of practice. A survey conducted by the University Health System Consortium, a large national consortium formed from the association of 103 academic medical centers, assessed use of APRNs in 25 organizations (Moote, Krsek, Kleinpell, & Todd, 2011). Productivity was reported as being measured using a variety of metrics, including patient encounters, number of procedures, gross charges, collections for professional fee, number of shared visits (Medicare), number of indirect billing visits (Blue Cross), and number of visits billed under the APRN provider number. Very few organizations had defined productivity targets, and despite significant investments in APRN models of care, most organizations reported that they did not measure the financial impact of employing APRNs or had done so in very limited areas. Most organizations (69%) did not track patient outcomes related to APRN care, primarily because of the inability to match patients to providers. A few organizations reported tracking several specific outcomes, often overall by service, including length of stay (15%), readmission rates (12%), family and patient satisfaction (12%), and specific clinical outcomes such as ventilator days (8%), urinary tract infection rates (4%), ventilator-associated event rates (4%), skin breakdown rates (4%), VTE prophylaxis rates (4%), and catheter-related bloodstream infection rates (4%) (Moote et al., 2011). The results of the study identify that even in institutions employing large numbers of APRNs (200 or more), a focused effort at assessing outcomes has not

been implemented. This study highlights the current need to reinforce the importance of assessing outcomes of APRNs as an essential component in their utilization and provides a call to action for APRNs to develop initiative and passion for this important work. Without capturing the impact of ARPN care, contributions to patient care as well as quality of care improvements, patient safety measures, and other salient measures such as family and patient knowledge and satisfaction remain unknown, challenging the overall contribution of APRNs in health care today.

Conceptual Models of Care Delivery Impact

Because APRNs usually work with other health professionals, their influence on care delivery outcomes can be difficult to assess. They may have a direct effect through their interactions with patients and families, and/or they may have an indirect effect through their enhancement of the performance of others. Moreover, a number of factors influence APRN practice irrespective of their direct or indirect efforts.

Models for Evaluating Outcomes Achieved by APRNs

A number of outcomes measurement and role impact models have been proposed, with several of these evolving from the original quality-of-care framework proposed by Donabedian (1966, 1980). Donabedian posited that quality is a function of the structural elements of the setting in which care is provided, processes used by care providers, and changes to the recipients of care (i.e., the outcomes) (see Chapter 2). Applying these concepts to APRN practice, structural variables relate to the components of a system of care. Process variables pertain to the behavior or actions of the APRN or the activities of an APRN-directed educational or care delivery program. Interactions among structures and processes result in outcomes. Structure (attributes of the setting in which care occurs), process (what is actually done in giving and receiving care), and outcome (describes the effects of care on the health status of patients and populations) variables, as defined by Donabedian, can be studied independently or as a model for overall APRN practice. The more complete the model (e.g., the inclusion of all or at least two of the components), the more likely is the successful identification of the APRN's impact on care delivery outcome. Two models are described below.

BOX 23.1 Examples of Health Care Outcome Measures by Organization

National Quality Forum Quality Measures Examples

- Acute otitis externa: percentage of patients age 2 years and older with a diagnosis of acute otitis externa who were not prescribed systemic antimicrobial therapy
- Adult major depressive disorder: percentage of patients age 18 years and older with a diagnosis of major depressive disorder who had a suicide risk assessment completed during the visit in which a new diagnosis or recurrent episode was identified
- Comprehensive diabetes care: percentage of members 18 to 64 years of age with diabetes (type 1 and type 2) whose most recent hemoglobin A_{1c} level is less than 7.0% (controlled)
- Urinary catheter–associated urinary tract infection for intensive care unit (ICU) patients
- ICU venous thromboembolism prophylaxis
- Provision of anticoagulation for patients with atrial fibrillation to prevent stroke

Agency for Healthcare Research and Quality Indicator Examples

- In-hospital fall with hip fracture rate
- Perioperative pulmonary embolism and deep venous thrombosis rate
- Pressure ulcer rate
- Percentage of ICU patients age 18 and older receiving mechanical ventilation who had an order on the first ventilator day for head-of-bed elevation (30-45 degrees)
- Sepsis: percentage of patients with severe sepsis/septic shock who had two sets of blood cultures collected within 24 hours following severe sepsis/septic shock identification

Centers for Medicare & Medicaid Services Hospital Value-Based Purchasing Program Examples

- Clinical Processes of Care Measures Examples
  - Influenza immunization
  - Acute myocardial infarction—aspirin prescribed at discharge

- Heart failure—discharge instructions
- Health care–associated infections—prophylactic antibiotics discontinued within 24 hours after surgery end time
- Hospital-Acquired Condition Measures Examples
  - Air embolism
  - Pressure ulcer stages 3 and 4
  - Vascular catheter-associated infection
  - Catheter-associated urinary tract infection
- Patient Experience of Care Measures
  - Communication with nurses
  - Communication with doctors
  - Responsiveness of hospital staff
  - Pain management
  - Communication about medicines
  - Discharge information

The Joint Commission National Patient Safety Goals Examples

- Reduce the likelihood of patient harm associated with the use of anticoagulant therapy.
  - Before starting a patient on warfarin, assess the patient's baseline coagulation status.
  - For all patients receiving warfarin therapy, use a current International Normalized Ratio to adjust this therapy.
- Reduce the risk of health care–associated infections.
  - Comply with either the current Centers for Disease Control and Prevention hand hygiene guidelines or the current World Health Organization hand hygiene guidelines.
  - Implement policies and practices aimed at reducing the risk of central line–associated bloodstream infections.
- Maintain and communicate accurate patient medication information.
  - Provide the patient (or family as needed) with written information on the medications the patient should be taking when he or she is discharged from the hospital or at the end of an outpatient encounter.

Outcomes Evaluation Model

This Donabedian-guided model, a classic outcomes evaluation model, was designed by Holzemer (1994). The value of this model is its program planning structure, which helps identify essential components of any outcomes evaluation plan (Table 23.2). In Holzemer's model, essential outcomes measurement components are defined in a table consisting of inputs/context (structure), processes, and outcomes, which are identified along the horizontal axis.

TABLE 23.2 Advanced Practice Registered Nurse Outcomes Planning Grid[a]

	Inputs/Context (Structure)	Processes	Outcomes

Patient	Age
	Gender
	Ethnicity
	Marital status, social supports
	Educational background
	Health status (current and past)
	Previous experience with health
	   system
	Special needs (e.g., visual, literacy,
	   hearing)
	Expectations of provider and health
	   system
	Access to care
	Insurance coverage
		Performance of self-care behaviors
		Ability
		Willingness
		Family involvement in care delivery
		   process
		Use of alternative or complementary
		   therapies
		Compliance with evidence-based
		   guideline recommended care for
		   discreet patient diagnoses
			Generic
			• Physical health
			• Mental health
			• Symptom control
			• Functional status
			• Perceived well-being
			• Patient perception of the quality
			  of health care services
			• Adherence to treatment regimen
			• Knowledge of condition, treatment
			  program, and expected outcomes
			Specific (dependent on patient condition
			  and need; representative examples)
			• Serum glucose level
			• Birth weight
			• Reinfarction rate
			• Transplant rejection rate
			• Smoking cessation rate
			• Length of stay
			• Ventilator days
			• Wound closure, wound healing

APRN provider	Educational preparation
	Specialty focus
	Years of experience
	Level of self-esteem
	Resourcefulness
	Assertiveness
		Expert practice
		Collaboration
		Communication patterns
		Interactions with other care
		   providers and staff
		Expert coaching
		Consultation
		Clinical and professional leadership
		Ethical decision making
		Evidence-based practice
		Case management
		Care delivery according to practice
		   standards
		Documentation
			Productivity
			Practice confidence
			Contributions to science: publications,
			   presentations

Setting	Geographic location (rural, urban,
	   mixed)
	Type of facility (academic health
	   center, acute care, clinic, industry)
	Diagnostic equipment
	Organizational culture and philosophy
	Administrative structure
	State regulations on advanced practice
	Policies and procedures
	Patient mix
	Type of care delivery model
	Availability of other services in vicinity
	Credentialing agency requirements
	State health department regulations
	Annual goals
	Annual budget
		Care provider credentialing process
		Quality improvement process
		Systems of care
		Communication patterns
		Governance process
		Care provider documentation
		   process
		Annual performance review process
		Provider credentialing process
			Length of stay
			Staff turnover rate
			Cost of services
			New program development
			Revenue generated
			Community satisfaction
			Provider satisfaction
			Staff satisfaction

[a]Components are not exhaustive of APRN-related outcomes planning but serve as a guide for planning activities.
Adapted from Holzemer, W. L. (1994). The impact of nursing care in Latin America and the Caribbean: A focus on outcomes. *Journal of Advanced Nursing, 20*, 5–12.

For the APRN, the patient is any recipient of APRN services (e.g., patients, families). The provider is the person (APRN) or interprofessional group providing the service and potentially could include trained community laypersons who assist with the provision of services. The setting is the local environment in which the services are delivered and includes the resources available to provide care. Table 23.2 contains an application of Holzemer's (1994) model to APRN outcomes assessment planning. Included in the table are potential variables that may facilitate assessment of the APRN's impact. Additional variables would be selected based on specialty service, population specifics, and additional characteristics of the provider, patient, or environment.

Nurse Practitioner Role Effectiveness Model

Sidani and Irvine (1999) have proposed a conceptual model designed to facilitate the evaluation of the acute care nurse practitioner (ACNP) role in acute care settings (Fig. 23.1). Developed in Canada, this model was adapted from a nursing role effectiveness model and is also a derivative of Donabedian's framework, with components focusing on structure (patient, ACNP, and organization), process (ACNP role components, role enactment, and role functions) and outcome (goals and expectations of the ACNP role). A concern with this model is the use of the term *goals and expectations* for outcome and the focus on quality of care, which is a dimension of care delivery process rather than outcome. Four processes (mechanisms) within the ACNP direct care component are expected to achieve patient and cost outcomes: (1) providing comprehensive care, (2) ensuring continuity of care, (3) coordinating services, and (4) providing care in a timely way (Sidani & Irvine, 1999). According to this model, the selection of outcome indicators is guided by the role and functions assumed by the ACNP, how the role is enacted, and the ACNP's particular practice model. Like the models before it, the usefulness of this framework for determining APRN impact is limited by its virtual absence of testing in clinical settings.

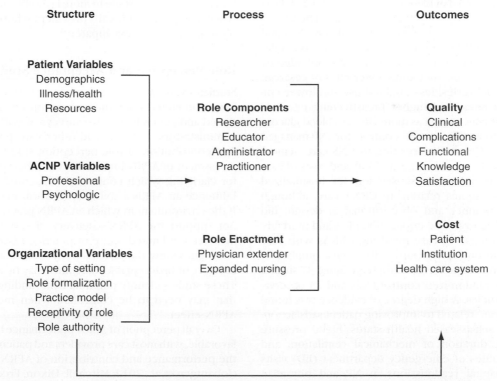

FIG 23.1 Nursing role effectiveness model for acute care nurse practitioners. *(From Sidani, S., & Irvine, D. [1999]. A conceptual framework for evaluating the nurse practitioner role in acute care settings.* Journal of Advanced Nursing, 30, *58-66.)*

Evidence to Date

A review of the literature suggests that increased attention is being given to the assessment of APRN performance. Several synthesis reviews highlighted that a number of studies had been conducted that focused on the evaluation of APRN roles and on the outcomes of APRN care (Hatem, Sandall, Devane, Soltani, & Gates, 2008; Laurant et al., 2005; Newhouse et al., 2011). These studies focused on all APRN roles, including NP, clinical nurse specialist (CNS), certified registered nurse anesthetist (CRNA), and certified nurse-midwife (CNM) care, and included two Cochrane Database reviews on the impact of primary care NPs (Laurant et al., 2005) and CNM care (Hatem et al., 2008).

Additionally, a synthesis review of the research conducted between 1990 and 2008 on the outcomes of APRN care focused on comparing APRN care with that of other providers (e.g., physicians, teams with APRNs); this study identified that care provided by APRNs has been demonstrated to affect outcomes positively (Newhouse et al., 2011). Of 107 studies focused on APRN care in NP, CNS, CNM, and CRNA roles, substantial evidence demonstrated that APRNs provide effective and high-quality care. The results of the review noted that care provided by NPs and CNMs in collaboration with physicians was similar to, and in some ways better than, care provided by physicians alone, including lower rates of cesarean section deliveries, less epidural use and lower episiotomy rates, and higher breastfeeding rates for CNM patients, as well as more effective blood glucose and serum lipid level control for NP-managed patients. The studies relating to CNS care demonstrated a decrease in length of stay and costs of care and high ratings of satisfaction for hospitalized patients. Studies relating to CRNA care, although few in number and observational in design, did suggest equivalent complication rates and mortality when comparing care involving CRNAs with care involving only physicians. The largest number of studies related to NP care; these included 37 studies with 14 randomized control trials and 23 observational studies. A high degree of evidence was found for NP care related to improving patient satisfaction, patient self-assessed health status, blood pressure control, duration of mechanical ventilation, and similar rates of emergency department (ED) visits and hospital readmissions in NP and physician comparison groups (Newhouse et al., 2011).

Studies related to the outcomes of APRN care and APRN performance and impact can be categorized according to whether they focus on role descriptions or practice characteristics, care delivery processes, process (or performance) improvement activities, program evaluation, disease management activities, outcomes management programs, or outcomes research.

Role Description Studies

Role description studies focus on defining and describing role components and job attributes of APRNs. These foundational studies assist in identifying the direct and indirect APRN actions that potentially influence care delivery outcome. As such, they provide information about the structure or process components of Donabedian's model (1966, 1980). Without information about the outcomes associated with the characteristics and role behaviors identified in these studies, however, little can be said about their impact on patient care. What these studies provide is evidence to guide the development of theories about which characteristics of APRN practice or aspects of the APRN role contribute to care delivery outcome. For example, do the APRN's expert coaching or collaboration processes contribute to more favorable outcomes when compared with care providers whose use of these processes is less apparent?

Role Perception and Acceptance Studies

Studies examining the acceptance of APRNs have been conducted since the various roles were introduced and generally involve surveys of staff nurses, administrators, patients, and other care providers. The contribution of role perception studies to the assessment of APRN impact lies with their potential for clarifying which contextual (structural) factors influence an APRN's ability to perform maximally. If the environment in which an APRN practices does not support the APRN's delivery of services—for instance if a limited scope of practice exists—or if colleagues view the APRN's performance as unsatisfactory or unacceptable, outcomes may be affected. These studies identify potential confounding factors that may need to be controlled when measuring APRN effect.

Overall perception of APRN performance has been favorable, with most care providers and patients rating the performance and contribution of APRNs highly (Johantgen et al., 2012; Mitchell, Dixon, Freeman, & Grindrod, 2001; Newhouse et al., 2011). Hardie and Leary (2010) explored patient perceptions of the value of the CNS role within a breast cancer clinic, finding in this small exploratory survey that the CNS improved respondents' clinic experience.

Care Delivery Process Studies

Studies evaluating care delivery processes often occur in combination with role definition research. The distinction between these studies and role definition explorations is their attention to what APRNs do as part of their roles. Examples include the delivery of preventive services (Counsell et al., 2007), management of ED patients (Lamirel et al., 2012), ordering of antibiotics (Goolsby, 2007), and inclusion of physical activity and physical fitness counseling in primary care practices (Buchholz & Purath, 2007). In these descriptive studies, information is provided about the direct and indirect actions taken by APRNs during the delivery of care. No statements can be made about the relationships between any of these processes and care delivery outcomes, although hypotheses can be generated based on study findings. As a result, these studies are useful as a preliminary step toward outcomes assessment.

In some studies, APRN care delivery processes were compared with those of physicians and other care providers. These studies generally examined NP care and have found that they are more likely than physicians and other community health providers to spend more time with patients (Seale, Anderson, & Kinnersley, 2005), informally manage patient care needs (Sidani et al., 2005, 2006), and discuss treatment options (Seale, Anderson, & Kinnersley, 2006). In one study, NPs were more likely to provide structural support for the emergency management of closed musculoskeletal injuries, although other interventions were similar to those of physician providers (Ball, Walton, & Hawes, 2007). In another study, residents spent significantly more time on coordination of care than NPs (Sidani et al., 2005, 2006). It is interesting to note that despite this difference, patients managed by NPs reported higher levels of coordination than those overseen by residents.

Other studies have examined clinical practice guideline use, demonstrating increased compliance among NP-led initiatives (Gracias et al., 2008) as well as impact on care coordination and patient and family knowledge (Fry, 2011). In a qualitative study describing barriers and facilitators to implementing a transitional care intervention for cognitively impaired older adults and their caregivers led by APRNs, identified themes included patients and caregivers having the necessary information and knowledge, care coordination, and caregiver experience (Bradway

et al., 2012). Additional studies are needed to highlight the impact of APRN-led care that is unique to various APRN roles to demonstrate further the unique features of APRN care that affect patient and health care outcomes.

"Process as Outcome" Studies

Among the process as outcome studies, several have focused on improving compliance with EBP and have demonstrated the benefit of APRN-led initiatives targeting hospitalized patients (Gracias et al., 2008) as well as primary care practice related to specialty care such as urinary incontinence (Albers-Heitner et al., 2012) and osteoporosis management (Greene & Dell, 2010).

An example of a case in which all the indicators described as outcomes were actually process focused is a retrospective medical record review of ACNP versus resident performance on patients admitted for cardiac catheterization (Reigle, Molnar, Howell, & Dumont, 2006). In this study, outcome indicators were defined as documentation of education and counseling for risk factors and discharge prescribing practices. Both these measures are indicators of care provider performance (process) rather than patient outcome. Differentiating process measures from outcome measures is an important distinction. While process measures can be used to evaluate APRN roles, such process measures, or those metrics reflecting the specific steps in a process, can have an impact on outcomes. In the study by Reigle et al. (2006), the findings demonstrated that ACNPs provided more education and counseling concerning dyslipidemia, exercise, and diabetes, whereas counseling for hypertension and smoking was comparable for both groups. The ACNPs also provided more appropriate medication prescriptions for management of heart disease postdischarge. Other studies comparing NP care with that of physician residents have demonstrated comparable medical management skills and improved staff and family satisfaction (Gershengorn et al., 2011; Lakhan & Laird, 2009).

Performance (Process) Improvement Activities

The focus on improving process or performance improvement activities is one aspect of outcomes assessment that focuses on the value-added complement to medical care provided by APRNs. O'Grady (2008) has highlighted the potential to demonstrate APRN importance by evaluating the impact of process improvement initiatives, including the focus on quality of care and patient safety. Several studies have focused on specific APRN role components that affected outcomes. The impact of a home-based APRN intervention for patients with psychiatric illness and human immunodeficiency virus was evaluated in a 4-year randomized controlled trial that studied 238 community residents. Over a 12-month period, those receiving the APRN intervention, which focused on case management and process improvements in the delivery of medical and mental health care, demonstrated improvements in depression and health-related quality of life compared with a control

group that received usual care (Hanrahan, Wu, Kelly, Aiken, & Blank, 2011).

Table 23.3 outlines examples of APRN-directed program evaluations. The focus area of the evaluation, target population, and brief study findings are outlined.

Disease Management Activities

There have traditionally been few formal reports of the APRN's role in disease management initiatives. The failure to identify disease management analyses may be, in part, because of their close linkages with

TABLE 23.3   Examples of Advanced Practice Registered Nurse (APRN)–Directed Program Evaluations

Study (Year)	Focus of Evaluation	Target Population	Findings
Albers-Heitner et al. (2012)	Urinary incontinence care	Primary care	Improved quality of life; improvement in incontinence severity; more cost-effective care
Anetzberger, Stricklin, Gaunter, Banozic, and Laurie (2006)	Achievement of program goals—service to at-risk groups and improved outcomes	High-risk older adults	Completed > 1600 visits to targeted population; number of referrals doubled; patients highly satisfied with service
Bissonnette (2011)	APRN-led program for kidney transplant patients	Kidney transplant patients	APRN-led interprofessional collaborative care model; improved care for patients with chronic kidney disease awaiting kidney transplantation
Brandon, Schuessler, Ellison, and Lazenby (2009)	Telephone follow-up program for heart failure patients	Primary care patients with heart failure	Reduced rates of rehospitalization and improved patient self-care behaviors
Callahan et al. (2006)	Collaborative care model for Alzheimer disease	Primary care patient	Improved behavioral and psychologic symptoms; less caregiver distress
Capezuti et al. (2007)	Consultation and educational services regarding side rail use	Long-term care nursing staff and patients	Reduction in side rail use varied by site; falls significantly reduced for site with reduced use of rails
Cheung et al. (2011)	Certified nurse-midwife–led normal birth unit	Obstetric patients undergoing childbirth	Significant differences in vaginal deliveries, rates of episiotomies and amniotomies (all decreased), and increased postdelivery mobility
Cibulka, Forney, Goodwin, Lazaroff, and Sarabia (2011)	Nurse practitioner (NP)–directed oral care program	Low-income pregnant women	Improved oral care, including improved frequency of brushing and flossing teeth, dental checkups, and marked reduction in intake of high-sugar drinks
Collins et al. (2014)	NP-directed care for trauma patients	Trauma patients transferred to step-down unit	Reduction in hospital length of stay and costs of care
Costa, Wallace, Barnato, and Kahn (2014)	NP-directed care for hospitalized patients	Intensive care unit patients	No difference in mortality rates compared to medical resident team
Dickerson, Wu, and Kennedy (2006)	Support groups	Patients receiving implantable cardioverter-defibrillators	No difference in quality-of-life scores for support group attendees
Greene and Dell (2010)	Disease management program	Patients with osteoporosis	Increased treatment of osteoporosis; decrease in hip fractures

TABLE 23.3   Examples of Advanced Practice Registered Nurse (APRN)–Directed Program Evaluations—cont'd

Study (Year)	Focus of Evaluation	Target Population	Findings
Hamilton and Hawley (2006)	Outpatient management of anemia	Patients with chronic renal disease	Significant improvement in quality of life
Kutzleb and Reiner (2006)	Patient education program	Patients with heart failure	Significant improvement in quality of life
Landsperger, Semler, Wang, Byrne, and Wheeler (2015)	NP-led team compared to resident-managed patients	Medical intensive care unit	No differences in mortality or hospital length of stay
Lowery et al. (2011)	Disease management model	Patients with chronic heart failure	Significantly fewer congestive heart failure and all-cause admissions at 1-year follow-up, lower mortality at both 1- and 2-year follow-ups
McCorkle et al. (2009)	Postsurgical care for gynecologic cancer	Women who had undergone gynecologic cancer surgery	Improved functional status, less symptom distress, less uncertainty
Morse, Warshawsky, Moore, and Pecora (2006)	Assessment of NP-led rapid response team	Hospitalized patients	Significant decrease in in-hospital cardiac arrests, decrease in mortality rates
Rideout (2007)	Care coordination	Hospitalized children with cystic fibrosis	Timeliness of nutrition and social work consultation improved significantly; length of stay declined by 1.35 days
Scherr, Wilson, Wagner, and Haughian (2012)	Comparison of NP-led program for rapid response teams compared with physician care	Hospitalized patients	No differences in number of cardiac arrests or mortality rates; nurses reported confidence in knowledge of NP team
Stolee, Hillier, Esbaugh, Griffiths, and Borrie (2006)	Role of NP	Long-term care nursing employees	Perception of positive impact; most staff reported improved skill levels
Sung, Huang, Ong, and Chen (2011)	NPs as coordinators of acute stroke team	Hospitalized patients with acute stroke onset	Time to computed tomography scan, time to neurology evaluation, and time to initiate thrombolytic therapy significantly improved
Wagner et al. (2007)	Consultation and educational services regarding side rail use	Long-term care patients	Five (median) recommendations per resident; median cost of intervention per resident was $135

other intervention and assessment activities. Studies have demonstrated improved disease management from NP care, including care for hypertension, cardiovascular disease, and diabetes (Newhouse et al., 2011) and specialty-based care such as Alzheimer disease management (Callahan et al., 2006), urology care (Albers-Heitner et al., 2012), cancer care (Cooper, Loeb, & Smith, 2009), and congestive heart failure care (Case, Haynes, Holaday, & Parker, 2010; Lowery et al., 2011). In a study assessing the quality of health care provided at a pediatric nurse–managed clinic, NP care provided to 500 patients was found to improve childhood immunization rates, improve treatment for children with upper respiratory infection, and increase children's access to primary care providers (Coddington, Sands, Edwards, Kirkpatrick,

& Chen, 2012). It is noteworthy that recent studies have focused on demonstrating the impact of APRN care in specialty-based care. This focus has implications to showcase further the impact of APRNs in a wide range of specialties.

Outcomes Management Activities

There are also few reports of APRN-directed outcomes management programs. The effectiveness of multidisciplinary NP-coordinated team visits to medically underserved patients with type 2 diabetes has demonstrated improvement in blood glucose and glycated hemoglobin levels and greater patient knowledge and self-efficacy (Jessee & Rutledge, 2012). In a study focusing on APRN care in psychiatry, admission rates to inpatient psychiatric facilities, visits to the ED, referral to rehabilitative services, occupational status, adherence to yearly routine blood tests and medications, and patient satisfaction were found to improve with APRN consultations (Cheng, 2012).

Impact of APRN Practice

In the last decade, an increasing number of studies examining the effect of APRN practice on patient and systems outcomes have been conducted. Table 23.4 organizes these studies by outcome indicator. Studies have investigated care delivery outcomes across providers and among different APRN types. In most cases, physician groups (including physician residents) have been used for comparison. As noted, this process is a concern because it implies that physician practice is the gold standard for APRNs and that it encompasses the full range of APRN activity. Actually, physician practice overlaps in some respects and diverges in others. In the process studies reviewed earlier, APRNs routinely used strategies that were not considered by physicians or were not

TABLE 23.4   Examples of APRN-Sensitive Outcome Indicators Tested in Practice

Outcome Indicator	Study (Year)	Study Design	Focus of Indicator[a]	Findings
Activities of daily living	Counsell et al. (2007)	Randomized controlled trial	Population-generic	Significantly improved
	Krichbaum (2007)	Randomized controlled trial	Population-generic	Significantly improved over control group
Adverse events, unplanned incidents, including drug reactions	Simonson, Ahern, and Hendryx (2007)	Retrospective comparison		Comparable to anesthesiologists
Amniotomy rates	Cheung et al. (2011)	Randomized controlled trial	Population-specific	Significant decreased rates compared with usual care
Anxiety, depression; mental health status; emotional state	McCorkle, Dowd, Pickett, Siefert, and Robinson (2007)	Secondary data analysis		Comparable to control group
Asthma control	Borgmeyer, Gyr, Jamerson, and Henry (2008)	Observational	Population-specific	Significantly improved
Blood pressure	Partiprajak (2012)	Observational	Population-specific	Significantly decreased
Cardiac arrest rates after rapid response team call	Morse, Warshawsky, Moore, and Pecora (2006)	Observational	Population-generic	Significantly decreased
	Scherr, Wilson, Wagner, and Haughian (2012)	Retrospective	Population-generic	Significantly decreased
Cesarean delivery	Cragin and Kennedy (2006)	Prospective descriptive cohort	Population-specific	Significantly lower than physician group
Cholesterol level	Paez and Allen (2006)	Randomized controlled trial	Population-generic	Significantly better than usual care group
Cost of care	Albers-Heitner et al. (2012)	Precomparison and postcomparison		Nurse practitioner (NP) care cost-effective for managing care for urinary incontinence
	Cowan et al. (2006)	Quasi-experimental comparison	Population-generic	Significantly improved compared with control
	Naylor et al. (2013)	Randomized controlled trial		Significantly less than control group
	Paez and Allen (2006)	Randomized controlled trial		Incremental costs offset by improved outcome
Depression management	Hanrahan, Wu, Kelly, Aiken, and Blank (2011)	Randomized controlled trial		Significantly improved

| TABLE 23.4 | Examples of APRN-Sensitive Outcome Indicators Tested in Practice—cont'd | | | |

Outcome Indicator	Study (Year)	Study Design	Focus of Indicator[a]	Findings
Door-to-needle time for thrombolytic therapy for acute stroke patients	Sung, Huang, Ong, and Chen (2011)	Parallel comparison	Population-specific	Significantly better than physician control group
Eczema flare-ups	Schuttelaar, Vermeulen, and Coenraads (2011)	Randomized controlled trial	Population-specific	Significantly lower rates than physician comparison group
Emergency department use	Smith, Pan, and Novelli (2016)	Case-control study	676 medical patients at high risk for readmission status after hospital discharge	Postdischarge home visit by NP resulted in decreased readmissions and fewer emergency department visits within 30 days postdischarge
Episiotomy rates	Cheung et al. (2011)	Randomized controlled trial	Population-specific	Decreased rates with certified nurse-midwife care
Functional status, ability	McCorkle et al. (2009)	Randomized controlled trial	Population-specific	Significantly improved
Hip fracture rate	Krichbaum (2007)	Care coordination program evaluation	Population-specific	Significantly decreased rate of fractures
Hip fractures with osteoporosis screening and treatment	Greene and Dell (2010)	Disease management program evaluation	Population-specific	Significantly decreased rate of fractures, increased rate of osteoporosis treatment
Hospitalizations, including readmissions	Brandon, Schuessler, Ellison, and Lazenby (2009)	Quasi-experimental comparison		Decreased readmissions, improved self-care behaviors
	Brandon, Schuessler, Ellison, and Lazenby (2009)	Telehealth program evaluation	Population-specific	Decreased readmission rates, improved patient self-care behaviors
Length of stay	Collins et al. (2014)	Precomparison and postcomparison	Population specific	Decreased hospital length of stay for trauma patients cared for by NP
	Fanta et al. (2006)	Randomized controlled trial		Significantly shorter than for residents
	Gershengorn et al. (2011)	Retrospective review		No difference in hospital mortality, length of stay (intensive care unit, hospital), and post–hospital discharge destination for NP care compared with physician care
	Rideout (2007)	Precomparison and postcomparison		No difference in precomparison and postcomparison
Mortality	Costa, Wallace, Barnato, and Kahn (2014)	Descriptive comparison	Population-generic	Comparable to physicians
	Landsperger, Semler, Wang, Byrne, and Wheeler (2015)	Descriptive comparison	Population-generic	Comparable to physicians
	Morse, Warshawsky, Moore, and Pecora (2006)	Observational	Population-generic	Significantly lower
	Scherr, Wilson, Wagner, and Haughian (2012)	Retrospective	Population-generic	Significantly decreased

Continued

TABLE 23.4   Examples of APRN-Sensitive Outcome Indicators Tested in Practice—cont'd

Outcome Indicator	Study (Year)	Study Design	Focus of Indicator[a]	Findings
Nurse satisfaction	McMullen, Alexander, Bourgeois, and Goodman (2001)	Program evaluation	Population-specific, organizational	Highly satisfied
	Rideout (2007)	Prcomparison- and postcomparison		Highly satisfied postintervention (no pre-intervention data)
	Simonson, Ahern, and Hendryx (2007)	Medical record review		Comparable to anesthesiologists
Patient, family satisfaction	Fanta et al. (2006)	Survey		Comparable to or significantly greater than residents
	Sidani et al. (2005, 2006)	Cross-sectional comparison		Significantly greater than residents
	Varughese, Byczkowski, Wittkugel, Kotagal, and Dean (2006)	Observational	Population-generic	Significantly improved
Physician satisfaction, perception of APRN performance	Rideout (2007)	Precomparison and postcomparison		Highly satisfied postcomparison (no precomparison data)
Pulmonary function	Rideout (2007)	Precomparison and postcomparison		No difference in precomparison and postcomparison
Quality of life	Hamilton and Hawley (2006)	Retrospective review		Significant improvement over time
	Kutzleb and Reiner (2006)	Quasi-experimental comparison		Significantly better than control group
	McCorkle et al. (2009)	Randomized controlled trial	Population-specific	Significantly improved
Readmission	Lowery et al. (2011)	Precomparison and postcomparison		Decreased heart failure readmissions
Time to service delivery	Reigle, Molnar, Howell, and Dumont (2006)	Medical record review	Population-generic, organizational	Significantly less than physicians
Urinary tract infection	Elpern et al. (2009)	Retrospective	Population-generic	Significantly reduced
Vaginal delivery rates	Cheung et al. (2011)	Randomized controlled trial	Population-specific	Significantly reduced
Ventilator-associated pneumonia	Quenot et al. (2007)	Observational	Population-generic	Significantly decreased rates of pneumonia
Weight	Rideout (2007)	Precomparison and postcomparison	Population-generic	No difference in precomparison and postcomparison

Note: Some indicators that were used with specific populations in studies have been labeled as generic because they can be applied to multiple patient groups. The outcome measures listed here are not uniformly consistent with the measure properties of similar indicators endorsed by the National Quality Forum.

[a]Definition of terms for the focus of the indicator:

Population-generic—indicators that could be used with any patient population.

Population-specific—indicators that are relevant to specific populations only.

incorporated to the extent evident in APRN practice. Ideally, attention should be directed at indicators that accurately measure all care providers' impact and those that can serve as benchmarks for APRN practice alone. In a recent study of the impact of granting APRNs full practice authority in the state of Ohio, the authors identified that access to health-care services would increase with possible increases in quality. Removing restrictive regulations that limit APRN scope of practice nationwide could therefore have a significant impact on a broader population scale (Martsolf, Auerbach & Arifkhanova. 2015).

Studies Comparing APRN to Physician and Other Provider Outcomes

Studies comparing APRNs with physicians have been reported in the United States, Canada, the British Isles, Europe, Australia, the Middle East, and elsewhere. As noted earlier, a synthesis review of US APRN roles has demonstrated that APRN care is equivalent to physician care and, for some outcomes, such as patient satisfaction, APRN care was rated higher (Newhouse et al., 2011). A number of studies comparing APRN care with physician care internationally have demonstrated similar results (Albers-Heitner et al., 2012; Scherr, Wilson, Wagner, & Haughian, 2012) and improved care in outcomes such as rates of vaginal deliveries and episiotomies (Cheung et al., 2011), eczema care (Schuttelaar, Vermeulen, & Coenraads, 2011), skilled procedures such as thoracostomy tube insertion (Bevis et al., 2008), and ophthalmic examination techniques in the ED (Lamirel et al., 2012). Alexandrov et al. (2009, 2011a, 2011b) have demonstrated that APRNs provided with postgraduate academic fellowship education and training in acute neurovascular care were able to diagnose acute ischemic stroke accurately through a combination of clinical localization and neuroimaging (multimodal computed tomography and magnetic resonance imaging) interpretation and make safe and effective tissue plasminogen activator (tPA) treatment decisions while also increasing the absolute number of tPA-treated stroke patients at their facility.

Nurse Practitioner Outcomes

A number of studies have examined the impact of care provided by NPs. A systematic review by Stanik-Hutt et al. (2013) identified data from 37 of 27,993 articles published from 1990 through 2009 that were summarized based on 11 aggregated outcomes of NP care. In comparison to physician care or teams without NPs, outcomes for NPs were comparable or better for all 11 outcomes reviewed. A high level of evidence identified better serum lipid levels in patients managed by NPs in primary care practices. A high level of evidence was also identified for patient outcomes related to satisfaction with care, health status, functional status, blood pressure control, blood glucose control, number of ED visits and hospitalizations, and mortality, all being similar for NP care compared to physician care (Stanik-Hutt et al., 2013).

A parallel synthesis review by Newhouse and associates (2011) confirmed the positive outcomes from NP care in comparison to physician care.

However, this focus of comparing NP outcomes with those of other care providers is probably no longer indicated because demonstrating the impact of the unique aspects of APRN care is more valuable. Other studies comparing care by NP-led teams to physician care have demonstrated no differences in care with respect to mortality rates, length of stay, or rehospitalization rates (Collins et al., 2014; Costa, Wallace, Barnato, & Kahn, 2014; Gershengorn et al., 2011; Landsperger, Semler, Wang, Byrne, & Wheeler, 2015).

Other recent studies related to NP care have demonstrated the benefit of specific role components such as NP-led rapid response teams (Barocas et al., 2014; Kapu, Wheeler, & Lee, 2014; Morse, Warshawsky, Moore, & Pecora, 2006; Scherr et al., 2012; Sonday & Grecsek, 2010); the impact of NP interventions such as a postdischarge home visit to high-readmission-risk medical patients (Smith, Pan, & Novelli, 2016) or to cardiac surgery patients (Sawatzky, Christie, & Singal, 2013); and specialty-based NP roles, including trauma care (Collins et al., 2014), emergency care (Li, Westbrook, Callen, Georgiou, & Braithwaite, 2013), inpatient medical services, geriatric inpatient care, cardiovascular care (Alexander-Banys, 2014; David, Britting, & Dalton, 2015; Kleinpell et al., 2015), and oncology and palliative care (Hutchinson, East, Stasa, & Jackson, 2014; Kilpatrick et al., 2014).

Clinical Nurse Specialist Outcomes

The impact of CNS care has been examined in several reviews, including a literature review on CNS competencies and outcome studies, highlighting the role of the CNS in specialty-based practice roles including chronic disease management, influence on the practice of nursing staff, and unit-level metrics such as pressure ulcer prevention, fall prevention, patient satisfaction, promotion of EBP, and staff turnover and satisfaction (Gordon, Lorilla, & Lehman, 2012). A number of studies have explored outcomes related to CNS care and CNS productivity (Urden & Stacy, 2012). Fulton (2012) reported on validating CNS core practice outcomes. In a survey of 427 CNSs using an international CNS list serve, the most frequently monitored outcomes related to APRN nursing interventions (68% in the patient sphere, 87% in the EBP sphere, and 86% in the nurse and organizational spheres). The least monitored outcomes related to diagnosing (range, 54%–57%) and cost and revenue (range 36%–55%). Other studies have focused on exploring outcomes related to specialty areas of care. Favorable outcomes have been seen for cancer patients managed by CNSs in outpatient settings (Dayhoff & Lyons, 2009). Other studies related to CNS outcomes in acute care have demonstrated reductions in hospitalization length of stay and costs (Dayhoff & Lyons, 2009; Newhouse et al., 2011). A recent systematic review on the effectiveness and cost-effectiveness of CNSs in outpatient roles identified 11 randomized controlled trials with evidence of reduced resource use and costs of care favoring CNS care (Kilpatrick et al., 2014).

The outcomes of CNS care have also been investigated in international models of care. Begley and colleagues (2010) assessed the impact of the CNS and midwifery roles in Ireland. APRNs, including CNSs and nurse-midwives, were found to improve service delivery by leading the development of new clinical services; taking responsibility for guideline development, implementation, and evaluation; and positively influencing quality patient care through formal and informal education.

Certified Nurse-Midwife Outcomes

A number of outcome studies have focused on the outcomes of CNM care and have demonstrated significant impact on vaginal delivery rates, decreased rates of episiotomies and amniotomies, less use of pain medication, and high satisfaction ratings, among other outcomes (Arthur, Marfell, & Ulrich, 2009; Cheung, et al., 2011; Johantgen, et al., 2012; Malloy, 2010). The American College of Nurse-Midwives (ACNM) conducts an annual benchmarking study to assess the impact of CNM outcomes by examining a number of metrics. This national benchmarking project enables CNM practices to identify and compare performance in a number of quality and best practice areas, including primary cesarean birth rate (goal, < 23.9%), preterm birth rate (goal, < 11.4%), and exclusive breastfeeding first 48 hours (goal, > 81%), among other metrics. The 2015 benchmarking study identified several categories, including the "Triple Aim" Best Practice, "4 Core" Best Practice, and best practices by volume (ACNM, 2016).

"Triple Aim" Best Practice recognizes practices that meet the Institute for Healthcare Improvement Triple Aim principles of improving the patient experience, reducing cost of care, and improving the health of populations. This is demonstrated by high breastfeeding rates, low preterm birth and cesarean rates, and reporting fiscal variables. Of the 285 practices participating in the 2015 ACNM Benchmarking Project, 71 were designated Triple Aim Best Practices (ACNM, 2016). The four core best practices are induction of labor (goal, <10%), primary cesarean birth rate (goal, < 15%), episiotomy (goal, < 2%), and exclusive breastfeeding first 48 hours (goal, > 75%).

A study of CNM outcomes used an optimality index to compare midwifery and physician practices according to the extent of preexisting conditions at the time of treatment (Cragin & Kennedy, 2006). The optimality index contained a list of 40 care delivery processes and outcome measures pertaining to pregnancy, parturition, and neonatal and maternal postpartum condition, which were scored according to level of optimality (0 = nonoptimal; 1 = optimal). Women cared for by physicians were 1.7 times as likely as those cared for by CNMs to have a cesarean section during delivery. Women seen by physicians in this study had a significantly greater proportion of chronic illness and drug abuse, although these differences did not explain the higher rate of cesarean section for the group.

A Cochrane Database systematic review comparing midwife-led care with other models of care examined 11 clinical trials and found that midwife-led models of care resulted in patients being less likely to experience antenatal hospitalization, regional analgesia, and episiotomy or instrumental delivery. Patients were more likely to experience no intrapartum analgesia or anesthesia, have spontaneous vaginal births, and initiate breastfeeding. There were no statistically significant differences between groups for cesarean births, but women who were randomized to receive midwife-led care were less likely to experience fetal loss before 24 weeks' gestation and hospital lengths of stay were shorter (Hatem, et al., 2008).

Certified Registered Nurse Anesthetist Outcomes

A recent Cochrane systematic review (Lewis, Nicholson, Smith, & Alderson, 2014) of CRNA studies identified six relevant studies, five of which were large observational studies. The reviewers identified that studies have demonstrated no difference in the number of people who died when given anesthetic by either a nurse anesthetist or a medically qualified anesthetist. One study found a lower rate of death with nurse anesthetists compared to medically qualified anesthetists. Other studies gave varied results, and overall there were variations between studies for the rates of complications for patients depending on their anesthetic provider. Several recent studies have demonstrated the impact of CRNA care on various outcomes, including cost-effectiveness (Dulisse & Cromwell, 2010; Hogan, Seifert, Moore, & Simonson, 2010; Kremer & Faut-Callahan, 2009). Studies of CRNA impact compared CRNA outcomes with those of anesthesiologists. One of these estimated costs was based on cases from four anesthesia services at four different hospitals—a large academic medical center, a large community hospital, a medium-sized community hospital, and a small community hospital (Cromwell & Snyder, 2000). Labor cost projections for 10,000 anesthetics delivered annually demonstrated that an all-CRNA care delivery model cost less than 50% of an all-anesthesiologist model. The cost savings for a mixed model composed of anesthesiologists and CRNAs in ratios of 1:1 to 1:4 ranged from 33% to 41% of the total costs for an all-anesthesiologist model.

Studies Comparing APRN and Physician Productivity

One of the most difficult and contentious elements of APRN outcomes measurement is the assessment of APRN productivity, which is an organizational rather than a patient outcome. Productivity is an indication of care provider efficiency rather than skill or capability and, as such, does not provide any guarantee of quality patient care. The issue with productivity is that reimbursement practices and the income generated by care providers are directly tied to productivity levels. Because APRNs have historically spent more time with patients, their overall productivity levels may result in changes in potential income for the organization or practice. Until reimbursement decisions are shifted to a care delivery outcomes approach, this will continue to be problematic for APRNs.

Relative Work Value of APRNs

Payment for services provided to Medicare patients is based on a resource-based relative value (RBRV) scale methodology, which incorporates an estimate for the amount of work, practice expense, and professional liability insurance associated with various procedures. The total relative value of each procedure is multiplied by a standard dollar conversion factor to determine the allowable service charge that providers can request for reimbursement of services (Sullivan-Marx, 2008). NP data have also been used to adjust the RBRVs for some payment codes, although considerable work is needed to clarify how NPs' work values differ from those of physicians (Sullivan-Marx, 2008). Demonstrating the quality and financial impact of APRN care is a priority area of focus but presents challenges in identifying the true impact of care on costs or through cost avoidance (Kapu, Kleinpell, & Pilon, 2014).

In the study by Sullivan-Marx (2008), to quantify the time required, NPs estimated preservice, intraservice, and postservice time in minutes. Complexity was measured by assessing mental effort, technical skill, physical effort, and the psychologic stress associated with an iatrogenic event related to the Current Procedural Terminology (CPT) code. In all cases, NPs' estimated relative work values were comparable to those established for physician practice, suggesting that practice patterns were similar for the scenarios described (Sullivan-Marx, 2008). Because the CPT codes and descriptors were designed with physicians in mind, however, other activities by APRNs may not have been included in the estimation process. Until these are well defined and marketed by APRNs, this process will potentially continue to underrepresent the APRN's actual relative value in the delivery of care. Tracking productivity and the work value of APRN care using productivity tools to capture outcomes has also been advocated (Steuer & Kopan, 2011). Other studies have continued to demonstrate comparable outcomes of APRN and physician care (Costa et al., 2014; Gershengorn et al., 2011; Landsperger et al., 2015; Newhouse et al., 2011).

A workload analysis of a CNS role in a specialty lung cancer practice found that the role was primarily used to support processes and administrative components. Restructuring the role to implement standardized care based on national practice guidelines led to proactive case management that resulted in a decrease in admissions for nonacute health care problems from 4/month to a mean of 0.3/month (Baxter & Leary, 2011). A study of postoperative patients with hypercholesterolemia involved a randomized clinical trial designed to compare the cost-effectiveness of services provided by an NP with that of usual care enhanced by feedback to a primary care provider (Paez & Allen, 2006). The incremental costs associated with the oversight of the NP included the costs of the NP's time and of the lipid-lowering medications and the laboratory monitoring activities of the NP. At 12 months after surgery, the incremental costs of the NP-managed group were $26 per 1-mg/dL decrease in cholesterol and $39 per percentage reduction of lipid level (in mg/dL). NP management was most intensive during the first 6 months of the year and medication costs were highest during this period, when NPs titrated dosages to achieve maximum effect. Although more costly during this initial period than for the usual care group, the ultimate outcome of achieving better lipid management offset the extra cost.

Internationally, the number of studies focusing on APRN outcomes has been increasing as APRN roles expand worldwide. Partiprajak (2012) followed 100 type 2 diabetes mellitus patients in Thailand to assess the impact of an APRN-led support group ($n = 44$) and a comparison group ($n = 56$). The results indicated that the APRN-led support group patients had lower systolic blood pressure, higher self-care abilities, and increased quality of life and satisfaction than the comparison group. Other international studies have demonstrated outcomes related to NP care (Ball et al., 2007), CNS care (Baxter & Leary, 2011; Begley et al., 2010; Oliver & Leary, 2010), and CNM care (Woods, 2007).

As noted, Table 23.4 provides a comprehensive summary of APRN outcome studies organized by outcome indicators. As outlined in the table, an impressive number of studies have been conducted that examined a number of specific outcomes. Most of the studies have demonstrated improved outcomes as a result of APRN care and/or comparable outcomes with other health care providers. As APRN roles continue to expand to different practice settings and to specialty-based practices, continued evaluation of the impact of APRN care is warranted to identify APRN contributions to care.

Future Directions for Using Outcomes in APRN Practice

The evidence of APRNs' impact on individual patient and organizational outcomes suggests that the quality of care that APRNs deliver is comparable or superior to that of other care providers in the specialty. Various studies have explored the direct and indirect processes that APRNs use to manage patient care and the outcomes achieved. All have determined that APRN practice overlaps that of other care providers in some respects and differs in others. These distinctions, and their potential to confound comparisons with other care providers, contribute to the complexity inherent in measuring the effect of APRNs. Moreover, the limited research linking specific APRN processes to care delivery outcomes makes it difficult to determine which role components achieved the effect. Difficult or not, a clear distinction is needed if APRNs are ever to receive the recognition they deserve or the financial reimbursement they are due.

This review of APRN outcome studies suggests that the quality and quantity of research pertaining to APRN outcomes has improved over time, with initial studies focusing primarily on role description and acceptance issues and more recent studies addressing performance and outcome considerations between APRN and other provider groups. A variety of research designs are now being used to measure APRN impact, with an increasing number of investigators using prospective designs and including comparison groups. Although medical record reviews continue to provide much of the data for these comparison studies, methods to control for differences in patient populations and the use of more sophisticated data analysis techniques are providing more reliable, replicable, and generalizable information.

Despite these improvements, intensive work is needed in several areas. The first of these involves the consistent use of a set of core outcome indicators relevant and sensitive to differences in APRN practice. An important step in this direction relates to the work performed by the NQF to establish a list of endorsed measures, many of which are applicable to the work of APRNs (NQF, 2017a). National leadership groups should assume responsibility for measure development and testing using the methods outlined by the NQF to guide their work; such a process would increase the number of measures in the domain of APRN practice and would ultimately facilitate standardized approaches to the evaluation of APRN effect and public reporting. Collaborations between APRNs and nurse researchers and the development of outcomes consortia also will facilitate this process. Bringing together clinical practice and research design and measurement experts from multiple locations and specialties is the best approach for the development and subsequent testing of reliable and valid indicators of the effect of APRN-directed and APRN-delivered care. Networks of APRN groups and institutions in which APRNs practice should also play an active role in the collection of data for measure testing to further the development of APRN-sensitive measures. An understanding of the important role that the NQF plays in relation to endorsing measures recognized by the CMS is essential, given the fact that other pathways to widespread measure adoption are lacking, particularly in regard to publicly reported measures. As noted, Table 23.4 lists examples of the various APRN-sensitive outcome indicators that have been used in previous studies; however, the conformity of these measures with the NQF-endorsed measures for use by the CMS, third-party payors, and public reporting is inconsistent. However, one consideration is the reporting burden that can result from requiring use of additional reporting metrics, an area of importance highlighted by the Institute for Healthcare Improvement in advocating for a reduction in the data-gathering burden (Institute for Healthcare Improvement, 2017).

Of additional importance is defining the specific role components of the APRN roles. A recent systematic review identified 43 randomized controlled trials evaluating the cost-effectiveness of APRNs using criteria that meet current definitions of the roles. Incomplete reporting of study methods and lack of details about the APRN roles create challenges in evaluating the evidence of the cost-effectiveness of these roles (Donald et al., 2014).

There is a need to also determine whether the increased patient and family satisfaction evident when APRNs spend extra time with patients and families also contributes to improvements in longer term care delivery outcomes. Because APRNs have traditionally spent more time with patients and provide additional teaching and healthy behaviors counseling, their impact may be most evident in the long-term prevention of diseases and the adverse outcomes commonly associated with poor health behaviors. Studies thus far have followed patient outcomes for relatively short periods, usually 6 to 12 months following APRN intervention. Additional longitudinal studies are needed to determine the true long-term impact of these early outcomes on overall lifestyle, quality of life, and health.

Another future direction for APRN outcomes is to focus on the unique contributions that APRNs make in their roles. Many studies have focused on comparing APRNs with other providers, particularly attending physicians, physician residents, or physician assistants. Although these studies are useful, they do not address the unique contributions of APRN care nor identify which outcome indicators are most sensitive to differences in APRN practices. The focus of outcomes assessment research needs to turn to the value of APRN care in patient and population outcomes, rather than comparison of care with other health care providers; however, when APRNs stretch the boundaries of their practice to incorporate new roles and responsibilities, comparisons to more traditional providers of these services are inevitable.

Additionally, evaluation of the value-added impact of APRNs in collaborative practice with physicians and other care providers is needed. Although the work of Newhouse and associates (2011) has highlighted that an impressive number of studies have been conducted that demonstrate outcomes of APRN care, additional research is needed as APRN roles continue to expand and as roles in novel practice areas develop. Because APRNs and physicians bring different perspectives about care and demonstrate distinct but complementary behaviors, studies are needed to determine how these combined practices reinforce and maximize the beneficial effects of one another. These studies may generate the data needed to demonstrate the value-added benefits of combining APRN and physician practices. By documenting favorable outcomes when a collaborative APRN-physician approach is used, the profession can more effectively argue for altered reimbursement procedures and reveal the contributions of APRNs to the public.

The literature also highlights the difficulties evident in generating widespread interest in measuring care delivery outcomes. Many APRNs view the ongoing assessment of care delivery impact as an additional burden to an already full agenda. Because APRN outcome measurement activities begin immediately when an APRN is hired, preparation for identifying target outcomes, collecting data, and managing and reporting findings is the minimum information required in graduate programs. In addition to clinically focused outcomes content, several individuals and groups have recommended including content on health care financing, health care information systems, database query, and statistics, particularly in Doctor of Nursing Practice education for APRNs (AACN, 2015). Developing APRN-associated metrics for outcomes assessment is a strategy that holds promise for future work highlighting the impact of APRN care (Kapu & Kleinpell, 2013). Dashboards can then be used to outline the metrics, assign data definitions, and enable data transfer and display to assess trends over time. In well-conceived electronic health records (EHRs), downloadable data can self-populate APRN dashboards to promote ready viewing of NP-led initiatives. For example, if promoting adherence to national quality guidelines such as VTE prophylaxis in hospitalized patients, tracking use of an EHR order set for eligible patients can enhance data capture and outline trends over time.

A number of strategies can be used to identify and develop APRN-associated outcomes metrics. These include identifying high-priority outcomes, outlining how these outcomes measure APRN core competencies, determining if currently existing data sets can be used to abstract metrics, and evaluating if informatics can be created to automatically collect the data (Kapu & Kleinpell, 2013). Ideally, APRNs should approach their regularly assigned duties, as well as newly initiated projects, with an eye to outcomes assessment, enabling development and ongoing refinement of metric-driven performance to ensure role value and evolution for years to come.

Conclusion

Focusing on the outcomes of APRN care is an essential component in demonstrating the impact of the role as well as contributions to quality and safe patient care. APRN care has been cited as being valuable but often invisible because APRNs traditionally have not focused on highlighting the impact of their care. This invisibility in the health care system further threatens the recognition of APRNs as viable and important providers of health care services. The current emphasis on quality of care and care effectiveness mandates that APRNs demonstrate their impact on patient care, health care outcomes, and systems of care. It is apparent that the need for well-designed, longitudinal assessments of APRN impact has never been greater. Assessing the outcomes of APRN care has become a necessary rather than an optional endeavor. It is only through demonstrating the outcomes of APRN care for patients, providers, and health care systems that the value of this care can be defined.

In addition, focusing on APRN-sensitive outcome indicators is important for highlighting the unique contributions of APRNs. Addressing APRN-sensitive outcome indicators will require focused attention on the continued development of EHRs that support the identification and tracking of process and outcome data in line with APRN contributions. An important component in this process is national agreement on a core set of outcome indicators relevant to APRNs, the initiation of standards that support the collection of APRN-sensitive data, testing of these core measures, and ultimately measure endorsement by the NQF.

This chapter has presented a review of concepts related to APRN outcomes and several frameworks for measuring and monitoring APRN practice. Other approaches are also available; the APRN should begin the process by selecting one and refining it to meet individual and organizational needs. The best approach is to begin small and expand activities over time. Networking with other APRNs is useful for identifying beneficial outcomes and sharing personal experiences about what does and does not work when integrating outcomes measurement into busy practices. Publishing and presenting on outcome evaluation initiatives are imperative to disseminating successful methods for assessing APRN outcomes and highlighting exemplars for replication.

Effective outcomes measurement requires APRNs to work collaboratively with others, plan and organize processes of care and assessment of quality in highly complex health services environments, and expose their individual practices to the scrutiny of others. Experience with organizational change behaviors and a willingness to seek information and assistance from others will help with this process. In the end, the quality and value of care will improve, as will the community's recognition of the APRN's positive impact on outcomes of care.

Key Summary Points

■ Performance indicators for APRN roles focus on two levels—the aggregate level, at which evidence addresses APRN role impact in one of the four APRN roles, and the individual level, with activities directed at the outcomes of a single APRN's practice.

■ Studies evaluating care delivery processes of APRN practice often occur in combination with role definition research. The distinction between these studies and role definition explorations is their attention to what APRNs do as part of their roles.

■ Various studies have explored the direct and indirect processes that APRNs use to manage patient care and the outcomes achieved. These studies identify that APRN practice overlaps that of other care providers in some respects and differs in others. These distinctions, and their potential to confound comparisons with other care providers, contribute to the complexity inherent in measuring the effect of APRNs.

■ Effective outcomes measurement requires APRNs to work collaboratively with others, plan and organize processes of care and assessment of quality in highly complex health services environments, and expose their individual practices to the scrutiny of others.

References

To access the references for this chapter, use your smartphone's QR code reader to scan the code below, or go to http://booksite.elsevier.com/ 9780323447751.

Using Health Care Information Technology to Evaluate and Improve Performance and Patient Outcomes

Marisa L. Wilson

"The only thing worse than being blind is having sight but no vision."

—*Helen Keller*

CHAPTER CONTENT

In 1965, Dr. Loretta Ford and Dr. Henry Silver developed the first pediatric nurse practitioner program at the University of Colorado. Since that time, the role and professional practice of the advanced practice registered nurse (APRN) have been well described (Archibald & Fraser, 2013; Honeyfield, 2009; Sackett, Spitzer, Gent, & Roberts 1974; Van Vleet & Paradise, 2015). The impact of APRN professional practice, as compared to similar care provided by physicians, has also been well described and has been demonstrated to be safe, of high quality, and cost effective (Mundinger et al., 2000; Stanik-Hutt et al., 2013; see Chapter 23).

The author would like to acknowledge the excellent work of Vicky A. Mahn-DiNicola in the previous edition of this chapter.

However, studies of comparison between providers individually or as a group have proven to have methodologic challenges due to inconsistencies in automated data collection as a by-product of care, lack of data specificity, and data storage. Despite these challenges and based on the available evidence, many state legislative bodies are following the recommendation of the Institute of Medicine (IOM) that all nurses, including APRNs, should practice at the top of their license. This is demonstrated as autonomous practice through the repeal of restrictive practice laws, which serves to increase access to quality care for millions of citizens (IOM, 2011; National Governors Association, 2012). Thus APRNs have seen increasing independence, authority, and responsibility. However, there remains a need to continue to demonstrate optimal comparable outcomes between and among providers.

Concurrent to work that has defined and evaluated the impact of APRN practice on care, there have been several decades of work that has been aimed at health care reform to improve quality and efficiency while containing escalating costs. This has generated much discussion on what the US health care system should look like and how it will be financially supported. This work has resulted in the Patient Protection and Affordable Care Act (ACA, 2010), which attempts to increase access to and quality of care for all citizens, and the creation of the Centers for Medicare & Medicaid Services (CMS) Innovation Center, which is designed to stimulate new ways to pay for and deliver care (https://innovation.cms.gov/index.html). Models have been offered, but there remains concern about which model will best achieve measureable progress on the challenges of containing and reducing cost while improving quality and efficiency. Innovative health care systems, such as Kaiser Permanente, Intermountain Healthcare, the Mayo Clinic, Geisinger Health System, and Bellin Health, have been on the forefront of developing and evaluating what the Institute for Healthcare Improvement (IHI) calls the Triple Aim: (1) provide effective, safe, and reliable care to individuals; (2) improve the health of populations by focusing on prevention, wellness, and improved management of chronic disease; and (3) decrease per capita costs (IHI, 2016). The evidence from these and other innovative systems has led to yet another refinement in overall care system goals. While it is likely that, in the current political climate, the existing ACA will change, it is reasonable to anticipate that health care reimbursement and regulation will continue to be focused on quality and outcomes. A current mandate is explored further in this chapter.

Despite the ongoing debates about what the health care system should look like and how it is to be financed, one component remains: a need for wider access to quality care that provides optimal outcomes. This can be addressed through expanded practice parameters and wider deployment of APRN services. The professional practice skills and expertise of the APRN, bolstered by evidence supporting comparable (or better) outcomes, is a necessary component regardless of which model is ultimately chosen. Currently, there exist impediments in the regulatory environment that place barriers to the full deployment of APRNs practicing to the full extent of their license uniformly across the nation. To reduce the impediments, practitioners, researchers, and evaluators require the ability to demonstrate, in a reliable and quantifiable manner, that quality and cost-effective care can be consistently delivered by APRNs as individual practitioners and as members/leaders of a care team. Not only is this information needed when working to lessen individual state regulatory restrictions to practice, it is needed by health care organizations to promote broader adoption and optimization of APRN professional services in their emerging health care delivery models. Recent final rules promulgated by the Department of Veterans Affairs (VA) recognizes the postive impact that APRNs can make on the almost 9 million veterans who receive care across a full spectrum of services in the United States. The VA has struggled recently to provide high quality care; to address this problem, the VA amended its regulations to permit full practice authority regardless of individual state practice regulations to Certified Nurse Practitioners, Clinical Nurse Specialists, and Certified Nurse Midwives practicing in VA facilities (Department of Veterans Affairs, 2016). These regulation omitted full practice authority for CRNAs.

The ability to evaluate the contributions of all care providers to positive outcomes will be required as the health care system transfers from payment based on quantity to one with payment based on quality. Finally, this information is needed by the public to help raise awareness that APRNs can deliver quality care in cost-effective ways. This means that it is every APRN's responsibility to engage fully in evaluative activities, not only to fulfill regulatory and reimbursement mandates but also to inform all stakeholders, including other APRNs, about the effectiveness of their practice.

Today, this is not uniformly occurring. Kapu and Kleinpell (2013) indicated that few organizations have defined productivity targets and most report that they do not measure the impact of APRN-led interventions, citing the difficulties with linking providers to patients or populations and also the difficulties of linking specific care provided to the measurement of outcomes. Kapu and Kleinpell (2013) also warned that even in institutions that employ large numbers of APRNs (i.e., 200 or more), no focused organizational efforts are being implemented to assess the outcomes. This situation is soon to change, and the APRN must be prepared to participate in the development and implementation of the evaluation activities using evidence, translation, informatics techniques, and information technology.

This chapter introduces the need for outcomes evaluation for APRNs, the regulatory and reimbursement mandates pushing this forward, and the informatics and information technology tools and processes required for conducting this work. The term *outcome evaluation* refers to three levels of activities: (1) that which evaluates individual APRN practice, such as peer review; (2) that which evaluates the collective value of all APRNs to an organization or population such as a research or demonstration project; or (3) that which evaluates outcomes in clinical populations served by all providers, including APRNs, in an organization or population. Depending on the nature of the outcome evaluation activity and metrics used to monitor performance, these activities may at times overlap *and* are not always mutually exclusive. For example, a performance indicator that examines the percentage of patients with diabetes who are evaluated annually to determine their hemoglobin A_{1c} (HbA$_{1c}$) level may be used to evaluate an individual APRN's compliance to a standard of care, or it could be used to illustrate the level to which populations are being managed by APRNs to determine if an acceptable rate of compliance has been achieved compared to physician providers. This same indicator could also be used by a health care organization to report overall provider compliance to this best practice standard to an external stakeholder to demonstrate an ability to monitor high-risk populations appropriately in their community or region (e.g., for public health reporting). Newer mandates are also going to require demonstration of improvement activities, which will require a measurement of the impact of a provider or a team of providers. To be able to highlight the contributions of an APRN, as an individual provider or as a member of a team, to patient or population outcomes will become very important in the transformation of care.

Informatics and Information Technology Supporting Improved Performance and Outcomes

Since the 1960s, providers and facilities have slowly been implementing a variety of technologies to support care and provide data for outcomes measurement. Over the last decade, this movement toward technology has accelerated. As of 2016, electronic health records (EHRs), patient portals, bar-code administration systems, point-of-care (POC) devices, physiologic device monitors with integration, and systems interoperability mechanisms are in use in over 90% of hospitals and over 75% of provider offices, affording a foundation for safe, quality, and efficient care (US Department of Health and Human

Services [DHHS], Office of the National Coordinator for Health Information Technology, 2017). The APRN must be aware of and able to manage the array of information systems and devices in use to collect patient data to evaluate fully the outcomes of care. The APRN has to be able to lead the process changes necessary to optimize the use of these tools from design to implementation to data extraction.

In 1999, the IOM issued the landmark report *To Err Is Human: Building a Safer Health System.* In this report, the IOM indicated that at least 44,000 people and perhaps as many as 98,000 people die in hospitals each year because of medical errors that could have been prevented. Medical errors were defined as failure of a planned action to be completed as intended or the use of a wrong plan to achieve an aim. In 2001, the IOM issued another report, *Crossing the Quality Chasm: A New Health System for the 21st Century,* in which the need for high-quality, evidence-based, standardized care for all was emphasized (IOM, 2001). Using studies published since the 1999 IOM report, Makary and Daniel (2016) extrapolated from annual inpatient death rates that medical error contributes to the deaths of 251,454 (9.5%) inpatients, making this the third-leading cause of death. While there has been some controversy as to the extrapolation methods used in the Makary and Daniels research, all of the studies utilized indicated that the main drivers of these care issues leading to medical errors were a lack of technologic infrastructure, uncoordinated care, communication errors, and lack of organization in a system that is complex, adaptive, and difficult to navigate and manage across multiple encounters and provider interactions. The IOM proposed that a fundamental component to address the problems found in health care in the United States was to increase the infiltration of advanced technology, specifically information technology (IT) such as EHRs. IT was determined to have the potential to transform the care delivery system and to assist care providers in reducing medical errors. At that time, health care had remained relatively untouched by the technology revolution that had already occurred in other sectors such as retail and banking.

However, the impact of IT infiltration on process and outcome is only as good as the ability of educated, engaged, and activated clinical personnel to use the IT to support optimized processes of care. The IOM added to the quality improvement calls and published *The Future of Nursing: Leading Chnage, Advancing Health*, which added a call for all nurses to be empowered to practice to the full extent of their education and training (IOM, 2011). This IOM report specified that APRNs, as full partners with physicians and other health care professionals, can contribute to the needed redesign of healthcare in the United States, in which information technology and informatics techniques are used efficiently and effectively to improve care and communication.

To achieve this technology revolution in health care, President Barack Obama in 2009 made an unprecedented move and mandated the use of EHRs by both health care providers and hospitals. This was not a new request; encouraging the use of EHRs had been previously recommended by President George W. Bush in 2004 when he specifically indicated, in his State of the Union address, the need for health care providers to implement the use of EHRs over 10 years to avoid medical mistakes, reduce costs, and improve care (The White House, 2004). However, there was no financial incentive or disincentive offered to motivate the health care community at large until the American Recovery and Reinvestment Act of 2009 was signed by President Obama. This act included the Heath Information Technology for Economic and Clinical Health (HITECH) Act, which allowed up to $29 billion for the adoption and utilization of EHRs in care facilities and also provided mandates for the technology vendors, along with implementation support and education. The Office of the National Coordinator for Health Information Technology, under the DHHS and the CMS, supports and manages the HITECH Act EHR incentive programs through the management of financial incentives and other support mechanisms for organizations that demonstrate meaningful use (MU) of EHRs to improve care and clinical outcomes (CMS, 2016). The HITECH Act represents one of the largest federal investments in health IT, demonstrating a broad and bipartisan commitment to realizing the potential of EHRs to transform care.

To be clear, MU did not mean simply implementing a system but also rethinking the way health care was provided with the infusion of health IT. To meet the requirements of MU, the providers or facilities must demonstrate: (1) the use of a certified EHR that has met defined criteria, (2) the ability to exchange standardized health data and information, (3) technology to advance clinical processes, and (4) the ability to report quality measures. The benefits of MU, upon implementation and deployment of EHRs, are to: (1) improve quality of patient care, (2) increase patients' participation and engagement in their own care, (3) improve accuracy of diagnoses and outcomes through decision support and guideline use, (4) improve care coordination through data and information exchange, (5) increase efficiency and cost savings by reducing duplication, and (6) improve public and population health through reporting, exchange, and analysis. To benefit from MU, hospitals and providers must demonstrate the ability to meet the mandates using technology and to have adapted and adjusted processes to improve outcomes.

EHRs are one form of IT used to support improved performance and outcomes. There are others that supplement the EHR and are also used to transform care to improve outcomes and efficiency. Exemplar 24.1 describes the technology-rich environment of a national urgent care center that is utilizing IT tools to manage outcomes, including EHRs with embedded guidelines and decision support tools along with patient-centered data from the use of kiosks.

One of the most commonly used ITs in hospitals is bar coding. Bar coding is used during medication administration, blood transfusions, patient tracking, equipment monitoring, and laboratory testing. Bar coding uses a reader to scan a data-embedded bar code that collects patient, product, and provider information. The database supporting the bar code application then is used to verify accuracy of the patient and the medication or laboratory order. The data collected can be used to validate administration of a medication or blood product or the completion of a laboratory test. Selected data elements can be incorporated into the individual patient record in the EHR. Process data can be collected as the reading is complete.

Additional technologies used to support quality care are POC testing devices. Among the most commonly used POC devices are blood glucose monitoring devices. Expansion of this technology includes other POC laboratory testing such as monitoring of electrolytes, troponins, cardiac markers, coagulation studies, hematocrit, blood gases, and proteins in the acute care and emergency areas. These devices, as an example, are used in urgent care, surgery centers, emergency departments, and other areas where time is an important factor in getting patients the care needed based on precise and accurate data. The benefits to POC testing are immediate access to results and a decrease in transcription error of the results, versus values coming from manual data entry. Data from POC devices can be integrated into the patient record in the EHR for data-sharing purposes and decision support.

Device integration is also expanding in scope and function across all EHR platforms. Device integration allows the ability to pull data from other source

| EXEMPLAR 24.1 | Walgreens Healthcare Clinics[SM] Make Advanced Practice Nursing Outcomes Transparent to the World[a] |

Walgreens has created an emerging market segment in health care delivery with its Healthcare Clinics. The care provided is acute, episodic, family-oriented care for patients older than 18 months. Although not positioned like an emergency or urgent care clinic, in which full laboratory and imaging resources are readily available, the care provided in the Healthcare Clinics helps patients without immediate access to primary care providers as well as providing preventive services such as immunizations. Common health complaints typically addressed with this service include upper respiratory infections (URIs), ear infections, minor sprains and injuries, school physicals, vaccinations, and screening and counseling services for hypertension, hyperlipidemia, and diabetes. More urgent conditions, such as sudden-onset chest pain, active bleeding, or trauma, are redirected to the nearest emergency care center. Patients can preschedule clinic visits online or walk in during hours of operation, which include extended evening and weekend hours. Clinics are located directly inside select Walgreens stores across the United States and, as of this writing, are staffed by over 1400 board-certified family nurse practitioners.

Advanced practice registered nurses (APRNs) who practice in a Walgreens Healthcare Clinic typically care for patients in an autonomous and technology-driven environment. Patients register at a touch-screen kiosk when they arrive, and services and pricing are visible via a liquid crystal display (LCD) screen outside the clinic. Patients are then seen in an examining room, which is generally located next to the pharmacy. During the visit, the APRN will interview the patient, entering information into a proprietary electronic health record (EHR) designed expressly for Walgreens with input from APRN end users. This EHR contains key information about the patient's health status and prompts the APRN to inquire about selected data elements necessary to compute various health care quality outcomes. It also tracks any prescribed medications and generates discharge instructions, which are printed out and provided to patients prior to their departure from the examination room, allowing the patient time and privacy to review instructions with the APRN. Finally, patients are invited to take a brief satisfaction survey in the kiosk outside the examination room following their visit, thus ensuring feedback immediately after the visit.

As part of the Walgreens quality improvement program, Healthcare Clinics use a tool known as HEDIS® (Healthcare Effectiveness Data and Information Set). HEDIS is a set of health care quality standards developed by the National Committee for Quality Assurance. HEDIS is used by hospitals, physician offices, and clinics across the country to measure the quality of care they provide. Three performance measures are publicly reported at https://www.walgreens.com/topic/healthcare-clinic/quality-scores.jsp:

- Percentage of children 18 months to 18 years of age who were diagnosed and appropriately treated for a URI
- Percentage of patients 18 to 64 years who were diagnosed and appropriately treated for bronchitis
- Percentage of children 2 to 18 years who appropriately received a group A *Streptococcus* (strep) test when prescribed an antibiotic for pharyngitis

Every month, each APRN is engaged in a professional peer review process whereby she or he receives randomly assigned electronic charts to review against best practice standards and quality documentation. Patient identifiers are stripped from the record, as is any information that will identify the individual APRN who delivered the care. APRNs then review their assigned records and enter their feedback into the computerized peer review application. In some cases, recommendations are offered to assist the growth and development of a fellow practitioner. For example, in one clinical review of a pediatric patient who presented with a URI, as well as childhood eczema, the reviewer offered a comment that it might be helpful to offer the family specific dietary counseling and skin care advice for improved management of the eczema as a comorbid condition. This recommendation later became part of a larger quality improvement strategy whereby patient educational materials on diet and skin care for pediatric eczema were developed and made available for use by all APRNs across the Walgreens network.

On completion of monthly peer review activities, results of the audits are returned to the APRN who completed the care; the identities of the reviewers are not disclosed. APRNs may then review and validate their scores and feedback. Although occurring very

Continued

EXEMPLAR 24.1   **Walgreens Healthcare Clinics**[SM] **Make Advanced Practice Nursing Outcomes Transparent to the World**[a]**—cont'd**

rarely, there is a process for an APRN to challenge the review findings by meeting with his or her local area APRN manager and, if needed, the medical provider assigned to the practice. In addition, each APRN has the ability to participate in monthly grand rounds, during which interesting and challenging cases are presented and discussed. Finally, all clinic quality and patient satisfaction scores are reported and discussed in quarterly market meetings, at which attendance is required for all Walgreens APRN employees nationally.

Quality scores for the HEDIS measures are consistently outstanding and significantly exceed published national benchmarks, thus meeting best practice standards in the treatment of URI, bronchitis, and pharyngitis in adult and pediatric populations. Patient satisfaction is reported by region using patient engagement score scores (1 to 5), in which responses typically average in the 4.4 to 4.78 range for all regions across the United States and are viewable for patients by region online. ◎

[a]The author wishes to thank Walgreens and Sandra Ryan, Chief Nurse Practitioner Officer for Walgreens Healthcare Clinics, for their generous time and support in describing the quality improvement process used by the APRN practices at Walgreens.

systems, such as cardiac monitors, anesthesia towers, ventilators, blood pressure monitors, and pulse oximetry devices, into an EHR. The data coming from the specific device goes through an integration and interface system where it is formatted for receipt into the EHR and into the specific patient's record. This eliminates manual entry issues, allowing providers to make clinical decisions based on accurate and timely patient data shared across a common platform.

Disparate system integration is also a key technology driver that supports improved outcomes through the transfer of patient data between systems and enterprises. This is known as interoperability. In 2016, the Office of the National Coordinator for Health Information Technology devised a 10-year interoperability road map that will lead to connected health and care for the nation. More information on this road map can be accessed on HealthIT.gov (https://www.healthit.gov/policy-researchers-implementers/interoperability). This integration can be internal, as in the case of a niche obstetrics system integrating data with the hospital-based EHR, or external, as in the case of a continuity-of-care record being electronically sent from one system and received by another as a patient is transferred between levels of care. However, not all technology vendors currently integrate with each other, which results in a fragmented data system as patients move between providers and systems. Therefore providers need to look to and support external information exchanges where a core set of patient data from disparate systems can be accessed by authorized care providers.

Health information exchanges (HIEs) have the potential to create widespread data sharing across the health care continuum and can change how providers practice and evaluate outcomes. Updated information about HIEs is available on HealthIT.gov at https://www.healthit.gov/providers-professionals/health-information-exchange/what-hie. HIEs can improve how patients experience their care by providing accurate and complete data wherever and whenever it is needed for care decisions. A HIE can be defined in several ways. First, a HIE is the activity of secure health data exchange between two or more authorized parties. For example, laboratory reports from a patient's recent hospital stay could be accessed in a clinic by an APRN who is conducting a follow-up assessment. Access to information in a HIE may often be viewed in a portal via the Internet so that all information is integrated in one application, even though it may be coming from multiple sources. In this example, the APRN could review information from a pharmacy indicating medications the patient had filled after being discharged from the hospital, if the pharmacy is part of the HIE. Use of HIEs may also require some level of data storage and warehousing.

To support data sharing among many different care settings, the concept of an HIE implies a standardized file format for specific data types, regardless of the technology vendor involved in the sending or receiving applications. This is necessary for interoperability. It simply means that there will finally be one set of technical rules for formatting data and moving them efficiently across the health care continuum so that they can be accessed wherever and whenever they are needed for the provision of care. HIE technologies also have the potential to make clinical information immediately accessible over the Internet via mobile devices such as cell phones, tablets, or laptop computers. As technologies progress, HIEs will enable information to be stored in a virtual environment, also referred to as a cloud platform, so that it can be uploaded and downloaded as needed to coordinate care effectively. APRNs may find an opportunity to expand services and interventions more effectively to other clinical settings, including nurse-managed community clinics, home care settings, church and parish nursing settings, school health areas, and retail health clinics. Using this technology will allow APRNs to extend access to preventive chronic care and episodic urgent care so that the Triple Aim objectives can be achieved.

A HIE can also refer to independent vendors or organizations who bring the information together on a common platform or who tag information to be accessed when needed. This type of HIE can also be referred to as a health information organization. HIEs can be created within a single health care provider system, region, or community. There has been significant growth in these organizations across the country; however, HIE sustainability is not without debate. There is much concern with the business and financial models that support these endeavors, and many regional HIEs have had significant starts and stops. Additional information on HIEs may be found in the HIE Toolkit (Healthcare Information and Management Systems, 2012). All APRNs should explore the availability of HIEs in their practice location. If established, the APRN should contact the HIE and gain access to the data.

One successful HIE to explore is the Chesapeake Regional Information System for Our Patients (CRISP), which serves Maryland and the District of Columbia. CRISP provides a query portal, drug monitoring services, encounter notification services, direct messaging, population health reporting, and single sign on for thousands of providers on hundreds of thousands of patients, with data coming from over 180 facilities. More information on current HIE participants can be obtained on the CRISP website (https://www.crisphealth.org/connected-providers).

Coding Taxonomies and Classification Systems

Fundamental to any technology that is built on databases with required reporting functions is the use of accurate terms to represent concepts of interest. These terms become the data. This is the foundation of any solid database model from which quality measures and evaluation processes will come. In the most concrete description, concepts of interest must be clearly described and uniformly named by all providers who use the terms. Although providers still prefer the free text note, concepts of interest should be coded and standardized across providers if the APRN is to use them in any evaluation process. Standards mandate how these concepts are named as data, which then allows comparisons to occur. Good data is the foundation of the data-information-knowledge continuum, which is a foundational model of informatics. One cannot form information and knowledge without a solid foundation of accurate and comparable data. APRNs must be able to articulate the type of data that they require to meet their information needs most effectively. In this regard, it is necessary for APRNs to understand how various coding taxonomies and terminology sets are used in health information management for documenting care and generating claims as well as how this information can be leveraged for purposes of outcome evaluation. For inpatient settings, this would include concepts within the International Classification of Diseases, 10th Revision (ICD-10). ICD-10 codes are used for documentation and billing of diagnoses and procedures as well as documenting cause of mortality from death certificates. ICD codes are alphanumeric designations given to almost every diagnosis, description of symptoms, and cause of death attributed to humans and are used worldwide. Concept standards also include the use of assessment and outcome terms housed within the Systematized Nomenclature of Medicine—Clinical Terms (SNOMED CT®) and the Logical Observation Identifiers Names and Codes (LOINC®), which are built into EHRs for seamless use. SNOMED CT is a systematically organized collection of over 300,000 medical concepts that are essential for documenting clinical concepts such as problem lists and patient histories. LOINC is a clinical standardized terminology important for laboratory test orders, results reporting, and other clinical observations. MU mandates the use of these standards within certified EHRs so that reporting and interoperability can occur.

APRNs practicing in acute care hospital settings must understand that for every claim there is a single principle ICD diagnosis code that indicates the primary reason for a patient's admission to the hospital. In addition, there may be multiple secondary ICD diagnosis codes that represent comorbid conditions that were present at the time of admission or conditions and complications that were acquired during the hospital stay. ICD procedure codes also have a designated principle procedure, which is typically the initial major procedure during the admission or care encounter. Many US hospitals code as many as 25 to 50 secondary ICD-10 diagnoses and procedure codes in the medical claim. In addition, the ICD diagnosis status flag of "present on admission" (POA) or "not present on admission" (NPOA) can be used to differentiate between hospital-acquired conditions and those acquired prior to hospitalization. This is useful when evaluating phenomena such as hospital-acquired pneumonia, pressure ulcers, acute renal failure, and sepsis. APRNs should become familiar with the coding practices in their practice settings because not all countries or organizations have adopted the use of the POA and NPOA status flags.

APRNs practicing in the United States should also have a strong working knowledge of the Medicare Severity Diagnosis-Related Groups (MS-DRGs). They should understand how clinical documentation by the APRN and medical providers directly affects MS-DRG assignments and ultimately reimbursement. Many US health care organizations are actively implementing clinical documentation improvement programs in their institutions for purposes of coaching and training medical providers and APRNs in improving their documentation skills for greater precision and accuracy in medical records coding and billing. Greater detail in the medical record can potentially lead to higher reimbursement and fewer denials and audits from payors, which are prevalent in the US health care payment system.

Finally, it may be useful for APRNs to understand other types of coding taxonomies and terminology sets that are available for purposes of quality reporting and research. Table 24.1 summarizes several common taxonomies used in inpatient and ambulatory settings. These taxonomies enable informaticians to take complex concepts and place them into databases for automated documentation, storage, and retrieval. As an example, the human brain can immediately form an image of the complex, multifactorial concept of acute abdominal pain, but a computer database cannot. This complex condition consists of three concepts: acute (versus benign), abdominal (as a specified location), and pain (as a phenomenon of interest). Each of these concepts would be separate entities in a database. With this level of granularity, an APRN looking for all patients with acute abdominal pain could locate them in the database.

Data that have alphanumeric identifiers such as ICD or SNOMED-CT codes that can be easily queried from a database are termed *discrete* or *structured data*. Data containing dictated sentences and phrases, such as radiology reports, operative summaries, or history and physical dictations, are termed *nondiscrete* or *unstructured*. Compiling and analyzing the unstructured data from free text notes is typically more challenging. Unless the organization has technology with a sophisticated reporting system containing a tool for natural language processing with a well-developed and tested rules engine, it is very difficult to mine information and knowledge from free text notes. As an example, it would be difficult to differentiate between patients with active pneumonia and those without because the narrative may contain phrases such as "pneumonia ruled out" or "no signs of pneumonia." If the APRN were trying to review data on the outcomes of patients with active pneumonia, free text mining may yield too many false-positives to be a reliable and valid screening tool.

Although it is not necessary for the APRN to understand the precision behind the coding processes, it is highly recommended that APRNs spend time interacting with a coder (also referred to as a health information management specialist) or an informatician to understand the timing and ways the various terminology sets are used. This is important to outcomes evaluation because some types of data are more useful than others, even though they represent similar concepts. For example, pneumonia could be captured from a claim (using an ICD-10 diagnosis or Current Procedural Terminology [CPT®] code), a laboratory culture and sensitivity report (using LOINC and RxNorm codes), a problem list in the EHR (using a SNOMED CT code), a chest imaging report (using natural language processing), or a dictated history and physical report (requiring manual chart abstraction). Although each source of information in the EHR may be correct, the APRN may have to determine the best source of information to address the nature of the inquiry in the most timely, efficient, and accurate manner. Exemplar 24.2 illustrates the critical evaluation of the various data types that an APRN would conduct when planning to deploy a new strategy to improve care as well as the collaborative process with quality and informatics specialists that will benefit the APRN in their outcome evaluation efforts.

TABLE 24.1   Coding Taxonomies and Terminology Sets Commonly Used in Outcomes

Coding Taxonomy	Description	Website
ICD-10-CM	International Classification of Diseases, Tenth Revision, Clinical Modification, published by the World Health Organization Based on the International Classification of Diseases, which houses unique alphanumeric codes to identify known diseases and other health problems Includes more than 68,000 diagnostic codes and reasons for visits	http://www.cdc.gov/nchs/icd/icd10cm.htm
ICD-10-PCS	The ICD-10 Procedure Coding System Contains approximately 87,000 procedure codes that are seven alphanumeric characters in length Used by most countries worldwide to classify procedures for inpatient hospital claims Coding set very specific, provides for precisely defined procedures and laterality	https://www.cms.gov/Medicare/Coding/ICD10/2018-ICD-10-PCS-and-GEMs.html
CPT	Current Procedural Terminology; CPT is a registered trademark of the American Medical Association and is considered a proprietary terminology set requiring licensure before using inside a health information technology application. Contains approximately 7800 codes for reporting medical, surgical, and diagnostic services in outpatient and office settings as well as acute care, emergency settings, ambulatory surgery, and inpatient procedures done in some hospitals outside the United States New codes are released each October	https://www.ama-assn.org/practice-management/cpt-current-procedural-terminology
HCPCS	Healthcare Common Procedure Coding System Two types of HCPCS codes: Level I and Level II Level 1 HCPCS codes: identical to CPT codes used for reporting services and procedures in outpatient and office settings to Medicare, Medicaid, and private health insurers Level II HCPCS codes: used by medical suppliers other than physicians such as ambulance services or durable medical equipment	https://www.cms.gov/Medicare/Coding/MedHCPCSGenInfo/index.html
SNOMED CT	Systematized Nomenclature of Medicine—Clinical Terms Developed by the College of American Pathologists and the National Health Service (Britain) Complex and highly hierarchical collection of over 1 million codes and medical terms that describe diseases, procedures, symptoms, findings, and more Used extensively throughout the world, SNOMED CT codes help organize content in the electronic health record (EHR) and cross to other terminologies such as ICD-9, ICD-10, and LOINC	http://www.snomed.org/snomed-ct
LOINC	Logical Observation Identifiers Names and Codes Universal standard containing 58,000 observation terms for identifying medical laboratory tests and clinical observations as well as nursing diagnosis, nursing interventions, outcomes classification, and patient care data sets Originally developed in the United States in 1994; international adoption expanding rapidly	https://loinc.org
RxNorm	Standardized nomenclature for clinical drugs produced by the National Library of Medicine; this data set is updated monthly to stay abreast of the rapidly changing pharmaceutical industry Contains links between national drug codes, which are used widely in EHRs and e-prescribing systems	https://www.nlm.nih.gov/research/umls/rxnorm/docs/index.html
MS-DRG	Medicare Severity Diagnosis-Related Group Each inpatient hospital stay in the United States is assigned one of over 750 MS-DRG codes, which are used for billing to Medicare and other payors; codes are derived from ICD diagnosis and procedure codes Many conditions are split into one, two, or three MS-DRGs based on whether any one of the secondary diagnoses has been categorized as a major complication or comorbidity (MCC), a complication or comorbidity (CC), or no CC, and are weighted accordingly to reflect severity and reimbursement; note there is a separate MS-DRG code set for long-term care Additional coding sets apply to other areas of care (e.g., resource utilization groups [RUGs] apply to skilled nursing and rehabilitation stays)	https://www.cms.gov/Medicare/Medicare-Fee-for-Service-Payment/AcuteInpatientPPS/index.html?redirect=/AcuteInpatientPPS/FFD/list.asp

EXEMPLAR 24.2   **Evaluating Data Types When Using Health Information Technology to Implement Practice Change**

An advanced practice registered nurse (APRN) working in a 400-bed, acute care setting needs to identify all inpatients with an active diagnosis of pneumonia to ensure that all best practice interventions have been implemented in a timely and appropriate manner. Although the performance in these areas is retrospectively monitored and reported periodically by the quality management department, the APRN wishes to engage in the process concurrently to influence outcomes for this population. The APRN's intervention is to perform clinical rounds several times a day on this population to ensure optimal delivery of best practice standards. These include antibiotic timeliness, appropriateness of antibiotic selection in intensive care unit (ICU) and non-ICU patients, smoking cessation advice and counseling, and influenza and pneumococcal vaccinations. The APRN wants to leverage the hospital's information systems to create a real-time alert notification system to identify and track patients with pneumonia immediately on any nursing unit and then monitor performance trends to reflect the impact of interventions on this population.

The APRN recognizes that there are multiple taxonomies and methodologies that could be used to identify pneumonia patients in her organization and begins to inventory the pros and cons of each data type and source to create the best technology solution for her requirements. International Classification of Diseases, Tenth Revision (ICD-10) diagnosis codes are a typical taxonomy for identifying patients with pneumonia. Although these codes are readily available, reliable, and robust population identifiers in other types of outcome evaluation measures used in the organization, such as length of stay, mortality, and readmissions, this approach would not be optimal because ICD-10 codes are typically not assigned until after the patient is discharged and the medical record is coded for the claim. This type of data element is retrospective and therefore not useable to identify patients with pneumonia on a real-time basis.

The APRN next considers a more concurrent coding methodology, which is based on the active problem lists in the electronic health record (EHR). In collaboration with a health information management specialist, a list of problem types and their corresponding Systematized Nomenclature of Medicine—Clinical Terms (SNOMED CT) codes is established, which can be used to identify patients with an active diagnosis of pneumonia. However, this approach is ruled out because medical provider adoption of the new EHR has not yet fully expanded to the critical care units at her hospital. In addition, she has observed that many medical providers in the organization do not update the problem list in the EHR until the patient is being discharged, which makes a real-time query unreliable.

The final option that the APRN considers to create automated alerts is the use of radiology and laboratory reports containing *pneumonia* or other related terms. In discussing this option with a nursing informatics specialist at her organization, she learns that the EHR has been fully implemented to report laboratory results for all clinical areas in the hospital and that this includes microbiology results. Using the Logical Observation Identifiers Names and Codes (LOINC) coding terminology set, patients with pneumonia can be identified as soon as the laboratory result transaction is received in the EHR. In addition, she learns of a pilot project in the Quality Department in which cardiac catheterization reports are being processed by a natural language processing engine to capture cardiac registry information. She asks about the potential to expand this pilot to include radiology reports to identify pneumonia patients. The Quality Department agrees to expand the project scope with the help of the APRN to begin formulating a list of phrases that will be used to identify pneumonia positively in a radiology report. The APRN collaborates with the medical director of radiology to create the final list of terms to be used in the pilot.

After 3 months of implementing the practice change, the APRN is able to demonstrate that performance in five best practice indicators for patients with pneumonia is almost 100% across the organization. She tracks the compliance rates in a statistical process control chart, which demonstrates a statistically significant favorable change in the process. Furthermore, she is able to use the organization's value-based purchasing calculator to demonstrate a financial contribution to the hospital's Medicare reimbursement program of almost $68,000 simply by improving performance. The APRN plans to make a formal recommendation to expand similar APRN interventions to other key populations influenced by so-called pay-for-performance initiatives, including cardiac, medical, orthopedics, and stroke. Thus the APRN is able to materially demonstrate the value-added benefit of APRN clinical interventions using financial and quality analytics. ◎

Regulatory Reporting Initiatives That Drive Performance Improvement

In the United States, legislative regulatory and reporting requirements are released by the CMS or DHHS and posted in the *Federal Register* numerous times each year (https://www.federalregister.gov). New requirements were released in November 2016 that significantly impact the mandate to evaluate performance and outcomes of providers, whether that provider is a physician or APRN, through mandated reporting requirements. This mandate is explored further in this section.

Current Reporting Requirements

The United States is evolving from a pay-for-service and pay-for-reporting culture to one of pay-for-performance. Many CMS reporting initiatives reuse the same measures, so it is possible for substandard performance in even a single measure to have significant financial impact across a health care organization. Failure to collect accurate and complete data, report it to the CMS by designated time frames, and achieve acceptable results in performance for even one required measure can result in sizeable reduction in payment to the hospital from the CMS.

Some measures, such as central line–associated blood stream infections, not only apply to multiple quality reporting programs in a single health care facility, they also apply to multiple care settings across the continuum, including acute care hospitals, cancer care hospitals, ambulatory surgery centers, and long-term care facilities. Failure to comply with reporting requirements has the potential to affect reimbursement across an entire health care system. Additional measurement and reporting requirements for specialized services and health care systems also exist. Box 24.1 illustrates a set of measures that are required for health care systems reorganizing as

BOX 24.1 Shared Savings Program for Accountable Care Organizations: Quality Measures

Consumer Assessment of Health Care Providers and Systems (CAHPS)*
- Getting timely care, appointments, and information
- How well your doctors communicate
- Patients' rating of doctor
- Access to specialists
- Health promotion and education
- Shared decision making
- Health status/functional status

Care Coordination and Patient Safety
- Ambulatory-sensitive conditions admissions—chronic obstructive pulmonary disease (COPD) and congestive heart failure (CHF) (Agency for Healthcare Research and Quality prevention quality indicator)
- Number of primary care providers (PCPs; %) who successfully qualify for an electronic health record incentive program payment
- Medication reconciliation after discharge from an inpatient facility
- Screening for fall risk

Preventive Health
- Influenza immunization
- Pneumococcal vaccination
- Adult weight screening and follow-up

- Tobacco use assessment and tobacco cessation intervention
- Depression screening
- Colorectal cancer screening
- Mammography screening
- Proportion of adults ≥ 18 yr who had their blood pressure measured within the preceding 2 yr

At-Risk Populations
- Diabetes composite (all or nothing scoring)—nonuse of tobacco, aspirin use
- Diabetes mellitus—hemoglobin A_{1c} poor control (>9%)
- Hypertension—blood pressure control
- Ischemic vascular disease—complete lipid profile and low-density lipoprotein control <100 mg/dL, use of aspirin or another antithrombotic
- Heart failure—beta blocker therapy for left ventricular systolic dysfunction (LVSD)
- Coronary artery disease (CAD) composite (all or nothing scoring)—angiotensin-converting enzyme inhibitor or angiotensin receptor blocker therapy for patients with CAD and diabetes and/or LVSD

*CAHPS asks patients to report on their experiences with a range of health care services at multiple levels of the delivery system. The survey asks about experiences with ambulatory care providers (e.g., health plans, physician offices, home care programs, mental health plans). For additional information, see https://www.ahrq.gov/cahps/surveys-guidance/index.html

Adapted from Centers for Medicare & Medicaid Services. (2016). Medicare program; Medicare shared savings program: Accountable care organizations (https://www.cms.gov/Medicare/Medicare-Fee-for-Service-Payment/sharedsavingsprogram/index.html).

accountable care organizations (ACOs). These measures focus on ambulatory populations and may overlap with several other reporting programs that exist simultaneously across an integrated health care organization, such as the measures required by the Health Resources and Services Administration for federal qualified health centers (Box 24.2) or those required by providers who care for patients within selected payor niches, such as the Medicaid Adult Health Care Quality Measures Program (Box 24.3).

In addition to payor-mandated reporting programs, health care organizations also have specific reporting requirements for their accreditation bodies, including The Joint Commission, the Healthcare Facilities Accreditation Program, and Det Norske Veritas Healthcare. It is not unusual for many of the measures required for accreditation to overlap with those reported to the CMS, although these measures typically reflect an all-payor population. What is important to note is that although many of these measures are similar across reporting programs, each program has specific requirements for data collection, data quality,

and data submission, to which health care organizations must strictly adhere in order to ensure proper accreditation, achieve financial incentives, or avoid financial penalties.

Given this broad array of reporting mandates, APRNs should become familiar with the regulatory reporting requirements of their organization. The National Quality Forum (NQF) Community Tool to Align Measurement is a useful tool for the APRN to review. This tool will help the APRN become familiar with the measures required for a specific practice setting. This tool organizes NQF-endorsed clinical quality measures associated with major national and state reporting initiatives for all practice settings into a single spreadsheet, which can then be sorted by various programs of interest. Hyperlinks are embedded in the spreadsheet so that it is easy to access the Quality Positioning System on the NQF website, on which measure definitions for each metric are maintained.

Traditionally, many reporting requirements were met by manual chart abstraction, along with an

---

BOX 24.2   Health Resources & Services Administration Uniform Data Set for Clinical and Financial Performance Measures[a]

Outreach and Quality of Care (%)
- Pregnant women beginning prenatal care in the first trimester
- Children age 2 yr during measurement year, with appropriate immunizations
- Women 21-64 yr of age who received one or more tests to screen for cervical cancer
- Patients 2-17 yr of age who had body mass index (BMI) percentile documentation, counseling for nutrition, and counseling for physical activity during the measurement year
- Patients ≥ 18 yr of age who had BMI calculated at last visit or within last 6 mo and, if overweight or underweight, had follow-up plan documented
- Percentage of women 21-64 yr of age who received one or more Papanicolaou tests to screen for cervical cancer
- Patients ≥ 18 yr of age who were queried about tobacco use 1 or more times within 24 mo
- Patients ≥ 18 yr of age who are tobacco users and who received advice to quit smoking or tobacco use

- Patients 5-40 yr of age with a diagnosis of persistent asthma who were prescribed the preferred long-term control medication or an acceptable alternative pharmacologic therapy during the current year

Health Outcomes and Disparities (%)
- Diabetic patients whose hemoglobin A_{1c} levels are < 7%, < 8%, ≤ 9%, or > 9%.
- Adult patients with diagnosed hypertension whose most recent blood pressure was less than 140/90 mm Hg
- Newborns weighing < 2500 g born to health center patients

Financial Viability and Cost
- Total cost per patient
- Medical cost per medical visit
- Change in net assets-to-expense ratio
- Working capital-to-monthly expenses ratio
- Long-term debt-to-equity ratio

[a]Required for federally qualified health centers.
Adapted from Bureau of Primary Health Care, Health Resources and Services Administration. (2016). Uniform data system reporting instructions for 2016 health center data (https://bphc.hrsa.gov/datareporting/reporting/2016udsreportingmanual.pdf).

BOX 24.3 **Centers for Medicare & Medicaid Services Medicaid Adult Health Care Quality Measures**

Prevention and Health Promotion
- Flu shots for adults ages 50–64 yr (collected as part of HEDIS CAHPS supplemental survey)
- Adult body mass index assessment
- Breast cancer screening
- Cervical cancer screening
- Medical assistance with smoking and tobacco use cessation (collected as part of HEDIS CAHPS supplemental survey)
- Screening for clinical depression and follow-up plan
- Plan all-cause readmission
- Diabetes, short-term complications admission rate
- Chronic obstructive pulmonary disease (COPD) admission rate
- Congestive heart failure admission rate
- Adult asthma admission rate
- Chlamydia screening in women ages 21–24 yr

Management of Acute Conditions
- Follow-up after hospitalization for mental illness
- Elective delivery
- Antenatal steroids
- Heart failure admission rates
- COPD or asthma in older adults admission rate

Behavioral Health and Substance Abuse
- Initiation and engagement of alcohol and other drug dependence treatment
- Antidepressant medication management
- Follow-up after hospitalization for mental illness

- Diabetes screening for people with schizophrenia and bipolar disorder
- Adherence to antipsychotics for individuals with schizophrenia
- Use of opioids at high dosage

Management of Chronic Conditions
- Annual HIV-AIDS medical visit
- Controlling high blood pressure
- Comprehensive diabetes care—low-density lipoprotein cholesterol screening, hemoglobin A_{1c} testing
- Antidepressant medication management
- Adherence to antipsychotics for individuals with schizophrenia
- Annual monitoring for patients on persistent medications

Family Experiences of Care
- CAHPS Health Plan Survey v. 5.0—adult questionnaire with CAHPS Health Plan Survey v. 5.0, National Committee for Quality Assurance supplemental Care Coordination Standards
- Care transition record transmitted to health care professional

Availability
- Initiation and engagement of alcohol and other drug dependence treatment
- Prenatal and postpartum care—postpartum care rate

HEDIS CAHPS, Healthcare Effectiveness Data and Information Set Consumer Assessment of Health Care Providers and Systems.
Adapted from Centers for Medicare & Medicaid Services. (2017). 2017 core set of adult health care quality measures for Medicaid (Adult Core Set). Retrieved from https://www.medicaid.gov/medicaid/quality-of-care/downloads/2017-adult-core-set.pdf

element of clinical judgment to determine the correct response to questions about whether or not a particular standard of evidence-based best practice was met. Questions such as "Did the patient get smoking cessation advice prior to discharge?" are typically abstracted by a review of patient education documentation in the medical record. However, questions such as "Was the patient eligible for ACE inhibitors at discharge?" may require a review and synthesis of multiple sources of information in the record, including the history and physical examination, cardiac imaging tests, or medical provider progress notes, before a determination can be made. These types of activities can be time consuming and often

are called into question regarding their reliability. APRNs may be engaged in many aspects of the data collection and analysis activities associated with chart-abstracted data. Today, through the MU provisions, EHRs need to demonstrate the ability for all providers, including APRNs, to electronically mine data and produce the needed reporting. However, even while the system can automate the reporting process, the data and results still need to be reviewed for accuracy of content and context, and this requires a human review. In addition, the quality reporting can only demonstrate outcomes. To produce true changes in outcomes, the APRN needs to engage in gap or need identification. From this, the APRN has to seek evidence, weigh and grade literature, translate findings, accommodate local need, develop and implement interventions, and then evaluate. The APRN needs to use quality improvement (QI) processes to truly address quality care and will need the tools of data and technology along with informatics support. Table 24.2 provides resources for QI activities that are needed to support the measures. For example, it is not enough just to report that smoking cessation advice was given to a proportion of patients based on a checkoff box frequency. The APRN needs to use evidence to build a process to address smoking cessation successfully with patients, including options for intervention and referral, and then use the data to evaluate the success of the outcome of the intervention.

Moreover, additional regulatory reporting requirements are beginning to emerge in the area of patient safety, an area in which APRNs can have significant impact. The Patient Safety and Quality Improvement Act of 2005 established a voluntary patient safety event reporting system and guidelines for the establishment of patient safety organizations (Agency for Healthcare Research and Quality [AHRQ], 2005). This act called for the standardization of data used for event reporting based on the common formats established and maintained by the AHRQ. Some of the initial risk events being reported include medication errors, patient falls, central line infections, and pressure ulcers.

New Reporting Requirements: MACRA

As of this writing, a new final rule began on January 1, 2017. In April 2015, the Medicare Access and CHIP Reauthorization Act (MACRA) became law. MACRA will substantially change how Medicare payments will be made to all providers, including physician assistants, nurse practitioners (NPs), clinical nurse specialists (CNSs), and certified registered nurse anesthetists (CRNAs). MACRA mandates that Medicare payments be based on quality and creates a new Quality Payment Program with two payment paths for designated providers: the Merit-based Incentive Payment System (MIPS) and the advanced Alternative Payment Model (APM) (https://www.cms.gov/Medicare/Quality-Initiatives-Patient-Assessment-Instruments/Value-Based-Programs/MACRA-MIPS-and-APMs/MACRA-MIPS-and-APMs.html).

MACRA will replace the traditional fee-for-service for provider payment and will instead base payment on and reward quality. This includes the quality of care and the outcomes for patients seen by APRNs as individual providers. This quality system is different than the current incentive programs, such as the Physician Quality Reporting System (PQRS). MACRA will become bigger than just reimbursement because it ties payment and reward to outcomes and quality of care. MACRA is set to consolidate three quality reporting programs: the PQRS, the Value-Based Payment Modifier, and MU. The start of MACRA is January 1, 2019; however, it is based on provider experiences starting on January 1, 2017.

Merit-Based Incentive Payment System

MIPS is one path of the new payment model that provides financial incentives and penalties based on the quality of care, outcomes, and efficiencies. Only providers who bill less than $30,000 or care for fewer than 100 patients will be exempt. Based on the current proposed rule, MIPS will attribute provider performance, inclusive of APRNs, across four categories:

1. **Quality** [50% of total MIPS score in year 1 (2019) and 30% thereafter]. The provider chooses six measures to report on from a list of options that align with patient population needs. The CMS will ensure that these options accommodate differences among specialties and practices. These must represent six quality measures, including an outcome measure for a minimum of 90 days. Table 24.3 lists the categories of MIPS Quality Measures along with an example measure. A complete listing of all 271 measures across all specialties is available on the Quality Payment Program website (https://qpp.cms.gov/measures/quality). It is important to note in reviewing the MIPS Quality Measures that many address issues of concern in primary and chronic illness care—areas in which APRNs have had a positive impact. In addition, there are some core measures that cross specialties, such as care planning for patients 65 years of age or older, in which providers have to document an advanced care plan or surrogate decision maker in the medical record. Another example of a measure that crosses specialties is documentation of current medications in the medical record.

2. **Advancing Care Information** (i.e., EHR MU) [24% of the total MIPS score in year 1 (2019) and beyond]. The provider will choose customizable measures reflecting daily technology

TABLE 24.2 Quality Improvement and Outcome Assessment Website Resources

Resource and Information Available	Website
Agency for Healthcare Research and Quality (AHRQ) • Supports evidence-based practice centers, outcomes and effectiveness trials, National Quality Measures Clearinghouse	https://www.ahrq.gov
American Society for Quality (ASQ) • Contains tools for cause analysis, evaluation and decision making, data collection and analysis, idea creation, project planning, and implementation • ASQ offers certification, training, and ongoing education in quality improvement (QI) techniques	http://asq.org/learn-about-quality/quality-tools.html
Centers for Medicare & Medicaid Services (CMS) Transforming Clinical Practice Initiative • Designed to help clinicians achieve large-scale health transformation to improve quality of patient care and manage costs	https://innovation.cms.gov/initiatives/Transforming-Clinical-Practices/
Institute for Healthcare Improvement (IHI) • Offers training and ongoing education in QI techniques • Promotes health care innovation through fellowships, the IHI Open School, and networking	http://www.ihi.org/Pages/default.aspx
Mind Tools • Excellent site for learning skills in change management, team building, brainstorming, straw man concept, strategy tools, leadership skills, and project management	http://www.mindtools.com
National Association for Healthcare Quality (NAHQ) • Promotes continuous improvement of quality in health care by providing educational and development opportunities and national certification as a Certified Professional of Healthcare Quality	http://www.nahq.org
National Committee for Quality Assurance (NCQA) • Developed the Healthcare Effectiveness Data and Information Set (HEDIS®) to measure quality of care delivered by US health plans • Offers online training and seminars on a wide range of quality-related topics	http://www.ncqa.org
National Database of Nursing Quality Indicators • Collects and evaluates unit-specific nurse-sensitive data from US hospitals	http://www.pressganey.com/solutions/clinical-quality/nursing-quality
National Network of Public Health Institutes, Public Health Learning Network • Dedicated to improving public health through innovation, QI, and education • Website includes QI tools and frameworks (e.g., aim statements, balanced scorecard templates, brainstorming, fishbone, cause-and-effect diagrams, force field analysis, Kaizen, Lean, story board, radar charts, tree diagrams, interrelationship diagrams, and others that may be useful in outcome evaluation)	https://nnphi.org/phln/
National Quality Forum (NQF), Community Tool to Align Measurement • Excel spreadsheet inventory of NQF-endorsed measures for one or more of the national reporting programs, including the Aligning Forces for Quality Alliances in regions across the United States • Also includes drill-down to the Quality Positioning System for quick access to measure definitions of NQF-endorsed measures • These resources are in the public domain and do not require membership	http://www.qualityforum.org/AlignmentTool/
Public Health Foundation, QI Quick Guide Tutorial • Online tutorial for review of the plan-do-check-act (PDCA) process, plus additional resources for population outcomes evaluation	http://www.phf.org/quickguide/LeftNavTwoPanel.aspx?Page=Introduction
The Joint Commission (TJC) • Maintains measure definitions for hospital quality reporting programs • Provides educational offerings for QI and accreditation standards • Expanding international presence	https://www.jointcommission.org

TABLE 24.3   Quality Patient Program Measure Categories With Example Measures

Specialty Measure Set	Example Measure
Allergy/immunology	Percentage of patients age 18 years and older with a diagnosis of acute sinusitis who were prescribed an antibiotic within 10 days after onset of symptoms
Anesthesiology	Percentage of patients, regardless of age, who undergo surgical or therapeutic procedures under general or neuraxial anesthesia of 60 minutes' duration or longer for whom at least one body temperature $\geq 35.5°C$ (or 95.9°F) was recorded within the 30 minutes immediately before or the 15 minutes immediately after anesthesia end time
Cardiology	Percentage of patients age 18 years and older with a diagnosis of coronary artery disease seen within a 12-month period who were prescribed aspirin or clopidogrel
Dermatology	Percentage of patients, regardless of age, with a current diagnosis of melanoma or a history of melanoma whose information was entered, at least once within a 12-month period, into a recall system that includes: • A target date for the next complete physical skin examination, AND • A process to follow up with patients who either did not make an appointment within the specified time frame or who missed a scheduled appointment
Diagnostic radiology	Percentage of final reports for computed tomography (CT) imaging studies of the thorax for patients age 18 years and older with documented follow-up recommendations for incidentally detected pulmonary nodules (e.g., follow-up CT imaging studies needed or that no follow-up is needed) based at a minimum on nodule size AND patient risk factors
Electrophysiology/cardiac specialist	Patients with physician-specific risk-standardized rates of procedural complications following the first time implantation of an implantable cardioverter-defibrillator
Emergency medicine	Percentage of children 3–18 years of age who were diagnosed with pharyngitis, ordered an antibiotic, and received a group A *Streptococcus* (strep) test for the episode
Gastroenterology	The percentage of patients 85 years and older who received a screening colonoscopy from January 1 to December 31
General oncology	Proportion of female patients age 18 years and older with breast cancer who are human epidermal growth factor receptor 2 (HER2)/neu negative who are not administered HER2-targeted therapies
General practice/family medicine	Percentage of patients age 2 years and older with a diagnosis of acute otitis externa (AOE) who were not prescribed systemic antimicrobial therapy
General surgery	Percentage of patients age 18 years and older who required an anastomotic leak intervention following gastric bypass or colectomy surgery
Hospitalists	Percentage of patients with sepsis due to methicillin-sensitive *Staphylococcus aureus* bacteremia who received a β-lactam antibiotic (e.g., nafcillin, oxacillin, or cefazolin) as definitive therapy
Internal medicine	Percentage of patients, regardless of age, who are active injection drug users who received screening for hepatitis C virus infection within the 12-month reporting period
Interventional radiology	Percentage of new patients whose biopsy results have been reviewed and communicated to the primary care/referring physician and patient by the performing physician
Mental/behavioral health	Percentage of individuals at least 18 years of age as of the beginning of the measurement period with schizophrenia or schizoaffective disorder who had at least two prescriptions filled for any antipsychotic medication and who had a Proportion of Days Covered of at least 0.8 for antipsychotic medications during the measurement period (12 consecutive months)
Neurology	Percentage of patients diagnosed with amyotrophic lateral sclerosis who were offered assistance in planning for end-of-life issues (e.g., advance directives, invasive ventilation, hospice) at least once annually
Obstetrics/gynecology	Percentage of women 50-74 years of age who had a mammogram to screen for breast cancer
Ophthalmology	Percentage of patients age 18 years and older who had surgery for primary rhegmatogenous retinal detachment who did not require a return to the operating room within 90 days of surgery
Orthopedic surgery	Percentage of patients 18 years of age and older with primary total hip arthroplasty who completed baseline and follow-up patient-reported functional status assessments
Otolaryngology	Percentage of patients age 2 years and older with a diagnosis of AOE who were prescribed topical preparations
Pathology	Percentage of esophageal biopsy reports that document the presence of Barrett epithelium that also include a statement about dysplasia

TABLE 24.3   Quality Patient Program Measure Categories With Example Measures—cont'd

Specialty Measure Set	Example Measure
Pediatrics	Percentage of children 2 years of age who had four diphtheria, tetanus, and acellular pertussis (DTaP); three inactivated poliovirus (IPV), one measles, mumps, and rubella (MMR); three *Haemophilus influenzae* type b (HiB); three hepatitis B (Hep B); one varicella zoster virus [chickenpox] (VZV); four pneumococcal conjugate (PCV); one hepatitis A (Hep A); two or three rotavirus (RV); and two influenza (flu) vaccines by their second birthday
Physical medicine	Percentage of visits for patients age 18 years and older with documentation of a current functional outcome assessment using a standardized functional outcome assessment tool on the date of the encounter AND documentation of a care plan based on identified functional outcome deficiencies on the date of the identified deficiencies
Plastic surgery	Percentage of patients age 18 years and older who had a surgical site infection
Preventive medicine	Percentage of patients 18–85 years of age who had a diagnosis of hypertension and whose blood pressure was adequately controlled (<140/90 mm Hg) during the measurement period
Radiation oncology	Percentage of visits for patients, regardless of age, with a diagnosis of cancer currently receiving chemotherapy or radiation therapy who report having pain with a documented plan of care to address pain
Rheumatology	Percentage of patients age 18 years and older with a diagnosis of rheumatoid arthritis who have an assessment and classification of disease prognosis at least once within 12 months
Thoracic surgery	Percentage of patients who underwent a nonemergency surgery who had their personalized risks of postoperative complications assessed by their surgical team prior to surgery using a clinical data-based, patient-specific risk calculator and who received personal discussion of those risks with the surgeon
Urology	Percentage of new patients whose biopsy results have been reviewed and communicated to the primary care/referring physician and patient by the performing physician
Vascular surgery	Percentage of asymptomatic patients undergoing carotid endarterectomy who are discharged to home no later than postoperative day 2

use to manage and share patient information. However, the CMS intends to emphasize interoperability and information exchange, with the goal of having patient records available across all systems, allowing providers needed access to patient data. Advancing Care Information also emphasizes patients' access to their own records and the engagement of patients in their own care and health management. There are six objectives with multiple measures in this category: protecting health information, electronic prescribing, patient electronic access, coordination of care through patient engagement, health information exchange, and public health and clinical data registry reporting. This MIPS category is a reconfiguration of the original MU measures. A complete list of specific measures can be found on the Healthcare Information and Management Systems Society MACRA Notice of Proposed Rulemaking Fact Sheet (http://s3.amazonaws.com/rdcms-himss/files/production/public/FileDownloads/MACRAFactSheet_MIPS_Advancing%20Care%20InformationPt3_050916.pdf).

3. **Clinical Practice Improvement** [15% of the total MIPS score in year 1 (2019) and beyond]. The provider will be rewarded for clinical practice improvement activities such as care coordination, patient engagement, and patient safety. This Clinical Practice Improvement category should be a focus of interest for APRNs because learning the tools and techniques to carry out these projects is an expectation of competency for doctorally prepared APRNs. There are nine categories: expanded practice access, beneficiary engagement, achieving health equity, population management, patient safety and practice assessment, emergency preparedness and response, care coordination, participation in an APM, and integrated behavioral and mental health. Under each category, there are multiple activities from which to choose. Table 24.4 lists example improvement activities under each of the nine categories. MIPS participants have to attest to completing four improvement activities for a minimum of 90 days. Improvement activities will also include the use of health IT functions

⚙ TABLE 24.4	Merit-Based Incentive Payment System Example Improvement Activities
Subcategory Name	**Improvement Activity**
Achieving health equity	Seeing new and follow-up Medicaid patients in a timely manner, including individuals dually eligible for Medicaid and Medicare.
Behavioral and mental health	Depression screening and follow-up plan: Regular engagement of MIPS-eligible clinicians or groups in integrated prevention and treatment interventions, including depression screening and follow-up plan (refer to NQF #0418) for patients with co-occurring conditions of behavioral or mental health conditions.
Beneficiary engagement	Engage patients, family, and caregivers in developing a plan of care and prioritizing their goals for action, documented in the certified EHR technology.
Care coordination	Implementation of practices/processes for care transition that include documentation of how a MIPS-eligible clinician or group carried out a patient-centered action plan for first 30 days following a discharge (e.g., staff involved, phone calls conducted in support of transition, accompaniments, navigation actions, home visits, patient information access, etc.).
Emergency response and preparedness	Participation in Disaster Medical Assistance Teams or Community Emergency Responder Teams. Activities that simply involve registration are not sufficient. MIPS-eligible clinicians and MIPS-eligible clinician groups must be registered for a minimum of 6 months as a volunteer for disaster or emergency response.
Expanded practice access	Collection of patient experience and satisfaction data on access to care and development of an improvement plan such as outlining steps for improving communications with patients to help understanding of urgent access needs.
Patient safety and practice assessment	Administration of the AHRQ Survey on Patient Safety Culture and submission of data to the comparative database (refer to AHRQ Surveys on Patient Safety Culture website at http://www.ahrq.gov/professionals/quality-patient-safety/patientsafetyculture/index.html)
Population management	Take steps to improve health status of communities such as collaborating with key partners and stakeholders to implement evidenced-based practices to improve a specific chronic condition. Refer to the local QIO for additional steps to take for improving health status of communities because there are many steps to select from for satisfying this activity. QIOs work under the direction of the CMS to assist MIPS-eligible clinicians and groups with quality improvement and review quality concerns for the protection of beneficiaries and the Medicare Trust Fund.

AHRQ, Agency for Healthcare Research and Quality; *CMS,* Centers for Medicare & Medicaid Services; *EHR,* electronic health record; *MIPS,* Merit-based Incentive Payment System; *NQF,* National Quality Forum; *QIO,* Quality Improvement Organization.

such as the capture of social, psychologic, and behavioral data as well as technology that can generate and exchange an electronic care plan to support these improvement activities. A complete listing of all current Improvement Activities is available on the Quality Payment Program website (https://qpp.cms.gov/mips/improvement-activities).

4. **Cost/Resource Use** [10% of the total MIPS score in year 1 (2019) and 30% thereafter]. A provider's score will be based on Medicare claims using episode-specific measures to account for differences among specialties. This category is based on the current Value-Based Payment Modifier.

In the MIPS model, accountability and scoring of care outcomes will be applied across an interprofessional team. Team members will then be scored individually. In the future, provider quality and cost

rankings will be publically available through mechanisms such as Physician Compare (https://www.medicare.gov/physiciancompare/). Everyone on the team will depend on high-quality care scores to achieve higher payment.

Alternative Payment Models

Providers can choose how they want to take part in MACRA. Providers deciding to participate in an advanced APM through Medicare Part B will earn incentive payments for participating in an innovative payment model and for using certified EHR technology. Practitioners wanting to participate as an APM will take on more than nominal risk because this means changing processes substantially. The CMS anticipates that there will be several types of programs that will be categorized as APMs: comprehensive end-stage renal disease care transformation programs, comprehensive primary medical care plus

TABLE 24.5	Advanced Alternative Payment Method Resource Types
Resource	**Website**
Comprehensive ESRD Care Model	https://innovation.cms.gov/initiatives/comprehensive-esrd-care/
Comprehensive Primary Care Plus	https://innovation.cms.gov/initiatives/comprehensive-primary-care-plus
Next Generation ACO Model	https://innovation.cms.gov/initiatives/Next-Generation-ACO-Model/
Shared Savings Program Track 2	https://www.cms.gov/Medicare/Medicare-Fee-for-Service-Payment/sharedsavingsprogram/index.html
Shared Savings Program Track 3	https://www.cms.gov/Medicare/Medicare-Fee-for-Service-Payment/sharedsavingsprogram/index.html
Oncology Care Model	https://innovation.cms.gov/initiatives/oncology-care/

models, advanced ACOs, shared savings programs, and new oncology care models. MACRA was built on the foundation of the ACA incentives that seek to transform care and delivery by rewarding the adoption of alternative payment models such as ACOs, bundled payment models, and patient-centered medical homes. In these models, providers accept the risk and reward for providing innovative, coordinated, high-quality, and efficient care. Most providers will participate in MACRA through the MIPS pathway; however, some will participate through an APM. Providers participating in one or more of the APMs will be exempt from participating in MIPS. Table 24.5 provides a listing of APM categories and resources that describe specific services in detail.

Relevance of Regulatory Reporting to Advanced Practice Nursing Outcomes

The national quality, patient safety, and accreditation reporting requirements are relevant to APRN outcome evaluation for several reasons. First, they are of critical interest to the organizations that employ APRNs. Many health care organizations are carefully tracking key performance measures that affect their financial bottom line in scorecards or dashboards, which are then communicated to all stakeholders, from clinical units to the board room. In many organizations, financial incentives and annual bonuses for those in strategic and operational leadership roles, as well as other key clinical staff, are based on achieving designated performance thresholds. Organizations monitor their performance against competitive market segments using comparative benchmarking systems so that they can ensure that their performance exceeds that of their peer groups. This is important not only to maintain their reputation within their community and market but also because CMS programs—specifically the current Value-Based Purchasing Program, the Hospital Readmission Reduction Program, and the MACRA program—base financial incentives on the organization's ranking across approximately 3000 US hospitals that are competing for incentive dollars in these programs.

The second and more compelling reason why national regulatory reporting initiatives are critical to APRN outcome evaluation is because so many of the clinical processes and outcomes reflected in these performance measures are directly sensitive to APRN intervention. Thus active participation in the data collection, data analysis, and resulting performance improvement initiatives provides a rich forum to make the value-added APRN contributions highly visible across the organization. In many organizations, key regulatory performance metrics are included in individual provider profiles and integrated into ongoing professional practice evaluation activities. Although the APRN has a direct and immediate opportunity to influence outcomes for many of these measures, linking APRNs to the performance trend is often a challenge, particularly in an acute care hospital environment in which many providers contribute to the management of a single patient's care episode. For example, medical orders for a patient with heart failure who is eligible for angiotensin-converting enzyme inhibitors at discharge could be written by the patient's attending physician, a cardiac specialist, a hospitalist, or an acute care NP who is accountable for overseeing the cardiac medical population.

The National Provider Identifier Number

Identifying the contributions of APRNs to outcomes of care, as a group or as an individual provider, is an essential element to ensuring that they can practice to the full extent of their license uniformly across the country. To accomplish this, there needs to be a data element that will identify the provider as an individual and as a type. The National Provider Identifier (NPI) number has been targeted as this data element. CMS began to issue NPIs in October 2006. Once assigned, an NPI should be permanent and remain with the provider regardless of job or location change. The NPI is a 10-digit numerical identifier for which the individual APRN should apply. In 2010, the American Nurses Association calculated that over 152,000 APRNs had obtained an NPI. This consisted of 5191 Certified Nurse Midwives, 35,996 Certified Registered Nurse Anesthetists, 105,958 Nurse Practitioners, and 4897 Clinical Nurse Specialists (American Nurses Association, 2010). Under MACRA, payment adjustments based on quality outcomes will be assigned at the level of the individual provider by pointing to the National Provider Identifier (NPI)/Tax Identification Number (TIN) combination. This means that all MIPS-eligible clinicians (physicians, NPs, physician assistants, CNSs, CRNAs) will be identified by the unique NPI and TIN combination. It will be imperative for information systems to capture the provider responsible for ordering individual medications or nonprocedural treatments. With MACRA, it will be essential for all providers to register for an NPI number so that all activity emanating from a singular provider across geography and time can be attributed to that provider and accounted for in a specific patient outcome. Having an NPI will allow comparisons of individual providers and provider groups and will allow for data to be rolled up into a team outcome. Registered providers can apply for an NPI through the CMS National Plan and Provider Enumeration System (https://nppes.cms.hhs.gov/NPPES/Welcome.do).

In addition, MACRA requires the CMS to maintain a list of patient relationship categories that will allow for the evaluation of human resources used during care episodes. This will also allow attribution of patients to physicians or practitioners who have primary responsibility for the patient, who consider themselves to be the lead provider, who furnish items and services to the patient on an ongoing basis, or who furnish items or services to a patient on an intermittent basis at the request of another provider. A discussion of the categories and codes describing patient relationships to providers is included in the CMS Patient Relationship Categories and Codes document https://www.cms.gov/Medicare/Quality-Initiatives-Patient-Assessment-Instruments/Value-Based-Programs/MACRA-MIPS-and-APMs/Patient-Relationship-Categories-and-Codes.pdf.

Providing individual NPI codes and relationship codes is going to allow for evaluation or comparison of outcomes and quality based on individual provider and/or specialties. This will provide opportunities to promote the value of the professional practice of APRNs using more efficient and accurate means.

Foundational Competencies in Managing Health Information Technology

At the heart of any performance measurement activity is the ability and competence to collect data and analyze results effectively so that one can reliably and accurately inform and educate stakeholders about an outcome or process. In health care, these outcomes typically consist of three types of information—clinical, financial, and administrative. Clinical data, such as a patient's medication list or laboratory results, are generally found in the EHR. In some cases, clinical data may be found in specialized registries such as the registry of the Society of Thoracic Surgeons, which collects data on open heart surgical outcomes and related cardiac diseases. Financial data, such as the cost of a given hospital stay or drug, are typically tied to a financial or billing system. Administrative data, such as a patient's age, gender, or address, are typically tied to a patient registration system (often referred to as an admission-discharge-transfer [ADT] system in acute care hospitals). The health information systems that store these data types also include the servers, cloud-based platforms, networks, clinical data warehouses, mobile applications, and POC devices. Minimum informatics competencies are required before one may access the various health information technology (HIT) applications in an organization.

Although APRNs directly engage with these technologies at various levels, not all APRNs are able to manipulate independently the various health information systems components to compile the data required to evaluate outcomes. More advanced skills from nurse informatics specialists or other expert report writers may be needed to capture necessary information such as creating a customized report or merging files from multiple databases to assemble the required information. However, stronger informatics competencies in HIT are needed by APRNs to design the evaluation strategy, validate the data, and interpret the findings effectively. For APRNs prepared at the Doctor of Nursing Practice (DNP) level, the expectation is that the APRN is prepared to "apply new knowledge, manage individual and aggregate level information, and assess the efficacy of patient care technology appropriate to a specialized area of practice" (American Association of Colleges of Nursing, 2006, p. 12). DNP graduates also design, select, and use information systems technology to evaluate programs of care, outcomes of care, and care systems. The expectations for being fluent in the use of technology are reflected in almost every

DNP competency (American Association of Colleges of Nursing, 2006). The DNP graduate also understands how to determine gaps in care or poor outcomes, search the literature, translate the evidence, and develop and implement a process to address the gap or problem. The DNP graduate uses the data to evaluate the new plan or uses a technology to address a gap.

TIGER Competencies for Use of Health Care Information Technology

Some competencies are applicable to all nurses. The Technology Informatics Guiding Education Reform (TIGER) Initiative was formed in 2004 to bring together nursing stakeholders to develop a shared vision, strategies, and specific actions for improving nursing practice, education, and the delivery of patient care through the use of HIT. The TIGER Informatics Competencies Collaborative (TICC) team was formed to develop informatics recommendations for all practicing nurses and graduating nursing students, including APRNs. The TIGER competency model consists of three parts—basic computer competencies, information literacy, and information management.

The first competency involves gaining comfort and skill with the actual hardware and software used in these processes. This includes understanding the basics behind managing a personal computer, smart phone or hand-held device; manipulating a software application and its functions; being familiar with social media; and using the Internet to find what is needed. The second competency involves information literacy. Information literacy is critical to incorporating evidence-based practice into nursing practice. The APRN must be able to determine what information is needed to assess outcomes of care, identify practice variation, and establish best practices. Furthermore, critical thinking and assessment skills are needed when evaluating or appraising the information and validating the source of the information.

The third competency involves information management, which is the underlying concept for performance measurement. This involves the process of collecting data, processing data, and presenting and communicating the processed data as meaningful information or knowledge. In addition, APRNs must understand and comply with their organization's Health Insurance Portability and Accountability Act of 1996 (HIPAA) policies and procedures, which provide for how and when patient protected health information (PHI) may be used and under what circumstances it must be de-identified (i.e., any unique patient identifiers, such as name, birth date, medical record numbers, social security number, and other personal information that could potentially identify specific individuals within a data set, must be removed). Breaches of information, such as an unintentional disclosure of PHI in an unencrypted email or a stolen laptop or device with PHI on it, must be immediately reported to the organization's compliance officer; this can result in financial fines and legal consequences for the health care organization. More information on the TIGER competencies can be found on the Healthcare Information and Management Systems Society (HIMSS) TIGER website (http://www.himss.org/professionaldevelopment/tiger-initiative).

In addition to the TIGER competencies, APRNs engaged in performance improvement activities may also require additional expertise in the information and quality management domains. These include an understanding of the various coding taxonomies and terminology sets used to classify health care data; proficiency with statistical tools, such as statistical process control (SPC) charts, which examine time-trended data; familiarity with benchmark data, data mining methods, and analytics; and knowledge about any risk adjustment methodologies that may pertain to the clinical populations being evaluated.

Although organizations such as the IHI and the National Association for Healthcare Quality can support the APRN in achieving competencies needed for successful outcome evaluation, developing such expertise in graduate programs is a challenge. Academic institutions that prepare APRNs must seek alliances with practice environments that not only exemplify or aspire to the best in professional nursing practice but also are learning organizations that are fully invested in the QI process. Institutional commitments to adopting best practices are essential if health care systems are to keep pace with new developments in performance measurement and outcomes evaluation. In addition, a robust, integrated, and reliable information systems infrastructure in the clinical environment is essential to assist the APRN student and graduate to achieve hands-on competencies in informatics and system evaluation.

Although most health care organizations have quality management departments with the expertise to build an outcome evaluation plan and conduct the actual data collection and reporting tasks, the APRN should understand these concepts to participate in, and in some cases lead, performance measurement activities throughout the full data-information-knowledge continuum. Without these competencies and skill sets, APRNs may find that their level of participation is often limited to routine data collection tasks that do not require critical thinking or clinical judgment. APRNs should be validating the accuracy of the data, monitoring performance trends, and ensuring that best practices are implemented and fully adopted by the interprofessional team. Exemplar 24.1 illustrates a scenario of appropriate APRN data collection activities associated with a professional peer review process for the purposes of outcome evaluation and performance improvement.

Descriptive, Predictive, and Prescriptive Data Analytics

Another component of outcomes evaluation in which APRNs need to become proficient involves understanding how data will ultimately be used to inform stakeholders about a phenomenon of interest. This may come in the form of performance metrics that describe historical trends for outcomes or processes that have happened in the past or tools that can be used in real time to alert providers to a potential trend or event. Collectively, the activities of designing the measurement process, collecting and analyzing the data, and presenting the data back to stakeholders in a timely and effective manner are termed *data analytics*. As EHR data become more standardized and broadly adopted, the methods for performing data analytics will continue to evolve toward more automated capture and compilation of

results, thus allowing data analytics to become more ingrained in every aspect of health care. Analytics in the health care industry can be organized into three main categories: descriptive, predictive, and prescriptive.

Descriptive Analytics

The term *descriptive analytics* essentially describes a retrospective trend or outcome. Typically, descriptive data are reported as percentages, rates, means, medians, ratios, or counts in which a value is assigned to inform the degree of positive or negative movement against a given target or norm. Another type of descriptive analytic would be time-trended comparison data, which could inform the audience about a hospital's overall and periodic fluctuations in performance related to readmissions compared with that of other hospitals. The limitations of both these analytic tools is that they do not illuminate the reasons behind a given pattern, suggest an improvement strategy, or help the audience understand the relative stability or predictability of the process that is currently producing outcomes to date.

One of the most effective methods for demonstrating that an intervention or process modification has resulted in meaningful change over time is SPC analysis. SPC analysis examines variation within an individual process as well as the timing in which a change in process occurred. SPC uses control charts, which visually display performance data against upper and lower control limits reflective of normal variation in a system. Fig. 24.1 provides an example of an SPC chart with upper and lower limits. In contrast to comparative reports, which display

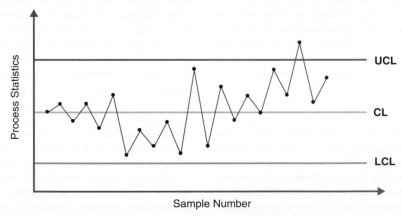

FIG 24.1 Example statistical process control chart. *CL,* Center line; *LCL,* lower control limit; *UCL,* upper control limit. *(From ProcessMA Resource, Statistical Process Control. Available at http://www.processma. com/resource/spc.php.)*

individual performance data compared with peer group performance, SPC charts display time-trended data only for individual performance data. No peer performance data are displayed in an SPC chart. Rather, the individual data are trended over time, with mathematically computed control limits that indicate the expected ranges for random variation within a given process. When data points within the time-trended process change in a manner indicative of a statistically significant change, a special cause signal is displayed in the SPC chart. Special cause signals can occur whenever a single data point exceeds the upper or lower control limits in the SPC chart. Additional trends in the data may also designate special cause signals such as eight data points in a row above or below the center line or six points in a row increasing or decreasing in a single direction.

SPC charts have the added advantage of being able to distinguish results achieved during a pre-intervention process from the results achieved following a process change that occurs as a result of an innovation or practice change. This is done by inserting a phase change line between the two different processes and computing new control limits to monitor for statistical process capability moving forward. A detailed discussion of these data analysis techniques is beyond the scope of this chapter, although a basic knowledge of control charts is useful for most situations. The reader is referred to the classic reference on SPC chart theory (Wheeler, 1993) or an online reference for basic SPC chart theory and application (Bauman, De Heck, Leonard, & Merrick, 2006).

To understand why a hospital has fluctuations in readmission performance data, or why a hospital's performance differs from that of others, the inquiry must progress further. Additional descriptive analytics may be used to look at specific details within the population, such as readmissions by gender, age, provider, payor, disease severity, and other related criteria. This type of inquiry that drills down to explore more specific patterns in data sets is termed *data mining*. APRNs are likely to be engaged in this sort of activity as they evaluate outcomes for their areas of interest. Typical tools that the APRN will use in data mining will likely involve Excel spreadsheets or other types of statistical software tools. Data patterns may then be displayed in charts to describe the patterns in the data. Table 24.6 lists several tools and techniques that are commonly used when working with descriptive analytics.

Predictive Analytics

Predictive analytics are rapidly emerging in the science of performance improvement. In contrast to descriptive analytics, which only describe a process after it has happened, predictive analytics provide insight on what might happen in the future based on past patterns or other criteria so that the appropriate interventions may be done to achieve desired outcomes. For example, there are several tools available to assist the APRN with predicting and reducing readmissions. The Agency for Healthcare Research and Quality (AHRQ) has published the *Hospital Guide to Reducing Medicaid Readmissions* (https://www.ahrq.gov/sites/default/files/publications/files/medread-tools.pdf). The Institute for Healthcare Improvement (IHI) provides access to multiple tools for reducing readmissions (http://www.ihi.org/Pages/default.aspx). In addition, the IHI provides the *Readmissions Diagnostic Worksheet* to assist the APRN with an in depth review of rehospitalization (http://www.ihi.org/resources/Pages/Tools/ReadmissionsDiagnosticWorksheet.aspx). The Health Research and Educational Trust developed the *Preventable Readmissions Change Package* (http://www.hrethiin.org/Resources/readmiins/16/HRETHEN_ChangePackage_Readmissions.pdf). An APRN engaged in activities aimed at decreasing readmissions would do well to review and critique these resources for use in the planning and evaluation of readmissions.

Currently, software engineers and clinical innovators are partnering to develop technology solutions that will assist in identifying individual patients at highest risk for readmissions, pressure ulcers, falls, and other hospital-acquired complications. Cerner Systems and Advocate Health Care have developed a predictive analytic for hospital readmissions based on 25 variables, including payor, race, prior hospitalization and emergency department use in the past 12 months, admission source, current use of insulin or warfarin, and 17 disease-related variables (Sikka, Gagen, Crayton, & Esposito, 2012). Most tools are not yet robust enough to have broad applicability to general populations; however, this area of performance improvement will likely accelerate particularly as Big Data techniques and visual analytics tools become more robust. Such development will allow measurement of more timely and proactive interventions to ensure that best practices are delivered at the right time for more high-risk patients. Kansagara and colleagues (2011) provided a systemic review of predictive analytics and risk predication models pertaining to hospital readmissions as of August 2011.

TABLE 24.6   Continuous Quality Improvement Tools and Techniques for Process Improvement

Tools and Techniques	Primary Function	Benefits
Flow chart	Displays the process	• Facilitates understanding of the process • Identifies stakeholders • Clarifies potential gaps and system breakdowns
Run chart	Displays performance over time	• Increases understanding of the problem • Identifies changes over time
Control chart	Displays how predictable the process is over time	• Identifies change in the process as a result of intentional or unintentional changes in the process • Identifies opportunities for improvement
Pie chart	Displays the percentage that each variable contributes to the whole	• Identifies variables affecting the process • Increases understanding of the problem
Bar chart	Compares categories of data during a single point in time	• Increases understanding of the problem • Identifies differences in variables • Compares performance with known standards
Pareto chart	Identifies the most frequent trend within a data set	• Identifies principal variables impacting the process • Identifies opportunities for improvement
Cause-and-effect diagram	Displays multiple causes of a problem	• Identifies root causes • Identifies variables affecting the process • Identifies opportunities for improvement • Plans for change
Scatter diagram	Displays relationship between two variables	• Increases understanding of the relationship between multiple variables
Brainstorming	Rapidly generates multiple ideas	• Promotes stakeholder buy-in • Increases understanding of the problem • Identifies variables affecting the process
Multivoting	Consolidates ideas	• Achieves consensus among stakeholders • Prioritizes improvement strategies
Nominal group technique	Rapidly generates multiple ideas and prioritizes them	• Identifies the problem • Achieves consensus among stakeholders • Prioritizes improvement strategies • Plans for change
Root cause analysis	Identifies the cause of the problem	• Increases understanding of the problem • Identifies multicause variables affecting the process • Identifies opportunities to improve • Plans for change
Force field analysis	Identifies driving and restraining forces that impact proposed change	• Identifies and lists variables affecting process • Plans for change
Consensus	Generates agreement among stakeholders	• Increases understanding of the problem • Reduces resistance to change • Plans for change

Adapted from *Powell, S. K. (2000). Advanced case management: Outcomes and beyond.* Philadelphia, PA: JB Lippincott.

Prescriptive Analytics

Finally, the term *prescriptive analytics* refers to tools that assist with modeling and longitudinal forecasting to inform users on how to respond to a given pattern in one's data. In prescriptive analytics, the evidence-based best practice is linked to the trend so that it indicates not only why there is a problem but what the most likely solutions would be to get a trend back on a desired course. With the use of computer science and machine learning, rapid acceleration and scientific innovation, will change how evidence-based practice is deployed in the clinical environment. APRN participation in collaborative learning with medical and nursing informatics specialists, clinical researchers, HIT vendors, and scientists may lead to transformational technologies within the next 5 to 8 years.

Foundational Competencies in Quality Improvement

APRNs must be able to participate in and lead interprofessional teams effectively toward data-based conclusions and process improvements. Data analysis is a specific skill for evidence-based practice. APRNs are required to have the ability to manipulate and interpret raw data, query information within a database containing clinical or financial information, and use an information system to collect data and trend performance. If it is not possible for the APRN to directly query, then the APRN must have the ability to work with an informatician or analyst to extract the correct data because the APRN has an appreciation for the content of the data needed and the context in which the data were collected. The purpose of this section is to elaborate on the specific skills that APRNs need to be knowledgeable participants and leaders in continuous quality improvement (CQI) efforts. APRN students need content on CQI knowledge and skills, and graduate APRNs should seek additional CQI training through reading, continuing education, and participation in formal QI training programs. A health care system's approach to CQI should be included in an APRN's orientation. If such programs are not in place, APRNs are strongly encouraged to include formal QI training in their performance and learning objectives within the first year of hire and to identify opportunities to initiate modest QI initiatives.

Continuous Quality Improvement Frameworks

There are numerous frameworks and related strategies for improving performance and evaluating outcomes in today's health care system. Some of these include the plan-do-study-act (PDSA) model used by the IHI, Six Sigma, and Lean Manufacturing techniques (Morgan & Brenig-Jones, 2012). APRNs can examine selected frameworks to understand the how-to mechanics of creating systems that are safe, effective, patient centered, timely, efficient, and equitable. Generally, the employer will have selected a framework or philosophy that guides CQI efforts across an organization. Many of these methodologies have evolved from the work of Drs. W. Edwards Deming and Joseph M. Juran, both considered to

be forefathers of modern day SPC theory. Although a detailed review of the various CQI frameworks is not included here, APRNs are highly encouraged to contact the quality management department in their organization and request an orientation to the CQI framework used in their practice settings. Marash, Berman, and Flynn (2003) have provided a comprehensive overview of the traditional QI methodologies discussed earlier.

Regardless of the type of QI approach an organization selects, the APRN should be competent in a variety of specific techniques, tools, and methodologies used to evaluate process performance and outcomes. Most approaches involve the use of different types of charts and analysis tools to examine findings and establish linkages. Some charts are easy to learn, such as flow charts. Other charts, such as Pareto charts, SPC charts, scatter diagrams, and cause-and-effect diagrams, also termed *fishbone* or *Ishikawa diagrams,* require specific training and expertise in statistical software. APRNs may also need to become familiar with the software used in their agencies to conduct CQI analyses and reports.

APRNs prepared at a master's level should achieve beginning-level competencies with these tools, including the ability to interpret the data in these reports and effectively participate in teams using CQI techniques. One exception is the CNS role, which has had expectations for leading QI efforts as part of system influence expectations embedded in their role; mastery is expected for any CNS, whether master's or DNP prepared. Other APRNs should achieve mastery of QI competencies at the DNP level, with full accountability for planning the CQI project; selecting and using appropriate tools and techniques, including being able to enter data and run the reports; synthesizing information from the reports; and coaching others in deriving meaning from the information and making decisions. QI training should also include techniques for analyzing how people and processes work. Root cause analysis is one popular approach to identifying underlying causes of problems and process failures in a particular system. This approach may be particularly useful for examining adverse events and other patient safety issues.

Organizational Structures and Cultures That Optimize Performance Improvement

APRNs who practice in a hospital or an integrated delivery network may find that their span of influence crosses many units, departments, and points of service within the system. Thus it is important to consider carefully the reporting structures that will best support their roles. In many organizations, APRNs report to nursing or medical executives. Regardless of organizational placement, APRNs should seek to work within a reporting structure that supports whole-system thinking and places a high value on innovation and process improvement. Conversely, APRNs should avoid reporting structures that constrain their practices to one unit's or department's interests or seem to place a particular emphasis on task-oriented activities. Optimally, the organization and its administrators should recognize that the APRN is in a unique position to promote excellence in clinical practice and system performance. To achieve these outcomes, the APRN may at times require the formal and tacit authority that come with the position and title of those to whom the APRN reports. Those who lead APRNs must be prepared to be responsible, if necessary, for changes perceived as coming from the APRN. Although APRNs will not need daily or even weekly supervision, they will need to be kept abreast of organizational issues that are likely to affect the practice and business environment. The APRN should have routine briefing sessions scheduled with his or her immediate supervisor to clarify goals and expected outcomes, identify any resource needs, discuss any barriers, and exchange information relating to pending contracts, changes in the product line, medical practice issues, or staff education needs.

Active membership on key medical and quality oversight committees and direct access to administrative decision makers are imperative. This access affords APRNs the opportunity to integrate clinical expertise with communication, negotiation, and leadership skills to promote effective and efficient clinical processes. For APRNs who contract independently, becoming familiar with the organizational structure and culture and becoming a trusted insider in the organization will be critical to successful contracting and service delivery. Exemplar 24.3 illustrates an APRN in a nurse-managed clinic working collaboratively with other quality leaders within a large health care system and influencing practice and systems by exercising leadership, QI skills, systems thinking, and use of informatics.

Strategies for Designing Quality Improvement and Outcome Evaluation Plans for Advanced Practice Nursing

As noted, much of health care practice in today's economic market is data driven, with APRNs assuming greater responsibility for collecting and using clinical, economic, and quality outcomes data. In particular, interprofessional QI teams are increasingly charged with improving care delivery outcomes or redesigning workflow processes for greater effectiveness or efficiency. Because APRNs routinely monitor and maintain clinical care delivery systems, they are in an ideal position to plan QI initiatives by leading or actively participating in interprofessional QI teams. As clinical experts, APRNs influence practice patterns and develop meaningful standards, practice protocols, clinical guidelines, health care programs, and health care policies that promote teamwork, improve clinical outcomes, and reduce costs. Moreover, APRNs' pattern recognition skills facilitate the identification of system inefficiencies, barriers to continuity of care, and other ineffective ways of delivering health care services. These in turn become opportunities for APRNs to influence processes and outcomes positively at both the individual patient and system levels. With these opportunities comes the responsibility to be knowledgeable in outcome evaluation. In the remainder of this chapter, a stepwise approach is proposed to developing and implementing an outcome evaluation plan that demonstrates an APRN's value and contribution to health care quality. Although the term *outcome evaluation* is used throughout this section, these steps can be applied to impact analysis, outcomes measurement, performance evaluation, process improvement, and program evaluation.

Phases of Preparing a Plan for Outcome Evaluation

There are three phases in the organizing framework to develop an effective outcome evaluation plan— defining the core questions that need to be answered, determining the data required to answer the questions, and interpreting the data and acting on the results. Box 24.4 lists the phases and related steps in developing and conducting an outcomes evaluation. A description of each step follows.

Define the Core Questions
Whether the APRN is designing an outcome evaluation project to assess her or his practice effectiveness or participating on an interprofessional team responsible for improving the care for a given clinical population, the first step is to clearly articulate and ask "What are the questions we are asking and why?" Clear questions will lay the foundation for an effective outcome evaluation and limit unintended project

Putting It All Together: Planning and Managing Quality Reporting at a Nurse-Managed Clinic[a]

Nancy Lawson (NL) is a nurse practitioner (NP) and clinical director of a nurse-managed health center (NMHC) in a large urban Midwestern city. Primary care services, including health promotion, preventive care, and chronic disease management, are provided to a diverse population consisting of college-age students, children, adolescents, and an increasing number of adults with chronic diseases such as hypertension and diabetes. The center's population has a mix of commercial, Medicare, and Medicaid payors, with some patients having little to no insurance. This NMHC is staffed by a practice of six primary care NPs, one administrative assistant, and a part-time information systems analyst, whose position is shared by the NMHC's sponsoring health care system. Although owned and operated by a school of nursing, the NMHC is also partnered with a large health care system, which is participating in the Centers for Medicare & Medicaid Services (CMS) demonstration project as a pioneering accountable care organization (ACO). The NMHC is also committed to supporting student placements at the undergraduate and graduate levels. As NL begins her annual review of the performance improvement plan, she creates a list of all quality and patient safety reporting requirements to which the NMHC must respond over the course of the next year. This year, the NMHC is planning to apply for status as a federally qualified health center, which will expand its quality reporting requirements. NL identifies four major quality reporting initiatives:

1. CMS Shared Savings Program for ACOs
2. Health Resources and Services Administration clinical and financial performance measures
3. CMS Medicaid adult quality reporting measures
4. Health information technology (HIT) functions associated with Meaningful Use

NL downloads the National Quality Forum (NQF) Community Tool to Align Measurement from the NQF website and filters the spreadsheet so that only measures associated with her clinic's programs of interest are listed. In addition, she includes a list of measures associated with the National Committee for Quality Assurance Healthcare Effectiveness Data and Information Set (HEDIS) Physician Measures and the CMS Physician Quality Reporting System so that she can get a complete inventory of all NQF-endorsed measures that might be applicable to the NMHC populations. In this manner, she can begin to see overlap in reporting requirements

and identify any gaps in terms of what is being collected and reported in the NMHC's current performance improvement plan (PIP). Knowing this information will also be useful to NL in her planning and prioritization for HIT enhancements that need to be implemented at the NMHC to reduce the data collection burden on her team.

Next, NL considers her professional practice team and their areas of interest. She calls a meeting to bring the stakeholders together, including her information technology (IT) analyst. NL then asks for input from the team to decide which measures they should select to meet their regulatory reporting requirements. She asks the stakeholders to consider the NMHC's population and mission as well as the value of knowing versus the burden of collection. The IT analyst contributes to this assessment by advising the team on whether their electronic health record and IT infrastructure is currently capable of capturing this information electronically or whether manual data collection methods would need to be incorporated to collect the necessary information. The IT analyst notes areas of future expansion and prioritizes these needs relative to quality reporting initiatives at the NMHC. This information will be shared in the upcoming meeting with the health care system's corporate HIT strategy team to build their integrated health care information system to support their work as an ACO.

Finally, NL asks the team to consider any other areas of interest that they would like to focus on over the course of the next year, that are not already captured in the must measure list and that will inform them about the quality, effectiveness, efficacy, and efficiency of the group's practice. They suggest that the average waiting time to be seen by a clinic provider and the number of patients who are admitted to the emergency department (ED) or hospital within 72 hours after being seen at the NMHC would be valuable information in the year ahead. In collaboration with their IT analyst, they determine the best ways to capture waiting time to be seen and 72-hour admissions.

As the team completes their final assessment, they raise concerns that although the value of knowing the patient satisfaction and patient experience data is high, the data collection effort will be intensive and likely require the assistance of additional staff or university students to collect and analyze this information. NL and the NPs in the practice suggest including the

Continued

Putting It All Together: Planning and Managing Quality Reporting at a Nurse-Managed Clinic[a]—cont'd

students from the college of nursing to partner with this project. NL schedules a meeting with the Dean of Academic Affairs to discuss internship opportunities for nursing students. With enthusiasm from the Dean that these would be good learning opportunities, these measures and the proposed data collection plan are added to the NMHC's performance improvement plan.

Finally, for each measure, the team identifies a target for their performance. Measures with known associated national benchmarks, such as the HEDIS process measure for diabetes care, which measures the percentage of diabetic patients receiving glycosylated hemoglobin (HbA_{1c}) tests in the reporting year, or the outcome measure that reports the percentage of diabetic patients with a controlled HbA_{1c} result, are set at higher percentiles of desired performance (e.g., 90%). Conversely, measures with which the relative goodness or badness of the phenomenon of interest is not established nationally, such as the number of patients admitted to the health care system's ED within 72 hours of a visit to the NMHC, may be set at lower thresholds of performance or have no specific target established until patterns in the performance data have been well established.

NL compiles the final list of measures to be reported, along with a data collection plan and schedule for periodic review and reporting to all stakeholders. She submits this PIP to the College of Nursing's Faculty Practice Plan group for feedback prior to submitting the plan to the sponsoring health care system's quality director for final review and approval. Over the course of the next year, the NMHC team monitors the results of their performance monthly. Measure rates and continuous variables are presented in a dashboard using statistical process control (SPC) charts so that trends can be rapidly visualized. For each measure a target is established so that all stakeholders reviewing the monthly dashboard can see at a glance any performance trends that are falling below desired targets.

Midway through the year, the NMHC team observes that their performance in mammography screening is substantially below the national median as reported by HEDIS. The team decides to review their performance stratified by payor (commercial, Medicare, Medicaid, and self-pay or uninsured) to see if any disparities might exist. No significant trends appear. However, when reviewing the inclusion and exclusion criteria for the measure, it is observed that the primary reason for failing to meet the criterion was that the results of the mammography were not reported back to the NMHC. The team quickly realized that to understand their effectiveness in this referral metric fully, they had to correct an underlying system issue and send the results of the mammography back to the referring NP provider.

NL organized a small team of stakeholders, which included the administrator for the contracted imaging facility, the medical director of the imaging facility, the oversight physician for the NMHC, and the IT systems analyst. During a 1-hour meeting, it was unanimously agreed by all parties that the NP provider ordering the mammogram required a copy of the results. It was further determined that the root cause for this omission was tied to the absence of the NP providers from the hospital information systems provider dictionary. The IT analyst was able to quickly add the six NPs to the required dictionary, enabling the admissions clerk at the imaging center to select the appropriate provider and route the results to her or him.

The next month, the performance trend for mammography referrals from the NMHC demonstrated a statistically significant increase. Using the SPC software function to designate a phase change within a time-trended process, NL modified the SPC chart in the dashboard by inserting a phase line to distinguish between the pre- and postprocess improvement periods. In this manner, she will be able to document the impact of the PIP initiative to have available for potential accreditation surveys and to detect any statistically significant changes in their new process moving forward that might indicate that they are not sustaining their improvements over time. NL makes a plan to reevaluate performance in mammography referrals monthly for the remainder of the year and at least once a quarter thereafter for the next 18 to 24 months, as long as the process appears to be stable. ◎

[a]The author wishes to thank Joanne Pohl, PhD, APRN-BC, for her contribution to the development of this exemplar based on her experiences with NMHCs nationally.

BOX 24.4   Summary of Outcome Evaluation Planning Process

Phase I: Define the Core Questions

I-1. Define the target population for study.
- Identify differences in patient characteristics within target population.
- Clarify relationships between APRN role behaviors and population needs and outcomes.
- Compare target group with other groups monitored through QI activities.
- Assess level of risk, complexity, and resource use of subpopulations within target group.

I-2. Identify the stakeholders.
- Facilitate participation by and input from key stakeholders.
- Isolate advanced practice registered nurse (APRN) interventions and actions from those of other care providers.
- Secure early buy-in from stakeholders.

I-3. Articulate program goals and interventions.
- Review literature for supportive evidence.
- Consider resources needed to implement and maintain the intervention.
- Formulate specific questions.
- Implement practice change or QI strategy.

Phase II: Define the Data Elements

II-1. Identify selection criteria for the population of interest.
- Clarify inclusion and exclusion criteria.
- Identify electronic data sources of information about the target population.

II-2. Establish performance and outcome indicators.
- Identify measures to determine evidence of APRN impact.
- Ensure alignment among program goals, proposed interventions, and outcome indicators.
- Consider the use of national databases for comparison and benchmarking purposes.

II-3. Identify and evaluate data elements, collection instruments, and procedures.
- Evaluate ease of collecting data and compare with need.

- Identify data resources available.
- Link use of intermediate outcome indicators to target goals and outcome achievement.
- Summarize the outcome evaluation plan.

Phase III: Derive Meaning From Data and Act on Results

III-1. Analyze data and interpret findings.
- Seek assistance from others, as needed.
- Select data analysis and reporting procedures.

III-2. Present and disseminate findings.
- Prepare reports according to audience and stakeholder needs and interests.
- Select software programs and other resources to support presentation approach.

III-3. Identify improvement opportunities.
- Work with stakeholders to identify most appropriate opportunity for improvement.
- Select most effective tools to facilitate performance improvement planning process.
- Conduct pilot studies to assess new program feasibility, cost, and resource needs.

III-4. Formulate a plan for ongoing monitoring and reevaluation.
- Summarize goals of performance improvement plan.
- Identify proposed interventions, responsible persons, and target dates for completion.
- Select indicators and measures based on goals and interventions identified.
- Provide education programs to support intervention, as needed.

III-5. Clarify the purpose of the APRN's role.
- Review organization's mission, vision, and goals.
- Clarify role expectations.
- Confirm clinical and reporting accountability.

scope creep. In formulating clear core questions, it is helpful to define the target population for study, identify the relevant stakeholders, and articulate specific program goals and interventions to be evaluated. It is also useful to understand any key business drivers tied to the outcome evaluation or performance improvement initiative. Once these foundational aspects have been established, the APRN can progress to the mechanics of how the data for the project will be collected.

Define the Target Population for Study

APRNs use a range of activities to manage heterogeneous clinical populations. When designing an outcome evaluation plan, it is necessary to focus on specific aspects of the practice with a particular patient group. This focus helps create a more manageable outcome evaluation plan and limits the impact of extraneous variables that could interfere with the interpretation of findings. Aspects of APRN activities used with the target population need to be identified and included in the design. Whenever possible, the target population should be comparable to other groups monitored through QI initiatives at the organizational or departmental level so that the vested interests of the organization's commitment to improving care and APRNs' activities are aligned. The decision to target subpopulations of patients may be based on a desire to evaluate patients who are high risk, are complex, or tend to use more services than others.

Other factors to consider when defining a target population include patient satisfaction and financial performance. For example, when a large pediatric medical group hires a pediatric NP to provide routine physical examinations and vaccinations, parent satisfaction is likely to be an important component of the outcome evaluation plan. Patient factors such as insurance provider, age, ethnicity, or comorbid conditions also may be used to define the target population at risk for adverse outcomes. Finally, some populations are targeted because of the need for organizations to determine their level of compliance with national care delivery guidelines, best practice standards, or regulatory requirements, as illustrated in Exemplar 24.3. Frequently, APRNs are involved in the care of several populations of interest and, as such, must prioritize which populations warrant first review and evaluation. APRNs must be sensitive to the resource requirements of any outcomes project, working closely with information systems, QI, and medical records staff for the support required to conduct the review.

Identify the Stakeholders

APRNs must identify the structures and processes of care for which they share accountability. Although APRNs are rarely the only or primary stakeholder in the provision of care to the populations they serve, they often serve as the glue that holds the team together. As such, they often move the team, health care agency, and/or system toward a shared vision of a desired outcome. Creating this vision is not an isolated APRN activity; APRNs must also facilitate the contributions, ideas, and creativity of professionals who participate in the care of the target population. Exemplar 24.4 demonstrates that small changes with multiple stakeholders using reminders within an EHR can make significant change. Stakeholders most commonly involved are physicians, physician assistants, other APRNs, registered nurses, pharmacists, administrators, and other members of the health care team. In some cases, APRNs will need to include stakeholders from outside their immediate practice settings. For example, a community-based APRN serving fragile older patients with chronic diseases may need to include stakeholders from managed care payors and insurers, primary care clinics, physicians' offices, skilled nursing facilities, home health care agencies, and hospitals. Although including all stakeholders in the development of an outcome evaluation plan may not be feasible or desirable, attention to the impact of primary stakeholders on care delivery outcomes will aid in the understanding and measurement of processes and outcomes interdependent with APRN practice.

Typically APRNs are only one component of a greater whole, so they cannot receive full credit for the positive results. Therefore, APRNs must articulate APRN-specific inputs and interventions that contribute to the team effect so that the value of the APRN to the organization can be documented and demonstrated. The need to carve out additional measures of role effectiveness results in a more complex outcomes plan, requiring multiple measurement methodologies, instruments, and analytic techniques. For example, part of an outcome evaluation plan may use quantitative methods to capture specific outcomes of treatment (e.g., average number of clinic visits by diabetic patients per year, total costs, number of diabetic patients with a normal HbA_{1c} level within 2 months of diagnosis). Another part of the plan may use a qualitative approach, using verbal or written feedback from physician and dietitian colleagues about APRN effectiveness in facilitating the development of new patient care

---

| EXEMPLAR 24.4 | Simple Changes Result in Substantial Improvement |

There is an identified need within an urban academic medical center to improve quality and outcomes related to heart failure 30-day readmission. A literature review by the advanced practice registered nurse indicates that it takes numerous transitions of care interventions to prevent the 30-day readmission of heart failure patients after discharge. One key intervention is to ensure that heart failure patients follow up with their primary care provider within 48 to 72 hours after discharge. The care team identified actions to increase use of this important intervention when it was discovered through data analytics that only 20% of heart failure patients had appointments scheduled prior to discharge. All clinicians were educated on how important the follow-up appointment was to improving overall outcomes. Patients were educated by the discharging nurse. The unit care team made checking on the status of the follow-up appointment part of discharge planning processes. In some cases, case managers were assigned the task of contacting the primary care provider to establish the appointment. The information system was adapted to capture follow-up appointment information, making it clear to patient and providers if this task was completed. A report was created listing all patients nearing discharge and the follow-up appointment information as a clinical decision support tool. All this information on follow-up was collected within the electronic health record so that results could be monitored. The net result was an increase in the number of conversations about follow-up appointments, an increase in the number of appointments made (up to 90% compliance), and a decrease in the 30-day preventable readmission rate. In addition, patient satisfaction scores for the heart failure clinic improved. ◎

---

guidelines to manage the diabetic population. Once the plan for an evaluation study has been shared with stakeholders, buy-in to any proposed change must be obtained to proceed. APRNs not only will be change recipients as a result of the outcome evaluation but also will serve as change implementers and change strategists for others and their organization. Involving stakeholders early in the process facilitates ongoing communication, reduces resistance to change, and promotes adoption of recommended changes.

Articulate Program Goals and Interventions

The easiest way to demonstrate positive outcomes of care is to do the right things, at the right times, for the right patients, in the right ways. The task of evaluation becomes an artful assembly of necessary data and information that reflect the outcomes and processes associated with the intervention. Determining which interventions to implement for a given population and which to include in an outcome evaluation plan may be based in part on the resources required to accomplish these interventions and maintain them in practice. To begin, APRNs should engage in a comprehensive literature review to examine all standards of care, regulatory requirements, national guidelines, and established or emerging evidence-based best practices relevant to their clinical population. The most current information may be found on websites that are relevant to the APRN's clinical specialty or through specialized fee-for-service vendor services that accumulate and organize best practice information and a meta-analysis of the literature for selected clinical topics, such as Zynx Health (http://www.zynxhealth.com).

Using information from the literature and experience, APRNs can identify appropriate interventions for managing populations. For example, interventions may include attention to early detection and diagnostic modalities, timeliness of interventions, drug appropriateness, or patient education. The organization's needs and any political agendas should also be considered. APRNs should limit the number of evaluated interventions to keep the project scope manageable. A commitment to multiple interventions at the same time or unrealistic data collection activities can overwhelm available resources and undermine or stall performance improvement and outcome evaluation initiatives.

Once the program goals and interventions have been defined, the APRN can begin to formulate specific questions of interest to stakeholders. Sketching out some basic questions serves as a useful exercise for establishing the outcome evaluation plan. The following are some sample questions:

- How cost effective is this program?
- How satisfied are patients with the services they received?
- How closely does the health care team adhere to best practice standards?
- How many patients experienced complications of care?

- What patient safety issues associated with this population should we examine?
- What can be done to reduce resource utilization and create efficiencies for this population?
- What do we need to do differently to become a center of excellence for this population?
- How has the APRN contributed to the training and development of other staff?
- What are the key business drivers behind the outcome evaluation project or performance improvement initiative?

Once the core questions have been formulated, the APRN can design the data collection methodology that will be used to answer key questions. Typically, this step occurs simultaneously with the actual implementation of a practice change or QI strategy. In the event that a pre-intervention baseline of performance measurement needs to be established, implementation of the improvement strategy would be deferred until after the baseline measurement has been established.

Define the Data Elements

After APRNs clarify the program goals, identify the key interventions to evaluate in the outcome evaluation plan, and determine the core questions to be answered, they are ready to define the outcome indicators and data elements they will use to measure the intervention's success. This phase in the outcome evaluation plan often poses the greatest challenge for APRNs, particularly for those who have had little or no exposure to QI principles and management information systems—both of which support outcome evaluation. There are three steps in this phase. First, APRNs decide how they will qualify patients or encounters of care for inclusion in the outcome evaluation; second, they identify which indicators they will use to answer the project's core questions; and third, they determine which data elements will be collected for each indicator chosen for the project. As noted, APRNs with limited expertise in these areas should seek assistance from other health care professionals with experience in CQI principles, health care statistics, nursing informatics, program evaluation, and/or nursing research.

Identify Selection Criteria for the Population of Interest

Although this may seem like an obvious step, it is important to consider which patient characteristics will be included in the evaluation. Identifying electronic data sources that contain information about the target population is generally the most efficient way to begin. For example, APRNs who practice in a physician's office or clinic may be able to retrieve a list of all patients seen within a given time frame. This is possible because the APRN's provider number, which identifies his or her patients in the claims database and generates the bill for services rendered, can be used to define the population of interest. The APRN could further reduce this list to patients seen for a specific diagnosis or symptom through the use of ICD-10 codes, CPT-4 codes, or ambulatory payment classification (APC) codes. In behavioral health settings, the use of the *Diagnostic and Statistical Manual of Mental Disorders,* 5th Edition (DSM-V) codes are generally more useful. Additional coding taxonomies and terminology sets relevant to this level of query are listed and described in Table 24.1.

In contrast, CNSs who practice in acute care environments may have a more difficult time obtaining a list of patients whose care they managed or influenced because CNSs do not typically bill directly for services. In this scenario, the population may be identified by non-electronic data sources such as a log or referral list. If the CNS's influence extends to a general clinical population, specified MS-DRG or ICD-10 diagnostic or procedure codes can be used to obtain a patient list if the outcome evaluation design is retrospective. CRNAs and certified nurse-midwives who contract with the hospital for their services may be able to identify patients for whom they have provided care from the procedure provider that corresponds to the procedure code; however, they should confirm that they are listed as the procedure provider in the final claim, rather than the medical provider assigned to their practice. This information is generally available from hospital information systems and is rapidly being enhanced through the adoption of the EHR and MU technologies (see earlier). As illustrated in Exemplar 24.2, APRNs should collaborate with health information management and nursing informatics specialists for this component of their analysis to ensure that the right inclusion variables have been identified to secure their population of interest.

Establish Performance and Outcome Indicators

Once the patient population has been defined, APRNs and their colleagues specify measures of performance that will be used to draw conclusions about how well the population was managed or the degree to which favorable outcomes were achieved. In general, descriptive measures are predominately classified into three types: (1) proportion measures (e.g., mortality rates, readmission rates, complication rates); (2) ratio measures (e.g., falls/1000 patient days, central line infections/1000 line days, restraint episodes per psychiatric patient days); and (3) continuous variable measures (e.g., median time to initial antibiotic administration, average length of stay). Some measures are direct counts of a particular phenomenon within a given time period, such as the number of allergic reactions in patients receiving antibiotics. Others are sums, such as total costs of care for a given population or total patient days. For rare events, such as ventilator-associated pneumonia in hospitals that have implemented aggressive protocols to prevent this phenomenon from occurring, the days between undesirable events may be a more effective way to track and monitor outcomes, with longer time intervals being the more desirable trend, rather than fewer events.

The type of measure selected is less important than how well it answers the core questions of the study, although ultimately the type of measure will determine the approach required for data analysis and presentation to stakeholders. The best approach is to create a draft list of indicators and obtain feedback from stakeholders about how well the indicators address their core questions and concerns. Only after stakeholder buy-in is secured should the APRN formally establish the indicators for the evaluation plan. When informing the stakeholders of the outcome evaluation plan, the APRN should keep in mind that if data collection is concurrent and involves the clinical practice patterns of the clinical stakeholders, the potential exists to bias the results simply because the providers know that they are being observed and their performance is being monitored. This reaction, termed the *Hawthorne effect,* is troublesome for process measurement. The data collection period should continue for a sufficient period to ensure that the novelty of the intervention has worn off and the changes in behaviors are a true reflection of intervention effect.

Alignment among program goals, interventions, and performance and outcome indicators is another important consideration when designing the outcome evaluation plan. This process ensures that the findings of the outcome evaluation can be traced back to APRN practice when appropriate. For example, if average length of stay is selected as one outcome indicator for a population of acute myocardial infarction patients under the direction of a hospital-based CNS, this variable should be linked in theory and in practice to an intervention for which the CNS has

or shares accountability (e.g., discharge planning or management of complications). Measures that reflect the subprocesses of other providers, such as time from first incision to the time the wire crosses the lesion in the coronary artery for patients undergoing angioplasty, may be of interest to invasive cardiologists and other stakeholders from the cardiac catheterization laboratory; however, they may have little to do with the APRN's direct practice role.

As noted earlier, APRNs are often lured into coordinating data collection for other providers as part of the performance monitoring process. APRNs may agree to perform these data coordination or data collection activities but must be careful not to become overburdened with tasks that diminish their own clinical effectiveness or assessment of intervention effect. If this happens, APRNs should examine other potential resources in the organization so they can continue to carry out their role and provide service to the institution. Staying focused on the interventions and specific program goals for which they are responsible will assist APRNs to formulate a meaningful and manageable outcome evaluation plan.

Identify and Evaluate Data Elements, Collection Instruments, and Procedures

To ensure an efficient data collection process, APRNs should evaluate the effort to collect each individual data element compared with the overall usefulness of the indicator. Data available only through specialized or resource-intensive instruments, such as phone surveys, home follow-up visits, or comprehensive chart reviews, are considered difficult to obtain and should be carefully evaluated before making a final decision to include them in the outcome evaluation plan. When data are obtained electronically, the specific source for each data element needs to be identified and understood. As noted earlier, running queries and reports from the EHR may or may not become an essential part of the APRN's role and, in most cases, expert resources are available in health care systems to assist APRNs in retrieving the information. However, in the era of the EHR, it is especially important that data obtained electronically be validated for accuracy before they can be reliably used. APRNs can collaborate with quality management and nursing informatics specialists to design a data validation strategy to ensure that data are complete, accurate, and sensitive to the issue of interest. This may involve the random review of records by expert clinicians and an inspection of an interface file by a technician in the IT department to ensure that all source systems are working as designed.

APRNs can avoid duplication of effort and data collection redundancy by becoming familiar with the many sources of data and information available in their respective organizations. This will require collaboration with interprofessional team members such as database administrators, report writers, data analysis experts, and administrators of the data warehouse. The APRN will be interacting with a variety of data storage systems. These may include registries, surgery scheduling systems, pharmacy or medication delivery systems, POC laboratory devices, quality management systems, case management systems, risk management systems, infection control systems, and cost accounting systems. In some cases, data from one information system might be cross-checked against another system with a similar data set. If differences between two similar data sets are identified, they should be closely examined to understand the discrepancy. For example, the number of infections captured by a laboratory system might be different than those captured by an infection control practitioner using an infection control information system, and different still from those captured in a medical record coding system. Common reasons for variance among similar HIT systems include variability in the start or end dates (or times) used to run the reports, a difference in the codes used to define the population of interest, or differences in how the data were captured in the source systems. In the case of medical records coding, variation is often the result of inconsistent documentation by medical and APRN providers. These types of variations should be understood during the design phase of the outcome evaluation plan so that the best data source can be selected to answer the core questions of the study.

In some cases, questions about the effective management of clinical populations can be answered only through longitudinal studies. For example, for a diabetic population, clinical outcomes such as reduced hospitalization, improved functioning, reduced evidence of retinopathy, and reduced limb amputations may be sound and reasonable for research purposes, but they are typically too long range to be useful for performance improvement or outcome evaluation activities. The link between APRN practice and outcomes may be difficult to assess over long periods, making intermediate outcomes assessment more desirable for a short-term evaluation.

When collecting patient identifiable data, APRNs should be cognizant of the restrictions on their use. HIPAA includes significant restrictions on the manner in which identifiable patient information may be used for research and QI activities. Typically, information used for QI and outcome evaluations is less restrictive. In some circumstances, particularly if they are contracted in a fee-for-service arrangement with the health care agency, APRNs may be required to sign a business associate agreement with the health care provider. For more information about HIPAA regulations and impact on evaluation activities, APRNs should refer to their organization's policies and procedures.

The APRN will have a full appreciation of the scope of the outcome evaluation project and resources required for successful completion only after all the indicators within the plan are evaluated. Once the indicators and the individual data elements have been finalized and the sources of data secured, APRNs should summarize the outcome evaluation plan in a concise document that describes the plan and communicate it to all stakeholders.

Derive Meaning From Data and Act on Results

The final phase of the outcome evaluation process involves evaluation and dissemination of the findings and identification of opportunities for improvement. In these final steps, results are transformed into meaningful information that can be used to improve quality, cost, and patient satisfaction and to evaluate the contributions of the APRN. The final step involves formulating a plan to implement and reevaluate changes that occur as a result of the study.

Analyze Data and Interpret Findings

Typically, data analysis is the responsibility of the APRN, although the inclusion of other peer reviewers is useful, especially when the APRN has a vested interest in the outcomes. Including others helps eliminate any perceived bias during the final data analysis and reporting phases. In some cases, the APRN may wish to enlist the support and guidance of a statistician or a nurse researcher to ensure that the end product is methodologically sound and contains the information necessary to convince others.

Comparing pre-intervention with postintervention performance data is one effective way to evaluate the degree of change resulting from APRN interventions. Pre-intervention performance data are commonly collected retrospectively and then compared with data collected during or after an APRN intervention. Retrospective data are generally available for measures constructed from electronic data sources. When electronic data are insufficient to provide adequate baseline information, APRNs may elect to collect more detailed data from noncomputerized medical records. Although this approach generally requires more effort, time, and planning, it may be warranted when specific processes of care are altered as part of the APRN's intervention. For example, a CRNA evaluating the frequency of intraoperative hypotensive episodes may have to review medical records because this phenomenon may not be contained in common electronic source data. In some cases, a baseline study must be conducted before the APRN intervention to ensure that appropriate baseline data are available for comparison. For example, a certified nurse-midwife who is implementing changes in clinic protocols to reduce waiting times for prenatal patients undergoing glucose tolerance testing may have to conduct a pre-intervention time and motion study to establish a baseline against which to compare postintervention results.

Although baseline information is useful for evaluating outcomes, not everything measured by APRNs will have suitable baseline data for comparison. In these cases, performance can be evaluated against a known standard of care or benchmark, especially when an area of practice is supported by evidence-based practice. When no best practice standard of performance is known, APRNs may use comparative data provided by a national database if the measures used for comparison are the same as those contained within the national database.

Present and Disseminate Findings

Effective communication of data-based findings, conclusions, and recommendations for future practice is an essential component of the outcome evaluation process. How the findings are presented depends on the audience. Nonclinical audiences with a business focus, such as boards of directors or operations teams, will require briefings that summarize pertinent findings, draw conclusions, and provide reasonable options or recommendations for consideration. Clinical audiences generally require additional detail about how the evaluation was conducted and a more extensive discussion of the clinical and statistical strengths of the evidence. Clinical audiences are becoming more sophisticated in their understanding of data analysis techniques and their assessment of the applicability of evidence to practice.

The APRN may be responsible for packaging the project's findings to present to stakeholders. Assistance from the facility's media or publications department may be required, depending on the final forum for communicating findings. Findings are commonly presented in committee meetings and formal presentations, although the APRN should also consider posters, newsletters, white papers, articles, bulk email communications, or list serve communities as additional ways to disseminate information.

Identify Improvement Opportunities

Once the outcome evaluation findings have been interpreted, the APRN begins to work closely with stakeholders to evaluate the effectiveness of the practice change or QI strategy. This step may occur very quickly following a practice change or intervention, depending on the QI project. Many health care organizations are adopting a rapid cycle of learning, in which they perform smaller tests of change, evaluate the results and then, if successful, expand to larger areas or populations. For example, an APRN intervention might be pilot-tested in one nursing unit before deploying the strategy across the hospital. If the intervention does not lead to the desired outcome in a timely manner, improvement opportunities are quickly identified and implemented and the results are reevaluated, with constant scrutiny on specific aspects of the care delivery processes, technology resources, or points in time that could be altered to achieve greater efficiency or effectiveness.

For example, an APRN working in an acute care hospital may identify opportunities to improve performance in teaching discharge instructions to patients with heart failure. For 1 week, a request report can be generated identifying patients who need heart failure instructions at discharge. The following week it is identified that during the weekends, there is a gap in the use of the report because the APRN is not available to request and review the report and make rounds. Rather than wait for a longer evaluation period to pass, an incremental improvement in the process is adopted whereby automated alerts are generated out of the HIT system to identify all patients with an active diagnosis of heart failure who are on the telemetry unit longer than 24 hours. Incremental improvement opportunities may be made over time until a larger and more sustaining strategy is identified and long-term adoption has been achieved. In this example, the most effective solution may ultimately be for the hospital to participate in the American Heart Association's Get With the Guidelines program, a national demonstration of best practice performance for the treatment of heart failure, acute myocardial infarction, stroke, and atrial fibrillation (http://www.heart.org/HEARTORG/). With this program, comprehensive Internet-based patient education materials are available to staff nurses and other clinicians, who can quickly customize the materials to meet the specific learning needs of individual patients. This solution may not have been part of the initial strategy at the onset of the project, but the APRN's stewardship of the process will assist team members to develop a shared vision of which intervention(s) to adopt and why. Bringing stakeholders together to review existing and ongoing processes of care and isolate any process failures or barriers that have contributed to suboptimal performance are essential in today's health care environment.

The process to identify opportunities for improvement is similar to any work redesign initiative. The APRN should identify champions and potential opponents of change. Change theory can serve as a useful foundation for APRNs responsible for preparing stakeholders and overcoming their resistance to new health care delivery practices. Issues such as level of difficulty with deploying the intervention should be addressed as well as projected costs and the human and technology resources required to implement and sustain the plan. Consideration should also be given to how much time the APRN will be engaged in the project and how this may affect other areas of practice. A staged pilot test approach is useful for new or large-scale projects. As noted, these smaller scale versions can help identify potential implementation problems and determine whether the intervention can achieve the desired effect.

Formulate a Plan for Ongoing Monitoring and Reevaluation

Once an acceptable outcome has been achieved and sustained for a period of time, a final summary of the performance improvement initiative should be documented. This type of documentation is useful to a health care organization during an accreditation survey so that it can demonstrate that a culture of quality has been established and that it is actively engaged in improving care. In addition, this information is also useful to demonstrate the APRN's value to her or his organization. Each goal should specify the primary interventions that were used to reach the goal, along with who was accountable for the actions required and the dates for completion. This reevaluation then becomes the basis for future outcome evaluation plans. Once performance in a

particular area is stabilized, the APRN may elect to discontinue monitoring a given area of performance or periodically revisit performance through intermittent monitoring.

Clarify Purpose of the APRN's Role

A final step in the process may include a thoughtful review of the APRN's role and her or his effectiveness in achieving desired outcomes. An APRN's role may change as a direct result of performance improvement and outcome evaluation studies. Findings may indicate that APRN interventions are better suited to other points of care across the continuum of services than originally envisioned or may reveal that care may be delivered more efficiently by other providers. Conversely, findings may support the effectiveness and efficiency of the APRN intervention, which could lead to program growth and expansion to other populations or points of care. In all cases, outcome evaluation, APRN role definition, and scope of practice go hand in hand. If the purposes of their roles are unclear, APRNs may need to identify and discuss reasonable and appropriate expectations with administrators and collaborators. It is not possible to decide which outcomes to measure without clarity about the APRN's clinical populations and their accountability for the structures and processes of care. Finally, employers may not recognize the APRN's full range of services or potential benefit to the organization. In such situations, the APRN may need to take the lead in identifying specific processes and areas of focus within the setting and set appropriate goals and performance objectives to meet them.

Although the strategies discussed in this chapter to evaluate outcomes and improve performance are integral to the success of the APRN in any organization, it is important to remember that data are ultimately a tool that can be used to foster learning, improve quality, and assist the nursing process to achieve its ultimate goal.

Conclusion

This chapter illustrates the interconnectivity among policy, regulation, health care information technology, information management, outcomes measurement, systems thinking, and performance improvement in every aspect of APRN practice. Effective outcomes measurement and management require APRNs to master information technologies, work collaboratively with others, plan and organize processes of care and assessments of quality in highly complex health services environments, and effectively manage change within their sponsoring organizations. Because reimbursement decisions are driven by evidence of organizational and individual provider performance, APRNs who lack reliable and valid data to substantiate their impact will struggle for equitable reimbursement for their services and possibly employment. For APRNs to be a visible and viable resource in tomorrow's health care delivery system, they must have visible and robust outcomes that demonstrate their value. APRNs in every practice setting must be willing and able to spearhead performance improvement initiatives in their institutions. Given the challenges of health care reform and the pioneering innovations of many health care systems across the United States and internationally, there are many opportunities to deploy APRNs to deliver primary, preventive, acute, and chronic care and episodic care services in a quality and cost-effective manner. It may be that APRNs who successfully steward safer care environments, improve clinical performance, and achieve greater efficiencies in caregiving processes will demonstrate their value more than they ever could have done in the past, but they must be involved in the development of information systems to help carry this out. APRNs who develop robust and ongoing outcome evaluation plans place themselves in the strongest position to demonstrate their impact on outcomes of care delivery. In so doing, they also render advanced practice nursing visible to patients, other providers, administrators, payors, and communities.

Given the many quality reporting initiatives that represent so many clinical specialty domains and care delivery settings, one must wonder why it has taken so long for the nursing profession to develop a quality data set that represents the best that advanced practice nursing has to offer to those we serve. In light of emerging HIT technologies, would it now be possible to develop a robust, reliable, and highly interoperable data set of clinical outcomes that are sensitive to APRN practice? Although these are important aspects of care, it seems long overdue to move beyond traditional measures such as pressure ulcers, falls, and medication errors, and actually examine the difference that APRN practice brings to patient outcomes, the patient experience, and the entire care delivery system. Is it not possible for APRNs to make a measurable difference in conditions such as childhood obesity, diabetes management, cardiac and pulmonary disease prevention, cancer treatment, acute and episodic care, and so much more? Through advanced education and clinical expertise, APRNs are in a unique position to lead the way to this new level of thought leadership and clinical practice that is sorely needed in today's health care ecosystem.

Key Summary Points

- Information technology is a necessary tool for collection and storage of data used to measure outcomes and improvement.
- Informatics is the combination of computer science, information science, and nursing science that allows the development of information and knowledge from the data collected.
- It will be mandatory for APRNs (and other providers) to be able to measure and report on care improvement and patient outcomes to benefit from a changing reimbursement structure that will pay for quality, and not quantity, of services performed.
- For APRNs to be able to practice at the top of their licenses uniformly across the nation, data collected in information systems must be adequate to demonstrate equal or better outcomes as compared to physician counterparts.

References

To access the references for this chapter, use your smartphone's QR code reader to scan the code below, or go to http://booksite.elsevier.com/ 9780323447751.

Index

Pages followed by *b, t,* or *f* refer to boxes, tables, or
figures, respectively.